ESSENCE OF
ANESTHESIA
PRACTICE

ESSENCE OF
ANESTHESIA
PRACTICE

SECOND EDITION

Michael F. Roizen, M.D.

Dean of the School of Medicine and Vice-President
for Biomedical Affairs
Professor of Internal Medicine and Anesthesiology
State University of New York Upstate Medical University
Syracuse, New York

Lee A. Fleisher, M.D.

Associate Professor
Department of Anesthesiology and Critical Care Medicine
Joint Appointments in Medicine (Cardiology), Biomedical
Information Sciences, and Health Policy and Management
Vice-Chairman for Clinical Investigation
Johns Hopkins University School of Medicine
Baltimore, Maryland

W.B. SAUNDERS COMPANY
A Harcourt Health Sciences Company
Philadelphia   London   New York   St. Louis   Sydney   Toronto

W.B. SAUNDERS COMPANY
A Harcourt Health Sciences Company

The Curtis Center
Independence Square West
Philadelphia, Pennsylvania 19106

Library of Congress Cataloging-in-Publication Data

Essence of anesthesia practice / [edited by] Michael F. Roizen, Lee A. Fleisher.—2nd ed.

p.   cm.

ISBN 0–7216–9267–2

1. Anesthesia—Handbooks, manuals, etc. 2. Anesthesiology—Handbooks, manuals, etc. I. Roizen, Michael F. II. Fleisher, Lee A.

RD82.2 .E87 2002

617.9′6—dc21   2001042046

Editor-in-Chief: Richard Lampert
Acquisitions Editor: Allan Ross
Developmental Editor: David Orzechowski
Manuscript Editor: Amy Norwitz
Production Manager: Norman Stellander
Book Designer: Lynn Foulk
Indexer: Dennis Dolan

ESSENCE OF ANESTHESIA PRACTICE   ISBN 0–7216–9267–2

Printed in the United States of America.

Last digit is the print number: 9   8   7   6   5   4   3   2   1

Dedication from Lee A. Fleisher:
To my wife, Renee, and my children, Jessica and Matthew,
for their unrelenting love and support despite the many late hours
devoted to the editing of these manuscripts.
To my parents, Lois and Lou,
for their lifelong encouragement
for me to follow my own goals.

Dedication from Michael F. Roizen:
To Nancy, Jeffrey, and Jennifer, whose support, sacrifices,
and love make working at home fun;
to Lee, who does so much, so well;
to the members of my prior and still loved department
(of Anesthesia and Critical Care) at the University of Chicago,
who allowed time and sacrificed their own interests
to the production of this work, and who encouraged it;
to my current dedicated department at SUNY Upstate,
which allows me to practice this art
and allows me to keep enjoying anesthesiology;
to my partners at the boards who stimulated this work
and invigorated me and it daily;
to the colleagues who garnered the expertise
embodied in these summaries.

Dedication from Michael and Lee:
To the many physicians and other practitioners
who must remember so much
to care so well for the many and diverse patients.

Therese K. Abboud, M.D.
Professor of Anesthesiology, University of Southern California Medical Center, Los Angeles, California
Eclampsia

Ezzat J. Abouleish, M.D.
Professor Emeritus of Anesthesiology, University of Texas–Houston Medical School, Houston, Texas
Cephalopelvic Disproportion (CPD)

Jerome H. Abrams, M.D.
Associate Professor of Surgery, Graduate Faculty, Biomedical Engineering, University of Minnesota; Staff Surgeon, Minneapolis VA Medical Center, Minneapolis, Minnesota
Nutritional Support

Anil Aggarwal, M.D.
Associate Professor, Department of Anesthesiology, Medical College of Wisconsin, Milwaukee, Wisconsin
Dobutamine

Charles Ahere, M.D.
Assistant Professor, University of Mississippi Medical Center, Jackson, Mississippi
Sleep Apnea, Obstructive

David B. Albert, M.D.
Director of Ambulatory Anesthesia, Hospital for Joint Diseases, New York, New York
Osteoporosis

Richard D. Alessi, Jr., M.D.
Assistant Professor, University of Chicago, Pritzker School of Medicine, Chicago, Illinois
Blalock-Taussig (BT) Shunt

Hassan H. Ali, M.B., B.Ch., M.D.,
Professor of Anesthesia, Harvard Medical School; Anesthetist, Massachusetts General Hospital, Boston, Massachusetts
Physostigmine Salicylate (Eserine, Antilirium)
Pyridostigmine Bromide

John C. Alverdy, M.D., F.A.C.S.
Associate Professor of Surgery, University of Chicago Hospitals, Chicago, Illinois
Gastric Bypass Stapling for Morbid Obesity

John R. Ammon, M.D.
Senior Lecturer, Department of Anesthesiology, University of Arizona, Tucson, Associate, Valley Anesthesiology Consultants, Ltd., Phoenix, Arizona
Diabetic Ketoacidosis (DKA)
Hyperosmolar Nonketotic Coma

Marvin L. Appel, M.D., Ph.D.
Assistant Professor, Department of Anesthesiology, Johns Hopkins University School of Medicine, Baltimore, Maryland
Cardiopulmonary Bypass

James F. Arens, M.D.
R. Lee Clark Professor and Chairman, Department of Anesthesiology, University of Texas, M.D. Anderson Cancer Center, Houston, Texas
Pulmonary Atresia

James Armstrong, M.D.
University of Ottawa, Heart Institute, Ottawa, Ontario, Canada
Treacher Collins Syndrome

Solomon Aronson, M.D.
Professor of Anesthesiology and Critical Care, Pritzker School of Medicine, University of Chicago; Director, Cardiothoracic Anesthesiology, University of Chicago Medical Center, Chicago, Illinois
Myxoma
Renal Function Testing

Takashi Asai, M.D., Ph.D.
Assistant Professor, Kansai Medical University, Moriguchi City, Osaka, Japan
Constipation

Rajkumari V. Asrani, M.D.
Clinical Professor of Anesthesiology and Director of Regional Anesthesia, University of Irvine Medical Center, Orange; Director of Anesthesia, Pain Clinic, VA Medical Center, Long Beach, California
Trigeminal Neuralgia (Tic Douloureux)

John L. Atlee, M.D.
Professor of Anesthesiology, Medical College of Wisconsin, Milwaukee, Wisconsin
Atrial Flutter
AV and Bifascicular Heart Block
Sick Sinus Syndrome (SSS)
Supraventricular Tachycardia (Tachyarrhythmias)
Ventricular Preexcitation Syndrome
Ventricular Tachyarrhythmias

Catherine R. Bachman, M.D., F.R.C.P.C.
Assistant Professor and Section Chief, Pediatric Anesthesia, University of Chicago, Chicago, Illinois
Rett Syndrome

Douglas R. Bacon, M.D.
Associate Professor of Anesthesiology, Mayo Medical School; Senior Associate Consultant, Mayo Clinic, Rochester, Minnesota
Sarcoma

Jeffrey M. Baden, M.D.
Professor, Department of Anesthesia, Stanford University School of Medicine, Stanford, California
Hepatic Encephalopathy

Andrew D. Badley, M.D.
Instructor in Medicine, Mayo Clinic and Foundation, Rochester, Minnesota
Cytomegalovirus (CMV) Infection

Peter L. Bailey, M.D.
Associate Professor, University of Utah Health Sciences Center, Salt Lake City, Utah
Nonsteroidal Anti-inflammatory Drugs (NSAIDs)

Jeffrey R. Balser, M.D., Ph.D.
Professor, Anesthesiology and Pharmacology, Vanderbilt University; Chairman, Department of Anesthesiology, Vanderbilt University Medical Center, Nashville, Tennessee
Paroxysmal Atrial Tachycardia
Wolff-Parkinson-White (WPW) Syndrome

Anis S. Baraka, M.D., F.R.C.A.
Professor and Chairman, Department of Anesthesiology, American University of Beirut, Beirut, Lebanon
Echinococcosis

Paul G. Barash, M.D.
Professor, Department of Anesthesiology, Yale University School of Medicine, New Haven, Connecticut
Aortic Regurgitation

Richard R. Bartkowski, M.D., Ph.D.
Professor of Anesthesiology, Jefferson Medical College, Thomas Jefferson University, Philadelphia, Pennsylvania
Urticaria, Cold

Christopher D. Beatie, M.D.
Assistant Clinical Professor of Anesthesiology, University of California, Los Angeles, School of Medicine, Los Angeles, California
Aspirin (Acetylsalicylic Acid)
Oral Hypoglycemics
Extracorporeal Shock Wave Lithotripsy (ESWL)

Charles Beattie, M.D., Ph.D.
Professor and Chairman and Anesthesiologist-in-Chief, Vanderbilt University Medical Center, Department of Anesthesiology, Nashville, Tennessee
Abdominal Aortic Aneurysm Repair

Robert F. Bedford, M.D.
Clinical Professor of Anesthesiology, University of Virginia School of Medicine, Charlottesville, Virginia and University of South Florida School of Medicine, Tampa; Consultant Anesthesiologist, James A. Haley Veterans Hospital, Tampa, Florida
Supratentorial Brain Tumors

Sean M. Berenholtz, M.D.
Assistant Professor, Department of Anesthesiology and Critical Care Medicine, Johns Hopkins University School of Medicine, Baltimore, Maryland
Glyburide, Oral Hypoglycemic Agents
Metformin (Glucophage)

David L. Berger, M.D.
Clinical Associate Professor of Anesthesiology, Stanford University School of Medicine, Stanford; Active Staff, Alta Bates — Summit Medical Center, Berkeley, California
Mitral Valve Replacement

Lauren Berkow, M.D.
Assistant Professor, Johns Hopkins University School of Medicine, Baltimore, Maryland
Transsphenoidal Surgery

M. Lawrence Berman, M.D., Ph.D.
Emeritus Professor of Anesthesiology and Associate Professor of Pharmacology, Vanderbilt University School of Medicine, Nashville, Tennessee
Hashimoto's Thyroiditis

Ralph L. Bernstein, M.D.
Professor of Clinical Anesthesiology, New York University School of Medicine, New York, New York
Scoliosis and Kyphosis
Scoliosis and Kyphosis Surgery

Wendy K. Bernstein, M.D.
Assistant Professor, and Director, Cardiothoracic Anesthesia Fellowship, University of Maryland, Baltimore, Maryland
Splenectomy

Michael J. Berrigan, M.D., Ph.D.
Chairman and Seymour Alpert Professor, Department of Anesthesiology and Critical Care Medicine, The George Washington University Medical Center, Washington, D.C.
Drug Abuse, Lysergic Acid Diethylamide (LSD)

Arnold J. Berry, M.D., M.P.H.
Professor of Anesthesiology, Emory School of Medicine and Hospital, Atlanta, Georgia
Hepatitis A
Hepatitis B
Hepatitis C

Frederic A. Berry, M.D.
Professor of Anesthesiology and Pediatrics, University of Virginia Health Science Center, Charlottesville, Virginia
Foreign Body Aspiration

Brian K. Bevacqua, M.D.
Visiting Associate Professor of Anesthesiology, Department of Anesthesiology, University of Wisconsin; Chief, Anesthesiology, and Director, Perioperative Services, Middleton VA Medical Center, Madison, Wisconsin
Diphtheria

Wendy B. Binstock, M.D.
Assistant Professor, Department of Anesthesia and Critical Care, Department of Pediatrics, University of Chicago, Chicago, Illinois
Omphalocele Surgery

David J. Birnbach, M.D.
Associate Professor, Departments of Anesthesiology and Obstetrics and Gynecology, College of Physicians and Surgeons of Columbia University; Director of Obstetric Anesthesiology, St. Luke's – Roosevelt Hospital Center, New York, New York
HELLP Syndrome

Michael J. Bishop, M.D.
Professor of Anesthesiology and Medicine (Pulmonary and Critical Care), University of Washington; Director, Headquarters Anesthesia Service and Director, Anesthesia/Operating Room Services, VA Puget Sound, Seattle, Washington
Asthma Drugs, New — Oral Antileukotriene Drugs (Accolate [Zafirlukast], Singulair [Montelukast], Zyflo [Zileuton])

Bruno Bissonnette, M.D.
Professor of Anesthesia and Director of Neuroanaesthesia and Cardiovascular Anesthesia Research, The Hospital for Sick Children, Toronto, Ontario, Canada
Opitz-Frias Syndrome (The G Syndrome)

Timothy M. Bittenbinder, M.D.
Interim Chairman, Department of Anesthesiology, Scott and White/Texas A&M College of Medicine, Scott and White, Temple, Texas
Geriatric Surgery

Jordan L. Blinder, M.D.
Assistant Professor of Anesthesiology, Tufts University School of Medicine, Boston; Neuroanesthesia Section Chief, Baystate Medical Center, Springfield, Massachusetts
Appendicitis, Acute

Brian M. Block, M.D., Ph.D.
Resident, Johns Hopkins University School of Medicine, Baltimore, Maryland
Calcium Deficiency / Hypocalcemia

Robert H. Bode, Jr., M.D.
Associate Professor of Anesthesiology, Boston University School of Medicine; Chairman, Department of Anesthesia, New England Baptist Hospital, Boston, Massachusetts
Amputation, Lower Extremity (LEA)

Thomas F. Boerner, M.D.
Assistant Professor of Anesthesiology and Critical Care Medicine, University of Pittsburgh School of Medicine, Pittsburgh, Pennsylvania
Tetracyclines

Lara Bonasera, M.D.
Resident, University of Chicago, Chicago, Illinois
Garlic (Allium sativum)

Cecil O. Borel, M.D.
Associate Professor, Anesthesiology and Neurosurgery, Duke University; Division Chief, Otolaryngology Head and Neck, and Medical Director, Neuro ICU, Duke University Medical Center, Durham, North Carolina
Myasthenia Gravis

Gregory H. Botz, M.D.
Associate Professor of Anesthesiology and Critical Care; Medical Director of Intensive Care, and Deputy Chairman, Department of Critical Care, University of Texas M.D. Anderson Cancer Center, Houston, Texas
Cardiomyopathy, Alcoholic
Cardiomyopathy, Ischemic

Charles D. Boucek, M.D.
Associate Professor of Anesthesiology and Internal Medicine, University of Pittsburgh School of Medicine; Staff Physician, UPMC Presbyterian University Hospital, Pittsburgh, Pennsylvania
Bone Marrow Transplantation (Harvest Procedure)

Denis L. Bourke, M.D.
Professor of Anesthesiology, University of Maryland; Chief, Anesthesiology Service, Baltimore Veterans Affairs Medical Center, Baltimore, Maryland
Transurethral Resection of Bladder Tumor
Ureteral Stent Placement

Gwendolyn L. Boyd, M.D.
Professor, University of Alabama at Birmingham, Birmingham, Alabama
Brain Death

Michelle Braunfeld, M.D.
Associate Clinical Professor, Department of Anesthesiology, University of California, Los Angeles, Center for the Health Sciences, Los Angeles, California
Diarrhea, Acute and Chronic
Drug Overdose, Rat Poison (Warfarin Toxicity)
Hypercalcemia

Caridad Bravo-Fernandez, M.D.
Assistant Professor, University of Florida College of Medicine, Department of Anesthesiology, Gainesville, Florida
Amputation, Above-Knee (AKA)

Peter H. Breen, M.D., F.R.C.P.C.
Associate Professor, Department of Anesthesiology, College of Medicine, University of California, Irvine, Irvine; Associate Professor and Vice Chair, Attending Anesthesiology, Department of Anesthesiology, UCI Medical Center, Orange, California
Carbon Monoxide (CO) Poisoning
Cyanide Poisoning

Marjorie P. Brennan, M.D.
Assistant Professor of Anesthesia, George
Washington University School of Medicine;
Attending Anesthesiologist, Children's
National Medical Center, Washington, D.C.
Carnitine Deficiency

Michael J. Breslow, M.D.
Associate Professor, Departments of
Anesthesiology and Critical Care
Medicine, Johns Hopkins University
School of Medicine, Baltimore, Maryland
Paroxysmal Atrial Tachycardia

Jay B. Brodsky, M.D.
Professor, Stanford University School of
Medicine; Section Chief, General OR
Group, Stanford University Medical
Center, Stanford, California
Guillain-Barré Syndrome

Burnell R. Brown, Jr., M.D., Ph.D.*
Former Professor and Chair, Department
of Anesthesiology, University of Arizona
College of Medicine, Tucson, Arizona
*Multiple Endocrine Neoplasia (MEN)
Types I and II*

Eli M. Brown, M.D.
Professor Emeritus, Wayne State
University; Honorary Staff, Detroit
Medical Center, Detroit, Michigan
Parathyroidectomy

Morris Brown, M.D.
Professor and Chair, Department of
Anesthesiology, Wayne State University
School of Medicine, Detroit, Michigan
Atrial Fibrillation

Sorin J. Brull, M.D.
Professor, University of Arkansas for
Medical Sciences, University of Arkansas
School of Medicine, Little Rock, Arkansas
*Cholecystectomy, Laparoscopic
Cholecystectomy, Open*

Claude Brunson, M.D.
Assistant Professor, Department of
Anesthesiology, University of Mississippi
School of Medicine, Jackson, Mississippi
Sleep Apnea, Obstructive

Yvon F. Bryan, M.D.
Assistant Professor of Anesthesia and
Critical Care, University of Chicago,
Chicago, Illinois
*Craniosynostosis
Otitis Media*

David Bui, M.D.
Clinical Assistant Professor of
Anesthesiology, State University of New
York at Buffalo, School of Medicine and
Biomedical Sciences, Buffalo, New York
IgA Deficiency

Michelle Burnett, M.D.
Assistant Professor, Department of
Anesthesia, Georgetown University School
of Medicine, Washington, D.C.
Eisenmenger's Syndrome

John Butterworth, M.D.
Professor of Anesthesiology and Head,
Section on Cardiothoracic Anesthesiology,
Wake Forest University School of
Medicine, Winston-Salem, North Carolina
Hypothyroidism

Jerry M. Calkins, M.D., Ph.D.
Professor of Clinical Anesthesiology,
University of Arizona, Tucson; Staff, Mayo
Clinic and Hospital, Scottsdale, Arizona;
Vice President of Medical Affairs,
Metasensors, Inc., Rockville, Maryland
*Gonorrhea
Reflex Sympathetic Dystrophy (Complex
Peripheral Pain Syndrome)*

Enrico Camporesi, M.D.
Professor and Chair, Department of
Anesthesiology, and Professor, Department
of Physiology, State University of New
York Upstate Medical University; Director,
Hyperbaric Treatment Unit, University
Hospital, Syracuse, New York
Burn Injury, Flame

Roy D. Cane, M.B., B.Ch.
Professor and Vice Chair, Northwestern
University Medical School, Chicago,
Illinois
Tetanus

Lisa A. Caramico, M.D.
Assistant Professor of Anesthesiology, Yale
University School of Medicine, Department
of Anesthesiology; Attending
Anesthesiologist, Yale-New Haven
Hospital, New Haven, Connecticut
Shy-Drager Disease

Ann M. Cartarius, R.N.
Research Nurse Coordinator, Department
of Anesthesiology and Critical Care
Medicine, Johns Hopkins University
School of Medicine, Baltimore, Maryland
Clopidogrel Bisulfate

Helmut F. Cascorbi, M.D., Ph.D.
Professor of Anesthesiology and
Psychiatry, Case Western Reserve
University, Cleveland, Ohio
Chloramphenicol (Chloromycetin)

Henry Casson, M.D.
Associate Professor, Anesthesiology,
Oregon Health Science University,
Portland, Oregon
Tetralogy of Fallot, Correction of

Charles B. Cauldwell, M.D., Ph.D.
Clinical Professor of Anesthesia,
University of California, San Francisco;
Chief, Division of Pediatric Anesthesia,
University of California, San Francisco,
Medical Center, San Francisco, California
Pierre Robin Syndrome

Andrei Cernea, M.D.
Staff Anesthesiologist, Providence
Hospital, Washington, D.C.
*Cleft Lip Repair
Cleft Palate*

Bernard R. Chaitman, M.D.
Professor of Medicine and Director,
Cardiovascular Research, St. Louis
University School of Medicine, St. Louis,
Missouri
Exercise Stress Testing

Susan Chan, M.D.
Assistant Clinical Professor, University of
California, Los Angeles, School of
Medicine, Los Angeles, California
Laparoscopy, Gynecologic

Bobby Su-Pen Chang, M.D.
Assistant Professor of Anesthesiology,
Cornell University Medical College, New
York, New York
Mycoplasma pneumoniae Infection

Alexandre N. Chapochnikov, M.D., Ph.D.
Cardiac Anesthesia Fellow, Department of
Anesthesia and Critical Care, University
of Chicago Hospitals, Chicago, Illinois
Vitamin D Deficiency

Mary L. Chavez, Pharm.D.
Associate Professor, Midwestern
University, Chicago College of Pharmacy,
Downers Grove, Illinois
Ginkgo

Ronald P. Chavez, M.D.
Assistant Professor of Anesthesia and
Critical Care, University of Chicago,
Chicago, Illinois
*Pregnancy, Maternal Physiology
Vitamin K Deficiency*

Eugene Y. Cheng, M.D., F.C.C.M.
Professor of Anesthesiology and Medicine
and Associate Program Director,
Anesthesiology, Medical College of
Wisconsin, Milwaukee, Wisconsin
Herpes, Type 1

Albert T. Cheung, M.D.
Associate Professor of Anesthesia,
Department of Anesthesia, University of
Pennsylvania School of Medicine,
Philadelphia, Pennsylvania
*Mitral Stenosis
Mitral Valve Prolapse*

Ashwani K. Chhibber, M.D.
Associate Professor of Anesthesiology and
Associate Professor of Pediatrics,
University of Rochester School of Medicine
and Dentistry; Director, Transplantation
Anesthesia Division, and Director,
Pediatric Anesthesia Division, Strong
Memorial Hospital, Rochester, New York
Liver Transplantation (Pediatric)

C. Daniel Chow, M.D.
Staff Anesthesiologist, Department of
Anesthesiology, Division of Cardiac
Anesthesia, Washington Hospital Center,
Washington, D.C.
Endoscopic Sinus Surgery (ESS)

*Deceased

Rose Christopherson, M.D., Ph.D.
Associate Professor, Oregon Health Science University; Staff Anesthesiologist, Portland Veterans Administration Medical Center, Portland, Oregon
Bypass Graft Procedure, Infrainguinal

Noel Lee Chun, M.D.
Associate Clinical Professor, Department of Anesthesiology, University of California, Los Angeles School of Medicine, Los Angeles, California
Burn Injury, Chemical
Radical Neck Dissection
Rotator Cuff Surgery

Richard B. Clark, M.D.
Professor of Emeritus, University of Arkansas for Medical Science, University of Arkansas College of Medicine; Anesthesiologist, University Hospital, Little Rock, Arkansas
Diabetes, Type III (Gestational Diabetes Mellitus)

Dennis W. Coalson, M.D.
Assistant Professor, Department of Anesthesia and Critical Care, University of Chicago, Chicago, Illinois
Kidney Transplantation
Pancreas Transplantation

Neal H. Cohen, M.D., M.P.H.
Professor Anesthesia and Medicine and Vice Dean, Academic Affairs, University of California, San Francisco; Director, Critical Care Medicine, UCSF Medical Center, San Francisco, California
Pneumocystis carinii *Pneumonia (PCP)*

Stephan J. Cohn, M.D.
Assistant Professor, Department of Anesthesia and Critical Care, University of Chicago, Chicago, Illinois
Raynaud's Phenomenon

Daniel J. Cole, M.D.
Professor of Anesthesiology, Loma Linda University School of Medicine; Director, Neurosurgical Anesthesiology, Loma Linda University Medical Center, Loma Linda, California
Amyotrophic Lateral Sclerosis (ALS)

Aisling Conran, M.D.
Clinical Assistant Professor of Anesthesia, University of Chicago, Pritzker School of Medicine; Staff Anesthesiologist, University of Chicago Hospitals, Chicago, Illinois
GI Endoscopy/EGD, Non–
Operating Room Anesthesia
Hepatitis, Halothane
Tacrolimus (FK-506)

Richard I. Cook, M.D.
Assistant Professor, University of Chicago, Chicago, Illinois
Doxorubicin (Adriamycin), Daunorubicin
(Cerubidine)
Duchenne Muscular Dystrophy
(Pseudohypertrophic Muscular Dystrophy)

Thomas Corbridge, M.D.
Assistant Professor of Medicine, Physical Medicine, and Rehabilitation, Northwestern University Medical School, Chicago, Illinois
Asthma, Acute

Randall C. Cork, M.D., Ph.D.
Professor and Chair, Department of Anesthesiology, Louisiana State University Medical Center, Shreveport, Louisiana
Intraoperative Recall

Vincent S. Cowell, M.D.
Assistant Professor of Anesthesiology, Medical College of Pennsylvania/Hahnemann University, Philadelphia, Pennsylvania
Cancer, Breast
Hemophilia

Paula A. Craigo, M.D.
Assistant Professor, Department of Anesthesia, Mayo School of Medicine; Senior Associate Consultant, Mayo Clinic, Rochester, Minnesota
Aspiration, Perioperative: Prevention and Management
Pneumonectomy

Roy F. Cucchiara, M.D.
Professor of Anesthesiology, University of Florida College of Medicine, Gainesville, Florida
Central Neurogenic Hyperventilation

David J. Cullen, M.D.
Professor of Anesthesiology, Tufts University School of Medicine; Chairman, Department of Anesthesiology, St. Elizabeth's Medical Center, Boston, Massachusetts
Delirium (Postanesthetic)

Anthony J. Cunningham, M.D., F.R.C.P.C.
Professor of Anaesthesia and Clinical Vice Dean, Royal College of Surgeons in Ireland; Consultant Anaesthetist, Beaumont Hospital, Dublin, Ireland
AV Graft for Hemodialysis

Nicola D'Attellis, M.D.
Director, Cardiovascular and Thoracic Anesthesia, Department of Anesthesiology and Intensive Care, Hôpital Européen Georges Pompidou, Paris, France
Congestive Heart Failure

Suanne M. Daves, M.D.
Associate Professor, University of Chicago, Chicago, Illinois
Extracorporeal Membrane Oxygenation (ECMO)

Peter J. Davis, M.D.
Professor of Anesthesia and Pediatrics, University of Pittsburgh School of Medicine; Anesthesiologist-in-Chief, Children's Hospital of Pittsburgh, Pittsburgh, Pennsylvania
Gastroschisis Surgery
Wilms' Tumor

Richard F. Davis, M.D.
Professor of Anesthesiology, Oregon Health Sciences University, Portland, Oregon
Buerger's Disease: Thromboangiitis Obliterans (TAO)

Ellise Delphin, M.D.
Associate Professor of Clinical Anesthesiology, Columbia University College of Physicians and Surgeons, New York, New York
Antithrombin III Deficiency

Sasha M. Demos, M.D., Ph.D.
Anesthesia Resident, University of Chicago Hospitals, Chicago, Illinois
Soy

Dawn P. Desiderio, M.D.
Associate Professor, Department of Anesthesiology, Cornell University Medical College, New York, New York
Cancer, Esophageal

Stanley Deutsch, M.D., Ph.D.
Professor of Anesthesiology, George Washington University School of Medicine and Health Sciences, Washington, D.C.
Diverticulosis

Charl de Wet, M.B., Ch.B.
Assistant Professor of Anesthesiology and Cardiothoracic Surgery, Washington University Medical Center, St. Louis, Missouri
Ephedrine
Epinephrine
Isoproterenol (Isuprel)
Lithium Carbonate

Bracken J. DeWitt, M.D., Ph.D.
Resident, Department of Anesthesiology and Critical Care Medicine, Johns Hopkins University School of Medicine, Baltimore, Maryland
Dehydroepiandrosterone (DHEA)
Ephedra (Ma-Huang)

Stephen F. Dierdorf, M.D.
Professor of Anesthesia, Indiana University School of Medicine, Indianapolis, Indiana
Rheumatoid Arthritis

Jeffrey Dodd-o, M.D.
Assistant Professor, Department of Anesthesiology and Critical Care Medicine and Department of Surgery, Johns Hopkins University School of Medicine, Baltimore, Maryland
Ulcerative Colitis, Chronic

Barbara A. Dodson, M.D.
Professor of Anesthesia, University of California, San Francisco, San Francisco, California
Cerebral Arteriovenous Malformations (AVMs)
Depression, Unipolar
Seizure Surgery

Karen B. Domino, M.D., M.P.H.
Professor of Anesthesiology, University of Washington; Staff Anesthesiologist, Harborview Medical Center, Seattle, Washington
Silicosis

John V. Donlon, Jr., M.D.
Associate Clinical Professor of Anesthesia, Harvard Medical School; Chief of Anesthesia, Massachusetts Eye and Ear Infirmary, Boston, Massachusetts
Glaucoma, Closed-Angle
Glaucoma, Open-Angle

Joseph Dooley, M.D.
Associate Resident, University of Rochester School of Medicine and Dentistry, Rochester, New York
Intracranial Hypertension (ICH)

Todd Dorman, M.D.
Associate Professor, Departments of
Anesthesiology and Critical Care
Medicine, Medicine, Surgery, and Nursing,
Johns Hopkins University School of
Medicine, Baltimore, Maryland
Deep Vein Thrombosis
Glyburide, Oral Hypoglycemic Agents
Metformin (Glucophage)

Frank W. Dupont, M.D.
Clinical Instructor of Anesthesia and
Critical Care, Department of Anesthesia
and Critical Care, University of Chicago,
Pritzker School of Medicine, Chicago,
Illinois
Aprotinin (Trasylol)
Dilated Cardiomyopathies (DCMs)
Epsilon-Aminocaproic Acid (EACA)
(Amicar)

Chadwick T. Dybowski, M.D.
Anesthesiology Resident, University of
Chicago, Pritzker School of Medicine,
Chicago, Illinois
Saw Palmetto (Serenoa repens, Sabal
berry, Serenoa repentis fructus, Sabal
serrulata berry

R. Blaine Easley, M.D.
Fellow in Pediatric Anesthesiology and
Pediatric Critical Care Medicine,
Department of Anesthesiology and Critical
Care Medicine, Johns Hopkins University
School of Medicine, Baltimore, Maryland
Creatine
Licorice (Glycyrrhiza glabra)

Thomas J. Ebert, M.D., Ph.D.
Professor of Anesthesiology and Adjunct
Professor of Physiology, Medical College of
Wisconsin; Staff Anesthesiologist, VA
Medical Center, Milwaukee, Wisconsin
Autonomic Hyperreflexia
Familial Dysautonomia (Riley-Day
Syndrome)

Paul D. Eckenbrecht, M.D.
Associate Professor, University of South
Carolina School of Medicine; Director of
Cardiac Anesthesia, Palmetto-Richland
Memorial Hospital, Columbia, South
Carolina
Implantable Cardioverters-Defibrillators
(ICDs), Implantation

Talmage D. Egan, M.D., Ph.D.
Associate Professor of Anesthesiology,
University of Utah School of Medicine;
Staff Physician, University Hospital, Salt
Lake City, Utah
Cigarette Smoking Cessation

Scott M. Eleff, M.D.
Professor and Chairman, Finch University
of Health Sciences, Chicago Medical
School, North Chicago, Illinois
Craniotomy

Nader El-Gamal, M.D.
Assistant Professor of Anesthesiology,
Alexandria University, Alexandria, Egypt
Eye Enucleation
Retinal Buckle Surgery

John Peder Erickson, M.D.
Assistant Clinical Professor of
Anesthesiology, University of Chicago,
Chicago; Medical Director, Midwest
Medical Center, Palos Height, Illinois
Pyloric Stenosis

Lucinda L. Everett, M.D.
Associate Professor, Department of
Anesthesiology, University of Washington;
Attending, Anesthesiology and Pain
Management, Children's Hospital—
Regional Medical Center, Seattle,
Washington
Inguinal Herniorrhaphy

Jane F. Eyrich, M.D.
Associate Professor, Department of
Anesthesiology, Louisiana State University
Health Sciences Center, New Orleans,
Louisiana
Gastrinoma

Nauder Faraday, M.D.
Assistant Professor of Anesthesiology and
Co-Director, Cardiac Surgical Intensive
Care, Johns Hopkins University School of
Medicine, Baltimore, Maryland
Thrombocytopenia

Michael Faulkner, M.D.
Fellow in Cardiac Anesthesiology and
Fellow in Critical Care Medicine, Johns
Hopkins University School of Medicine,
Baltimore, Maryland
CREST Syndrome

Thomas W. Feeley, M.D.
Helen Shafer Fly Distinguished Professor
of Anesthesiology and Head, Division of
Anesthesiology and Critical and Palliative
Care, University of Texas M.D. Anderson
Cancer Center, Houston, Texas
Multisystem Organ Failure, Lung
Dysfunction in

James J. Fehr, M.D.
Assistant Professor, Department of
Anesthesiology, Division of Pediatric
Anesthesiology and Pain Management,
Washington University School of Medicine,
St. Louis Children's Hospital, St. Louis,
Missouri
Mucopolysaccharidoses

James M. Feld, M.D.
Assistant Professor of Anesthesiology,
University of Illinois College of Medicine,
Chicago, Illinois
Hypomagnesemia

Kenneth B. Fickling, M.D.
University of Rochester School of Medicine
and Dentistry, Rochester, New York
Myringotomy and Tympanostomy

Leonard Firestone, M.D.
Professor and Chair, Department of
Anesthesiology and Critical Care
Medicine, University of Pittsburgh School
of Medicine, Pittsburgh, Pennsylvania
Heart Transplant (Adult)
Heart Transplant (Pediatric)

Susan Firestone, M.D.
Associate Professor of Anesthesiology and
Critical Care Medicine, University of
Pittsburgh School of Medicine, Pittsburgh,
Pennsylvania
Heart Transplant (Pediatric)

Stephen P. Fischer, M.D.
Assistant Professor of Anesthesiology,
Stanford University School of Medicine,
Stanford, California
Addison's Disease
Conn's Syndrome (Hyperaldosteronism,
Primary)

Lee A. Fleisher, M.D.
Associate Professor, Department of
Anesthesiology and Critical Care
Medicine; Joint Appointments in Medicine
(Cardiology), Biomedical Information
Sciences, and Health Policy and
Management; Vice-Chairman for Clinical
Investigation; Johns Hopkins University
School of Medicine, Baltimore, Maryland
Angina, Chronic Stable
Chromium
Clopidogrel Bisulfate
Dipyridamole Thallium Imaging
Nitroglycerin
Phytosterols
Radical Prostatectomy (Retropubic)
Scleroderma
Sildenafil Citrate (Viagra)
Splenectomy
Varicella-Zoster Virus

Pierre Foëx, M.D.
Nuffield Professor of Anaesthetics,
University of Oxford; Honorary
Consultant, Radcliffe Infirmary, Oxford,
United Kingdom
Hypertension

Joseph F. Foss, M.D.
Assistant Clinical Professor, University of
Chicago; Director, Perioperative Screening
Clinic; Director, Integrated Anesthesia
Laboratory; University of Chicago,
Chicago, Illinois
Arteritis, Takayasu's
Cisplatin

Nancy K. France, M.D.
Associate Professor, Medical College of
Wisconsin, Milwaukee, Wisconsin
Arnold-Chiari Syndrome

Steven M. Frank, M.D.
Assistant Professor, Department of
Anesthesiology and Critical Care
Medicine, Johns Hopkins University
School of Medicine, Baltimore, Maryland
Liver Resection

Marc B. Freeman, M.D.
Anesthesia Resident, University of
Chicago, Chicago, Illinois
Pyruvate

Edward J. Frink, Jr., M.D.
Associate Professor of Anesthesiology,
Pennsylvania State University College of
Medicine, Hershey, Pennsylvania
Liver Function Tests
Multiple Endocrine Neoplasia (MEN)
Types I and II

William R. Furman, M.D.
Associate Professor of Anesthesiology,
University of North Carolina—Chapel
Hill, Chapel Hill, North Carolina
Emphysema

Angela Gailey, M.D.
Anesthesia Resident, Johns Hopkins
University School of Medicine, Baltimore,
Maryland
Office-based Anesthesia

Robert Gaiser, M.D.
Associate Professor of Anesthesiology and
Pharmacology, University of Pennsylvania
School of Medicine; Director of Obstetric
Anesthesia, Hospital of the University of
Pennsylvania, Philadelphia, Pennsylvania
Split-Thickness Skin Graft

T. James Gallagher, M.D.
Professor of Anesthesiology and Surgery
and Chief, Critical Care Medicine,
University of Florida College of Medicine,
Gainesville, Florida
Respiratory Distress Syndrome

Kristin K. Galli, M.D.
Assistant Professor, University of
Pennsylvania School of Medicine;
Children's Hospital of Philadelphia,
Department of Anesthesia, Philadelphia,
Pennsylvania
*Total Anomalous Pulmonary Venous
    Return Correction*

David R. Gambling, M.B., B.S., F.R.C.P.C.
Associate Clinical Professor, Department
of Anesthesiology, University of California,
San Diego; Staff Anesthesiologist, Sharp
Mary Birch Hospital for Women, San
Diego, California
Hypermagnesemia

Abraham C. Gaupp, M.D.
Resident House Staff, University of
Chicago—Anesthesia, Chicago, Illinois
*Psyllium, Bulk-Forming Laxatives
    (Plantago isphagula, Plantago ovata)*

Brian K. Gehlbach, M.D.
Fellow in Pulmonary and Critical Care,
University of Chicago Hospitals, Chicago,
Illinois
*Acute Respiratory Distress Syndrome
    (ARDS)*
Asthma, Acute

Jeremy M. Geiduschek, M.D.
Associate Professor, Department of
Anesthesiology, University of Washington
School of Medicine; Attending Physician,
Department of Anesthesiology, Children's
Hospital and Regional Medical Center,
Seattle, Washington
Kearns-Sayre Syndrome
*Leigh Syndrome (Subacute Necrotizing
    Encephalopathy)*

Simon Gelman, M.D., Ph.D.
Leroy D. Vandam/Benjamin G. Covino
Professor of Anesthesia, Harvard Medical
School; Chairman, Department of
Anesthesiology, Perioperative and Pain
Medicine, Brigham and Women's Hospital,
Boston, Massachusetts
Liver Transplantation

Ghaleb A. Ghani, M.D.
Associate Professor of Anesthesiology,
Emory University School of Medicine,
Atlanta, Georgia
Glomus Jugulare Tumors

Charles P. Gibbs, M.D.
Professor Emeritus, University of Colorado
Health Sciences Center; Staff
Anesthesiologist, University of Colorado
Hospital, Denver, Colorado
Abruptio Placentae

Kevin J. Gingrich, M.D.
Assistant Professor of Anesthesiology,
Pharmacology, and Physiology, University
of Rochester School of Medicine and
Dentistry, Rochester, New York
Intracranial Hypertension (ICH)

D. David Glass, M.D.
Professor of Anesthesiology and Medicine
and Chairman, Department of
Anesthesiology, Dartmouth Medical School,
Dartmouth Hitchcock Medical Center,
Lebanon, New Hampshire
*Disseminated Intravascular Coagulation
    (DIC)*

Barbara S. Gold, M.D.
Associate Professor of Anesthesiology,
University of Minnesota School of
Medicine; Staff Anesthesiologist, Twin
Cities Anesthesia Associates, Fairview-
University Medical Center, Minneapolis,
Minnesota
HIV Testing

Randolph B. Gorman, M.D.
Staff Anesthesiologist, Greater Baltimore
Medical Center, Towson, Maryland
Abdominoperineal Resection

Alexander W. Gotta, M.D.
Professor Emeritus of Anesthesiology,
State University of New York Downstate
Medical Center, Brooklyn, New York
Trauma

Alexandru Gottlieb, M.D.
Associate Professor, Ohio State University,
Columbus; Staff Physician, Cleveland
Clinic Foundation, Cleveland, Ohio
Bypass, Femoral-Femoral
Endovascular Aortic Stent Repairs

Ori Gottlieb, M.D.
Assistant Professor, Ohio State University,
Department of General Anesthesia,
Cleveland, Ohio
*Melatonin (N-acetyl-5-methoxytryptamine,
    Bevitamil, Vitamist, Melatonex)*

Nishan G. Goudsouzian, M.D.
Professor of Anaesthesia, Harvard Medical
School; Director, Pediatric Anaesthesia,
Massachusetts General Hospital, Boston,
Massachusetts
Atropine
Kasai Procedure

George J. Graf, M.D.
Clinical Assistant Professor, Department
of Anesthesiology, University of California,
Los Angeles, School of Medicine, Los
Angeles, California
Diabetes Insipidus

Gilbert J. Grant, M.D.
Assistant Professor of Anesthesiology, New
York University School of Medicine, New
York, New York
Tubal Ligation

Nikolaus Gravenstein, M.D.
The Jerome H. Modell, M.D., Professor
and Chairman of Anesthesiology,
University of Florida College of Medicine,
Gainesville, Florida
Diuretics

William J. Greeley, M.D.
Professor and Chairman, Department of
Anesthesiology and Critical Care
Medicine, Children's Hospital of
Philadelphia, Philadelphia, Pennsylvania
Marfan's Syndrome
*Total Anomalous Pulmonary Venous
    Return Correction*

James A. Greenberg, M.D.
Assistant Professor of Anesthesiology and
Pediatrics, University of Pittsburgh School
of Medicine, Pittsburgh, Pennsylvania
Down Syndrome

George A. Gregory, M.D.
Professor of Anesthesia and Pediatrics,
University of California, San Francisco,
School of Medicine, San Francisco,
California
Patent Ductus Arteriosus

Alan W. Grogono, M.D.
Professor, Department of Anesthesiology,
Tulane University School of Medicine,
New Orleans, Louisiana
Acidosis, Lactic/Metabolic

Brett B. Gutsche, M.D.
Professor Emeritus of Anesthesiology and
Obstetrics and Gynecology, University of
Pennsylvania School of Medicine,
Philadelphia, Pennsylvania
Magnesium Sulfate

J. Michael Haering, M.D.
Instructor in Anaesthesia, Harvard
Medical School, Boston, Massachusetts
Cardiomyopathy, Hypertrophic (HCM)

Jonathan D. Halevy, M.D.
Attending Anesthesiologist, Neurosensory
Institute, Wills Eye Hospital, Philadelphia,
Pennsylvania
Burr Hole

Jesse B. Hall, M.D.
Professor of Medicine, University of
Chicago; Section Chief, Pulmonary and
Critical Care Medicine, and Director,
Respiratory Therapy, University of
Chicago, Chicago, Illinois
*Acute Respiratory Distress Syndrome
    (ARDS)*
Asthma, Acute

Rukaiya K.A. Hamid, M.D.
Clinical Professor of Pediatric
Anesthesiology, University of California,
Irvine, Orange, California
*Syndrome of Inappropriate Antidiuretic
    Hormone Secretion (SIADH)*

Long K. Han, M.D.
Assistant Professor of Anesthesia and Critical Care, University of Chicago, Chicago, Illinois
Atrial Septal Defect—Ostium Primum
Atrial Septal Defect—Ostium Secundum

Raafat S. Hannallah, M.D.
Professor of Anesthesiology and Pediatrics, George Washington University; Chairman of Anesthesiology, Children's National Medical Center, Washington, D.C.
Anhidrosis (Congenital Anhidrotic Ectodermal Dysplasia)
Carnitine Deficiency

C. William Hanson, III, M.D.
Professor of Anesthesia, Surgery and Internal Medicine, Hospital of the University of Pennsylvania, Department of Anesthesia, Philadelphia, Pennsylvania
Bronchitis, Chronic

Charles B. Hantler, M.D.
Professor, University of Texas Health Science Center at San Antonio, San Antonio, Texas
Adrenal Insufficiency, Acute or Secondary

Andrew P. Harris, M.D., M.H.S.
Associate Professor, Department of Anesthesiology and Critical Care Medicine and Department of Obstetrics and Gynecology; Chief, Division of Obstetric Anesthesia, Johns Hopkins University School of Medicine, Baltimore, Maryland
Cesarean Section, Planned

Stephen N. Harris, M.D.
Associate Clinical Professor, Yale University Department of Anesthesia, Yale University School of Medicine, New Haven; Staff Anesthesiologist, Danbury Hospital, Danbury, Connecticut
Pericarditis, Constrictive

Laura A. Hastings, M.D.
Assistant Professor, Department of Anesthesiology and Critical Care Medicine, Johns Hopkins University School of Medicine, Baltimore, Maryland
Single (Including Common) Ventricle

Martin Hautkappe, M.D.
Physician, Klinik fuer Anaesthesiologie, Technische Universitaet, University of Munich, Munich, Germany
Capsaicin

John K. Hayes, Ph.D.
Department of Anesthesiology, University of Utah College of Medicine, Salt Lake City, Utah
Hyponatremia
Hypernatremia

Stephen O. Heard, M.D.
Associate Professor of Anesthesiology and Surgery, University of Massachusetts Medical Center, Worcester, Massachusetts
TMJ Arthroscopy

James E. Heavner, D.V.M., Ph.D.
Professor and Director of Research, Department of Anesthesiology, and Professor, Department of Physiology, Texas Tech University Health Sciences Center, Lubbock, Texas
Dibucaine Number (Atypical Cholinesterase)

James R. Hebl, M.D.
Assistant Professor, Department of Anesthesiology, Mayo Clinic, Rochester, Minnesota
Subphrenic Abscess

Amr R. Hegazi, M.D.
Senior Resident, Department of Anesthesiology, Texas Tech Medical Center, Lubbock, Texas
Androstenedione

Eugenie Heitmiller, M.D.
Associate Professor, Department of Anesthesiology and Critical Care Medicine, Johns Hopkins University School of Medicine, Baltimore, Maryland
Patent Ductus Arteriosus, Ligation of

Mark Helfaer, M.D.
Associate Professor of Anesthesiology, Critical Care Medicine, and Pediatrics, University of Pennsylvania School of Medicine; Chief, Critical Care Medicine, Children's Hospital of Philadelphia, Philadelphia, Pennsylvania
Friedreich's Ataxia

Lori B. Heller, M.D.
Assistant Professor, Department of Anesthesiology and Critical Care, University of Chicago, Chicago, Illinois
Atorvastatin (Lipitor)
Cardiopulmonary Bypass
Pseudoephedrine

Mitzi K. Hemstreet, M.D., Ph.D.
Instructor, Department of Anesthesiology and Critical Care Medicine, Division Neuroanesthesiology and Neurosciences Critical Care, Johns Hopkins University School of Medicine, Baltimore, Maryland
Carnitine
Hormone Replacement Therapy

Ian A. Herrick, M.D., F.R.C.P.C.
Associate Professor of Anesthesiology and Clinical Pharmacology, University of Western Ontario, London, Ontario, Canada
Occlusive Cerebrovascular Disease

Michael S. Higgins, M.D.
Assistant Professor, Vanderbilt University School of Medicine, Nashville, Tennessee
Ileostomy

Roberta L. Hines, M.D.
Professor and Chair, Department of Anesthesiology, Yale University School of Medicine; Chief, Department of Anesthesiology, Yale-New Haven Hospital, New Haven, Connecticut
Beta-Adrenergic Receptor Antagonists (Blockers)

Irving A. Hirsch, M.D.
Assistant Professor, Case Western Reserve University School of Medicine; Medical Director, Metro Health Outpatient Surgery Center of Metro Health Medical Center, Cleveland, Ohio
Hyperkalemia
Hypokalemia

Michael Ho, M.D.
Assistant Professor of Anesthesiology, Baylor University School of Medicine, Houston, Texas
Conversion Disorder
Schizophrenia

Charles W. Hogue, Jr., M.D.
Associate Professor of Anesthesiology and Chief, Division of Cardiothoracic Anesthesia, Washington University School of Medicine, St. Louis, Missouri
Atrial Septal Defect, Repair of
Chagas' Disease

Kenneth J. Holroyd, M.D.
Executive Vice President and Chief Business Officer, Genaera Corporation, Plymouth Meeting, Pennsylvania
Amyloidosis

William Hope, M.D., Ph.D.
Instructor of Anesthesiology, Medical College of Wisconsin, Milwaukee, Wisconsin
Familial Dysautonomia (Riley-Day Syndrome)

Philippe Housmans, M.D.
Associate Professor of Anesthesiology, Mayo Medical School, Rochester, Minnesota
Procainamide

Wendy Stevens Howard, M.D.
Assistant Professor of Anesthesiology, State University of New York at Syracuse, Veterans Administration Medical Center, Syracuse, New York
Burn Injury, Flame

Simon J. Howell, M.D.
Consultant Senior Lecturer in Anaesthesia, University of Bristol; Consultant Senior Lecturer and Honorary Consultant Anaesthetist, United Bristol Healthcare Trust, Bristol, United Kingdom
Hypertension

Michael B. Howie, M.D.
Professor and Vice Chair, Department of Anesthesiology, The Ohio State University Medical Center, Columbus, Ohio
Quinidine

Cindy Hughes, M.D.
Associate Professor of Anesthesiology, Albany Medical College, Albany, New York
Ventricular Septal Defect, Repair of

Catherine Huraux, M.D.
Research Fellow, Emory University School of Medicine, Atlanta, Georgia
Anticoagulation, Preoperative

Stefan A. Iantchoulev, M.D.
Fellow, Cardiothoracic Anesthesia, Department of Anesthesiology, Washington University School of Medicine, St. Louis, Missouri
Chagas' Disease

Lorna L. Im, M.D.
Physician, Department of Anesthesia and Critical Care, University of Chicago Hospitals, Chicago, Illinois
Trimethaphan

Robert M. Insoft, M.D.
Attending Neonatologist, Massachusetts General Hospital; Instructor in Pediatrics, Harvard Medical School, Boston, Massachusetts
Necrotizing Enterocolitis

Shiroh Isono, M.D.
Assistant Professor, Department of Anesthesiology (B1), Graduate School of Medicine, Chiba University, Chiba, Japan
Swallowing Disorders

Eric Jacobsohn, M.B., Ch.B., F.R.C.P.C.
Associate Professor, Anesthesiology and Surgery, Washington University School of Medicine; Director, Cardiothoracic Critical Care, Barnes–Jewish Hospital, St. Louis, Missouri
Ephedrine
Epinephrine
Isoproterenol (Isuprel)
Lithium Carbonate

Subhash Jain, M.D.
Chief, Pain Service and Department of Anesthesiology and Critical Care Medicine, Memorial Sloan-Kettering Cancer Center, New York, New York
Leukemia

Uday Jain, M.D., Ph.D.
Clinical Associate Professor, Stanford University School of Medicine, Stanford; Partner, San Francisco Anesthesia Medical Group, San Francisco, California
Hypercholesterolemia
Hypertriglyceridemia
Lipidemias

Roger A. Johns, M.D.
Professor and Chair, Department of Anesthesiology and Critical Care Medicine, Johns Hopkins University School of Medicine, Baltimore, Maryland
Bretylium Tosylate

Madelyn Kahana, M.D.
Professor of Clinical Anesthesia and Professor of Clinical Pediatrics, University of Chicago; Medical Director, Pediatric Intensive Care Unit, University of Chicago Children's Hospital, Chicago, Illinois
Meningomyelocele Repair
Spinal Fusion

Zeev N. Kain, M.D.
Assistant Professor of Anesthesiology and Pediatrics, Yale University School of Medicine, New Haven, Connecticut
Cocaine
Neurofibromatosis

Surinder K. Kaller, M.D.
Professor, Medical College of Virginia/Virginia Commonwealth University, Richmond, Virginia
Inguinal Herniorrhaphy

Helen W. Karl, M.D.
Associate Professor of Anesthesiology, University of Washington School of Medicine; Attending Anesthesiologist, Children's Hospital and Regional Medical Center, Seattle, Washington
Tonsillectomy and Adenoidectomy

Jeffrey Katz, M.D.
Professor and Chairman, Department of Anesthesiology, University of Texas–Houston Medical School, Houston, Texas
Encephalopathy, Hypertensive

Jeffrey A. Katz, M.D.
Professor of Clinical Anesthesia, University of California, San Francisco, School of Medicine, San Francisco, California
Candidiasis
Pemphigus

Sandy Kaufmann, M.D.
Fellow/Resident, Department of Anesthesiology and Critical Care Medicine, Johns Hopkins University School of Medicine, Baltimore, Maryland
Beckwith-Wiedemann Syndrome

Shubjeet Kaur, M.D.
Associate Professor of Clinical Anesthesiology, University of Massachusetts Medical School; Clinical Vice Chair, Anesthesiology, University of Massachusetts Memorial Hospital, Worcester, Massachusetts
Cromolyn Sodium

Adam M. Kaye, Pharm.D., F.A.S.C.P.
Assistant Clinical Professor of Pharmacy Practice, University of the Pacific, School of Pharmacy and Health Sciences, Stockton, California
Androstenedione

Alan D. Kaye, M.D., Ph.D.
Chairman and Professor, Department of Anesthesiology, Texas Tech University Health Sciences Center, Lubbock, Texas
Androstenedione
β-Sitosterol
Headache, Migraine
S-Adenosyl-L-Methionine (SAMe)

Nancy B. Kenepp, M.D.
Associate Professor, Department of Anesthesiology, Temple University School of Medicine, Philadelphia, Pennsylvania
Epidermolysis Bullosa

Mary A. Keyes, M.D.
Associate Professor, Department of Anesthesiology, University of California, Los Angeles, Los Angeles, California
Bronchopulmonary Dysplasia (BPD)
Latex Allergy
Physiologic Anemia and the Anemia of Prematurity
Reye's Syndrome

Woo Chan Kim, M.D.
Physician, Department of Anesthesia and Critical Care, University of Chicago, Chicago, Illinois
Herpes, Type 2

Kimberly M. King, M.D.
Resident, Department of Anesthesiology and Critical Care Medicine, Johns Hopkins University School of Medicine, Baltimore, Maryland
Dandelion

Jerome M. Klafta, M.D.
Assistant Professor, Clinical Anesthesia and Critical Care, University of Chicago, Pritzker School of Medicine, Chicago, Illinois
Blebs and Bullae

P. Allan Klock, Jr., M.D.
Assistant Professor, Department of Anesthesia and Critical Care, University of Chicago, Chicago, Illinois
Amniotic Fluid Embolism
Terbutaline

Arthur J. Klowden, M.D.
Clinical Assistant Professor, Department of Anesthesiology, University of Illinois College of Medicine; Attending Anesthesiologist, Illinois Masonic Medical Center and Shriners Hospital for Children, Chicago, Illinois
Myotonia Dystrophica (Myotonic Dystrophy, Steinert's Disease)

Paul R. Knight III, M.D., Ph.D.
Professor and Chair, Department of Anesthesiology, State University of New York at Buffalo, School of Medicine and Biomedical Sciences, Buffalo, New York
IgA Deficiency
Immune Suppression
Q Fever
Rocky Mountain Spotted Fever

Donald D. Koblin, M.D., Ph.D.
Professor of Anesthesia, University of California, San Francisco; Staff Anesthesiologist, Department of Veterans Affairs, San Francisco, California
Fluoxetine (Prozac)
Haloperidol (Haldol)
Vitamin B_{12}/Folate Deficiency

W. Andrew Kofke, M.D.
Professor, Department of Anesthesia, University of Pennsylvania School of Medicine; Director of Neuroanesthesia, Hospital of the University of Pennsylvania, Philadelphia, Pennsylvania
Seizures, Epileptic

Anne C. Kolker, M.D.
Assistant Professor, Department of Anesthesiology, Cornell University Medical College, New York, New York
Cancer, Esophageal

Tracy Koogler, M.D.
Assistant Professor, Department of Anesthesia and Critical Care and Pediatrics, University of Chicago, Chicago, Illinois
Post Transplant Lymphoproliferative Disease
Reye's Syndrome

Vincent J. Kopp, M.D.
Associate Professor of Anesthesiology and
Pediatrics and Adjunct Associate Professor
of Social Medicine, School of Medicine,
University of North Carolina at Chapel
Hill; Medical Director, Precare, University
of North Carolina Hospitals, Chapel Hill,
North Carolina
Pertussis (Whooping Cough)

Fayez Kotob, M.D.
Clinical Instructor of Anesthesiology, State
University of New York Downstate
Medical Center, Brooklyn, New York
Pregnancy Testing

Vandana Kulkarni, M.D.
Assistant Professor of Anesthesia and
Critical Care, University of Chicago,
Chicago, Illinois
Phenytoin

C. Dean Kurth, M.D.
Associate Professor, Department of
Anesthesia and Pediatrics, University of
Pennsylvania School of Medicine; Senior
Anesthesiologist, Children's Hospital of
Philadelphia, Philadelphia, Pennsylvania
Cleft Palate Repair

Carol L. Lake, M.D., M.B.A., M.P.H.
Professor and Chair, Associate Dean for
Continuing Medical Education, University
of Louisville Health Sciences Center,
Louisville, Kentucky
Calcium-Channel Blockers
Double Aortic Arch
Endocardial Cushion Defect

George H. Lampe, M.D.
Staff Physician, Good Samaritan Hospital,
San Jose, California
Cushing's Syndrome

William L. Lanier, M.D.
Professor of Anesthesiology, Mayo Medical
School; Consultant in Anesthesiology,
Mayo Clinic, Rochester, Minnesota
Hyperglycemia

Lawrence O. Larson, M.D.
Private practice, Bloomfield, Michigan
Lesch-Nyhan Syndrome

John P. Lawrence, M.D.
Assistant Professor of Anesthesiology and
Clinical Director, Cardiovascular
Anesthesia, University of Cincinnati,
Cincinnati, Ohio
Folic Acid

Jesse A. Leak, M.D.
Associate Professor of Anesthesiology,
University of Texas M.D. Anderson Cancer
Center, Houston, Texas
Nutraceuticals

Charles Lee, M.D.
Assistant Professor of Anesthesiology,
Loma Linda University School of
Medicine, Loma Linda, California
Carotid Sinus Syndrome (CSS)

Keith K. Lee, D.O.
Resident Physician, Anesthesiology, Johns
Hopkins University School of Medicine,
Baltimore, Maryland
Chondroitin Sulfate

Michael K. Lee, M.D.
House Staff, University of Chicago,
Chicago, Illinois
*Ginseng (Panax ginseng, Panax
quinquefolius)*
St. John's Wort (Hypericum perforatum)

David Eric Lees, M.D.
Professor and Chair, Anesthesia,
Georgetown University Medical Center;
Chief of Service, Anesthesia, Georgetown
University Hospital, Washington, D.C.
Dementia
Do Not Resuscitate (DNR) Orders

George S. Leisure, M.D.
Assistant Professor of Anesthesiology,
University of Virginia Health Sciences
Center, Charlottesville, Virginia
Bleomycin Sulfate Toxicity
Bretylium Tosylate

William A. Lell, M.D.
Benjamin Carraway Professor of
Anesthesiology, University of Alabama,
Birmingham, Birmingham, Alabama
Bronchiolitis Obliterans (BO)

Mark J. Lema, M.D., Ph.D.
Professor and Chair, Department of
Anesthesiology, State University of New
York at Buffalo, School of Medicine and
Biomedical Sciences; Chair, Department of
Anesthesiology and Pain Medicine,
Roswell Park Cancer Institute, Buffalo,
New York
Alkylating Agents
Bleomycin

Harry J. M. Lemmens, M.D., Ph.D.
Associate Professor, Stanford University
Medical Center, Department of Anesthesia,
Stanford, California
*Benzodiazepines (Midazolam, Lorazepam,
Diazepam)*

W. Casey Lenox, M.D.
Assistant Professor, Johns Hopkins
University School of Medicine, Baltimore,
Maryland
Orchiopexy

Irene E. Leonard, M.B., F.F.A.R.C.S.I.
Lecturer in Anaesthesia, Royal College of
Surgeons in Ireland; Beaumont Hospital,
Dublin, Ireland
AV Graft for Hemodialysis

Jacqueline M. Leung, M.D., M.P.H.
Associate Professor of Anesthesia and
Perioperative Care, University of
California, San Francisco, School of
Medicine; Attending Anesthesiologist,
University of California, San Francisco,
Medical Center, San Francisco, California
Atherosclerotic Disease
Peripheral Vascular Disease

Jerrold H. Levy, M.D.
Professor of Anesthesiology, Division of
Cardiothoracic Anesthesiology and Critical
Care, Emory University School of
Medicine, Atlanta, Georgia
Allergy
Anticoagulation, Preoperative

Hong Li, M.D.
Anesthesia and Critical Care Resident,
University of Chicago Hospital, Chicago,
Illinois
Goldenseal (Hydrastis canadensis)

J. Lance Lichtor, M.D.
Professor, Department of Anesthesia and
Critical Care and Pediatrics, University of
Chicago, Chicago, Illinois
Pyloric Stenosis Repair

Kevin P. Limp, M.D.*
Formerly, Assistant Professor, Department
of Anesthesiology and Critical Care
Medicine, Johns Hopkins University
School of Medicine, Baltimore, Maryland
Colostomy

Karen S. Lindeman, M.D.
Associate Professor, Department of
Anesthesia and Critical Care Medicine,
Johns Hopkins University School of
Medicine, Baltimore, Maryland
Placenta Previa

Ronald S. Litman, D.O.
Associate Professor of Anesthesiology,
University of Pennsylvania School of
Medicine; Children's Hospital of
Philadelphia, Philadelphia, Pennsylvania
Imperforate Anus Repair
Klippel-Feil Syndrome
Strabismus Surgery
Testicular Torsion Surgery
Thalassemia

Maywin Liu, M.D.
Chief, Division of Chronic Pain
Management, Department of Anesthesia,
St. Joseph Medical Center, Towson,
Maryland
Autonomic Hyperreflexia

Terrence H. Liu, M.D.
Research Fellow, Critical Care Department
of Surgery, University of Minnesota
Hospitals and Clinics, Minneapolis,
Minnesota
Nutritional Support

Wen-Shin Liu, M.D.
Professor of Anesthesiology,
Northeastern Ohio Universities College of
Medicine, Rootstown; Medical Staff, Mercy
Medical Center, Canton, Ohio
Cancer, Prostate

Aaron Lloyd, M.D.
Resident, Department of Anesthesiology,
Johns Hopkins University School of
Medicine, Baltimore, Maryland
Ventriculoperitoneal Shunt

Martin J. London, M.D.
Professor of Clinical Anesthesia,
University of California, San Francisco;
Attending Anesthesiologist, San Francisco
VA Medical Center, San Francisco,
California
Diagnostic 12-Lead ECG

*Deceased

Sandra V. Lowe, M.D.
Assistant Professor of Anesthesiology and Pediatrics, Department of Pediatric Critical Care and Anesthesiology, Vanderbilt University School of Medicine, Nashville, Tennessee
Achondroplasia, Dwarfism

Edward Lowenstein, M.D.
Henry Isaiah Dorr Professor of Anaesthesia and Professor of Medical Ethics, Harvard Medical School; Provost, Department of Anesthesia and Critical Care, Massachusetts General Hospital, Boston, Massachusetts
Cardiomyopathy, Hypertrophic (HCM)

Jeffrey K. Lu, M.D.
Associate Professor of Anesthesiology, University of Utah Medical School, Salt Lake City, Utah
Phenothiazines

Philip D. Lumb, M.B., B.S., F.C.C.M.
Professor and Chairman, Department of Anesthesiology, Keck School of Medicine, University of Southern California, Los Angeles, California
Lyme Disease

Carl Lynch III, M.D., Ph.D.
Professor and Chair of Anesthesiology, University of Virginia Health System, Charlottesville, Virginia
Pacemaker Implantation for Sick Sinus Rhythm

Anne Marie Lynn, M.D.
Professor, Anesthesiology and Pediatrics, University of Washington School of Medicine, Seattle, Washington
Jeune Syndrome (Asphyxiating Thoracic Dystrophy)

Tetsuji Makita, M.D.
Lecturer, Nagasaki University Hospital, Division of Intensive Care Unit, Nagasaki, Japan
Allergy

Vinod Malhotra, M.D.
Professor of Clinical Anesthesiology, Weill Medical College of Cornell University; Vice-Chair for Clinical Affairs, Clinical Director of Operating Rooms, Department of Anesthesiology, New York Presbyterian Hospital–Weill Cornell Center, New York, New York
Nephrectomy/Radical Nephrectomy

Andrew M. Malinow, M.D.
Professor of Anesthesiology, Obstetrics, Gynecology, and Reproductive Sciences, University of Maryland School of Medicine; Director, Obstetric Anesthesiology and Associate Vice-Chair, Development, Department of Anesthesiology, University of Maryland Medical Center, Baltimore, Maryland
Preeclampsia

Dennis T. Mangano, M.D., Ph.D.
Director and Founder, McSPI Research Group, San Francisco, California
Myocardial Ischemia (MIsch)

Srinivas Mantha, M.D.
Additional Professor, Nizam's Institute of Medical Sciences, Hyderabad, India
Hyperparathyroidism
Malnutrition

Jonathan B. Mark, M.D.
Associate Professor of Anesthesiology and Assistant Professor of Medicine, Duke University Medical Center; Chief, Anesthesiology Service, Veterans Affairs Medical Center, Durham, North Carolina
Cardiomyopathy, Alcoholic
Cardiomyopathy, Ischemic

H. Michael Marsh, M.B., B.S., B.Sc.(Med)
Professor and Chair of Anesthesiology, Wayne State University; Specialist-in-Chief, Detroit Medical Center, Detroit, Michigan
Bronchiectasis
Methemoglobinemia

Jackie Martin, M.D.
Associate Professor, Johns Hopkins University School of Medicine, Baltimore, Maryland
Subclavian Steal Syndrome

J.A. Jeevendra Martyn, M.D.
Professor of Anesthesiology and Critical Care, Harvard Medical School; Anesthestist and Director, Clinical and Biochemical Pharmacology Laboratory, Massachusetts General Hospital, Boston, Massachusetts
Burn Injury, Electrical

Douglas Martz, Jr., M.D.
Assistant Professor of Anesthesiology, University of Maryland School of Medicine, Baltimore, Maryland
Narcolepsy

Gertie F. Marx, M.D.
Professor, Albert Einstein College of Medicine, Bronx, New York
Cesarean Section, Emergent

Donald D. Mathes, M.D.
Assistant Professor of Anesthesiology, Department of Anesthesiology, University of Virginia Health Sciences Center, Charlottesville, Virginia
Bleomycin Sulfate Toxicity

M. Jane Matjasko, M.D.
Professor and Chair of Anesthesiology and Clinical Chief of Anesthesiology, University of Maryland School of Medicine, Baltimore, Maryland
Encephalitis

Lynne G. Maxwell, M.D.
Associate Professor, Department of Anesthesiology and Critical Care Medicine, Johns Hopkins University School of Medicine, Baltimore, Maryland
Duodenal Atresia

John P. McCarren, M.D.
Associate Clinical Professor of Anesthesiology, University of California, San Diego; Medical Director of Perioperative Services, Department of Anesthesiology, Thornton Hospital, La Jolla, California
Cancer, Bronchial

William A. McDade, M.D., Ph.D.
Assistant Professor, Department of Anesthesia and Critical Care, University of Chicago, Chicago, Illinois
Sickle Cell Disease

Susan B. McDonald, M.D.
Fellow, Cardiothoracic Anesthesia, Washington University School of Medicine, St. Louis, Missouri
Atrial Septal Defect, Repair of

Kathryn E. McGoldrick, M.D.
Professor and Chairman, Department of Anesthesiology, New York Medical College; Director of Anesthesiology, Westchester Medical College, Valhalla, New York
Blowout Orbital Fracture
Cataract ± IOL

Brian J. McGrath, M.D.
Associate Professor of Anesthesiology and Critical Care Medicine and Associate Dean for Admissions and Financial Aid, George Washington University School of Medicine; Attending Anesthesiologist, George Washington University Medical Center, Washington, D.C.
Fat Embolism

Charles H. McLeskey, M.D.
Professor and Chairman, Department of Anesthesiology, Texas A&M University Health Science Center, Temple, Texas
Geriatric Surgery

Thomas M. McLoughlin, Jr., M.D.
Clinical Associate Professor of Anesthesia, Penn State University College of Medicine; Chief, Division of Cardiac Anesthesia, Lehigh Valley Hospital, Allentown, Pennsylvania
Coagulopathy, Factor IX Deficiency
Von Willebrand's Disease

Robert McPherson, M.D.*
Formerly, Associate Professor, Department of Anesthesiology and Critical Care Medicine; Johns Hopkins University School of Medicine, Baltimore, Maryland
Craniotomy

William L. Meadow, M.D., Ph.D.
Associate Professor, Department of Pediatrics, University of Chicago, Chicago, Illinois
Apnea of the Newborn

Robert G. Merin, M.D.
Professor of Anesthesiology, Medical College of Georgia School of Medicine, Augusta, Georgia
Coronary Artery Spasm (CAS)
Digitalis

William T. Merritt, M.D., M.B.A.
Associate Professor, Division of Critical Care Anesthesia, Johns Hopkins University School of Medicine, Baltimore, Maryland; President, International Liver Transplantation Society
Jaundice

Scott Metzger, M.D.
Director, Metzger Pain Management, Shrewsbury, New Jersey
Alcohol Abuse

*Deceased

Leslie Newberg Milde, M.D.
Professor of Anesthesiology, Mayo Medical School, Scottsdale, Arizona, and Rochester, Minnesota; Chair, Department of Anesthesiology, Mayo Clinic, Scottsdale, Scottsdale, Arizona
Carbamazepine (Tegretol)

Edward D. Miller, Jr., M.D.
Professor of Anesthesiology and Critical Care Medicine, and Dean of the Medical Faculty, CEO, Johns Hopkins Medicine, Johns Hopkins University School of Medicine, Baltimore, Maryland
Hypertension, Uncontrolled, with Cardiomyopathy

Lisa F. Miller, M.D.
Senior Resident, Department of Anesthesia and Critical Care, University of Chicago Hospitals, Chicago, Illinois
Glycine

Matthew K. Miller, M.D.
Assistant Professor and Clinical Department Head, Department of Anesthesiology, Louisiana State University School of Medicine, New Orleans, Louisiana
Acetaminophen
Hyperaldosteronism (Secondary)

Marek A. Mirski, M.D., Ph.D.
Associate Professor of Surgery and Medicine, University of Hawaii John A. Burns School of Medicine, Honolulu, Hawaii
Seizures, Grand Mal (Tonic-Clonic)
Seizures, Petit Mal (Absence)

Scott Mittman, M.D., Ph.D.
Assistant Professor, Department of Anesthesiology and Critical Care Medicine, Johns Hopkins University School of Medicine, Baltimore, Maryland
Carpal Tunnel Release

Roy Mongkolpradit, M.D.
Resident, Department of Anesthesia and Critical Care, University of Chicago, Chicago, Illinois
Glucosamine Sulfate

Constance L. Monitto, M.D.
Assistant Professor, Department of Anesthesiology and Critical Care Medicine, Johns Hopkins University School of Medicine, Baltimore, Maryland
Ureteral Reimplantation

Terri G. Monk, M.D.
Associate Professor, Department of Anesthesiology, Washington University School of Medicine, St. Louis, Missouri
Urinary Lithiasis

Richard E. Moon, M.D.
Professor of Anesthesiology; Associate Professor of Pulmonary Medicine; Medical Director, Hyperbaric Center; Medical Director, Divers Alert Network; Duke University Medical Center, Durham, North Carolina
Carbon Monoxide (CO) Poisoning
Gas Embolism

Laurel E. Moore, M.D.
Assistant Professor, Department of Anesthesiology, Johns Hopkins University School of Medicine, Baltimore, Maryland
Anterior Cervical Fusion
Electroconvulsive Therapy (ECT)

Roger A. Moore, M.D.
Clinical Associate Professor, University of Medicine and Dentistry, Newark; Chair, Department of Anesthesia, Deborah Heart and Lung Center, Browns Mills, New Jersey
Anomalous Pulmonary Venous Drainage
Cancer, Lung Parenchyma

Jeffrey P. Morray, M.D.
Professor, Department of Anesthesiology, University of Washington School of Medicine; Director, Department of Anesthesiology, Children's Hospital and Regional Medical Center, Seattle, Washington
Truncus Arteriosus

Jonathan Moss, M.D., Ph.D.
Professor of Anesthesia and Critical Care and Vice Chairman for Research, University of Chicago Medical Center, Department of Anesthesia and Critical Care, Chicago, Illinois
Anaphylaxis
Syndrome X

John R. Moyers, M.D.
Professor, Department of Anesthesia, University of Iowa College of Medicine, University of Iowa Hospital and Clinics, Iowa City, Iowa
Mesothelioma

Jesse J. Muir, M.D.
Assistant Professor of Anesthesiology and Director of Pain Clinic, Mayo Clinic, Scottsdale, Scottsdale, Arizona
Insulinoma

John M. Murkin, M.D., F.R.C.P.C.
Professor of Anesthesiology, University of Western Ontario; Director, Cardiac Anesthesia, University Campus, London Health Sciences Centre, London, Ontario, Canada
Thyroid Supplements

Jane M. Murphy, R.N., M.S.
Clinical Nurse Specialist, Surgical Programs; Children's Hospital, Boston, Boston, Massachusetts
Blue Cohosh (Caulophyllum thalictroides)
Chitosan

Phillip Mushlin, M.D.
Associate Professor, Harvard Medical School, Boston, Massachusetts
Liver Transplantation

Laura Myers, M.D.
Professor of Anesthesiology, University of Pennsylvania School of Medicine, Philadelphia, Pennsylvania
Marfan's Syndrome

Michael L. Nahrwold, M.D.
Professor of Anesthesiology, Indiana University School of Medicine, Indianapolis, Indiana
Hyperparathyroidism

Mohammad Naqibuddin, M.B., B.S., M.P.H.
Research Fellow, Department of Anesthesiology and Critical Care Medicine, Johns Hopkins University School of Medicine, Baltimore, Maryland
Sildenafil Citrate (Viagra)
Statins

Rosa M. Navarro, M.D.
Physician, Department of Anesthesia and Critical Care, University of Chicago, Chicago, Illinois
Herpes, Type 2

Stephan P. Nebbia, M.D.
Clinical Assistant Professor of Anesthesiology, State University of New York at Buffalo, School of Medicine and Biomedical Sciences, Buffalo, New York
Sarcoma

Philippa Newfield, M.D.
Assistant Clinical Professor, Anesthesia and Neurosurgery, University of California San Francisco; Attending Anesthesiologist, California Pacific Medical Center, San Francisco, California
Syndrome of Inappropriate Antidiuretic Hormone Secretion (SIADH)

Thai Nguyen, M.D.
Fellow/Assistant Resident, Department of Anesthesiology and Critical Care Medicine, Johns Hopkins University School of Medicine, Baltimore, Maryland
ACE Inhibitors

Susan C. Nicolson, M.D.
Professor of Anesthesia, University of Pennsylvania School of Medicine; Director, Cardiothoracic Anesthesia, Children's Hospital of Philadelphia, Philadelphia, Pennsylvania
Tricuspid Atresia
Upper Respiratory Tract Infection

Joan M. Niehoff, M.D.
Assistant Professor of Anesthesiology, Washington University School of Medicine, St. Louis, Missouri
Diaphragmatic Hernia (Congenital)

Dolores B. Njoku, M.D., F.A.A.P.
Assistant Professor, Anesthesiology and Critical Care Medicine, Johns Hopkins University School of Medicine, Baltimore, Maryland
Subclavian Steal Syndrome

Mary J. Njoku, M.D.
Associate Professor of Anesthesiology and Critical Care, University of Maryland School of Medicine, Baltimore, Maryland
Encephalitis

Judith Nolan, M.B., B.S., M.R.C.P., F.R.C.A.
Consultant Paediatric Anaesthetist, Bristol Royal Hospital for Sick Children, Bristol, United Kingdom
Cerebral Palsy

Carol Norred, C.R.N.A., M.H.S.
Clinical Instructor, School of Medicine,
Certified Registered Nurse Anesthetist,
Department of Anesthesiology; Doctoral
Student, School of Nursing, University of
Colorado Health Sciences Center, Denver,
Colorado
Dehydroepiandrosterone (DHEA)
Echinacea (Echinacea angustifolia, E.
pallida, *or* E. purpurea)
Valerian (Valeriana officinalis L.)

Edward J. Norris, M.D., M.B.A.
Assoicate Professor, Department of
Anesthesiology and Critical Care
Medicine; Attending Anesthesiologist,
Section Head, Vascular Anesthesia, Johns
Hopkins University School of Medicine,
Baltimore, Maryland
Whipple Procedure
(Pancreaticoduodenectomy)

Mark C. Norris, M.D.
Staff Anesthesiologist, Department of
Anesthesiology, Henry Medical Center,
Stockbridge, Georgia
Retained Placenta, Removal of

Michael Nugent, M.D.
Professor and Chairman, Department of
Anesthesiology, Medical College of Ohio,
Toledo, Ohio
Coarctation of the Aorta

Ramon Nuñez-Hernandez, M.D.
Assistant Professor, Department of
Anesthesia and Critical Care, University
of Chicago Hospitals, Chicago, Illinois
Alpha₂-Adrenergic Agonists

Daniel Nyhan, M.D.
Associate Professor and Chief, Division of
Cardiac Anesthesia, Johns Hopkins
University School of Medicine, Baltimore,
Maryland
Single (Including Common) Ventricle

Dorene A. O'Hara, M.D., M.S.E.
Associate Professor of Anesthesiology, New
York Medical College, Valhalla, New York
Transurethral Resection of Prostate
(TURP)

Irene B. O'Hara, M.D.
Lecturer, Department of Anesthesia,
University of Pennsylvania School of
Medicine, Philadelphia, Pennsylvania
Transposition of the Great Vessels (TGV),
Repair of

Nancy E. Oriol, M.D.
Associate Professor of Anesthesia, Harvard
Medical School, Boston, Massachusetts
Vaginal Delivery, Normal

Maureen M. O'Rourke, M.D.
Assistant Professor, University of
Pennsylvania School of Medicine,
Philadelphia, Pennsylvania
Botulism
Kartagener's Syndrome

Andreas M. Ostermeier, M.D.
Physician, Clinic for Anesthesiology,
University of Munich, Munich, Germany
Sleep Apnea, Central and Mixed

Andranik Ovassapian, M.D.
Professor, Anesthesia and Critical Care,
and Director, Airway Study and Training
Center, University of Chicago, Chicago,
Illinois
Bronchoscopy, Fiberoptic
Bronchoscopy, Rigid
Laryngoscopy

Kent Z. Ozkum, M.D.
Staff Anesthesiologist, Providence
Hospital, Washington, D.C.
Monoamine Oxidase Inhibitors; Reversible
Inhibitors of Monoamine Oxidase

Richard J. Palahniuk, M.D.
Professor, Department of Anesthesiology,
University of Minnesota, Minneapolis,
Minnesota
Anemia, Hemolytic
Pregnancy, Intra-abdominal

Susan K. Palmer, M.D.
Professor of Anesthesiology and
Preventive Medicine, Faculty of Program
in Heathcare Ethics, Humanities, and
Law, University of Colorado Health
Sciences Center, Denver, Colorado
Pregnancy-Induced Hypertension

Barbara W. Palmisano, M.D.
Associate Professor, Anesthesiology and
Pediatrics, Medical College of Wisconsin;
Attending Staff, Children's Hospital of
Wisconsin, Milwaukee, Wisconsin
Cri du Chat Syndrome (5p Syndrome)

Sally C. Palmon, M.D.
Instructor, Johns Hopkins University
School of Medicine, Baltimore, Maryland
Lumbar Laminectomy

Wei Pan, M.D.
Resident, Department of Anesthesiology,
University of Chicago, Chicago, Illinois
Ginger (Zingiber officinale)

Robert K. Parker, D.O.
Assistant Professor of Anesthesiology,
Obstetrics, and Gynecology, Tufts
University School of Medicine, Boston,
Massachusetts
Hysterectomy, Vaginal

Jonathan L. Parmet, M.D.
Staff Anesthesiologist, Hospital of the
University of Pennsylvania, Philadelphia,
Pennsylvania
Joint Replacement Cementing
(Methylmethacrylate Cementing)

K. Gage Parr, M.D.
Assistant Professor, Department of
Anesthesiology and Critical Care
Medicine, Johns Hopkins University
School of Medicine, Baltimore, Maryland
Bretylium Tosylate

L. Reuven Pasternak, M.D., M.P.H.
Associate Professor of Anesthesiology,
Johns Hopkins University School of
Medicine, Baltimore, Maryland
Chest X-ray

Ronald W. Pauldine, M.D.
Associate Professor, Department of
Anesthesiology and Critical Care
Medicine, Baltimore, Maryland
Esophagectomy

Carlos V. Paya, M.D., Ph.D.
Professor of Medicine and Immunology,
Mayo Medical School and Clinic,
Rochester, Minnesota
Cytomegalovirus (CMV) Infection

Ronald G. Pearl, M.D., Ph.D.
Professor and Chairman of Anesthesia,
Stanford University, Stanford, California
Pulmonary Embolism

Michael J. Peck, M.D.
Staff Physician, Suburban Healthcare,
Metropolitan Anesthesia Group, Bethesda,
Maryland
Endoscopic Sinus Surgery (ESS)

John Penner, M.D.
Assistant Professor, Anesthesia and
Critical Care, University of Chicago
Hospitals, Chicago, Illinois
Ludwig's Angina

Azriel Perel, M.D.
Associate Professor and Chairman,
Deparment of Anesthesiology and
Intensive Care, Sheba Medical Center, Tel-
Hashomer, Israel
Mastocytosis

Edelberto Perez, M.D.
Assistant Professor, Rush Medical College
of Rush University, Chicago, Illinois
Phenylephrine (Neo-Synephrine)
Ventricular Tachycardia

Charise T. Petrovitch, M.D.
Chair and Director, Department of
Anesthesia, Providence Hospital,
Washington, D.C.
Warfarin (Coumadin)

Patricia H. Petrozza, M.D.
Professor and Section Head,
Neuroanesthesia, Wake Forest University
School of Medicine, Winston-Salem, North
Carolina
Brain Cortex Resection (for Epilepsy)

Evan G. Pivalizza, M.B., Ch.B., F.F.A.S.A.
Associate Professor of Anesthesiology,
University of Texas–Houston; Assistant
Medical Director, Operating Room,
Hermann Hospital, Houston, Texas
Purpura, Immune Thrombocytopenic (ITP)
Purpura, Thrombotic Thrombocytopenic
(TTP)

Susan L. Polk, M.D., M.S.Ed.
Associate Professor of Clinical Anesthesia
and Critical Care, University of Chicago,
Chicago, Illinois
Morbid Obesity
Pickwickian Syndrome

Vivian H. Porche, M.D.
Associate Professor of Anesthesiology and
Associate Anesthesiologist, Division of
Anesthesiology, Critical and Palliative
Care, University of Texas M.D. Anderson
Cancer Center, Houston, Texas
Radiotherapy / CT Scan

Kamla K. Prasad, M.D.
President/Vice Chairman, Fair Oaks
Anesthesia Associates, P.C., Department of
Anesthesiology, Inova Fair Oaks Hospital,
Fairfax, Virginia
*Hereditary Hemorrhagic Telangiectasia
   (Osler-Weber-Render Disease)*
Multiple Myeloma
Waldenström's Macroglobulinemia

Margaret G. Pratila, M.D.
Associate Professor of Clinical
Anesthesiology, Cornell University Medical
College, New York, New York
Chemotherapeutic Agents

Vasilios Pratilas, M.D.
Associate Professor of Clinical
Anesthesiology, Mount Sinai School of
Medicine of the City University of New
York, New York, New York
Chemotherapeutic Agents

Hugh L. Preas II, M.D.
Assistant Professor of Anesthesiology,
Department of Anesthesiology, University
of Maryland School of Medicine,
Baltimore; Senior Staff Physician,
Department of Anesthesia and Surgical
Services, Warran G. Magnuson Clinical
Center, National Institutes of Health,
Bethesda, Maryland
Histiocytosis

Johnathan L. Pregler, M.D.
Associate Clinical Professor, Department
of Anesthesiology, University of California,
Los Angeles; Director, UCLA Surgery
Center, Los Angeles, California
Hepatitis, Alcoholic
Hypopituitarism
Rifampin

Richard C. Prielipp, M.D., F.C.C.M.
Professor, Cardiac Anesthesiology, and
Section Head, Critical Care, Bowman Gray
School of Medicine, Wake Forest
University, Winston-Salem, North Carolina
Dopamine

Donald S. Prough, M.D.
Professor of Anesthesiology, Neurology, and
Pathology, and Chair, Department of
Anesthesiology, The University of Texas
Medical Branch, Galveston, Texas
Renal Failure, Chronic

G.B. Racz, M.D.
Professor and Chairman, Department of
Anesthesiology, Texas Tech University
Health Sciences Center, Lubbock, Texas
Headache, Migraine

Bronwyn R. Rae, M.D.
Assistant Professor, Northwestern
University, Evanston; Attending
Anesthesiologist, Children's Memorial
Hospital, Chicago, Illinois
Congenital Methemoglobinemia

Chandra Ramamoorthy, F.F.A.R.C.S.
Assistant Professor, Department of
Anesthesiology, University of Washington
School of Medicine, Seattle, Washington
Truncus Arteriosus

Vidya T. Raman, M.D.
Fellow/Assistant Resident and Department
of Anesthesiology and Critical Care
Medicine, Johns Hopkins University
School of Medicine, Baltimore, Maryland
Angiotensin II Receptor Antagonists

Sivam Ramanathan, M.D.
Professor of Anesthesiology and Critical
Care Medicine, University of Pittsburgh
School of Medicine, Pittsburgh,
Pennsylvania
Labor, Peripheral Blocks

Ira J. Rampil, M.D.
Associate Professor of Anesthesia,
University of California, San Francisco,
School of Medicine, San Francisco,
California
Laser Surgery of Airway
Pituitary Tumors

James G. Ramsay, M.D., F.R.C.P.C.
Professor of Anesthesiology, Emory
University School of Medicine;
Anesthesiology Service Chief, Emory
University Hospital, Atlanta, Georgia
Aortic Valve Replacement

Earl S. Ransom, Jr., M.D.
Staff Anesthesiologist, Durham Regional
Hospital, Durham Anesthesia Associates,
Durham, North Carolina
Amphetamines

Russell C. Raphaely, M.D.
Clinical Professor of Anesthesiology,
Jefferson Medical College, Thomas
Jefferson University, Philadelphia,
Pennsylvania; Co-Director, Nemours
Cardiac Center, Pediatric
Anesthesiologist/Intensivist, A. I. duPont
Hospital for Children, Wilmington,
Delaware
Botulism
Kartagener's Syndrome

Athos J. Rassias, M.D.
Assistant Professor of Anesthesiology,
Dartmouth Medical School;
Anesthesiologist/Intensivist, Dartmouth-
Hitchcock Medical Center, Lebanon, New
Hampshire
*Disseminated Intravascular Coagulation
   (DIC)*

Leila L. Reduque, M.D.
Resident, Johns Hopkins University
School of Medicine, Baltimore, Maryland
Evening Primrose

David L. Reich, M.D.
Professor of Anesthesiology, Mount Sinai
School of Medicine; Co-Director of
Cardiothoracic Anesthesia, Mount Sinai
Medical Center, New York, New York
Ventricular Septal Defect (Congenital)
*Ventricular Septal Rupture (Defect), Post
   Myocardial Infarction*

J.G. Reves, M.D.
Dean and Vice President for Medical
Affairs and Professor of Anesthesiology,
Medical University of South Carolina,
Charleston, South Carolina
*Coronary Artery Disease (Left Main and
   Non-Left Main Disease)*

Christine S. Rinder, M.D.
Associate Professor of Anesthesiology and
Laboratory Medicine, Yale University
School of Medicine; Attending Physician,
Yale-New Haven Hospital, New Haven,
Connecticut
Complement Deficiency
Transfusion-Related Acute Lung Injury

Brian J. Robinson, Ph.D.
Director, National Patient Simulation
Training Centre, Wellington Hospital,
Wellington South, New Zealand
Autonomic Function

David M. Robinson, M.D.
Assistant Professor, Department of
Anesthesiology, Medical College of
Pennsylvania/Hahnemann University,
Philadelphia, Pennsylvania
Systemic Lupus Erythematosus

Peter Rock, M.D.
Professor, Departments of Anesthesiology
and Medicine; Vice-Chair, Department of
Anesthesiology: Co-Director, In-Patient
Operating Room; Director, Division of
Critical Care; Medical Director, Critical
Care Stepdown Unit, University of North
Carolina, Chapel Hill, North Carolina
Flow-Volume Loops
Spirometry

Michael F. Roizen, M.D.
Dean of the School of Medicine and Vice-
President for Biomedical Affairs, Professor
of Internal Medicine and Anesthesiology,
State University of New York Upstate
Medical University, Syracuse, New York
Adrenalectomy for Pheochromocytoma
Cimetidine
Diabetes, Type I (Insulin Dependent)
Diabetes, Type II (Noninsulin Dependent)
Hyperthyroidism
Myocardial Ischemia (MIsch)
Phenoxybenzamine
Pheochromocytoma
Propylthiouracil—Antithyroid Drugs
*Retropharyngeal and Peritonsillar
   Abscess Drainage in Adults*
Sickle Cell Trait
Sleep Apnea, Central and Mixed
Sleep Apnea, Obstructive
Thyroidectomy for Hyperthyroidism
Total Hip Arthroplasty

Joseph Rosa III, M.D.
Assistant Clinical Professor of
Anesthesiology and Director, Rarlery
Training Program, University of
California, Los Angeles, Los Angeles,
California
Appendectomy
Pregnancy, Ectopic

Robert J. Rose, M.D.
Associate Professor of Anesthesiology, Dartmouth Medical School, Hanover; Faculty, Department of Anesthesiology and Pain Management Program, Dartmouth-Hitchcock Medical Center, Lebanon, New Hampshire
Bulimia

David A. Rosen, M.D.
Professor of Anesthesia and Pediatrics and Director of Pediatric Cardiac Anesthesia, West Virginia University, Morgantown, West Virginia
Intestinal Obstruction
Intussuscepted Bowel Repair

Kathleen R. Rosen, M.D.
Associate Professor of Anesthesia, West Virginia University, Morgantown, West Virginia
Intestinal Obstruction
Intussuscepted Bowel Repair

Michael Rosen, C.B.E., F.R.C.A.
Past President, Royal College of Anaesthesiology, United Kingdom
Constipation

Stanley H. Rosenbaum, M.D.
Professor of Anesthesiology, Medicine, and Surgery, and Vice Chairman for Academic Affairs, Department of Anesthesiology, Yale University School of Medicine, New Haven, Connecticut
Carcinoid Syndrome
Diabetes, Type II (Noninsulin Dependent)

Andrew D. Rosenberg, M.D.
Clinical Instructor, Department of Anesthesiology, New York University School of Medicine, New York, New York
Cervical Disk Disease (Cervical Spine Disease)
Sarcoidosis

Andrew L. Rosenberg, M.D.
Robert Wood Johnson Clinical Scholar, Department of Anesthesiology and Critical Care Medicine, University of Michigan, Ann Arbor, Michigan
Myocardial Contusion

Henry Rosenberg, M.D.
Professor of Anesthesiology and Vice Chair for Academic Affairs, Jefferson Medical College, Thomas Jefferson University; Anesthesiologist, Thomas Jefferson University Hospital, Philadelphia, Pennsylvania
Malignant Hyperthermia (MH) and Other Anesthetic-Induced Myodystrophies (AIMs)

Jeffrey Rosenberg, M.D., Ph.D.
Assistant Professor, Department of Anesthesiology and Critical Care Medicine, Johns Hopkins University School of Medicine, Baltimore, Maryland
Mediastinal Masses

Meg A. Rosenblatt, M.D.
Clinical Associate Professor of Anesthesiology, Mount Sinai School of Medicine, New York, New York
Hip Fracture Repair
Jehovah's Witness Patient

William H. Rosenblatt, M.D.
Assistant Professor of Anesthesiology, Yale University School of Medicine, New Haven, Connecticut
Cancer, Bladder

Myer H. Rosenthal, M.D.
Professor of Anesthesia, Stanford University School of Medicine, Stanford, California
Septic Hyperdynamic Shock; Systemic Inflammatory Response Syndrome (SIRS)

Steven Roth, M.D.
Associate Professor, Department of Anesthesia and Critical Care, University of Chicago, Chicago, Illinois
OKT3 (Muromonab-CD3)
Postoperative Encephalopathy, Metabolic

Franklin J. Ruiz, M.D.
Assistant Professor, Department of Anesthesiology, The Medical College of Wisconsin; Section of Pediatric Anesthesiology, Children's Hospital of Wisconsin, Milwaukee, Wisconsin
Arnold-Chiari Syndrome

Judith Ruiz-Lachica, M.D.
Department of Anesthesia, University of Chicago, Chicago, Illinois
Uterine Rupture

Winnie Y. Ruo, M.D.
Assistant Professor, Department of Anesthesia and Critical Care, University of Chicago, Chicago, Illinois
Tetralogy of Fallot

Stephen M. Rupp, M.D.
Associate Clinical Professor, University of Washington; Chief, Department of Anesthesiology, Virginia Mason Medical Center, Seattle, Washington
Pituitary Resection, Transsphenoidal Approach

Renata Rusa, M.D.
Assistant Professor, Department of Anesthesiology, Oregon Health and Sciences University, Portland, Oregon
Cerebrovascular Transient Ischemic Attack (TIA)

Garfield B. Russell, M.D., F.R.C.P.C.
Eric A. Walker Professor and Chair, Pennsylvania State University College of Medicine, Hershey, Pennsylvania
Herniated Nucleus Pulposus

W. John Russell, M.B., F.R.C.A., F.A.N.Z.C.A., Ph.D.
Associate Professor, Department of Anesthesia and Intensive Care, University of Adelaide, Adelaide, South Australia
Familial Periodic Paralysis (Hyperkalemic)
Familial Periodic Paralysis (Hypokalemic)

Thomas A. Russo, M.D., C.M.
Assistant Professor, Department of Medicine, University of Buffalo, Buffalo, New York
Q Fever
Rocky Mountain Spotted Fever

Thomas Ryan, M.D.
Director of Echocardiography, Duke University Medical Center, Durham, North Carolina
Dobutamine Stress Echocardiography

Alar Saaremets, M.D.
Staff Anesthesiologist, Lake Tahoe, Nevada
Fish Oil

Lloyd R. Saberski, M.D.
Associate Professor of Anesthesiology, Yale University School of Medicine, New Haven, Connecticut
Reflex Sympathetic Dystrophy (Complex Peripheral Pain Syndrome)

Denis Safran, M.D.
Professor of the Universities—Hospital Expert, Anesthesiology, Hospital Broussais, Paris, France
Congestive Heart Failure

M. Ramez Salem, M.D.
Clinical Professor of Anesthesiology, University of Illinois College of Medicine; Chair, Department of Anesthesiology, Advocate Illinois Masonic Medical Center, Chicago, Illinois
Bilirubinemia of the Newborn

Kevin V. Sanborn, M.D.
Associate Professor of Clinical Anesthesiology, College of Physicians and Surgeons, Columbia University; Associate Director of Anesthesiology, St. Luke's—Roosevelt Hospital Center, New York, New York
ORIF of Hip

Ted J. Sanford, Jr., M.D.
Clinical Professor of Anesthesiology, University of Michigan, Ann Arbor, Michigan
Hypoxemia

Mukesh C. Sarna, M.D.
Fellow, Obstetric Anesthesia, Beth Israel Deaconess Medical Center, Harvard Medical School, Boston, Massachusetts
Vaginal Delivery, Normal

Patricia Satitpunwaycha, M.D.
Fellow/Assistant Resident and Department of Anesthesiology and Critical Care Medicine, Johns Hopkins University School of Medicine, Baltimore, Maryland
Aortic Valve Replacement

Paul D. Schanbacher, M.D.
Chairman, Department of Anesthesiology, Resurrection Medical Center, Chicago, Illinois
Bilirubinemia of the Newborn

Randall M. Schell, M.D.
Associate Professor of Anesthesiology and Director, Medical Student and Resident Education in Anesthesiology, Loma Linda University School of Medicine, Loma Linda, California
Carotid Sinus Syndrome (CSS)

Michelle Schlunt, M.D.
Assistant Professor of Anesthesiology, Loma Linda University School of Medicine, Loma Linda, California
Amyotrophic Lateral Sclerosis (ALS)

Armin Schubert, M.D.
Professor of Anesthesiology, Cleveland Clinic Health Sciences Campus of The Ohio State University; Chairman, Department of General Anesthesiology, Cleveland Clinic Foundation, Cleveland, Ohio
Cerebral AVM Repair
Multiple Sclerosis

Alan Jay Schwartz, M.D., M.S.Ed.
Clinical Professor of Anesthesiology, University of Pennsylvania School of Medicine; Director of Education, Department of Anesthesiology and Critical Care Medicine, Children's Hospital of Philadelphia, Philadelphia, Pennsylvania
Advanced Cardiac Life Support (ACLS)
Transportation of the Great Vessels (TGV), Repair of

Jeffrey J. Schwartz, M.D.
Associate Clinical Professor, Department of Anesthesiology, Yale University School of Medicine, New Haven, Connecticut
Pancreatitis, Acute
Pancreatitis, Chronic

Joseph L. Seltzer, M.D.
Professor and Chairman of Anesthesiology, Jefferson Medical College, Thomas Jefferson University, Philadelphia, Pennsylvania
Autoimmune Disease, Cold

Valerie Sera, M.D.
Assistant Professor, Department of Anesthesiology and Critical Care Medicine, Johns Hopkins University School of Medicine, Baltimore, Maryland
CREST Syndrome

Michael A. Seropian, M.D., F.R.C.P.C.
Assistant Professor, Department of Anesthesiology, School of Medicine, Orgeon Health Sciences University, Doernbecher Children's Hospital, Portland, Oregon
Tetralogy of Fallot, Correction of

Daniel I. Sessler, M.D.
Assistant Vice-President for Health Affairs, Associate Dean for Research, Outcomes Research™ Institute, University of Louisville, Louisville, Kentucky
Hypothermia, Mild (Core Temperature 34–36°C)

Navil F. Sethna, M.B., Ch.B.
Associate Professor of Anesthesia, Harvard Medical School; Associate Director, Pain Treatment Service and Senior Associate in Anesthesia, Children's Hospital, Boston, Massachusetts
Prader-Willi Syndrome

Amar Setty, M.D.
Resident Physician, Department of Anesthesiology, Johns Hopkins University School of Medicine, Baltimore, Maryland
Psyllium, Bulk-Forming Laxatives (Plantago isphagula, Plantago ovata)

Ferne B. Sevarino, M.D.
Associate Professor, Yale University School of Medicine; Chief, Section of Obstetrical Anesthesiology, Yale-New Haven Hospital, New Haven, Connecticut
Total Abdominal Hysterectomy

Paul W. Shabaz, M.D., Ph.D.
Assistant Professor of Anesthesiology, University of Rochester Medical Center, Rochester, New York
Placenta Previa

Maneesh Sharma, M.D.
Resident Physician, Department of Anesthesiology and Critical Care Medicine, Johns Hopkins University School of Medicine, Baltimore, Maryland
Insulin Receptor Modifiers

Michael D. Sharpe, M.D., F.R.C.P.C.
Associate Professor, Department of Anesthesia, University of Western Ontario; Site Chief, Intensive Care Unit, London Health Sciences Center, University Campus, London, Ontario, Canada
Parkinson's Disease (Paralysis Agitans)

Nigel E. Sharrock, M.B., Ch.B.
Associate Professor, Weill Medical College of Cornell University; Attending Anesthesiologist, Hospital for Special Surgery, New York, New York
Knee Arthroscopy

Joanne Shay, M.D.
Assistant Professor of Anesthesiology, George Washington University School of Medicine and Health Sciences, Washington, D.C.
Anemia, Aplastic

John G. Shutack, D.O.
Associate Professor, Department of Anesthesiology, Medical College of Pennsylvania/Hahnemann University, Philadelphia, Pennsylvania
Malignant Hyperthermia and Other Anesthetic-Induced Myodystrophies (AIMs)

Frederick E. Sieber, M.D.
Associate Professor, Johns Hopkins University School of Medicine, Baltimore, Maryland
Cerebral Aneurysm Clipping

Daniel Siker, M.D.
Associate Professor of Anesthesiology, Medical College of Wisconsin; Staff Physician, Children's Hospital of Wisconsin, Milwaukee, Wisconsin
Cherubism
Treacher Collins Syndrome

J. Christopher Sill, M.D.
Associate Professor, Mayo Clinic and Foundation, Rochester, Minnesota
Tissue Plasminogen Activator

Brett A. Simon, M.D., Ph.D.
Associate Professor, Department of Anesthesiology and Critical Care Medicine, Johns Hopkins University School of Medicine, Baltimore, Maryland
Lung Volume Reduction Surgery (Pneumoplasty)

Raymond S. Sinatra, M.D., Ph.D.
Professor of Anesthesiology, Yale University School of Medicine; Attending Anesthesiologist and Director, Pain Management Service, Yale-New Haven Hospital, New Haven, Connecticut
Labor, Epidural Block

Robert N. Sladen, M.B., Ch.B., M.R.C.P., F.R.C.P.C.
Professor of Anesthesiology and Vice-Chair, Department of Anesthesiology, Columbia University College of Physicians and Surgeons; Director, Cardiothoracic and Surgical ICUs, Columbia Presbyterian Center at New York Presbyterian Hospital, New York, New York
Renal Failure, Acute (ARF)

Douglas A. Snyder, M.D.
Assistant Professor, Department of Anesthesiology and Critical Care Medicine, Johns Hopkins University School of Medicine, Baltimore, Maryland
Herniorrhaphy

Sophia Socaris, M.D.
Associate Professor of Surgery and Anesthesiology, Albany Medical College, Albany, New York
Lyme Disease

Martin D. Sokoll, M.D.
Professor, Department of Anesthesia, University of Iowa College of Medicine and University of Iowa Hospitals and Clinics, Iowa City, Iowa
Gold (Auranofin, Aurothioglucose, Aurothiomalate)

James M. Sonner, M.D.
Associate Professor, Department of Anesthesia and Perioperative Care, University of California, San Francisco, San Francisco, California
Candidiasis
Pemphigus

Donat R. Spahn, M.D.
Professor and Chair, Department of Anesthesiology, University Hospital, Lausanne, Switzerland
Anemia, Chronic Disease

Bruce D. Spiess, M.D.
Professor and Vice Chair, Department of Anesthesiology; Director, Cardiothoracic Anesthesia; Director, VCURES (Shock Center), Virginia Commonwealth University/Medical College of Virginia, Richmond, Virginia
Pericardial Effusion

Peter S. Staats, M.D.
Associate Professor, Department of Anesthesiology and Critical Care Medicine and Oncology, and Director, Division of Pain Medicine, Johns Hopkins University School of Medicine, Baltimore, Maryland
Spasmodic Torticollis

Theodore H. Stanley, M.D.
Professor, Department of Anesthesiology, University of Utah Health Sciences Center, Salt Lake City, Utah
Phenothiazines

Stanley W. Stead, M.D.
Professor, Department of Anesthesiology, University of California, Davis, School of Medicine; Director of Perioperative Services, University of California, Davis, Medical Center, Sacramento, California
Blindness
Circumcision
Prilocaine (Citanest)

Randy H. Steadman, M.D.
Assistant Clinical Professor, Department of Anesthesiology, University of California, Los Angeles, School of Medicine, Los Angeles, California
Bicarbonate Sodium
Carcinoid, Excision of
Ventricular Fibrillation

Linda Stehling, M.D.
Formerly Professor of Anesthesiology and Pediatrics, State University of New York Health Science Center, Syracuse, New York
Blood Components

Keith L. Stein, M.D.
Physician Executive Consultant, APM, Inc., New York, New York
Mitral Regurgitation

John K. Stene, M.D., Ph.D.
Professor of Anesthesiology, Pennsylvania State University College of Medicine; Co-director, Anesthesia/Surgery Intensive Care Unit, Milton S. Hershey Medical Center, Hershey, Pennsylvania
Riboflavin (Vitamin B₂)
Vitamin B₁₂ (Cyanocobalamin)

Wendell C. Stevens, M.D.
Professor Emeritus, Department of Anesthesiology, Oregon Health Sciences University; Volunteer Faculty (Clinical), Oregon Health Sciences University Hospital; Anesthesia Staff, Portland Veterans Administration Medical Center, Portland, Oregon
Tetralogy of Fallot, Correction of

David J. Steward, M.B., B.S., F.R.C.P.C.
Professor, Department of Anesthesiology, University of Southern California; Senior Anesthesiologist, Children's Hospital, Los Angeles, California
Preterm Infant

Kevin Stierer, M.D.
Clinical Assistant Professor, Department of Anesthesiology, Uniformed Services University of Health Sciences, Bethesda, Maryland
Bowel Resection

Tracey L. Stierer, M.D.
Assistant Professor, Department of Anesthesiology and Critical Care Medicine, Johns Hopkins University School of Medicine, Baltimore, Maryland
Oral Contraceptives

Bryant W. Stolp, M.D., Ph.D.
Assistant Professor, Department of Anesthesiology, Duke University Medical Center, Durham, North Carolina
Carbon Monoxide (CO) Poisoning
Gas Embolism

David F. Stowe, M.D., Ph.D.
Professor of Anesthesiology and Physiology, Medical College of Wisconsin; Senior Staff in Anesthesiology, Froedert Memorial Hospital and VA Medical Center, Milwaukee, Wisconsin
Serotonin: Agonists, Antagonists, and Reuptake Inhibitors

Scott C. Streckenbach, M.D.
Instructor in Anesthesia, Harvard Medical School; Chief, Cardiac Anesthesia, Massachusetts General Hospital, Boston, Massachusetts
Mycoplasma pneumoniae *Infection*

Theodore W. Striker, M.D.
Professor of Anesthesia and Pediatrics, University of Cincinnati; Anesthesiologist-in-Chief and Director, Department of Anesthesia, Children's Hospital Medical Center, Cincinnati, Ohio
Cystic Fibrosis
Eisenmenger's Syndrome

Cheri A. Sulek, M.D.
Assistant Professor of Anesthesiology, University of Florida College of Medicine, Gainesville, Florida
Central Neurogenic Hyperventilation

Tommy Symreng, M.D., Ph.D.
Staff Anesthesiologist, St. Mary's Hospital, Evansville, Indiana
Steroids

Zuhayr A. Tabbarah, M.D.
Associate Clinical Professor of Medicine (Infectious Diseases), American University of Beirut Medical School, Beirut, Lebanon
Echinococcosis

René Tempelhoff, M.D.
Professor of Anesthesiology and Neurological Surgery, Washington University School of Medicine; Director of Neuroanesthesia, Chief, Barnes–Jewish Hospital, South Campus, Division of Anesthesiology, St. Louis, Missouri
Seizures, Intractable

John E. Tetzlaff, M.D.
Residency Program Director, Division of Anesthesiology and Critical Care Medicine, Cleveland Clinic Foundation, Cleveland, Ohio
Ankylosing Spondylitis
Degenerative Disk Disease

Stephen J. Thomas, M.D.
Professor and Vice Chair, Department of Anesthesiology, New York Hospital—Cornell Medical Center, New York, New York
Aortic Stenosis

Alisa C. Thorne, M.D.
Associate Professor of Clinical Anesthesiology, Weill Medical College of Cornell University; Director, Ambulatory Anesthesia, Memorial Sloan-Kettering Cancer Center, New York, New York
Lymphomas
Thyroid Neoplasms

Daniel M. Thys, M.D.
Professor, Department of Anesthesiology, Columbia University College of Physicians and Surgeons; Chairman, Department of Anesthesiology, St. Luke's–Roosevelt Hospital Center, New York, New York
Coronary Artery Bypass Graft
Transesophageal Echocardiography (TEE)

Joseph R. Tobin, M.D.
Associate Professor, Departments of Anesthesiology and Pediatrics, and Section Head on Pediatric Anesthesiology and Pediatric Critical Care, Wake Forest University School of Medicine, Winston-Salem, North Carolina
Hydrocephalus

Michael J. Tobin, M.D.
Assistant Professor of Anesthesiology, Northwestern University Medical School; Attending Anesthesiologist and Director of the Sedation Services, Children's Memorial Hospital, Chicago, Illinois
Tracheoesophageal Fistula Repair

I. David Todres, M.D.
Professor of Pediatrics (Anesthesia), Harvard Medical School, Boston, Massachusetts
Necrotizing Enterocolitis

Alan S. Tonnesen, M.D.
Professor of Anesthesiology, University of Texas Medical School–Houston, Houston, Texas
Hypophosphatemia

Thomas J. Toung, M.D.
Associate Professor, Department of Anesthesiology, Johns Hopkins University School of Medicine, Baltimore, Maryland
Craniotomy, Sitting Position
Venous Air Embolism

Karen B. Traber, M.D.
Staff Anesthesiologist, Main Line Health, Jefferson Health System, Bryn Mawr, Pennsylvania
Tuberculosis (TB)

Mark F. Trankina, M.D.
Associate Professor, Department of Anesthesiology, Division of Cardiothoracic Anesthesia, University of Alabama at Birmingham, Birmingham, Alabama
Pacemakers

Kevin K. Tremper, M.D., Ph.D.
Professor and Chair, Department of Anesthesiology, University of Michigan Medical Center, Ann Arbor, Michigan
Cigarette Smoking

Kenneth J. Tuman, M.D.
The Max Sadove, M.D., Professor of Anesthesiology, Rush Medical College; Vice-Chair, Department of Anesthesiology, Rush-Presbyterian–St. Lukes Medical Center, Chicago, Illinois
Phenylephrine (Neo-Synephrine)
Ventricular Tachycardia

Avery Tung, M.D.
Assistant Professor of Anesthesia and
Critical Care, University of Chicago,
Chicago, Illinois
Aminophylline
Necrotizing Fasciitis

Rebecca Twersky, M.D.
Professor of Clinical Anesthesiology and
Vice Chair for Research, State University
of New York Health Science Center at
Brooklyn; Associate Attending in
Anesthesiology, Long Island College
Hospital, Brooklyn; Attending
Anesthesiologist, King's County Hospital
Center, Brooklyn, New York
Pregnancy Testing

Nolan Tzou, M.D.
Medical Director, Huntington Center for
Pain Treatment, Huntington, New York
Leukemia

John A. Ulatowski, M.D., Ph.D.
Associate Professor and Vice Chairman,
Clinical Affairs, Department of
Anesthesiology and Critical Care
Medicine, Johns Hopkins University
School of Medicine, Baltimore, Maryland
Transverse Myelitis

Michael Urban, M.D., Ph.D.
Assistant Clinical Professor of
Anesthesiology, Cornell University Medical
College, New York, New York
Total Knee Arthroplasty

Manuel C. Vallejo, M.D.
Assistant Professor, Magee Women's
Hospital, Department of Anesthesiology
and Critical Care Medicine, University of
Pittsburgh School of Medicine, Pittsburgh,
Pennsylvania
Labor, Peripheral Blocks

Carole Vannier, M.D.
Assistant Professor of Anesthesiology and
Critical Care Medicine, Johns Hopkins
University School of Medicine, Baltimore,
Maryland
Intra-aortic Balloon Counterpulsation
(IABCP)

Garry V. Walker, M.D.
Assistant Professor of Anesthesiology,
Vanderbilt University Medical School and
Center, Nashville, Tennessee
Abdominal Aortic Aneurysm Repair

Russell T. Wall III, M.D.
Professor of Anesthesiology, Georgetown
University School of Medicine,
Washington, D.C.
Acromegaly
Anorexia Nervosa

David C. Warltier, M.D., Ph.D.
Professor of Anesthesiology, Cardiology,
and Pharmacology, Medical College of
Wisconsin, Milwaukee, Wisconsin
Dobutamine

Toni Anne Washington, M.D.
Anesthesia Fellow, Children's Hospital of
Philadelphia, Philadelphia, Pennsylvania
Hirschsprung's Disease
Otitis Media

Lucy Waskell, M.D., Ph.D.
Professor of Anesthesia, Department of
Anesthesiology, University of Michigan
Medical Center, Ann Arbor, Michigan
Penicillins

W. David Watkins, M.D., Ph.D.
Professor and Vice Chairman, Department
of Anesthesiology and Critical Care
Medicine, University of Pittsburgh School
of Medicine, Pittsburgh, Pennsylvania
Tetracyclines

Lisa M. Weavind, M.B., B.Ch.
Assistant Professor, Critical Care and R.C.
Support Services, University of Texas M.D.
Anderson Cancer Center, Houston, Texas
Multisystem Organ Failure, Lung
Dysfunction in

Michael Webb, M.D.
Staff Anesthesiologist, Anne Arundel
General Hospital, Annapolis, Maryland
Gastrectomy

Denise J. Wedel, M.D.
Professor of Anesthesiology, Mayo Medical
School, Rochester, Minnesota
Osteoarthritis

William B. Weems, M.D.
Fellow, Department of Anesthesia and
Critical Care, University of Chicago,
Chicago, Illinois
Tranexamic Acid

Herbert D. Weintraub, M.D.
Professor of Anesthesiology, George
Washington University School of Medicine
and Health Sciences, Washington, D.C.
Drug Abuse, Lysergic Acid Diethylamide
(LSD)

Eric Weissend, M.D.
Resident, Department of Anesthesiology,
Wilford Hall Medical Center, San Antonio,
Texas
Klippel-Feil Syndrome
Strabismus Surgery
Testicular Torsion Surgery
Thalassemia

Charles Weissman, M.D.
Professor and Chair, Department of
Anesthesiology and Critical Care
Medicine, Hebrew University, Hadassah
School of Medicine, Jerusalem, Israel
Encephalopathy, Metabolic
Encephalopathy, Postanoxic
Protein C Deficiency

M. Emily White, M.D.
Resident, Department of Anesthesiology
and Critical Care Medicine, Johns
Hopkins University School of Medicine,
Baltimore, Maryland
Hypospadias Repair

Roger S. Wilson, M.D.
Professor of Anesthesiology, Weill Medical
College of Cornell University; Chairman,
Department of Anesthesiology and Critical
Care Medicine, Memorial Sloan-Kettering
Cancer Center, New York, New York
V/Q Scan (Split Lung Function)

Bernard Wittels, M.D., Ph.D.
Assistant Professor of Clinical Anesthesia
and Critical Care, Department of
Anesthesia and Critical Care, University
of Chicago, Chicago, Illinois
GIFT Procedure

David Wlody, M.D.
Clinical Associate Professor of
Anesthesiology, State University of New
York Downstate Medical Center, Brooklyn,
New York
Hysteroscopy

David H. Wong, Pharm.D., M.D.
Clinical Professor, University of California,
Irvine, Irvine; Chief of Anesthesiology,
Long Beach Veterans Hospital, Long
Beach, California
Cryptococcus Infection

Kuang C. Wong, M.D., Ph.D.
Professor and Chairman, Department of
Anesthesiology, University of Utah College
of Medicine, Salt Lake City, Utah
Cigarette Smoking Cessation
Hypernatremia
Hyponatremia

Eveltna Worwag, M.D.
Assistant Professor, University of Chicago;
Director of Pain Services, Weiss Memorial
Hospital, Chicago, Illinois
Glossopharyngeal Neuralgia

Zheng Xie, M.D., Ph.D.
Clinical Assistant Professor, Department
of Anesthesia and Critical Care,
University of Chicago; Attending
Physician, University of Chicago
Hospitals, Chicago, Illinois
Transjugular Intrahepatic Portosystemic
Shunt (TIPS)

Ron Yaniv, M.D.
Clinical Instructor, Dermatology, Sackler
School of Medicine, Tel Aviv University,
Tel Aviv, Israel
Mastocytosis

Kelvin Yee, M.D.
Assistant Professor, Department of
Anesthesiology and Critical Care
Medicine, Johns Hopkins University
School of Medicine, Baltimore, Maryland
Crohn's Disease

Christopher C. Young, M.D.
Assistant Professor of Anesthesiology and
Chief of Division of Critical Care
Medicine, Department of Anesthesiology,
Duke University Medical Center, Durham,
North Carolina
Thoracic Aortic Repair

Christopher J. Young, M.D.
Clinical Lecturer, Southwest Missouri
School of Anesthesia, Southwest Missouri
State University; Director of Cardiac
Anesthesia, St. John's Regional Health
Center, Springfield, Missouri
Nicotine (Tobacco, Cigarettes, Snuff, Spit
Tobacco) and Nicotine Replacement
Therapies (Gum, Inhaler, Nasal Spray,
Patch)

Marie L. Young, M.D.
Medical Director, Wills Surgery Center
Wilmington, Wilmington, Delaware
Infratentorial Tumors

John A. Youngberg, M.D.
Professor of Anesthesiology, Tulane
University School of Medicine, New
Orleans, Louisiana
Carotid Endarterectomy

Chun-Su Yuan, M.D., Ph.D.
Assistant Professor, Department of
Anesthesia and Critical Care, University
of Chicago, Pritzker School of Medicine,
Chicago, Illinois
*Ginseng (Panax ginseng, Panax
quinquefolius)*
St. John's Wort (Hypericum perforatum)

Francine S. Yudkowitz, M.D., F.A.A.P.
Assistant Professor of Anesthesiology and
Pediatrics, Mount Sinai School of
Medicine; Director, Pediatric Anesthesia,
Mount Sinai Medical Center, New York,
New York
*Congenital Bronchogenic Cyst/Pulmonary
Cyst/Lobar Emphysema*
Gastroesophageal Reflux in Children
Moyamoya

Nina Zachariah, M.D.
Chief Resident, Division of Anesthesia,
Boston University Medical Center, Boston,
Massachusetts
Cardiomyopathy, Hypertrophic (HCM)

James P. Zacny, Ph.D.
Associate Professor, Department of
Anesthesia and Critical Care, University
of Chicago, Chicago, Illinois
Marijuana
*Nicotine (Tobacco, Cigarettes, Snuff, Spit
Tobacco) and Nicotine ZReplacement
Therapies (Gum, Inhaler, Nasal Spray,
Patch)*
Phencyclidine (PCP)

James R. Zaidan, M.D.
Professor of Anesthesiology and Interim
Chair and Associate Dean for Graduate
Medical Education, Emory University
School of Medicine, Atlanta, Georgia
*Mobitz I (Second Degree Atrioventricular
Block)*
*Mobitz II (Second Degree Atrioventricular
Block)*

Paul Zanaboni, M.D., Ph.D.
Assistant Professor, Department of
Anesthesiology, Washington University
School of Medicine; Staff, Barnes—Jewish
Hospital, St. Louis, Missouri
Cor Pulmonale

Warren M. Zapol, M.D.
Professor, Anesthetist-in-Chief,
Department of Anesthesia and Critical
Care, Massachusetts General Hospital,
Harvard Medical School, Boston,
Massachusetts
Nitric Oxide, Inhaled

Shuomin Zhu, M.D., Ph.D.
Assistant Professor, University of Chicago,
Department of Anesthesia and Critical
Care, Chicago, Illinois
Cholestin
Cranberry

William Zimmerman, M.D.
Assistant Professor, Department of
Anesthesia and Critical Care, University
of Chicago, Chicago, Illinois
Parkinson's Disease (Paralysis Agitans)

Ross H. Zoll, M.D., Ph.D.
Partner, Anesthesia Associates of
Springfield; Mercy Hospital, Springfield,
Massachusetts
Cardioversion

Howard Alan Zucker, M.D.
Assistant Professor of Pediatrics and
Anesthesiology, Columbia University
College of Physicians and Surgeons, New
York, New York
Aortopulmonary Window

Rhonda Zuckerman, M.D.
Assistant Professor, Department of
Anesthesiology and Critical Care
Medicine, Johns Hopkins University
School of Medicine, Baltimore, Maryland
Pregnant Surgical Patient

Maurice S. Zwass, M.D.
Professor of Anesthesia and Pediatrics,
University of California, San Francisco;
Associate Director, Pediatric Critical Care
Medicine; Co-Director, Fellowship in
Pediatric Critical Care Medicine; Director,
Fellowship in Clinical Pediatric
Anesthesia, University of California, San
Francisco, and Moffitt—Long Hospital,
San Francisco, California
Croup (Laryngotracheobronchitis)
Epiglottitis

Michael Roizen and Lee Fleisher have updated and expanded the first edition of *Essence of Anesthesia Practice,* which ingeniously encapsulated information important for any anesthesia consultant. Having been their associates at SUNY Upstate and at Yale, we respect their clinical judgments, the fruit of years of experience in the practice of anesthesia. This book reflects the innovative yet comprehensive approach that they often take. They are no ivory tower practitioners—they work "in the trenches." We think that they have succeeded well in summarizing the pertinent aspects of the disease process, as well as the procedures, drugs, alternative medicines, and tests that are considered before a patient is anesthetized. Each chapter succinctly points the reader toward optimal care of a patient, by exploring the pathophysiology of a disease process and the management appropriate to specific conditions, clinical situations, and drug interactions. The intent is to help the physician rapidly and comprehensively plan perioperative management.

This is not a how-to-do-it book or "recipes" for perioperative care. Rather, it suggests that the pathophysiology of a disease or the physiologic imbalance caused by an operation should influence our thinking about therapeutic options. It offers a method for setting priorities to facilitate exemplary performance as a consultant in anesthesia. *Essence of Anesthesia Practice* has proven useful not only to anesthesiologists but also to our colleagues in other specialties who interface with the surgical patient.

The second edition expands on their previous success by including additional topics and a section on alternative medicines. Interaction between herbal medicines and anesthetics is becoming increasingly important, and this text will serve as a handy reference. The availability of some of the key portions of the text for the Palm Pilot should further enhance its value.

The editors are to be congratulated for improving on their innovative clinical and educational format to serve both novice residents and experienced practitioners.

PAUL G. BARASH, M.D.
PROFESSOR, DEPARTMENT OF ANESTHESIOLOGY
YALE UNIVERSITY SCHOOL OF MEDICINE
NEW HAVEN, CONNECTICUT

RONALD D. MILLER, M.D.
ADVISOR
CHAIRMAN, DEPARTMENT OF ANESTHESIA
UNIVERSITY OF CALIFORNIA, SAN FRANCISCO
SAN FRANCISCO, CALIFORNIA

Preface to the Second Edition

The goal of *Essence of Anesthesia Practice* was and is to provide a concise one-page summary of the pathophysiology of conditions rarely or often seen in the perioperative period. These summaries highlight important concerns facing those practitioners caring for patients in this critical time period. No one can keep current on all advances and fields in medicine, and in the rush of the perioperative environment, we ourselves found useful reminders and triggers to call attention to important aspects. So we enrolled over 500 experts to distill their wisdom for you. That you, the practitioner, made the first edition a bestseller in seven languages, and that over 500 physicians expert in some aspect of care again committed to contribute to this substantially revised and improved edition, attest to the need for such summaries.

This edition improves and updates all the material that went before. We deleted some sections you didn't find useful, and we added an important section on perioperative concerns with alternative medications. For those of you who asked for an electronic version, we hope the optional Palm Program meets your desires. To create it, we extracted and highlighted elements related to the preoperative evaluation and preparation of the patient based on co-existing disease, chronic medication usage (including alternative medications), and planned surgical procedure. Specifically, the sections entitled Overview, Perioperative Risks, Worry About, and Preoperative Preparation are included. We also included the different systemic effects from the assessment table, but not how they can be assessed by history/physical examination or testing. For that aspect of the evaluation, you will need to use the book. Our goal is to provide what many of you who e-mailed, wrote, and spoke to us told us you wanted—the essence of the preoperative evaluation in a readily accessible form on the Palm Pilot—while the more complete evaluation and management can be obtained from the printed version of *Essence of Anesthesia Practice*.

We wish to thank Allan Ross, our editor at Harcourt Health Sciences, who has continued in the tradition of Lewis Reines in ensuring that our book received appropriate editing and development and providing the relentless support for this book to be published in a timely fashion. We also wish to thank Juliane Tarr and Juanita Taylor in our offices for their tireless work in ensuring that all of the manuscripts were received, collated, and properly prepared for the publisher. Lee would also like to acknowledge Ann Cartarius, R.N., his research coordinator, for her efforts in ensuring that his laboratory continued to run smoothly during preparation of this book.

MICHAEL F. ROIZEN

LEE A. FLEISHER

Preface to the First Edition

It was in 1986 that the idea of a one-page summary of the pathophysiology of diseases and their implications for anesthesia was conceived. Drs. Charise T. Petrovitch and Michael F. Roizen were formulating questions at that time to assess whether candidates for Board certification could qualify as consultants. That an anesthesiologist can deliver anesthesia safely for the majority of patients is assessed by the Board's multiple-choice test and the Clinical Competence Committee in their training program. But as a consultant, the anesthesiologist must be able to convey an understanding that many diseases cause pathophysiologic disturbances that may affect perioperative management. Awareness of those disturbances and an ability to integrate that knowledge in clinical care to minimize their consequences separates the merely good anesthetic practitioner from the master practitioner or consultant.

We thought that the implications of disease, chronic drug therapy, procedures, and abnormalities on diagnostic tests for perioperative care could be most easily understood and remembered if they were summarized on one page. The summaries presented in this book review the pathophysiologic implications of specific diseases, including suggestions for evaluation of patients, the effective medications for the disease, the implications of anesthesia for operative procedures, and the pathophysiologic implications of a diagnostic test abnormality. These summaries are not substitutes for textbooks of medical specialties but are offered as brief overviews of the essentials to be reviewed in caring for the patient.

The book is divided into four sections: Diseases, Procedures, Drugs, and Tests. In all sections, each topic is outlined on a single page divided into three sections.

The top section presents an overview of information about a disease, chronic drug therapy, procedure, or test. This section lists the etiology of the condition, indications, and usual treatments. For diseases or procedures, perioperative risk and potential problems during the perioperative period are outlined. The objective is to assist the practitioner in choosing topics to discuss with a patient in the preanesthetic interview and tailoring an anesthetic plan to reduce risk. Indications for drugs and tests and alternative treatments or procedures are also suggested. An ICD-9-CM code has been included for diseases and the primary underlying pathology for many operations. Since a wide range of codes can be ascribed to particular conditions, we have included the most common ICD-9-CM codes; these codes can help the practitioner locate the most applicable one for each individual patient but are not meant to be definitive.

The middle section is arranged in table format. The table outlines the effects of a procedure, disease, drug therapy, or test implication on an organ system. The contributors have identified aspects from a patient's history and physical examination that can be used to diagnose each effect. Finally, tests that may be used to further assess the probability of morbidity are suggested. These tests should be performed only if indicated by a patient's history or physical examination. Such tests are by no means intended to be part of every evaluation, nor are they the only laboratory tests to be considered.

The bottom section is devoted to perioperative implications. Again, the pathophysiologic approach is emphasized for management. Finally, there is a subsection on anticipated problems and concerns during the postoperative period.

Publication of *Essence of Anesthesia Practice* required assistance from many individuals. We especially acknowledge the efforts of Dr. Charise Petrovitch; Lewis Reines, President of W.B. Saunders, who took a personal interest in the project; and John Cooke, Evelyn Adler, Constance Burton, Linda R. Garber, and Joan Slowinski of W.B. Saunders, for translating our ideas into a workable text. Our secretaries, Kelle Martin, Elaine Lowery, and Annette Y. Hargrave, worked with a combination of over 600 contributors and manuscripts. While all of us try to ensure brevity, accuracy, consistency of style (both of us edited each summary page at least twice), and freedom from typographical errors, we are sure that some errors have eluded us. We hope you will write or e-mail us (roizenm@upstate.edu *or* lfleishe@jhmi.edu) so that should future printings or editions be warranted, we may correct our errors. If you notice an omission from any of the four sections, we would appreciate having the omission called to our attention. Further, although we tried to prepare the summaries in a format ready for electronic media, most people do not yet have screens big enough to show the full page. We believe that will soon be corrected.

Although Dr. Petrovitch's family and other obligations forced her to drop out of working on this project, we, Drs. Roizen and Fleisher, and the contributors have tried to convey in this work the essence of the pathophysiologic implications of acute or chronic conditions, drug therapies, procedures, and test abnormalities. *Essence of Anesthesia Practice* is not intended to be a "cookbook" of anesthesiology. While some people with expertise in one area were approached to write or contribute a page on the conditions that they know most about, some initially refused, saying that they did not want to be involved in a "cookbook." Most later accepted after we further explained the concept to them. This book and each summary is anything but a "cookbook"; in fact, it is close to the opposite. It assumes that the practitioner knows how to deliver anesthesia. It is intended to highlight concisely the pathophysiologic derangements and perioperative implications of diseases, procedures, drugs, and test abnormalities in an ordered fashion. This book was designed for the novice and consultant alike to help each one function better. We believe that our patients have already benefited from the work done on this book. We hope that you will feel that you and your patients have benefited also.

MICHAEL F. ROIZEN

LEE A. FLEISHER

Contents

Section II
PROCEDURES

Section III
DRUGS

SECTION IV
ALTERNATIVE MEDICINE

List of Abbreviations

SYMBOLS

±	plus or minus
?	questionable
~	approximately
°C	degrees centigrade
°F	degrees Fahrenheit
1°	primary; first degree
2°	secondary; second degree
3°	third degree

A

A/G	albumin-globulin
A-a	alveolar-arterial
AA	arachidonic acid
AAA	abdominal aortic aneurysm
A-aDO$_2$	alveolar-arterial oxygen delivery
AAT	automatic atrial tachycardia
abd	abdomen; abdominal
ABF	aorto-bifemoral bypass
ABG	arterial blood gas
ABI	aorto-bi-iliac bypass
abn	abnormal; abnormality
ACAS	Asymptomatic Carotid Atherosclerosis Study
ACE	angiotensin-converting enzyme
ACG	angle-closure glaucoma
ACh	acetylcholine
AChE	acetylcholinesterase
ACL	anterior cruciate ligament
ACLS	advanced cardiac life support
ACOG	American College of Obstetricians and Gynecologists
ACS	acute confusional state
ACT	activated clotting/coagulation time
ACTH	adrenocorticotropic hormone
ADH	antidiuretic hormone
ADHD	attention-deficit hyperactivity disorder
ADI	atlas-dens interval
ADL	activities of daily living
admin	administration; administered
ADP	adenosine diphosphate
AED	automated external defibrillator
AFIB	atrial fibrillation
AFLT	atrial flutter
A/G	albumin/globulin
AH	autonomic hyperreflexia
AI	aortic insufficiency
AICD	automatic implantable cardioverter defibrillator
AIDS	acquired immunodeficiency syndrome
AIMs	anesthetic-induced myodystrophies

AKA	above-knee amputation; also known as
alb	albumin
alk phos	alkaline phosphatase
ALL	acute lymphoblastic leukemia
ALT	alanine aminotransferase
Alv	alveolar
AM	morning
AML	acute myelogenous leukemia
AMP	adenosine monophosphate
ampl	amplitude
amt	amount
ANA	antinuclear antibody
angio	angiogram
ANS	autonomic nervous system
ant	anterior
anticoag	anticoagulation
AP	accessory pathway; action potential; anterior-posterior
API	alkaline protease inhibitor
apo B	apolipoprotein class B
approx	approximate; approximately
APTT	activated partial thromboplastin time
APUD	amine precursor uptake and decarboxylation
AR	aortic regurgitation
ARDS	acute respiratory distress syndrome
ARF	acute renal failure
art	arterial
AS	aortic stenosis
ASA	acetylsalicylic acid; Adams-Stokes attack; American Society of Anesthesiologists
ASAP	as soon as possible
ASCVD	atherosclerotic cardiovascular disease
ASD	atrial septal defect
assoc	associated
AST	aspartate aminotransferase
AT	antithrombin
AT1	angiotensin receptor 1
ATG	anti-thymus globulin
ATN	acute tubular necrosis
ATP	adenosine triphosphate; antitachycardia pacing
Au	gold
AV	atrioventricular
AVHB	atrioventricular heart block
AVM	arteriovenous malformation
AVR	aortic valve replacement

B

β-hCG	beta human chorionic gonadotropin
BAER	brainstem auditory evoked response
BBB	bundle branch block; blood-brain barrier

BCNU	nitrosourea (carmustine)		CHO	carbohydrate
BF	bifascicular; blood flow		CI	cardiac index; confidence interval
BFHB	bifascicular heart block		CIN	cervical intraepithelial neoplasia
bid	twice per day		circ	circulation; circulatory
BIG	botulism immune globulin		cis-DDP	cis-diamminedichloroplatinum
bilat	bilateral		CK	creatine kinase
BKA	below-knee amputation		CK-MB	isoenzyme of creatine kinase with muscle and brain subunits
bleo	bleomycin			
BLS	basic life support		CLL	chronic lymphocytic leukemia
BM	bowel movement		CLR	chlorambucil
BMI	body mass index		CML	chronic myelogenous leukemia
BMR	basal metabolic rate		$CMRO_2$	cerebral metabolic rate of oxygen
BMT	bone marrow transplantation		CMV	cytomegalovirus
BO	bronchiolitis obliterans		CN	cranial nerve; cyanide
BOOP	bronchiolitis obliterans with cryptogenic organizing pneumonia		CNH	central neurogenic hyperventilation
			CNS	central nervous system
BP	blood pressure		CO	carbon monoxide; cardiac output
BPD	bronchopulmonary dysplasia		CO_2	carbon dioxide
BPH	benign prostatic hyperplasia/hypertrophy		coag	coagulation
bpm	beats per minute		COHb	carboxyhemoglobin
BS	breath sounds		COM	chronic otitis media
BSA	body surface area		COMT	catechol-o-methyltransferase
BT	bleeding time; Blalock-Taussig (shunt)		conc	concentration
BUN	blood urea nitrogen		COPD	chronic obstructive pulmonary disease
Bx	biopsy		COX	cyclooxygenase
			COX-2	cyclooxygenase-2
C			cP	centipoise
			CP	cerebral palsy; cerebellopontine (angle)
CA	cancer; cold agglutinins		CPAP	continuous positive airway pressure
ca.	about (L., circa)		CPB	cardiopulmonary bypass
Ca^{2+}	calcium		CPD	cephalopelvic disproportion
CAB	coronary artery bypass		CPP	cerebral perfusion pressure
CABG	coronary artery bypass graft		CPR	cardiopulmonary resuscitation
CAD	coronary artery disease		CPT	carnitine palmityl transferase
CAHS	central alveolar hypoventilation syndrome		CPZ	chlorpromazine
cAMP	cyclic adenosine monophosphate		Cr	creatinine
CaO_2	arterial oxygen concentration		CrCl	creatinine clearance
cardiopulm	cardiopulmonary		CRI	chronic renal insufficiency
CAS	coronary artery spasm		cryo	cryoprecipitate
CASS	Coronary Artery Surgery Study		CS	chondroitin sulfate
CATCH 22	cardiac defect; abnormal facies; thymic hypoplasia; cleft palate; hypocalcemia (syndrome)		C-section	cesarean section
			CSF	cerebrospinal fluid
			CSH	carotid sinus hypersensitivity
cath	catheter; catheterization		CSM	carotid sinus massage
CBC	complete blood count		C-spine	cervical spine
CBF	cerebral blood flow		CSS	carotid sinus syndrome
CBV	cerebral blood volume		CT	computed tomography; connective tissue
CCNU	nitrosourea (lomustine)		CTX	cyclophosphamide (Cytoxan)
CD4	antigenic marker on helper/inducer T cells		CV	cardiovascular
$CD4^+$	presence of CD4		CVA	cerebrovascular accident
CDC	Centers for Disease Control and Prevention		CVD	cerebrovascular disease
			CVP	central venous pressure
CEA	carotid endarterectomy		CVS	cardiovascular status
CGL	chronic granulocytic leukemia		CXR	chest x-ray
cGMP	cyclic guanosine monophosphate		CYP	cytochrome P450
C-GSF	granulocyte colony–stimulating factor		cysto	cystoscopy
CHB	complete heart block			
CHD	congenital heart disease; congenital heart defect		**D**	
ChE	cholinesterase		2,3-DPG	2,3-diphosphoglyceric acid
ChemoRx	chemotherapy		2D	two-dimensional
CHF	congestive heart failure		d	day

D and T	diphtheria and tetanus		ECMO	extracorporeal membrane oxygenation
D&C	dilatation and curettage		ECoG	electrocorticography
D/C	discontinue(d)		ECT	electroconvulsive therapy
D_5	dextrose 5% in water		ED_{50}	median effective dose
DA	dopamine		EDAS	encephalodural arteriosynangiosis
DBP	diastolic blood pressure		EDTA	ethylenediaminetetraacetic acid
DC	direct current		EDV	end-diastolic volume
DCM	dilated cardiomyopathy		EEC	ectrodactyly-ectodermal dysplasia, cleft (syndrome)
DDAVP	1-deamino(8-D-arginine) vasopressin; desmopressin acetate		EEG	electroencephalogram
DDT	dichlorodiphenyltrichloroethane		EENT	eyes, ears, nose, throat
DEA	Drug Enforcement Agency		EF	ejection fraction
DEB	dystrophic epidermolysis bullosa		EGD	esophagogastroduodenoscopy
deriv	derivative(s)		E-L	Eaton-Lambert
derm	dermatology		ELBW	extremely low birth weight
DFA	direct immunofluorescent assay		ELISA	enzyme-linked immunosorbent assay
DFT	defibrillation threshold		EMD	electromechanical dissociation
DGL	deglycyrrhized licorice		EMG	electromyography
DGLA	dihomo-γ-linolenic acid		EMI	electromagnetic interference; electromechanical interference
DHA	docosahexaenoic acid			
DHEA	dehydroepiandrosterone		EMLA	eutectic mixture of local anesthetics
DHT	dihydrotestosterone		endo	endocrine
DI	diabetes insipidus		ENT	ear, nose, and throat
DIC	disseminated intravascular coagulation		EP	electrophysiologic
diff	differential		EPA	eicosapentaenoic acid
Dig	digoxin		EPI	epinephrine
DJD	degenerative joint disease		EPO	evening primrose oil
DKA	diabetic ketoacidosis		EPS	electrophysiologic study
DL_{CO}	carbon monoxide diffusion capacity in the lungs		ER	emergency room
			ERCP	endoscopic retrograde cholangiopancreatography
DM	diabetes mellitus			
DMD	Duchenne muscular dystrophy		ERV	expiratory reserve volume
DMT	dimethyltryptamine		ES	Eisenmenger's syndrome
DNR	do not resuscitate		es	estimated
Do_2	oxygen delivery		ESM	ethosuximide
DOB	dobutamine		esp	especially
DOE	dyspnea on exertion		ESR	erythrocyte sedimentation rate
dP/dT	ratio of change in ventricular pressure to change in time		ESRD	end-stage renal disease
			ESS	endoscopic sinus surgery
DPNB	dorsal penile nerve block		ESV	end-systolic volume
dSSEP	dermatomal somatosensory evoked potentials		ESWL	extracorporeal shock wave lithotripsy
			ET	endotracheal
DTIC	dimethyltriazenoimidazole carboxamide (dacarbazine)		$ETCO_2$	end-tidal carbon dioxide
			ETN_2	end-tidal nitrogen
DTPA	diethylenetriaminepenta-acetic acid		ETOH	ethanol
DTR	deep tendon reflex		ETT	endotracheal tube; exercise tolerance test
DTs	delirium tremens		eval	evaluation
DVT	deep vein thrombosis		Ex	exercise
Dx	diagnosis; diagnostic		exam	examination
			ext	exterior

E

EACA	epsilon-aminocaproic acid			
EBL	estimated blood loss		**F**	
EBV	Epstein-Barr virus			
EC	eclampsia		5-FU	5-fluorouracil
ECA	ethacrynic acid		F	female(s)
ECC	extracorporeal circulation		Fa/Fi	fraction alveolar/fraction inspired
ECD	endocardial cushion defect		Fab	fragment, antigen-binding
ECFV	extracellular fluid volume		FAD	flavin adenine dinucleotide
ECG	electrocardiogram		FBS	fasting blood sugar
ECHO	echocardiogram		FDA	Food and Drug Administration
			FDP	fibrin-degradation product
			Fe	iron

Fe^{2+}	ferrous
Fe^{3+}	ferric
FEN_a	excreted fraction of filtered sodium
FES	fat embolism syndrome
FEV	forced expiratory volume
FEV_1	FEV in 1 second
FFA	free fatty acid
FFP	fresh frozen plasma
FHF	fulminant hepatic failure
FHR	fetal heart rate
FHT	fetal heart tone
FIO_2	fractional inspired oxygen
FIX	factor IX
FMN	flavin mononucleotide
FOB	fiberoptic bronchoscopy
FRC	functional residual capacity
freq	frequent; frequency
FSBG	fingerstick blood glucose
FSH	follicle stimulating hormone
FSP	fibrin split products
FT_4E	free thyroxine estimate
FTT	failure to thrive
FUDR	floxuridine
FVC	forced vital capacity
FVIII	factor VIII
Fx	fracture

G

G	gauge
G6PD	glucose-6-phosphate dehydrogenase
GA	general anesthesia
GABA	γ-aminobutyric acid
GBL	gamma butyrolactone
G-CSF	granulocyte colony-stimulating factor
GDM	gestational diabetes mellitus
GE	gastroesophageal
GER	gastroesophageal reflux
GERD	gastroesophageal reflux disease
GETA	general endotracheal anesthesia
GFR	glomerular filtration rate
GGTP	gamma-glutamyl-transpeptidase
GH	growth hormone
GHB	gamma hydroxybutyrate
Gi	inhibitory G protein
GI	gastrointestinal
GIFT	gamete intrafallopian transfer
GLA	γ-linolenic acid
glu	glucose
GMP	guanosine monophosphate
Gn-RH	gonadotropin-releasing hormone
GRAS	generally recognized as safe
GTP	guanosine triphosphate
GTT	glucose tolerance test
GU	genitourinary
GVHD	graft vs. host disease
gyn	gynecologic

H

5-HIAA	5-hydroxyindoleacetic acid
5-HT	5-hydroxytryptamine
h	hour
H & N	head and neck
H & P	history and physical
H_1	histamine receptor type 1
H_2	histamine receptor type 2
H_2O	water
HAF-PCM	hypoalbuminemic form of protein-calorie malnutrition
HAV	hepatitis A virus
HB	heart block
HbA_{1c}	glycosylated hemoglobin
HbAA	hemoglobin homozygous for A
HbM	hemoglobin Milwaukee
HbO_2	oxyhemoglobin
HbsAg	hepatitis B surface antigen
HbSS	homozygosity for hemoglobin S (sickle cell anemia)
HBV	hepatitis B virus
HCFA	Health Care Financing Administration
hCG	human gonadotropic hormone
HCM	hypertrophic cardiomyopathy
HCO_2	bicarbonate
Hct	hematocrit
HCV	hepatitis C virus
HD	heart disease; Hodgkin's disease
HDL	high-density lipoprotein
HDL-C	HDL cholesterol
He	helium
HEENT	head, eyes, ears, nose, throat
HELLP	hemolysis, elevated liver enzymes, and low platelet count (syndrome)
heme	hematology
Hg	mercury
Hgb	hemoglobin
HGPRT	hypoxanthine-guanine-phosphoribosyl-transferase
HHV-3-6	human herpesviruses
HIV	human immunodeficiency virus
HLA	human leukocyte antigen
hLH	hemophagocytic lymphohistiocytosis
HLHS	hypoplastic left heart syndrome
HMD	hyaline membrane disease
HMG CoA	3-hydroxy-3-methylglutaryl
HN_2	nitrogen mustard
hosp	hospitalization
HPV	hypoxic pulmonary vasoconstriction
hr	hour(s)
HR	heart rate
HSV	herpes simplex virus
HSV-1	HSV type 1
HSV-2	HSV type 2
ht	height
Htn	hypertension
HUS	hemolytic uremic syndrome
Hx	history

I

I & D	incision and drainage
I/O	intake-output
IABCP	intra-aortic baloon counterpulsation
IABP	intra-aortic balloon pump

IADH	inappropriate antidiuretic hormone
IBD	inflammatory bowel disease
IBS	irritable bowel syndrome
ICA	internal carotid artery
ICD	implantable cardioverter-defibrillator
ICGA	immunochromatographic assay
ICH	intracranial hypertension
ICMA	immunochemiluminometric assay
ICP	intracranial pressure
ICU	intensive care unit
ID	infectious disease
IDCM	idiopathic dilated cardiomyopathy
IDDM	insulin-dependent diabetes mellitus
IDL	intermediate-density lipoprotein
I:E	inspiratory:expiratory ratio
IFN	interferon
Ig	immunoglobulin
IGF	insulin-like growth factor
IGF-I	insulin-like growth factor I
IHD	ischemic heart disease
IHSS	idiopathic hypertrophic subaortic stenosis
IL	interleukin
IM	intramuscular
immuno	immunologic
in.	inch
incl	including
inf	inferior
info	information
INH	isoniazid
INR	International Normalized Ratio
insp	inspiratory
intox	intoxication
intraop	intraoperative
IOL	intraocular lens
IOP	intraocular pressure
IP	impedance plethysmography; intraperitoneal; intraperitoneally
IPPB	intermittent positive pressure breathing
IPPV	intermittent positive pressure ventilation
IQ	intelligence quotient
IRDS	infant respiratory distress syndrome
IRMA	immunoradiometric assay
ITP	immune thrombocytopenic purpura
I-V	interventricular
IV	intravenous
IVC	inferior vena cava
IVF	intravascular fluid; intravenous fluid
IVH	intracranial/intraventricular hemorrhage
IVP	intravenous pyelogram

J

JCAHO	Joint Commission on Accreditation of Healthcare Organizations
JEB	junctional epidermolysis bullosa
JV	jugular vein
JVD	jugular venous distention
JVP	jugular venous pressure

K

K^+	potassium
Kr	krypton

KSS	Kearns-Sayre Syndrome
KUB	kidney, ureter, bladder

L

L	left
L→R	left to right
LA	left atrial; left atrium; linoleic acid; local anesthetic
lab	laboratory
LAD	left anterior descending (coronary artery)
LAFB	left anterior fascicular block
LAO	left anterior oblique
LAP	left atrial pressure
lat	lateral
LBBB	left bundle branch block
LBO	large-bowel obstruction
LCAT	lecithin-cholesterol acyltransferase
LCH	Langerhans cell histiocytosis
LDH	lactate dehydrogenase
LDL	low-density lipoprotein
LDL-C	LDL cholesterol
LE	lower extremity
LEA	lower extremity amputation
LES	lower esophageal sphincter
LFT	liver function test
LGL	Lown-Ganong-Levine syndrome
LH	luteinizing hormone
LLQ	left lower quadrant
LMA	laryngeal mask airway
LMP	last menstrual period
LMW	low molecular weight
LMWH	low molecular weight heparin
LOC	level of consciousness; loss of consciousness
LOS	length of stay
LP	lumbar puncture
Lp(a)	lipoprotein(a)
L-PAM	melphalan (Alkeran)
LPFB	left posterior fascicular block
LPO	left posterior oblique
LR	lactated Ringer's (solution)
LRI	lower respiratory tract infection
LSB	lumbar sympathetic block
LSD	lysergic acid diethylamide
LTB_4	leukotriene B_4
LUQ	left upper quadrant
LV	left ventricle
LVAD	left ventricular assist device
LVEDP	left ventricular end-diastolic pressure
LVEF	left ventricular ejection fraction
LVET	left ventricular ejection time
LVF	left ventricular failure
LVH	left ventricular hypertrophy
LVOT	left ventricular outflow tract
lytes	electrolytes

M

M	male(s)
M:F	male to female ratio

M2	muscarinic		MW	molecular weight
MAC	minimum alveolar concentration; monitored anesthesia care		MYL	Myleran (busulfan)
MALA	metformin-associated lactic acidosis		**N**	
MAO	monoamine oxidase			
MAOI	MAO inhibitor		N	nitrogen
MAP	mean arterial pressure		n.	nerve
MAST	medical antishock trousers		n-MPTP	1-methyl-4-phenyl-1,2,3,6-tetrahydropyridine
MAT	multiform atrial tachycardia			
max	maximum; maximal		N/A	not applicable
MBC	maximal breathing capacity		N/S	normal saline
MCA	middle cerebral artery		N/V	nausea/vomiting
MD	muscular dystrophy		N_2O	dinitrogen monoxide (nitrous oxide)
MEA	multiple endocrine adenomas		Na^+	sodium
mech	mechanical; mechanism		NAC	N-acetyl-L-cysteine
med	medication		NADH	nicotinamide adenine dinucleotide, reduced form
MEN	multiple endocrine neoplasia		NADPH	nicotinamide adenine dinucleotide phosphate, reduced form
MEN I	MEN type I			
MEN II	MEN type II		NAPA	N-acetyl procainamide
MEP	motor/multimodality evoked potential		NB	nota bene (note well)
MET	metabolic equivalent		NCV	nerve conduction velocity
metab	metabolism; metabolic		Nd:YAG	neodymium:yttrium-aluminum-garnet
metHb	methemoglobin		NE	norepinephrine
mets	metastases		NEC	necrotizing enterocolitis
MF-PCM	marasmic form of PCM		neg	negative
Mg^{2+}	magnesium		neuro	neurologic
$MgSO_4$	magnesium sulfate		NF	neurologic findings
MH	malignant hyperthermia		NF-1	neurofibromatosis
MI	myocardial infarction		NFL	National Football League
MIDCAB	minimally invasive direct coronary artery bypass		NG	nasogastric
min	minimal; minimum; minute		NH_3	ammonia
MIsch	myocardial ischemia		NHL	non-Hodgkin's lymphoma
mIU	milli-International unit		NHR	non−hemodynamically related
MIV	mivacurium		NIBP	noninvasive blood pressure
MLAP	mean left atrial pressure		NICU	neonatal intensive care unit
MLD	median lethal dose		NIDDM	non−insulin-dependent diabetes mellitus
MMEFR	maximal midexpiratory flow rate		NIF	negative inspiratory force
MMR	masseter muscle rigidity		NIH	National Institutes of Health
mo	month		NK	natural killer (cell)
mo wt	molecular weight		NM	neuromuscular
MODS	multiorgan dysfunction syndrome		NMB	neuromuscular blockade
MP	mucopolysaccharide		NMDA	N-methyl-D-aspartate
MPAP	mean pulmonary artery pressure		NMEPs	neuromuscular evoked potentials
MPD	mast cell proliferative disorder		NMJ	neuromuscular junction
MR	mitral regurgitation		nml	normal
MRA	magnetic resonance angiography		NMS	neuroleptic malignant syndrome
MRI	magnetic resonance imaging		NO	nitric oxide
MS	mental status; mitral stenosis; multiple sclerosis; musculoskeletal		no.	number
			nondep	nondepolarizing
ms	milliseconds		NP	nasopharyngeal
MSLT	Multiple Sleep Latency Test		NPH	neutral protamine Hagedorn
MSOF	multisystem organ failure		NPO	nil per os (nothing by mouth)
MTX	methotrexate		NPPB	normal perfusion pressure breakthrough (syndrome)
MU	million units			
mucocut	mucocutaneous		NRI	nutritional risk index
MUGA	multiple gated acquisition		NS	normal saline (solution)
musc	muscular		NSAID	nonsteroidal anti-inflammatory drug
MVD	microvascular decompression		NSR	normal sinus rhythm
MVI	multiple vitamin infusion		NT	nasotracheal
Mvo_2	minute venous oxygen		NTG	nitroglycerin
MVP	mitral valve prolapse		NTP	nucleoside triphosphate

NVD	nausea, vomiting, and diarrhea		PEF	peak expiratory flow
NYHA	New York Heart Association		PEP	positive expiratory pressure
			periop	perioperative
O			PET	positron emission tomography
			$PETCO_2$	end-tidal partial pressure of carbon dioxide
O/P	output		PFO	patent foramen ovale
O_2	oxygen		PFT	pulmonary function test
OA	osteoarthritis		PG	prostaglandin
OB	obstetric		PGD_2	prostaglandin D_2
OB/GYN	obstetrics and gynecology		PGE_1	alprostadil (prostaglandin E_1)
OC	oral contraceptive		pharm	pharmaceutical; pharmacy
OD	overdose		pheo	pheochromocytoma
OG	orogastric		physiol	physiologic
OKT3	Ortho Kung T cell (muromonab-CD3)		P_i	inorganic phosphate
OLD	obstructive lung disease		PID	pelvic inflammatory disease
OM	otitis media		PIH	pregnancy-induced hypertension
OMIM	Online Mendelian Inheritance in Man		PIP	peak inspiratory pressure
OPCAB	off-pump coronary artery bypass		pK_a	negative logarithm of the dissociation constant of an acid
ophthal	ophthalmologic			
OPO	Organ Procurement Organization		plt	platelet
OR	operating room		pM	picomolar
ORIF	open reduction internal fixation		PMI	posterior myocardial infarction; point of maximal intensity
Osm	osmole; osmolality			
OTC	over-the-counter		PMN	polymorphonuclear
			PMS	premenstrual syndrome
P			PND	paroxysmal nocturnal dyspnea
			PNS	peripheral nervous system
P	phosphorus		PO	per os
$P(A-a)O_2$	alveolar-arterial oxygen difference		PO_2	oxygen partial pressure
PA	plasma aldosterone; pulmonary artery		PO_4	phosphate
PAC	premature atrial contraction		POAG	primary open-angle glaucoma
$PaCO_2$	partial pressure of carbon dioxide, arterial		pos	positive
PACU	postanesthesia care unit		poss	possible; possibly
PAF	platelet activating factor		postop	postoperative
PAIR	puncture-aspiration-injection-reaspiration		PPAR	peroxisome proliferator-activated receptor
palp	palpation of		PPD	purified protein derivative (tuberculin)
PaO_2	partial pressure of oxygen in arterial blood		PPH	persistent pulmonary hypertension
PAOP	pulmonary artery occlusion pressure		Pplat	plateau pressure
PAP	pulmonary artery pressure		ppm	parts per million
PAPVD	partial anomalous pulmonary venous drainage		PPV	positive predictive value; positive pressure ventilation
PAT	paroxysmal atrial tachycardia		PR	per rectum
Paw	mean airway pressure		PRA	plasma renin activity
PAWP	pulmonary artery wedge pressure		prb	problem
PBF	pulmonary blood flow		PRBCs	packed red blood cells
PCA	patient-controlled analgesia		preg	pregnancy; pregnant
PCFS	posterior cranial fossa surgery		premed	premedication
PCM	protein-calorie malnutrition		preop	preoperative
PCO	polycystic ovary		prep	preparation
PCO_2	partial pressure of carbon dioxide		PRL	prolactin
PCP	phencyclidine		prn	as needed
PCR	polymerase chain reaction		PS	pulmonary stenosis
PCV	packed cell volume		PSA	prostate-specific antigen
PCWP	pulmonary capillary wedge pressure		PSVT	paroxysmal supraventricular tachycardia
PD	peritoneal dialysis		psych	psychological
PDA	patent ductus arteriosus		pt	patient
PDE III	phosphodiesterase III (inhibitors)		PT	physical therapy; prothrombin time
PDI	pituitary diabetes insipidus		PTCA	percutaneous transluminal coronary angioplasty
PDR	Physicians' Desk Reference			
PE	physical examination; preeclampsia; pressure equalization; pulmonary embolism		PTH	parathyroid hormone
			PTLD	post transplant lymphoproliferative disease
PEEP	positive end-expiratory pressure			

pts	patients
PTSS	posttraumatic stress syndrome
PTT	partial thromboplastin time
PTU	propylthiouracil
PUD	peptic ulcer disease
pulm	pulmonary
PUVA	psoralens plus ultraviolet A
PVC	polyvinyl chloride; premature ventricular contraction
PVD	peripheral vascular disease
PVO_2	partial pressure of oxygen, venous
PVR	pulmonary vascular resistance

Q

Q	perfusion
q	every
q.a.m.	every morning
q.n.	every night
q.p.m.	every evening
qhs	every hour of sleep
qid	four times per day
Qp:Qs	ratio of pulmonary blood to systemic blood flow
QRS	Q wave, R wave, S wave

R

R	right
R/O	rule out
RA	rheumatoid arthritis; right atrium
RAAS	renin-angiotensin-aldosterone system
RAD	reactive airway disease
RAE	right atrial enlargement
RAH	right atrial hypertrophy
RAI	resting ankle index
RAO	right anterior oblique
RAP	right atrial pressure
RAST	radioallergosorbent test
RBBB	right bundle branch block
RBC	red blood cell
RBF	renal blood flow
RCM	congenital methemoglobinemia of the recessive type
RDA	recommended daily allowance
RDS	respiratory distress syndrome
reg	regular
rehab	rehabilitation
REM	rapid eye movement
reprod	reproductive (system)
resp	respiratory
RH	releasing hormone
RHD	rheumatic heart disease
RHF	right heart failure
RIA	radioimmunoassay
RIJ	right internal jugular
RIMA	reversible inhibitor of monoamine
RIND	reversible ischemic neurological deficit
RLD	restrictive lung disease
ROM	range of motion
ROP	retinopathy of prematurity
ROS	review of systems

ROSC	return of spontaneous circulation
RPO	right posterior oblique
RR	respiratory rate
R→L	right to left
RSD	reflex sympathetic dystrophy
RSV	respiratory syncytial virus
RT	radiation therapy
RTA	renal tubule acidosis
RUQ	right upper quadrant
RV	residual volume; right ventricle
RVE	right ventricular enlargement
RVEDP	right ventricular end-diastolic pressure
RVH	right ventricular hypertrophy
Rx	therapy; treatment; therapeutic

S

S	Svedberg unit
S/P	status post
SA	sinoatrial; beta S/beta A globin gene
SAH	subarachnoid hemorrhage
SAM	systolic anterior motion
SAMe	S-adenosyl-L-methionine
SaO_2	oxygen saturation in arterial blood
SAP	systemic arterial pressure
SAS	sleep apnea syndrome
sat	saturation
SBE	standard base excess; subacute bacterial endocarditis
SBO	small-bowel obstruction
SBP	systolic blood pressure
SCD	sudden cardiac death
SCH	succinylcholine
SD	standard deviation(s)
SEB	simplex epidermolysis bullosa
sec	second(s)
SEP	sensory evoked potential
seroneg	seronegative
SG	specific gravity
SGOT	serum glutamic-oxaloacetic transaminase
SGPT	serum glutamate pyruvate transaminase
SIADH	syndrome of inappropriate secretion of antidiuretic hormone
SICU	surgical ICU
SIDS	sudden infant death syndrome
SIRS	systemic inflammatory response syndrome
SL	sublingual
SLE	systemic lupus erythematosus
SMA	superior mesenteric artery
SMA-20	Sequential Multiple Analyzer
SNS	sympathetic nervous system
SOB	shortness of breath
soln	solution
SPECT	single-photon emission computed tomography
SPK	simultaneous pancreas-kidney
SpO_2	oxygen saturation as measured by pulse oximetry
spont	spontaneously
SQ	subcutaneous; subcutaneously
SSEP	somatosensory evoked potential
SSRI	selective serotonin reuptake inhibitor

SSS	sick sinus syndrome		TP	total protein
STD	sexually transmitted disease		t-PA	tissue plasminogen activator
STP	2,5-dimethoxy-4-methylamphetamine		TPN	total parenteral nutrition
STSG	split-thickness skin graft		TR	tricuspid regurgitation
Stz	streptozocin		TRH	thyrotropin-releasing hormone
sup	superior		TRUS	transrectal ultrasonography
surg	surgery; surgical		TSH	thyroid stimulating hormone
SV	stroke volume		TT	thrombin time
SVC	superior vena cava		TTE	transthoracic echocardiography
SVO$_2$	mixed venous continuous oxygen saturation		T-TEPA	triethylene-thiophosphoramide (thiotepa)
SVR	systemic vascular resistance		TTP	thrombotic thrombocytopenic purpura
SVT	supraventricular tachycardia		TURBT	transurethral resection of bladder tumor
Sx	signs and symptoms		TURP	transurethral resection of the prostate
Sz	seizure		TV	tidal volume
			TVH	total vaginal hysterectomy
T			Tx	transplant; transfusion
			TXA$_2$	thromboxane A$_2$
^{99m}Tc	technetium 99m		TXA$_3$	thromboxane A$_3$
T	temperature		TXB$_2$	thromboxane B$_2$
T&C	type and crossmatch			
T$_{1/2}$	half-life		**U**	
T$_3$	triiodothyronine			
T$_4$	thyroxine		UA	urinalysis
TA	tricuspid atresia		UE	upper extremity
TAH	total abdominal hysterectomy		UGI	upper gastrointestinal
TAPVD	total anomalous pulmonary venous drainage		UK	United Kingdom
			U-lytes	urine electrolytes
TB	tuberculosis		UO	urine output
TCA	tricyclic antidepressant		UP	urticaria pigmentosa
TCD	transcranial Doppler		UPJ	ureteropelvic junction
TDP	torsades de pointes		URI	upper respiratory tract infection
TEE	transesophageal echocardiography		urol	urology; urologic
TEF	transesophageal fistula		US	ultrasound
TEG	thromboelastography		USA	United States of America
temp	temperature		UT	urinary tract
TENS	transcutaneous electrical nerve stimulation		UTI	urinary tract infection
			UV	ultraviolet
tet	tetralogy of Fallot			
TFA	trifluoroacetic acid		**V**	
TFT	thyroid function test			
TGA	transposition of the great arteries		V	ventilation
TGV	transposition of great vessels		V/Q	ventilation-perfusion
THC	delta-9-tetrahydrocannabinol		VACTERL	vertebral, anal, cardiac, tracheal, esophageal, renal, and limb
THR	total hip replacement		VAE	venous air embolism
TIA	transient ischemic attack		VALI	ventilator-associated lung injury
tid	three times per day		VAS	Visual Analogue Scale
TIPS	transjugular intrahepatic portosystemic shunt		vasc	vascular
			VATER	vertebral anomalies, anal atresia, tracheoesophageal fistula, esophageal atresia, radial dysplasia
TKR	total knee replacement			
TLC	total lung capacity/compliance		VC	vital capacity; vocal cord
Tm	maximal tubular excretory capacity (of kidney)		VCO$_2$	carbon dioxide consumption per unit time
			V$_d$	volume of distribution
TM	temporomandibular		Vd$_{ss}$	volume of distribution in a steady state
TMEP	telangiectasia macularis eruptiva perstans		vent	ventilation
			VFIB	ventricular fibrillation
TMJ	temporomandibular joint		VFP	ventricular filling pressure
TMP/SMX	trimethoprim/sulfamethoxazole		VIPoma	vasoactive intestinal peptide-secreting tumors
TN	trigeminal neuralgia			
TNF	tumor necrosis factor			
TNM	tumor, nodes, and metastasis		vit	vitamin
TOF	train-of-4; tetralogy of Fallot		VLBW	very low birth weight

VLDL	very low density lipoprotein		**W**	
VM-26	teniposide			
VMA	vanillylmandelic acid		w/	with
VO_2	oxygen consumption per unit time		w/o	without
vol	volume		WBC	white blood cell
VP-16	etoposide		wk	week(s)
VPA	valproic acid		WNL	within normal limits
VR	venous return		WPW	Wolff-Parkinson-White syndrome
VS	vital signs		wt	weight
vs.	versus			
VSD	ventricular septal defect		**XYZ**	
VSM	vascular smooth muscle			
VTach	ventricular tachycardia		Xe	xenon
VUR	vesicoureteral reflux		XS	excessive
VVB	venovenous bypass		y	year(s)
VVI	ventricular inhibited			
vWF	von Willebrand factor			

SECTION I

DISEASES

ABRUPTIO PLACENTAE

Charles P. Gibbs, M.D.

RISK

• People within USA: ~1% of the 4 million pregnancies/y
• Race with highest prevalence: ?
• Increased prevalence with cocaine use, trauma, increased age and parity, smoking, premature rupture of membranes, and prior abruption

PERIOPERATIVE RISKS

• Maternal: Antepartum and postpartum hemorrhage; DIC
• Fetal: Hypoxia due to maternal hypotension and/or decreased area for placental exchange

WORRY ABOUT

• Concealed hemorrhage behind the placenta that does not manifest as vaginal bleeding—may be considerable
• Fetal distress

• Postpartum hemorrhage refractory to usual oxytocic agents
• Need for cesarean hysterectomy

OVERVIEW

• Along with placenta previa, a major cause of antepartum hemorrhage and maternal mortality
• Perinatal mortality also high: 30–40%
• Abruptio placentae is the most common cause of DIC in pregnant patients; 20% with clinically significant abruption develop clotting defects
  – DIC probably due to release of thromboplastin by damaged tissues at abruption site
  – Postpartum hemorrhage correlates directly with severity of coagulopathy
  – Blood and clot in muscle fibers may inhibit ability of uterus to contract, leading to more blood loss

ICD-9-CM Code: 641.2

ETIOLOGY

• Etiology unknown
• Htn; smoking, cocaine use, trauma, increased age and parity, premature rupture of membranes, and history of previous abruption are predisposing factors

USUAL TREATMENT

• Maintenance of volume status and fetal surveillance
• If fetus premature and hemorrhage not great, careful observation would be appropriate to allow for fetal growth
• If at term and volume status OK, labor with vaginal delivery optimal
• If hemorrhage continues and/or fetal distress occurs, C-section is necessary

ASSESSMENT POINTS

SYSTEM	EFFECT	ASSESSMENT BY HX	PE	TEST
CV	Hemorrhage	Vaginal bleeding and abdominal pain	Vaginal bleeding and firm, tender uterus; hypotension, tachycardia, low CVP and wedge pressures, decreased UO	Hematocrit
HEME	Hypovolemia Acute anemia	Bleeding diathesis	Hypotension, tachycardia, bleeding from puncture sites, easy bruisability	Hgb, Hct, clotting evaluation that includes platelets, fibrinogen, and FSP
RENAL	Oliguria and/or acute renal failure	UO	Signs of hypovolemia	Urinalysis to include specific gravity and sodium excretion, possibly in addition to central hemodynamic monitoring values
UTERUS/ VAGINA	Abruption Hemorrhage	Painful vaginal bleeding	Tender, firm uterus; vaginal bleeding may be < CV signs and symptoms, indicating concealed hemorrhage	Hct and hemodynamic monitoring values
FETUS	Fetal distress and/or demise	Presence or absence of fetal movement	Fetal movement, heart rate	Electronic fetal monitoring

Key Reference: Mayer DC, Spielman FJ: Antepartum and postpartum hemorrhage. *In* Chestnut DH (ed): Obstetric Anesthesia: Principles and Practice, 2nd ed. St. Louis, Mosby, 1999, pp 725–748.

PERIOPERATIVE IMPLICATIONS—FOR LABOR AND VAGINAL DELIVERY

Preinduction/Induction/Maintenance

• Optimize CV and fetal status and evaluate coag system
• Epidural analgesia appropriate if volume status can be maintained and if hemorrhage controllable
• Technique not different from that for normal labor and vaginal delivery except that the smallest effective doses should be utilized; combined spinal/epidural with narcotics and local anesthetic may be useful
• Electronic fetal monitoring essential
• CV monitoring appropriate for volume and bleeding status

PERIOPERATIVE IMPLICATIONS—FOR CESAREAN SECTION

• Optimization of CV and fetal status, usually by means of appropriate volume replacement

Monitoring

• All cases will require electronic fetal monitoring
• UO

• Hct and clotting studies as above
• Consider CVP and/or PA catheter depending upon severity of hemorrhage; decreased UO not responsive to simple fluid challenges

General Anesthesia

Preinduction/Induction: Probably required for massive hemorrhage and/or acute fetal distress
• Aspiration prophylaxis
• Rapid-sequence induction with cricoid pressure
• Consider ketamine 1 mg/kg and large-bore lines
Maintenance: Watch for continued hemorrhage after delivery of infant. Uterus may not respond to usual tocolytic agents.
• Oxytocin 20–40 mU in 1 L of balanced salt solution
• Methergine 0.2 mg IM; *not* in the presence of Htn
• Prostaglandin $F_{2\alpha}$ 250 μg IM or intramyometrial
• Hypogastric artery ligation
• Cesarean hysterectomy
Extubation: Awake extubation required

Regional Anesthesia

In the absence of severe hemorrhage and/or acute fetal distress
• Aspiration prophylaxis

• Optimize volume status
• Epidural preferred over spinal because can raise level *slowly*
• Treat hypotension early and vigorously
• Watch for continuing uterine hemorrhage

Postoperative Period

• Patient needs to be in an appropriately staffed and equipped recovery/SICU area
• Be alert for continuing uterine hemorrhage and/or development of coagulopathy
• Continue intraoperative monitoring

ANTICIPATED PROBLEMS/CONCERNS

• Amount of bleeding may be considerably greater than what is evident per vagina. A significant amount of blood can be trapped behind the abrupted placenta.
• Be alert to the need for immediate C-section for fetal distress and/or dramatic increase in hemorrhage
• Best therapy for DIC is removal of the placenta by C-section or vaginal delivery
• Hemorrhage may continue post partum from an atonic uterus that is refractory to the usual oxytocic agents
• C-section hysterectomy may be necessary—may be accompanied by large blood loss

ACHONDROPLASIA, DWARFISM
Sandra V. Lowe, M.D.

RISK

- People within USA: 1 million
- 28/1 million in Northern Ireland
- 1:26,000 live births
- Most common type of dwarfism

PERIOPERATIVE RISKS

- Foramen magnum and cervical spine stenosis. Small rib cage, abnormal spinal curvatures may impair respiratory function.
- Persistent thoracolumbar kyphosis can compress the spinal cord

WORRY ABOUT

- Paresthesia or paraplegia
- Cauda equina syndrome
- Small intervertebral foramina can cause compression of individual nerve root
- Central apnea
- Cervicomedullary compression

OVERVIEW

- Results from failure in development and premature fusion of bones, which ossify in cartilage. Short arms and legs, trident hands, prominent frontal region with bridge of nose depression.
- Small, flat chest; lumbar lordosis. Vertebrae of skull base fuse prematurely; foramen magnum is small and funnel-shaped.
- Lateral diameter of spinal cord is narrowed
- Compression of neural tissue by bone can occur at three levels: foramen magnum, thoracolumbar, and lumbar spine
- Trunk length, intelligence, and life span are normal
- Mean adult height is 52 inches in males, 48 inches in females
- Mean adult weight is 120 lbs (55 kg) for males and 100 lbs (45 kg) for females
- Obesity is often present in both sexes

ICD-9-CM Code: 756.4

ETIOLOGY

- Autosomal dominant skeletal dysplasia primarily of endochondral bone
- >80% are new mutations: children born to parents of average height
- Achondroplastic parent has 50% chance of an affected child
- Both achondroplastic parents have 75% penetrance
- Homozygous form is usually fatal within first few weeks of life from respiratory insufficiency
- A change in the genetic information for fibroblast growth factor receptor 3 has been identified
- Spontaneous mutation of X chromosome linked to advanced paternal age (>37 y)

USUAL TREATMENT

- Myringotomy and tube placement, suboccipital craniectomy, various orthopedic procedures, laminectomy, ventricular-peritoneal shunts, C-section, tracheostomy, dental
- GH not effective

ASSESSMENT POINTS

SYSTEM	EFFECT	ASSESSMENT BY HX	PE	TEST
HEENT	Choanal stenosis Tongue thrust Prominent forehead and mandible Flattened midface with saddle nose Hearing loss from chronic otitis media Long narrow mouth with high-arched palate	Apnea with cyanotic spells Speech problems	Nasopharyngoscopy Limited head extension	Flexion/extension neck films
CV	Pulmonary artery hyperplasia Right ventricular hypertrophy RV strain			ECG CXR ECHO
RESP	Restrictive disease from constrictive thoracic cage Encroachment of upper airways Hypoxemia, hypercapnia	Apnea with cyanotic spells Loud snoring Recurrent pneumonia Cyanotic episodes/apnea		ECG ABGs
GI	Obesity	Reflux symptoms		
ENDO	Rule out other causes for growth failure			Growth hormone assay
CNS	Hyperreflexia, sustained clonus Hypertonia, paresis, asymmetry of movement or strength, abnormal plantar response Obstructive sleep apnea	Pyramidal signs Paresis Snoring, restless sleep Enuresis Daytime somnolence	Increased lateral ventricular size Increased extracerebral CSF Small foramen magnum Craniocervical stenosis Absent posterior subarachnoid space	Axial head CT SSEPs Polysomnography
PNS	Atropine fever	Increased sweating		
MS	Decrease in overall limb length Hyperlordosis Rhizomelia Kyphoscoliosis Tibial bowing		Kyphosis of thoracolumbar spine Proximal segments of limbs shorter than distal segments	Bone scan Bone x-ray

Key Reference: Berkowitz I, Raja S, Bender K, Kopits S: Dwarfs: pathophysiology and anesthetic implications. Anesthesiology 1990; 73:739–759.

PERIOPERATIVE IMPLICATIONS

Preoperative Preparation

- Consider metoclopramide/ranitidine in obesity
- Assess respiratory, CV, CNS status
- Assess airway and assume C-spine stenosis

Monitoring

- Difficult IV access
- Respiratory status may require arterial line
- SSEP for spinal cord procedures

Airway

- Difficult mask fit
- No guidelines for endotracheal tube size and length
- Difficult direct laryngoscopy
- Avoid hyperextension or hyperflexion
- Consider awake fiberoptic intubation
- Laryngeal mask airway

Induction

- General anesthesia with controlled airway
- Conduction anesthesia may cause neurologic impairment

Maintenance

- Controlled ventilation
- Consider SSEP in spinal surgery

Postoperative Period

- Respiratory insufficiency
- Pain control
- ICU monitoring

ANTICIPATED PROBLEMS/CONCERNS

- Increased incidence of SIDS (3%)
- Postop ventilation
- Neurologic impairment

ACIDOSIS, LACTIC/METABOLIC

Alan W. Grogono, M.D.

RISK

- Incidence requiring surgery in USA: unknown
- Gender/race predilection: unknown

PERIOPERATIVE RISKS

- Contributes to cardiovascular instability
- Inhibits local anesthetic solution uptake
- Diminishes effect of morphine and meperidine by decreasing availability of lipophilic, uncharged base
- ↑ Extracellular potassium

WORRY ABOUT

- ↓ Effect of vasopressors, inotropes, and vasodilators
- ↓ Oxygen uptake in lung by ↓ affinity for hemoglobin

OVERVIEW

- All body acids are "metabolic" except CO_2
- A pH that is more acidic than appropriate for PCO_2
- Cell membranes enclose 70% of body water; transfer of respiratory acid (CO_2) is rapid, but transfer of polar, ionized substances (e.g., metabolic acids) is slow
- Extracellular [H^+], 40 nmol/L, pH 7.4 is one quarter of the intracellular 160 nmol/L, pH 6.8; this gradient favors H^+ elimination from cell; counterbalanced by intracellular potential of − 60 mV, which attracts H^+ into cell

ICD-9-CM Codes: 276.2 (Acidosis; metabolic, mixed, or lactic); 276.4 (Mixed acid-base disorder); 250.1 (Diabetic ketoacidosis)

ETIOLOGY

- Accumulation of nonrespirable acids (e.g., lactic, pyruvic, ketoacids) at a rate too great for correction by renal elimination or hepatic metabolism
- Use of normal salt solution for long operative procedures (as opposed to a lactated Ringer's or similar solutions)

USUAL TREATMENT

- Treat the underlying disease because neutralizing metabolic acid does not cure diabetes, ischemia, etc.
- Bicarbonate therapy (e.g., 1 mEq/L) may be indicated during resuscitation or with some other cause of CV instability

ASSESSMENT POINTS

Measurement: Several techniques have been used to estimate a metabolic abnormality, e.g., the *standard pH* and the *standard bicarbonate,* both measured at normal body temperature and $PCO_2 = 40$ mmHg; today, two techniques are in widespread use.

Standard Base Excess (SBE): SBE is normally 0; blood base (total base) is about 48 mmol/L, depending mostly on Hgb concentration; changes are termed *excess* or *deficit.* *"This patient has an SBE of minus 10"* means *"this patient has a metabolic acid excess (acidosis) of plus 10 mEq/L."* SBE estimates amount of treatment required to fully neutralize metabolic acidosis (or alkalosis).

Bicarbonate: In acid-base determinations the concentration (in mEq/L) of the bicarbonate ion (HCO_3^-) is a calculated value derived from PCO_2 and pH. Both respiratory and metabolic components affect bicarbonate level; it cannot, therefore, be an ideal measure of either. In practice, changes in bicarbonate ion concentration may be used as a rough guide to metabolic change.

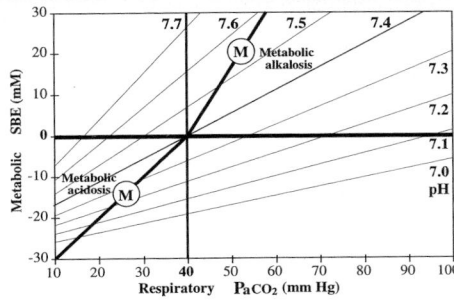

Characteristic Compensation: The figure illustrates that metabolic disturbances are usually accompanied by a characteristic degree of respiratory compensation. In practice, the pH lies approximately halfway between no respiratory compensation ($PCO_2 = 40$ mmHg) and complete compensation (pH = 7.4).

Treatable Volume: Extracellular fluid is 20% of body weight (e.g., 14 L). For therapy, treatable space is calculated as 30% (e.g., 21 L) because some equilibration occurs between intra- and extracellular fluid; treatable volume, therefore, tends to appear to be somewhat greater. In addition, further change may occur during the period of therapy, because the body may be either correcting the abnormality or making it worse.

Bicarbonate Therapy: This may be indicated when metabolic acidosis accompanies difficulty in resuscitating an individual or in maintaining cardiovascular stability. A typical dose of bicarbonate is 1 mEq/kg of body weight followed by repeated blood gas analysis. Bicarbonate's effect can be anticipated by calculating the dose that would be required for complete correction: **dose (mEq) = 0.3 × wt (kg) × SBE (mEq/L).** This dose would return the metabolic disturbance to about 0. This full dose is rarely recommended. It is customary either to give a small standard dose (1 mEq/L) and re-evaluate or to give about half the calculated dose and then expect about half the effect.

Key References: Schlichtig R, Grogono AW, Severinghaus JW: Current status of acid-based quantitation in physiology and medicine. Anesthesiol Clin North Am 1998; 16:211–233; Acid-base teaching Website: Grogono AW: Available at http://www.acid-base.com

PERIOPERATIVE IMPLICATIONS

- Correction of acid-base balance becomes more critical in patients with compromised cardiovascular stability:
  - In myocardial ischemia
  - Following cardiopulmonary bypass
  - Following any prolonged cardiac arrest
- Metabolic acidosis may also be a compensatory mechanism for chronic hyperventilation (e.g., in hyperventilation syndrome) or an adaptive response to high-altitude exposure for many days. This compensatory metabolic response rarely requires therapy.

ANTICIPATED PROBLEMS/CONCERNS

- Caution when administering bicarbonate: give only when clinically required, and then give small dose
- Bicarbonate initially injected into plasma volume (3 L) instead of into the calculated treatable space (21 L)
- Bicarbonate converted to CO_2 and has to be eliminated; each 100 mEq yields ~ 2.24 L of CO_2, which has to be exhaled (~ 10 min of normal production)
- CO_2 enters cells freely, unlike bicarbonate ions that have been administered

- Bicarbonate ions are accompanied by sodium ions, which increase osmolality of extracellular fluid; with other Rx, such as IV glucose, hyperosmolality may cause coma; in neonates, rapid bicarbonate infusion may distort vascular structures and result in intracranial hemorrhage
- After recovery, when the body has dealt with metabolic acidosis, bicarbonate Rx leaves residual metabolic alkalosis, hypernatremia, and hyperosmolality

ACROMEGALY

Russell T. Wall III, M.D.

RISK

• People within USA:
– Prevalence is 40/million; incidence is 3/million/y
– Occurs with equal frequency in men and women and most frequently in 4th and 5th decades of life

PERIOPERATIVE RISKS

• Common conditions increasing perioperative risk include airway abnormalities, cardiovascular dysfunction (Htn), respiratory impairment (obstructive sleep apnea), endocrine abnormalities (hyperglycemia)

WORRY ABOUT

• Difficulty in or inability to ventilate/intubate
• Extent of cardiovascular disease
• Postop airway obstruction

OVERVIEW

• Acromegaly is an endocrinopathy resulting from excess secretion of growth hormone, usually from pituitary gland, characterized by enlargement of extremities of skeleton (nose, jaw, fingers, toes)

ICD-9-CM Code: 253.0

ETIOLOGY

• >99% of cases result from primary pituitary adenoma

USUAL TREATMENT

• Surgery—primary therapy
– Transsphenoidal pituitary microsurgery vs. transcranial; transsphenoidal more common, with less morbidity. Smaller tumors (<10 mm diameter) yield probable cure.
• Pituitary radiation—reserved for persistent postsurgical disease
• Medical—adjunctive therapy or for nonsurgical candidates
– Dopamine agonists—bromocriptine
– Somatostatin analogue—octreotide

ASSESSMENT POINTS

SYSTEM	EFFECT	ASSESSMENT BY HX	PE	TEST
HEENT	Bone and soft tissue overgrowth of head and neck	TMJ arthritis Hoarseness	Enlarged frontal, nasal bones Macroglossia Prognathism Vocal cord thickening Subglottic narrowing	Indirect laryngoscopy Lateral neck x-rays CT of neck
CV	PVD LV dysfunction (?cardiomyopathy)	Htn CHF Dysrhythmias	Htn CHF Dysrhythmias Cardiomegaly	CXR ECG ECHO
RESP	Airway soft tissue overgrowth	Obstructive sleep apnea	Kyphoscoliosis	PFTs (if indicated)
RENAL	↑ (GI) Ca^{2+} absorption ↑ Intravascular volume	Urolithiasis	↑ Total body Na^+, plasma vol	
ENDO	↑ BMR Hyperprolactinemia Hyperthyroidism (3–7%) Glucose intolerance (30–45%) (10–20% overt DM) Hypertriglyceridemia (20–45%)	Heat intolerance ↓ Libido, impotence Menstrual abnormalities	Hyperhidrosis Goiter	To diagnose acromegaly: ↑ 24 h GH levels ↑ serum IGF I Oral glucose tolerance test (GH levels do not ↓) Thyroid function Glucose
CNS	Pituitary mass effect	Hypersomnolence Visual field defects		CT MRI
PNS	Carpal tunnel syndrome	Paresthesias	Median nerve compression	EMG, NCVs
MS	Bone and soft tissue overgrowth Osteoporosis Myopathy	Arthralgias/arthritis (knees, hips, shoulders, LS spine) Fatigue, weakness	Enlarged hands and feet Muscle weakness	X-rays

Key Reference: Schmitt H, Buchfelder M, Radespiel-Troger M, Fahlbusch R: Difficult intubation in acromegalic patients: incidence and predictability. Anesthesiology 2000; 93:110–114.

PERIOPERATIVE IMPLICATIONS

Preoperative Preparation
• Optimize hemodynamics—BP control, no CHF

Monitoring
• Pulse oximeter may be difficult to fit (large fingers, toes); if A-line, brachial or femoral preferable

Airway
• Large masks, airways, blades available
• Consider awake fiberoptic endotracheal intubation

Induction
• If GA, anticipate airway obstruction

Maintenance
• For transsphenoidal approach—surgical use of cocaine
• If preop pneumoencephalography, do not use nitrous oxide

Extubation
• Anticipate airway obstruction

Adjuvants
• If myopathy, cautious use of muscle relaxants
• If sleep apnea, cautious use of narcotics

• If peripheral neuropathy, document prior to regional

Postoperative Period
• Diabetes insipidus <5% of patients
• CSF rhinorrhea <5% of patients
• Anterior pituitary insufficiency (ACTH, TSH, gonadotropins)
• Meningitis, sinusitis, hematoma, cranial nerve palsy <1% each

ANTICIPATED PROBLEMS/CONCERNS

• Airway management
• Hemodynamic stability

ACUTE RESPIRATORY DISTRESS SYNDROME (ARDS)

Brian K. Gehlbach, M.D.
Jesse B. Hall, M.D.

RISK

- Risk as high as 75 per 100,000 population/y. Many predisposing conditions occur in perioperative setting (e.g., aspiration, hemorrhagic shock, sepsis); acute lung injury as high as 30–40%.
- Racial predominance: none
- Mortality improving to 30% overall but strongly influenced by associated conditions (e.g., higher when associated with sepsis, liver disease, and advanced age; lower with drug overdose or other easily reversed conditions)

PERIOPERATIVE RISKS

- Profound hypoxemia following any ↓ in cardiac output (intraoperative fluid shift, ↑ PEEP, myocardial depression) due to mixed venous O_2 desaturation in presence of large intrapulmonary shunt
- ↑ FIO_2 requirements and worsened shunt due to dependent lung atelectasis, large intraoperative fluid requirements

WORRY ABOUT

- Inability of standard operating room ventilators to deliver minute ventilation and inspiratory pressures often required
- Maintaining required PEEP during manual bag ventilation and patient transport
- Minimizing fluid to avoid edemagenesis on one hand, and inadequate cardiac output, and oxygen delivery, on the other

OVERVIEW

- Defined as acute onset of lung dysfunction with Pao_2/FIO_2 ≤ 200 mmHg (regardless of PEEP level), bilateral infiltrates on CXR, PCWP ≤ 18 when measured, or no clinical evidence of left atrial Htn
- Precipitants include pneumonia, sepsis, aspiration, hypertransfusion during resuscitation from shock, pancreatitis, trauma (fat embolism), opiate or cocaine overdose, CNS injury, air embolism, CPB
- Differentiated from focal pulmonary processes (e.g., lobar pneumonia) because standard Rx for ARDS (e.g., PEEP) may worsen gas exchange in focal disease
- Clinically useful to distinguish two phases: exudative (first 7–10 days) and proliferative (10 days to several weeks). Exudative phase characterized by pulmonary capillary leak best treated with low tidal volumes to ↓ ventilator-associated lung injury, ↑ PEEP to reduce shunt, and fluid restriction (as permitted by CO and BP) to limit edemagenesis. Proliferative phase marked by progressive fibrosis causing ↑ dead space and high minute volume requirements; PEEP less helpful, but high FIO_2 requirements may persist.
- Most deaths are from sepsis or MSOF

ICD-9-CM Code: 518.81 (With respiratory failure)

ETIOLOGY

- Direct (e.g., aspiration) and indirect (e.g., sepsis) lung injury cause endothelial and epithelial cell injury leading to ↑ microvascular permeability and formation of protein-rich exudate and hyaline membranes. Progression to proliferative phase is marked by fibrosing alveolitis and increased risk of death.

- Mechanical ventilation may worsen lung injury through alveolar distention and shear forces from cyclic opening and closing of collapsed alveoli

USUAL TREATMENT

- Respiratory: NIH trial demonstrated lower mortality in patients with lower TVs. Aim for plateau pressure ≤ 30 cm H_2O through use of lower TVs (6–8 ml/kg) and higher respiratory rates (watch for autoPEEP), and accept ↑ CO_2 if respiratory acidosis is not extreme (e.g., pH ≥ 7.20). Apply PEEP to achieve O_2 saturation ≥ 90% on nontoxic FIO_2; higher levels of PEEP than mandated by gas exchange end points ("open-lung" approach) beneficial but not proven. Pressure-control ventilation helpful in achieving ventilator goals and may improve oxygenation in some patients. Prone positioning improves oxygenation in 2/3 of patients but must be weighed against surgical constraints.
- Circulatory: Seek least filling pressure that provides adequate CO and mixed venous oxygenation; inotropes and transfusion to Hct 30–35 may be helpful in patients with severe hypoxemia. ↓ O_2 consumption through fever reduction, sedation, and judicious use of paralytics. Proliferative phase may require ↑ filling pressures because of ↑ dead space.
- Diagnosis and Rx of underlying condition and prevention of complications (superinfection, barotrauma, GI bleeding, protein-calorie malnutrition, MSOF)

ASSESSMENT POINTS

SYSTEM	EFFECT	ASSESSMENT BY HX	PE	TEST
CV	↓ CO	Hypotension, hypoxemia, ↓ mental status, urine output	Cool extremities, narrow pulse pressure	PA catheter, MvO_2 sat, urine electrolytes
	Pulm Htn		↑ P_2, RV heave, peripheral edema	PA catheter, ECHO
RESP	Barotrauma	Hypotension, hypoxemia, ↑ Paw	Absent breath sounds, tracheal deviation	CXR, blood and sputum culture
	Pneumonia	Fever, ↑ WBC/bandemia, purulent tracheal aspirate	Focal rales, hyperdynamic circulation	Bronchoscopy
GI	Hemorrhage	↓ Hct	Melena, bloody NG output	Guaiac stool, esophagogastroduodenoscopy
GU	↓ Function	↓ CO, urine output Nephrotoxic drugs, multisystem organ failure		Cr Urine electrolytes
MS	Prolonged weakness	Pharmacologic paralysis High-dose steroids	Polyneuropathy, myopathy	Electromyography, muscle biopsy

Key References: Ware LB, Matthay MA: The acute respiratory distress syndrome. N Engl J Med 2000; 342:1334–1349.

PERIOPERATIVE IMPLICATIONS

Preoperative Preparation

- Re-evaluate least PEEP required to maintain adequate arterial saturation
- Have proper ventilator available in OR
- Correct hypovolemia, fluid overload
- Use PEEP valve for transport; consider use of mechanical ventilation during transport
- Meticulous attention to aseptic technique

Monitoring

- PA catheter, particularly in exudative phase, when fluid shifts produce marked hypoxemia
- TEE may be useful in estimating adequate cardiac filling and cardiac output

Airway

- Avoid suctioning, unnecessary ETT disconnection. Even transient loss of PEEP may result in lung derecruitment and severe hypoxemia that may take minutes to hours to correct.

Preinduction/Induction

- Expect worsening shunt with loss of hypoxemic pulmonary vasoconstriction and/or V/Q mismatch with ↑ FIO_2 requirements

Maintenance

- Attention to fluid management to avoid worsening pulmonary edema from excessive fluid administration, or inadequate CO and mixed venous O_2 sat from inadequate fluids
- Maintain adequate circulating hemoglobin

Postoperative Period

- Close monitoring of volume status, PEEP requirements
- Reduce FIO_2 to nontoxic levels as soon as possible

ANTICIPATED PROBLEMS/CONCERNS

- Maintaining adequate oxygenation on nontoxic FIO_2 requires attention to volume status
- Complications of mechanical ventilation (O_2 toxicity, barotrauma, ↓ CO, pneumonia)
- Superinfection, MSOF

ADDISON'S DISEASE

Stephen P. Fischer, M.D.

RISK

- People within USA: 1 per 100,000
- Race/gender predominance: none

PERIOPERATIVE RISKS

- Increased risk of circulatory collapse 2° to inability to respond to stress
- Postop instability may be greater than intraoperative

WORRY ABOUT

- Addisonian crisis
- ↓ Response to circulating catecholamines
- Severe hypotension with ↓ SVR and ↓ LV stroke index
- Cardiac conduction abnormalities, including hyperkalemic arrest
- Volume status/electrolyte imbalance

OVERVIEW

- Primary adrenal insufficiency with cortex destruction
- Glucocorticoid/mineralocorticoid deficiency (especially if bilateral)
- Perioperative stress increased with magnitude of surgery
- Dx by ACTH stimulation test
- Clinical Sx usually insidious over months
- Proper treatment should result in normal life expectancy if no associated diseases

ICD-9-CM Code: 255.4

ETIOLOGY

- Autoimmune destruction of adrenal cortex (80% of nonexogenous steroid-induced cases)
- Associated with Hashimoto's, TB, sepsis, adrenal hemorrhage (anticoagulants)
- Congenital adrenal hyperplasia (rare); autosomal recessive
- Associated with suppression of adrenocortical function due to exogenous steroids

USUAL TREATMENT

- Surgical excision of adrenal gland(s)
- Glucocorticoid/mineralocorticoid replacement

ASSESSMENT POINTS

SYSTEM	EFFECT	ASSESSMENT BY HX	PE	TEST
HEENT	Severe dental caries	Pain, loose teeth	Teeth for structural stability	
CV	Hypotension/hypovolemia Cardiopenia ↓ Response to catecholamines Arrhythmias if ↑ K+	Orthostatic Sx		BP change on standing CXR ECG, K+
RESP	Possible resp muscle weakness	Exercise tolerance	2-flight walk	
GI	Dehydration/hypovolemia Abdominal pain/cramping	Nausea/emesis/diarrhea Orthostatic Sx		Na+, Cl−, K+ BP change on standing
RENAL	Azotemia			BUN/Cr
ENDO	↓ Na+, ↓ Cl−, ↓ glucose, ↑ K+			Na+, Cl−, K+, glucose
HEME	Hemoconcentration Lymphocytosis/eosinophilia			CBC
CNS		Nervous/mental irritability		
MS	Muscle weakness Weight loss	Fatigue Anorexia	Strength (ability) to rise from chair without using hands	K+ Albumin

Key Reference: Roizen MF: *In* Miller RD (ed): Anesthesia, 4th ed. New York, Churchill Livingstone, 2000, pp 918–924.

PERIOPERATIVE IMPLICATIONS

Preoperative Preparation

- Correct hypovolemia, hyperkalemia, hyponatremia, hypoglycemia
- Stress steroid coverage: up to 300 mg/d hydrocortisone/70 kg body wt (usual 100 mg/d)
- For mineralocorticoid treatment: 0.05–0.1 mg PO fludrocortisone
- Benzodiazepine premed OK

Monitoring

- Consider arterial and pulmonary artery catheterization if cardiac filling pressures indicated/major surgery

Airway

- No change from usual

Induction

- No specific anesthesia regimen superior

Maintenance

- May not see changes in HR despite ↓ SVR
- Check electrolytes, glucose intraoperatively

Extubation

- Prolonged emergence possible

Adjuvants

- Avoid etomidate: causes adrenal suppression
- Myocardial sensitivity to drugs (narcotics/barbiturates)
- Muscle weakness/wt loss may require a reduced muscle relaxant dose

Postoperative Period

- CXR for pneumothorax if adrenalectomy: up to 20% postop
- ↑ Pancreatitis with left adrenalectomy
- Perioperative steroids may ↓ wound healing, ↑ infections, ↑ stress ulcers, ↑ glucose intolerance, ↑ BP
- Postop stress greater than intraop

ANTICIPATED PROBLEMS/CONCERNS

- Addisonian crisis/circulatory collapse both intra- and postop. Consider ICU observation postop.
- Cardiac arrhythmias with hyperkalemia

ADRENAL INSUFFICIENCY, ACUTE OR SECONDARY

Charles B. Hantler, M.D.

RISK

- Risk of adrenal insufficiency 1/1000–1/10,000 (if steroids used in prior year)
- With steroids >20 mg/d (cortisol equivalent), >7–14 days within 1 y (Large variability in patient response to dose duration and timing of prior steroid use)
- Clinical signs worse with stress, such as trauma, surgery, or infection

PERIOPERATIVE RISKS

- Increases cardiovascular instability, fever, CHF, electrolyte abnormalities
- High cardiac output failure, or low-output state (hypovolemia) with signs of tissue hypoperfusion
- Often evidence of systemic vasodilation with decreased reactivity to vasopressors

WORRY ABOUT

- GI; N/V; dehydration and risk of aspiration
- Anemia, neutropenia with androgen deficiency: rare
- CV response; ↓ SVR, ? cardiac reserve, and ↓ vascular responsiveness to maintain perfusion pressure; steroids necessary for blood vessel responsiveness to catecholamines
- Hyperkalemia with or without hyponatremia (usually aldosterone deficiency); hypoglycemia, acidosis, hypercalcemia, and anemia; cardiac conduction abnormalities

OVERVIEW

- Adrenal insufficiency due to exogenous steroid administration leads to inadequate production of glucocorticoids (cortisol), mineralocorticoids (aldosterone), and androgens
- Primary adrenal insufficiency; Addison's disease, infectious, autoimmune, trauma, and metastatic disease
- May present without symptoms until stress
- Chronic adrenal insufficiency from use of steroids in prior year may manifest as weakness, fatigue, nausea, emesis, weight loss, and a variety of psychiatric disturbances
- Inadequate mineralocorticoid production can cause hyperkalemia, hyponatremia, and metabolic acidosis, with or without signs of dehydration
- Inadequate glucocorticoid production may cause signs of hemodynamic instability (hypotension) during stress
- Abdominal trauma and/or sepsis may cause signs of adrenal corticoid insufficiency, which resolve within hours of steroid administration
- Anecdotal evidence exists of restoration of circulatory function (e.g., normalization of cardiac output and SVR) following steroid administration in cases of trauma, and of possible synthetic glucocorticoid–induced adrenal suppression that resolved with the intraoperative administration of synthetic glucocorticoid

ICD-9-CM Code: 255.4

See also Addison's Disease in Diseases section

ETIOLOGY

- Inadequate replacement of synthetic glucocorticoids
- Renin deficiency (hypoaldosterone) rare

USUAL THERAPY

- Normal conditions: 12–15 mg/m² of hydrocortisone replacement daily
- Minor stress (minor surgery): 50–75 mg or about 2× normal production for 1 or 2 days postoperatively
- Major stress (major trauma, major surgery): 150–200 mg of hydrocortisone per day 2 or 3 days postoperatively, followed by taper to usual dose
- Aldosterone deficiency (manifested by abnormalities in Na⁺/K⁺ or dehydration): fludrocortisone (Florinef), 50–200 μg/d

ASSESSMENT POINTS

SYSTEM	EFFECT	ASSESSMENT BY HX	PE	TEST
CV	Dehydration Hypotension High-output failure	Postural symptoms Fatigue Wt loss, Hx of surgery on adrenals, pituitary	Low BP, postural drop Signs of dehydration	Hct(?), BUN/Cr, adrenal, ACTH stimulation, insulin tolerance, metyrapone test
RESP	CHF (high or low output)	DOE, SOB	S_3, rales	CXR
GI	Dehydration, nausea, emesis	Appetite Hx of emesis	See CV	Lytes
HEME	Anemia Neutropenia		Hyperpigmentation (excess corticotropin)	Hct WBC
CNS	Depression, confusion, psychosis			Reverses with replacement
MS	Weakness, potentiation of neuromuscular blockage			Nerve stimulator

Key Reference: Oelkers W: Adrenal insufficiency. N Engl J Med 1996; 335:1206–1212.

PERIOPERATIVE IMPLICATIONS

Preoperative Preparation
- Consider perioperative steroid coverage if benefits outweigh risks if high index of suspicion of adrenal depression (e.g., supraphysiologic doses of steroids for >1 wk within last year)
- Correct electrolyte abnormalities, hypoglycemia, and dehydration prior to elective surgery
- Fludrocortisone with resistant aldosterone (K⁺ and Na⁺) abnormalities; glucose for hypoglycemia

Monitoring
- ECG for signs of abnormal conduction (QRS duration, u waves)
- Consider CVP, PCWP, or TEE if fluid/electrolyte abnormalities
- Sodium, potassium, bicarbonate, and glucose

Airway
- None

Premedication/Induction
- Consider volume status with regard to hydration and choice of agents

Maintenance
- No hemodynamic instability: follow electrolytes and glucose as needed
- Hemodynamic instability (hypotension):
  – R/O other causes, then consider hydrocortisone hemisuccinate, 25–100 mg IV then 100 mg q 12–24 h for 2 or 3 days
  – Fluid resuscitation as needed

Extubation
- Possible potentiation of nondepolarizing muscle relaxants with use of high-dose steroids; ensure adequate muscle relaxant reversal

Adjuvants
- Glucose, fluids, careful monitoring of temperature to avoid hyperthermia

Postoperative Period
- Stress steroids poss required several days postop
- High steroid doses may be assoc with ↓ wound healing and immunosuppression with infection risk
- Consider prolonged steroid coverage if severe stress continues (e.g., severe trauma with multiple operations)
- Mineralocorticoid administration as needed; usually glucocorticoids have significant mineralocorticoid action

ANTICIPATED PROBLEMS/CONCERNS
- Severe resistant hypotension, hyperthermia, and CNS abnormalities, such as confusion, coma, lethargy, may occur intraoperatively or postoperatively and may be unpredictable
- Syndrome may occur in severely traumatized patients without history of steroid use, with clinical picture of sepsis and associated abnormalities in adrenal function; Rx is lifesaving

ALCOHOL ABUSE

Scott Metzger, M.D.

RISK

- People within USA: 15 million
- Alcoholic physicians in USA: 22,000
- Third leading cause of death and disability
- Male gender and family Hx major risk factors

PERIOPERATIVE RISKS

- Severe malnutrition as significant as ethanol-induced end-organ injury
- Risk of Htn, stroke, diabetes, GI disease
- Liver most severely affected organ
- Dilated cardiomyopathy
- Withdrawal symptoms can themselves be life-threatening

WORRY ABOUT

- Concomitant use of amphetamines, cocaine, diazepam
- Chronic smoking and COPD
- Vasopressor effect of ETOH or its withdrawal may cause Htn
- Avoid all medications with ETOH, including skin prep solutions
- Withdrawal symptoms

OVERVIEW

- Large number of individuals have the disease characterized by addiction (compulsion and craving despite consequences) to alcohol
- Clinical syndromes related to direct effect of ETOH and secondary adaptive response to excess ETOH exposure
- ETOH rapidly absorbed and metabolized

- Hepatic dysfunction usually takes 10–15 y to develop
- Cirrhosis may develop after 1 or more acute episodes

ICD-9-CM Code: 303.0 (Acute)

ETIOLOGY

- Unknown: has environmental, genetic, and psychosocial components

USUAL TREATMENT

- Recovery involves almost all of the following:
  - Disulfiram (Antabuse): acetaldehyde dehydrogenase inhibitor
  - Alcoholics Anonymous
  - Psychiatric counseling

ASSESSMENT POINTS

SYSTEM	EFFECT	ASSESSMENT BY HX	PE	TEST
CV	Cardiomyopathy Arrhythmias Hypertension	Orthopnea, nocturnal urination, coughing, and leg swelling	Dyspnea BP lying and standing HR	ECG, ECHO Electrolytes
GI	Erosive gastritis Hepatic cirrhosis Acute hepatitis	Hx of bleeding Easily bruised Anorexia, N/V	 Ascites, jaundice Hepatomegaly, "spider" angiomas	Upper endoscopy, stool guaiac LFTs LFTs
	Pancreatitis Fatty liver		Abd pain Abd pain, hepatomegaly	Serum amylase Mg^{2+}; K^+
ENDO	Gynecomastia, testicular atrophy, irregular menses			
HEME	Leukopenia, anemia, thrombocytopenia			CBC with differential
CNS	Wernicke's syndrome Korsakoff's syndrome Peripheral polyneuropathy Cerebellar degeneration	Amnesia, impaired reasoning	Sixth nerve palsy, ataxia CNS exam Distal numbness and paresthesias Unsteady gait	 MRI or CT scan

Key Reference: Lieber CS: Medical disorders of alcoholism. N Engl J Med 1995; 333:1058–1065.

PERIOPERATIVE IMPLICATIONS

Preoperative Preparation

- Gastric prophylaxis
- Blood ETOH and toxicology screen if indicated

Monitoring

- Routine
- Consider invasive monitors for severe cardiomyopathy and hepatic dysfunction

Airway

- Consider full stomach in acute intoxication

Preinduction/Induction

- Consider long-acting benzodiazepine or barbiturate
- Anesthetic doses increased in chronic disease
- Decreased dose in acute intoxication

- Rapid-sequence in acute intoxication
- Consider Rx of nutritional/metabolic deficiencies

Maintenance

- Requirements vary by age, general health, nutrition and hydration states, concomitant disease

Extubation

- Ensure return of airway reflexes

Postoperative Period

- Provide adequate analgesia in PACU
- Anxiety can worsen withdrawal symptoms
- Withdrawal syndrome may develop within 6–8 h; treat with IV ETOH, β-adrenergic agonist, α_2-adrenergic agonist, benzodiazepines, PO ETOH
- DTs develop in 5% of patients in withdrawal

- 10% mortality secondary to hypotension, arrhythmias; treat with diazepam, β-adrenergic agonist

Adjuvants

- Long-term consumption of ETOH impairs hepatic metabolism
- Short-term consumption inhibits drug metabolism
- Polyneuropathy a relative contraindication to regional anesthesia
- Consider clonidine patch perioperatively

ANTICIPATED PROBLEMS/CONCERNS

- Recognition and treatment of withdrawal important, as significant mortality occurs if inadequately treated

ALLERGY

Tetsuji Makita, M.D.
Jerrold H. Levy, M.D.

RISK

- 5% of adults in USA are allergic to one or more drugs
- The incidence of perioperative anaphylaxis is 1/4500, with a mortality of 6%
- Females > males (1.6:1)

PERIOPERATIVE RISKS

- Intensity of Sx variable: from an isolated cutaneous eruption to CV collapse and death
- CV, cutaneous, respiratory systems are mostly involved
- Increased morbidity and hospitalization time if intensive care required

WORRY ABOUT

- Patient's Hx: Knowledge of prior allergic event leads to avoiding drugs or other components involved
- Hypotension, bronchospasm, and swelling may become life-threatening events

OVERVIEW

- IgE anaphylaxis (type I immediate hypersensitivity reaction): Adverse response of host; mediated by antibodies: the antigen bridges with two IgE on the surface of basophils and mast cells; can be reproduced if foreign substance reinjected
- Anaphylactoid reaction or histamine release: Describes a clinically indistinguishable syndrome, probably involving similar mediators but not mediated by IgE antibody and not necessarily requiring previous exposure to the inciting substance, associated with vancomycin, benzylisoquilinium-derived muscle relaxants

ICD-9-CM Codes: 995.3 (Allergic reaction); 477.0–477.9 (Inhaled allergen)

See also Anaphylaxis in Diseases section

ETIOLOGY

- Clinical history of allergy or perianesthetic allergic reaction considered to put patient at increased risk for a reaction, from neuromuscular blocking agents, induction agents

USUAL TREATMENT

- "Preventive therapy" with corticosteroids and antihistamines is of unproven value
- Severe allergic therapy: Stop antigen; maintain the airway with 100% O_2 and intubate if necessary; discontinue all anesthetic drugs; volume expansion; epinephrine (5–10 μg IV boluses as starting doses and titrate upward); antihistamines; β_2-sympathomimetic if bronchospasm; phosphodiesterase inhibitors for RV dysfunction, airway evaluation prior to extubation; ICU observation

ASSESSMENT POINTS

SYSTEM	EFFECT	PE	TEST
CV	Hypotension Tachycardia, dysrhythmias Pulmonary hypertension Cardiac arrest	BP	ECG PA pressure
RESP	Dyspnea, sneezing Coughing, wheezing Laryngeal edema Fulminant pulmonary edema Acute respiratory failure	Chest exam	CXR PA catheter End-tidal CO_2 ABGs
DERM	Urticaria, flushing Perioral, periorbital edema	Skin exam	

Key Reference: Levy JH: Anaphylactic Reactions in Anesthesia and Intensive Care, 2nd ed. Boston, Butterworth-Heinemann, 1992.

PERIOPERATIVE IMPLICATIONS

Preoperative Preparation

- Prick tests, intradermal testing: Anesthetic drugs (muscle relaxant)
- Most of the allergic reactions are unexpected. In case of established allergy, those drugs or latex should be strictly avoided.

Monitoring

- Routine if major anaphylaxis occurs. Consider pulmonary and radial arterial catheterization to guide therapeutic interventions.

Airway

- None, except specific care for the asthmatic patient

Preinduction/Induction/Maintenance/Extubation

- Slow injection of drugs. Avoid histamine-releasing drugs in high-risk patients.

ANTICIPATED PROBLEMS/CONCERNS

- Consider for each patient who has a perioperative allergic reaction evaluation 1 mo after with skin testing, antigen-specific IgE level dosage (radioallergosorbent test, ELISA)
- Latex allergy incidence is increasing and Hx has to be evoked at the preanesthetic evaluation

AMNIOTIC FLUID EMBOLISM

P. Allan Klock, Jr., M.D.

- Prevalence: 0.8 to 5 cases/100,000 live births

PERIOPERATIVE RISKS

- Amniotic fluid embolism accounts for approximately 9% of maternal deaths in USA
- Mortality is approximately 86%

WORRY ABOUT

- Hypoxia
- Cardiopulmonary collapse
- Right heart failure
- DIC—occurs in nearly all survivors of the initial catastrophic event
- Hemorrhage—40% of amniotic fluid embolism–associated deaths are due to hemorrhage

OVERVIEW

- Amniotic fluid going to central circulation
- There are three necessary conditions:
  - Amniotomy (rent in the membranes)
  - Laceration of endocervical or uterine vessels
  - Pressure gradient (intrauterine pressure > CVP or uterine venous pressure)
- Although not a common disease of pregnancy amniotic fluid embolism has a significant impact on health care providers because it is usually fatal and often presents without warning

ICD-9-CM Code: 673.1

ETIOLOGY

- Postulated mechanism of action: Powerful contractions force amniotic fluid into the maternal circulation through a defect in the fetal membranes, placenta, or elsewhere
- Risk factors: Advanced maternal age; multiparity (88% of patients with amniotic fluid embolism are multiparas); meconium (present in 75% of cases); cervical laceration (present in 50% of cases); intrauterine fetal demise (present in 40% of cases); very strong, frequent, or "tetanic" contractions; sudden fetal expulsion; uterine rupture; chorioamnionitis; macrosomia

USUAL TREATMENT

- Treatment is usually supportive
- Case reports of successful treatment with cardiopulmonary bypass and thrombectomy
- Employ left uterine displacement to prevent aortocaval compression
- Stop oxytocin infusion if present
- Cardiopulmonary resuscitation (100% O_2 with PEEP)
- Pressors and inotropes will often be required
- Delivery of fetus as soon as is practical; may require operative or cesarean delivery
- Replacement of clotting factors if patient develops DIC

ASSESSMENT POINTS

SYSTEM	EFFECT	ASSESSMENT BY HX	PE	TEST
CV	Tachycardia Hypotension			HR BP
RESP	Hypoxia Pulmonary edema	Dyspnea	Tachypnea Cyanosis Frothy pink sputum	Pulse oximetry Aspirate blood from PA or renal artery Stain buffy coat for cells and mucin
GI		Nausea	Vomiting	
HEME	DIC		Excessive bleeding Thrombolysis (bleeding from IV sites)	PT, PTT, plt, fibrinogen, FSP
CNS		Anxiety	Convulsions Shivering Sweating	

Key Reference: Davies S: Amniotic fluid embolism: a review of the literature. Can J Anaesth 2001; 48:88–98.

PERIOPERATIVE IMPLICATIONS

- Usually this disease presents as sudden CV collapse

Preoperative Preparation

- Maximize maternal oxygen delivery
- Place several large-bore IVs
- Notify blood bank of anticipated coagulopathy and cross-match for several units of packed RBCs and FFP
- Consider preparing for cardiopulmonary bypass, if an option

Monitoring

- If amniotic fluid embolism is suspected, consider PA catheter to aspirate blood; hemodynamic management

Maintenance

- Usually resuscitative with support of breathing and circulation
- Case reports of use of CPB

Extubation

- If patient survives, keep intubated until stable

ANTICIPATED PROBLEMS/CONCERNS

- Not all sudden deaths during the peripartum period are due to amniotic fluid embolism. The pathologic diagnosis is quite specific (finding hair, mucin, or nucleated squamous cells in the maternal circulation), but its sensitivity is unknown.
- The emotional impact on caregivers can be tremendous. One should confirm the pathologic diagnosis and share the results of the postmortem examination with those who helped care for the deceased. While surgeons and anesthesiologists occasionally witness an intraoperative death, labor and delivery nurses are not accustomed to having their patients die. Psychological counseling may be helpful for those who have difficulty after the event.

AMYLOIDOSIS

Kenneth J. Holroyd, M.D.

RISK

- People within USA: 50,000
- Race with highest prevalence: unknown

PERIOPERATIVE RISKS

- Increased risk of perioperative renal failure, CHF; bleeding from coagulopathy
- Autonomic neuropathy

WORRY ABOUT

- Signs of CHF
- Decreasing urine output

OVERVIEW

- Extracellular deposition of amyloid type proteins
- Congo red stain of tissue reveals green birefringence in a polarizing microscope
- Associated end-stage renal, myocardial, and neuropathic disease
- Best diagnosed by subcutaneous abdominal fat pad aspirate or rectal biopsy

ICD-9-CM Code: 277.3

ETIOLOGY

- Both acquired and hereditary forms exist
- Major risk factors for acquired disease: multiple myeloma, chronic infectious or inflammatory disease (osteomyelitis, rheumatoid arthritis)
- Hereditary forms very rare

USUAL TREATMENT

- Acquired: treat underlying disease
- Hereditary: colchicine, liver transplantation

ASSESSMENT POINTS

SYSTEM	EFFECT	ASSESSMENT BY HX	PE	TEST
HEENT	Macroglossia Tracheal stenosis	Enlarged tongue Dyspnea	Macroglossia Stridor	CT scan Flow-volume loop
CV	Restrictive myopathy LV and RV dysfunction Conduction abnormalities	Exercise tolerance Dyspnea Syncope	S_3 Bradycardia	ECHO ECG
RESP	CHF Lung nodules	Cough Chest wall pain	Rales	CXR
GI	Autonomic dysfunction	Wt loss Diarrhea		Biopsy
HEME	Factor X deficiency	Bruising	Periorbital bruises	Factor X assay
RENAL	Decreased renal perfusion Nephrotic syndrome			BUN/Cr Urine
CNS	Autonomic neuropathy	Inability to sweat; hoarseness; early satiety; postural dizziness	Orthostasis	Biopsy

Key Reference: Noguchi T, Minami K, Iwagaki T, Takura H, Sata T, Shigematsu A: Anesthetic management of a patient with laryngeal amyloidosis. J Clin Anesth 1999; 11:339−341.

PERIOPERATIVE IMPLICATIONS

Preoperative Preparation

- Optimize treatment of heart failure
- Avoid dehydration (renal failure)

Monitoring

- Consider PA catheter for large fluid shift operations or patients with severe LV dysfunction

Airway

- Macroglossia or tracheal stenosis
- Increased risk of bleeding into airway from capillary fragility and possible coagulopathy

Preinduction/Induction

- May develop reduced CO and hypotension
- Coagulopathy may contraindicate regional anesthesia

Maintenance

- No agent or technique shown superior
- Maintain adequate urine output

Extubation

- Patient fully awake to minimize risk of reintubation
- Caution with nasal airway—may cause hemorrhage

Postoperative Period

- Close monitoring of CV and renal status
- Consider ICU setting for postop care

Adjuvants

- Avoid digoxin—not usually helpful in treating amyloid CHF, associated with increased arrhythmias

ANTICIPATED PROBLEMS/CONCERNS

- Difficult airway
- CHF
- Hypotension
- Renal failure

AMYOTROPHIC LATERAL SCLEROSIS (ALS)

Michelle Schlunt, M.D.
Daniel J. Cole, M.D.

RISK

- Annual incidence: 0.8–1.5/100,000
- Prevalence: 4–6:100,000
- Age (most common) at onset: 55–60 y
- Male:female incidence: 1.5:1
- Minimal racial/geographic variation: ↓ incidence African-Americans (?), ↑ prevalence in Guam and regions of Japan

PERIOPERATIVE RISKS

- Aspiration
- Respiratory failure
- Infection

WORRY ABOUT

- Hyperkalemia after succinylcholine
- Prolonged response to nondepolarizing muscle relaxants
- Respiratory failure postoperatively

OVERVIEW

- A degenerative process causing upper and lower motor neuron death with denervation and atrophy of corresponding muscle fibers.

The classic clinical signs include asymmetrical muscle weakness, hyperreflexia, fasciculations, and muscle atrophy. If the condition is limited to the motor cortex, disease is termed *primary lateral sclerosis;* with limitation to brainstem nuclei, *pseudobulbar palsy;* with limitation to spinal cord, *progressive muscular atrophy.* Typically, extraocular muscles, bowel/bladder sphincters, sensory system, movement coordination, and intellect remain intact. ALS may be associated with malignant tumors.

- Laboratory aids in diagnosis:
  - ↑ Serum creatinine kinase in ~$\frac{2}{3}$ of pts
  - Abnormal acetylcholine receptor antibody
  - ↓ Compound muscle action potential
  - EMG evidence of denervation with reinnervation
  - Abnormal evoked responses
  - Abnormalities on MRS, MRI, and CT
- Progressive course leading to death within 3–5 y (50% of cases)

ICD-9-CM Code: 335.20

ETIOLOGY

- Genetic predisposition in <5% of cases (autosomal dominant gene). Other hypotheses:
  - Autoimmune, apoptotic (programmed cell death), viral, and neurotoxic mechanisms (glutamate, calcium, free radicals)

USUAL TREATMENT

- Supportive care:
  - Psychological support, exercise, pharmacotherapy for spasticity and sialorrhea
    - Pyridostigmine sometimes ↑ strength
    - Tube feedings if difficulty swallowing
    - Chest physical therapy, bronchodilators, bilevel positive airway pressure or tracheostomy with mechanical ventilation
- Riluzole (Rilutek) is the only FDA-approved drug for the treatment of ALS; not curative but prolongs survival time; acts by inhibiting glutamate release; metabolized in the liver; may increase liver enzymes during Rx
- Many investigational pharmaceutical therapies in clinical trials. See <http://www.alsa.org/research/drugdev.cfm>

ASSESSMENT POINTS

SYSTEM	EFFECT	ASSESSMENT BY HX	PE	TEST
HEENT	Dysfunction of pharyngeal muscles, dysphagia, dysarthria, sialorrhea	Dysphagia, dysarthria, sialorrhea	Gag reflex	
CV	Vagal dysfunction		Tachycardia	
RESP	Respiratory impairment from muscle weakness and diaphragm paralysis; susceptible to infection and aspiration	Dyspnea, restlessness, fatigue, lethargy, apnea, regurgitation, cough, fever, sputum	↓ Breath sounds and excursion, wheezing	CXR (to rule out current infection) PFTs (optional) ABGs
GI	Poor nutrition	Caloric intake Infection		Serum albumin/transferrin Skin test anergy
ENDO	Abnormal glucose/Ca^{2+} metabolism, thyroid dysfunction, B$_{12}$ and hexosaminidase A deficiency, dysproteinemia, vasculitis, ganglioside antibodies			Hyperglycemia Hypercalcemia Fractures on x-ray
CNS	Motor cell loss in cortex, brainstem, spinal cord	Dysarthria, dysphagia, labile emotional expression, dementia (<5% of cases)		Abnormal evoked responses
MS	Loss of large myelinated fibers in ventral roots with abnormalities of the motor end-plate	Muscle weakness and atrophy	Spasticity Fasciculations Hyperreflexia	↑ Serum creatinine kinase, ↓ muscle action potential, denervation with evidence of reinnervation on EMG, abnormal evoked responses

Key Reference: Miller RG, Rosenberg JA, Gelinas DF, et al: Practice parameter: the care of the patient with amyotrophic lateral sclerosis (an evidence-based review)—report of the Quality Standards Subcommittee of the American Academy of Neurology. Neurology 1999; 52:1311–1323.

PERIOPERATIVE IMPLICATIONS

Preoperative Preparation
- Maximize respiratory status. Treat any superimposed respiratory condition.

Monitoring
- Routine

Airway
- Management of secretions

Induction
- Local or regional anesthesia if possible
- If general anesthetic necessary, avoid succinylcholine (hyperkalemic response) and expect an exaggerated response and response duration to nondepolarizing muscle relaxants
- May be susceptible to aspiration

Maintenance
- No technique shown to be superior (in theory, local or regional technique preferable)

Extubation
- Low risk for postop mechanical ventilation if peak inspiratory pressure >30 cm H$_2$O, vital capacity >1.5 L, and no concurrent problems
- Moderate risk for postop mechanical ventilation if peak inspiratory pressure 20–30 cm H$_2$O, vital capacity 1.0–1.5 L, or mild hypercarbia
- High risk for postop mechanical ventilation if peak inspiratory pressure <20 cm H$_2$O, vital capacity <1.0 L, hypercarbic, hypoxic, or a concurrent problem

Adjuvants
- Avoid succinylcholine (hyperkalemic response)
- Pyridostigmine to ↑ muscle strength

Postoperative Period
- Monitor for resp failure or complications
- Pain management may be critical for return of baseline motor function
- Glucose management
- Communication difficulties

ANTICIPATED PROBLEMS/CONCERNS

- Respiratory insufficiency with potential requirement for prolonged mechanical ventilation. Treat concurrent conditions (e.g., pneumonia) that may exacerbate respiratory status.
- Aspiration from weak pharyngeal muscles. Extubate when patient completely awake with full return of baseline muscle function.
- Possible deterioration of neurologic status postoperatively
- High incidence of hepatotoxicity and unknown anesthetic interactions of riluzole

ANAPHYLAXIS

Jonathan Moss, M.D., Ph.D.

RISK

- Approximately 1 in 5000 anesthetic procedures
- Females outnumber males 3:1.
- No prospective data to suggest an increased risk of generalized allergy, although Hx of atopy is overrepresented in several series of life-threatening anaphylaxis to anesthetic agents

PERIOPERATIVE RISKS

- Significant risks of life-threatening airway compromise, CV collapse, and bronchospasm—particularly severe in patients on β-blockers

WORRY ABOUT

- Patients with pre-existing ASCVD tolerate CV sequelae poorly
- Patients with Hx of allergy to anesthetics.
- Antibodies to muscle relaxants may persist for > 25 y

OVERVIEW

- The body's response to what is perceived to be a foreign substance
- Although itching, cutaneous manifestations, and a feeling of doom are present in the awake patient, CV collapse is the most common and serious presentation under general anesthesia
- Bronchospasm occurs in < 50% of life-threatening cases of anaphylaxis
- Usually occurs during induction of anesthesia and within 10 min of drug administration
- Often confused with anaphylactoid reactions (e.g., vancomycin) that involve chemically mediated histamine release. These are common, related to drug dose and speed of injection, blocked by H_1/H_2 antihistamines.

ICD-9-CM: 995.0

ETIOLOGY

- IgE binds to mast cells and causes a degranulation, releasing many vasoactive substances, including histamine. Although patients may not have been exposed to anesthetics, there may be common epitopes between cosmetics and myorelaxants.
- Risk factors for latex allergy include meningomyelocele and other congenital defects. Also allergy to figs, papayas, and avocados.
- Is most commonly associated with administration of muscle relaxants, particularly succinylcholine. Can be caused by all muscle relaxants, even those that do not release histamine chemically (e.g., rocuronium).
- The second most common cause appears to be latex allergy
- Rarely due to opiates or local anesthetics

USUAL TREATMENT

- IV fluids (put in large-bore IV), often to 7 L in adults
- Epinephrine even in the face of significant tachycardia
- O_2 and supportive measures
- Possible H_1 and H_2 antagonists

ASSESSMENT POINTS

SYSTEM	EFFECT	ASSESSMENT BY HX	PE	TEST
HEENT	Head and neck swelling and potential glottic edema	Will occur suddenly	Swelling	Clinically obvious
CV	↑ HR; ↓ BP and SVR; ↑ ectopy; change in PR interval; coronary vasospasm		Hypotension, tachycardia	ECG may reveal PVCs or change in P-R interval; CV collapse may ensue
RESP	Bronchospasm		Wheezing	↑ Peak insp pressure; ↓ O_2 saturation
SKIN	Urticaria or other cutaneous manifestations; generalized edema with fluid leakage		Body rash	Not needed CVP or PA pressures or TEE

Key Reference: Bouaziz H, Laxenaire M-C: Anaesthesia for the allergic patient. Curr Opin Anaesthesiol 1998; 11:339–344.

PERIOPERATIVE IMPLICATIONS

Monitoring

- It is important to distinguish from drug effects or mechanical problems
- CV collapse with or without associated bronchospasm or cutaneous manifestations during induction, but without evidence of mechanical problems, suggest anaphylaxis
- Prophylactic H_1 and H_2 antagonists may attenuate the severity, although not the incidence
- The airway may swell, making intubation very difficult

Induction

- Reactions usually occur during induction. Give antibiotics in the preop holding area rather than during induction.

Maintenance

- Perpetuation of reaction can occur, particularly if due to latex
- Significant cross-reactivity between myorelaxants (approaching 80%)
- Avoid all muscle relaxants if necessary to proceed with the operation

Extubation

- Stable from a cardiorespiratory viewpoint
- Assess for airway edema

Adjuvants

- Epinephrine is drug of choice in true anaphylaxis, even in the face of tachycardia

Postoperative Period

- Blood should be drawn for possible tryptase levels. Although histamine measurements during the acute event can assist in Dx, they can be difficult to perform. Tryptase can be drawn up to 2 h afterward and may be positive in anaphylaxis but is not elevated in chemically mediated reactions. Skin testing may be done several weeks after initial event to assess etiologic agent.

ANTICIPATED PROBLEMS/CONCERNS

- Advise patients exactly what drugs they have received

RISK

- 2000 new cases/y in USA
- 1.1 per million up to age 9 y
- Southeast Asia and South Africa have 10–20 × higher incidence
- Within USA, related to agricultural areas or petrochemical industry and chemical exposures

PERIOPERATIVE RISKS

- Infection
- Hemorrhage
- LV dysfunction due to high-output state and fluid overload

WORRY ABOUT

- Sepsis
- Co-existing congenital anomalies, especially renal and cardiac
- Concomitant GI and intracranial hemorrhage
- Difficulty cross-matching blood products after previous multiple transfusions

OVERVIEW

- Self-perpetuating disorder resulting in pancytopenia due to a congenital or acquired loss of hemopoietic pluripotent stem cells
- Fanconi anemia is congenital familial marrow hypoplasia associated with mental retardation, kidney, spleen, and skeletal hypoplasia
- Estren-Dameshek anemia is inherited marrow hypoplasia without physical abnormalities
- Pathophysiology: reduction or dysfunction of pluripotent stem cells or their microenvironment from toxic or immunologic causes
- Prognosis for long-term survival has ↑ to 40–75% in those treated with antilymphocyte serum and 60–80% in those treated with bone marrow transplantation (BMT)
- Two forms of drug-induced aplastic anemia possible:
  – Hypersensitivity: not related to dose or duration
  – "Reversible" reaction: often resolves with discontinuation; severity proportional to dosage

ICD-9-CM Code: 284.9

ETIOLOGY

- 50–75% of cases idiopathic
- Fanconi anemia demonstrates autosomal recessive inheritance with heterozygote frequency of 1 in 300,000–600,000 in USA
- Drug-induced: chloramphenicol, NSAIDs, antiepileptics, gold and sulfa group–containing compounds
- Environmental toxins including aromatic hydrocarbons (benzene, naphthalene, toluene), pesticides (DDT, indane), and radiation
- Infectious causes include hepatitis C, CMV, EBV, HIV, TB, and toxoplasmosis
- Sequelae of other processes such as pancreatitis, pregnancy, and lupus erythematosus

USUAL TREATMENT

- Patients <55 y are managed with HLA-matched BMT
- Patients >55 y or those unable to find HLA-matched donor receive immunosuppression and immunomodulation Rx including ATG, cyclosporine, steroids, androgens, and G-CSF

ASSESSMENT POINTS

SYSTEM	EFFECT	ASSESSMENT BY HX	PE	TEST
HEENT	Epistaxis Oral/mucosal friability	Headache	Stomatitis	CBC, differential, plt PT, PTT, CT scan
RESP	Pulmonary embolism Pneumonia Interstitial pneumonitis Pulmonary edema	Dyspnea	Tachypnea Lung field consolidation Wheezing	CXR, V/Q scan CT scan ABGs, bronchoscopy ± bronchoalveolar lavage, biopsy
CV	LV failure ASD/VSD	Dyspnea Lethargy	Tachycardia, S_3 Displaced posterior MI	ECG Echocardiography
GI	GI bleeding GI GVHD Hepatic veno-occlusive disease	N/V, diarrhea Melena	Acute abdomen Hypoactive bowel sounds Jaundice	Endoscopy, bleeding scan Selective angiography Albumin, transferrin LFT, liver biopsy
CNS	Microcephaly Meningitis Intracranial hemorrhage	Irritability, lethargy Headache, seizures	Meningismus Papilledema	Lumbar puncture after coagulopathy treated, head CT, MRI
HEME	Pancytopenia Leukemia Paroxysmal nocturnal hemoglobinuria	Bleeding gums, infections Easy bruisability Fatigue	Petechiae Retinal hemorrhage Pallor	CBC, differential Reticulocyte count, BM biopsy Ham's test
METAB	Electrolyte abnormalities Glucose intolerance Hypoproteinemia	Long-term hyperalimentation GI GVHD		Electrolytes Ca^{2+}, Mg^{2+}, phosphate, albumin, transferrin

Key Reference: Kojima S, Nakao S, Tomonaga M, Hows J, Marsh J, Gerard S, Macigalupo A, Mizoguchi H: Consensus Conference on the Treatment of Aplastic Anemia. Int J Hematol 2000; 72:118–123.

PERIOPERATIVE IMPLICATIONS

Preoperative Preparation
- Reverse isolation precautions
- Adequacy of blood products
- Severe neutropenia, co-existing congenital heart disease (HD) may warrant prophylactic antimicrobial therapy
- Avoid IM and rectal sedation
- Concomitant steroid therapy and necessity of "stress" doses should be considered

Monitoring
- Arterial line if indicated
- Consider CVP or PA catheter as indicated
- Urine output for new-onset hemoglobinuria as first sign of transfusion reaction

Airway
- Avoidance of nasal manipulation

- Use extreme caution with friable oral and pharyngeal mucosal surfaces

Preinduction/Induction
- May exhibit hypotension and excessive fluid requirements to maintain adequate CO
- Central neuraxial blockade contraindicated in ongoing thrombocytopenia requiring transfusion
- Peripheral neural blockade may be approached cautiously if coagulation status is judged adequate

Maintenance
- PEEP assures adequate tissue oxygenation at lower FIO_2 as hyperoxia depresses normal erythropoietin synthesis and marrow function
- Nitrous oxide depresses bone marrow function even after brief exposure; best to use O_2-air mixture
- Normothermia promotes coagulation

- Chronically anemic patients may tolerate lower Hct; adequacy of tissue O_2 must be addressed if CV decompensation ensues
- Avoid induced hypotension in anemic patients

Extubation
- Period with greatest O_2 demands

Postoperative Period
- Continued monitoring of coagulation status
- Transfusion requirements >normal
- Increased susceptibility to infection
- Pain management improves pulmonary toilet

ANTICIPATED PROBLEMS/CONCERNS

- Age of RBC in patients with aplastic anemia is older than usual, with lower 2,3-DPG levels inside cells resulting in increased O_2 binding by Hgb (shift to the right) and decreased delivery of oxygen to tissues for same SaO_2

ANEMIA, CHRONIC DISEASE

Donat R. Spahn, M.D.

RISK

- People within USA: ~ 10%
- Race with highest prevalence: African-Americans
- Gender with higher prevalence: Age < 55 y: F 8–15%, M 3–5%. Age > 55 y: progressively increasing in both sexes; at age ≥ 80 y: F 9–20%, M 15–40%.

PERIOPERATIVE RISKS

- Related to underlying disorders
- Anemia per se not an additional risk as long as minimal Hgb level and compensatory mechanisms maintained in perioperative period
- Minimal Hgb level is individual; in general, this level is not higher than the preop Hgb level in chronic anemia

WORRY ABOUT

- Underlying diseases and their perioperative complications
- Compensatory mechanisms aimed at maintaining O_2 delivery to tissue despite low Hgb and arterial O_2 content

OVERVIEW

- WHO definition of anemia: Children 6 mo–6 y: Hgb < 11 g/dl; 6–14 y: Hgb < 12 g/dl; nonpregnant females: Hgb < 12 g/dl; pregnant females: Hgb < 11 g/dl; males: Hgb < 13 g/dl
- Chronic anemia may itself be a disease but more often is secondary manifestation of another primary disorder (see Etiology)
- Symptoms of anemia depend on the underlying disease, severity and chronicity (time of development) of anemia, adequacy of compensatory mechanisms, and secondary manifestation of anemic state, e.g., angina pectoris, intermittent claudication, and transient cerebral ischemia due to local obstructive vascular disease

ICD-9-CM Code: 285.9 (Nonspecific)

ETIOLOGY

- Chronic blood loss, particularly in GI tract
- Iron, folic acid, cobalamin deficiencies
- Due to other primary disorders, e.g., chronic infections, malignancies, chronic renal failure, endocrine failure such as hypothyroidism
- Hemolytic anemia
- Aplastic anemia

USUAL TREATMENT

- Treatment of underlying disease
- Iron, folic acid, cobalamin supplementation
- Human recombinant erythropoietin
- Rarely, allogeneic blood transfusion

ASSESSMENT POINTS

SYSTEM	EFFECT	ASSESSMENT BY HX	PE	TEST
CV	Hyperdynamic circulation Myocardial ischemia CHF	Palpitation Pounding pulse Angina Sx, dyspnea Exercise intolerance	Tachycardia Wide pulse pressure	ECG Exercise ECG
RESP		Dyspnea		
GI	Chronic blood loss Hypoperfusion	Blood in stool Angina equivalent (pain, nausea, indigestion)		Occult blood in stool See CV
HEME	Hgb below WHO definition level (see Overview)	↓ Exercise tolerance		Hgb
RENAL	Chronic renal failure	Decreased urine output Dialysis	Shunt	Cr K^+
CNS	Decreased cerebral O_2 delivery	Dizziness Headache Transient cerebral ischemia		
MS	Low exercise capacity	Fatigability		

Key Reference: Roizen MF: Anesthetic implication of concurrent diseases. *In* Miller RD (ed): Anesthesia. New York, Churchill Livingstone, 2000, pp 903–1015.

PERIOPERATIVE IMPLICATIONS

Preoperative Preparation
- None

Monitoring
- Temperature
- UO
- CVP, Hgb, electrolytes
- ST-segment analysis in patients with signs of CAD
- PA catheter for large fluid shifts or patients with signs of LV dysfunction or advanced renal failure
- ABG in patients with severe anemia

Airway
- None

Preinduction/Induction
- Prehydrate liberally if CV status will tolerate
- Avoid marked reduction in CO
- Choose drugs according to renal function

Maintenance
- Aim at high PaO_2. Use FIO_2 of 1.0.
- Avoid hyperventilation or acute alkalosis
- Aim at high CO
- Avoid hypovolemia
- Keep patient warm
- Maintain Hgb above critical level. This level is individual, not above preop Hgb.

Extubation
- Keep patient warm
- Maintain high PaO_2

- In patient with CAD, this is the period of greatest risk for ischemia

Postoperative Period
- Keep patient warm, prevent shivering
- Maintain high PaO_2

Adjuvants
- According to underlying disorder

ANTICIPATED PROBLEMS/CONCERNS

- Myocardial ischemia/infarction or CHF in patients with concomitant CAD
- Deterioration of renal function in patients with moderate renal failure
- Prolonged effects of drugs in patients with impaired renal and/or hepatic function

ANEMIA, HEMOLYTIC

Richard J. Palahniuk, M.D.

RISK

- Up to 1% of USA population
- Highest prevalence in African-Americans (sickle cell disease, G6PD deficiency)

PERIOPERATIVE RISKS

- Increased risk of tissue hypoxia intraoperatively
- May have pre-existing renal or hepatic dysfunction

WORRY ABOUT

- Maximizing FIO_2
- Maintaining adequate alveolar ventilation
- Maintaining normal body temperature unless hypothermia is intended

OVERVIEW

- Hemolytic anemias occur from a variety of causes with a variety of perianesthetic implications
- Patients with previous splenectomy may be at increased risk of perioperative infection
- Acute hemolytic crises require a different therapeutic approach from that for chronic slow hemolysis

ICD-9-CM Code: 283.9

ETIOLOGY

- Acquired hemolytic anemias
  – Hypersplenism, immune hemolysis, microangiopathic hemolytic anemia, infection (malaria), paroxysmal nocturnal hematuria, spur cell anemia
- Hereditary hemolytic anemias
  – Membrane defects (spherocytosis), enzyme defects (G6PD deficiency, pyruvate kinase deficiency), thalassemias, hemoglobinopathies (sickle cell disease)

USUAL TREATMENT

- None
- Some disorders respond to splenectomy
- Cholecystectomy may be indicated if cholelithiasis is a problem
- Repeated transfusion may be necessary in some disorders
- Erythropoietin prior to operation can be considered even if only 3 days

ASSESSMENT POINTS

SYSTEM	EFFECT	ASSESSMENT BY HX	PE	TEST
GI	Acute hemolytic crisis	Abdominal pain	Splenomegaly Hepatomegaly	
HEME	Hemolytic anemia			Hgb Reticulocyte count Peripheral blood smear Serum haptoglobin ^{51}Cr RBC half-life

Key Reference: Ballas SK: The pathophysiology of hemolytic anemias. Tranfus Med Rev 1990; 4:236–256.

PREOPERATIVE IMPLICATIONS

Preoperative Preparation

- Preop transfusion should be utilized judiciously, usually after consultation with a hematologist. Erythropoietin is often prescribed even if only 3 d preoperatively.
- Acute drops in Hgb to <8 g/dl and chronic reductions to below 6 g/dl should be considered for preop packed cell transfusion

Monitoring

- Core temperature
- Consider arterial line and PA catheter for cases with even a modest risk of blood loss

Airway

- None

Preinduction/Induction

- Maintain supplemental FIO_2, adequate alveolar ventilation
- No agent or technique specifically indicated or contraindicated

Extubation

- Routine

Postoperative Period

- Maintain supplemental oxygen

Adjuvants

- None

ANTICIPATED PROBLEMS/CONCERNS

- Inadequte tissue O_2 delivery if SaO_2 falls, blood loss occurs, or cardiac output falls
- Variation in oxygenation, acid-base balance, and/or body temperature may promote hemolysis in some disorders

ANGINA, CHRONIC STABLE

Lee A. Fleisher, M.D.

RISK

- People within USA: 3 million
- Race with highest prevalence: ?
- African-Americans have highest death rates

PERIOPERATIVE RISKS

- Increased risk of perioperative MI and death varies, depending on study (3–12%)
- Risk of LV dysfunction, hypotension, myocardial infarction

WORRY ABOUT

- Increasing frequency of symptoms
- Signs of LV dysfunction with ischemia
- Silent myocardial ischemia

OVERVIEW

- Chronic stable angina identifies patients at risk for developing myocardial ischemia and MI
- Angina is present in < 25% of episodes of myocardial ischemia
- Symptoms should be stable for previous 60 d for "stable" diagnosis
- Can result from
  – Inadequacy of myocardial oyxgen supply in patients with critical coronary artery stenosis
  – Coronary vasospasm
  – Inadequacy of myocardial oxygen supply 2° to increased demand from ventricular hypertrophy
  – Endothelial cell-mediated vasoconstriction
- Thrombosis overlying unstable plaque can lead to unstable angina/MI

ICD-9-CM Code: 413

ETIOLOGY

- Acquired disease with genetic predisposition
- Patients with diabetes have higher incidence of CAD, frequently silent
- Other risk factors include Htn, hyperlipidemia, advanced age, tobacco use, homocystinemia

USUAL TREATMENT

- Medical therapy—β-adrenergic receptor antagonist, Ca^{2+}-channel antagonists, nitrates, aspirin, folate, lipid-reducing agents
- Angioplasty
- CABG

ASSESSMENT POINTS

SYSTEM	EFFECT	ASSESSMENT BY HX	PE	TEST
CV	Myocardial ischemia LV dysfunction	Angina Sx Angina-equivalent Sx Dyspnea Exercise tolerance	Displaced posterior MI S_3	ECG Exercise ECG Exercise radionuclide scintigraphy Pharmacologic stress testing ECHO Coronary angiography
RESP	CHF	Dyspnea; nighttime cough Orthopnea Chest tightness	S_3 Rales Wheezing	CXR
GI		Angina-equivalent Sx –LUQ pain –Nausea, indigestion		See CV Assessment
RENAL	↓ Renal perfusion	↑ UO at night		Cr
CNS	Syncope	Syncope with chest pain		Exercise stress test
MS		Angina-equivalent Sx –Arm pain/neck pain		See CV Assessment

Key Reference: Eagle KA, Brundage BH, Chaitman BR, et al: Guidelines for perioperative cardiovascular evaluation for noncardiac surgery. Circulation 1996; 93:1278–1317.

PERIOPERATIVE IMPLICATIONS

Preoperative Preparation

- Preop β-adrenergic receptor antagonist associated with a lower incidence of myocardial ischemia/infarction

Monitoring

- ST-segment analysis
- PA catheter for large fluid shift operations or patients with signs of LV dysfunction
- TEE most sensitive, but technical issues of real-time interpretation

Airway

- None

Preinduction/Induction

- May develop reduced CO and hypotension with ischemia
- Avoid tachycardia, hypotension

Maintenance

- Myocardial ischemia may manifest as
  – CV instability
  – Intraoperative myocardial ischemia
  – Reduced CO, increased PCWP
- No one agent or technique shown superior
- Maintain normothermia, adequate hematocrit (≥ 28%)

Extubation

- Period at greatest risk for developing ischemia
- CABG patients frequently left intubated until warm

Postoperative Period

- Pain management may be critical

Adjuvants

- β-adrenergic receptor antagonist, nitroglycerin, Ca^{2+}-channel blockers

ANTICIPATED PROBLEMS/CONCERNS

- Patients with angina who develop dyspnea on exertion are at greatest risk for developing perioperative cardiac complications
- Exercise tolerance may be the best predictor of perioperative risk. Patients with a good exercise tolerance may not require further evaluation for less-invasive procedures.

ANHIDROSIS (CONGENITAL ANHIDROTIC ECTODERMAL DYSPLASIA)

Raafat S. Hannallah, M.D.

RISK

- Rare

PERIOPERATIVE RISKS

- Impaired thermoregulation (risk of hyperthermia in infants)
- Postop chest infections

WORRY ABOUT

- Impaired thermoregulation
- Abnormal pain perception

OVERVIEW

- Absent sebaceous and sweat glands; heat loss by evaporation is impaired
- Absent mucous glands from respiratory tract and esophagus; frequent respiratory infections
- Partial or complete absence of teeth
- Hypotrichosis (absent hair)
- Characteristic facies: prominent supraorbital ridges, depressed bridge and root of nose, large deformed ears, thick lips, underdeveloped maxilla and mandible

ICD-9-CM Code: 705.0

ETIOLOGY

- Sex-linked recessive disorder
- Full expression only in males; carrier females may be mildly affected

USUAL TREATMENT

- Protect from risks of hyperpyrexia due to infection, hot weather, vigorous exercise

ASSESSMENT POINTS

SYSTEM	EFFECT	ASSESSMENT BY HX	TEST
HEENT	Airway anomalies	Snoring Difficult breathing	
RESP	Decreased mucus	Repeated infections	
OPHTHAL	Decreased lacrimation	Dryness, ulceration	
METAB	Hyperpyrexia		Record/monitor temp

Key Reference: Okuda K, Arai T, Miwa T, Hiroki K: Anesthetic management of children with congenital insensitivity to pain with anhidrosis. Paediatr Anaesth 2000; 10:545–548.

PERIOPERATIVE IMPLICATIONS

Preoperative Preparation

- Avoid anticholinergic premedication

Monitoring

- Routine
- Temperature

Airway

- Awkward mask fit
- Laryngoscopy and intubation may be difficult.

Maintenance

- Regional anesthesia may be preferable when possible
- Warm and humidify anesthetic gases

Extubation

- Vigorous postop chest physical therapy

Adjuvants

- Protect eyes with tape and ophthalmic ointment (lacrimation is reduced)

ANTICIPATED PROBLEMS/CONCERNS

- Difficult airway (mask and/or intubation)
- Hyperthermia
- Postop chest infections

ANKYLOSING SPONDYLITIS

John E. Tetzlaff, M.D.

RISK

- 1:2000 incidence in Caucasians, rare in non-Caucasians
- M:F 10:1; more severe in males
- 18–50% incidence in Native Americans

PERIOPERATIVE RISKS

- Difficult airway, atlantoaxial instability
- "Bamboo spine" with potential for fracture during airway manipulation
- Rigid chest with difficult ventilation, myocarditis, myocardial conduction defects
- Increased blood loss due to abnormal chest structure, mechanics

WORRY ABOUT

- Inability to intubate, spine fracture, arrhythmia, inability to ventilate, massive blood loss

OVERVIEW

- An arthritic process, seronegative for rheumatoid factor, that attacks ligamentous attachments of the spinal column
- Characterized by low back pain, sacroiliitis, multiplane rigidity of spine, chest stiffness, uveitis, and insidious onset at <40 y of age
- Autosomal dominant and strongly prevalent among first-degree relatives

ICD-9-CM Code: 720.00

ETIOLOGY

- Etiology unknown
- Genetic transmission led to discovery of a genetic marker, HLA-B27
- Infectious origin speculated; one species of *Klebsiella* reported to be associated with some cases

USUAL TREATMENT

- Symptomatic, with exercise, NSAIDs, immunosuppression can be tried in severe cases
- Wedge osteotomy is a drastic surgical intervention

ASSESSMENT POINTS

SYSTEM	EFFECT	ASSESSMENT BY HX	PE	TEST
HEENT	Uveitis	Visual disturbance	Funduscopic exam	
	TMJ arthritis, arytenoid deviation	Limited mouth opening, jaw pain, voice abnormality	Airway exam, indirect laryngoscopy	Fiberoptic nasopharyngoscopy
CV	Cardiomyopathy, conduction defects	SOB, chest pain, palpitation	Distant heart sounds, rales, arrhythmia	ECG, CXR, ECHO
RESP	Pleuritic inflammation, chest rigidity	Chest pain, limited exercise tolerance	Decreased breath sounds, chest excursion	Pulmonary function tests, CXR
GI	IBS	Abdominal pain, bowel dysfunction	Abdominal pain	
GU	Chronic prostatitis	Pain with urination	Rectal exam	
CNS	Atlantoaxial subluxation, occult spine fracture	Long tract signs, sphincter abnormality; sometimes no symptoms	Basic neurologic exam	Cervical spine x-ray with flexion-extension
PNS	Radiculopathy	Radiating pain in extremities	ROM of the extremity	EMG (medicolegal use)
MS	Back pain, sacroiliitis, joint ankylosis, kyphosis ("chin on chest"), "bamboo spine," spondylodiskitis	Review of skeletal function	Spine, skeleton	Radiologic studies

Key Reference: Calin A: Ankylosing spondylitis. *In* Kelly WN, Harris ED Jr, Ruddy S, Sledge CB (eds): Textbook of Rheumatology, 3rd ed. Philadelphia, WB Saunders, 1989.

PERIOPERATIVE IMPLICATIONS

Preoperative Preparation

- Airway evaluation, pulmonary function assessment; consider positioning difficulties. Antisialagogue for awake intubation.

Monitoring

- ST-segment analysis; pulmonary artery catheter if severe myocardial dysfunction

Airway

- Inability to intubate possible, owing to cervical spine fusion, distortion. Fiberoptic intubation may be necessary. Cervical spine instability possible. Spine fracture possible with airway manipulation. Occult spine fracture may already be present.

Induction

- If general anesthesia, any approach acceptable. If limited cardiac reserves, avoid depressants of myocardial contractility. If regional, skeletal abnormality can make the block difficult to perform, and response to injection is unpredictable. If local anesthetic toxicity, airway management can be difficult.

Maintenance

- With positive pressure ventilation, decrease tidal volume and increase rate
- High ventilating pressure may predict large blood loss

Extubation

- Awake is preferable

Adjuvants

- None

Postoperative

- Comfortable position, pain control without airway embarrassment

ANTICIPATED PROBLEMS/CONCERNS

- Airway control
  - The extreme distortion of the spine, especially the neck, may make intubating trachea and ventilating patient very difficult
  - Any airway compromise or depression of ventilation can result in catastrophe
  - Depression of ventilation with opiate analgesics can be dangerous
- Pulmonary function
  - Owing to abnormal mechanics of the thorax and neck, the ability to ensure normal oxygenation during surgery and in the postop period can be a potential problem
- Regional anesthesia
  - Placement of spinal, epidural, or caudal block could be technically very difficult. Action of local anesthetics in the central axis could be unpredictable.
  - Strongly consider paramedian approach to central block

RISK

- 1% of all congenital heart defects
- Total anomalous pulmonary venous drainage (TAPVD), the severe form, or partial anomalous pulmonary venous drainage (PAPVD), the less severe form, exists when pulmonary veins drain into the venous circulation.
- 4:1 male-female ratio in infradiaphragmatic type

PERIOPERATIVE RISKS

- Rapid CV deterioration secondary to acidosis
- Sudden pulmonary Htn and right heart failure during hypoventilation
- Mortality: 2–20% depending on preop status

WORRY ABOUT

- Air bubbles entering the venous circuit
- Polycythemic hyperviscosity attack with
  - Perioperative dehydration
  - Cold OR environment

OVERVIEW

- TAPVD incompatible with life unless an ASD allows R→L shunting of blood. TAPVD patients with small ASDs are more critically ill. Some cyanosis, usually with O_2 saturations of 85–95%.
- Increased flow through pulmonary vascular beds, resulting in pulmonary Htn
- Four types of TAPVD:
  - Supracardiac—pulmonary veins connect to the left innominate vein via an anomalous "vertical vein" or connect to right SVC via an anomalous "short connecting vein," or connect to the left SVC (45%)
  - Cardiac—pulmonary veins drain into coronary sinus or directly into the right atrium (23%)
  - Infracardiac—pulmonary veins drain into IVC, portal veins, hepatic veins, or ductus venosus (21%)
  - Mixed—combined supracardiac, cardiac, and infracardiac connections (11%)

ICD-9-CM Code: 747.41

ETIOLOGY

- Embryologic atresia or malformation of the common pulmonary venous system resulting in persistence of abnormal connections

USUAL TREATMENT

- Severe TAPVD with little systemic shunt needs immediate cardiac correction after birth. Most children with TAPVD require cardiac correction before 1 y of age.
- Cardiac correction of PAPVD may be postponed into childhood

ASSESSMENT POINTS

SYSTEM	EFFECT	ASSESSMENT BY HX	PE	TEST
HEENT	Hypoxemia	Snoring	Airway class	
CV	CHF	Decreased activity level	Rales	ECG—RVH, RAH
	Hypoxemia	Dyspnea	Cyanosis	ECHO; catheterization
				Cardiac consultation
	Monitoring problems	Anomalous peripheral vessels	Pulses and blood pressures in all 4 extremities	
RESP	Hypoxemia	Bronchospasm	Wheezing	CXR
		Shortness of breath	Tachypnea	Granular lung fields
		Pulmonary edema		
HEME	Sludging	Polycythemia	Clubbing	Hgb
	DIC	Bleeding or bruising	Bruises	PT, PTT, bleeding time
CNS		Previous stroke	Complete neurologic evaluation	CT scan if neurologic findings
MS		Feeding difficulty	Ht, wt, head circumference	Plot of growth curves
		Failure to thrive		

Key Reference: Caldarone CA, Najm HK, Kadletz M, Smallhorn JF, Freedom RM, Williams WG, Coles JG: Surgical management of total anomalous pulmonary venous drainage: impact of coexisting cardiac anomalies. Ann Thorac Surg 1998; 66:1521–1526.

PERIOPERATIVE IMPLICATIONS

Preoperative Preparation

- Desired hemodynamics: Preload—normal (CVP 10–12 mmHg); afterload—low; PVR—normal; HR—normal to high; contractility—normal
- Liberal oral fluids preoperatively
- Avoid heavy premedication
- Subacute bacterial endocarditis prophylaxis

Monitoring

- Absolute air bubble precautions
- Arterial catheter
- CVP catheters
- Others as per ASA routine

Airway

- Associated congenital syndromes with airway anomalies
- Cricoid ring limiting diameter of airway
- Primary need to maintain airway and avoid increased Pa_{CO_2}

Induction

- If IV in place use fentanyl or ketamine with pancuronium or vecuronium.
- If no IV
  - If unstable, ketamine IM
  - If stable, slow inhalational induction with sevoflurane (avoid high sevoflurane levels until IV placed)
- Actively avoid hypoventilation and agents that produce myocardial depression

Maintenance

- Positive pressure ventilation usually improves oxygenation
- Use narcotics in conjunction with inhalational agents as tolerated
- Avoid nitrous oxide
- Use high FIO_2
- Capnographic end-tidal CO_2 will not accurately reflect Pa_{CO_2}
- Avoid hypothermia

Extubation

- Do not attempt deep or early extubation
- Prior to extubation assess adequacy of ventilation with inspiratory pressures of at least −20 mmHg and adequate tidal volumes

Postoperative Period

- Close monitoring of ventilation and pulse oximetry
- Active warming with avoidance of shivering
- Be prepared for immediate reintubation

Adjuvants

- Inotropic support with dopamine or dobutamine

ANTICIPATED PROBLEMS/CONCERNS

- If pulmonary hypertensive crisis occurs
  - Hyperventilate
  - 100% Inspired oxygen
  - Consider prostaglandin E_1, tolazoline, amrinone, isoproterenol, or nitric oxide

ANOREXIA NERVOSA

Russell T. Wall III, M.D.

RISK

- Primarily in white adolescent females from middle- or upper-class families
- 0.4–1.5/100,000 population
- Age of onset from prepuberty to mid-20s

PERIOPERATIVE RISKS

- Predisposing conditions include cardiovascular dysfunction (bradycardia, hypotension), acid-base abnormalities (both acidosis and alkalosis are possible), lyte abnormalities ($\downarrow K^+$, $\downarrow Mg^{2+}$, $\downarrow Ca^{2+}$, $\downarrow P$), hematologic abnormalities ($\downarrow$ Hgb, $\downarrow$ WBC, $\downarrow$ fibrinogen, $\downarrow$ Plt), hypothermia, delayed gastric emptying, and renal dysfunction (prerenal azotemia)

WORRY ABOUT

- Degree of malnutrition (excess protein depletion = impaired cellular function)
- Greater weight loss = greater risk

OVERVIEW

- Anorexia nervosa
  - Obsessive fear of being fat
  - Radical restriction of caloric intake
  - Wt loss $\geq 15\%$ of ideal wt
  - Risk of death high if wt loss $\geq 35\%$ of ideal weight
- Bulimia
  - Obsessive fear of being fat
  - Irresistible urge to overeat
  - Wt control by vomiting, diuretic and laxative use
  - Wt loss less than in anorexia

ICD-9-CM Code: 307.1

ETIOLOGY

- Unknown
- Possibly hypothalamic dysfunction or psychiatric cause

USUAL TREATMENT

- No specific treatment
- Therapies offered
  - Psychotherapy
  - Behavior modification
  - Antidepressants
  - Nutritional (1500–2500 calories/d, metoclopramide or bethanechol for gastric emptying, benzodiazepine before meals)
  - Relaxation exercises
- If severe: hospitalization, with tube feedings or hyperalimentation

ASSESSMENT POINTS

SYSTEM	EFFECT	ASSESSMENT BY HX	PE	TEST
CV	$\downarrow$ Response to SNS		Bradycardia	
	Hypovolemia		Hypotension (<70 mmHg systolic)	
	LV dysfunction			
	$\quad \downarrow$ LV wall thickness	CHF symptoms	CHF	CXR
	$\quad \downarrow$ LV cavity size			ECHO
	MV prolapse		Murmur	
	Cardiomyopathy			
	Conduction abnormalities		Dysrhythmias (ventricular tachydysrhythmias, AV blocks)	ECG
RESP	Aspiration pneumonia	Vomiting	Bradypnea (<15/min)	CXR
GI	Delayed gastric emptying	Constipation		
	Esophagitis, esophageal/gastric rupture	Vomiting		
RENAL	Prerenal azotemia			BUN 60–70 mg/dl
	Acid-base abnormalities	Starvation	Muscle weakness	ABGs
		Vomiting	Edema	
	Lyte abnormalities	Diuretics		Serum lytes
	$\quad \downarrow K^+$, $\downarrow Ca^{2+}$, $\downarrow Mg^{2+}$, $\downarrow P$, Cl^-			
	Impaired concentrating ability	Polyuria		
	Hypoalbuminemia			
ENDO	$\downarrow$ BMR			
	Hypothermia (<96.6°F rectally)		Vasoconstriction	
	Depressed immune function	Amenorrhea		
	Abn glucose tolerance			Serum glucose
CNS	Brain atrophy	Starvation		
	Depression	Illicit drug, alcohol use		
	Diabetes insipidus			
MS	Osteoporosis			
			Peripheral edema	

Key Reference: Cerami R: Anesthetic considerations with anorexia nervosa. AANA J 1993; 61:165–169.

PERIOPERATIVE IMPLICATIONS

Preoperative Preparation

- Delay elective surgery until patient is medically stable
- Optimize hemodynamics, acid-base status, lytes
- Consider metoclopramide to promote gastric emptying

Monitoring

- ABGs, lytes
- A-line, CVP, PA catheters may be indicated

Airway

- Induction
  - Consider rapid-sequence induction
  - Cautious dosing because of possible LV dysfunction and hypovolemia

Maintenance

- Aggressively avoid hypothermia
- Probably avoid halothane (dysrhythmias)
- Cautious use of potent inhalation agents
- Excess fluids may precipitate pulmonary edema

Extubation

- Consider awake extubation

Adjuvants

- Cautious use of muscle relaxants ($\downarrow$ muscle mass, lyte and acid-base abnormalities)

ANTICIPATED PROBLEMS/CONCERNS

- Temperature control
- Hemodynamic stability
- Acid-base and lyte management

ANTICOAGULATION, PREOPERATIVE

Catherine Huraux, M.D.
Jerrold H. Levy, M.D.

RISK

- Pts with mechanical heart valves, atrial fibrillation, pulmonary embolism, recent venous thrombosis
- Oral anticoagulant therapy may → potential risks in elective or emergency surgery
- Other populations are pts who receive heparin IV before vascular or cardiac surgery and pts undergoing cardiac surgery with extracorporeal circulation

PERIOPERATIVE RISKS

- Balance between risk of bleeding vs. thromboembolic complication is major periop risk
- Risk increases with major and emergency vs elective surgery

WORRY ABOUT

- Excessive allogeneic transfusions, either to correct effects of warfarin or for risk of excessive bleeding
- In pts with valvular heart disease, concomitant hepatic dysfunction due to HF may produce abnormal PT and/or thrombocytopenia
- Can be associated with heparin therapy due to acute administration or prolonged use (7–10 days)
- Use of protamine to reverse heparin after bypass may lead to CV dysfunction and anaphylactoid reactions

OVERVIEW/PHARMACOLOGY

Heparin (Standard Unfractionated)

- For preventive therapy and acute management, binds to antithrombin III and factor X to inhibit their effects
- Variability in response to heparin depends on
  - Prep of heparin administered
  - Individual characteristics of pts
  - Duration of therapy (due to ↓ antithrombin III levels)
- Duration of action depends on dose and method of administration
  - 100U/kg: $T_{1/2}$ 56 min
  - IV: 60 min
  - 400U/kg: $T_{1/2}$ tripled
  - Subcutaneous: 3 h
- Depolymerized in endothelial cells
- Eliminated in urine
- Heparin resistance (many proteins neutralize anticoagulant therapy; prolonged therapy can lower antithrombin III levels)
- Monitoring of the anticoagulant effect: PTT

Heparin (LMW)

- $T_{1/2}$ 4–7 h
- Higher and more predictable bioavailability: 100%
- Removed by renal filtration

Warfarin

- Oral anticoagulant
- Member of the coumarin family
- Vit K antagonist causing inactivation of factors II, VII, IX, X and anticoagulants C, S
- Used for thromboembolic complication prevention
- Peak plasma concentration reached 1–4 h after ingestion
- $T_{1/2}$: 36–42 h
- International Normalized Ratio (INR) required: 2–3
- Stop for surgery and replace with heparin

Warfarin Reversal Treatment

- Vit K: 10–20 mg PO, IM, or IV; IV form potentially associated with anaphylactoid reactions
- Normalization of INR within 24 h
- Fresh frozen plasma starting with 2 U

Heparin Reversal Treatment

- Protamine reversal according to the ratio heparin:protamine 1:1.3 (or start with 50–100 mg and check the ACT)
- Monitoring: ACT in cardiac surgery

ASSESSMENT POINTS

SYSTEM	EFFECT	ASSESSMENT BY HX
ENDO	Risk of protamine reactions is 10- to 30-fold higher in diabetics receiving protamine-containing insulin	History of insulin use

Key Reference: Douketis JD, Crowther MA, Cherian SS: Perioperative anticoagulation in patients with chronic atrial fibrillation who are undergoing elective surgery: results of a physician survey. Can J Cardiol 2000; 16:326–330.

PERIOPERATIVE IMPLICATIONS

Preoperative Preparation

- Elective surgery/warfarin therapy
  - Stop warfarin 5 days before surgery
  - Replace with heparin in checking INR, PTT, platelet count
  - Stop heparin 60–90 min before surgery
- Reversal for emergency surgery
  - Warfarin therapy can be acutely reversed with FFP, and heparin therapy can be reversed with protamine
- Consider avoiding regional anesthesia
- Approach anticoagulation reversal cautiously in the anticoagulated patient

Postoperative Period

- Restart heparin therapy immediately after surgery (PTT, platelet count, blood cell count, bleeding)

ANTICIPATED PROBLEMS/CONCERNS

- Introduction of epidural or spinal anesthesia requires minimum 60–120 min between stopping and restarting heparinization; consider removing catheter at least 120 min after stopping heparinization and complete restoration of normal clotting time

ANTITHROMBIN III DEFICIENCY

Ellise Delphin, M.D.

Key Reference: Vinazzer HL: Hereditary and acquired antithrombin III deficiency. Semin Thromb Hemost 1999; 25:257−263.

RISK

- Incidence in USA: 1 in 2000−1 in 5000 (may be higher)
- Race with highest prevalence: Caucasian

PERIOPERATIVE RISKS

- Risk of postoperative thromboembolic phenomena; 40−70% most common (in descending order): deep vein thrombosis, pulmonary embolus, mesenteric thrombosis, highest risk in those with antithrombin III (AT III) levels <50% of normal
- Heparin resistance is common

WORRY ABOUT

- Hypercoagulable state perioperatively
- Thrombus formation on indwelling catheters

- Pulmonary emboli or DVT with immobility
- Mesenteric, inferior vena caval, or CNS thrombosis
- Withdrawal of warfarin sodium preoperatively, as patients may be heparin-resistant

OVERVIEW

- AT III is an α_2-globulin capable of inactivation of thrombin and factor x_a in blood; AT III deficiency results in an unusual susceptibility to thromboembolic disease
- Heparin resistance may be problematic during surgery
- Massive thromboembolism can occur perioperatively with AT III levels <50%

ICD-9-CM Code: 286.5

ETIOLOGY

- Genetic: reduced AT III synthesis inherited as an autosomal dominant trait, manifests as thromboembolism in late teens to early 30s
- Acquired: secondary to consumption of AT III due to massive thromboembolic disease, disseminated intravascular coagulation, renal disease with proteinuria (esp nephrotic syndrome), chronic liver disease, prolonged heparin therapy, increased protein catabolism
- Conflicting data about role of oral contraceptive use, pregnancy, and CAD

USUAL TREATMENT

- Medical therapy: sodium warfarin or combination of oral anticoagulants and platelet suppression (aspirin or dipyridamole)
- Perioperatively: fresh frozen plasma, cryoprecipitate, AT III concentrate, heparin; heparin resistance can be treated with FFP

ASSESSMENT POINTS

SYSTEM	EFFECT	ASSESSMENT BY HX	PE	TEST
CV	CAD		Angina, dyspnea	ECG, CXR Angiography
PERIPHERAL VASC	DVT Arterial occlusion		Gangrene, absent pulses	
RESP	Pulmonary embolus	Dyspnea Exercise tolerance decreased	SOB	CXR V/Q scan
GI	Mesenteric artery/vein occlusion Decreased AT III	Abdominal pain Chronic liver disease symptoms	Rectal bleeding Jaundice, hepatomegaly	Serum albumin, AT III level
HEME	Bleeding and thrombosis	DIC	Petechiae, purpura, thrombosis	FDP, PT, PTT, AT II, AT III level
GU	Decreased albumin and AT III levels	Nephrotic syndrome, proteinuria	Edema	Urinalysis, serum albumin
CNS	CVA	Sudden onset, Hx of other embolic disease	Seizure, loss of vision, loss of motor function	CT scan, angiogram

Key Reference: Vinazzer HL: Hereditary and acquired antithrombin III deficiency. Semin Thromb Hemost 1999; 25:257−263.

PERIOPERATIVE IMPLICATIONS

Preoperative Preparation

- Assess whether congenital or acquired; if acquired, treat primary disease if possible
- Stop oral anticoagulation and substitute FFP or AT III concentrate to bring AT III level to 70−80% normal
- Heparin to provide PTT of 40−60 sec

Monitoring

- Careful attention to temperature
- Volume status, respiratory variables
- PTT, AT III levels

Airway

- None

Induction

- None

Maintenance

- Maintain normothermia to avoid hyperviscosity
- Maintain intravascular volume
- IV heparin effect should be monitored
- Careful evaluations of hypotension or change in $ETCO_2$

Adjuvants

- No special concerns with adjuvant agents

Postoperative Period

- Consider ICU for monitoring
- Continue anticoagulation
- Early mobilization

- Remove indwelling catheters as soon as possible
- Oral anticoagulation might be reintroduced ASAP

ANTICIPATED PROBLEMS

- Embolic phenomena can occur intraoperatively
- Monitoring lines may be foci for thrombus formation
- Perioperative thromboembolic events major concern; continuous anticoagulation is required, as is operative prophylaxis with FFP and heparin

AORTIC REGURGITATION

Paul G. Barash, M.D.

RISK

- 100,000 aortic valve operations/y
- 20–30% of aortic valve replacements have AR
- 12–30% of aortic valve replacements have combined AR and stenosis
- Gender predominance: male > female, 3:1
- Racial predominance: none known

PERIOPERATIVE RISKS

- Left ventricular failure
- Right ventricular failure
- Subendocardial ischemia
- Splanchnic ischemia

WORRY ABOUT

- Aspiration pneumonitis (acute AR)
- Avoid hypertension, which ↑ AR and ↓ cardiac output
- Avoid bradycardia, which ↑ AR and ↓ cardiac output

OVERVIEW

- Long latency period between onset of hemodynamic changes and symptoms (~ 20–30 y)
- Myocardial ischemia uncommon
- Abdominal pain manifestation of splanchnic ischemia

ICD-9-CM Code: 424.1

ETIOLOGY

- Damage to leaflets
- Aortic root dilatation
- Loss of commissural support

TREATMENT

- Medical: digoxin, diuretic, vasodilator
- Surgical: prosthetic valve

ASSESSMENT POINTS

SYSTEM	EFFECT	ASSESSMENT BY HX	PE	TEST
CV	Aortic valve dysfunction		High-pitched, early diastolic, decrescendo blowing murmur Mid-diastolic low-pitched murmur (Austin Flint) Widened arterial pulse pressure (water-hammer) To and fro bobbing of head (de Musset's sign)	CXR ECHO
	LV dysfunction	Dyspnea with exercise Nocturnal dyspnea	Displaced posterior MI S₃	ECG CXR ECHO Cardiac catheterization
RESP	CHF	Dyspnea Nocturnal dyspnea	Rales S₃	CXR
GI	Splanchnic ischemia	Abdominal pain	Distended abdomen	

Key Reference: Braunwald E: Valvular heart disease. *In* Braunwald E (ed): Heart Disease: A Textbook of Cardiovascular Medicine, 4th ed. Philadelphia, WB Saunders, 1992, pp 1043–1053.

PERIOPERATIVE IMPLICATIONS

Preoperative Preparation

- Consider optimizing LV performance with vasodilators, inotropes, and diuretic
- Avoid reduction in aortic diastolic pressure
- Emergent procedures (acute AR): full-stomach precautions

Monitoring

- Arterial catheter
- ECG leads II/V5 and ST-segment analysis
- Consider PA catheter or TEE

Preinduction/Induction

- Elective: consider narcotic induction with inhalation supplement (0.25–50% MAC); nondepolarizing muscle relaxant devoid of bradycardic effects
- Emergency (acute AR with aortic dissection): consider rapid-sequence technique with ketamine, etomidate, or low-dose narcotic plus amnestic agent

- ↓ Aortic diastolic pressure ↓ coronary perfusion pressure and may lead to subendocardial ischemia
- Bradycardia and Htn ↑ regurgitant fraction and ↓ cardiac output

Maintenance

- During period until institution of cardiopulmonary bypass, consider maintaining LV function with minimum of anesthetic interventions
- PCWP may underestimate LVEDP due to premature closure of mitral valve
- PCWP may overestimate LVEDP in patients with combined AR and MR

Extubation

- Consider extubation for patients undergoing valve replacement in ICU after respiratory and hemodynamic criteria are met

Postoperative Period

- Consider augmenting preload to maintain and preserve filling volume of still-dilated, hypertrophic LV

- Inotropic support may be required to maintain CO if inadequate intraoperative myocardial preservation
- Evaluation for neurologic injuries 2° to embolism during valve replacement

ANTICIPATED PROBLEMS/CONCERNS

- Prolonged Trendelenburg position poorly tolerated during PAC insertion
- Intra-aortic balloon counterpulsation contraindicated before valve replacement
- Atrial fibrillation or other supraventricular tachycardias poorly tolerated and require aggressive treatment
- Retrograde cardioplegia (not anterograde) may be required for myocardial protection
- Associated diseases may present difficult intubation, e.g., rheumatoid arthritis, Marfan's syndrome, trauma (acute aortic dissection)

AORTIC STENOSIS

Stephen J. Thomas, M.D.

RISK

• Bicuspid aortic valve in 1% of population; 5–15% may become stenotic
• Isolated aortic stenosis 3× more common in men

PERIOPERATIVE RISKS

• Increased risk of perioperative MI following noncardiac surgery if stenosis is severe
• ↑ Risk of CNS dysfunction following aortic valve replacement if, in addition to the valve itself, the aorta is heavily calcified

WORRY ABOUT

• If patient is symptomatic, probably needs AVR prior to noncardiac surgery
• Differentiate systolic dysfunction (impaired contractility) from diastolic dysfunction (reduced ventricular compliance); diastolic change is common, but true contractile failure occurs only late in the disease

OVERVIEW

• Chronic obstruction to left ventricular outflow due to LVH
• LVH results in
  – Reduced ventricular compliance; ventricular filling pressures (VFPs) ↑; small ↑ in ventricular volume are associated with wide swings in VFP
  – Potential myocardial ischemia; ↑ muscle mass requires increased basal flow; coronary reserve ↓; O_2 supply may be compromised by low aortic diastolic pressure combined with elevated LVEDP
  – Stroke volume is preserved

ICD-9-CM Code: 424.1

ETIOLOGY

• In patients <60 y, AS develops on a congenitally deformed valve—usually bicuspid
• Patients >60 y usually have calcific degeneration of a previously normal valve

USUAL TREATMENT

• Careful follow-up after murmur noted; usually with Doppler ECHO
• Aortic valve replacement following onset of symptoms
• From onset of angina, syncope, or CHF, 50% mortality at <5, 3, and 2 y without surgical treatment

ASSESSMENT POINTS

SYSTEM	EFFECT	ASSESSMENT BY HX	PE	TEST
CV	Progression of stenosis	Symptoms (angina, dyspnea) appear	Murmur; S_4 gallop	Doppler ECHO for valve gradient
	Myocardial ischemia	Angina		ECG, coronary angiography
	LV dysfunction	Dyspnea, fatigue	S_3 gallop	CXR, ECHO
	Arrhythmias	Palpitations, syncope		ECG, ? Holter
	Syncope	Exertional arrhythmias		ECG, Holter
CNS	Stroke, syncope	Stroke, ± residua	Neuro exam	
			Carotid bruit	Carotid Doppler

Key Reference: Jackson JM, Thomas SJ: Valvular heart disease. *In* Kaplan JA (ed): Cardiac Anesthesia, 4th ed. Philadelphia, WB Saunders, 1999, ch 22.

PERIOPERATIVE IMPLICATIONS

Preoperative Preparation

• Continue antiarrhythmic drugs
• In prosthetic aortic valve, evaluate for anticoagulation status, risk of endocarditis

Monitoring

• ECG: ST-segment analysis ideal; may be difficult due to pre-existing changes of LVH
• Arterial line helpful to continuously follow arterial pressure
• PA catheter much less helpful; wide swings in filling pressure may lead to overtreatment
• TEE: not usually necessary, but can easily differentiate systolic from diastolic failure

Preinduction/Induction

• Avoid tachycardia, hypotension
• Because of sensitivity to volume depletion (low-compliance ventricle doesn't fill) and hypotension (poor coronary filling), hemodynamic changes should be either prevented or identified early and managed appropriately

Maintenance

• Fear of myocardial depression often overstated: contractility usually well preserved; however, volatile anesthetics associated with junctional rhythm, which ↓ stroke volume, cardiac output, and BP
• Bradycardia can cause hypotension; thick ventricle of limited distensibility, and excessively prolonging diastole does not improve ventricular filling

Extubation

• Period of potential ischemia

Postoperative Period

• Adequate pain relief helps to prevent undesirable tachycardia.

ANTICIPATED PROBLEMS/CONCERNS

• Prevent potential hemodynamic spiral of hypovolemia, hypotension, and tachycardia by careful attention to fluid requirements, pain relief, resolution of any sympathetic block
• Development of supraventricular arrhythmias, including AFIB, deleterious; early identification and treatment can be crucial

APNEA OF THE NEWBORN   William L. Meadow, M.D., Ph.D.

RISK

- Full-term infants with neurologic disorders
- Premature infants, ± neurologic disorders

PERIOPERATIVE RISKS

- More prone to apnea during local or epidural anesthesia
- More prone to apnea postoperatively

WORRY ABOUT

- Unexpected apnea in recovery room
- Unexpected apnea in hours after outpatient procedures
- Unexpected apnea on ward hours after inpatient procedures

OVERVIEW

- Apnea in term infant never "physiologic"
- Apnea in preterm infants may signal CNS disorder or developmental immaturity
- Sudden onset of apnea in any infant may also reflect sepsis or hypoglycemia
- Relationship to subsequent SIDS unclear
- Utility of pneumogram screening controversial
- Indications for home apnea monitoring controversial

ICD-9-CM Code: 770.8

ETIOLOGY

- Term or preterm infants:
  – CNS disorders (seizures, bleeds, structural changes)
  – Systemic disorders (hypoglycemia, sepsis, GE reflux)
- Preterm infants:
  – Same as term infants
  – If full evaluation is negative, "physiologic" apnea of prematurity diagnosed

USUAL TREATMENT

- Theophylline
- Oxygen
- Transfusion
- CPAP

ASSESSMENT POINTS

SYSTEM	EFFECT	ASSESSMENT BY HX	PE	TEST
CV	Congenital heart disease leads to desaturation; PDA may cause CHF	Congenital heart disease, PGE$_1$ treatment	Murmur; cyanosis	ECHO
RESP	Children with bronchopulmonary dysplasia may be prone to apnea	Hx of hyaline membrane disease or other parenchymal lung disorder	Abnormal pulmonary compliance or O$_2$ requirement	CXR; ABGs; O$_2$ sat
GI	GE reflux may cause vagal overload	Hx of reflux	None obvious	pH study; barium swallow
CNS	Seizures may cause apnea; structural abnormalities may create ineffective respiratory drive	Hx of seizures or change in neurologic development	Exam for seizures or neurologic change	EEG, head ultrasound; CT; MRI

Key Reference: Henderson-Smart DJ, Steer P: Postoperative caffeine for presenting apnea in preterm infants. Cochrane Database Syst Rev 2000; CD000048.

PERIOPERATIVE IMPLICATIONS

Monitoring
- Routine

Airway
- Not usually a problem; obstructive apnea may occur but is rare
- Bronchospasm may occur in infants with bronchopulmonary dysplasia

Maintenance
- Usually no problem during procedure; vigilance required postoperatively

Extubation
- Watch for intermittent inadequate respiratory effort for hours

Adjuvants
- No special concerns

ANTICIPATED PROBLEMS/CONCERNS

- Perioperatively not complex; vigilance regarding care and assessment in postoperative period

APPENDICITIS, ACUTE

Jordan L. Blinder, M.D.

RISK

- Incidence 6–7% of population
- Highest in 2nd and 3rd decades
- Usual male:female ratio is 1 : 1, but there is a 2:1 male predominance from age 15–25 y
- Most common extrauterine surgical emergency during gestation, occurring in 1:2000 deliveries

PERIOPERATIVE RISKS

- Mortality: <1% for nonperforated, 2% for perforated
- Risks increase with perforation and peritonitis
- Risk of sepsis if perforated
- Fetal mortality range: 2.0–8.5% overall but as high as 35% in perforation with peritonitis

WORRY ABOUT

- Aspiration of gastric contents
- Development of septic shock
- Antibiotic coverage
- Conversion to more extensive intra-abdominal surgery, e.g., for obstruction
- Carcinoid of the appendix

OVERVIEW

- The most common acute surgical condition of the abdomen
- Physical signs vary depending upon anatomic location and stage of disease
- Over 50% of deaths from appendicitis are in patients over age 60 y, although this group represents only 10% of patients with appendicitis; concomitant disease, late diagnosis contribute
- Mild dehydration and fever are common, but significant electrolyte disturbance and symptomatic dehydration are rare

ICD-9-CM Code: 540.9

ETIOLOGY

- Obstruction of the appendiceal lumen by enlarged lymphoid tissue or fecalith
- Bacterial proliferation and fluid accumulation produce distention of hollow viscus with increased intraluminal pressure, leading to bacterial invasion of mucosal layer
- Gangrenous infarction and eventual perforation may result in frank peritonitis

USUAL TREATMENT

- Laparoscopic appendectomy
- Open appendectomy still used in 20% of cases
- For ruptured appendix with frank periappendiceal abscess, high-dose antibiotics followed by elective appendectomy at 6–12 wk is an option

ASSESSMENT POINTS

SYSTEM	EFFECT	ASSESSMENT BY HX	PE	TEST
CV	Tachycardia	Review hospital record	Resting pulse Orthostatic signs	
RESP	V/Q mismatch, including Mvo_2	Dyspnea Tachypnea	Splinting Observation	Pulse oximetry
GI	Ileus	Anorexia Vomiting	Abdominal auscultation	Electrolytes (if protracted)
	Perforation		Rebound tenderness Guarding	Upright CXR (rarely needed)
RENAL	Dehydration	Oliguria	Skin turgor Orthostatic signs	Urine specific gravity (rarely needed) BUN/Cr (rarely needed)
CNS	Somnolence/confusion	Rule out sepsis	Mental status exam	WBC
METAB	Metabolic acidosis	Prolonged period before presentation		ABGs

Key Reference: Nguyen DB, Silen W, Hodin, RA: Appendectomy in the pre- and postlaparoscopic eras. J Gastrointest Surg 1999; 3:67–73.

PERIOPERATIVE IMPLICATIONS

- Replace fluid and electrolyte deficits
- Antibiotic coverage
- Aspiration prophylaxis: nonparticulate antacid and H_2 blocker
- Metoclopramide avoided if obstruction suspected

Monitoring
- Routine

Airway
- Assess for rapid-sequence induction vs. awake intubation; assume full stomach
- Secure airway with cuffed endotracheal tube
- Laryngeal mask airway is contraindicated (use ASA Difficult Airway Algorithm)

Induction
- Minimal depressant premedication
- Intravenous rapid-sequence induction

- Anticipate hypotension due to hypovolemia/peripheral vasodilation in early sepsis
- Consider regional anesthetic in exceptional circumstances

Maintenance
- Requires profound skeletal muscle relaxation for dissection followed by fast recovery for brief closure
- Intermediate-duration nondepolarizing relaxant or succinylcholine infusion for shorter cases
- Analgesic requirements for somatic pain not great once offending organ is removed
- Laparoscopic procedures ~ 15 min longer

Extubation
- Assure that patient is awake and responsive
- Assure full return of neuromuscular function
- Vomiting common

Postoperative Period
- PCA a cost-effective option
- Laparoscopic procedures result in shorter length of stay

Adjuvants
- Antibiotic interaction with nondepolarizers; "recurarization" rare
- Recrudescence of fever in postop period is common
- Differential diagnosis: postop sepsis vs. malignant hyperthermia

ANTICIPATED PROBLEMS/CONCERNS

- Concern for aspiration
- Need for intense muscle relaxation and rapid wound closure, along with potential interaction of muscle relaxants with antibiotics, increases likelihood of incomplete reversal of NMB
- Overall morbidity related to stage of disease at presentation, not surgical technique

ARNOLD-CHIARI SYNDROME

Nancy K. France, M.D.
Franklin J. Ruiz, M.D.

RISK

- Most common anomaly involving cerebellum
- Present in all children with myelomeningocele
- Frequently asymptomatic
- >50% of those who require treatment will present before 3 mo of age
- In older children and adults commonly associated with syringomyelia
- Stridor due to bilateral vocal cord paralysis is usually the most common sign on presentation

PERIOPERATIVE RISKS

- Most common causes of perioperative death are respiratory failure, meningitis, and ventriculitides
- Swallowing difficulties cause pooling of oral secretions; GER; GERD, increased risk of aspiration
- Gag reflex may be diminished or absent
- Mortality increased in those who rapidly progress to vocal cord paralysis, arm weakness, or cardiorespiratory arrest
- Potential air embolism during posterior fossa surgery

WORRY ABOUT

- Bulbar symptoms preop; these may influence postop airway management
- Procedure performed prone with the neck in flexion; extreme head flexion can cause brainstem compression. Prepare for difficult airway/intubation.
- Abnormal responses to hypoxia and hypercarbia because of cranial nerve and brainstem dysfunction; may persist after surgery
- Prone to apneic episodes

OVERVIEW

- Malformation characterized by caudal displacement of lower brainstem portions
- Results in frequent brainstem compression and complete obstruction of foramina of Luschka and Magendie → progressive hydrocephalus and dilation of cervical central canal (hydromelia)
- Multiple cranial n. defects (6, 7, 9–12)
- Presenting Sx: vocal cord paralysis with stridor and respiratory distress, apnea, ↓ gag reflex, abn swallowing and pulmonary aspiration, opisthotonos, cranial nerve deficits, and upper arm weakness

ICD-9-CM Code: 741.0

ETIOLOGY

- Complex developmental anomaly appears early in life
- Associated with myelomeningocele
- Malformation consists of elongation of cerebellar vermis that results in herniation of caudal vermis and choroid plexus through the foramen magnum with kinking of medulla and upper cervical cord
- Medullary or cervical cord compression can occur

USUAL TREATMENT

- Surgical therapy: posterior fossa decompression with upper cervical laminectomy and opening of the dura to decompress the herniated cerebellar tongue and cervical cord; may include plugging obex and myelotomy

ASSESSMENT POINTS

SYSTEM	EFFECT	ASSESSMENT BY HX	PE	TEST
HEENT	Brainstem compression Cranial n. deficit	Vocal cord paralysis	Stridor, resp distress	SpO$_2$, PFT
CV	Brainstem compression		Arrhythmias Tachy/bradycardia, sinus arrest	ECG
RESP	Brainstem compression Cranial n. deficit	Swallowing difficulties ↓ Gag reflex	↑ Secretions Aspiration pneumonitis	CXR
RENAL	Dehydration		↓ Skin turgor	↓ UO, ↑ urine SG
GI	GER	Vomiting, cough, apnea		
CNS	Associated myelomeningocele, hydrocephalus	Possible ↑ ICP Central sleep apnea	Lower extremity paresis/paralysis Lyte imbalance and contraction of intravascular volume	
MS	Cervical cord compression Scoliosis		Upper extremity weakness and sensory changes	

Key Reference: Nel MR, Robson V, Robinson PN: Extradural anaesthesia for caesarean section in a patient with syringomyelia and Chiari type I anomaly. Br J Anaesth 1998; 80:512–515.

PERIOPERATIVE IMPLICATIONS

Preoperative Preparation

- Preop glycopyrrolate to ↓ secretions
- Consider chronic lung disease 2° to recurrent aspiration pneumonitis
- Prone position for procedures in the posterior cranial fossa or upper cervical spine

Monitoring

- Precordial Doppler, ETN$_2$, or transesophageal ECHO to detect air embolism; SEP; MEP

Airway

- Nasal ET tube may be better secured for prone position and for prolonged postop airway control
- Extreme neck flexion may cause endobronchial intubation or brainstem compression
- Extreme head extension drives brainstem downward

Preinduction/Induction

- Preoxygenation, rapid-sequence IV induction; preserve CPP, avoid ICP elevation, provide adequate depth of anesthesia

or

mask induction with volatile agent; mask PEEP diminishes stridor
- Prone: pad face; eyes free of compression, pressure points padded

Maintenance

- Any anesthetic technique; frequent choices are remifentanil/propofol, fentanyl/isoflurane and a nondepolarizing muscle relaxant
- Maintain adeqate CPP, avoid CP elevation
- Controlled ventilation
- ICP reduced by hyperventilation (Paco$_2$ 28–32 mmHg), mannitol, furosemide; consider steroids

Extubation

- Endotracheal tube postop if vocal cord paresis and depressed gag reflex remain
- Consider extubation over a fiberoptic scope to evaluate VC
- Examination of VC

Postoperative Period

- Stridor frequently improved; pts require close monitoring for several days post surgery
- Neuro exam as soon as possible

ANTICIPATED PROBLEMS/CONCERNS

- Some with vocal cord paralysis and diminished gag reflex may require tracheostomy and gastrostomy

ARTERITIS, TAKAYASU'S

Joseph F. Foss, M.D.

Joseph F. Foss, M.D.

RISK

- People within USA: rare (<24:100,000)
- Presents at <50 yr of age, often in adolescence
- Race and sex prevalence: Asian; female > male

PERIOPERATIVE RISKS

- Acute laryngeal edema seen in related syndromes (polyarteritis nodosa and temporal arteritis)
- Difficult arterial access
- Major organ ischemia or thromboembolism

WORRY ABOUT

- Pulmonary vasculitis in 50% of patients, resulting in pulmonary hypertension

- Renal function
- High cardiac afterload
- Hyperextension of neck may compromise cerebral blood flow

OVERVIEW

- Chronic occlusive panarteritis of medium and large vessels, including pulmonary vasculature
- Renal artery involvement induces neurovascular hypertension (most frequent cause of hypertension in Asian children)
- Pulmonary dysfunction may be present

ICD-9-CM Code: 446.7

ETIOLOGY

- Immune-complex mechanism is hypothesized

USUAL TREATMENT

- Steroids
- Cyclophosphamide as second-line treatment
- PTCA for stenosis
- Endovascular stenting
- Platelet inhibitors (low-dose aspirin) or anticoagulants to decrease thromboembolic risk
- ACE inhibitors for hypertension

ASSESSMENT POINTS

SYSTEM	EFFECT	ASSESSMENT BY HX	PE	TEST
HEENT	Head pain	Head pain	Pain on pressure of inflamed artery	Biopsy of affected artery
CV	Multiple occlusions of peripheral arteries Ischemic heart disease (ostial occlusion) Cardiac valve dysfunction (aortic regurgitation) Cardiac conduction defects Hypertension (2° to renal artery occlusion) in 50% of patients	Angina, especially in younger patient with no other risk factors	Diminished peripheral pulses Difference in BP of >10 mmHg between arms Hypertension Murmur or bruits	ECHO
RESP	Pulmonary hypertension Hypoxemia 2° to V/Q mismatching			Arterial hypoxemia
HEME	Elevated ESR Anemia Elevated immunoglobulins			ESR Hct, Hgb
RENAL	Renal artery stenosis		Hypertension	BUN/Cr
CNS	Cerebral ischemia or infarction 2° to carotid involvement CVAs in 15% of patients	Vertigo Visual disturbances Syncope, seizures	Carotid or subclavian bruits Ocular changes	
MS	Ankylosing spondylitis Rheumatoid arthritis	Pain in head Pain in joints		

Key Reference: Henderson K, Fludder P: Epidural anaesthesia for caesarean section in a patient with severe Takayasu's disease. Br J Anaesth 1999; 83:956–959.

PERIOPERATIVE IMPLICATIONS

Preoperative Preparation

- Noninvasive evaluation of carotid or coronary vessels if symptomatic

Monitoring

- Noninvasive BP and pulse oximeters may be ineffective
- Arterial access may require cut-down
- Pulmonary artery catheter may be useful, but placement may fail in up to 50% of cases

Airway

- Avoid extension of neck in symptomatic patient

Induction

- Routine

Maintenance

- Maintain intraoperative BP within range usually seen for patient; hypotension may be associated with higher risk of ischemia or thrombosis of major organs
- Sympathomimetics may be used to maintain BP while correcting underlying causes of hypotension
- Avoid low CO_2 due to hyperventilation and use agents that maintain cerebral blood flow, especially with carotid involvement

Extubation

- Routine

Adjuvants

- Perioperative steroid replacement may be indicated

Postoperative Period

- Routine

ANTICIPATED PROBLEMS/CONCERNS

- Postoperative cardiorespiratory failure due to pulmonary hypertension
- Adrenal deficiency state if steroid supplementation or replacement does not occur in steroid-dependent patient
- Acute airway edema from disease

ASPIRATION, PERIOPERATIVE: PREVENTION AND MANAGEMENT

Paula A. Craigo, M.D.

RISK

- Risk of significant aspiration: 1.36 to 15 per 10,000 anesthetized patients
- Mortality: 0.2 to 0.3 per 10,000
- Loss of protective reflexes and sphincter function
- Obstructed or abnormal GI motility
- Increased GI contents
- Trauma, emergency/night surgery, pregnancy, difficult airway

PERIOPERATIVE RISKS

- Mortality after aspiration: 5%; higher if ASA > 2

WORRY ABOUT

- 20% of patients who aspirated had no risk factor: of these, 66% had difficult intubation
- Rapid-sequence induction in cardiac patients leads to tachycardia, hypertension, hypotension

OVERVIEW

- Aspiration has no definitive treatment. Prevention best. How to prevent it and in whom to prevent it?
- Vast majority of patients with risk factor(s) do not aspirate
- Consider aspiration in differential diagnosis of bronchospasm with hypoxemia

ICD-9-CM Codes: 997.3 (Aspiration pneumonia after procedure); 668.0 (Aspiration, peripartum)

ETIOLOGY

- Loss of protective reflexes: sedation, neuromuscular disorders/relaxants, altered mental status, reflux
- Obstructed or abnormal motility: achalasia, gastroparesis, pain, opioids
- Increased GI contents: bleeding, obstruction, feeds
- Other: difficult airway, pregnancy, obesity, emergency surgery

USUAL TREATMENT

- Suctioning: bronchoscopy if obstructing particles
- Lavage, steroids not helpful; surfactant investigational
- Empiric antibiotics may confuse cultures: consider if compromised patient, fulminant course, high bacterial load

ASSESSMENT POINTS

SYSTEM	EFFECT	ASSESSMENT BY HX	PE	TEST
HEENT (airway)	Awake intubation in difficult airway	Hx difficult airway, head and neck surgery/radiation, diabetes	Airway exam Palm or prayer signs	X-rays, CT scan, OR records as available
CV	Rapid-sequence intubation may lead to ischemia with tachycardia, hyper/hypotension; myocardial depression	Anginal Sx, exercise intolerance, Hx CHF, CAD Age, sex, risk factors	S_3, rales, displaced PMI	ECG, ECHO in selected patients
RESP	Rapid-sequence intubation may lead to bronchospasm	Hx pulmonary disease, wheezing with URI, smoking	Wheezing, prolonged expiratory phase	CXR
GI	Abnormal sphincters, motility, acidity	Hx peptic ulcer disease, reflux Sx, diabetes, scleroderma		
NM	↑ ICP leads to vomiting; depressed protective reflexes; muscle weakness		Neurologic exam	

Key Reference: Engelhardt T, Webster NR: Pulmonary aspiration of gastric contents in anesthesia. Br J Anesth 1999; 83:453–460.

PERIOPERATIVE IMPLICATIONS

Preoperative Preparation

- NPO status
  - Currently, for healthy elective-surgery patients, no solids allowed for 6 h, clear liquids allowed up to 2 h preop
- Prophylaxis in selected patients:
  - ↑ Gastric pH: antacid, H_2 blockers, proton pump inhibition
  - ↓ GI contents: prokinetics, NG suction

Monitoring

- Routine

Airway

- Protect airway with ETT or maintain protective reflexes
- Awake intubation in difficult airway
- LMA not protective against aspiration

Preinduction/Induction

- Regional associated with aspiration if ↓ BP → ↓ consciousness or seizures
- GA: highest risk at induction

- Denitrogenation with 100% O_2
- Check optimal patient position, table height, drugs and tools available, suction at hand
- Rapid-sequence induction; cricoid pressure on until ETT placement assured by ET CO_2

Maintenance

- Care with level of sedation during sedation/regional cases

Extubation

- Return of muscular strength/coordination/consciousness adequate to protect airway if emesis occurs
- If emesis, head-down or right-side tilt, thoroughly suction oropharynx and trachea

Postoperative Period

- If no symptoms in 2 h, significant aspiration extremely unlikely
- If chemical pneumonitis occurs, initial postoperative CXR may be normal, proceeding to "white-out" in a few to 24 h

- PEEP redistributes lung water, improves oxygenation; higher PEEP may ↓ cardiac output and ventilation
- Maintaining low filling pressures may limit lung fluid accumulation, but may worsen negative effects of PEEP

Adjuvants

- Muscle relaxants—must be dependably rapid-acting
- Regional drugs—avoid oversedation, hypotension
- Drug interactions between anesthetic drugs and 1 or 2 doses of aspiration prophylaxis not significant

ANTICIPATED PROBLEMS/CONCERNS

- Must balance concern for aspiration risk against airway quality, cardiopulmonary reserve, feasibility and, most significant, tolerance for regional techniques

ASTHMA, ACUTE

Brian K. Gehlbach, M.D.
Thomas Corbridge, M.D.
Jesse B. Hall, M.D.

RISK

- 14.5 million in USA have asthma, but only a small fraction exhibit severe acute asthma
- Increased prevalence and severity in African-Americans, adult females
- Prevalence increasing since early 1980s
- Increased risk in atopic individuals

PERIOPERATIVE RISKS

- Increased risk of exacerbation and barotrauma
- Risk may be related to degree of preop control
- Risk of myocardial failure

WORRY ABOUT

- Bronchospasm from airway manipulation
- Lung hyperinflation during mechanical ventilation
- Medication side effects, including hypokalemia (β_2-adrenergic agonists)
- Adrenal insufficiency in prior oral corticosteroid users

- Airways may be hyperreactive for up to 6 wk following a respiratory infection

OVERVIEW

- Characterized by bronchial wall inflammation, airway hyperreactivity, and variable degrees of reversible airflow obstruction resulting in wheeze, dyspnea, and cough
- Airflow obstruction results from airway inflammation, intraluminal mucus, and bronchoconstriction
- Severe airway obstruction may lead to dynamic hyperinflation
- Attacks may be slowly progressive or explosive in onset
- Intubation almost always increases airway resistance

ICD-9-CM Code: 493.9

ETIOLOGY

- Host factors: genetic predisposition; atopic individuals at risk

- Environmental factors: risk may be increased by childhood exposure to tobacco, pollutants, viruses. Occupational exposures include grain dust, plastics, fumes.
- Attacks usually triggered by respiratory tract infections or noncompliance

USUAL TREATMENT

- Medical therapy
  – First-line drugs: oxygen, inhaled albuterol, systemic corticosteroids. Subcutaneous epinephrine or terbutaline for patients unable to take inhaled drugs or not responding adequately to inhaled Rx. Terbutaline preferred in pregnant patients since epinephrine may ↓ placental blood flow and ↑ congenital malformations.
  – Second-line drugs: ipratropium bromide, theophylline, helium/oxygen (to decrease resistive work of breathing)
- Mechanical ventilation: indicated for arrest, obtundation, impending ventilatory failure (somnolence, slumped posture, progressive hypercapnia)

ASSESSMENT POINTS

SYSTEM	EFFECT	ASSESSMENT BY HX	PE	TEST
HEENT	Sinusitis, nasal polyposis	Nasal congestion, post-nasal drip, headaches, decreased sense of smell	Nasal mucosal erythema or edema, nasal polyps, granular pharyngitis	Sinus CT or sinus x-ray
CV	Tachyarrhythmias, possible pulmonary hypertension	Palpitations, heart rate	Tachycardia, irregular rhythm, loud P_2	ECG ECHO
RESP	Airflow obstruction Decreased lung elastance, hyperinflation, hypoxemia, hypercapnia Variations in peak flow	Dyspnea, cough, wheeze, chest tightness, nighttime awakenings, exercise-induced symptoms Peak flow diary	Prolonged I:E, decreased breath sounds, wheezes Pulsus paradoxus	Pulmonary function tests, CXR, ABGs
ENDO	Steroid-induced hyperglycemia, adrenal insufficiency (prior < 1 y steroid users)	Polyuria, polydipsia, weakness	Hypotension in adrenal insufficiency	Glucose, electrolytes, cortisol, ACTH stimulation test
MS	Steroid myopathy, steroid-paralytic myopathy	Difficulty climbing stairs or rising from chair Difficulty weaning from mechanical ventilation	Proximal muscle weakness in steroid myopathy Possible quadriplegia in steroid-paralytic myopathy	Measurement of inspiratory muscle force, CPK, EMG, muscle biopsy

Key Reference: Corbridge T, Hall J: The assessment and management of adults with status asthmaticus. Am J Resp Crit Care Med 1995, 151:1296–1316.

PERIOPERATIVE IMPLICATIONS

Preoperative Preparation

- Assess preoperative control
- Optimize medical treatment (acute attacks require systemic corticosteroids and more frequent inhaled β-agonists)
- Consider alternatives to ETT and GA
- Halothane, isoflurane, and enflurane may cause bronchodilation during (but usually not after) their administration
- Assess risk of adrenal insufficiency

Monitoring

- Airway peak-to-plateau gradient (as determined by an inspiratory pause) is a useful measure of airway resistance at a constant flow for time-to-time comparison
- Plateau pressure (Pplat) serves as a measure of lung hyperinflation and may be best predictor of complications of hypotension and barotrauma. Peak pressure does not predict complications

- Aim for Pplat < 30 cm H_2O by prolonging expiratory time (e.g., ↓ minute ventilation and/or ↑ inspiratory flow; use square flow waveform)

Airway

- Large oral tubes to ↓ airway resistance and aid mucus clearance. Nasal intubation may be preferred in awake patients. Problems with nasal tubes include need for smaller tube and high incidence of polyps and sinusitis.

Induction

- Postintubation hypotension may result from lung hyperinflation, hypovolemia, and sedation. Significant lung hyperinflation mimics tension pneumothorax. A trial of hypoventilation improves cardiopulmonary status within 30–60 sec in former. Volume challenge is indicated for hypotensive patients.

Maintenance

- Rising peak-to-plateau pressure gradient suggests ↑ airway resistance
- Rising Pplat suggests worsening lung hyperinflation

- Consider keeping Pplat < 30 cm H_2O by prolonging expiratory time. May need to accept hypercapnia.

Extubation

- May precipitate exacerbation. Inhaled β-agonists may be needed more frequently post extubation.

Adjuvants

- Muscle relaxants + systemic corticosteroids may cause acute myopathy
- Ketamine, halothane, isoflurane, and enflurane are bronchodilators

Postoperative Period

- Observe for asthma exacerbation

ANTICIPATED PROBLEMS/CONCERNS

- Hypokalemia from β_2-agonist administration
- Hypotension or pneumothorax from lung hyperinflation
- ↑ Risk of tension pneumothorax. Clinical features of lung hyperinflation mimic tension pneumothorax. If trial of hypoventilation does not quickly achieve hemodynamic stability, consider chest tube placement.

ATHEROSCLEROTIC DISEASE
Jacqueline M. Leung, M.D., M.P.H.

RISK
- Prevalence: 2,000,000 persons in USA
- 56,000,000 persons have some form of cardiovascular disease

PERIOPERATIVE RISKS
- CAD ↑ the risk of developing postoperative myocardial ischemia
- Presence of CAD in vascular surgical patients increases operative and long-term mortality

WORRY ABOUT
- ↑ Risk of perioperative myocardial ischemia and perioperative cardiac complications
- ↑ Risk of CVA not evident after nonvascular surgery
- Aortic dissection in cases of aneurysm requiring emergency surgery

OVERVIEW
- Thickening and hardening of the medium-sized and large arteries accounts for large proportion of heart attacks and cases of IHD
- Also leads to strokes, PVD, and aneurysm of lower abdominal aorta
- Blood vessels affected include coronary, carotid, basilar, and vertebral arteries, as well as aorta and iliac arteries

ICD-9-CM Code: 414.0 (Atherosclerotic heart disease)

ETIOLOGY
- Multifactorial
- Risk factors: hyperlipidemia, Htn, cigarette smoking, male sex, diabetes mellitus

USUAL TREATMENT
- Primary prevention includes modification of risk factors, especially in high-risk individuals, and prophylaxis with aspirin
- Atherosclerotic heart disease: antianginal Rx is employed for symptomatic persons; other treatment includes angioplasty and CABG surgery
- Carotid artery disease: carotid endarterectomy
- Other cerebrovascular insufficiency: extracranial-intracranial bypass sometimes performed
- Peripheral vascular insufficiency: angioplasty or revascularization of lower extremities
- AAA: abdominal aortic aneurysmectomy

ASSESSMENT POINTS

SYSTEM	EFFECT	ASSESSMENT BY HX	PE	TEST
CV	Hypertension Coronary artery stenoses MI	Usually asymptomatic Angina, may be asymptomatic	Normal if treated S_3 and/or S_4 Cardiomegaly	Vital signs ECG ECG exercise treadmill Pharmacologic stress test, coronary angiography, ECHO, radionuclide studies
	Ventricular dysfunction (systolic and/or diastolic)	Exercise intolerance Sx of heart failure	S_3 and/or S_4 Cardiomegaly	Determine LV ejection fraction and function by ECHO, radionuclide studies Diastolic function by Doppler ECHO
RESP	COPD (many are smokers)	Dyspnea on exertion	Decreased breath sounds, prolonged expiration, wheezes	ABGs PFTs (if indicated)
CNS	Cerebrovascular insufficiency Cerebral infarct	TIAs Syncope Strokes	Carotid bruits Focal neurologic deficits	Doppler or angiogram (if indicated)
PERIPHERAL ARTERIES	Occlusive lesions Abdominal aortic aneurysm	Claudication Abdominal pain, may be asymptomatic	Decreased pulses Pulsatile abdominal mass	Angiogram (if indicated) Aortogram (if indicated) MRI (if indicated)
GI	Intestinal ischemia	Abdominal pain Occult blood in stool or gastric contents Leukocytosis Serum amylase may be elevated	Abdominal exam may be paradoxically normal	Mesenteric angiography

Key Reference: Adler Y, Levinger U, Koren A, et al: Association between mitral annulus calcifications and peripheral arterial atherosclerotic disease. Angiology 2000; 51:639–646.

PERIOPERATIVE IMPLICATIONS

Preoperative Preparation
- Stabilize cardiac Sx medically
- Continue antianginal Rx
- Attention to and stabilization of co-existent diseases
- Consider perioperative β-blockade to ↓ myocardial ischemia

Monitoring
- Cardiovascular
  - ECG with appropriate lead placement, ST trending
  - Consider CVP or PA catheterization to monitor preload, esp in patients with Hx of CHF
  - Consider TEE, esp in patients with uninterpretable ECG (e.g., ventricular pacemaker or LBBB)
- Cerebrovascular
  - In carotid endarterectomy, measurement of stump pressure, EEG, and SEPs have been used
  - CSF pressure monitoring and drainage in thoracoabdominal aneurysmectomy

Airway
- None

Preinduction/Induction
- Preventing tachycardia (use of short-acting β-blockers desirable)
- Treat BP changes aggressively

Maintenance
- No one anesthetic agent or technique superior, maintaining HR at low level and hemodynamic stability more important
- For peripheral vascular surgery, regional anesthesia in combination with postop epidural analgesia may ↓ incidence of graft thrombosis (see also Peripheral Vascular Disease)
- For carotid endarterectomy, maintaining cerebral perfusion pressure important goal
- For abdominal aortic surgery, optimizing loading conditions, detecting and treating myocardial ischemia and ventricular dysfunction are important, particularly during and after aortic clamping

Extubation
- Same concerns as during induction
- Rapid awakening to allow neurologic assessment after carotid endarterectomy

Adjuvants
- β-blocking agents and other antihypertensives useful in hyperdynamic situations
- Prophylactic nitroglycerin and Ca^{2+}-channel blockers to treat myocardial ischemia not conclusively proven effective
- Caution in use of vasoconstrictors, such as α-adrenergic agonists, to ↑ BP in cases of heart failure

ANTICIPATED PROBLEMS/CONCERNS
- Postoperative myocardial ischemia and other cardiac complications
- Graft occlusion (with peripheral revascularization procedures)
- Heart failure (with a history of CHF)
- Paraplegia, particularly after surgery for thoracoabdominal aneurysms
- Renal dysfunction in cases of aortic surgery

ATRIAL FIBRILLATION

Morris Brown, M.D.

RISK

- Affects >1% of those >60 y
- 0.4% of adult population
- Racial predominance: none
- ↑ Prevalence with ↑ age

PERIOPERATIVE RISKS

- Rapid ventricular response in CHF
- Myocardial ischemia
- Embolization

WORRY ABOUT

- ↓ Cardiac output
- Myocardial ischemia
- Embolization

OVERVIEW

- Develops over 2 decades in 2% of patients >30 y
- Related to left atrial size, underlying heart disease, and abnormal electrophysiology
- Incidence ↑ with age
- Most affected people have underlying cardiac disease
- Common after cardiac surgery, particularly valve surgery

ICD-9-CM Code: 427.31

ETIOLOGY

- CAD
- Rheumatic heart disease
- Cardiomyopathy
- Mitral stenosis
- Hypertensive CV disease
- Pericarditis
- Hypoxia
- Heart failure
- Pulmonary emboli
- Hyperthyroidism
- Subarachnoid hemorrhage
- Sarcoidosis/amyloidosis
- Idiopathic

USUAL TREATMENT

- Cardioversion for hemodynamic instability
- Digitalis
- β-blockers
- Calcium antagonists
- Quinidine (with digitalis)

ASSESSMENT POINTS

SYSTEM	EFFECT	ASSESSMENT BY HX	PE	TEST
CV	CHF Angina Stroke	Palpitations Chest pain Dyspnea Orthopnea	Variation in intensity of 1st heart sound; absence of A waves in jugular venous pulse; irregularly irregular ventricular rhythm	ECHO (if indicated)
RESP	CHF Pulm embolism	Dyspnea Orthopnea Chest pain Tachypnea	S_3 Rales Wheezing	CXR V/Q scan (if suspicion of pulmonary embolism)
GI	Ischemic bowel from low flow or embolization	Abdominal pain	Acute abdomen	ABGs/electrolytes
RENAL	↓ Renal perfusion	↓ Urine output		BUN/Cr
CNS	Syncope, lightheadedness, fatigue, dizziness	Stroke	Neurologic deficit	Head CT
MS		Anginal equivalent		See CV

Key Reference: Hogue CW, Hyder ML: Atrial fibrillation after cardiac operation: risks, mechanisms and treatment. Ann Thorac Surg 2000; 69:300–306.

PERIOPERATIVE IMPLICATIONS

Preoperative Preparation

- Search for precipitating causes—new onset may signify acute disease process, which may delay surgery
- Control ventricular response or convert to normal sinus rhythm if unstable

Monitoring

- ECG with ST-segment analysis
- PA line in patients with low cardiac output

Airway

- None

Preinduction/Induction

- Avoid excessive sympathetic stimulation
- Maintain oxygenation/ventilation

Maintenance

- Monitor oxygenation, maintain normocarbia
- Control ventricular response

Extubation

- Avoid excessive sympathetic stimulation

Adjuvants

- Digitalis: little effect of anesthetic agents
- Ca^{2+} antagonists: can ↓ AV conduction; can ↑ NM blockade

- β-blocker agents: can cause ↓ AV conduction
- Quinidine (with digitalis): ↑ NM blockade

Postoperative Period

- Maintain adequate analgesia
- New onset may require prompt treatment

ANTICIPATED PROBLEMS/CONCERNS

- Rapid ventricular response may result in significant fall in cardiac output
- Direct current (DC) cardioversion establishes sinus rhythm in >90%

ATRIAL FLUTTER

John L. Atlee, M.D.

RISK

- Atrial flutter (AFLT) occurs rarely in the general population and infrequently in patients with heart disease, < 1/10 as often as atrial fibrillation (AFIB)
- AFLT develops more frequently as patients age and acquire significant heart and pulmonary disease
- Patients with AFLT more likely to have CAD, sometimes complicated by Htn
- AFLT occurs relatively frequently after cardiac surgery but seldom after noncardiac surgery including thoracotomy

PERIOPERATIVE RISKS

- Circulatory insufficiency or ischemia from extremes of HR in patients with CAD
- Cerebral, coronary, or systemic embolism from left atrial mural thrombus

WORRY ABOUT

- Associated disease, especially adequacy of CV and pulmonary function
- Ventricular rates > 200 bpm with quinidine, vagolytics, β-agonists
- Dangerously rapid ventricular rates in patients with WPW or Lown-Ganong-Levine syndromes and AFLT

OVERVIEW

- Clinical EP studies have established that most cases of AFLT are due to right atrial re-entry. Many patients are cured with radiofrequency catheter ablation to endocardium between the IVC orifice and tricuspid valve.
- Type I AFLT: regular atrial rates 240–340 bpm with fixed (often 2:1) AV conduction
- Type II AFLT: regular atrial rates 350–450 bpm with variable or fixed AV conduction
- Differential: type I AFLT is, and type II AFLT and AFIB are not, pace-terminable
- About $\frac{1}{4}$ of patients with AFLT have left atrial thrombi, especially those with low ejection fraction ($\leq 40\%$). The incidence of thromboembolism with AFLT is unknown.

ICD-9-CM Codes: 427.31 (Atrial fibrillation); 427.32 (Atrial flutter)

ETIOLOGY

- AFLT is acquired, with no specific cause beside pulmonary or structural heart disease
- Many antiarrhythmic drugs convert AFIB to AFLT, sometimes in the course of restoring sinus rhythm. Alcohol intoxication produces AFLT $\sim \frac{1}{2}$ as often as AFIB ("holiday heart syndrome").

USUAL TREATMENT

- Drugs for ventricular rate reduction (β-blocker, Ca^{2+}-channel blocker) or chemical conversion (ibutilide, procainamide, amiodarone); catheter ablation is definitive therapy
- Value of anticoagulation has not been established for patients with AFLT, except for those with previous thromboembolic events
- Prophylactic amiodarone and β-blockers ↓ incidence of AFLT after cardiac surgery
- Atrial pacing at 120–150% of the flutter rate for type 1 AFLT (flutter rate < 350 bpm) using atrial or esophageal indirect atrial pacing leads frequently converts AFLT to sinus rhythm. Type II AFLT (flutter rate > 350 bpm) is not terminated by atrial overdrive pacing.
- Consider early cardioversion if AFLT poorly tolerated

ASSESSMENT POINTS

SYSTEM	EFFECT	ASSESSMENT BY HX	PE	TEST
CV	AFLT–AFIB	Palpitations, dizziness, weakness, lethargy	Irregular pulse, pulse deficit, S_1–S_2 intensity vary S_3, rales, wheezes	ECG, Holter monitoring, EP studies
	LV function CAD severity	CHF, exercise intolerance Sx of angina		ECHO, exercise ECG, MRI, cardiac catheter Stress ECG, dipyridamole scintigraphy, angiography
RESP	CHF, COPD	Dyspnea, orthopnea, cough	S_3, rales, wheezes	CXR, pulmonary function testing
GI	↓ Perfusion	GI distress, diarrhea		
RENAL	↓ Perfusion	Polyuria (nocturnal)		BUN/Cr
CNS	Ischemia or stroke	Syncope, mental changes, paresis/paralysis, dementia	Neurologic or mental deficits	See CV assessment

Key Reference: Kastor JA: Arrhythmias, 2nd ed. Philadelphia, WB Saunders, 2000, pp 131–163.

PERIOPERATIVE IMPLICATIONS

Preoperative Preparation

- Adequate ventricular rate control (80–100 bpm) with β-blockers or Ca^{2+}-channel blockers
- Treat CHF if present; otherwise, optimize cardiopulmonary function
- If acute onset AFLT (≤ 3 days), consider cardioversion, anticoagulation

Monitoring

- ECG with ST–T trending and strip-chart recorder for documentation of new arrhythmias
- Consider direct arterial and PA catheter monitoring with significant LV dysfunction

Induction

- LV dysfunction and AFLT increase risk of severe hypotension during induction with agents such as thiopental or propofol
- Desflurane, ketamine, and pancuronium may accelerate ventricular rate with AFLT

Maintenance

- Expect ↑ circulatory instability and less tolerance of large fluid shifts or blood loss
- No anesthetic drugs are especially contraindicated; caution with drugs that speed conduction

Extubation

- Possibly at ↑ risk for thromboembolism with hyperdynamic circulatory state

- Use drugs/means to reduce/avoid effects of airway stimulation and hyperdynamic circulation

Adjuvants

- Sympathomimetic or antimuscarinic drugs may accelerate ventricular rate

ANTICIPATED PROBLEMS/CONCERNS

- Patients with acute or chronic AFLT appear at ↑ risk of embolic stroke
- Dangerous acceleration of ventricular rate to > 300 bpm with WPW or Lown-Ganong-Levine syndrome
- Increased proarrhythmia risk with drugs for chemical conversion with underlying CAD

ATRIAL SEPTAL DEFECT, OSTIUM PRIMUM

Long K. Han, M.D.

RISK

- People within USA: 60,000 with ostium primum ASD (30% of ASDs)
- Gender prevalence: female > male, 2:1
- ↑ Incidence in high altitude
- ↑ Incidence in Down syndrome
- Association with AV canal defect

PERIOPERATIVE RISKS

- Perioperative mortality rate: 1%
- Late in course, associated with atrial dysrhythmias and CHF with L→R shunt
- ↑ Risk of atrial dysrhythmias, heart block, and air embolus with surgical repair

WORRY ABOUT

- Risk of infectious endocarditis and air embolization with IV access

OVERVIEW

- Failure of inferior septum to close—usually an endocardial cushion defect associated with mitral and tricuspid valve abnormalities
- Usually asymptomatic early in life
- L→R shunt causes ↑pulmonary blood flow
- Late in course: CHF and shunt reversal
- Frequently associated with tricuspid regurgitation and/or mitral regurgitation
- Life expectancy without repair ~40 y. Risks of death are 25% by 27 y, 50% by 36 y, 75% by 50 y, 90% by 60 y.
- Diagnosis by echocardiography

ICD-9-CM Code: 745.61

ETIOLOGY

- Failure of septum primum to fuse with endocardial cushion to close ostium primum

USUAL TREATMENT

- Digitalis and diuretics for child with CHF
- Antiarrhythmics occasionally needed for atrial dysrhythmias
- Surgery or umbrella repair indicated when Qp:Qs ratio ± 1.5:1, if ASD >25 mm diameter, if anomalous pulmonary venous return, if CHF, if significant cardiomegaly
- Endocarditis prophylaxis not indicated after successful simple surgical closure

ASSESSMENT POINTS

SYSTEM	EFFECT	ASSESSMENT BY HX	PE	TEST
HEENT	Difficult intubation	Down syndrome	Down syndrome facies	
CV	Atrial dysrhythmias	Palpitation SOB, frequent fatigue Cyanosis (rare)	Irregular rate and rhythm	ECG (RVH, LAD) ECHO
	Right-sided heart failure		Right heart enlargement	Angiography
	L→R shunting (rare) Hypertrophic RA and RV		Loud S$_1$, fixed S$_2$, and crescendo-decrescendo systolic murmur	Dye dilution study
RESP	↑ Pulmonary blood flow ↑ PVR	SOB Frequent URIs	Rales, wheezing	CXR
GI	Hepatic dysfunction if severe CHF	Jaundice	Hepatomegaly	LFTs, PT
CNS	Embolic stroke from chronic AFIB	Various neurologic changes		Head CT, cardiac ECHO if emboli suspected
MS			Enlarged left costal cartilage	
RENAL	Renal dysfunction if severe CHF			Cr, BUN

Key Reference: Findlow D, Doyle E: Congenital heart disease in adults. Br J Anaesth 1997; 78:416–430.

PERIOPERATIVE IMPLICATIONS

Preoperative Medications

- Narcotics and anticholinergics
- Antibiotic prophylaxis
- Continue digoxin if used for rate control

Monitoring

- Routine monitors, arterial line, CVP; TEE helpful in assessing anatomy before CPB; check for air and residual shunting after CPB; central and peripheral temperature monitoring; ECHO and fluoroscopic control a necessity for umbrella repairs

Induction

- IV induction theoretically slowed by L→R shunt; inhalational induction not significantly affected
- Epidural with loss of resistance to saline technique to avoid air embolism

Maintenance

- Avoid nitrous oxide to minimize size of air bubbles; any other techniques appropriate; watch for shunt reversal with hypothermia, hypercarbia, hypoxemia

Extubation

- Usually mechanically ventilated at end of any operative procedure, especially if heart block is present

Adjuvants

- Watch for dysrhythmia from hypokalemia if patient is on digoxin and diuretics

Postoperative Period

- Adequate analgesia for sternotomy or thoracotomy pain; pacemakers available for transient heart block

ANTICIPATED PROBLEMS/CONCERNS

- Air emboli with vascular access
- Dysrhythmia (5–10% if no prerepair dysrhythmia)
- Heart failure
- Heart block after CPB
- Sternal infection (rare)
- Endocarditis (rare)

ATRIAL SEPTAL DEFECT, OSTIUM SECUNDUM

Long K. Han, M.D.

RISK

- People within USA: 140,000 with ostium secundum ASD (70% of ASDs)
- Gender prevalence: female > male, 2:1
- Familial incidence: significant if associated with P-R prolongation or forearm and hand abnormalities (Holt-Oram syndrome)
- ↑ Incidence in high altitude

PERIOPERATIVE RISKS

- Perioperative mortality rate: 1%
- Late in course, associated with atrial dysrhythmias and CHF with L→R shunt
- ↑ Risk of atrial dysrhythmias, heart block (rare), and air embolus with surgical repair

WORRY ABOUT

- Risk of infectious endocarditis and air embolization with IV access

OVERVIEW

- Failure of closure of midseptal fossa ovalis
- Usually asymptomatic early in life
- L→R shunt causes ↑ pulmonary blood flow
- Late in course: CHF and shunt reversal
- Life expectancy without repair ~40 y. Risks of death are 25% by 27 y, 50% by 36 y, 75% by 50 y, 90% by 60 y.
- 15% incidence of associated noncardiac anomalies
- Diagnosis by echocardiography

ICD-9-CM Code: 745.5

ETIOLOGY

- Failure of septum secundum to fuse with septum primum to form interatrial septum

USUAL TREATMENT

- Digitalis and diuretics for child with CHF
- Antiarrhythmics occasionally needed for atrial dysrhythmias
- Surgery or transcatheter closure is indicated when Qp:Qs ratio ≥ 1.5:1
- Surgery also indicated if ASD >25 mm diameter or if anomalous pulmonary venous return is present
- Endocarditis prophylaxis not indicated after successful simple surgical closure

ASSESSMENT POINTS

SYSTEM	EFFECT	ASSESSMENT BY HX	PE	TEST
CV	Atrial dysrhythmias	Palpitation SOB, DOE	Irregular rate and rhythm	Echocardiogram Angiography Dye dilution study
	Right-sided heart failure L→R shunting		Right heart enlargement Loud S_1, fixed S_2, and crescendo-decrescendo systolic murmur	
RESP	↑ Pulmonary blood flow ↑ PVR	SOB Frequent URIs	Rales, wheezing	CXR
GI	Hepatic dysfunction if severe CHF	Jaundice	Hepatomegaly	LFTs, PT
RENAL	Renal dysfunction if severe CHF			Cr, BUN
CNS	Embolic stroke from chronic AFIB	Various changes		Head CT, cardiac ECHO if suspected emboli
MS			Holt-Oram syndrome Large left costal cartilage	

Key Reference: Findlow D, Doyle E: Congenital heart disease in adults. Br J Anaesth 1997; 78:416–430.

PERIOPERATIVE IMPLICATIONS

Preoperative Medications
- Narcotics and anticholinergics
- Antibiotic prophylaxis
- Continue digoxin if used for rate control

Monitoring
- Routine monitors, arterial line, CVP; TEE helpful in assessing anatomy before CPB, and check for air, and residual shunting after CPB; central and peripheral temperature monitoring

Induction
- IV induction theoretically slowed by L→R shunt; inhalational induction not significantly affected
- Epidural with loss of resistance to saline technique to avoid air embolism

Maintenance
- Avoid nitrous oxide to minimize size of air bubbles; any other techniques appropriate; watch for shunt reversal with hypothermia, hypercarbia, hypoxemia

Extubation
- Controversial; usually can be extubated at the end of case if hemodynamically stable

Adjuvants
- Watch for dysrhythmia from hypokalemia if patient is on digoxin and diuretics

Postoperative Period
- Adequate analgesia for sternotomy or thoracotomy pain

ANTICIPATED PROBLEMS/CONCERNS
- Air emboli with vascular access
- Dysrhythmia (5–10% if no prerepair dysrhythmia)
- Heart failure
- Heart block after CPB (rare)
- Sternal infection (rare)
- Endocarditis (rare)

AUTOIMMUNE DISEASE, COLD

Joseph L. Seltzer, M.D.

RISK

- Rare
- Autoimmune hemolytic anemias occur in 1 of 80,000 persons; of these, 17.3% are due to cold antibodies

PERIOPERATIVE RISKS

- Acute hemolysis due to cold
- Hemoglobinemia
- Hemoglobinuria
- Rarely, vascular occlusion

WORRY ABOUT

- Cooling to 28–31°C will cause hemolysis
- These temperatures can be reached in extremities in the OR or during cardiopulmonary bypass

OVERVIEW

- In two circumstances antibodies will react in the cold to produce hemolysis:
  – IgG antibodies associated with mononucleosis, *Mycoplasma* pneumonia
  – IgM antibodies are found in the idiopathic form of the disease and in lymphoproliferative disease
- Hemolysis usually occurs at temperatures below 31°C

ICD-9-CM Code: 283.0

ETIOLOGY

- Idiopathic
- Lymphoid malignancy
- Infections: *Mycoplasma* pneumonia, mononucleosis

USUAL TREATMENT

- Keep warm, folic acid
- For severe cases, chlorambucil or cyclophosphamide
- Plasmapheresis
- Prednisone

ASSESSMENT POINTS

SYSTEM	EFFECT	PE	TEST
HEME	Mild to moderate anemia	Hgb	Blood bank antiglobulin tests
GU	Hemoglobinuria		

Key Reference: Beebe DS, Bergen L, Palahniuk PJ: Anesthetic management of a patient with severe cold agglutinin hemolytic anemia utilizing forced air warming. Anesth Analg 1993; 76:1144–1146.

PERIOPERATIVE IMPLICATIONS

Perioperative Preparation

- Routine

Monitoring

- Temperature
- Urine output

Maintenance

- Keep warm, including extremities
  – Consider forced air warming
- Normothermic cardiopulmonary bypass
- No preferred agent or technique
- Consider hemodilutional autologous transfusion or other techniques to avoid homologous transfusion and formation of new antibody

ANTICIPATED PROBLEMS/CONCERNS

- Hemolysis if temperature falls
- Renal dysfunction due to hemoglobinuria

AUTONOMIC HYPERREFLEXIA

Maywin Liu, M.D.

RISK

- Those with spinal cord transection at T7 or above have a 65–85% risk of developing autonomic hyperreflexia (AH) following resolution of spinal shock
- Develops 2–3 wk after initial injury
- Risk with lower transections

PERIOPERATIVE RISKS

- Severe Htn and bradycardia with stimulation below level of transection. Placement of a Foley catheter a common trigger.
- Difficult airway due to possible unstable neck/limited mobility of cervical spine
- Muscle spasms during period of abd closure can cause evisceration of abd contents

WORRY ABOUT

- AH in postop period
- Severe bradycardia due to postop inability to void or defecate

OVERVIEW

- AH can cause severe Htn and bradycardia, which can lead to arrhythmias, pulmonary edema, CV collapse, cerebral hemorrhage, seizures, and death
- Common triggers are hot and cold stimuli, surgery, manipulation of hollow viscus, and labor (OB)
- Any stimulus below the level of transection can trigger AH
- Pathophysiology is unopposed reflex sympathetic activity. Normally sympathetic activity is modulated by inhibitory impulses from supraspinal centers. With a transected cord, inhibitory impulses cannot travel below the transection.

ICD-9-CM Code: 344.61

ETIOLOGY

- Most common cause is trauma
- Can also occur due to infectious or oncologic causes

USUAL TREATMENT

- Stop initiating stimulus, if possible
- Can ↓ or prevent by use of neuraxial blockade (spinal ≫ epidural)
- When signs of AH are evident, administer ganglionic blockers (trimethaphan), direct vasodilators (nitroprusside) or α-antagonists (phentolamine), or GA or spinal anesthesia
- Centrally acting hypotensive agents (e.g., clonidine) are *not* effective
- Tachyarrhythmias may be treated with β-blockers in combination with antihypertensives

ASSESSMENT POINTS

SYSTEM	EFFECT	ASSESSMENT BY HX	PE	TEST
HEENT	Possible difficult airway	C-spine trauma/surgery Hx difficult intubation	↓ C-spine ROM, ↓ mouth opening	C-spine x-ray
CV	May have orthostatic hypotension; may have baseline hypotension	Dizziness going to upright position	BP, orthostatic hypotension, tachycardia, bradycardia	ECG
RESP	↓ Resp reserve/vol Atelectasis, pneumonia, hypoxemia Impaired cough reflex, possible PE	SOB, pain on inspiration	Pain on palp ribs Tachypnea, cyanosis, ↓/unequal BS	CXR ABGs PFTs
GI	Possible full stomach from GI atonicity	Reflux complaints		
RENAL	Possible UTI, renal stones, renal failure		Chronic Foley cath	UA BUN/Cr
ENDO	May have ACTH deficiency			
CNS	Bowel and bladder dysfunction May have thermoregulation prb with high lesions, may have chronic pain, altered MS (with Hx of severe head trauma)	Incontinence on chronic opioids, NSAIDs, other drugs for pain	Hyperreflexic below level of transection Babinski's sign present	Temp
PNS	Insensate below level of transection, possible pain at level of transection		Sensory demarcation on sensory exam	
MS	Paralysis, muscle atrophy below level of transection, osteoporosis, muscle spasms Possible sacral decubiti	Paraplegia or quadriplegia	Muscle atrophy Sacral decubiti	

Key Reference: Amzallog M: Autonomic hyperreflexia. Int Clin Anesth 1993; 31:87–102.

PERIOPERATIVE IMPLICATIONS

Preoperative Preparation
- Assess adequate CV and pulm function, volume status
- Nifedipine can be used for prophylaxis, given 30 min prior to procedure likely to trigger AH

Monitoring
- Consider intra-arterial catheter
- Consider CVP/PA catheter if vol changes expected and if poor cardiac reserve present (esp with high lesions) and/or renal problems

Airway
- May require fiberoptic intubation

Induction
- Use nondepolarizing muscle relaxants. Succinylcholine can cause severe hyperkalemia, esp in injuries >6 mo old.
- Consider nitroprusside before induction

Maintenance
- GA with volatile agent may be better than N₂O/opioids for prevention/treatment of AH

Regional Anesthesia
- Anesthetic technique of choice if possible
- Spinal highly effective in preventing AH during surgery
- Difficult to assess height of neuraxial blockade due to sensory deficits below transection, resulting in either inadequate coverage to prevent AH or too-high block
- Use of epidural appears effective for preventing AH in laboring patients

Extubation
- May be difficult to extubate due to resp impairment with high transections

Adjuvants
- Require muscle relaxants with GA due to muscle spasticity

Postoperative Period
- AH can occur during recovery from anesthesia, esp if pt has distended bladder or rectum
- With severe Htn and difficulty awakening, consider possible cerebral bleed

ANTICIPATED PROBLEMS/CONCERNS

- AH can occur with placement of Foley cath
- Hyperkalemia with use of succinylcholine due to ↑ number of receptors in muscles below level of transection

AV AND BIFASCICULAR HEART BLOCK
John L. Atlee, M.D.

RISK

• Most acquired AV and bifascicular (BF) heart block (HB) is due to idiopathic fibrosis of the conducting system rather than to coronary heart disease. AVHB is also a complication of AV nodal ablation for supraventricular tachycardia.
• Prevalence of high-degree AVHB increases with age, with acquired complete (3°) AVHB most commonly appearing in the 7th decade of life and in males
• Congenital 3° AVHB occurs in 1:20,000–1:25,000 live births and more commonly in females

PERIOPERATIVE RISKS

• Circulatory compromise due to bradycardia and escape rhythms with advanced 2° and 3° AVHB
• Unlikely progression of lesser AVHB or BFHB to high-degree AVHB

WORRY ABOUT

• Status of associated CV disease, especially coronary, congenital, or other heart disease

• If patient has pacemaker, indication(s) for device and perioperative malfunction
• Adverse effects of chronotropic drugs used to treat bradycardia due to heart block

OVERVIEW

• Fascicular block: left anterior/posterior fascicles (LAFB, LPFB); right bundle branch block (RBBB)
• Bifascicular heart block (BFHB): LBBB or RBBB + LAFB or RBBB + LPFB
• No studies show ↑ risk of BFHB progressing to high-degree AVHB during surgery
• Anesthetic drugs may transiently increase ratio of dropped beats (6:5 → 4:3) with type I (Wenckebach) 2° AVHB
• Possibly, anesthetics or adjuvant drugs may slow or enhance instability of escape rhythms

ICD-9-CM Codes: 426.10 (AV heart block); 426.53 (bifascicular heart block)

ETIOLOGY

• 1°, 2°, and 3° AVHB occur in 9%, 5%, and 7% of patients with acute MI, respectively

• 3° AVHB develops in 12% of patients with inferior MI and 2% with anterior MI
• AVHB, usually only 1° AVHB, occasionally occurs with mitral valve prolapse. A few patients with aortic stenosis, and less frequently mitral stenosis or regurgitation, develop AVHB from extension of valvular calcification into the AV conducting system.
• Most patients with RBBB and LAFB, but without symptoms of bradycardia, do not acquire advanced degrees of AVHB. About 10% of patients with RBBB and LPFB develop high-degree AVHB.
• Patients with bundle branch and fascicular blocks develop complete AVHB during acute MI more frequently than do patients with normal intraventricular conduction (~40% with RBBB + LAFB or LPFB; ~18% with LPFB or RBBB (~12% with LBBB)

USUAL TREATMENT

• With disadvantageous bradycardia or escape rhythms, positive chronotropic drugs may be used as temporary measure to increase heart rate, although temporary or permanent pacing is definitive treatment

ASSESSMENT POINTS

SYSTEM	EFFECT	ASSESSMENT BY HX	PE	TEST
CV	Bradycardia, escape beats, or rhythms	Dizziness, syncope (2° rare, advanced 2° or 3° common), fatigue, weakness, lethargy, exercise intolerance, CHF, palpitations, angina rare with high 2° or 3° AVHB, mental status changes, no symptoms	Slow, full pulse with high-degree AVHB, S_1, and variation in pulse amplitude with variable atrial filling, cannon A waves	ECG, Holter monitor, His bundle ECG and programmed extrastimulation, exercise testing
	Heart disease	Angina, symptoms of CHF	Edema, ascites, liver enlargement, rales	ECHO, scintigraphy, MRI, coronary angiograms
	Pacemaker	Sx of arrhythmias suggest pacemaker malfunction	If inhibited, magnet or vagal maneuvers to ascertain function	Pacemaker system analyzer/programmer
RESP	COPD	Dyspnea, cough	Rhonchi, wheezes	CXR
GI	↓ Perfusion	GI distress, diarrhea		
RENAL	↓ Perfusion	Polyuria		BUN/Cr
CNS	Ischemia/stroke	Syncope, dementia, mental status changes, paralysis	Neurologic or mental deficits	Tilt table testing to R/O neurogenic (vasodepressor) component

Key Reference: Kastor JA: Arrhythmias, 2nd ed. Philadelphia, WB Saunders, 2000, pp 509–565.

PERIOPERATIVE IMPLICATIONS

Preoperative Preparation

• With AVHB-BFHB and symptomatic bradycardia, prophylactic perioperative pacing indicated
• BFHB without symptomatic bradycardia or acute MI not indication for temporary/permanent pacing
• For pacemaker patients, check function and inactivate or reprogram device if electrocautery to be used
• Transport of patient with temporary pacer: caution handling leads; have chronotropes available

Monitoring

• ECG and strip-chart recorder
• Consider direct arterial and PA catheter monitoring
• Arterial pulse waveform (oximetric, direct) if patient has permanent or temporary pacer

Induction/Maintenance/Extubation

• Have chronotropes available in case of unexpected bradycardia or pacemaker malfunction
• Be prepared for pacemaker malfunction (e.g., inappropriate inhibition or triggering of output) due to sensed electromagnetic interference (EMI) or myopotentials

Adjuvants

• Atropine has little effect on lower escape pacemakers; direct acting β-adrenergic agonists more reliable

Postoperative Period

• Check for proper pacemaker function following surgery or exposure to EMI

ANTICIPATED PROBLEMS/CONCERNS

• For patients with pacemakers: what is intended device function, does it function as intended, and what is potential for perioperative malfunction?
• Chronotropes used to treat bradycardia may be ineffective or cause paroxysmal tachycardia

BECKWITH-WIEDEMANN SYNDROME
Sandy Kaufmann, M.D.

RISK

- 1/13,700
- No association with race or gender

PERIOPERATIVE RISKS

- Difficult airway secondary to macroglossia
- Metabolic perturbations: hypoglycemia, polycythemia, hypocalcemia

WORRY ABOUT

- Persistent hypoglycemia: may exacerbate problems with mental capacity. Need to administer glucose infusion and check levels frequently
- Difficult airway
- High index of suspicion in those presenting with omphalocele
- May have impaired drug excretion

OVERVIEW

- Overgrowth syndrome characterized by macroglossia, macrosomia, omphalocele, visceromegaly, hemihypertrophy, characteristic earlobe creases, and pancreatic cell hypertrophy
- 50% born prematurely
- Association with multiple tumors: nephoblastoma, hepatoblastoma, neuroblastoma, adrenal cortical carcinoma, rhabdomyosarcoma, gonadoblastoma, and renal medulla dysplasia

ICD-9-CM Code: 759.89

ETIOLOGY

- Complex genetic inheritance
- Variety of mutations in chromosome 11p15.5 region
- Mutation near gene for IGF-II

USUAL TREATMENT

- Screen for tumors early in childhood
- Surgical resection of most operative tumors
- Surgical repair of omphalocele; possible partial glossectomy

ASSESSMENT POINTS

SYSTEM	EFFECT	ASSESSMENT BY HX	PE	TEST
HEENT	Macroglossia	Hx of difficult intubation	Determine extent by PE, previous anesthesia Hx	No testing
CV	VSD, ASD, cardiomegaly, TOF possible	SOB, DOE	Cardiac exam for murmurs	ECHO
ENDO	Assume hypoglycemia	Shaking		Glucose
RENAL	Renal medullary dysplasia	Hx of renal tumors/previous resections	Palpate for masses	BUN/Cr

Key Reference: Kim Y, Shibutani T, Itirota Y, Mahbub SF, Matsuura H: Anesthetic considerations of two sisters with Beckwith-Wiedemann syndrome. Anesth Prog 1996; 43:24–28.

PERIOPERATIVE IMPLICATIONS

Preparation

- Carefully review lab results for polycythemia, hypocalcemia, and hypoglycemia
- Review cardiac work-up if available

Monitoring

- Standard monitoring appropriate for surgical procedure
- Check glucose frequently

Airway

- Assume difficult airway
- Have appropriate staffing and equipment available
- Tube size should be age appropriate

Induction

- Care with oxygenation. Combination of low FRC, high oxygen consumption, and difficult airway may lead to desaturation quickly.

Extubation

- Be conservative with extubation criteria

ANTICIPATED PROBLEMS/CONCERNS

- Difficult airway
- Hypoglycemia

BILIRUBINEMIA OF THE NEWBORN

Paul D. Schanbacher, M.D.
M. Ramez Salem, M.D.

RISK

• 3–7% of newborns have physiologic jaundice
• Low birth weight, premature neonates, breast fed, maternal diabetes ↑ incidence
• East Asian, Native American, and population in some areas of Greece have ↑ bilirubin levels
• Perinatal events: delayed cord clamping, delivery by vacuum extraction/forceps, breech delivery, oxytocin, maternal bupivacaine analgesia, cephalohematoma, bruising, Rh/ABO incompatibility

PERIOPERATIVE RISKS

• Must consider pathophysiologic conditions present in premature or low birth weight infants, e.g., RDS, sepsis
• ↑ Risk for CNS injury with high levels of unconjugated bilirubin, e.g., >20–25 mg/dl or lower values in ill preterm neonate

WORRY ABOUT

• Factors that increase blood-brain barrier permeability to unconjugated bilirubin: hypoxia, hypercarbia, acidosis, hyperosmolality, Htn, seizure activity, sepsis
• Increasing free fraction of bilirubin from drugs, e.g., sulfonamides, moxalactam, radiocontrast dye
• Surgically induced increases in heme degradation, e.g., hematoma absorption
• Liver dysfunction
• Hemolytic anemia

OVERVIEW

• Unconjugated hyperbilirubinemia is a CNS toxin; however, kernicterus occurs in only a small fraction of hyperbilirubinemic neonates—usually in sick newborns
• Difficult to predict at what bilirubin level injury occurs or which newborn will suffer neurologic damage for a given bilirubin value
• Probable safe bilirubin level in the healthy, nonstressed, full-term neonate is <20 mg/dl in the first 48 h of life; after 48 h <25 mg/dl
• Probable safe bilirubin level for ≥1500-g healthy preterm neonate <15 g/dl for the first week of life
• Hemolysis and other co-existing illness lower threshold and above values for CNS toxicity
• Clinical features of hyperbilirubinemia are lethargy, anorexia, nausea, vomiting, icteric skin and sclerae
• Clinical features of kernicterus (very rare):
  – *Acute:* Opisthotonic posturing, muscle rigidity, seizure, oculogyric crisis
  – *Chronic:* Sensorineural hearing loss, choreoathetoid cerebral palsy, dysarthria, dysphagia, autonomic dysfunction, hyperactivity, ↓ intellectual development

ICD-9-CM Code: 774

ETIOLOGY

• Multifactorial: genetic, maternal, and perinatal events, inborn errors of metabolism
• Besides "physiologic jaundice," hemolytic disease, intestinal obstruction, and sepsis are common causes of unconjugated hyperbilirubinemia
• ↑ Bilirubin load, ↓ glucuronyltransferase activity, and ↑ enterohepatic circulation of bilirubin are common factors

USUAL TREATMENT

• Phototherapy for moderate hyperbilirubinemia
• Exchange blood transfusion for more severe levels of serum bilirubin (e.g., bilirubin concentration >20–25 mg/dl in a healthy full-term neonate; lower values for premature infants or infants with hemolysis, sepsis, and other co-existing illnesses and rapidly rising bilirubin levels)
• Heme oxygenase inhibitors and phenobarbital—rarely used

ASSESSMENT POINTS

SYSTEM	EFFECT	ASSESSMENT BY HX	PE	TEST
RESP	Pleural effusion, pulmonary edema possible in hydrops fetalis	Maternal prenatal history	Respiratory distress	CXR
HEME	Hemolysis	Rh/ABO maternal-fetal incompatibility	Anemia, possible hepatosplenomegaly, hyperbilirubinemia	Peripheral blood smear Direct Coombs' test Reticulocyte count
CNS	Bilirubin toxic to CNS cells	High levels of bilirubin	Abnormal posture, tonicity, and reflexes	

Key Reference: Avery GB: Neonatology, 5th ed. Philadelphia, JB Lippincott, 1999, pp 764–819.

PERIOPERATIVE IMPLICATIONS

Preoperative Preparation

• Active efforts to lower bilirubin levels
• Address co-existing disease states
• Consider atropine 0.1 mg IV to help prevent bradycardia

Monitoring

• Arterial blood sampling may be indicated

Airway

• Neonatal airway concerns

Induction

• Maintain normal hemodynamics

Maintenance

• No one agent or technique preferred
• Few data reflecting effects of anesthetic agents on bilirubin levels
• Adjust for FIO_2 to SaO_2 90–95%
• Supplemental glucose and calcium
• Maintain normothermia

Extubation

• Maintain intubation if infant ill or premature or for extensive surgical procedure

Adjuvants

• Chloral hydrate and pancuronium associated with hyperbilirubinemia
• Maternal epidural bupivacaine associated with neonatal jaundice

Postoperative Period

• Apnea/bradycardia possible
• Monitor bilirubin levels

ANTICIPATED PROBLEMS/CONCERNS

• Small, ill premature neonates with hyperbilirubinemia are at particular risk for kernicterus. Perioperative phototherapy and/or exchange blood transfusion needed to reduce bilirubin load.
• Dual concern: Avoid factors known to increase blood-brain barrier permeability, and treat associated neonatal diseases

BLEBS AND BULLAE

Jerome M. Klafta, M.D.

RISK

- Smokers with COPD
- Male predominance, 3:1

PERIOPERATIVE RISKS

- Concurrent COPD
- Pulmonary hypertension and RV failure

WORRY ABOUT

- Expiratory obstruction and air trapping
- Deadspace ventilation
- Expansion of bullae
- Rupture of bullae leading to tension pneumothorax

OVERVIEW

- Destruction of lung parenchyma with resultant formation of air-filled, thin-walled space within lung
- Walls of bullae may be connective tissue septa, compressed lung, or pleura
- "Bleb" connotes subpleural collection of air within layers of visceral pleura due to ruptured alveoli

ICD-9-CM Code: 492.0 (Emphysematous bleb)

ETIOLOGY

- Usually emphysematous in origin
- Minority familial and occur in younger patients
- Air cysts similar but have epithelial lining

USUAL TREATMENT

- Surgical resection of 1 or more bullae (bullectomy) done for ↑SOB or recurrent pneumothorax
- Bullectomy performed via thoracoscopic, thoracotomy, or median sternotomy approach and may involve laser ablation

ASSESSMENT POINTS

SYSTEM	EFFECT	ASSESSMENT BY HX	PE	TEST
CV	CAD, pulmonary hypertension, RV failure	Angina, DOE	Signs of RV failure (palpable PA, peripheral edema)	ECG, stress test, ECHO
RESP	Expiratory obstruction, air trapping V/Q mismatch Hypoxia, hypercarbia Pneumothorax	Exercise tolerance Cough	Pursed-lip breathing, tachypnea	CXR, ABGs, chest CT, V/Q scan
ENDO	Possible steroid use			Glucose
MS	Barrel-chested			

Key Reference: Benumof JL: Anesthesia for Thoracic Surgery, 2nd ed. Philadelphia, WB Saunders, 1995, pp 542–548.

PERIOPERATIVE IMPLICATIONS

Preoperative Preparation

- Control of bronchospasm
- Treatment of concurrent infection

Monitoring

- Consider arterial catheter (for frequent ABGs and rapid identification of hemodynamic embarrassment if tension pneumothorax develops)
- Consider precordial stethoscope over hemithorax at risk (if feasible)

Airway

- Double-lumen endotracheal tube extremely useful for differential treatment

Induction

- Keep airway pressures low
- Consider spontaneously breathing induction if Hx of pneumothorax

Maintenance

- Keep airway pressures low
- Have high index of suspicion for tension pneumothorax and plan for treatment (needle or tube thoracostomy)
- Avoid nitrous oxide, which can lead to expansion of poorly ventilated bullae
- Have contingency plan for development of bronchopleurocutaneous fistula: a pressure-cycled, high inspiratory flow ventilator (e.g., Siemens Servo 900C)
- Consider regional anesthetic, if feasible

Extubation

- May require postoperative ventilation
- Continued avoidance of high airway pressures ("fighting the ventilator")

ANTICIPATED PROBLEMS/CONCERNS

- Underlying lung disease with hypoxia, hypercarbia, dyspnea
- Rupture of bullae leading to bronchopleural fistula or tension pneumothorax

BLEOMYCIN SULFATE TOXICITY

Donald D. Mathes, M.D.
George S. Leisure, M.D.

RISK

• Pulmonary fibrosis from damaged alveolar pneumocytes, increased alveolar macrophage migration, and collagen synthesis
• Occurs in 11–30% of patients treated with bleomycin; may or may not be reversible
• Pulmonary toxicity increases with total dose >450 units, CrCl <35 ml/min, concurrent cyclophosphamide use, or prior or concurrent chest radiation therapy

PERIOPERATIVE RISKS

• Postoperative hypoxemia and potential lethal ARDS
• High perioperative risk if evidence of bleomycin pulmonary injury on PFTs or recent bleomycin exposure within 2 mo combined with hyperoxia exposure, vigorous fluid administration, or blood transfusions

WORRY ABOUT

• Development of interstitial pneumonitis leading to pulmonary fibrosis
• Perioperative exposure with >30% FIO_2
• Large amounts of fluid administration and blood transfusions are associated with postoperative ARDS
• Patients with evidence of bleomycin pulmonary damage clinically or on PFTs and/or recent exposure to bleomycin within 2 mo are particularly the subgroup at risk in the OR

OVERVIEW/PHARMACOLOGY

• Antitumor antibiotic isolated from the fungus *Streptomyces verticillus* used predominantly in germ cell tumors of the testes; squamous cell carcinoma of the head, neck, and esophagus; Hodgkin's and non-Hodgkin's lymphoma
• Often used in combination with myelotoxic chemotherapy agents because of its minimal myelotoxicity

• The enzyme bleomycin hydrolase inactivates bleomycin
• Lung and skin have the lowest level of bleomycin hydrolase and thus are the predominant sites of injury
• Cleared principally by renal excretion: Renal insufficiency with CrCl <35 ml/min leads to ↑ risk of toxicity

ICD-9-CM Code: E930.7 (Bleomycin—therapeutic)

ETIOLOGY

• Clinical symptoms of pulmonary toxicity such as dyspnea, tachypnea, and nonproductive cough can occur before significant changes occur on PFTs or CXR
• ↓ Carbon monoxide diffusion capacity (DLco) may be the earliest marker of pulmonary damage, followed by restrictive changes on spirometry

ASSESSMENT POINTS

SYSTEM	EFFECT	ASSESSMENT BY HX	PE	TESTS
RESP	Pulmonary fibrosis	Dyspnea Dry cough	Fine rales	↓ DLco, restrictive spirometry, ↓ O_2 sats, interstial thickening on CXR (may occur late in the disease process)
MUCOCUT	Skin tenderness, erythema, stomatitis, pruritus, alopecia			
HEME	Minimal bone marrow toxicity			

Key Reference: Mathes DD: Bleomycin and hyperoxia exposure in the operating room. Anesth Analg 1995; 81:624–629.

PERIOPERATIVE IMPLICATIONS

Preoperative Preparation

• Dyspnea, tachypnea, dry cough, or fine rales on auscultation should be evaluated prior to surgery
• Review most recent spirometry and DLco (these studies are done frequently during bleomycin administration)
• Any patient with abnormal pulmonary studies or who is clinically symptomatic should be considered high risk for postoperative hypoxia and ARDS
• Any recent exposure within 2 mo should be considered high risk

Intraoperative Management

• For those patients identified as high risk, limit FIO_2 exposure to <30% if possible and avoid excessive fluid or blood administration
• Consider use of PEEP to reduce FIO_2 and intravascular monitoring where larger fluid administration is expected

• Regional anesthesia may be preferred when appropriate to avoid administering hyperoxic inspired gases
• In high-risk patients in whom hyperoxia exposure is anticipated (i.e., 1 lung ventilation) pretreatment with corticosteroids (1 mg/kg prednisone) may be helpful in limiting postoperative ARDS. (No controlled study has been done to verify the benefits of corticosteroid pretreatment.)
• Restrict fluid administration in fashion appropriate to condition of patient and extent of surgery (hypotension might be treated with vasopressors rather than vigorous fluid administration)

Postoperative Period

• Verify adequate oxygenation on or near normoxic inspired gas
• Auscultate for rales

Postoperative Period

• Avoid excessive oxygen exposure
• For postoperative hypoxia, use PEEP or nasal CPAP to limit FIO_2 exposure; diurese if evidence of excessive lung water; and add methylprednisolone >1.0 mg/kg daily if developing ARDS
• Monitor O_2 saturation for a sustained period (12 h) if GA used

ANTICIPATED PROBLEMS/CONCERNS

• Association of postoperative hypoxia and ARDS with preoperative residual bleomycin pulmonary injury or recent exposure to bleomycin within 2 mo
• Inspired oxygen concentrations >30%, large amounts of fluid administration, and blood transfusions combined with preoperative bleomycin pulmonary injury or recent bleomycin exposure place patients at particular risk for postoperative hypoxia and ARDS

BLINDNESS

Stanley W. Stead, M.D.

RISK

• Eye injuries represent 3% of claims analyzed in the ASA Closed Claims Project
• Most common injury with GA is corneal abrasion, which is rarely associated with blindness
• Blindness can result from injury to the eye, its surrounding structures (eyelid and conjunctiva), blood supply, and optic nerve
• Injuries that may indirectly lead to blindness may involve the extraocular muscles and occipital lobe of the brain

PERIOPERATIVE RISKS

• Procedures associated with blindness:
  – Cardiopulmonary bypass
  – Neurosurgical procedures
  – Plastic surgery of the face
• Intraocular procedures, procedures around the eye, prone position with padding around the face and eyes, exophthalmos or ophthalmic nerve blocks
• 1.5% glycine irrigation during TURP and transurethral bladder procedures

WORRY ABOUT

• Pressure or contact with eye by foreign objects or solutions
• Positioning of patient, especially prone
• Posterior ischemic optic neuropathies secondary to prolonged hypotension
• Operations in physical proximity to the eyes
• During ophthalmic surgery:
  – Movement of patient under either MAC or GA during intraocular surgery
  – Trauma to optic nerve, retinal artery, or vein during orbital or sinus surgery
  – Coughing or substantial Valsalva maneuvers by patient following intraocular surgery
• During ophthalmic nerve block:
  – Perforation of globe
  – Trauma to the optic nerve, retinal artery, and vein

OVERVIEW

• Unless associated with glycine irrigating solution, blindness is an irreversible complication following anesthesia and surgery
• Blindness is most often associated with injury to the eye, its surrounding structures (eyelid and conjunctive), blood supply, and optic nerve

ICD-9-CM Codes: 369.00 (Acquired); 950.9 (Due to nerve injury); 368.12 (Transient)

ETIOLOGY

• Conditions that can result in blindness following anesthesia include
  – Corneal abrasion, vitreous loss, hemorrhage, movement of patient while operating upon or in the eye, chemical injury to the cornea or conjunctiva from cleaning materials on the anesthetic mask, spillage of prep solution into the eye, and direct trauma to the eye due to OR table padding, needle used in retrobulbar block, anesthetic mask pressure upon the globe or foreign body falling into eye. Additionally, prone position, hypoxemia following cardiac arrest, prolonged hypotension resulting in central retinal artery occlusion, increased intraocular pressure, and embolization, occlusion, thrombosis, or spasm of the retinal artery.
• Following absorption of glycine irrigating solution during TURP. Glycine distribution similar to that of γ-aminobutyric acid, an inhibitory neurotransmitter. Levels of glycine > 143 mg/L associated with transient blindness.

USUAL TREATMENT

• In the case of glycine, supportive treatment is indicated until plasma glycine levels < 143 mg/L. When actual blindness occurs from other causes, there is no treatment.

ASSESSMENT POINTS

SYSTEM	EFFECT	ASSESSMENT BY HX	PE	TEST
OVERALL	Retinal artery occlusion	Migraines Coagulopathies Hemoglobinopathies Oral contraceptives ↑ IOP		
HEENT	Ischemic retinopathy	Hypotension Hypoxemia Shock	Funduscopic: A normal retina but optic nerve head is swollen and ischemic	
	Orbital pressure		Funduscopic: An edematous retina with dilated arterioles and engorged veins	
GU	Transient blindness during or after TURP	TURP with glycine irrigating solution		Plasma glycine level (nml 13–17 mg/L)

Key Reference: Roth S, Thisted RA, Erickson JP, Black S, Schreider BD: Eye injuries after nonocular surgery: a study of 60,965 anesthetics from 1988 to 1992. Anesthesiology 1996; 85:1020–1027.

INTRAOPERATIVE MANAGEMENT

Monitoring

• Proper positioning essential
• If prone, adequate padding so no pressure transmitted to either globe or nasal bridge
• When face is completely draped, consider use of a metallic Fox shield to protect eye from inadvertent pressure

• In ophthalmic nerve blocks, needle does not enter globe or retinal artery, vein, or nerve. Avoid excessive volume of local anesthetic, which increases IOP and may compromise vascular supply of globe.

Airway

• Anesthetic masks may injure eye, either through inadequate drying and application of cleaning solution to eye or through direct pressure.

Surgical Stages

• Hypotension and hypoxemia implicated in cases of retinal artery occlusion.

Closure/Postoperative Considerations

• Protection of unoperated eye with the Fox shield is useful.
• When recovered in prone position, ensure that there is no pressure upon orbit or globe.

BOTULISM

Russell C. Raphaely, M.D.
Maureen M. O'Rourke, M.D.

RISK

- Infant botulism
  - Infants within USA: >1000 confirmed cases since first recognized as distinct clinical entity in 1976
  - Regional preponderance: California, Pennsylvania, Utah, and Hawaii
  - Gender predilection: none
  - Average age at onset of Sx: 3–4 mo

PERIOPERATIVE RISKS

- Autonomic dysfunction may cause hemodynamic instability
- Muscle weakness results in vulnerability to aspiration, pulmonary infection, and respiratory failure

WORRY ABOUT

- Autonomic dysfunction
- Gastroparesis
- Respiratory gas exchange

OVERVIEW

- Three forms: food-borne, wound, and infant
- Food-borne botulism intoxication results when improperly preserved food allows germination and toxin production by contaminating spores of *Clostridium botulinum;* consumption of food with preformed toxin results in absorption of potent neurotoxin; with education and control of food industries, food-borne botulism has been uncommon in USA in last 50 years
- Wound botulism, a rare entity, results when *C. botulinum* organisms contaminating traumatized tissue cause local infection and produce toxin that is absorbed
- Infant botulism is much more common; concepts described for infant botulism are referable to food-borne and wound forms
- Botulinum toxin binds irreversibly to synaptic membrane of cholinergic nerves and subsequently prevents release of acetylcholine

ICD-9-CM Code: 005.1

ETIOLOGY

- Infant: Ingestion of *C. botulinum* spores into intestinal tract that is transiently permissive to germination, subsequent colonization, elaboration of toxin, absorption into circulation, and delivery to acetylcholine receptors
- Food-borne: Consumption of preformed toxin with food
- Wound: Local infection with produced toxin causing symptoms after absorption

USUAL TREATMENT

- Nutritional support. Lactulose with glycerin suppositories for goal of daily defecation
- Insertion of artificial airway
- Mechanical ventilation
- Human botulism immune globulin (BIG)—www.infantbot.org

ASSESSMENT POINTS

SYSTEM	EFFECT	ASSESSMENT BY HX	PE	TEST
RESP	Pharyngeal constrictor and genioglossal hypotonia, paralysis of respiratory musculature	Drooling Poor feeding Decreased respiratory effort	Poor head control Absent gag	Negative inspiratory force; crying VC
	Infection	Increased secretions	Fever Rhonchi Rales	WBC CXR
	Atelectasis	Poor color	Cyanosis Tracheal secretions	SpO$_2$ CXR
GI	Constipation	No bowel movement Irritability	Palpable stool Abdominal distention	
RENAL	UTI	Foul-smelling urine		Urine culture
CNS	SIADH		Diminished urine flow	Serum/urine Na Serum/urine osmolality
	Seizures	Twitching Altered consciousness	Seizure activity	EEG
	Cranial neuropathies	Ptosis Expressionless face Feeble cry	Fixed and dilated pupils Facial palsy Poor cough and gag	
PNS	Spinal neuropathies	Limp limbs	Hypotonia	EMG

Key Reference: Wohl DL, Tucker JA: Infant botulism: considerations for airway management. Laryngoscope 1992; 102:1251–1254.

PERIOPERATIVE IMPLICATIONS

Preoperative Preparation

- Insert NG tube and apply vacuum to reduce retained gastric secretion volume
- Perform chest physical therapy
- Treat infection

Monitoring

- ECG, SpO$_2$, SAP

Airway

- Select appropriately sized uncuffed tracheal tube

- Monitor pressures at which gas escapes from between inner wall of airway and outer wall of gasway and change tracheal tube to obtain acceptable value (may reduce laryngeal injury)

Induction

- Expect variability in HR and BP
- Anticipate alveolar hypoventilation

Maintenance

- Recognize sensitivity to neuromuscular blockers and administer them guided by evoked motor response
- Differentiate between blood loss, anesthetic effect, and autonomic dysfunction as causes for hemodynamic abnormalities

Extubation

- Examine for genioglossal tone
- Assess gag and cough reflex
- Observe and test for sufficient respiratory muscle strength (inspiratory force and crying vital capacity)
- Consider peri-extubation steroids
- Employ aerosolized vasoconstrictor to control laryngeal swelling

ANTICIPATED PROBLEMS/CONCERNS

- Respiratory failure from airway obstruction, bellows muscle weakness, chemical or infectious pneumonia, and fluid overload, added neuromuscular dysfunction associated with aminoglycosides

BRAIN DEATH

Gwendolyn L. Boyd, M.D.

RISK

- People within USA: 29,000/y
- Potential organ donors 10–12,000
  - Lack of recognition by the hospital
  - Call Organ Procurement Organization (OPO) for all acute patients with Glasgow Coma Scale ≤ 5
- Cadaveric organ donors 5748 (1998 data)
- Racial distribution of organ donors
  - Caucasian   80%
  - African-American 15%
  - Hispanic   5%

PERIOPERATIVE RISKS

- Hemodynamically unstable
- Hypothermia
- Coagulopathy
- Diabetes insipidus
- Electrolyte imbalance

WORRY ABOUT

- Maintaining optimal organ function until procurement
- Ask for OPO assistance *prior* to approaching family for consent for organ donation

OVERVIEW

- Irreversible cessation of all functions of entire brain: including brainstem
- There must be no evidence of hypothermia or depressant drugs as known cause of death
- One factor in the failure of organ procurement is inadequate knowledge of the pathophysiology of brain death
- Donor management should be considered the beginning of organ preservation
- While the quality of organs from diseased donors should conform to that of the living, the pathophysiologic changes associated with brain death intervene

- Diagnosed by cerebral unresponsiveness, absence of motor activity and brainstem reflexes, absent cough after deep tracheal suctioning, no HR response to atropine (2 mg), no respiratory response on apnea testing (Pco_2 >60 mmHg), and electrical silence without hypothermia, metabolic encephalopathy, or depressant drugs

ICD-9-CM Code: 348.8

ETIOLOGY

- Massive intracranial trauma or primary CNS tumor
- Occurs when ICP exceeds systolic BP within 12–24 h of injury

USUAL TREATMENT

- Supportive until organ procurement

ASSESSMENT POINTS

SYSTEM	EFFECT	ASSESSMENT BY HX	PE	TEST
RESP	Neurogenic pulmonary edema Hypoxemia Infections DVT and pulmonary embolism		Rales	ABGs, CXR
CV	CNS ischemia response Hypovolemia Ventricular dysfunction Depletion of myocardial substrates Unstable vasomotor center Brain herniation Nonfunctional sympathetic system Lack of ADH	Need for inotrope support		BP Cardiac filling pressures Atropine resistance (2 mg) TEE for heart donors
HEME	Coagulopathy Anemia			Coagulation studies Hct
GU	Diabetes insipidus			UO >3 ml/kg/h Lytes SG <1.0005 Serum osmolality >310 mOsm
CNS	Lack of cerebral and brainstem function	Hx of drug ingestion, metabolic encephalopathy, and/or hypothermia excluded		Nonreaction of pupils to light Loss of corneal reflexes Oculocephalic or doll's eyes Oculovestibular Gag or cough absent Apnea to Pco_2 >60

Key Reference: Fitzgerald RD, Dechtyar I, Templ E, Fridrich P, Lackner FX: Cardiovascular and catecholamine response to surgery in brain-dead organ donors. Anaesthesia 1995; 50:388–392.

PERIOPERATIVE IMPLICATIONS

Monitoring
- Temperature
- A-line
- CVP or PA catheter
- UO
- ABGs for lung donors

Airway
- ETT already in place
- 5 cm H_2O PEEP

Maintenance
- Rule of 100s:
  - Pao_2 >100 mmHg

  - UO >100 ml/h
  - Systolic BP >100 mmHg
- Keep warm
- Hemodynamic states:
  - Keep dopamine <10 µg/kg/min
- Good blood volume
- Muscle relaxant to facilitate surgery
- Drugs per procurement team, e.g., heparin, chlorpromazine

Extubation
- Not done
- Ventilation discontinued when cross-clamp:
  - Ascending aorta for heart-lung donors

  - Descending aorta for liver-kidney donors above SMA and celiac artery

Adjuvants
- None

ANTICIPATED PROBLEMS/CONCERNS

- Expect an increase in BP and HR with incision—does not obviate criteria for brain death
- Knowledge of sequelae of brain death

BRONCHIECTASIS

H. Michael Marsh, M.B., B.S., B.Sc.(Med)

RISK

- People within USA: < 1/10,000 hospital admissions
- Gender prevalence: none
- Socioeconomic or ethnic prevalence: inbreeding and primitive health care, particularly lack of immunization and poor treatment of childhood bronchitides, increase the prevalence. Ciliary deformities have been shown in a Polynesian population.
- Occasionally seen in children:
  – Bronchial cartilage deficiency (Williams-Campbell syndrome)
  – Tracheobronchomegaly (Mounier-Kuhn's syndrome)
  – Inherited immunoglobulin deficiencies, impaired phagocytosis, complement deficiency
  – α_1-Antitrypsin deficiency
- Occasionally seen in adults with acquired γ-globulin deficiency:
  – Cystic fibrosis
  – Rheumatoid arthritis
  – Pulmonary ciliary dyskinesias (Kartagener's syndrome)

PERIOPERATIVE RISKS

- Spillage of infected secretions from bronchiectatic regions to normal lung → pneumonitis, retention of secretions
- Risk from bacteremia, after manipulation

- Risk of secondary acute respiratory failure
- Massive hemoptysis
- Pneumothorax

WORRY ABOUT

- Exacerbation of asthma
- Amount of sputum produced and its nature
- Fever, hemoptysis: acute pulmonary infection
- Right heart function
- Check frequency of cough and daily sputum volume; culture and smear for composition; check body temp and WBC count for acute infection
- Exercise tolerance will indicate associated impairment or disability. Right heart function may need assessment.

OVERVIEW

- Abnormal widening or dilatation of one or more branches of the bronchial tree. Widened segments commonly filled with purulent secretions; mucosa is swollen and inflamed and may be ulcerated with granulation tissue exposed. Extensive collateral flow occurs in these chronically inflamed bronchi (3–12% of CO).

ICD-9-CM Codes: 494; 748.61 (Congenital); 011.5 (Tuberculous)

ETIOLOGY/PATHOGENESIS

- Exact etiology for acquired form remains unclear but often involves necrotizing infection in tracheobronchial wall. Five mechanisms may predispose: (1) bacterial, viral, or fungal bronchopulmonary infections, including TB, pertussis, and measles; (2) bronchial obstruction; (3) immunodeficiency states, including IgG deficiency, IgA deficiency, and leukocyte dysfunction; (4) hereditary defects in ciliary-mucosal clearance, including Kartagener's syndrome, α_1-antitrypsin deficiency, and cystic fibrosis; and (5) miscellaneous disorders, including recurrent aspiration, inhaled irritants, Young's syndrome, and bronchiolitis obliterans following heart-lung transplantation.

USUAL TREATMENT

- Medical therapy—postural drainage, deep breathing and assisted coughing, antibiotics, bronchodilators, and fluids/humidity. Drainage of sinuses.
- Surgical therapy—resection indicated for uncontrolled hemoptysis; or lobar closely confined disease, age > 20 y. Bronchopulmonary lavage under GA with divided airway (double-lumen tube).

ASSESSMENT POINTS

SYSTEM	EFFECT	ASSESSMENT BY HX	PE	TEST
HEENT	Sinusitis	Postnasal drip Stuffiness, headache	Translucency	X-ray
CV	Clubbing, cyanosis CHF (cor pulmonale)	Exercise tolerance Pulm Htn, edema		ABGs Loud P_2 Right heart studies
	Kartagener's syndrome	Chronic sinusitis	Situs inversus	Immotile spermatozoa
RESP	Bronchiectasis	Cough, sputum	Rhonchi CXR—93% tram lines, 7% normal	Smear, culture, high-resolution CT, bronchogram
		Hemoptysis Wheezing		Bronchoscopy PFTs
HEME	Immunodeficiency Infection			IgG, IgA, WBC
CNS	Brain abscess			CT/MRI

Key Reference: O'Brien C, Guest PJ, Hill SL, Stockley RA; Physiological and radiological characterization of patients diagnosed with chronic obstructive pulmonary disease in primary care. Thorax 2000; 55:635–642.

PERIOPERATIVE IMPLICATIONS

Monitoring
- Routine: consider PA catheter for cor pulmonale or CHF

Airway
- Careful frequent suctioning and humidification of inspired gases

Induction
- Avoid asthma exacerbation
- Consider regional anesthesia when possible

Maintenance
- Routine

Extubation
- Depends upon degree of pulmonary and cardiac dysfunction

Adjuvants
- Routine

Postoperative Period
- Use stir-up regimen; monitor for retained secretions and respiratory failure

- Check for platypnea—orthodeoxia if right atrial pressures become elevated

ANTICIPATED PROBLEMS/CONCERNS

- Retained secretions, secondary respiratory failure
- Right heart decompensation if hypoxemia persists
- Bacteremia from airway manipulations

BRONCHIOLITIS OBLITERANS (BO)

William A. Lell, M.D.

RISK

- People within USA: 1/40,000
- Racial predilection: none

PERIOPERATIVE RISKS

- Hypoxemia
- Pulmonary infection

WORRY ABOUT

- Pulmonary dysfunction
- Pulmonary infection
- Steroid coverage
- Other effects of etiologic agents

OVERVIEW

- A nonspecific pulmonary inflammatory response affecting bronchiolar epithelium of small conducting airways and adjacent alveoli, sparing the interstitium
- Two histopathologic types: (1) the more common proliferative form—organized connective tissue proliferating into the respiratory bronchioles and alveoli resulting in a reversible, restrictive ventilation defect; (2) the rarer constrictive type—extensive scarring and fibrosis of the more proximal conductive bronchioles resulting in a permanent obstructive abnormality. It may result from longer exposure to a more intense etiologic agent.

ICD-9-CM Code: 491.8

ETIOLOGY

- Diverse agents can trigger the BO response, including
  – Inhalation: Toxic dusts, grains, gases (smoke inhalation, nitrogen dioxide from inhaled nitric oxide therapy)
  – Post infections: Viral (most common cause in children), mycoplasmal, bacterial
  – Connective tissue diseases: Virtually all, but rheumatoid arthritis in particular
  – Drugs: Amiodarone, cephalosporin, gold, free-base cocaine, many others
  – Post organ transplantation: Especially lung, heart-lung, bone marrow; possible liver, pancreas
  – Idiopathic: BO with cryptogenic organizing pneumonia (BOOP)

USUAL TREATMENT

- Varies with etiology and histopathology
- Mainly supportive with oxygen, chest physical therapy
- Steroids controversial (usually effective with BOOP and toxic fume inhalation)
- Bronchodilators usually ineffective
- Specific antibiotics for active infection

ASSESSMENT POINTS

Use classification above to determine possible cause of BO. Then look for other manifestations of underlying disease (e.g., impaired joint mobility in patient with BO due to rheumatoid arthritis). (See other Diseases.)

SYSTEM	EFFECT	ASSESSMENT BY HX	PE	TEST
GENERAL	Active infection	Fever	↑ Temperature, tachycardia	WBC
RESP	*Proliferative Type* Restrictive defect (common) *Constrictive Type* Obstructive defect (rare)	Progressive, dry cough with dyspnea	Dry, inspiratory rales Wheezes (more common with constrictive type)	CXR ABGs Spirometry V/Q scan Bronchoalveolar lavage Lung biopsy (for diagnosis)

Key Reference: Takahashi M, Murata K, Takazakura T, Nakahara T, Shimizu K, Minese M, Itoh H: Bronchiolar disease: spectrum and radiological findings. Eur J Radiol 2000; 35:15–29.

PERIOPERATIVE IMPLICATIONS

Preoperative Preparation

- Treat active infections
- Consider prophylactic antibiotics, supplemental O$_2$
- Premedication useful but avoid excessive resp depression
- Steroid coverage if indicated

Monitoring

- Routine
- Consider arterial catheter if oximetry inadequate

Airway

- Prevent additional mechanical obstruction
- Increase FIO$_2$
- Use aseptic tracheal suction technique

Induction

- Use short-acting agents to avoid prolonged CNS, resp depression

Maintenance

- Avoid fluid overload

Extubation

- Delay until adequate ventilation assured

Adjuvants

- Consider regional technique for anesthesia/perioperative analgesia

Postoperative Period

- Monitor for and aggressively treat resp depression and infection
- Continue steroids if indicated

ANTICIPATED PROBLEMS/CONCERNS

- Many patients with resting hypoxia come to OR for diagnostic lung biopsy. A thoracoscopic technique may be impossible owing to adhesions post heart/lung transplantation or inability to tolerate 1-lung anesthesia.
- Anticipate further perioperative resp decompensation after open-lung biopsy and treat aggressively

BRONCHITIS, CHRONIC

C. William Hanson III, M.D.

RISK

- People within USA: 8 million
- Race with highest prevalence: Caucasian
- Male:female ratio 2:1
- Smoking, occupational exposure to pulmonary toxic substances (radon, coal, asbestos)

PERIOPERATIVE RISKS

- Bronchospasm

WORRY ABOUT

- Airway stimulation at light levels of anesthesia
- Laryngospasm (due to secretions and hyperreactivity)
- Hypoxia
- Hypercarbia

OVERVIEW

- Chronic productive cough with periodic exacerbations
- Enlargement of the mucus-secreting glands in the airways with excessive sputum production
- Expiratory airways obstruction
- Derangement in V/Q relationships
- Chronic hypoxia with right heart failure
- Exacerbations with intercurrent bacterial or viral infections

ICD-9-CM Code: 491.9

ETIOLOGY

- Acquired, usually due to smoking
- May also be due to asthma or frequent childhood respiratory infections

USUAL TREATMENT

- Cessation of smoking (preferably >8–10 wk prior to elective surgery)
- Antibiotics for acute exacerbations; inefficacious for prophylactic treatment
- Glucocorticoids of uncertain benefit; trial appropriate in acute exacerbations
- Bronchodilators, when response can be demonstrated by changes in either PFT or Sx

ASSESSMENT POINTS

SYSTEM	EFFECT	ASSESSMENT BY HX	PE	TEST
HEENT			Short, fat neck	
CV	Right heart failure	Exercise tolerance	RV heave Dependent edema	ECG ECHO
	Pulmonary Htn			PA catheter
RESP	Airways obstruction	Smoking Hx (current, recent, remote) Number and severity of recent exacerbations	Cyanosis	PFT, DLco, ABGs
MS			Clubbing of fingers	

Key Reference: Mitchell CK, Smoger SH, Pfeifer MP, Vogel RL, Paudit MK, Donnelly PJ, Garrison RN, Rothschild MA: Multivariate analysis of factors associated with postoperative pulmonary complications following general elective surgery. Arch Surg 1998; 133:194–198.

PERIOPERATIVE IMPLICATIONS

Preoperative Preparation

- Smoking cessation
- Antibiotics to decrease sputum production
- Respiratory conditioning

Monitoring

- Consider arterial line to monitor blood gases
- Consider pulmonary artery catheter for large fluid shift operations

Airway

- Often, truncal obesity (especially with corticosteroids); may have redundant soft tissue in airway or short, fat neck

Preinduction/Induction

- Avoid stimulating the airway while in light levels of anesthesia; may precipitate bronchospasm (although less likely than with asthma)
- Regional anesthesia may be preferable

Maintenance

- Frequent suctioning of endotracheal tube
- Limit narcotic administration (danger of perioperative CO_2 retention)
- Adjuvant regional anesthesia for procedures that affect respiratory mechanics (e.g., intercostal nerve blocks, epidural analgesia)

Extubation

- Administer intratracheal bronchodilator in responsive patients prior to extubation
- Consider intravenous lidocaine prior to extubation

ANTICIPATED PROBLEMS/CONCERNS

- Postop respiratory complications (secretions, mucus plugging, atelectasis, pneumonia, prolonged requirement for mechanical ventilation)

BRONCHOPULMONARY DYSPLASIA (BPD) Mary A. Keyes, M.D.

RISK

• Severe resp distress at birth requiring prolonged mechanical ventilation and supplemental O_2
• Hyaline membrane disease (HMD) incidence inversely proportional to gestational age and weight (60–80% <28 wk, 15–30% between 32–36 wk, and rarely in term infants)
• Diabetic mothers, multiple gestations, C-section delivery, pulmonary infection with *Ureaplasma urealyticum,* asphyxia, and prior affected siblings

PERIOPERATIVE RISKS

• Cardiopulmonary abnormalities in the first years include ↑ airway reactivity, ↑ airway resistance, ↑ FRC; ↑ arterial Pco_2, ↓ arterial Po_2, right or left ventricular hypertrophy, and pulmonary and systemic Htn. Tracheomalacia and bronchomalacia may be present.
• Pulmonary function generally improves with age.

WORRY ABOUT

• Adequate oxygenation and ventilation during intraoperative period and transport (hand ventilation to assess changes in compliance)
• Endotracheal tube dislodgment
• Retinopathy of prematurity (ROP)
• ↑ Airway reactivity exacerbated by ETT
• Association between SIDS and BPD

OVERVIEW

• Chronic lung disease in premature infants treated for resp distress with mechanical ventilation
• Have characteristic CXR—almost complete opacification with air bronchograms or of small, lucent areas alternating with areas of irregular density
• Severe maldistribution of ventilation
• Prolonged mechanical ventilation, pulmonary Htn, cor pulmonale, and prolonged O_2 dependence are poor prognostic indicators
• Most common chronic lung disease in infants in USA

ICD-9-CM Code: 770.7

ETIOLOGY

• O_2 toxicity
• Barotrauma from PPV
• Genetic predisposition
• Inflammation
• Excessive fluid administration

USUAL TREATMENT

• Bronchodilators, including aerosolized β_2-adrenergic agents and theophylline
• Diuretics and fluid restriction as needed
• Steroids improve ability to wean from mechanical ventilation but increase risk of Htn and infection
• Nifedipine for infants with elevated PAP
• Prophylactic administration of human recombinant antioxidant enzymes

ASSESSMENT POINTS

SYSTEM	EFFECTS	ASSESSMENT BY HX	PE	TEST
CV	Cor pulmonale LV failure	Inability to wean from ventilator Poor feeding and weight gain Dyspnea in extubated infant	Tachypnea Sternal retractions Nasal flaring Hepatomegaly Cardiomegaly Pulmonary rales	CXR ± ECHO
RESP	↑ Airway reactivity ↑ FRC ↑ $Paco_2$ ↓ Pao_2	Inability to wean from supplemental O_2 or ventilator Poor feeding and weight gain Frequent URI associated with bronchospasm	Tachypnea Sternal retractions Nasal flaring Wheezing Rhonchi	CXR ABGs

Key Reference: Avery AB, Fletcher MA, MacDonald MG (eds): Neonatology, Pathophysiology and Management of the Newborn, 5th ed. Philadelphia, Lippincott Williams & Wilkins, 1999, pp 509–531.

PERIOPERATIVE IMPLICATIONS

Preoperative Preparation

• Optimal management of pulmonary and cardiac systems
• If URI, postpone all but life-and-death emergency surgery

Monitoring

• Routine
• ABG monitoring indicated if tenuous cardiac or pulmonary status or major surgery

Airway

• Routine

Preinduction/Induction

• Ensure adequate anesthetic depth (once the cycle of bronchospasm and desaturation has been initiated, it is difficult to recover)

Maintenance

• Routine

Extubation

• Awake with good respiratory pattern
• Postoperative apnea monitoring

Adjuvants

• Spinal anesthesia acceptable alternative in suitable procedures (avoiding endotracheal intubation may improve outcome)

ANTICIPATED PROBLEMS/CONCERNS

• Tenuous pulmonary status that is challenged during anesthesia and surgery
• Older child with Hx of BPD at risk for ↑ airway reactivity

BUERGER'S DISEASE: THROMBOANGIITIS OBLITERANS (TAO)

Richard F. Davis, M.D.

RISK

- People within USA: 8–10/100,000 Caucasian males aged <45 y but up to 90–100/100,000 in 1950s Mayo Clinic data of entire age range
- Peak age 25–40 y, before appearance of occlusive atherosclerotic disease
- Male:female, 10–100:1
- Racial predisposition: Most common among males of Eastern European, Jewish, Indian, and Asian heritage
- Ten-year survival rate from Dx is approximately ⅔ that for the general population

PERIOPERATIVE RISKS

- No clinical data describing perioperative risks

WORRY ABOUT

- Enhanced temperature-related vasoconstrictor responsiveness
- Concurrent pulmonary disease due to tobacco abuse
- Co-existent thrombophlebitis

OVERVIEW

- Clinical common denominator is distal extremity ischemia, including gangrenous changes
- Dx established only by histopathology showing active vascular inflammatory lesion
- Vascular lesions most common in peripheral arteries of upper and lower extremities
- Lesions may occur in mesenteric, coronary, and cerebral vasculature
- Pathologic lesion includes a highly cellular organizing luminal thrombus with a panangiitis including venous involvement
- Significant association with tobacco abuse
- Significant temperature sensitivity

ICD-9-CM Code: 443.1

ETIOLOGY

- Entirely unknown, although a dramatic association with tobacco abuse exists together with marked temperature-related vasoconstriction.

USUAL TREATMENT

- Treatment is palliative
- Pentoxifylline 400 mg tid or Ca^{2+}-channel blocker
- Steroids often offered to diminish an acute inflammatory exacerbation
- Debridement and/or amputation frequently necessary owing to gangrene

ASSESSMENT POINTS

SYSTEM	EFFECT	ASSESSMENT BY HX	PE	TEST
CV	Coronary lesions and resultant myocardial ischemia	Angina, MI, CHF		ECG; more advanced testing guided by Hx
RESP	Concomitant cold	Cough, dyspnea, sputum production	Distant BS, coarse rhonchi, expiratory flow rate (match test)	Obstructive pattern on PFT
GI	Mesenteric ischemia	"Intestinal" angina	Abdominal bruit	
HEME	Carbon monoxide producing carboxyhemoglobin	Smoking		Blood gases with co-oximetry
CNS	Extra- or intracranial vascular disease leading to CNS ischemia	TIA, reversible ischemic neurodefecit, syncope	Carotid bruit	Carotid US to assess severity if extracranial disease suspected
EXTREMITIES	Digital ischemia; gangrene	Pain; cold intolerance	Poor capillary refill; hair loss; poor pulses; skin tropic changes	Doppler, plethysmography, arteriography

Key Reference: Mills JL, Porter JM: Buerger's disease: a review and update. Semin Vasc Surg 1993; 6:14–23.

PERIOPERATIVE IMPLICATIONS

Monitoring
- Temperature control
- Positioning with pressure point padding

Airway
- Routine

Maintenance
- Maintain normothermia
- Maintain normal to high cardiac output
- Be wary of myocardial ischemia issues
- Regional anesthesia acceptable choice

Recovery
- Avoid vasoconstrictor stimuli (hypothermia, hypovolemia)

Adjuvants
- None of specific importance

ANTICIPATED PROBLEMS/CONCERNS

- Thrombophlebitis, gangrene, ulcerations
- Impaired pulmonary function

BULIMIA

Robert J. Rose, M.D.

RISK

• Affects 5–18% of adolescent girls and young women
• Bulimic symptoms can be part of anorexia nervosa syndrome

PERIOPERATIVE RISKS

• Increased risks (which have not been quantified) of hypotension, cardiac arrhythmias, hypothermia, and aspiration of gastric contents, and their consequences

WORRY ABOUT

• Reduced cardiac muscle mass with ↓ chamber size, impaired myocardial contractility with ↓ cardiac output, and relative hypotension
• Mitral valve prolapse and its arrhythmogenic effects
• Starvation, dehydration, hyponatremia, and hypokalemia
• Alterations (hypofunction) in autonomic nervous system function and a hypervagal state
• Abnormal temperature regulation
• ↓ Gastric emptying, gastric dilatation, aspiration of gastric contents, and gastric rupture
• Suicide

OVERVIEW

• Eating disorder characterized by binge-eating episodes followed by self-induced vomiting, fasting, and use of diuretics or laxatives
• Greatest perioperative risks are associated with low cardiac output and cardiac arrhythmias

• Hx is characterized by denial and is often unreliable

ICD-9-CM Codes: 783.6; 307.51
See also Anorexia Nervosa in Diseases section

ETIOLOGY

• Unknown; thought to be largely emotional

USUAL TREATMENT

• Tricyclic antidepressants and fluoxetine (Prozac) (60 mg q.a.m.) have been found effective in some patients

ASSESSMENT POINTS

SYSTEM	EFFECT	ASSESSMENT BY HX	PE	TEST
CV	Cardiomyopathy, mitral valve prolapse, arrhythmia, ipecac cardiomyopathy	Exercise intolerance, syncope	Heart sounds, BP, pulse	ECG, ECHO
GI	Gastric dilatation, diarrhea	Usually unreliable		Lytes
	Hepatic dysfunction Inanition			Hepatic enzymes Serum glucose
ENDO	Amenorrhea, "euthyroid sick," ↓ norepinephrine, ↓ vasopressin secretion, abn temp regulation	Cold intolerance		
HEME	Pancytopenia			CBC, plt
RENAL	↓ GFR on basis of dehydration			BUN/Cr
CNS	Depression, ↓ CSF norepinephrine			
MS	Muscle mass	Marked weight fluctuation	Thin	

Key Reference: Arnold AE, Rose RJ, Stoddard P: Intraoperative cardiac dysrhythmias in a patient with bulimic anorexia nervosa. Anesthesiology 1987; 67:1003–1005.

PERIOPERATIVE IMPLICATIONS

Perioperative Preparation

• Assess cardiac, lyte, volume status

Monitoring

• Routine
• Arrhythmia, volume status, myocardial function
• Temperature monitoring important

Airway

• May have ↑ risk of aspiration of gastric contents

Induction

• Hypovolemia, myocardial dysfunction, ANS dysfunction may make for CV instability

Maintenance

• CV instability, volume and lyte status, temperature should dictate anesthetic regimen

Extubation

• Awake due to GI motility dysfunction
• Autonomic hypofunction may lead to sudden postop collapse

Adjuvants

• Vary if lyte, renal, or hepatic dysfunction exists

ANTICIPATED PROBLEMS/CONCERNS

• Gastric volume changes may increase risk of aspiration
• Volume status, lyte, CV, and ANS changes increase risk of hypotension, arrhythmia, and sudden postoperative collapse
• Habitus and metabolic changes may predispose to hypothermia

BURN INJURY, CHEMICAL

Noel Lee Chun, M.D.

RISK

- >25,000 different chemicals can cause burns
- Compose ~10% of total burn population
- 85% of chemical burns are industrial and 75% occur in men 20–45 y from factories or labs
- USA Poison Control Centers report 15,000 caustic ingestions/y; 80% involve children, mostly <5 y
- Majority of adult caustic ingestions are suicidal gestures and more severe burns; majority of caustic ingestions in children are accidental and less severe burns

PERIOPERATIVE RISKS

- If involve ≤30% BSA, less problematic; if >40% BSA, hypotensive shock, lyte abn, sepsis, arrhythmias, myoglobinemia, ATN, and compartment syndromes can occur
- Serious ingestion burns can cause injury to entire aerodigestive tract, including oropharyngeal injury, esophageal/gastric perforation, aspiration, and ARDS
- 40% BSA burns have 40% mortality in 60–75 y (90% survival in <45 y)

WORRY ABOUT

- Significant number of patients do not present until many hours after injury
- Chemical burns often look deceptively benign, often having a smooth, suntanned appearance
- Extent cannot be assessed for 2–3 days. Immediate treatment is irrigation with large amounts of sterile saline to dilute and wash away the agent.

OVERVIEW

- The reaction of an acid or base with tissue liberates heat, damaging tissue
- Other agents injure by liquefaction necrosis (alkalis), delipidation (petroleum products), and vesicle formation (vesicant gases)
  - Mortality rare in <40% BSA burns and related to the extent of injury
  - Morbidity includes disfiguration and loss of function of tissue damaged, infection, loss of joint mobility due to scarring, and, particular to caustic ingestion, esophageal and gastric stricture/perforation

ICD-9-CM Codes: 949.0; 941 (Burn, face)

ETIOLOGY

- Majority fall into two categories: accidental skin burns at work usually involving the extremities; caustic ingestions, accidentally by children or as suicidal gesture by adults

USUAL TREATMENT

- Immediate care usually focuses on the burn (occasional large BSA burns treated like large thermal burns, i.e., fluid resuscitation 3–4 ml/kg/% BSA over 24 h). Irrigate with sterile saline for at least 30 min to dilute agent, and cleanse wound.
- Treat lyte abn, arrhythmias, ATN, ARDS
- Strict asepsis in dressing wounds, usually early debridement and tangential excision with flap reconstructions or skin grafting

ASSESSMENT POINTS

SYSTEM	EFFECT	ASSESSMENT BY HX	PE	TEST
HEENT	Chemical may burn eyes, oropharynx, trachea, esophagus, stomach	Consistent Hx, visual disturbances, dysarthria, dysphagia, chest/abdominal pain	Inspection for evidence of same, ocular analgesics, dye, slit-lamp exam	Early endoscopic exam; Contrast x-ray
CV	Hypotensive shock, arrhythmias, myocardial depression	Hx dyspnea/orthopnea, palpitations or chest pain	Chest exam	CXR; ECG; Electrolytes
RESP	Aspirated chemical, ARDS	Hx dyspnea/SOB, chest pain, mental status changes	Chest exam	CXR; ABGs
GI	Gastric, esophageal burns/perforation	Hx ingestion with chest or abdominal pain; Hematemesis	Pharyngeal, chest, and abdominal exam	Endoscopic exam, contrast x-rays
RENAL	ATN from myoglobin, hypotension	Hx massive tissue injury, prolonged hypotension	Oliguria–anuria	BUN/Cr; Cr clearance; Serum/urine myoglobin
EXTREMITIES	Compartment syndrome	Hx circumferential extremity burns	Weak pulses, neurologic deficits	Transduce compartment pressures

Key Reference: Carlotto RC, Peters WJ, Negligan PC, Douglas LG, Beeston J: Chemical burns. Can J Surg 1996; 39:205–211.

PERIOPERATIVE IMPLICATIONS

Preoperative Preparation
- Stabilize first
- Most common operative procedures are panendoscopy, escharotomies/fasciotomies emergently, and debridements with tangential excisions of eschar, flap reconstructions, and skin grafting procedures days and weeks later

Monitoring
- Attempt to minimize invasive lines to avoid sepsis; however, use whatever monitors necessary to manage patient's medical status; staple ECG leads on; staple pulse oximeter on

Airway
- If aerodigestive tract involvement, anticipate airway management problems and ARDS

Induction
- In more severely injured, considerations similar to those for thermal burns. Acute phase: anticipate homeostatic problems; electrolyte abn; hypovolemia. Chronic phase: scarring causing loss of function and positioning problems, infection, hyperkalemic response to succinylcholine, poor nutritional status, NMB resistance.

Maintenance
- Cardiorespiratory stability is important to avoid renal and other organ dysfunction
- Significant blood loss can occur with debridements
- Avoid hypothermia (warm room and all fluids—warm air heating)

Extubation
- Assess resp status carefully; if in doubt, monitor patient and reassess later

Adjuvants
- NMB: consider avoiding succinylcholine; resistant to NM blockers
- Inhalation: patient may be esp sensitive to depressant/arrhythmogenic effects of halothane

Postoperative Period
- Monitor cardiorespiratory status
- Heat loss in transfer to/from OR

ANTICIPATED PROBLEMS/CONCERNS
- Level of concern related to degree of injury
- Easy to underestimate extent of injury, esp early on, and undertreat these patients

BURN INJURY, ELECTRICAL

J.A. Jeevendra Martyn, M.D.

RISK

• About 1% of the 100,000 accidental deaths or approximately 3% of the 150,000 burns in USA are caused by electrical or natural lightning injury
• Low-voltage (< 1000 V) injury usually occurs in the household; high-voltage (> 1000 V) typically occurs in industry or in contact with high-tension wires

PERIOPERATIVE RISKS

• Immediate sequelae are momentary or prolonged unconsciousness, temporary paralysis (including quadriplegia), and autonomic disturbances (arterial spasm and pupillary abnormalities)
• Possible destruction of muscle or visceral tissues, pancreatitis, diabetes, gastric stress ulceration, coagulation abnormalities
• Possible fractures because of either intense muscle contraction or fall from height

WORRY ABOUT

• Injury to CNS, fractures, visceral injuries, pneumothorax, renal shutdown due to myoglobinemia and hemoglobinemia, and cardiac arrhythmias

OVERVIEW

• Injuries caused by either the current or its arc (flash burn). Burns can occur directly because of the flame or hot gases that are heated by the arc. Since electrical current chooses the shortest pathway between the contact points, any vital organs in its path will be damaged during its passage. Characteristic entry and exit wounds usually signal destruction of deeper tissues, severity of which cannot be predicted.
• Loss of vascular volume into damaged and undamaged tissue occurs
• Injury to underlying tissues may necessitate amputation, excision of large amounts of muscle, and release of deep fascial compartments

ICD-9-CM Code: 948

ETIOLOGY

• Heat produced is directly proportional to the resistance and the square of the current. Heat production, $J = I^2 \cdot RT$ where I is the current, R is the resistance, and T is the time of contact. Poor conductors of electricity develop heat when transmitting electrical energy. Thus, tissues such as the bone, which are poor conductors, damage the surrounding muscle owing to the heat developed.
• Skin and subcutaneous tissues, being better conductors, are damaged less severely, and such injury may not reflect organ/muscle damage

ASSESSMENT POINTS

SYSTEM	EFFECT	ASSESSMENT BY HX	PE	TEST
DERM	Burn injury, loss of intravascular volume, edema	↓ Urine ↓ BP	↑ Heart rate	CVP Tilt table test
CV	VFIB, tachycardia, or cardiac arrest initially; arrhythmias and conduction abnormalities, nonspecific ECG changes, myocardial rupture; blood loss due to visceral injury from fall	Hemodynamic instability ↓ Hct		↑ CK-myocardial bands > 4% Increases in CK-MB do not necessarily correlate with severity of cardiac damage
	Arterial or venous thrombosis, aneurysms, hemolysis	Will vary depending on site		Angiography
RESP	Pleural effusion, tracheobronchitis, bronchopleural fistula, pneumothorax			X-rays, scans
NEURO	Unconsciousness, coma, paralysis, cerebral hemorrhage, spinal paralysis, transverse myelitis, neuropathies	Will vary depending on type of injury		X-rays, CT, or MRI C-spine injury
RENAL	Oliguria, albuminuria, myoglobinuria, acute renal failure			Urine volume, urine myoglobin
GI	Nausea, vomiting, paralytic ileus, Curling's ulcer, perforated bowel, pancreatitis	Peritonitis		Blood sugar, exploratory laparotomy
INFECTIONS	Local and systemic, anaerobic and aerobic			
MS	Release of myoglobin and CK from muscle, fractures, or dislocation of bones			See above

Key Reference: Ge S, Yang Y, Bai G: Treatment of severe electrical burns. Ann N Y Acad Sci 1999; 888:60–74.

PERIOPERATIVE IMPLICATIONS

• Complications can occur acutely, during intermediate, and during late periods
• Scans or x-rays needed to exclude CNS or bone damage
• Measure UO because of high incidence of renal shutdown due to myoglobinuria
• Monitor sensorium for any deterioration in consciousness
• Continuous vigilance for evidence of perforation or visceral damage

• Monitor ECG if there is evidence for myocardial damage
• Therapy for Curling's ulcer
• Watch for direct injury to chest wall, pleural damage with hydrothorax, aspiration or pneumonia, or frank bronchial perforation and mediastinal compression
• Vascular damage to arteries and veins and evidence of thrombosis should be assessed

MANAGEMENT OF ELECTRICAL INJURIES

• Basic or advanced life support for cardiac or respiratory arrest
• IV fluids to maintain urine ≥ 1 ml/kg/h
• Furosemide and mannitol with alkalinization of urine may be indicated to maintain UO and prevent renal shutdown
• Therapy for cardiac and neurologic dysfunction may be necessary
• Monitor BUN, Hgb, blood gases
• Administer anticlostridrial prophylaxis, including penicillin
• Post-traumatic stress disorder of electrical injury has also been reported

BURN INJURY, FLAME

Wendy Stevens Howard, M.D.
Enrico Camporesi, M.D.

RISK

- >2.5 million/y in USA seek medical care for flame burn injury
- >100,000 require hospitalization
- Burn injuries are the second cause of accidental death, behind motor vehicle accidents
- High-risk groups include the young and the old

PERIOPERATIVE RISKS

- Mean burn size with 50% mortality ranges from 65–75% BSA
- Inhalation injury significantly increases mortality by 30–40%
- Burn eschar readily supports infection, leading to high mortality due to systemic sepsis
- Aggressive early excision and grafting after 48-h stabilization ↓ mortality

WORRY ABOUT

- Inadequate fluid resuscitation will leave significant hypovolemia

- Underlying medical condition (e.g., epilepsy, CVA), drug or alcohol overdose may have caused the burn
- Possibility of associated injuries (e.g., bone fractures, closed head injuries, spinal injuries, or blunt internal injuries)

OVERVIEW

- Cause loss of microvascular integrity with consequent ↑ capillary permeability, fluid accumulation, ↓ perfusion
- Generalized edema results; maximal losses occur in the first 8–12 h
- Deep burns can constrict an extremity or chest wall causing circulatory or ventilatory insufficiency
- Inhalation injury may be associated with massive pulmonary edema

ICD-9-CM Codes: 940–949 (948—burn classified by % body affected)

See also Carbon Monoxide (CO) Poisoning in Diseases section and Cyanide Toxicity in Diseases section

ETIOLOGY

- Hot liquid scalds, residential fires, ignition of clothing, and cigarettes

USUAL TREATMENT

- Initially as a multiple trauma patient with a thorough systematic evaluation; first priority given to airway, ventilation, and then circulation
- Large-bore IV access–ideally avoiding burnt skin
- Rule of nines for rapid assessment of BSA burnt
- IV fluid calculated with Parkland formula: 4 ml/kg/%burn in the first 24 h, half in first 8 h from time of injury (50% burn to 70 kg person — 14L/24h)
- Maintain warm environment and body temperature
- Better to intubate earlier than later when edematous

ASSESSMENT POINTS

SYSTEM	EFFECT	ASSESSMENT BY HX	PE	TEST
HEENT	Airway damage	Enclosed space Toxic fumes Dysphagia Lengthy exposure	Soot or burn to nose or mouth Stridor or cough	ABGs CXR Carboxyhemoglobin level
CV	Hypovolemic shock Ischemia	Burn extent Associated injuries May be asymptomatic	Hypotension	CVP PVR ECG
RESP	Lung injury	Inhalation injury	See HEENT	See HEENT
RENAL	↓ Renal perfusion	Hypovolemic shock Massive tissue injury	Decreased UO	Creatinine Myoglobinuria
CNS	Hypoxia	Inhalation injury	Altered LOC	ABGs Carboxyhemoglobin level
MS	Massive tissue injury	Burn extent	Myoglobinemia	

Key Reference: Schultz AM, Werba A, Wolrab C: Early cardiorespiratory patterns in severely burned patients with concomitant inhalation injury. Burns 1997; 23:421–425.

PERIOPERATIVE IMPLICATIONS

Preoperative Preparation

- Elevate room temperature
- Consider use of warming devices: blankets, fluid, ventilator
- Secure adequate venous access

Monitoring

- Routine monitors
- If anticipating large blood losses, consider CVP, arterial line (for repeated lab work), and UO measurement
- Consider PA catheter or TEE if underlying CV disease or hemodynamically unstable (sepsis or shock)
- Consider suturing or stapling ECG leads and oximeter probe to attachment sites

Airway

- Anticipate difficulty due to generalized body edema

Preinduction/Induction

- Hypermetabolic state with high cardiac output, high O_2 demand, ↑ CO_2 output, and low PVR
- May be hypovolemic or have unrecognized sepsis
- Low serum albumin and protein binding

Maintenance

- Replace fluid losses rapidly (both evaporation and blood losses)
- Liberally transfuse blood and consider albumin or other plasma volume expanders (e.g., Hespan)
- Avoid hypothermia
- Consider tourniquet to reduce blood loss

Extubation

- Consider postop intubation if large fluid losses or suspected airway edema
- High risk of pulmonary edema and respiratory distress

Adjuvants

- Often rapidly metabolize drugs or increase binding sites for nondepolarizing muscle relaxants
- High narcotic demands
- Avoid succinylcholine owing to possibility of ↑ K^+

ANTICIPATED PROBLEMS/CONCERNS

- Avoid succinylcholine. Massive tissue damage associated with excessive K^+ release and CV collapse. Significant for unknown time, possibly for 6 mo.
- Airway difficulty due to burn or to inhalation injury. At risk of pulmonary edema.
- Hypovolemia 2° to fluid loss from burn and generalized edema due to vascular permeability
- High blood levels of epinephrine with topical application used to reduce blood loss

CALCIUM DEFICIENCY/ HYPOCALCEMIA

Brian M. Block, M.D., Ph.D.

RISK

- Suspect in critically ill and malnourished patients, including alcoholics

PERIOPERATIVE RISKS

- Exacerbation secondary to anesthetic management

WORRY ABOUT

- Accentuated hypotension from anesthetic agents
- Bradydysrhythmias and long QT—associated dysrhythmias
- Postop respiratory failure/laryngospasm

OVERVIEW

- Chronic calcium (Ca^{2+}) deficiency in adults associated with disordered parathyroid hormone (PTH) or vitamin D function, malnutrition, and hyperphosphatemia
- Acute hypocalcemia can also be induced in the operating room by common anesthetic and surgical procedures
- Neonatal hypocalcemia observed in the first week of life, particularly in premature infants, infants born to diabetic mothers, and those after birth asphyxia

ICD-9-CM Code: 275.4

ETIOLOGY

Acute Hypocalcemia

- Alkalosis/hyperventilation: ↑ binding to albumin, ↓ ionized Ca^{2+}
- Transfusion of large amounts of citrated blood (>30 ml/kg/h), effects worsened by liver dysfunction, hypothermia
- Cardiopulmonary bypass
- Sepsis
- Thyroidectomy or parathyroidectomy
- Pancreatitis
- Hyperphosphatemia, when severe and acute; as seen in tumor lysis syndrome, hepatic failure, rhabdomyolysis, necrotizing fasciitis, trauma

Chronic Ca^{2+} Deficiency

- Malnutrition: may lead to actual calcium deficiency from lack of vitamin D and calcium intake or apparent hypocalcemia (with normal ionized calcium) from hypoalbuminemia
- Chronic renal failure, leads to hyperphosphatemia and defective vitamin D metabolism
- Vitamin D deficiency secondary to inadequate nutrition and sun exposure, malabsorption, anticonvulsant therapy (particularly Dilantin)

- Hypomagnesemia, seen with serum Mg^{2+} < 1 mg/dl
- Hypoparathyroidism, hereditary or acquired: hereditary hypoparathyroidism may be isolated or as part of a syndrome; acquired hypoparathyroidism is usually postparathyroidectomy
- Rickets
- Pseudohypoparathyroidism: hereditary, some forms associated with Albright's osteodystrophy

Neonatal

- Neonatal kidneys respond poorly to PTH, ↓ phosphate excretion → ↓ Ca^{2+}

USUAL TREATMENT

- Acutely: calcium gluconate or calcium chloride IV. 10% calcium gluconate has 94 mg elemental Ca^{2+}/10 ml while $CaCl_2$ has 272 mg/10 ml
- Correct any alkalosis
- Chronic: vitamin D and calcium supplementation, thiazide diuretics, restricted phosphate intake

ASSESSMENT POINTS

SYSTEM	EFFECT	ASSESSMENT BY HX	PE	TEST
CV	Long QT Hypotension Bradycardia	Syncope Palpitations	None BP HR	ECG Serum Ca^{2+}
PULM	Laryngospasm	Dyspnea	Stridor	Serum Ca^{2+}
NEURO	Neuromuscular irritability	Circumoral numbness Muscle cramps/tetany Seizures Chorea	Chvostek's sign Trousseau's sign Hyperactive reflexes	Serum Ca^{2+}
PSYCH	Anxiety Dementia Depression			Serum Ca^{2+}

Key Reference: Aguilera IM, Vaughn RS: Calcium and the anaesthetist. Anaesthesia 2000; 55:779–790.

PERIOPERATIVE IMPLICATIONS

Preoperative Preparation

- Check serum ionized Ca^{2+}, or total Ca^{2+} and total protein (corrected Ca^{2+} = measured Ca/(0.6 + [total protein/8.5]); normal total Ca^{2+} = 8.8–10.4 mg/dl, ionized = 1.13–1.32 mmol/L
- Correct underlying etiology if possible
- ↑Ca^{2+} and vitamin D supplementation
- Digitalis is less effective

Monitoring

- Ionized Ca^{2+} levels: line for blood sampling

- CV: ECG for ↑QT interval: consider A-line or PA catheterization if severe hypocalcemia and/or major procedure, given possible ↓ SVR and ↓ CO

Preinduction/Induction

- Beware ↓ BP and/or ↓ HR
- Thiobarbiturates may induce less hypotension than other agents
- Avoid hyperventilation and resulting alkalosis

Maintenance

- Potent inhalation agents have potentiated negative inotropic effects; consider turning off and giving Ca^{2+} if ↓ BP and/or ↓ HR occur

- Maintain normocapnia
- Consider giving Ca^{2+} if transfusing blood at >30 ml/kg/h. Maintain normothermia to maintain hepatic blood flow and citrate clearance.

Extubation

- Anticipate laryngospasm, treat with Ca^{2+} if it occurs
- Possible respiratory muscle weakness, potentiated muscle relaxation, reintubation

ANTICIPATED PROBLEMS/CONCERNS

- Hypotension/bradycardia
- Laryngospasm
- Respiratory muscle weakness

CANCER, BLADDER

William H. Rosenblatt, M.D.

RISK

- Primary risk factor is smoking
- Incidence 0.7/1000
- M:F 4:1, Caucasian > African-Americans
- Aged 60–85 y
- Quitting smoking decreases risk over time (normal in 5–8 y)

PERIOPERATIVE RISKS

- Risk varies based on surgical procedure and co-existing disease
- Chemotherapy: pulmonary fibrosis, renal and cardiac dysfunction
- Fatty infiltration of liver in those with poor nutritional status
- Protein-calorie malnutrition due to cancer, metabolism, and anorexia: anemia, hypoalbuminemia

WORRY ABOUT

- Significant blood loss
- Hyperextension of lumbar spine/pelvis and compression of iliac veins results in reduced venous return of blood volume
- Monitoring of UO difficult after ligation/division of ureters

OVERVIEW

- Transitional cell cancer generally systemic disease at time of Dx—60% will die of metastatic complications
- Patients are typically elderly with long Hx of smoking, thereby promoting concurrent disease: COPD, lung CA, atherosclerosis, angina, CAD, CHF, Htn
- Chemotherapy/radiation therapy may be used preoperatively, thus complicating perioperative period

ICD-9-CM Code: 188.9

ETIOLOGY

- Exposure to aromatic amines (arylamines): β-naphthylamine in cigarette smoke causes bladder cancer in mice
- Work-related exposure: β-naphthylamine and benzene in the manufacture of rubber products, arylamines in synthetic textile and hair dyes, paint pigments
- Drivers of diesel trucks
- "Slow acetylators" (homozygous, autosomal recessive) may be at higher risk—N-acetyltransferase may detoxify aromatic amines

USUAL TREATMENT

- Chemotherapy
  – Doxorubicin/bleomycin/cyclophosphamide/cisplatin/methotrexate; -5-fluorouracil/vinblastine/teniposide
- Radiation therapy
- Transurethral fulgeration
- Radical surgery

ASSESSMENT POINTS

SYSTEM	EFFECT	ASSESSMENT BY HX	PE	TEST
CV	Doxorubicin (Adriamycin) toxicity: cardiomyopathy	>550 mg/m^2, prior or concurrent mediastinal radiation therapy	CHF	Endomyocardial biopsy, serial ECHO; radionuclide angiography, DL$_{CO}$ ECG
	5-Fluorouracil: myocardial ischemia (rare)	Angina		ECG
	Cyclophosphamide: pericarditis with effusion	CHF	CHF	ECHO
RESP	Smoking-related injury	Cough, sputum, infections	Wheezes, rhonchi, barrel chest	CXR PFT
	Bleomycin or cyclophosphamide toxicity: pulmonary fibrosis	>500 mg (bleo), cough, dyspnea	Rales, fever	CXR
	Methotrexate: inflammation		Pulm edema, effusions, infiltrates	CXR
RENAL	Cisplatin: ATN	Occurs 3–5 days after course		BUN, Cr, proteinuria, hyperuricemia
	Methotrexate: renal failure			Hematuria, proteinuria
HEPATIC	Methotrexate: fibrosis			SGPT
CNS	Methotrexate: encephalopathy	Confusion, somnolence, ataxia, tremors, focal signs		

Key Reference: Whalley DG, Berrigan MJ: Anesthesia for radical prostatectomy, cystectomy, nephrectomy, pheochromocytoma, and laparoscopic procedures. Anesthesiol Clin North Am 2000; 18:899–917.

PREOPERATIVE IMPLICATIONS

Preoperative Preparation
- Rehydration after bowel prep

Monitoring
- Renal perfusion difficult to judge after division of ureters: consider CVP or PA catheter or TEE
- Consider aterial catheter

Anesthesia Technique
- Consider combined general-epidural anesthesia to treat postop incisional pain and reduce blood loss and fluid requirements for cystectomy

Induction
- May be volume depleted from bladder prep

Maintenance
- Avoid high concentrations of oxygen in pulmonary fibrosis
- Consider avoiding N$_2$O (bowel surgery)
- Maximize efforts to prevent hypothermia

Postoperative Considerations
- Consider overnight ventilation if long procedure, significant blood loss/fluid resuscitation. Epidural catheter can optimize pulmonary toilet and recovery.
- Fluid shifts occur during first 48 h
- EBL: TURBT, 200 ml; cystectomy, 500–1000 ml
- Pain score: 7–9 (cystectomy)

CANCER, BREAST

Vincent S. Cowell, M.D.

RISK

- Occurs predominantly in women: female > male, ~ 100:1
- 1 in 8 women develop breast cancer, most common cancer in USA for women
- Aging: About 77% of women with breast cancer are over age 50 y at time of diagnosis
- Racial predilection: Caucasians > African-Americans > Asians, Hispanics, and Native Americans
- African-Americans are more likely to die of breast cancer because their cancers are often diagnosed at an advanced stage
- 10% of breast cancer cases are directly due to inherited mutations of the BRCA1 and BRCA2 gene
- >80% of breast cancers are diagnosed in women with no family Hx
- ↑Risk: Family history among close blood relatives, personal history ↑ risk of developing a new cancer in the other breast
- Associated ↑ risk: Obesity and high-fat diets

PERIOPERATIVE RISKS

- Mortality very rare
- Lymphedema of arm following axillary node dissection
- Ipsilateral brachial plexus injury from extensive abduction of the arm
- Injury to long thoracic and/or thoracodorsal n. during surgical dissection of axilla

- Rare incidence of unrecognized pneumothorax
- Breast surgery is associated with postop N/V, incidence as high as 60%

WORRY ABOUT

- Systemic or regional impact of metastasis to lung, brain, or bones
- High incidence of postop N/V
- NMB and identification of major n.
- Access to an upper extremity may be restricted or limited
- Potential adverse effects of chemotherapeutic drugs and chest radiation therapy

OVERVIEW

- Abnormal growth of adenomatous tissue that results in systemic symptoms and metastasizes to liver, bone, lung, and brain
- Early detection of breast cancer ↑ time of survival
- Women >40 y benefit from screening mammography
- Physical examination and mammography are complementary
- Needle biopsies and incisional or excisional breast biopsy provides histologic Dx
- Presurgical needle localization may be necessary for nonpalpable lesions
- Most breast biopsies yield benign diagnosis

ICD-9-CM Code: 174

ETIOLOGY

- Cause of most breast cancers is still not known
- BRC genetic mutations

USUAL TREATMENT

- Noninvasive breast cancer: lumpectomy or partial mastectomy with sentinel node Bx and/or axillary node dissection with radiation and/or hormonal therapy (e.g., tamoxifen)
- Invasive breast cancer: total (with axillary node dissection) or modified radical mastectomy and poss radiation with chemotherapy and/or hormonal therapy (e.g., tamoxifen)
- Radical mastectomy rarely performed
- Reconstructive surgery integral part of management

PROGNOSIS

- An est 41,200 deaths (40,800 women, 400 men) in 2000; ranks 2nd among cancer deaths in women
- 5-y relative survival rates by stage at diagnosis: 96.3% localized, 76.6% regional, 21.3% distant, 52.5% unstaged

ASSESSMENT POINTS

SYSTEM	EFFECT	ASSESSMENT BY HX	PE	TEST
CHEST	Lung lesions	Nipple discharge Chest pain or discomfort	Breast asymmetry Nipple discharge, erythema, crusting, or erosion Nipple retraction Skin dimpling	Physical exam Mammography Fine-needle aspiration biopsy CXR
GI	Liver metastasis	Fatigue, abdominal pain	Enlarged or nodular liver	Liver US or CT scan
HEME	Bone metastasis	Lethargy, SOB	Anemia, pancytopenia	CBC
CNS	Brain metastasis	Change in mental status, seizures	Neurologic exam	Head CT
MS	Bone metastasis Pathologic fractures	Severe pain Immobility Arm swelling	Deformities Pain on palpation Axillary adenopathy	Bone scan X-rays Physical exam

Key Reference: http://cancernet.nci.gov/cancer_types/breast_cancer.shtml#tocO

PERIOPERATIVE IMPLICATIONS

Preoperative Preparation

- Optimal preop preparation, in response to associated anxiety, which can be achieved through both pharmacologic and nonpharmacologic means

Monitoring

- Routine with attention to placement of ECG leads
- IV site and BP cuff on contralateral arm

Airway

- Table arrangements may warrant a secure airway
- Nasal O_2 or LMA may be appropriate

Induction

- Thoracic epidurals, intercostal nerve blocks; and local infiltration have successfully been administered as primary anesthetics and adjuvants to GA

Maintenance

- Consideration for the high incidence of postop N/V
- Incision over operative breast that can also include axilla
- Dissection can include breast areolar tissue, muscle down to chest wall, and extension into axilla
- Identification of thoracodorsal and long thoracic n. often requires stimulation that contraindicates presence of NM blocking agents
- Surgical field will be in view and allow for monitoring of active blood loss
- Surgical team leaning on chest can affect ventilatory performance

CLOSURE/POSTOPERATIVE CONSIDERATIONS

- BL varies from minimal for breast biopsy to 500–1000 ml for radical procedure
- Pain score: 2–6
- Pain adequately managed with PCA or regional block
- Communicate with PACU that no venous "sticks" or BP measurements should be performed on arm of operative side when axillary lymph node dissection is involved

ANTICIPATED PROBLEMS/CONCERNS

- Anxiety associated with the fear of breast cancer and altered body image can be quite significant

CANCER, BRONCHIAL

John P. McCarren, M.D.

RISK

- 160,000 cases/y in USA
- Race with highest prevalence: ?
- Tobacco consumption is the major risk factor; males > females but this difference is decreasing as gender ratio of smokers of long duration is equalizing

PERIOPERATIVE RISKS

- Respiratory insufficiency from severe COPD or from lung resection

WORRY ABOUT

- Endobronchial obstruction: obstructive pneumonitis, consolidation, atelectasis, or localized air trapping
- Metastasis: brain, bone, adrenal glands, pericardium, pleural

- Paraneoplastic syndromes: Cushing's, SIADH, hypercalcemia, neuromuscular (Eaton-Lambert, neuropathy, myelopathy, polymyositis), hematologic (migratory thrombophlebitis, marantic endocarditis, DIC)

OVERVIEW

- Malignancy of squamous cell, adenocarcinoma, large cell, and small cell types.
- Leading cause of cancer deaths in USA for both men and women, with an overall 1-y survival of 20% and a 5-y survival of 8%
- Cigarette smoking major risk factor for both lung cancer and COPD; hence, high incidence of COPD in patients with lung cancer
- Severe COPD affects perioperative management and may limit lung resection
- Paraneoplastic syndromes are rarely manifested

ICD-9-CM Code: 162.9

ETIOLOGY

- 85% related to cigarette smoking, 24% excess risk from passive smoking; asbestos, radiation, heavy metal exposure, genetics contributing factors

USUAL TREATMENT

- Surgical resection of localized disease for non–small cell carcinoma
- Chemotherapy, radiation therapy for small cell carcinoma
- Unresectable endobronchial or endotracheal tumors treated with external beam radiation and/or bronchoscopic laser resection

ASSESSMENT POINTS

SYSTEM	EFFECT	ASSESSMENT BY HX	PE	TEST
HEENT	Possible tracheal fixation or obstruction by tumor	Dyspnea, cough, rhonchi	Poor air flow SOB	PFT CXR
CV	Pericardial effusion SVC syndrome	Dyspnea, cough	Dilated neck veins and facial swelling	ECHO CXR
RESP	Lung mass, airway consolidation and atelectasis, pleural effusion	Dyspnea, cough, feverish	Rhonchi Fever Dullness to percussion	CXR ABGs DLco
GI	Rarely pancreatitis from hypercalcemia	Anorexia, nausea, vomiting, constipation		Serum Ca^{2+}
CNS	Brain metastasis	Headache, visual changes, unsteady gait, sensory or motor symptoms	Funduscopic or neurologic findings	
	Paraneoplastic syndrome	Optic neuritis, subacute cerebellar degeneration, peripheral neuropathy		
	Superior sulcus tumor (Pancoast tumor)	Upper extremity pain, Horner's syndrome		
MS	Bone metastasis Eaton-Lambert syndrome Polymyositis with activity	Bone pain Fatigue and weakness Muscle soreness	Bone tenderness Decreased DTRs Improved strength	

Key Reference: Carr DT, Holoye PY, Hong WK: Bronchogenic carcinoma. *In* Murray J, Nadel J (eds): Textbook of Respiratory Medicine. Philadelphia, WB Saunders, 1994, pp 1528–1596.

PERIOPERATIVE IMPLICATIONS

Preoperative Preparation

- Adequate hydration, correction of electrolyte abnormalities, bronchodilators for bronchospasm, antimicrobials if infected, steroid coverage for adrenal insufficiency, if present
- Instruction in incentive spirometry

Monitoring

- Consider arterial line for lung resections

Airway

- Determine need for left- or right-sided double-lumen ETT

Preinduction/Induction

- Bronchodilators when appropriate
- Judicious use of neuromuscular blockers if Eaton-Lambert syndrome

Maintenance

- No one agent or technique is superior
  - Halogenated agents decrease bronchomotor tone and permit high FIO_2 but minimally decrease HPV
- CPAP and PEEP as needed

Extubation

- Change to single-lumen ETT if will remain intubated

Adjuvants

- Consider bronchodilators

Postoperative Period

- Consider epidural catheter for pain management

ANTICIPATED PROBLEMS/CONCERNS

- Potentially life-threatening postop problems include bronchial disruptions, cardiac herniation, tension pneumothorax, cardiac dysrhythmias
- Adequate analgesia beneficial if severe COPD

CANCER, ESOPHAGEAL

Dawn P. Desiderio, M.D.
Anne C. Kolker, M.D.

RISK

- People within USA: 6 in 100,000 men, 1.6 in 100,000 women
- African-Americans three times greater incidence than Caucasians
- Increased in patients with tobacco abuse, excessive alcoholic intake

PERIOPERATIVE RISKS

- Reflux as a risk for aspiration
- Malnutrition with dehydration due to swallowing dysfunction
- 30% 30-day serious morbidity and 1–3+% 30-day operative mortality

WORRY ABOUT

- Pulmonary compromise due to either chronic aspiration or extensive tobacco history

- Hydration status
- Airway protection at time of anesthesia induction and postop
- Alcohol withdrawal syndromes

OVERVIEW

- Primarily either squamous cell from esophageal squamous epithelium or adenocarcinomas of gastric origin
- Usually 55 to 65 y, with a long-standing Hx of tobacco and alcohol intake
- Dysphagia and weight loss are initial symptoms, often present for 3–4 mo
- Characterized by extensive local growth and lymphatic involvement before becoming widely disseminated

ICD-9-CM Code: 150.9

ETIOLOGY

- Achalasia of 25 y or longer, tobacco use, excessive alcohol intake, lack of aspirin use are associated with an increased incidence of squamous cell cancer
- Reflux esophagitis (Barrett's esophagus) is associated with adenocarcinoma
- Nutritional factors and ingestion of hot liquids have been implicated

USUAL TREATMENT

- Treatment depends on extent of disease and patient's medical status
- Surgery with or without chemotherapy the only possibly curative option
- Patients who are unacceptable surgical risks or with advanced disease may benefit from radiation
- Palliative placement of an internal esophageal stent allows for swallowing of liquids and secretions

ASSESSMENT POINTS

SYSTEM	EFFECT	ASSESSMENT BY HX	PE	TEST
CV	Alcohol abuse–induced cardiomyopathy	DOE Exercise tolerance		ECG ECHO
RESP	Tobacco abuse Chronic aspiration Radiation/chemotherapy	Pneumonias; RV Htn Cough, dyspnea Sputum	Wheezing RV heave	CXR PFTs, diffusion capacity ABGs
GI	Obstruction Reflux Malnutrition	Difficulty swallowing Unable to sleep flat Weight loss	Debilitated	UGI Endoscopy
CNS	Alcohol abuse Delirium tremens	Last alcohol ingestion and amount		
MS	Weakness	Poor nutrition	Muscle wasting	Serum albumin
RENAL	Dehydration	Limited intake		Lytes, Cr, BUN

Key Reference: Baue AE (ed): Glenn's Thoracic and Cardiovascular Surgery. Norwalk, CT, Appleton & Lange, 1991, pp 767–827.

PEROPERATIVE IMPLICATIONS

Preoperative Preparation

- Premedication not to obtund a patient at risk for aspiration
- Antisialagogue (atropine 0.4 mg or glycopyrrolate 0.2 mg)
- Premedication with H_2 blocker for acid aspiration prophylaxis plus metoclopramide to promote gastric emptying
- Steroids given if recently used

Monitoring

- Central venous or PA catheter placement for volume assessment and replacement, and for volume loading prior to surgical compression of the mediastinal structures
- Arterial line for BP monitoring and ABGs

Airway

- Rapid-sequence induction or awake fiberoptic intubation
- The surgical need for one-lung ventilation if thoracoabdominal approach requires a double-lumen endotracheal tube, a bronchial blocker, or a Univent tube and proper positioning

Induction

- Hypovolemia often results in BP fluctuation
- Aspiration risk during intubation

Maintenance

- No one agent or technique shown superior
- Volume requirements due to mediastinal compression, blood loss, and initial dehydration status
- Oxygenation concerns during one-lung ventilation, the use of 100% O_2 and chemotherapy Hx (bleomycin, mitomycin), prior pulmonary compromise due to tobacco history
- Hypothermia of concern in long procedures
- Placement of nasogastric tube with surgical guidance

Extubation

- Continuing risk of aspiration
- Extubation after postop ventilation to allow for prior resp problems to be resolved and adequate pain control
- Patients with double-lumen endotracheal tubes in place should be reintubated or bronchial blockers pulled back (Univent) or removed

- Reintubation difficult because of edema and fluid shifts. With solid paralysis and pharyngeal suctioning, double-lumen tube withdrawn under direct vision and replaced with a styletted single-lumen tube.
- In difficult patients, a tube exchanger (Cook Airway Exchanger Catheter 5mm) can be inserted in the tracheal lumen, the double-lumen tube withdrawn, and a single-lumen tube threaded

Adjuvants

- Patients who have received chemotherapy (mitomycin or bleomycin) might be administered an O_2 concentration of 28% or as low as possible (see Bleomycin in Drugs section)

Postoperative Period

- Epidural analgesia may be beneficial

ANTICIPATED PROBLEMS/CONCERNS

- Airway management: aspiration risk, reintubation problems, extubation criteria
- Volume status in a dehydrated patient undergoing a lengthy surgical procedure with mediastinal compression

CANCER, LUNG PARENCHYMA
Roger A. Moore, M.D.

RISK
- 172,000 new cases/y
  - 75 deaths/100,000 males/y
  - 30 deaths/100,000 females/y
  - Asbestos exposure increases risk 5-fold
  - Smoking increases risk 15-fold
- Radon exposure—50% increased risk

PERIOPERATIVE RISKS
- Associated coronary artery disease
- Pulmonary insufficiency following lung tissue resection

WORRY ABOUT
- Optimization of preop pulmonary status
- Myasthenic syndrome (Eaton-Lambert) with oat cell carcinoma
- Massive hemoptysis with cancer invasion of bronchial arteries
- Active pneumonia in pulmonary parenchyma distal to obstructed bronchioles

OVERVIEW
- Four primary types of lung cancers: (1) epidermoid or bronchogenic; (2) adenocarcinoma; (3) alveolar cell carcinoma; (4) undifferentiated carcinoma (large cell, small cell [oat cell])
- Oat cell metastasizes early
- 70% with COPD need extra postop pulmonary care
- Patients often nutritionally depleted
- Many have alcohol abuse history
- Preop pulmonary state may limit option of lobectomy
- Hormonal imbalances common
  - 3% of patients are cushingoid
  - 70% of bronchogenic carcinomas have increased ACTH or pro-ACTH
  - Up to 60% with lung cancer have inappropriate ADH
- Myasthenic syndrome occurs owing to decreased release of nerve-ending acetylcholine → increased sensitivity to *all* muscle relaxants

ICD-9-CM Code: 162.9

ETIOLOGY
- Environmental factor important (i.e., smoking, asbestos exposure, radon exposure)
- Higher incidence in areas located near oil refineries

USUAL TREATMENT
- Oat cell cancer frequently treated with radiation and chemotherapy (need good renal function)
- Lobectomy or pneumonectomy common approaches in other types of lung cancers; DL_{CO} of <60% predicts 75% mortality; >100% predicts 100% survival

ASSESSMENT POINTS

SYSTEM	EFFECT	ASSESSMENT BY HX	PE	TEST
CV	Myocardial ischemia	Angina SOB	S_3 gallop	Exercise stress test
	Arrhythmia	Palpitations	Irregular pulse	ECG
	Cor pulmonale	SOB	Distended neck veins	Catheterization ECHO
RESP	Pneumonia	Productive cough	Rhonchi—rales	CXR
	Bronchospasm	Wheezing	Wheezes	PFTs: MBC; MMEFR; DL_{CO}
	COPD	SOB, dyspnea	Decreased BS	ABGs
ENDO	SIADH	Lethargy, ↑ weight, ↓ urine Thin skin; poor wound healing	Hypometabolic	Electrolytes Elevated urine sodium (rarely needed)
	↑ ACTH	Weight gain; striae	Cushingoid; ↑ BP	Cortisone level (rarely needed)
NM	Eaton-Lambert (myasthenic)	↓ Muscle weakness	↓ Muscle strength with exercise	EMG (rarely needed)
NUTRITION	Wasting	Weight loss	Cachexia; BMI change	Liver function tests (esp albumin)
	DTs	Alcohol abuse	↑ Liver size	

Key Reference: Ferguson MK, Little L, Rizzo L, Popovich KJ, Glonek GF, Leff A, Manjoney D, Little AG: Diffusing capacity predicts morbidity and mortality after pulmonary resection. J Thorac Cardiovasc Surg 1988; 96:894–900.

PERIOPERATIVE IMPLICATIONS

Preoperative Preparation
- Respiratory optimization with bronchodilatation, antibiotics, pulmonary hygiene, and smoking cessation
- Correction of lyte imbalances

Monitoring
- Routine monitors
- Intra-arterial line and possible pulmonary catheter
- Neuromuscular blockade monitor

Airway
- Double-lumen tube needed—usually left-sided
- Fiberoptic bronchoscope available

Induction
- Anesthetic choice dependent on associated medical problems
- Light premedication to decrease CO_2 retention
- When right-sided double-lumen tube used, ensure right upper lobe ventilation (easiest with fiberoptic bronchoscope)

Maintenance
- Nerve damage with lateral position
  - Use axillary roll
  - Brachial plexus injury with arm hyperextension
  - Pad all pressure points
- Substantiate pulse oximetric and capnographic readings with ABGs
- If oxygen saturation falls during one-lung ventilation, PEEP on dependent lung may help. If not, CPAP on nondependent lung may help.

Extubation
- At end of procedure, double-lumen tube should be switched to single-lumen tube
- Extubation should be determined by adequacy of respiratory variables

Adjuvants
- Bronchodilators for intraoperative use, inotropes for myocardial depression, antiarrhythmics for post—lobectomy-pneumonectomy arrhythmias (some advocate prophylactic digoxin—but conflicting reported results)

Postoperative Period
- Adequate pain management usual for recovery of pulmonary function
  - PCA effective
  - Thoracic epidural most efficacious
- Be watchful for DTs, inappropriate ADH, and ↓ neuromuscular strength

ANTICIPATED PROBLEMS/CONCERNS
- Intensive pulmonary toilet postoperatively
- Careful suctioning of bronchial stump because of possibility of rupture
- Bronchopleural fistula or tension pneumothorax should be anticipated

CANCER, PROSTATE

RISK

- The second leading cause of cancer death in men after lung cancer
- Use of prostate-specific antigen (PSA) led to an increase in earlier-stage detection
- The incidence increases with age; more than 75% of cancers diagnosed are in men older than age 65

PERIOPERATIVE RISKS

- Perioperative mortality for radical prostatectomy is 0.3%
- Complications of radical retropubic prostatectomy include excessive blood loss, rectal laceration, ureteral injury, wound infection, DVT, pulmonary embolus, anastomotic leak, myocardial infarction, and later lymphocele, incontinence, impotence, and anastomotic stricture
- Radical perineal prostatectomy is for patients with well to moderately differentiated prostate cancer. Less blood loss, less postop discomfort. But patients with large prostates, narrow inferior pubic rami angles, or significant hip problems are not good candidates for this approach.

WORRY ABOUT

- Increased prevalence of age-related, multiple concomitant diseases and a decline in basic organ function in these elderly men
- Perioperative complications

OVERVIEW

- Localized disease—rarely causes symptoms
- Locally advanced or metastatic disease—obstructive voiding and irritative voiding symptoms, bone pain
- TNM classification and Whitmore-Jewett classification are the most commonly used clinical staging classification systems. The most prominent grading system is Gleason Scoring System.
- Early Dx by the triad of (1) digital rectal exam, (2) serum PSA, and (3) transrectal ultrasound (TRUS)–guided prostate biopsies
- Heterogeneous tumors (usually acinar adenocarcinomas) composed of hormone-sensitive and hormone-insensitive cells

ICD-9-CM Code: 185

ETIOLOGY

- Genetic predisposition, hormonal influences, dietary and environmental carcinogenic influences, infectious agents

USUAL TREATMENT

- Quality-of-life issues and co-morbid condition help to guide treatment choices
- Watchful waiting—especially if other diseases present or age >70 y with moderately differentiated, low-volume cancer, and a life expectancy of fewer than 10 y
- Radical prostatectomy (retropubically or perineally)—in selected patients with clinically confined prostate cancer, usually for those <70 y. Rate of radical prostatectomy has increased over past decade because of PSA screening and development of nerve-sparing technique to reduce sexual impotence.
- Radiation therapy—external-beam radiotherapy or interstitial radioactive seed implantation
- Hormonal therapy—for locally advanced or metastatic cancer: (1) estrogens, (2) bilateral orchiectomy, (3) LH-RH agonists, (4) anti-androgens, (5) combined androgen blockade
- Others—cytotoxic chemotherapy; cryosurgery

ASSESSMENT POINTS

SYSTEM	EFFECT	ASSESSMENT BY HX	PE	TEST
RESP	Age-related changes			CXR
CV	Age-related changes	Exercise tolerance		ECG
HEME	In advanced stages: anemia, azotemia, uremia		Anemia in extensive metastases	Serum PSA ↑; serum acid phosphatase ↑ in 75% of pts with bone metastases
GU	Early—asymptomatic; Late stages—hesitancy, intermittency, urgency, frequency, retention, infection, impotence, hematospermia	Pathologic finding in prostate tissue in TURP for BPH	Rock-hard nodule on digital rectal exam	Digital rectal exam; TRUS-guided biopsy
METAB	Malnutrition	Malaise	Wt loss in extensive metastases	
CNS	Metastases to spine		Neurologic deficits in lower limbs	
MS	Metastases to spine	Bone pain (commonly in lumbosacral area)	Pathologic fracture (uncommon)	Radionuclide bone scans

Key Reference: Hahnfeld LE, Moon TD: Prostate cancer. Med Clin North Am 1999; 83:1231–1245.

PERIOPERATIVE IMPLICATIONS

Preoperative Preparation

- Use of Allen stirrups
- Leg pumps or compression stockings or low-dose Coumadin to reduce DVT
- Autologous blood donation, although some question cost-effectiveness

Anesthetic Technique

- General, epidural, or spinal for radical prostatectomy
- Consider patient's concomitant diseases, position on the operating table, intraoperative blood loss, and possible thromboembolic events in choosing anesthetic technique
- Consider hemodilution

Monitoring

- Consider arterial line
- Consider CVP and/or PA catheter for expected excessive blood loss and/or severe co-existing disease

Adjuvants

- Increased risk of adverse drug effects in elderly patients
- Hormonal therapy causes abnormal liver metabolism

ANTICIPATED PROBLEMS/CONCERNS

- Air embolism from prostatic fossa during surgery in Trendelenburg position
- Intraoperative hemorrhage—especially with retropubic approach

- In radical prostatectomy—injury to obturator nerve, ureter, or rectum; immediate postop DVT and pulmonary embolism; symptomatic pelvic lymphocele; wound or urinary tract infections; perioperative main CV complications—MI and postop arrhythmias; long-term surgical complications—incontinence and impotence
- For nonprostate surgery—worry about effects of chemotherapeutic agents, hormones, or radiation on hematologic, liver, renal, and vascular systems

CANDIDIASIS

James M. Sonner, M.D.
Jeffrey A. Katz, M.D.

RISK

- Current or recent broad-spectrum antibiotic treatment
- Immunosuppression (e.g., AIDS, neutropenia, drugs)
- Breach of epithelial barriers (e.g., by surgery, indwelling catheters, burns)
- Lengthy critical illness
- IV hyperalimentation
- Incidence: There were 3.8 fungal infections per 1000 hospital discharges in 1990. *Candida* accounts for about 3% of all nosocomial infections.

PERIOPERATIVE RISKS

- Increased mortality (>50%) with candidemia
- Sequelae of sepsis

WORRY ABOUT

- Metastatic disease to brain, heart, lung, liver, kidney, bone may be involved with corresponding organ dysfunction
- Side effects of amphotericin treatment: hypotension, fever, azotemia, hypokalemia, emesis, thrombophlebitis
- Septic shock

OVERVIEW

- Clinical spectrum ranges from mild mucosal overgrowth of organisms to life-threatening disseminated infection. The former is easier to diagnose and treat; the latter, much more difficult.
- Any organ can be affected. Mucosal surfaces are usually overgrown but may be invaded with microabscess formation and fungemia. *Candida* in solid organs reflects abscesses from disseminated disease.

ICD-9-CM Code: 112.5 (Systemic)

ETIOLOGY

- Fungal infection due to *Candida* species. Disease occurs when normally commensal yeasts overgrow tissues that they colonize, e.g., thrush, or when *Candida* invades tissues (e.g., abscess).
- Infection facilitated by disruption of mucocutaneous barriers, immunosuppression, and following antibiotic treatment (kills bacterial flora that normally check *Candida* growth)

USUAL TREATMENT

- PO nystatin, clotrimazole, or ketoconazole for oral or esophageal candidiasis
- Topical antifungals for vaginal or cutaneous candidiasis
- IV amphotericin B for systemic candidiasis; fluconazole (fungistatic) for mild to moderate infection or refractory disease; IV flucytosine added for persistent or metastatic fungemia or septic shock
- IV and arterial catheters removed or replaced for candidemia
- Surgical excision for infected prostheses, endocarditis, thrombophlebitis
- Fluconazole in selected cases
- Amphotericin bladder irrigation for urinary bladder infections

ASSESSMENT POINTS

SYSTEM	EFFECT	ASSESSMENT BY HX	PE	TEST
HEENT	Endophthalmitis Thrush	↓ Visual acuity Dysphagia	Cottonball lesions on funduscopy White plaque in oropharynx	
CV	Endocarditis Myocardial invasion Shock		Murmur, hypotension Fever	ECHO ECG CVP, PCWP, CO
RESP	Pneumonia ARDS	Dyspnea, cough Cyanosis	Signs of consolidation not uniformly present	CXR
GI	Esophagitis Enteritis Peritonitis Intra-abdominal abscess	Dysphagia Abdominal pain	Hepatomegaly Splenomegaly Peritoneal signs Ileus	Endoscopy LFTs CT or MRI
RENAL	Bladder infection Kidney abscess	Urinary frequency Dysuria	Costovertebral tenderness	Urinalysis BUN/Cr, CT
CNS	Meningitis Brain abscess	Altered mental status	Altered mental status Meningeal signs	Lumbar puncture CT or MRI
MS	Osteomyelitis	Pain over bone	Tender over bone	X-ray, bone scan

Key Reference: McNeil MM, Lasker BA, Lott TJ, Jarvis WR: Postsurgical *Candida albicans* associated with an extrinsically contaminated intravenous anesthetic agent. J Clin Microbiol 1999; 37:1398–1403.

PERIOPERATIVE IMPLICATIONS

Preoperative Preparation
- Continue antifungal therapy
- Assess for presence of septic shock, impaired gas exchange, neurologic or cardiac involvement
- Check K+, Cr if on amphotericin therapy
- Determine age of IV lines for possible changing in OR

Monitoring
- If septic shock is present, close monitoring of cardiac filling pressures, arterial pressure, ABGs, UO is required.

Airway
- None

Preinduction/Induction
- If sepsis is present ↑ risk of hypotension 2° to hypovolemia and myocardial depression
- With pulmonary involvement, rapid oxygen desaturation may occur

Maintenance
- Hypotension may be present because of sepsis and may be worsened by superimposing negative inotropic or vasodilating agents

Extubation
- Respiratory function can be compromised by pulmonary candidiasis or ARDS; may require postop ventilatory support

Adjuvants
- Depends on organ damage from disease or its treatment; often ↓ renal function and modification of anesthetic and neuromuscular blockers due to this organ impairment

ANTICIPATED PROBLEMS/CONCERNS
- Fever and hypotension are associated with candidemia and its treatment; mortality is high
- Septic shock or multiple organ involvement may be present

CARBON MONOXIDE (CO) POISONING

Peter H. Breen, M.D., F.R.C.P.C.
Richard E. Moon, M.D.
Bryant W. Stolp, M.D., Ph.D.

RISK

- Most frequent toxic gas in smoke
- Major cause of death
- CO produced by all internal combustion engines, incomplete oxidative combustion (e.g., house fires, charcoal and gas grills, malfunctioning butane/propane stoves), and endogenous sources (e.g., by liver from exogenous exposure to paint stripper)
- During GA, use semiclosed circuits, esp when machine has not been used for 2–3 days
- No odor, taste, or color; nonirritating
- Toxicity potentiated by low inspired O_2 concentration (e.g., smoke inhalation)
- In carbon dioxide absorbers of anesthesia machines (esp on Monday mornings)

PERIOPERATIVE RISKS

- Main target organs: heart and brain
- Heart: can resemble ischemia; potentiated by CAD
- Brain: acute loss of consciousness; after initial improvement, up to 30% risk of secondary syndrome: chronic psychiatric dysfunction and cerebral and cerebellar syndromes

WORRY ABOUT

- Seek other smoke inhalation injury
- Consider concomitant cyanide poisoning that potentiates CO toxicity
- Be alert for CO poisoning in donor for organ transplantation

OVERVIEW

- CO, a colorless nonirritating and odorless gas, is a natural byproduct of combustion
- CO binds avidly to Hgb ($> 200 \times O_2$) to form carboxyhemoglobin (COHb), which carries no O_2 and causes left shift in oxyhemoglobin dissociation curve ($\downarrow O_2$ off-loading to tissues)
- CO binds to intracellular hemoproteins such as myoglobin and cytochrome aa_3 (especially cardiac) to inhibit O_2 uptake and metabolism
- "Classic" cherry-red complexion rarely observed
- COHb level correlates poorly with clinical condition
- Treatment should be guided by symptoms and signs, not by blood COHb concentration

ICD-9-CM Code: 986

ETIOLOGY

- CO produced by incomplete oxidative combustion (e.g., house fires, malfunctioning butane/propane stoves, home heaters, and all internal combustion engines)
- Suicide attempts

USUAL TREATMENT

- Normobaric oxygen: $T_{1/2}$ of COHb decreases from 3.5 h (air-breathing) to 0.75 h (O_2-breathing)
- General supportive care, especially for other aspects of smoke inhalation injury
- Hyperbaric O_2 (2.5 atm) $\downarrow$ COHb $T_{1/2}$ to 20 min and has been shown to $\downarrow$ probability of development of delayed neurologic complication; for patients with neurologic Sx (including impaired consciousness), evidence of myocardial ischemia, fetal distress (if pregnant), poisoning in pediatric patient, or other Sx of significant exposure (e.g., COHb $>25\%$), hyperbaric O_2 is recommended if feasible, within 6–8 h of exposure

ASSESSMENT POINTS

SYSTEM	EFFECT	ASSESSMENT BY HX	PE	TEST
HEENT	Thermal/toxic upper airway injury	Fire exposure/ smoke inhalation	Perioral burns Airway edema	Laryngoscopy/ bronchoscopy
RESP	CO diffuses rapidly into blood → COHb Thermal/toxic airway and parenchymal injury	Dyspnea, tachypnea	Bronchoconstriction and pulm edema	Co-oximetric COHb: Po_2 usually normal CXR Bronchoscopy
CV	$\downarrow$ Blood O_2 content and $\downarrow$ tissue O_2 unloading	Possibly angina or evidence of heart failure; tachycardia	Cardiac failure	ECG: ischemic ST-T changes; CXR
METAB	Tissue hypoxia → acidosis			Lactic acidosis
CNS	Coma, cerebral edema	Temporal headache, N/V, restlessness	Muscle weakness, altered mental status	Abnormal neuropsychometric testing
	Neuropsychiatric syndrome	Cerebral, cerebellar		Can occur after initial recovery

Key Reference: Breen PH, Isserles SA, Westley J, Roizen MF, Taitelman UZ: Combined carbon monoxide and cyanide poisoning: a place for treatment? Anesth Analg 1995; 80:671–677.

PERIOPERATIVE IMPLICATIONS

Preoperative Preparation
- Continuous 100% O_2
- Document CNS status
- Consider hyperbaric O_2 if mental status altered or patient has myocardial ischemia or is pregnant

Monitoring
- Routine monitors
- Pulse oximetry (SpO_2) unreliable in presence of COHb (SpO_2 overestimates oxyhemoglobin)
- Arterial cannula for frequent blood sampling
- Venous and arterial COHb levels are almost identical

Airway
- Airway injury and edema often occur during smoke inhalation → may require emergent airway management

Induction
- Avoid cardiac depressant agents

Maintenance
- 100% O_2 (no N_2O)
- Assess muscle weakness to guide muscle relaxant dosage

Extubation
- Ensure CNS status permits natural airway maintenance and protection

Adjuvants
- Consider treatment for concomitant cyanide poisoning (see under Cyanide Poisoning in Diseases section)

Postoperative Period
- Maintain 100% O_2
- Consider hyperbaric O_2

ANTICIPATED PROBLEMS/CONCERNS

- Heart and brain affected most
- Follow CNS function carefully
- Seek concomitant smoke inhalation injury and cyanide toxicity
- CO toxic in trace quantities (breathing 0.1% inspired CO for 1 h results in significant toxicity, with COHb ~ 30%); CO not detectable with conventional gas analysis instruments (e.g., capnographs, mass spectrometers)
- Pulse oximeters do not specifically measure COHb, and O_2 sat readings are only minimally affected, even by severe CO poisoning

CARCINOID SYNDROME

Stanley H. Rosenbaum, M.D.

RISK

- Most common GI endocrine tumor
- 15 cases/1 million population per year

PERIOPERATIVE RISKS

- Associated with patient's ability to tolerate abrupt hemodynamic change and/or bronchospasm

WORRY ABOUT

- Abrupt hypertension or hypotension with stress
- Right-sided valvular heart disease
- Bronchospasm

OVERVIEW

- Endocrinologically active tumor from GI mucosa
- May release histamine-like substances leading to hypotension and bronchospasm, or may release serotonin leading to hypertensive reactions (and hypovolemia)
- Commonly in ileum (especially appendix) or rectum, less so in pancreas and lung
- Systemically active when metastatic to liver, or when released substances avoid metabolism by liver (carcinoid syndrome)

ICD-9-CM Codes: 199.1 (Tumor); 259.2 (Syndrome)

ETIOLOGY

- Acquired disease
- May be associated with other ectopic humoral tumors, such as MEN I syndrome

USUAL TREATMENT

- Surgery or arterial embolization to reduce tumor burden
- Histaminic effects blocked only partially by H_1 and H_2 blockers
- Serotonin synthesis blocked by parachlorophylalamine and effects blocked by ketanserin
- Octreotide blocks humoral release
- No specific medical Rx for established valvular heart lesions
- Catecholamines may ↑ humoral release and worsen symptoms

ASSESSMENT POINTS

SYSTEM	EFFECT	ASSESSMENT BY HX	PE	TEST
HEENT	Cutaneous flushing, lacrimation Pellagra-like skin lesions	Episodic flushing induced by stress, eating, alcohol consumption	Hyperkeratosis, hyperpigmentation	
CV	Histamine-induced hypotension Serotonin-induced Htn Endomyocardial fibrosis, especially in right heart	Sx of right-sided CHF	Murmurs of pulmonic stenosis, tricuspid regurgitation Ascites, edema	Echocardiogram Cardiac catheterization
RESP	Bronchospasm Endobronchial tumor with obstruction	Episodic asthma poorly responsive to medication Focal wheeze at site of obstructing tumor	Wheezing associated with episodes of flushing	
GI	Diarrhea Obstructing tumor	Episodic watery diarrhea		Bowel films Hepatic CT, ultrasound, angiograms
ENDO	Serotonin secretion			Urinary 5–HIAA levels elevated in most patients Occasionally need to measure plasma histamine
RENAL	Dehydration from chronic vasospasm or diarrhea			BUN/Cr, electrolytes
CNS	Hemodynamic instability, vasodilation	Hypertensive headache Syncope with flushing		
MS	Cutaneous flushing, lacrimation Pellagra-like skin lesions	Episodic flushing, induced by stress, eating, alcohol consumption	Hyperkeratosis, hyperpigmentation	

Key Reference: Buckley FP. *In* Barash PG, Cullen BF, Stoelting RK (eds): Clinical Anesthesia, 3rd ed. Philadelphia, Lippincott Raven, 1992, pp 986–987.

PERIOPERATIVE IMPLICATIONS

Preoperative Preparation

- Assess adequacy of fluid balance
- Assess right-sided valvular status
- Somatostatin analogue (octreotide) available; its use has dramatically decreased hazards of anesthesia for patients with carcinoid syndrome

Monitoring

- Expect rapid fluctuation of BP
- Central venous pressures may not correlate well with fluid volumes

Airway

- Risk of stress-induced wheezing (Rx: somatostatin analogue)

Induction

- Chronic vasoconstriction and diarrhea may cause hemodynamic instability

Maintenance

- Volume assessments complicated by changing vascular tone
- Cardiac function limited by right-sided valvular lesions

Extubation

- Possible stress-induced hemodynamic instability (Rx: somatostatin analogue)

Adjuvants

- Caution! Catecholamines may increase humoral release and worsen symptoms
- Somatostatin analogue for hypo- or hypertension or bronchospasm has dramatically ↓ anesthesia risk for pts with carcinoid syndrome

Postoperative Period

- Humoral effects of hemodynamically active metastatic carcinoid usually not eliminated by surgery

CARDIOMYOPATHY, ALCOHOLIC

Gregory H. Botz, M.D.
Jonathan B. Mark, M.D.

RISK

- People within USA: 15 to 20 million chronic heavy ethanol users
- As much as 50% of dilated cardiomyopathy may be ethanol related
- Population at risk: unclear; likely includes chronic ethanol users with at least 5 oz daily ETOH for at least 5 y
- Gender: male predominance

PERIOPERATIVE RISKS

- Alcohol withdrawal
- CHF
- Dysrhythmias common: AFIB, PAC, PVC

WORRY ABOUT

- Myocardial ischemia: supply < demand (CAD rare)
- Abnormal systolic and diastolic function
- Chronic alcohol use alters myocardial response to inotropes
- Alcohol withdrawal symptoms

OVERVIEW

- Insidious onset; Sx uncommon unless severely stressed until late in course
- Dilated cardiomyopathy: ventricular hypertrophy early, chamber dilation later
- Low-output cardiac failure (as compared with high-output failure in cirrhosis and beriberi)
- Malnutrition often co-exists

ICD-9-CM Code: 425.5

ETIOLOGY

- Direct myocardial damage by ethanol and its metabolites
- Progressive chamber dilation and ventricular hypertrophy; microscopic fibrinoid deposition
- Possible intracellular calcium dysregulation
- Possible muscle excitation-contraction impairment

USUAL TREATMENT

- Abstinence—ventricular function improves markedly after abstinence
- Pharmacologic management—digitalis, diuretics, vasodilators
- Address nutritional deficits—thiamine, folate, multivitamin

ASSESSMENT POINTS

SYSTEM	EFFECT	ASSESSMENT BY HX	PE	TEST
HEENT	Plethora, reflux, esophageal varices, friable mucosa	Reflux Sx Hematemesis	Spider angiomata	Endoscopy
CV	LV dysfunction CHF Myocardial ischemia Dysrhythmia	Fatigue, orthopnea PND Rare angina Palpitations	Narrow pulse pressure Cardiomegaly S_3, S_4, murmur JVD, peripheral edema	ECG ECHO Stress testing
RESP	Pulmonary edema	Dyspnea Cough	Rales	CXR
GI	Hepatic congestion	Poor appetite, distention	Hepatomegaly	PT, albumin, LFTs
HEME	Coagulopathy Anemia	Abnormal bleeding	Pallor Ecchymosis	CBC PT/PTT, plt
RENAL	↓ Renal perfusion	Oliguria		Cr, FENa
CNS	Poor perfusion	Confusion	Abn mental status	
MS	Proximal muscle weakness		Proximal limb weakness and muscle atrophy	

Key Reference: Tonnesen H, Kehlet H: Preoperative alcoholism and postoperative morbidity. Br J Surg 1999; 86:869–874.

PERIOPERATIVE IMPLICATIONS

Preoperative Preparation
- Pharmacologic management of CHF

Monitoring
- ECG with ST-segment analysis
- Consider arterial pressure catheter, pulmonary artery catheter, TEE depending on surgery and ventricular function

Airway
- None

Preinduction/Induction
- May have intravascular volume depletion

Maintenance
- Avoid tachycardia, increased sympathetic activity
- Avoid depression of myocardial contractility

Extubation
- Routine

Postoperative Period
- Consider monitoring in critical care unit
- Observe for ethanol withdrawal

Adjuvants
- Multivitamins, thiamine, B_{12}, folate continued
- Consider benzodiazepines, α_2 agonists for prophylaxis against withdrawal symptoms
- Volume of distribution may be increased; consider adjusting drug dosages

ANTICIPATED PROBLEMS/CONCERNS

- Postop ventricular dysfunction and CHF can occur
- Alcohol withdrawal symptoms can develop

CARDIOMYOPATHY, HYPERTROPHIC (HCM)

Nina Zachariah, M.D.
J. Michael Haering, M.D.
Edward Lowenstein, M.D.

RISK

• Incidence: 2% reported incidence between 0.025–1%
• Inherited as autosomal dominant with high degree of penetrance and variable expressivity

PERIOPERATIVE RISKS

• Dynamic outflow obstruction (either provoked or baseline) seen in 25–50% of patients with HCM
• ↑ Risk for myocardial ischemia due to profound LVH, high intraventricular pressures, and abnormal intramyocardial coronary arteries
• Little data to support worse perioperative outcome

WORRY ABOUT

• Worsening dynamic outflow obstruction with resultant hypotension due to
  – ↓ In preload and afterload, esp with sudden volume loss or induction of anesthesia
  – ↑ In LV contractility
• Myocardial ischemia
• Diastolic dysfunction
• Supraventricular and ventricular dysrhythmias; AFIB and resultant loss of atrial contribution to ventricular filling

OVERVIEW

• Definition: presence of hypertrophied, nondilated LV in absence of other cardiac or systemic causes for LVH
• Myocardial disarray on histopathology
• Septum usually disproportionately affected
• Vigorous LV function and hypertrophied myocardium may physically obstruct left ventricular outflow tract (LVOT) during systole, resulting in dynamic outflow tract gradient
• Anterior leaflet of mitral valve may contribute to dynamic obstruction as it is "drawn" into LVOT during systole (systolic anterior motion [SAM] of the mitral valve leaflet)
• Associated mitral regurgitation often present
• May present as sudden death
• Other symptoms include dyspnea, syncope, and angina
• Diagnosis is made echocardiographically and can be confirmed with biopsy; genetic tests likely to be available in the future
• LVOT gradient can be demonstrated with echocardiography and at cardiac catheterization

ICD-9-CM Code: 425.1 (Hypertrophic obstructive cardiomyopathy)

ETIOLOGY

• Genetically heterogeneous; mutations in genes that encode for cardiac sarcomeric proteins (myosin, myosin binding protein, troponin, tropomyosin)

TREATMENT

• Medical: reduce LV contractility (β-blockers: Ca^{2+}-channel blockers), avoid physiologic changes that reduce LV cavity size (maintain preload and afterload, avoid tachycardia)
• Measures to reduce LVOT gradient
  – Surgical: septal myotomy-myomectomy, mitral valve replacement, mitral valve plication
  – Nonsurgical: dual-chamber pacing, septal ablation by alcohol injection
• ICD in patients at high risk of sudden death
• Screen all first-degree relatives

ASSESSMENT POINTS

SYSTEM	EFFECT	ASSESSMENT BY HX	PE	TEST
CV	Myocardial ischemia	Angina		ECG, exercise tests
	LVOT obstruction	Dyspnea, syncope, dizziness	Systolic murmur accentuated by Valsalva	ECHO
	Mitral regurgitation	Dyspnea	Holosystolic murmur	ECHO
	Dysrhythmias	Syncope, sudden death		ECG, Holter
	Diastolic dysfunction	Dyspnea	Rales, wheeze, edema	ECHO, CXR
RESP	Pulmonary congestion	Dyspnea	Rales, wheeze	CXR
CNS	Syncope	Syncope, presyncope		

Key Reference: Spirito P, Seidman CE, McKenna WJ, Maron BJ: The management of hypertropic cardiomyopathy. N Engl J Med 1997; 336:775–785.

PERIOPERATIVE IMPLICATIONS

Preoperative Preparation

• Replace any preoperative fluid deficit, ensure adequate ventricular volumes
• Consider pre- and perioperative β-blocker or Ca^{2+}-channel blockade
• Sedate adequately to prevent anxiety-induced sympathetic stimulation

Monitoring

• Consider invasive arterial pressure monitoring
• Consider pulmonary artery catheter
• Transesophageal ECHO when blood loss or volume shifts are anticipated

Airway

• None

Preinduction/Induction

• Phenylephrine infusion prepared, as worsening dynamic outflow tract gradient may be anticipated with any ↓ in SVR
• Avoid ketamine as induction agent

• Avoid prolonged laryngoscopy with attendant sympathetic stimulation
• Insertion of CVP/PAC may induce atrial or ventricular dysrhythmias

Maintenance

• Volatile agents that ↓ LV contractility without dramatic vasodilation desirable; halothane is the classic example
• Consider β-blockade or Ca^{2+}-channel blockade for tachycardia worsening LVOT obstruction
• Avoid agents that ↓ preload and afterload (e.g., nitroglycerin, nitroprusside), or any agent with significant histamine release
• Avoid agents that directly or indirectly ↑ HR and contractility (e.g., pancuronium, atropine, epinephrine, ephedrine)
• Hypotension treated with
  – Volume expansion
  – Pure α-adrenergic agonist (e.g., phenylephrine)
• Blood loss to be replaced promptly
• Spinal and epidural anesthesia may be associated with hypotension due to sympatholysis
• Consider early electrical cardioversion for atrial fibrillation

Extubation

• Avoid sympathetic stimulation
• Anticipate subendocardial ischemia

Postoperative Period

• Aggressive postop pain management

ANTICIPATED PROBLEMS/CONCERNS

• Myocardial ischemia
• Profound hypotension in setting of hypovolemia, ↓ preload/afterload, or ↑ contractility
• Dysrhythmias
• Diastolic dysfunction

CARDIOMYOPATHY, ISCHEMIC

Jonathan B. Mark, M.D.
Gregory H. Botz, M.D.

RISK

- Approximately 1:1000 incidence per year
- Men > women (2:1)

PERIOPERATIVE RISKS

- Most important perioperative risk factor for cardiac morbidity and mortality
- Risk of CHF, hypotension, pulmonary edema, myocardial ischemia and infarction, renal insufficiency, arrhythmias
- Left ventricular ejection fraction (LVEF) important for prognosis, perioperative complications. LVEF may not correlate with symptoms or exercise tolerance.

WORRY ABOUT

- CHF exacerbation, pulmonary edema, hypotension, myocardial ischemia and infarction, renal insufficiency, inability to tolerate fluid shifts associated with major surgery, arrhythmias

OVERVIEW

- Severe impairment of LVF leading to CHF; that arising from myocardial ischemia and infarction has extremely poor prognosis, with 30–50% 2-y mortality
- Patients may benefit from intensive medical therapy for underlying ischemia (nitrates, β-blockers, calcium antagonists, aspirin), CHF (ACE inhibitors, hydralazine, digoxin, diuretics), and prevention of cardiac thrombus (warfarin)
- Associated mitral regurgitation, left ventricular aneurysm, and ventricular arrhythmias may have specific perioperative considerations

ICD-9-CM Code: 414.8

ETIOLOGY

- Acquired disease with genetic predisposition
- Risk factors include associated hypertension, diabetes, hyperlipidemia, cigarette smoking, advanced age, peripheral vascular disease

USUAL TREATMENT

- Medical therapy (as indicated in Overview)
- Myocardial revascularization (percutaneous coronary angioplasty, atherectomy, stent or laser coronary bypass surgery, or transmyocardial laser revascularization)
- Cardiomyoplasty (generally experimental)
- Cardiac transplantation
- Associated cardiac surgery (mitral valve replacement/repair, left ventricular aneurysmectomy, implantation of AICD [automatic implantable cardioverter defibrillator])

ASSESSMENT POINTS

SYSTEM	EFFECT	ASSESSMENT BY HX	PE	TEST
CV	Myocardial ischemia Arrhythmias CHF	Angina Dyspnea, PND Palpitations	S_3, S_4, loud P_2 Narrow pulse pressure Displaced point maximal impulse	ECG Stress testing Echocardiogram Cardiac catheterization
RESP	Pulm congestion/edema	Dyspnea on exertion Orthopnea Cough	Rales Wheezes	CXR
GI	Ascites	Abdominal distention	Shifting dullness Fluid wave Hepatomegaly	Liver function tests PT Albumin
CNS	Embolic stroke due to cardiac thrombosis	Weakness Vision problems Confusion	Altered mental status Focal deficits	CT or MRI
MS	Peripheral edema	Swollen ankles Weakness	Pitting edema	
RENAL	Insufficiency (prerenal)	Oliguria		Cr, BUN Excreted fraction of filtered sodium

Key Reference: Vlay SC: Innovations in the management of ischemic cardiomyopathy. Am Heart J 1994; 127:235–242.

PERIOPERATIVE IMPLICATIONS

Preoperative Preparation
- Pharmacologic control of myocardial ischemia and CHF

Monitoring
- ECG (V_5 or multilead) with ST-segment analysis
- Arterial catheter (close BP monitoring, ABGs)
- Consider PA catheter or TEE for major operations and/or poor medical condition

Airway
- None

Preinduction/Induction
- Avoid tachycardia and increased afterload to prevent ischemia and reduced cardiac output

- Hypovolemia may result from diuretic therapy

Maintenance
- Limited ability to increase cardiac output in response to stress
- Attention to fluid balance PAWP to avoid pulmonary edema or low cardiac output
- High doses of inhaled anesthetics may be poorly tolerated because of myocardial depression superimposed on cardiomyopathy

Extubation
- May be time of greatest stress for developing myocardial ischemia or LV dysfunction
- Consider postoperative mechanical ventilation if a large fluid resuscitation was required intraoperatively

Adjuvants
- Extensive preoperative medical therapy may have circulatory consequences
- Preoperative anticoagulation may preclude regional anesthesia

Postoperative Period
- Epidural pain management techniques may limit stress if operation was major (beware of warfarin therapy)
- Intensive care and hemodynamic monitoring may prevent complications if operation was major

ANTICIPATED PROBLEMS/CONCERNS

- Perioperative myocardial ischemia and CHF remain paramount concerns

CARNITINE DEFICIENCY

Raafat S. Hannallah, M.D.
Marjorie P. Brennan, M.D.

RISK

- Rare

PERIOPERATIVE RISKS

- Hypoglycemia
- Massive rhabdomyolysis and cardiac arrest described following GA and succinylcholine. The response may be confused with malignant hyperthermia.

WORRY ABOUT

- Perioperative hypoglycemia: avoid prolonged fast; IV glucose should be administered
- Neurologic and cardiopulmonary status: determine if a cardiomyopathy is present

OVERVIEW

- Carnitine is essential cofactor in enzymatic transport of long-chain fatty acids into mitochondria, in which they are oxidized
- When carnitine deficient, peripheral tissues cannot use fatty acids for energy production and the liver cannot adequately make ketone bodies as an alternative substrate
- The tissues become glucose dependent, and their metabolism exceeds liver's capacity for glucose production
- This glucose dependency can lead to severe liver failure (↑ hepatic enzymes, lactic acidosis, hepatic encephalopathy) and hypoglycemia

ICD-9-CM Code: 791.3

ETIOLOGY

- Rare inherited condition associated with lipid storage disorders ascribed to defect in hepatic biosynthesis of carnitine (systemic form) or reduced carnitine transport into muscle cells (myopathic form)
- Differentiate from carnitine palmityl transferase (CPT) deficiency, which results in impaired transfer of fatty acids into mitochondria
  – CPT deficiency associated with rhabdomyolysis and higher incidence of renal insufficiency

USUAL TREATMENT

- Dietary supplementation with L-carnitine and high-carbohydrate diet to prevent hypoglycemia.

ASSESSMENT POINTS

SYSTEM	EFFECT	ASSESSMENT BY HX	TEST
CV	Cardiomyopathy		ECHO
HEPATIC	Hypoglycemia Hepatomegaly with fatty infiltration	Lethargy	Blood glucose Bilirubin Liver function tests
HEME	Coagulopathy	Bleeding	Hypoprothrombinemia
CNS	Encephalopathy	Vomiting, diarrhea	Hyperammonemia
RENAL	Renal insufficiency	Recurrent myoglobinuria	BUN/Cr

Key References: Lucas M, Hinojosa M, Rodriguez A, Garcia-Guasch R: Anaesthesia in lipid myopathy. Eur J Anaesthesiol 2000; 17:461–462; Rowe RW, Helander E: Anesthetic management of a patient with systemic carnitine deficiency. Anesth Analg 1990; 71:295–297.

PERIOPERATIVE IMPLICATIONS

Preoperative Preparation

- Continue daily carnitine therapy
- Glucose infusion preoperatively
- Avoid protracted preoperative fasting
- For emergency surgery while in metabolic crisis, rehydrate; correct glucose, acid-base, and electrolyte imbalances, use IV carnitine if necessary, treat hypoprothrombinemia with FFP

Monitoring

- Blood glucose

Airway

- Best to avoid succinylcholine for intubation

Maintenance

- IV glucose infusion, frequent monitoring of serum glucose level
- Muscle weakness may be present and requires careful titration of muscle relaxant dosing

Extubation

- No unusual concerns

Adjuvants

- Consider antiemetic prophylaxis to speed resumption of oral intake

ANTICIPATED PROBLEMS/CONCERNS

- Perioperative hypoglycemia

CAROTID SINUS SYNDROME (CSS)

Randall M. Schell, M.D.
Charles Lee, M.D.

RISK

- Carotid sinus hypersensitivity (CSH) may occur in $\approx$ 10% of adults
- True incidence is controversial
- >50 years of age and male
- Underdiagnosed cause of dizziness, falls, syncope
- Often associated with CAD, Htn
- Known complication of carotid endarterectomy

PERIOPERATIVE RISKS

- Potential for syncope, dizziness, falls
- CV causes of syncope carry ~30% mortality and in cases of unexplained syncope ~6% per annum; probably similar to standardized mortality for this age group

WORRY ABOUT

- High incidence of associated vascular disease (coronary, cerebrovascular) and aortic valvular disease
- Perioperative bradycardia, cardiac dysrhythmias, hypotension
- Associated with extravascular triggers (coughing, sneezing, micturition, acute biliary tract disease), classic triggers (neck hyperextension, forced head turning), and pathologic changes adjacent to carotid sinus (thyroid tumors, carotid body tumors)

OVERVIEW

- Cardinal symptom is syncope or near-syncope

- Diagnosed if 5 sec of carotid sinus massage (CSM), in a patient with otherwise unexplained syncope or presyncope, produces either asystole >3 sec or, in the absence of asystole, a decrease in systolic BP >50 mmHg
  - Type I *cardioinhibitory:* asystole >3 sec with CSM
  - Type II *vasodepressor:* ↓ systolic BP >50 mmHg independent of heart rate slowing
  - Type III *mixed:* characteristics of both types I and II
- Cardioinhibitory type (80%) most common
- Difference between CSS and CSH is lack of spontaneous symptoms in the latter; only ~5–20% with CSH demonstrate spontaneous symptoms

ICD-9-CM Code: 337.0

ETIOLOGY

- Exaggeration of normal activity of baroreceptors in response to mechanical stimulation
- Symptoms (syncope, dizziness) result from baroreflex-mediated cerebral hypoperfusion due to bradycardia/asystole (cardioinhibitory), hypotension (vasodepressor), or both (mixed)
- Transmitted via branches of glossopharyngeal nerve to medulla; cardioinhibitory reflex is mediated by the vagus nerve, leading to asystole/bradycardia; the vasodepressor component is mediated by inhibition of sympathetic nervous system vasomotor tone, leading to ↓ SVR and ↓ BP

USUAL TREATMENT

- Asymptomatic CSH → No treatment
- CSS
  - Single episode → ?no treatment
  - Recurrent episodes → treatment
- Controversial—surgical (carotid sinus denervation, pacemaker implantation, glossopharyngeal nerve transection), carotid sinus irradiation, and medical (vasopressors, anticholinergics, avoidance of cervical pressure, mineralocorticoid)
- Cardioinhibitory
  - VVI or DDD cardiac peacemaker
  - Dual-chamber cardiac pacing is more effective and protects against pacemaker syndrome
  - Atrial pacing contraindicated because of high incidence of AV block in addition to sinus arrest during carotid sinus reflex activation
- Vasodepressor—cardiac pacemaker or if refractory to cardiac pacing, surgical ablation of carotid sinus
- Glossopharyngeal nerve block is alternative treatment in patients with CSS refractory to drug or pacemaker therapy
- Intraoperative
  - Cardiac pacemaker: external vs. internal
  - Drugs: atropine, isoproterenol, epinephrine
  - Other: infiltration of local anesthetic around carotid sinus, glossopharyngeal nerve block

ASSESSMENT POINTS

SYSTEM	EFFECT	ASSESSMENT BY HX	PE	TEST
HEENT	Bradycardia Hypotension	Syncope/near-syncope Falls with mechanical stimulation of neck	CSM	CSM (monitored) Electrophysiologic study
CV	See HEENT			
CNS	Syncope Stroke	See HEENT	Carotid bruit	Imaging studies of carotid artery
MS	Soft tissue injury Fx bone	Hx of falls		

Key Reference: Strasberg B, Sagie A, Erdman S, et al: Carotid sinus hypersensitivity and the carotid sinus syndrome. Prog Cardiovasc Dis 1989; 31:379–391.

PERIOPERATIVE IMPLICATIONS

Preoperative Preparation

- Evaluate for co-existing CAD and aortic valvular disease
- Evaluate cardiac pacemaker if in place to assure normal functioning (see under Pacemakers)

Monitoring

- Consider invasive BP monitoring

Positioning

- Avoid neck hyperextension, forced head turning, and pressure over carotid sinus (surgical preparation)

Airway

- Avoid neck hyperextension with intubation

Maintenance

- CSS may present as bradycardia/asystole, hypotension, or both
  - Esophageal pacing of the atria not expected to be of benefit

Adjuvants

- Digitalis, α-methyldopa, clonidine, and propranolol can enhance response to CSM
- Have epinephrine, atropine, and isoproterenol immediately available

- ?External pacemaker in OR
- Pancuronium may offer some advantages if muscle relaxant required
- Local anesthetic (lidocaine) available for infiltration around carotid sinus during carotid endarterectomy

ANTICIPATED PROBLEMS/CONCERNS

- Associated coronary, valvular, and/or cerebrovascular disease

CENTRAL NEUROGENIC HYPERVENTILATION

Cheri A. Sulek, M.D.
Roy F. Cucchiara, M.D.

INCIDENCE

- True central neurogenic hyperventilation (CNH) exceedingly rare; exact incidence unknown
- In patients with neurologic injury, not rare and most often associated with pulmonary dysfunction or shunting (aspiration, pneumonia, pulmonary edema, baseline disease)
- No association with age or gender

OVERVIEW

- A diagnosis of exclusion in neurologic disorders and hyperventilation
- Associated primarily with brainstem tumors with inconsistent involvement of midbrain, pons, and/or medulla

- CNS lymphomas and astrocytomas most common tumor types
- Gliomas, lymphomatoid granulomatosis, medulloblastoma, metastatic tumors also reported
- Effects of GA unknown

ETIOLOGY

- Exact etiology and level of brainstem dysfunction not known
- Probable etiology:
  - Loss of descending inhibitory control of ventilation by cerebral cortex with brainstem lesion
  - Postulated to be due to mesencephalic or pontine injury

- Ultimate control of respiration may lie in medulla (dorsal and ventral respiratory groups) with fine control from the pneumotaxic center of the pons with input from cerebral cortex, hypothalamus, chemo- and mechanoreceptors, and vagal nerve
- Stimulation of most areas of cerebral cortex except motor/premotor areas, which inhibit respiration
- Unlikely etiology:
  - Tumor pH: in vivo is alkalotic; does not appear to contribute to respiratory control
  - Mid- to caudal pontine lesions produce apneustic breathing, not CNH
  - Destructive lesions of midbrain or pons do not produce CNH, but animal models may not simulate the human brain

ASSESSMENT POINTS

SYSTEM	EFFECT	ASSESSMENT BY HX	PE	TEST
RESP	Tachypnea	Tachypnea that persists during sleep and is unpleasant to conscious patient	Resp rate Normal inspiratory and expiratory excursion	ABGs (all must be present to diagnose): • PCO_2 (low) • pH (alkalotic) • PaO_2 (increased for age) • Decreased bicarbonate Alveolar-to-arterial gradient not larger than normal
CNS		Patient cannot volitionally inhibit hyperventilation	Focal or nonfocal CNS findings	CSF pH may be normal CT/MRI

Key References: Jaeckle KA, Digre KB, Jones CR, et al: Central neurogenic hyperventilation: Pharmacologic intervention with morphine sulfate and correlative analysis of respiratory, sleep and ocular motor dysfunction. Neurology 1990; 40:1715–1720; Siderowf AD, Balcer LJ, Kenyon LC, Nei M, Raps EC, Galetta SL: Central neurogenic hyperventilation in an awake patient with a pontine glioma. Neurology 1996; 46:1160–1162.

DIFFERENTIAL DIAGNOSIS FOR HYPERVENTILATION

- Anxiety
- Psychogenic
- Drug toxicity (salicylates, theophylline, cyanide)
- Pulmonary pathology with hypoxemia (pneumonia, pulmonary embolus, pulmonary edema, restrictive or obstructive lung disease)
- Cardiac (CHF, valvular disease)
- High altitudes
- Sepsis
- Hepatic dysfunction/encephalopathy
- Hyperthyroidism
- Pregnancy
- Metabolic acidosis
- Must exclude other etiologies for respiratory alkalosis with appropriate lab/Dx testing

ADVERSE EFFECTS

- Respiratory alkalosis shifts oxyhemoglobin curve to left
- Hypocapnia is a potent cerebral vasoconstrictor, subsequently decreasing cerebral blood flow and volume
- Hypocapnia in injured brains may result in ischemic insults
- Effect of severe hypocapnia in normal brains is less clear and may produce ischemia when combined with Bohr effect

TREATMENT

- No completely effective or consistent treatment
- Narcotics may attenuate respiratory rate and improve blood gases but will not correct rate or alkalosis

- Increasing dead space ventilation, administration of supplemental oxygen and benzodiazepines are not effective
- Treatment of tumor with steroids, chemotherapy, or radiation therapy; however, not always effective
- Mechanical ventilation with neuromuscular blockade and sedation during treatment of tumor has been attempted

OUTCOME

- Death from progressive neurologic deterioration or other complications (aspiration, pneumonia) likely
- Improvement with treatment of tumor or long-term narcotics

CEPHALOPELVIC DISPROPORTION (CPD) Ezzat I. Abouleish, M.D.

RISK

- 3% of pregnant population

PERIPARTUM RISKS

- Increased maternal and fetal mortality and morbidity
  - Protracted labor
  - Arrested labor
  - Ruptured uterus
  - Higher rate of C-section
  - Higher rate of forceps delivery

WORRY ABOUT

- Increased need for operative delivery (including abdominal surgery)
- Increased incidence of fetal distress and need for emergency (stat) C-section

OVERVIEW

- Leads to abnormal labor pattern with subsequent high incidence of operative delivery
- Operative delivery associated with higher incidence of mortality and morbidity to mother and fetus
- Anesthesia: complete system exam, esp airway (for possible GA for "stat" section or failure of regional anesthesia), and landmarks at back (for regional anesthesia for labor and operative delivery)

ICD-9-CM Code: 660.1 (Obstructing labor)

ETIOLOGY

- Maternal causes: abnormality of mother's pelvis, e.g., android pelvis, scoliosis, old poliomyelitis, previous pelvis fracture
- Fetal causes: macrosomia

USUAL TREATMENT

- Obstetric: proper evaluation before and during labor
- Anesthesia: usually regional, for pain relief during labor and operative delivery, if required

ASSESSMENT POINTS

CPD can be diagnosed by clinical evaluation, radiographic cephalopelvimetry (rarely by x-ray, mostly by sonography), and failure of adequate response to oxytocin augmentation

Key Reference: Creasy RK, Resnik R: Maternal–Fetal Medicine, 3rd ed. Philadelphia, WB Saunders, 1994, pp 526–557.

PERIOPERATIVE IMPLICATIONS

- *Labor* usually more prolonged and painful than in absence of CPD
- Regional anesthesia adequate without interfering with course of labor

Anesthetic Technique

- Epidural analgesia: low concentration of bupivacaine supplemented with an opioid
- Combined spinal and epidural analgesia. *In early labor:* 10 μg sufentanil or 25 μg fentanyl with 1 ml of 0.20% ropivacaine intrathecally followed by continuous epidural infusion of 0.2% ropivacaine, 10 ml/h. If ropivacaine is not available, 0.25% bupivacaine can be used in the same volume. *In late labor:* The initial intrathecal injection of local anesthetic and opioid is often sufficient for remainder of first stage + second stage. In delay of labor or if C-section required, epidural catheter can be used to administer epidural analgesia or anesthesia.

- *C-section:* In all cases: Anesthesia machine checked. Left uterine displacement, apply all monitors, e.g., BP, ECG, pulse oximeter, and capnograph with GA
- *Elective C-section:* Spinal anesthesia, prehydration 15 ml/kg within 20 min; bupivacaine injected at L2–L3. Supine with left uterine displacement. BP maintained >90% or original level with ephedrine drip. Increments of 50 to 100 μg phenylephrine can supplement ephedrine when hypotension is resistant to treatment or if significant tachycardia is present.

- *Emergency C-section:* Following labor without fetal distress (failure to progress): If patient already has reliable epidural block, epidural anesthesia is extended using 3% chloroprocaine + 75 μg fentanyl epidurally. If patient has not had epidural block during labor, spinal anesthesia can be used.
- *Following labor with fetal distress:* If patient has epidural, use as above. If patient has no epidural and airway is acceptable, perform GA.

ANTICIPATED PROBLEMS/CONCERNS

- If airway is expected to be difficult and no epidural catheter is in place, use spinal anesthesia or perform awake intubation. Fiberoptic and laryngeal mask airway (LMA) must be available.

CEREBRAL ARTERIOVENOUS MALFORMATIONS (AVMs)

Barbara A. Dodson, M.D.

RISK

- Prevalence estimated at 0.2–0.5% of general population
- Account for ~1% of acute subarachnoid hemorrhages (SAHs)

PERIOPERATIVE RISKS

- ↑ ICP, seizures, neurologic deficits
- 4–10% perioperative mortality
- 4–10% incidence of associated aneurysms

WORRY ABOUT

- ↑ Risks for new neurologic deficits, rebleed, severe intraoperative bleeding, and postop cerebral edema and hemorrhage (i.e., hyperemic complications)

OVERVIEW

- Neurovascular lesions with SAH as most common (80%) initial presentation and occurs in 50% of the lesions. Morbidity and mortality from initial hemorrhage are 23–80% and 10–29%, respectively, and ↑ with each rebleed. Risk of recurrent hemorrhage is 6–18% the 1st year and 2–12% thereafter.
- May produce seizures and severe headaches. High-flow low-resistance shunt associated with AVMs can be severe enough to produce focal neurologic deficits 2° to hypoperfusion or systemic effects (CHF is most common presentation for vein of Galen malformations in neonates).

ICD-9-CM Code: 747.81

ETIOLOGY

- Usually congenital, arising during primitive vasculature development
- Symptoms usually first occur between 2nd and 4th decades of life. Exceptions are great vein of Galen malformations.

USUAL TREATMENT

- Surgical removal, often with endovascular embolization, is treatment of choice
- Inoperable (because of size or location) AVMs may be treated with radiation therapy or endovascular embolization

ASSESSMENT POINTS

SYSTEM	EFFECT	ASSESSMENT BY HX	PE	TEST
HEENT	Loss of airway protection, change in pupil size, facial weakness	Aspiration, pupil size, facial asymmetry	Gag reflex, pupillary response	Testing of cranial nerve function
CV	ECG changes, cardiac arrhythmias, CHF	Sx CHF, Sx angina	Heart rate, S_3, rales	ECG, ECHO CXR
RESP	Hypoxia		Resp rate	ABGs
ENDO	Diabetes insipidus Syndrome of inappropriate antidiuretic hormone secretion		Volume status, BP	Serum and urine lytes and osmolality
CNS	Mass effect, CBF steal, neurologic deficits, aneurysmal bleed	Headaches, ataxia, seizures, LOC	Neurologic exam	CT, MRI, cerebral angiogram

Key Reference: Dodson BA: Interventional neuroradiology and the anesthetic management of patients with arteriovenous malformation. *In* Cotrell JE, Smith DS (eds): Anesthesia and Neurosurgery, 4th ed. St. Louis, Mosby-Year Book, 2001.

PERIOPERATIVE IMPLICATIONS

Preoperative Preparation

- Determine baseline neurologic status and evaluate for signs of mass effect
- Review results of preop endovascular procedures (embolization)
- Review medical status

Monitoring

- Invasive arterial pressure monitoring
- Continuous end-tidal CO_2 and N_2 to detect venous air embolism, as applicable to surgical position
- Consider CVP or pulmonary artery catheter

Airway

- May require early intubation if patient is hypoxic, with ↓ airway reflexes, ↑ ICP or otherwise obtunded

Maintenance

- Tight BP control to prevent ↑ CPP (↑ mass effect or aneurysmal rupture) or ↓ CPP (ischemia in hypoperfused areas)
- Anesthetic technique dependent on medical and neurologic status, need for intraoperative neurologic testing, desire for early neurologic evaluation
- Deliberate hypotension or high-dose barbiturates should be considered

Extubation

- Need for tight BP control to prevent rebleeding

Adjuvants

- Nitroprusside, nitroglycerine, and/or β-blockers to prevent ↑ BP
- Consider hypothermia, barbiturates, propofol, etomidate for brain protection

Postoperative Period

- Changes in CBF following AVM shunt removal can result in cerebral edema and hemorrhage due to (1) rebleeding from incomplete hemostasis or resection; (2) venous thrombosis or obstruction; (3) inability of previously hypoperfused areas to autoregulate at normal CPP (i.e., normal perfusion pressure breakthrough)

ANTICIPATED PROBLEMS/CONCERNS

- New neurologic deficits
- Severe intraoperative blood loss
- Hyperemic complications

CEREBRAL PALSY
Judith Nolan, M.B., B.S., M.R.C.P., F.R.C.A.

RISK

- 2 per 1000 live births in developed countries
- Incidence has not decreased despite improved perinatal care because of increased survival in premature neonates
- Leading cause of childhood motor disability

PERIOPERATIVE RISKS

- Dehydration
- Electrolyte imbalance
- Hypothermia
- Delayed recovery

WORRY ABOUT

- Difficult intubation
- Gastroesophageal reflux and aspiration
- Associated respiratory impairment
- Drug interactions
- Latex allergy

OVERVIEW

- Nonprogressive disorder of motion and posture
- Associated cognitive impairment, visual and hearing disturbances, seizures, and behavioral disturbance to varying degrees
- Often have normal intellect (esp dyskinetic group)
- Other systems involved: GI/respiratory
- Classified as spastic (70%), dyskinetic (10%), ataxic (10%), and mixed (10%)

ICD-9-CM Code: 343.9

ETIOLOGY

- Mostly unknown
- Antenatal cerebral events causing complications at time of delivery, e.g., periventricular hemorrhage and infection
- Postnatal events such as trauma and infection
- All causes result in damage to CNS during early brain growth

USUAL TREATMENT

- Anticonvulsants, antispasmodics (benzodiazepines, baclofen, dantrolene), antidepressants, antireflux agents, laxatives, anticholinergics
- Often intramuscular botulinum toxin injections and orthopedic procedures (tendon releases and osteotomies), fundoplication for reflux, and dental extractions

ASSESSMENT POINTS

SYSTEM	EFFECT	ASSESSMENT BY HX	PE	TEST
HEENT	Tongue thrusting Poor dentition Salivary drooling	Difficulty swallowing	Dental malocclusion Dental caries	Formal airway assessment usually difficult
RESP	Restrictive defect Aspiration pneumonia Recurrent chest infections	Cough Dyspnea (difficult to detect if mobilization limited)	Often normal Reduced air entry Bronchial breathing Wheeze	Pulmonary function tests ABGs CXR
CV	Right-sided heart failure from restrictive lung disease	Often normal Dyspnea	Tachycardia S_3 or S_4 Distended JVP Hepatomegaly	ECG ECHO
GI	GE reflux Esophageal dysmotility	Poor swallowing Night wakening	Dehydration Pallor Malnutrition	CBC Electrolytes ±Endoscopy
MS	Spasticity Dyskinesia Ataxia	Muscle pain and spasms	Increased muscle tone Contractures Tremor	Gait analysis performed before major orthopedic surgery
CNS	Epilepsy (30%) Visual and hearing defects	Tonic-clonic and complex-partial seizures	Myopia Visual field defects Strabismus	Not usually relevant
HEME	Iron-deficiency anemia	Fatigue	Pallor	CBC, differential
METAB	Electrolyte imbalance	Laxative use Fatigue	Dehydration Malnutrition	UA Albumin

Key Reference: Nolan J, Chalkiadis GA, Low J, Olesch CA, Brown TO: Anaesthesia and pain management in cerebral palsy. Anaesthesia 2000; 55:32–41.

PERIOPERATIVE IMPLICATIONS

Preoperative Preparation

- Can have normal intellect
- Involve parents in management, as parents have good insight into perioperative care
- Avoid unfamiliar faces if possible
- Optimize respiratory status (bronchodilators, antibiotics, physical therapy)
- Optimize nutrition; fix lyte imbalance
- Continue medical RX, esp anticonvulsants
- May need antireflux, antisialagogue, or sedative premed (cautious doses of sedatives)
- Topical local anesthetic for venipuncture
- Discuss perioperative analgesia (often regional technique for lower limb surgery)

Monitoring

- Core temp (susceptible to hypothermia)
- Neuromuscular blockade
- Airway pressures

Airway

- ETT is better sized to age, not weight
- Salivary secretions may make ventilation difficult
- Overbite may make intubation difficult

Induction

- Rapid-sequence may be required but often impractical
- Cannulation often difficult
- Inhalation sometimes favored (in semisitting position if concerns of reflux)

Maintenance

- Careful positioning
- Consider antiemetics
- IV fluids
- MAC may be lower in cerebral palsy
- Use warming devices
- Consider regional (epidural) techniques for lower limb surgery

Extubation

- Awake if prone to reflux

Drug considerations

- Baclofen should not be stopped abruptly but may cause postoperative bradycardia and hypotension
- Resistance to nondepolarizing NMB (probably not clinically significant)
- Ketamine and methohexitone may be avoided in epileptic pts
- N_2O and opiates may worsen nausea

Postoperative Period

- Maintain normothermia
- Susceptible to nausea and vomiting
- Avoidance/treatment of muscle spasm (intravenous diazepam, epidural clonidine)

ANTICIPATED PROBLEMS/CONCERNS

- Latex allergy
- Hypothermia
- Prolonged recovery time
- Postoperative NIV (worse with opiates)
- Postoperative muscle spasms
- Retention of secretions and postoperative chest infection

CEREBROVASCULAR TRANSIENT ISCHEMIC ATTACK (TIA)

Renata Rusa, M.D.

See also Carotid Endarterectomy in Procedures section

RISK

- Incidence in USA: 1/100,000 for age <45 y, 293/100,000 for age ≥75 y
- Gender and race factors: extracranial disease more prevalent in Caucasians; intracranial disease in African-Americans and Asians
- People at increased risk: Caucasian males
- Male > female 3:1 at age 75 y in 1990; female risk not decreasing as fast as male (thought because of increased cigarette usage in females)

PERIOPERATIVE RISKS

- Increased risk of CVA during CABG in patients with symptomatic carotid artery disease
- Increased risk for perioperative CVA in noncardiac noncarotid artery surgery: asymptomatic patients 0.0–3.0% vs. patients with TIAs: 0.0–17%
- Risk of co-existing heart disease (HD)

WORRY ABOUT

- Crescendo TIAs
- Critical carotid stenosis
- Impending basilar artery occlusion

OVERVIEW

- An episode of focal, nonconvulsive, neurologic deficit due to inadequate perfusion that is completely reversible in 24 h
- Disease of the carotid or vertebrobasilar system most often responsible
- Incidences of a stroke: 10%/y for first 3 y after TIA
- 50% survival time after first TIA is 7–8 y
- HD the leading long-term cause of death
- Patients with TIA/CVA have 40% frequency of significant CAD
- Recommended by some that elective surgery be postponed for 6 wk after TIA
- Most perioperative CVAs in general surgery occur postop. Predictors: Htn, PVD, cerebrovascular and heart disease.

ICD-9-CM Code: 435.9

ETIOLOGY

- Atherosclerosis—risk factors: Htn, DM, heart disease, smoking, hyperlipidemia
- Cardioembolic—e.g., recent MI, AFIB, valvular heart disease
- Other—traumatic, mechanical compression, steal syndromes, nonatherosclerotic vasculopathy
- Carotid endarterectomy

USUAL TREATMENT

- Risk factor management
- Antiplatelet agents or anticoagulants if not a bleeding diathesis
- Carotid endarterectomy for >60–70% stenosis

ASSESSMENT POINTS

SYSTEM	EFFECT	ASSESSMENT BY HX	PE	TEST
HEENT		Trauma to neck	See CV	
CV	Cerebrovascular disease Other major artery disease	TIA Sx, previous CVA	Funduscopic exam; carotid pulse, bruit; BP in both arms	Carotid duplex transcranial Doppler MRA or angio: carotid, vertebrobasilar, aortic arch
	CAD	History of MI, arrhythmias Poor exercise tolerance Atherosclerotic risk factors	Heart murmur, irregular heart beat S_3	ECG, Holter, stress test TTE or TEE
GI		Nausea, vomiting can accompany other signs of brainstem ischemia		
CNS	Amaurosis fugax	Transient monocular blindness	Ischemic retina Presence of microemboli	See CV
	Transient focal neurologic deficit	Speech, language difficulties; visual disturbance, weakness, paresthesia, ataxia, vertigo, diplopia in combination with some other Sx	Neuro exam usually nml between attacks; disturbance of consciousness rare with TIAs	CT or MR brain scan

Key Reference: Fine-Edelstein JS, Wolf PA, O'Leary PH, Poehlman H, Belanger AJ, Kusc CS, D'Agostino RB: Precursors of extracranial carotid atherosclerosis in the Framingham study. Neurology 1994; 44:1046–1050.

PERIOPERATIVE IMPLICATIONS

Preoperative Preparation

- Determine range of BP tolerated from both neuro and cardiac standpoint
- Avoid excessive sedation
- Need for preop work-up depends on risk assessment of perioperative CVA, cardiac morbidity, urgency of current procedure

Monitoring

- ECG, ST-segment analysis
- Consider invasive monitors for major procedures if significant atherosclerosis of major arteries or organs
- Use of intraoperative EEG has been limited, probably not practical in general surgery setting
- No data on sensitivity or specificity of transcranial Doppler

Airway

- Avoid extreme rotation and extension of neck during intubation, as such can impair flow through the vertebrobasilar system

Preinduction/Induction

- Maintain normal hemodynamics and adequate cerebral perfusion pressure
- Realize that cerebral autoregulation curve is shifted to the right in Htn patients

Maintenance

- Maintain glucose <200 mg/dl; avoid glucose in IV solutions
- Maintain slight hypocarbia to normocarbia for patient
- Weigh potential neuroprotective benefits of mild hypothermia against cardiac risk
- Theoretical advantage of isoflurane: allows lowest CBF before evidence of ischemia develops on EEG and is the least potent cerebral vasodilator; sevoflurane similar to isoflurane

Extubation

- Extubate deep to avoid Htn and tachycardia, or awake to ensure that patient can follow commands, protect airway, and is free of major neurologic deficit that could later result in significant cerebral edema

Postoperative Period

- Period of greatest risk for CVA in general surgery
- Resume antiplatelet and anticoagulation therapy ASAP

Adjuvants

- Barbiturates not clinically useful in prevention of perioperative stroke

ANTICIPATED PROBLEMS/CONCERNS

- TIA is marker for both cerebrovascular and cardiac disease

CERVICAL DISK DISEASE (CERVICAL SPINE DISEASE)

Andrew D. Rosenberg, M.D.

RISK

- 12,000 deaths in USA/y; 70 million in USA with cervical disk disease, spondylosis, or trauma
- Disk disease—a consequence of aging (3rd–5th decades)
- Present in rheumatoid arthritis (RA), ankylosing spondylitis, other rheumatic disorders
- Trauma, esp motor vehicle accidents
- Male > female (3:2)

PERIOPERATIVE RISKS

- Mortality (acute) 1–5% (depending on associated injuries)
- Spinal cord damage with C-spine movement
- Difficulty intubating or reintubating postextubation
- After neck surgery, swelling or hematoma can cause obstruction of airway
- Steroid-induced complications

WORRY ABOUT

- Airway management; C-spine movement during or after intubation
- Exacerbating or causing spinal cord damage with neck motion
- Osteoarthritis with osteophytes impinging on nerve roots

OVERVIEW

- Neck pain present in 30% of adults in USA
- Can cause radiculopathy, which can be aggravated by neck extension
- Root: C3—Unusual; C4—numbness rare, pain at root of neck; C5—numb over shoulder to lateral aspect of upper arm ("epaulet" area); C6—second most common radiculopathy: pain across top of neck, along biceps muscle into tips of thumb and index finger as well as biceps muscle weakness; C7—most common herniation: pain across back of shoulder triceps, and into middle finger as well as loss of triceps reflex; C8—numb small finger, interossei weak

ICD-9-CM Codes: 952.0 (Cervical spine injury); 756.19 (Cervical spondylosis)

ETIOLOGY

- Disk disease—a process of aging
- Inflammatory arthropathy or trauma: in trauma, can have fractures, dislocations, or ligamentous damage causing spinal cord paralysis; can get swelling of soft tissues of neck

USUAL TREATMENT

- Neck should be stabilized, not forced into position: any movement can cause damage
- In patients with atlantoaxial subluxation, avoid flexion. Can have superior migration of odontoid as well as subaxial subluxation.
- Stabilization and time to heal, repair
- Shoulder and strap muscle strengthening exercises
- Epidural steroids for recent disk disease
- Steroids for acute spinal cord injury

ASSESSMENT POINTS

SYSTEM	EFFECT	ASSESSMENT BY HX	PE	TEST
HEENT	Numbness and pain In RA: superior migration of odontoid, atlantoaxial subluxation, atlas-dens interval (ADI) increased (>4 mm unstable), subaxial subluxation Cricoarytenoid arthritis Airway abnormalities Trauma Swelling	Hoarseness, snoring	In RA: TMJ problems, hypoplastic mandible	In RA: neck x-ray flexion and extension (measure ADI) Evaluate bones, ligament alignment, soft tissue swelling, motion
CV	Trauma: possible cardiac contusion/injury, spinal shock		Heart sounds distant Unstable BP	ECG, ECHO
RESP	Rheumatologic disorders: fibrosis, honeycombing Ankylosing spondylitis: restrictive pattern Trauma: diaphragm function (C3–C5), pneumothorax, hemothorax, contusion, aspiration, rib fractures	SOB	In trauma: dyspnea, paradoxical ventilation, flail chest, breath sounds absent with pneumothorax	CXR, ABGs
GI	Ulcers 2° to aspirin for RA			
HEME	RA: anemia 2° to medications		Trauma: look for signs of bleeding	Hgb
CNS	Vertebral artery compression: dizziness, vertigo, nausea, blurred vision			

Key Reference: Wong JK, Tongier WK, Ambruster SC, White PF: Use of the intubating laryngeal mask airway to facilitate awake orotracheal intubation in patients with cervical spine disorders. J Clin Anesth 1999; 11:346–348.

PERIOPERATIVE IMPLICATIONS

- Assess neck in disk disease, rheumatic diseases, trauma
- Consider intubation with neck stabilized by assistant to avoid flexion or extension or awake fiberoptic intubation
- Consider intubating with laryngeal mask airway or light wand
- Avoid premedication (e.g., midazolam) that might interfere with spinal cord monitoring

Monitoring

- Acute spinal cord shock may require arterial and PA catheters or TEE to facilitate monitoring and treating hemodynamic disturbances

Induction

- Consider not initiating irreversible steps (e.g., muscle relaxants) until airway is secured

Extubation

- Consider not extubating until patient able to maintain airway without threat of swelling or airway obstruction

Adjuvants

- Steroids reduce injury in acute traumatic spinal cord injury

Postoperative Period

- Observe for neck swelling, hoarseness, airway obstruction
- Assess neurologic status

ANTICIPATED PROBLEMS/CONCERNS

- Anticipate difficulty intubating patients due to abnormal anatomy or limitation of motion. Prepare patient for fiberoptic intubation.
- Associated traumatic injuries—cardiac, brain, lung, abdomen, bladder, long bones—and their consequences
- ARDS from aspiration in preop traumatic event

CHAGAS' DISEASE

Stefan A. Iantchoulev, M.D.
Charles W. Hogue, Jr., M.D.

RISK

- 16–18 million infected worldwide
- Rare in Southern USA; chronic disease more likely in emigrants from endemic regions
- More than 50,000 die each year
- Laboratory workers and personnel exposed to blood products

PERIOPERATIVE RISKS

- Not defined
- Related to CV dysfunction
- Esophageal changes due to megaesophagus and reflux
- Associated with myasthenia gravis
- CNS symptoms—meningoencephalitis (particularly in immunocompromised patients)

WORRY ABOUT

- LV dysfunction and CHF
- Conduction abnormalities (complete AV block)
- Ventricular arrhythmias
- Megaesophagus, achalasia, risk of pulmonary aspiration
- Blood transmission and infections

OVERVIEW

- Acute infection, asymptomatic in $2/3$ of patients, followed by chronic disease after latency of >2 decades
- In endemic areas, mild forms of disease common with benign course
- Pathogenesis to chronic, progressive end-organ disease poorly understood; autoimmunity, microvascular dysfunction, autonomic neuropathy implicated
- Cardiac involvement most serious end-organ manifestation; colon and esophagus also affected
- In USA, Dx usually not considered; presentation as CAD or dilated cardiomyopathy, or with AV heart block, CHF, ECG conduction abnormalities, sustained VTach
- Serologic test for Dx
- Continues to cardiac involvement—decapillarization of the myocardium
- Downregulation of the nicotinic ACh receptors and associated myasthenia gravis symptomatology

ICD-9-CM Code: 086.0

ETIOLOGY

- *Trypanosoma cruzi*
- Transmission to humans by reduviid bug
- Transmission by blood transfusion possible
- Central and South America endemic areas

USUAL TREATMENT

- Nifurtimox (limited efficacy): for acute disease; usefulness for indeterminate phase or chronic disease not established
- Benznidazole (similar efficacy as nifurtimox) second agent
- Recent success with protriptyline in the acute and chronic form
- Allopurinol for the cutaneous form

ASSESSMENT POINTS

SYSTEM	EFFECT	ASSESSMENT BY HX	PE	TEST
CV	Conduction abnormalities LV dysfunction and aneurysm	Syncope, DOE, orthopnea, fatigue	JVD, edema, rales, cardiomegaly	ECG ECHO MUGA Cardiac catheter
	Ventricular arrhythmias	Syncope, palpitations	Biventricular enlargement	Holter Electrophysiologic study, TTE, TEE
GI	Megaesophagus, megacolon	Dysphagia, GE reflux, constipation	Abdominal distention	Barium studies CXR Endoscopy

Key Reference: Hagar JM, Rahimtoola SH: Chagas' heart disease in the United States. N Engl J Med 1991; 325:763–768.

PERIOPERATIVE IMPLICATIONS

Preoperative Preparation

- LV function optimization with diuretics, ACE inhibitors, consider β-blockers and Ca^{2+}-channel blockers. Consider amiodarone in cases of VTach/VFIB.
- Prophylaxis against pulmonary aspiration
- Assessment of conduction abnormalities, arrhythmias

Monitoring

- Dictated by degree of LV dysfunction and proposed procedure; consider PA catheter or TEE. On TEE may see biventricular enlargement, thinning of ventricular walls, apical aneurysm, intramural thrombus.

- ECG during entire perioperative period. Often see long QT interval, AV block, bundle branch block. Can have VTach/VFIB.

Preinduction/Induction

- Consider temporary pacing if symptomatic AV block
- Caution with negative inotropic drugs
- Awake or rapid-sequence intubation
- Consider judicious use of muscle relaxants

Maintenance

- Technique dictated by preferences, procedure, degree of cardiac involvement
- Avoid hypoxemia (facilitates ischemic myocardial changes on capillary level, which can further progress to wall thinning and aneurysm formation)

Postoperative Period

- Continued monitoring depends on pre-existing LV dysfunction and operative procedure
- ECG monitoring for ventricular arrhythmias and AV conduction block

CHERUBISM

RISK
- >200 cases in world literature
- Cherubs have a 40% chance of a cherub offspring

PERIOPERATIVE RISKS
- Swelling of lower face causing airway obstruction
- Displacement of ocular orbit and lower eyelid causing visual changes
- Excessive blood loss from curettage of vascular lesions
- Association with Noonan syndrome

WORRY ABOUT
- Pulmonary valve stenosis (Noonan syndrome)
- Undiagnosed hyperparathyroidism
- Convex, V-shaped hypertrophied hard palate
- Small mouth opening and mild trismus

OVERVIEW
- Progressive symmetric fullness of cheeks and jaw, with retraction of lower eyelids exposing an inferior rim of sclera
- Onset age 2–12 y
- These round-faced, upwardly gazing infants look like Renaissance art "cherubs" (Jones)
- Diagnostic biopsy of mandible shows multinucleated giant cells
- Associated problems with speaking, breathing, swallowing, chewing
- Pathognomonic x-ray of jaw demonstrates radiolucent lesions

ICD-9-CM Code: 526.89

ETIOLOGY
- Familial—autosomal dominant
- Penetrance—100% for boys, 50% for girls
- Unknown but named alternatively familial fibrous dysplasia, bilateral giant cell tumors, familial multilocular cystic disease
- Multilocular cystic malformation of mandible and maxilla with painless submandibular lymphadenopathy

USUAL TREATMENT
- Operative curettage, removal of displaced teeth, cortical reshaping of mandible
- Selective embolization with operative excision of vascular lesions
- Bone grafts

ASSESSMENT POINTS

SYSTEM	EFFECT	ASSESSMENT BY HX	PE	TEST
HEENT	Orbits shifted	Loss of binocular vision	Upward gaze	
	Enlargement	Photo review by age	Painless jaw swelling	Jaw series
			Lymphadenopathy	
	Poor opening	Moderate trismus	Soft tissue swelling	
			Concave palate	
	Malocclusion	Absence of third molar	Loose teeth	X-ray
CV	If associated with Noonan syndrome	Pulmonic valve disease	Pulmonary valve stenosis	ECHO
RESP	Generally unaffected	Obstructive airway		Sleep study
ENDO	Rule out hyperparathyroidism	Onset at older age		Normal Ca^{2+}, K^+
CNS	Midparental intelligence	No developmental delay, except with Noonan syndrome		
MS	Long bone lesions		Humerus, anterior ribs, femoral neck	

Key Reference: Battaglia A, Merati A, Magit A: Cherubism and upper airway obstruction. Otolaryngol Head Neck Surg 2000; 122:573–574.

PERIOPERATIVE IMPLICATIONS

Preoperative Preparation
- Rule out parathyroid disease
- Available blood for curettage replacement

Monitoring
- Routine

Airway
- Difficult airway protocol

Preinduction/Induction
- Spontaneous ventilation
- Laryngeal mask airway

Maintenance
- Consider hypotensive technique for minimizing blood loss

Extubation
- May require ICU admission for prolonged intubation

Adjuvants
- Routine

Postoperative Period
- Extubation awake with confirmation of no bleeding

ANTICIPATED PROBLEMS/CONCERNS
- Nasal intubation for oral procedures may be problematic, similar to Pierre Robin, Goldenhar's, and Treacher Collins syndromes. As mandibular rami approach midline, no space for visualization of airway.

CIGARETTE SMOKING

Kevin K. Tremper, Ph.D., M.D.

- People within USA: 50 million
- No racial predilection
- Males > females (3:2); young females fastest-growing group

PERIOPERATIVE RISKS

- Increased risk of CAD × 2.0 of nonsmokers of same age
- Postop pulmonary complications × 6 of nonsmoker
- Carboxyhemoglobin (COHB) ↑ (up to 15%)
- Hyperreactive airway

WORRY ABOUT

- CAD, COPD, PVD, productive cough, reactive airway
- Increases physiologic age by 8 y (30 pack-years) relative to nonsmoker

OVERVIEW

- Addictive habit. Cigarette smoke contains >3000 identifiable constituents, many of which have toxic or tumorigenic effects. Acute effects relate to CO and nicotine.
- Nicotine stimulates the sympathetic ganglia, causing release of catecholamines from the adrenal medulla and sympathetic nerve endings, increasing BP, HR, and SVR, that persists for 30 min after one cigarette.
- Associated with ↓ MAO and ↑ dopamine levels in brain
- Inhaled CO produces up to 15% COHb. Combined effects of nicotine and COHb put diseased myocardium at risk.
- An irritant to pulmonary system, increasing mucus production while decreasing ciliary activity and mucus flow, markedly impairing tracheobronchial secretion clearance
- Chronic use associated with CAD, Htn, COPD, peripheral vascular disease, numerous cancers
- Cessation of smoking the night before surgery will reduce the COHb and nicotine levels to that of nonsmokers

- Cessation of smoking for ≤8 wk has controversial additional benefits; cessation of >8 wk has demonstrated decreased incidence of postop pulmonary complications. Cessation for 2 y reduces risks of myocardial infarction to that of the nonsmoking population.
- Considered to be the cause of 1 of every 6 deaths in the USA and is the leading cause of preventable mortality (400,000 preventable deaths/y)

ICD-9-CM Code: 305.1 (Tobacco abuse)

ETIOLOGY

- Habituation

USUAL TREATMENT

- Nicotine patch and clonidine, Smokers Anonymous, or self-withdrawal
- Cessation for a minimum of 12–24 h. Decrease in COHb and nicotine.
- Cessation for ≥8 wk will reduce postop pulm complications
- Cessation for ≥2 y decreases risk of MI

ASSESSMENT POINTS

SYSTEM	EFFECT	ASSESSMENT BY HX	PE	TEST
HEENT	Oral, pharyngeal, head and neck cancers		Lesions on exam or intubation	Usually not needed
CV	↑ Heart rate, SVR, coronary vascular resistance → myocardial ischemia ↑ PVR ↑ Blood viscosity	Exercise tolerance, angina (see Coronary Artery Disease in Diseases section)	Two-flight walk	ECG
RESP	↑ COHb, COPD, ↓ FEV$_1$/FVC ↑ Secretion ↓ Clearance ↑ Airway reactivity	Exercise tolerance, chronic productive cough, character of sputum	Auscultation	CXR if symptomatic Hct, sputum (see COPD)

Key Reference: Moores LK: Smoking and postoperative pulmonary complications. Clin Chest Med 2000; 21:139–146.

PERIOPERATIVE IMPLICATIONS

Preoperative Preparation

- Cessation overnight will ↓ COHb and nicotine
- Cessation for 8 wk will ↓ postop pulmonary complications
- If chronic productive cough, consider preop antibiotic treatment

Monitoring

- Routine
- SpO$_2$ monitoring, may read higher SpO$_2$ than actual if COHb present (SpO$_2$ = % HbO$_2$ + % COHb)
- Consider invasive monitoring if symptomatic pulmonary or cardiac disease

Airway

- None

Premedication/Induction

- Consider deep induction if history of reactive airway disease

Maintenance

- Routine unless symptomatic cardiac or pulmonary disease

Extubation

- Consider deep extubation if severe reactive airway disease but is easy to intubate and ventilate, with no aspiration risk

Adjuvants

- Routine; smoking ↑ metabolism of theophylline, ↓ half-life from 265 to 180 min

Postoperative Period

- Epidural analgesia may be beneficial in decreasing complications of hypercoagulability, CAD, or COPD

ANTICIPATED PROBLEMS/CONCERNS

- Long-standing Hx of smoking with symptomatic pulmonary disease leads to high risk of developing postop pulmonary complications (pneumonia) due to ↑ mucus production and ↓ ciliary function. Cessation for 8 wk is recommended.
- Airway reactivity significantly increased in smokers; abstinence for 24 h does not change this reactivity. Reactivity starts reducing after 24–48 h and reduces to near level of nonsmokers after 10 days of cessation.
- Risk of myocardial infarction decreases to that of nonsmokers after several years of cessation

CIGARETTE SMOKING CESSATION

Talmage D. Egan, M.D., Ph.D.
K.C. Wong, M.D., Ph.D.

RISK

• Adults within USA: nearly $1/4$ smoke cigarettes
• Higher prevalence of smoking among lower socioeconomic classes
• Prevalence among teens and women increasing

PERIOPERATIVE RISKS

• Risk not well defined through controlled studies; 25 pack-year Hx increases physiologic age 8 y in those 40–65 y
• ↑ Perioperative morbidity and mortality related to smoking-associated diseases
• ↑ Risk of postop lung complications

WORRY ABOUT

• Undiagnosed or poorly treated smoking-related disease that may require modification of the anesthetic plan (e.g., CAD, COPD)
• Propensity for bronchospasm and mucus plugging

• ↓ O_2 content 2° to high carboxyhemoglobin levels
• ↑ Autonomic activity (↑ heart rate and BP) 2° to nicotine in patients who have smoked just prior to anesthesia
• Recent evidence suggests that exposure to environmental cigarette smoke (i.e., "passive smoking") is a risk factor predisposing to perioperative pulmonary complications in children

OVERVIEW

• Smoking results in acute changes in cardiopulmonary function even in otherwise asymptomatic patients. With long-term use, smoking causes chronic changes in cardiopulmonary function that eventually culminate in irreversible cardiopulmonary disease.
• Acute changes include carbon monoxide–mediated decreases in O_2 content and nicotine-induced increases in heart rate and BP. Nicotine-mediated effects are relatively short-lived, whereas carboxyhemoglobin per-

sists for many hours.
• Chronic changes include a gradual decline in lung function consisting of ↓ FEV_1, ↓ mucociliary activity, ↓ gas exchange surface, and ↓ pulmonary macrophage activity
• Associated diseases include CAD, COPD, and numerous cancers (e.g., lung, laryngeal, oral)

ICD-9-CM Code: 305.1 (Tobacco dependence)

ETIOLOGY

• Acquired behavior that is generally viewed as addiction
• Highest risk factors are low education level, low socioeconomic status

USUAL TREATMENT

• Counseling
• Group therapy (e.g., "12-step" program)
• Pharmacologic adjuncts such as nicotine patches/gum, anticraving pill, exercise, and emotional support

ASSESSMENT POINTS

SYSTEM	EFFECT	ASSESSMENT BY HX	PE	TEST
HEENT	Oral/laryngeal cancer	Hoarseness	Oral exam (and inspection during direct laryngoscopy)	
CV	CAD (± altered LV function)	Exertional chest pain, dyspnea, poor exercise tolerance, orthopnea, paroxysmal nocturnal dyspnea	S_3 gallop, dysrhythmia	ECG, stress test, ECHO, angiography
RESP	COPD	Dyspnea, poor exercise tolerance	Tachypnea, rales, wheezing, pursed lip breathing	CXR, ABGs
OTHER	↑ Carboxyhemoglobin (with recent smoking)	Dyspnea	Tachycardia, tachypnea	ABGs with co-oximetry

Key Reference: Egan TD, Wong KC: Perioperative smoking cessation and anesthesia—a review. J Clin Anesth 1992; 4:63–72.

PERIOPERATIVE IMPLICATIONS

Preoperative Preparation

• Advise smoking cessation for at least 12 h before operation (so that carboxyhemoglobin levels fall to near-normal)
• Advise that a much longer period of cessation (i.e., ~2 mo) is necessary to achieve a decrease in postop pulmonary morbidity; may rarely be worthwhile in true pulmonary cripples undergoing major procedures and very worthwhile for long-term motivation
• Suggest that this is an excellent time to quit smoking (and reduce future aging-related wrinkles and physiologic aging changes)
• Recent evidence suggests that in-hospital smoking-cessation programs consisting only of a brief education and counseling visit, self-help "take-home" materials, and a follow-up phone call are cost-effective in promoting cessation

Monitoring

• Routine
• Current pulse oximeters cannot discriminate between carboxyhemoglobin and oxyhemoglobin. Significant levels of carboxyhemoglobin may exist without ↓ in pulse oximeter SpO_2 reading.

Airway

• Smokers vulnerable to bronchospasm or mucus plugging obstruction anytime

Induction

• Avoid instrumentation of airway until deep level of anesthesia
• Provide complete preoxygenation since less tolerance of apnea

Maintenance

• Routine; ensure adequate depth of anesthesia to avoid bronchospasm

Extubation

• Consider deep extubation if other considerations permit in order to avoid bronchospasm (e.g., empty stomach, easy laryngoscopy)

Postoperative Period

• Monitor for respiratory complications (e.g., pneumonia, bronchospasm)
• Encourage permanent smoking cessation

ANTICIPATED PROBLEMS/CONCERNS

• Propensity for bronchospasm
• ↓ O_2 content secondary to high carboxyhemoglobin levels

CLEFT PALATE

Andrei Cernea, M.D.

- ~1/800 live births
- Racial predominance: Caucasian
- Frequently associated with cleft lip
- Gender predominance: cleft lip/palate more common in males (2:1); isolated cleft palate more common in females (3:1)

PERIOPERATIVE RISKS

- Morbidity and mortality extremely low; only 5 life-threatening cases of postoperative airway obstruction described in literature

WORRY ABOUT

- Difficult airway when associated with syndromes such as Mohr, Shprintzen, 4P, or Pierre Robin

- Intrainduction laryngospasm and airway obstruction due to chronic URIs, chronic otitis media, and/or tongue becoming wedged in cleft
- Difficult intraoperative oxygenation due to chronic aspiration syndrome
- ↑ Risk for transfusion if anemic due to poor ability to feed
- Intraoperative airway obstruction and extubation by Dingman gag
- Intraoperative dysrhythmias caused by surgical infiltration of epinephrine
- Postoperative airway obstruction by forgotten pharyngeal packs and severe lingual edema
- Undiagnosed associated congenital heart and renal diseases

OVERVIEW

- Congenital condition occurs by 7th–12th wk of intrauterine life (associated with benzodiazepine usage)
- Cleft palate repaired at 12–18 mo
- Usually not associated with severe blood loss
- Postoperative airway obstruction may occur more frequently in prolonged procedures

ICD-9-CM Code: 749.00

USUAL TREATMENT

- If child is in otherwise good health, a palatoplasty is performed electively; all children with cleft palate should have repair by 18 mo to ensure
  - Normal speech development
  - Appropriate social integration
  - Normal growth of maxilla

ASSESSMENT POINTS

SYSTEM	EFFECT	ASSESSMENT BY HX	PE	TEST
HEENT	Otitis media	Ear pain	Temporomandibular exam	
	Clear rhinorrhea			
	Difficult airway	Snore, grunt	Airway exam (micrognathia)	
CV	Associated congenital heart disease	SOB, cyanosis, poor growth	CV exam, club feet	ECG, ECHO
RESP	URI	Cough, fever	Chest exam	
		Congestion		
	Aspiration	SOB, cyanosis	Chest exam	CXR
GI	Impaired deglutition	Nasal regurgitation		Observe feeding
	Malnutrition	Poor growth		
HEME	Anemia	Malnutrition	Pallor	Hgb/Hct
RENAL	Associated congenital defects	UTI	Club feet	UA, BUN/Cr

Key Reference: Hodges SC, Hodges AM: A protocol for safe anesthesia for cleft lip and palate surgery in developing countries. Anaesthesia 2000; 55:436–441.

PERIOPERATIVE IMPLICATIONS

Preoperative Preparation

- Recognize possibility of multiple future procedures and attempt to minimize stress during induction: consider oral premedication

Anesthetic Technique

- GA usually induced via mask using ↑ concentrations of volatile agent in oxygen
- Oral airway or gauze packing of cleft may help manual ventilation by preventing tongue from lodging in cleft
- Intubation, often with RAE endotracheal tube secured to mandible, as access to airway may be severely limited

Monitoring

- Precordial stethoscope
- Maintain normocapnia if epinephrine injection and halothane inhalation

Postoperative Considerations

- Significant risk for airway obstruction due to edema
- Often obligate mouth breathers
- Transfusion usually not required for cleft palate repair
- Rectal Tylenol frequently sufficient

ANTICIPATED PROBLEMS/CONCERNS

- Airway difficulty during induction and intubation, especially when associated with other facial anomalies
- Postoperative airway obstruction due to forgotten pharyngeal pack, severe lingual edema, or obligate mouth breathing

COAGULOPATHY, FACTOR IX DEFICIENCY

Thomas M. McLoughlin, Jr., M.D.

RISK

- People within USA: 3000–4000 (15% of all hemophiliacs). Incidence = 1:25,000–50,000 males.
- Race with highest prevalence: none
- Gender with highest prevalence: overwhelmingly male

PERIOPERATIVE RISKS

- Increased risk of hemorrhagic complications from any and all operations

WORRY ABOUT

- Excessive and/or uncontrollable hemorrhage
- Tendency for recurrent hemorrhage after initial control
- Expansive deep and soft tissue hematomas
- Increased risk if hepatic dysfunction present from prior plasma product transfusions

OVERVIEW

- Also called hemophilia B or Christmas disease
- Clinically indistinguishable from hemophilia A (classic hemophilia)
- Hemarthroses account for 75% of bleeding episodes; chronic debilitating arthritis is a common development
- Soft tissue hematomas and hematuria also common
- Intracranial hemorrhage is common fatal complication, accounting for death in 25%
- Severity of disease proportional to circulating factor IX activity (<1% normal activity = severe disease, >5% = generally mild disease)

ICD-9-CM Code: 286.1

ETIOLOGY

- Sex-linked recessive disorder

USUAL TREATMENT

- Restoration of circulating factor IX activity
- Solvent/detergent-treated pooled factor IX concentrates (AlphaNine SD, Alpha Therapeutic, Los Angeles, CA)
- Recombinant factor IX concentrate now available (BeneFix, Genetics Institute, Cambridge, MA). Dose (IU) = body weight (kg) × desired factor IX activity increase (%) × 1.2 IU/kg.
- Prothrombin complex concentrates and FFP are alternatives for life-threatening hemorrhage if concentrates unavailable

ASSESSMENT POINTS

SYSTEM	EFFECT	ASSESSMENT BY HX	PE	TEST
GI				LFTs if hepatitis Hx
HEME	Coagulopathy	Dental extractions, menses, lacerations, epistaxis	Ecchymoses, hematomas	Prolonged PTT; PT, TT, plt count usually normal
RENAL	Hematuria; eventual clot formation can obstruct collecting system	Discolored urine		BUN/Cr, urine dipstick or microscopic exam
CNS	Intracranial hemorrhage	Headache	Neurologic exam	
PNS	Discrete peripheral neuropathies	Hx of compressive hematoma	Sensory and motor exam	
MS	Hemarthroses, chronic arthritis	Painful, warm joints	↓ ROM	X-rays usually not necessary

Key Reference: McIntyre AJ: Blood transfusion and haemostatic management in the perioperative period. Can J Anaesth 1992; 39:R101–114.

PERIOPERATIVE IMPLICATIONS

Preoperative Preparation

- Collaboration with consulting hematologist
- Schedule surgery early in wk to allow optimal laboratory support of postop assessment of hemostasis; if multiple procedures are contemplated in near future, schedule simultaneously
- Assess preop factor IX activity; determine goal as guided by magnitude of hemostatic challenge (15–30% factor IX activity for minor lacerations/hematomas; 30–50% for hemarthroses or major hemorrhage, 50–75% for perioperative coverage or life-threatening bleeding)
- Units factor IX needed = (2)(wt in kg) (plasma volume in ml/kg)(fractional increase in factor IX activity desired); once-daily dosing is sufficient for maintenance

Monitoring

- *Confirm* expected increase in factor IX activity after preop dose but before incision

Airway

- Laryngoscopy to avoid tissue trauma, consider mask ventilation
- Nasotracheal route best avoided

Maintenance

- Consider tourniquets and local cooling to minimize blood loss

Extubation

- Avoid coughing on endotracheal tube
- Cautious oropharyngeal suction, best done under direct vision

Adjuvants

- Regional anesthesia not absolutely contraindicated but consider with caution; successful brachial plexus blockade at the axilla has been described
- Postop factor IX activity requirement: 15–40%

ANTICIPATED PROBLEMS/CONCERNS

- Excessive perioperative blood loss, hematoma formation
- Potential for delayed or recurrent bleeding after initial control
- Increased likelihood of infectious bloodborne disease (HIV, hepatitis)

COARCTATION OF THE AORTA
Michael Nugent, M.D.

RISK
- 1 in 12,000 children
- Males > females, 2–5 : 1

PERIOPERATIVE RISKS
- Neonate: 10% mortality (preoperative CHF and associated cardiac anomalies)
- Children: 0.4% mortality

WORRY ABOUT
- Closure of ductus arteriosus causing severe CHF and hypoperfusion to body below coarctation
- Severe upper body hypertension in older children

- Risk of paraplegia: 0.5%
- Post-coarctectomy syndrome or mesenteric arteritis marked by abdominal pain, abdominal distention, N/V, and hypertension (postoperative day 1–3) treated with gastric decompression, IV fluids, and control of systemic hypertension

OVERVIEW
- Congenital constriction of aorta opposite insertion of ductus arteriosus
- Associated with bicuspid aortic valves, complex congenital anomalies, and aneurysms of circle of Willis (8–10%)

ICD-9-CM Code: 747.10

ETIOLOGY
- Aortic ampulla of ductus constricts obstructing aortic flow

USUAL TREATMENT
- Early surgical repair when diagnosed to minimize residual postoperative hypertension
- Subclavian flap used in coarctation repair of neonate
- Some prefer elective repair of asymptomatic children at age of 4–6 y to ↓ rate of re-coarctation

ASSESSMENT POINTS

SYSTEM	EFFECT	ASSESSMENT BY HX	PE	TEST
HEENT	Upper body hypertension	Older children may complain of headache and epistaxis		
CV			Decreased lower extremity pulses	2-D ECHO usually diagnostic
Neonates	Severe CHF	Poor feeding, irritability	Tachycardia, hepatomegaly	ABG: metabolic acidosis from hypoperfusion
Children >5 y	Collateral vessel formation	Older children asymptomatic	Visible or palpable collateral vessels	Rib notching on CXR
RESP	CHF (neonate)		Tachypnea Grunting Retractions	CXR of CHF: Cardiomegaly Pulmonary edema Pleural effusion "Figure 3" configuration of aorta
GI	Poor feeding in neonate			
RENAL	Renal failure 2° to CHF and poor distal aortic perfusion in neonate			Urinary catheter Electrolytes Creatinine
MS	Lower body hypoperfusion	Children may complain of lower extremity fatigue		

Key Reference: Findlow D, Doyle E: Congenital heart disease in adults. Br J Anaesth 1997; 78:416–430.

PERIOPERATIVE IMPLICATIONS

Preoperative Preparation
- Stabilize CHF in neonate using prostaglandin E₁ to reopen ductus arteriosus; severe CHF requires positive pressure ventilation, inotropic support, diuresis, and bicarbonate infusion

Monitoring
- Consider right radial arterial catheter and lower extremity BP cuff (arterial catheter if poor collateral circulation below coarctation)
- Temperature: incidental hyperthermia in neonate may predispose to paraplegia; moderate hypothermia to 34°C advocated in older children
- Consider evoked potentials, particularly if high gradient and poorly developed collateral circulation

Airway (Left Thoracotomy)
- Consider double lumen endotracheal in older patients

Induction
- Consider IV narcotic/relaxant-based anesthetic or slow induction with halothane and 50% nitrous oxide (< 1% halothane) with severe CHF

Maintenance
- Nitroprusside often used to control hypertension during aortic crossclamping (minimizes doses with labetalol)
- Hand ventilation when left lung retracted for exposure
- Prior to crossclamp release, consider discontinuing inhalation agent and nitroprusside and administering volume
- Consider ABGs after crossclamp release and bicarbonate as needed

Extubation
- Older children can be extubated at end of procedure
- Neonates in CHF generally remain intubated and ventilated; wean when CHF improves

ANTICIPATED PROBLEMS/CONCERNS
- Paroxysmal hypertension postoperatively
- Post-coarctectomy syndrome
- Paraplegia (0.5%)
- Newer techniques with intravascular (closed) repair using stents—similar problems and concerns

COMPLEMENT DEFICIENCY

Christine S. Rinder, M.D.

RISK

- Incidence: <0.1% of general population
- Male-female ratio: 1:6
- Higher (6%) in patients with autoimmune disease (see Immune Suppression in Diseases section)
- Patients with Hx of *Neisseria* meningitis have incidence of 15%

PERIOPERATIVE RISKS

- ↑ Risk of postoperative infection, particularly if the deficiency affects the early complement components, C1–C3
- Risk for inflammatory complications, e.g., glomerulonephritis, vasculitis

WORRY ABOUT

- ↑ Infectious risk

OVERVIEW

- May affect any component of classical pathway, alternate pathway, or terminal common pathway
- Virtually all deficiencies show some ↑ risk of infection and/or autoimmune disease
- Deficiencies in early complement components, namely C1, C2, and C3, associated with immunocompromise, resulting in recurrent life-threatening infections due to a variety of organisms
- ↑ Risk of autoimmune diseases
- Deficiency in any of the terminal components C5–C8 show selective risk of recurrent neisserial infections, usually not life-threatening

ICD-9-CM Code: 279.8

ETIOLOGY

- All complement proteins inherited in autosomal fashion, with possible exception of properdin, which appears to be X-linked

USUAL TREATMENT

- No specific therapy indicated
- Antibiotic treatment dictated by specific infection

ASSESSMENT POINTS

SYSTEM	EFFECT	TEST
IMMUNO	Infectious risk for all systems	CH50 screening test for complement-mediated lysis of sheep erythrocytes; tests for specific complement components available at reference laboratories. Assess other specific organs as indicated by autoimmune disease (renal for SLE, etc.)

Key Reference: Ross SC, Densen P: Complement deficiency states and infection: epidemiology, pathogenesis and consequences of neisserial and other infections in an immune deficiency. Medicine 1984; 63:243–273.

PERIOPERATIVE IMPLICATIONS

Preoperative Preparation
- Sterile technique strictly observed

Monitoring
- Routine
- Coagulation profile
- Minimize invasive lines

Airway
- Routine

Induction
- Routine

Maintenance
- Routine

Extubation
- Extubate and remove all lines at earliest opportunity

Postoperative Period
- Maintain sterile techniques

ANTICIPATED PROBLEMS/CONCERNS

- Meticulous sterile technique to minimize risk of infection

CONGENITAL BRONCHOGENIC CYST/PULMONARY CYST/LOBAR EMPHYSEMA

Francine S. Yudkowitz, M.D., F.A.A.P.

RISK

- Cause of cardiorespiratory compromise
- 10–15% associated with congenital heart disease

PERIOPERATIVE RISKS

- May develop worsening of cardiorespiratory status
- Contamination of unaffected lung by infected material from cyst

WORRY ABOUT

- Associated congenital anomalies
- Tension pneumothorax
- Cardiorespiratory compromise

OVERVIEW

Congenital Bronchogenic Cyst/Pulmonary Cyst

- Centrally located cysts in the mediastinum produce obstruction by mass effect
- Carinal cysts cause obstruction by ball-valve effect
- Hilar or lung cysts cause respiratory infections and may result in abscess formation

Lobar Emphysema

- Accumulation of air in one lobe. Most commonly occurs in the left upper lobe, followed in frequency by the right middle and then the right upper lobe.
- Preterm infants on mechanical ventilation develop emphysema in the right upper lobe
- Chest x-ray shows emphysematous lobe crossing midline, mediastinal shift, atelectasis of lower lobe and possibly contralateral lung. The presence of bronchovascular markings distinguishes this from pneumothorax and congenital cysts.

ICD-9-CM CODE: 748.4 (Congenital bronchogenic/Pulmonary cyst); 770.2 (Congenital lobar emphysema)

ETIOLOGY

Congenital Bronchogenic Cyst/Pulmonary Cyst

- May be bronchogenic, alveolar, or a combination of both
- Anomalous development of bronchopulmonary system at stage of terminal bronchiolar or early alveolar development. Expiratory obstruction from bronchiolar narrowing.
- Acquired cysts are more common

Lobar Emphysema

- Extrinsic bronchial obstruction from abnormal vessels or enlarged lymph nodes
- Intrinsic bronchial obstruction from deficient bronchial cartilage, bronchial stenosis, or redundant bronchial mucosa

USUAL TREATMENT

- Surgical removal

ASSESSMENT POINTS

SYSTEM	EFFECT	ASSESSMENT BY HX	PE	TEST
RESP	↓ Lung volume	Cyanosis, dyspnea, grunting, coughing	Tachypnea, retractions, wheezing, ↓ BS, asymmetric chest expansion	CXR CT scan
CV	Mediastinal shift, ↓ CO VSD, PDA	Irritability, poor feeding	↓ Heart sounds Murmur	CXR ECG, ECHO

Key Reference: Davis PJ, Hall S, Deshpande JK, Spear RM: Anesthesia for general, urologic, and plastic surgery. *In* Motoyama EK, Davis PJ (eds): Smith's Anesthesia for Infants and Children, 6th ed. St. Louis, Mosby–Year Book, 1996.

PERIOPERATIVE IMPLICATIONS

Preoperative Preparation

- Assess the severity of cardiopulmonary compromise
- Identify associated congenital anomalies
- Optimize respiratory infection if patient is stable
- Aspirate cyst prior to induction if there is cardiac compromise or airway obstruction

Monitoring

- Arterial line for blood pressure monitoring and blood gas analysis

Induction

- Avoid positive pressure ventilation until thorax is opened to avoid expansion of cyst or lobe
- Avoid N_2O, which will expand the lobe or cyst
- Inhalation induction with 100% oxygen
- Intubate without the use of muscle relaxants
- May need to isolate the affected lung. In small infants and children this may be accomplished by using a bronchial blocker or doing a main stem intubation.
- Surgeon should be available to open the chest immediately if deterioration should occur during induction of anesthesia

Maintenance

- No one anesthetic preferred
- Maintain spontaneous ventilation or assist with low airway pressures until the thorax is opened
- Once the pathology is removed, N_2O may be used
- If history of repeated lung infections (cysts), there may be large blood losses

Extubation/Postoperative Period

- May be extubated after uncomplicated surgery and when cardiopulmonary function is adequate
- Analgesia to allow sufficient ventilation and avoid atelectasis

ANTICIPATED PROBLEMS/CONCERN

- Patients with altered cardiopulmonary reserve before surgery may require postoperative intubation and ventilation
- If pneumonectomy performed; there will be overinflation of the remaining lung with a decrease in vital capacity. These children may have significant exercise intolerance for a prolonged period after surgery.
- To avoid postoperative atelectasis, coughing and early ambulation or increase in activity important
- Altered pulmonary mechanics (decreased forced vital capacity and delayed forced expiration) may be present throughout childhood.

CONGENITAL METHEMOGLOBINEMIA

Bronwyn R. Rae, M.D.

RISK

- Navajo Indians, Alaskan Indians, people of Puerto Rican and Cuban ancestry
- Normal life span (except for recessive congenital methemoglobinemia [RCM] type II)

PERIOPERATIVE RISKS

- No data available
- Pregnancies not compromised

WORRY ABOUT

- Measurement of SpO_2
- Oxidant drugs, e.g., prilocaine, benzocaine, nitroglycerin, sulfonamides, contraindicated

OVERVIEW

- Due to deficient reducing capacity of oxidized heme:
  - RCM types I and II: Deficient reducing capacity due to NADH cytochrome b5 reductase (diaphorase) deficiency. Shift of O_2 dissociation curve to left leads to mild erythrocytosis. Normal RBC life span.
  - RCM type I defect restricted to red cell soluble cytochrome b5 reductase only. Cyanosis is sole clinical symptom.
  - RCM type II: Defect in all tissues; involves both soluble and microsomal forms of cytochrome b5 reductase. Mental retardation, spasticity, opisthotonos, microcephaly, growth retardation. Death by 2–3 y.
- Due to structural abnormality in globin moiety:
  - HbM variations: Amino acid substitutions create abnormal environment for heme residues, displacing the equilibrium toward ferric state. Alpha chain variants affected from birth, beta chain variants by 3–6 mo of age. Mild hemolytic anemia.

ICD-9-CM Code: 289.7

ETIOLOGY

- RCM types I and II—autosomal recessive inheritance. Heterozygotes have increased susceptibility to metHb formation after exposure to oxidant drugs and chemicals.
- HbM variants—autosomal dominant inheritance

USUAL TREATMENT

- RCM types I and II: Reducing agents, e.g., riboflavin 20–60 mg orally, methylene blue 1 mg/kg IV. Effect lasts 10–14 days.
- May require exchange transfusion
- HbM variants: Treatment not possible or indicated

ASSESSMENT POINTS

SYSTEM	PE	TEST
RESP	Look cyanosed but more "blue" than "sick"	15–30% metHb
HEME		RCM types I and II: mild erythrocytosis HbM variants: mild hemolytic anemia

Key Reference: Dotsch J, Demirakca S, Kratz M, Repp R, Knerr I, Rascher W: Comparison of methylene blue, riboflavin, and N-acetylcysteine for the reduction of nitric oxide-induced methemoglobinemia. Crit Care Med 2000; 28:958–961.

PERIOPERATIVE IMPLICATIONS

Preoperative Preparation

- Can give reducing agents to patients with RCM type I but no data on whether treatment is indicated prior to anesthesia

Monitoring

- Pulse oximeter overestimates at low SpO_2 and underestimates at high SpO_2. In practice reads between 80–85% regardless of true saturation.
- May need to measure ABGs, and estimate SpO_2 from ABG

Airway

- None

Preinduction/Induction

- None

Maintenance

- Prilocaine, benzocaine, EMLA cream contraindicated
- Lidocaine, bupivacaine, nitrous oxide, volatile agents OK

Adjuvants

- None

Postoperative Period

- Avoid acetanilids for pain relief; narcotics OK

ANTICIPATED PROBLEMS/CONCERNS

- Avoid oxidant drugs in both homozygotes and heterozygotes
- Pulse oximetry is inaccurate; use ABGs

CONGESTIVE HEART FAILURE

Nicola D'Attellis, M.D.
Denis Safran, M.D.

RISK

- Complication and/or evolution of most cardiac disease
- 4.6 million in USA; 550,000 new cases annually. Primary discharge diagnosis in 1 million patients.
- Median survival after onset is 1.7 y in men and 3.2 y in women

PERIOPERATIVE RISKS

- CHF is a major determinant of perioperative risk
- EF <40% associated with ↑ operative risk
- Single greatest risk factor for cardiac surgery: Use congestive heart failure score (CASS): Hx of CHF = 1; Rx digitalis = 1; Rales = 1; If overt symptoms after treatment = 1; Total 0–4: If score = 4, operative risk is 8× greater.

WORRY ABOUT

- Ventricular dysfunction preop; associated with increased operative mortality
- Diastolic dysfunction leads to increased left atrial pressures with pulmonary congestion
- Dysrhythmias due to cardiac ischemia (sudden cardiac death)
- Associated acute or chronic mitral insufficiency
- Volume status
- Prolonged effect of ACE inhibitors

OVERVIEW

- Different types of failure (left vs. right; acute vs. chronic; systolic vs. diastolic; low output vs. high output)
- Heart unable to pump blood to meet metabolic demands.
- Acute ischemia can lead to global diastolic dysfunction and CHF
- Papillary muscle ischemia may lead to severe mitral regurgitation and pulmonary congestion
- New York Heart Association classification: I: no limitation; II: slight limitation; III: marked limitation; IV: inability to carry out any physical activity. Overall 1-y mortality for classes III and IV 34–58%.

ICD-9-CM Code: 428.0

ETIOLOGY

- *Acquired, acute or chronic:* CHD, MI; cardiomyopathy (idiopathic, hypertrophic, hypertrophic obstructive, congestive, alcoholic). Valvular heart disease: arrhythmias, severe Htn.
- *Congenital:* Congenital heart disease, L → R shunts; intracardiac (ASD, VSD, atrioventricular canal), extracardiac (PDA, anomalous pulmonary venous connection). Obstructive (coarctation of the aorta, aortic stenosis). Complex (Ebstein's anomaly).
- *Multiple precipitating causes:* Noncompliance with medications (digitalis, diuretics), excessive Na⁺; excessive IV fluids; drugs (β-blockers, doxorubicin, corticosteroids, disopyramide, nortriptyline, NSAIDs, androgens and estrogens). Pulmonary embolism: High-output states (pregnancy, fever, hyperthyroidism, sepsis, AV fistula, anemia).

USUAL TREATMENT

Chronic

- Physical activity encouraged
- Restriction of sodium intake
- Chronic β-blockade may lead to substantial clinical benefit
- Inhibit renin-angiotensin-aldosterone system (RAAS) (ACE inhibitors, angiotensin receptor blockers, aldosterone inhibitors)
- Improvement in systolic heart failure (digitalis)
- Diuretics, vasodilators (ACE inhibitors)

Acute

- Optimize pre- and afterload before starting inotropes and vasodilators
- Inotropes (dobutamine, milrinone, amrinone)
- Vasodilators (intravenous)
- Acute β-blockade may intensify heart failure

Special Measures

- Stimulation therapy (biventricular pacing + ICD)
- Surgical correction (CABG, CHD, valvular surgery, cardiomyoplasty, cardiac transplantation)
- Assist devices (IABP, LV assist, artificial heart)

ASSESSMENT POINTS

SYSTEM	EFFECT	ASSESSMENT BY HX	PE	TEST
CV	Inadequate cardiac output, congestion	Tachycardia, arrhythmias	Peripheral edema Facial edema (infants/young children) Cardiomegaly, pulsus alternans, distended neck veins, Kussmaul's sign, abdominojugular reflex	Exercise testing ECG, CXR Circulation time
RESP	Pulmonary congestion, decreased lung compliance, VC, TLC, pulmonary diffusion capacity	Breathlessness (exertional dyspnea, orthopnea, paroxysmal nocturnal dyspnea) Frequent respiratory infections	Rales and wheezes Pleural effusions Expectoration: frothy blood-tinged sputum	PFT ABGs CXR
GI	Hepatic and intestinal congestion	Nausea, bloating, fullness	Congestive hepatomegaly, ascites, icterus, cachexia	Liver enzymes
RENAL	Decreased GFR, activation RAAS	Nocturia, oliguria	Ankle edema	BUN/Cr, K⁺, Na⁺ Proteinuria Specific gravity
CNS	Hypoperfusion	Confusion, impairment of memory	Mental status exam	
PNS	Increased sympathetic tone	Cool extremities	Peripheral vasoconstriction, pallor, diaphoresis, tachycardia, clubbing	

Key Reference: Ryckwaert F, Colson P: Hemodynamic effects of anesthesia in patients with ischemic heart failure chronically treated with angiotensin-converting enzyme inhibitors. Anesth Analg 1997; 84:945–949.

PERIOPERATIVE IMPLICATIONS

Preoperative Preparation

- Stabilize patient by treating CHF before surgery
- Continue inotropic support
- Continue cardiac medications (ACE inhibitors may cause hypotension on induction)

Monitoring

- Consider arterial line
- Consider CVP, PA catheter, or TEE
  - CVP may be inaccurate in assessing volume

Airway

- Frothy secretions may lead to difficult visualization

Induction

- Preop therapeutic regimen (diuretics) causes hypovolemia, hypokalemia, and hyponatremia, which are potential problems before surgery
- Judicious volume replacement (avoid dehydration and overhydration)
- Avoid myocardial contractility depressants (e.g., barbiturates, inhalation agents)

Maintenance

- Maintain myocardial contractility, reduce afterload, and normalize PVR

Extubation

- May be delayed owing to CV and pulmonary insufficiencies

Adjuvants

- Rx inotropes; digitalis, diuretics
  - May be less responsive to catecholamines
- Regional anesthesia debated and not recommended by some (sympathectomy, volume status) or preferred (reduce preload) by others

Postoperative Period

- Inotropic support and mechanical assistance may be needed
- Pulmonary edema develops in 2–16% of patients

ANTICIPATED PROBLEMS/CONCERNS

- Pulmonary edema may necessitate prolonged ventilation with high FIO₂
- RV and/or LV failure in the postop period

CONN'S SYNDROME (HYPERALDOSTERONISM, PRIMARY)

Stephen P. Fischer, M.D.

RISK

- People within USA: 0.5–1% of Htn patients without known etiology
- Female:male 2:1
- Age onset usually 30–50 y

PERIOPERATIVE RISKS

- ↑ Risk of CHF 2° to hypervolemia
- ↑ Risk of ischemic heart disease
- ↑ Diastolic Htn with LVH

WORRY ABOUT

- Volume/electrolyte imbalance, especially hypokalemia
- Nephropathy may impair renal function
- Pathologic fractures with positioning 2° to osteoporosis

OVERVIEW

- Primary aldosteronism; mineralocorticoid excess
- K^+ depletion, Na^+ conservation with ↑ extracellular volume
- Dx by ↑ urinary aldosterone and K^+ with ↓ plasma renin
- Proper treatment results in normal life expectancy

ICD-9-CM Code: 255.1

ETIOLOGY

- Unilateral adrenal functional adenoma (66%)
- Bilateral adrenocortical hyperplasia (33%)
- Adrenal carcinoma (<1%)
- Excess secretion of aldosterone

USUAL TREATMENT

- Initial treatment: K^+ supplement and competitive aldosterone antagonist (e.g., spironolactone 25–100 mg bid)
- Surgical excision of adrenal gland(s)
  – Open laparoscopic technique

ASSESSMENT POINTS

SYSTEM	EFFECT	ASSESSMENT BY HX	PE	TEST
HEENT		Visual disturbances		
CV	Cardiomegaly, diastolic Htn Arrhythmias 2° to ↓ K^+ ↑ Preload 2° to hypervolemia		BP ↑ JVD	CXR, ECG K^+
RESP	Hypoventilation Resp muscle weakness	Truncal obesity possible ↓ Exercise tolerance		
RENAL	Hypokalemic metabolic alkalosis Polyuria, polydipsia, nocturia Nephropathy, renal Htn			K^+, ABGs Glucose BUN/Cr
GI	Hyperacidity	Reflux Hx		
SKIN	Atrophic	Easy bruising		
ENDO	Hyperglycemia (50% of patients) Hypernatremia, hypokalemia			Glucose, K^+, Na^+
HEME	Hypercoagulability with thromboembolism ↑ Infection susceptibility			
CNS		Headache		
PNS	Paresthesias			K^+
MS	Muscle weakness, fatigue, tetany Osteoporosis	Pathologic fractures		K^+

Key Reference: Winship SM, Winstanley JH, Hunter JM: Anaesthesia for Conn's syndrome. Anaesthesia 1999; 54:569–574.

PERIOPERATIVE IMPLICATIONS

Preoperative Preparation

- Correct hypervolemia, hypokalemia, hypernatremia, hyperglycemia
- Treat hyperacidity: cimetidine/bicitrate

Monitoring

- Consider arterial or pulm artery catheter if suspect CV impairment, ↑ CO, or major surgery

Airway

- Tracheal intubation may be difficult with obesity

Induction

- No specific anesthesia technique for adrenalectomy

Maintenance

- Monitor intraoperative glucose, acid-base status, fluid balance
- Avoid hyperventilation: ↑ metabolic alkalosis and ↓ K^+

Extubation

- Prolonged emergence possible

Adjuvants

- Hypokalemia may potentiate response to muscle relaxants

- Use of enflurane questionable if hypokalemic nephropathy and polyuria

Postoperative Period

- CXR for pneumothorax; up to 20% postop if adrenalectomy

ANTICIPATED PROBLEMS/CONCERNS

- ↑ Pancreatitis with left adrenalectomy

CONSTIPATION

Takashi Asai, M.D., Ph.D.
Michael Rosen, C.B.E., F.R.C.A.

RISK

- Incidence in USA: 2–25%
- Higher prevalence in elderly and in females

PERIOPERATIVE RISKS

- Increased risk of nausea, vomiting, abdominal pain, headache

WORRY ABOUT

- A possibility of increased risk of pulmonary aspiration of gastric contents
- Pseudo-obstruction of the intestine
- High airway pressure, decreased vital capacity, and decreased FRC due to elevated diaphragm

OVERVIEW

- Can cause nausea, vomiting, and abdominal pain
- By itself does not affect life expectancy

ICD-9-CM Code: 564.0

ETIOLOGY

- Idiopathic in most cases
- In some cases associated with congenital (e.g., Hirschsprung's disease) or acquired (whether genetic or not) diseases (diabetes mellitus, multiple sclerosis)

USUAL TREATMENT

- Ingestion of dietary fiber
- Laxatives and enemas
- Colectomy and ileorectostomy

ASSESSMENT POINTS

SYSTEM	EFFECT	ASSESSMENT BY HX	TEST
RESP	Elevated diaphragm Increased airway pressure	Abdominal distention	CXR
GI	Intestinal obstruction Nausea and vomiting Gastroparesis	Abdominal distention	Abdominal x-ray
CNS	Headache		

Key Reference: Stewart RB, Moore MT, Marks RG, Hale WE: Correlates of constipation in an ambulatory elderly population. Am J Gastroenterol 1992; 87:859–864.

PERIOPERATIVE IMPLICATIONS

Monitoring
- Airway pressure

Airway
- Decreased FRC

Induction
- Awake or rapid-sequence induction if there is an obstruction of the intestine

Maintenance
- Avoid using nitrous oxide if there is an obstruction of the intestine

Extubation
- Extubate after the airway reflexes have recovered

Adjuvants
- Opioids or atropine, but not NSAIDs, delay gastrointestinal transit

ANTICIPATED PROBLEMS/CONCERNS

- Gaseous distention of gut and elevated diaphragm may be present. Avoid using nitrous oxide in such patients.
- Gastrointestinal transit may be delayed. Consider Rx enemas.

CONVERSION DISORDER

Michael Ho, M.D.

RISK

- Reported prevalence varies widely (11–300/100,000); may account for as much as 1–3% of outpatient psychiatric referrals
- Reported to be more common in rural populations, developing areas, lower socioeconomic groups, those less medically sophisticated

PERIOPERATIVE RISKS

- No definite association with increased perioperative morbidity or mortality, as long as patient's symptoms are due only to conversion disorder

WORRY ABOUT

- Presence of undiagnosed neurologic or general medical illnesses, which could take years to become evident
- Appearance of conversion symptoms mimicking medical disturbances, drug effects, or anesthetic or surgically related complications
- Malingering, factitious disorder, drug abuse, confabulation

OVERVIEW

- DSM-IV: Conversion disorder is one of 7 somatoform disorders (disorders whose physical symptoms suggest the presence of, but are not fully explained by, a general medical illness)
- Diagnosis based on involuntary appearance of one or more symptoms affecting voluntary motor or sensory function that suggest (but are not explained by) a neurologic or general medical condition ("pseudoneurologic" symptoms)
- Symptoms cannot be intentional or feigned, attributable to culturally sanctioned or religious experiences, limited to pain or sexual dysfunction, or better explained by another mental disorder, and must cause clinically significant distress or impairment in functioning
- Although individual symptoms are of short duration (< 2 wk), recurrence is common (20% within 1 y)
- Patients may undergo numerous examinations, diagnostic procedures, and hospitalizations, potentially causing morbidity; diagnosis is usually tentative and provisional

ICD-9-CM Code: 300.11

ETIOLOGY

- Hypothesis that somatic symptoms represent symbolic resolution of an unconscious psychologic conflict by reducing anxiety and removing the conflict from awareness
- Although validity of hypothesis not essential, associated psychologic factors must be present
- Symptoms more frequently found among relatives of conversion disorder patients; risk is greater in monozygotic than dizygotic twins
- $1/4$ to $1/2$ of patients initially diagnosed actually have general medical conditions

USUAL TREATMENT

- First line: reassurance and relaxation
- Second line: amobarbital interview, hypnosis, behavior therapy, psychotherapy or psychoanalysis
- Anecdotal use of phenothiazines, lithium, ECT
- Direct confrontation not recommended

ASSESSMENT POINTS

SYSTEM	EFFECT	ASSESSMENT BY HX	PE	TEST
CNS	Four subtypes: 1. Motor: impaired coordination or balance, paralysis or localized weakness, aphonia, difficulty swallowing or sensation of lump in the throat, urinary retention 2. Sensory: loss of touch or pain sensation, double vision, blindness, deafness, hallucinations 3. Seizures or convulsions 4. Mixed presentation	Differential diagnosis includes almost any medical condition (e.g., myasthenia gravis, multiple sclerosis, porphyria, diabetic neuropathy, hyperparathyroidism, tumors, idiopathic or substance-abuse dystonias)	Findings do not conform to known anatomic pathways or physiologic mechanisms, symptoms inconsistent, e.g., unacknowledged strength in antagonistic muscles; normal muscle tone, intact reflexes; equal difficulty swallowing solids and liquids "Paralyzed" extremity moves on own with dressing: arm held over patient's head by examiner and dropped will not fall on head; stocking-glove anesthesia without proximal to distal gradient; equal loss of touch, temperature, and pain at sharply demarcated anatomic landmarks rather than dermatomes	Absence of expected findings (including EEG, EMG, lumbar puncture, CT, MRI, SPECT scan, nerve conduction velocity, drug screen) suggest and confirm diagnosis
GENDER		Gender tendencies: Men—antisocial personality, work-related or military injury Women—more common, especially on left side of body. Children < 10 y: seizures, gait disturbances.		

Key Reference: Diagnostic and Statistical Manual of Mental Disorders. Washington, DC, American Psychiatric Association, 1994, pp 452–457.

PERIOPERATIVE IMPLICATIONS

Perioperative Preparation
- Careful history and PE, carefully documenting any pre-existing neurologic deficits
- Confer with previous physicians (e.g., internist, neurologist, psychiatrist) when necessary
- Verify that tests are negative to rule out misdiagnosis
- Consider possibility that reason for surgery in patient with multiple procedures may involve conversion symptom

Monitoring
- Routine

Airway
- None

Premedication/Induction/Maintenance
- No specific technique clearly superior
- Regional anesthesia not contraindicated

Extubation
- None

Adjuvants
- Sedatives as appropriate

Postoperative Period
- Watch for reappearance of conversion symptoms
- Conversion symptoms may represent previously undiagnosed medical disease, unmasked by stresses of anesthesia and surgery

ANTICIPATED PROBLEMS/CONCERNS

- Previously undiagnosed medical disease is probably common among patients with psychiatric disease. The anesthesiologist may be the first to suggest the presence of both psychiatric disease and related medical conditions. In order to properly treat patients with somatic complaints, a preoperative screening clinic should be employed whenever possible and appropriate consultation sought whenever necessary.

COR PULMONALE

Paul Zanaboni, M.D., Ph.D.

RISK

• Third most common cardiac Dx after age 50 y
• 10–20% of all CHF admissions have some aspect of right heart failure
• Gender predominance: male > female

PERIOPERATIVE RISKS

• ↑ Risk for respiratory failure, right heart failure (≥10% if cor pulmonale Dx made preoperatively)
• Risk of prolonged postoperative ventilatory support

WORRY ABOUT

• ↑ Pulmonary vascular resistance (PVR) may cause systemic hypotension
• Hypoxia, hypoxemia, hypercarbia, and acidosis intraoperatively or in early postoperative period, which ↑ PVR
• Underlying CAD, LV dysfunction

OVERVIEW

• Alteration in RV structure (hypertrophy) and function
• Most common cause: COPD (↑ PVR 2° to chronic hypoxia and structural changes)
• Any disease that ↑ PVR chronically can induce RV changes, including idiopathic pulmonary hypertension and toxin-induced pulmonary hypertension, pulmonary fibrosis
• Prognosis: favorable for those who can maintain a near-normal PaO_2; unfavorable for those with structural changes

ICD-9-CM Code: 416.9

ETIOLOGY

• COPD: smoking or severe asthma
• Primary pulmonary hypertension: Pulmonary fibrosis; either drug-induced or idiopathic; chronic pulmonary embolism

USUAL TREATMENT

• ↓ PVR toward normal levels by ↑ PaO_2 to 60 mmHg (beware of depression of hypoxic drive to breathe; may have desensitized hypercarbic drive to breathe 2° to chronic ↑ $PaCO_2$); giving diuretics, digoxin to relieve symptoms of CHF (caution: diuretics may increase Hct by hemoconcentration; if Hct already ↑ 2° to ↓ PaO_2, this may further ↑ viscosity of blood, increasing risk for sludging and microemboli)
• Vasodilators (only ⅓ of patients improve); inhaled nitric oxide; other vasodilators, such as calcium-channel blockers, have been tried; use caution because may ↓ SVR in face of fixed ↑ PVR, causing severe systemic hypotension (unable to increase CO)
Antibiotics for prompt treatment of infection

ASSESSMENT POINTS

SYSTEM	EFFECT	ASSESSMENT BY HX	PE	TEST
CV	RV failure ↑ PVR Tricuspid regurgitation	DOE Effort-related syncope Chest pain	Accentuated pulmonary S_2 Diastolic or systolic murmur Dependent edema	CXR ECHO Right heart catheterization
RESP	COPD	DOE Chronic cough, sputum	Hyperinflated lungs Wheezing, rhonchi	CXR PFTs
GI	Passive congestion of liver, spleen		Hepatosplenomegaly	LFTs Albumin PT
RENAL	Impaired ability to excrete Na^+, H_2O	Edema	Edema	Urinary Osm Urine specific gravity
CNS	Stimulation of sympathetic nervous system 2° to hypoxia		Tachycardia	

Key Reference: Ceccarelli P, Bigatello LM, Hess D, Kwo J, Melendez L, Horford WE: Inhaled nitric oxide delivery by anesthesia machines. Anesth Analg 2000; 90:482–488.

PERIOPERATIVE IMPLICATIONS

Preoperative Preparation

• Treat underlying infections
• Maximize treatment of reversible airway disease
• Maximize pulmonary toilet to expand airways and ↓ secretions
• Avoid preoperative medications that will depress ventilation

Monitoring

• Consider arterial line for ABG
• Consider pulmonary arterial catheter to monitor PA pressures, CVP monitoring for evaluation of RV function for large fluid shift reoperations

Airway

• Potential for bronchospasm

Induction

• Try to ↑ SVR in face of fixed ↑ PVR
• Deep anesthesia for intubation may ↓ incidence of bronchospasm and sympathetic stimulation, which ↑ PVR

Maintenance

• Potent inhalational agents for bronchodilation
• Consider avoiding nitrous oxide (which may ↑ PVR) and large doses of narcotics (which may cause postoperative hypoventilation)
• Although positive pressure ventilation may ↑ PVR 2° to alveolar expansion, it can ↓ PVR 2° to better oxygenation
• Aggresively prevent hypercarbia, hypoxemia, and hypothermia, all of which may cause ↑ in PVR
• Consider the use of β-adrenergic agents such as dobutamine or epinephrine to support RV cardiac output if faced with hemodynamic instability
• Consider the use of inhaled NO to treat ↑ PVR
• Can also consider use of prostaglandin E_1 to ↓ PVR (beware of ↓ SVR, which may require treatment with an α-adrenergic agonist)

Extubation

• Bronchospasm may occur during emergence

Adjuvants

• Regional anesthesia an option, but high level may cause ↓ SVR in face of fixed ↑ PVR
• Nitric oxide increasing in use

Postoperative Period

• Postoperative pain management with either low-dose epidural local anesthetics with low-dose opioids or low-dose intrathecal opioids can minimize respiratory depression

ANTICIPATED PROBLEMS/CONCERNS

• ↑ PVR and RV dysfunction from hypoxia/hypercarbia or hypothermia

CORONARY ARTERY DISEASE
(LEFT MAIN AND NON–LEFT MAIN DISEASE)

J.G. Reves, M.D.

RISK

- Incidence: 11 million in USA
- 1.5 million patients per year with CAD will have an acute MI; one third of these will die
- CAD responsible for 51% of deaths in men and 49% in women (largest single disease cause in both)
- Male predominance < 55 y, M = F > 55 y
- Risk factors: Htn, diabetes, smoking, familial incidence, hyperlipidemia, and high cholesterol

PERIOPERATIVE RISKS

- Presence of disease by coronary anatomy is good predictor of survival with CAD
- Presence of left main disease with high degree of stenosis is life-threatening
- Recent MI ↑ risk, but revascularization interventions protect patient
- Impaired ventricular function, unstable anginal pattern, major surgery, and emergency surgery ↑ risk
- ↑ Risk if reoperation for bypass surgery

WORRY ABOUT

- Myocardial ischemia can lead to MI
- Postop MI carries very high mortality (> 50%) in noncardiac surgical patients
- Atherosclerosis in other vascular beds (CNS, renal, mesentery)
- Increased bleeding during and after surgery if patient is taking an anticoagulant for prevention of MI

OVERVIEW

- Atherosclerosis of vessels supplying blood to heart results in ↓ blood flow by limitation of flow due to anatomy or due to vasoactive dysfunction (spasm, etc.)
- Single greatest cause of death in USA population (500,000 deaths/y)
- Most prevalent form of cardiovascular disease: > 11 million of USA population has CAD
- Leading cause of death in major noncardiac surgery

ICD-9-CM Code: 414.0

See also Angina, Chronic Stable, in Diseases section

ETIOLOGY

- Atherosclerosis and obstructive deposits in coronary artery
- Interaction of genetics, diet, and environment: hypertension, cigarette smoking, and diabetes are three common predisposing factors
- Myocardial oxygen delivery does not meet myocardial oxygen demands: causes myocardial ischemia
- Myocardial oxygen supply does not reach myocardium after thrombosis of coronary artery: causes MI

USUAL TREATMENT

- Medical: nitroglycerin, β-blockers, calcium-channel blockers (low dose and in vasospastic component), diet, antihyperlipidemia drugs, aspirin, exercise, weight loss, antioxidants
- Catheter-based interventional cardiology (indicated in ≤ 2-vessel CAD): PTCA (has 30% 3-mo closure rate), intracoronary stent (has good angiographic result and lower closure rate, but event-free survival is little different from PTCA)
- CABG surgery (indicated in ≥ 2-vessel CAD). CABG indicated before noncardiac surgery in left main CAD.

ASSESSMENT POINTS

CONCERN	EFFECT	ASSESSMENT BY HX	PE	TEST
Noncardiac Surgery				
Ischemia	Causes ventricular dysfunction Can herald and/or cause MI	Angina		Holter monitor, ECG exercise radionuclide, treadmill stress ECHO
Infarction	Indicates severe CAD Causes death			ECG, CK-MB and troponin enzyme release
Impaired function	Heart failure, shock	Activity history Stair climbing	Orthopnea gallop Neck veins	Ejection fraction (cath, ECHO, radionuclide)
Cardiac Surgery				
Cardiac function	Best predictor of outcome	Activity history, stair climbing		Ventricular angiogram (EF > 50% = good risk)
Coronary anatomy	Extent of disease and overall long-term survival			Coronary angiography
Renal function	↑ Risk if impaired			Cr ≥ 2.0 denotes ↑ risk
CNS	↑ Risk of stroke	Hx of TIA, symptomatic bruits		Carotid Doppler study

Key Reference: Eagle KA, Guyton RA, Darrdoff R, et al: ACC/AHA guidelines for coronary artery bypass graft surgery: executive summary and recommendations—a report of the American College of Cardiology/American Heart Association Task Force on Practice Guidelines. Circulation 1999; 100:1464–1480.

PERIOPERATIVE IMPLICATIONS

Preoperative Preparation

- Supportive preoperative interview to ↓ stress and anxiety
- Consider analgesic (opioid) if pain or likelihood of pain prior to anesthesia
- Give morning cardiac medications, especially the β-blockers
- Nitroglycerin at bedside

Monitoring

- Consider systemic arterial BP (invasive and continuous in unstable patients or in cases where BP swings are anticipated)
- Consider CVP and/or PA catheters; in cardiac surgical patients, EF ≤ 30% should trigger consideration of catheter, or use of TEE

Anesthesia

- Principle is to maintain O_2 supply and to minimize myocardial O_2 consumption
  – Maintain O_2 sat and Hgb concentration (O_2 carrying capacity)
  – Maintain diastolic BP (perfusion pressure)
  – ↓ HR, contractility, and wall tension (O_2 consumption)
- No outcome difference demonstrated among general anesthetics
- Regional and conduction anesthesia with postoperative analgesia may be beneficial
- Transient periods of hypertension are well tolerated; prolonged periods of hypotension, tachycardia, and anemia are not well tolerated

Adjuvants

- Nitroglycerin, sublingual or (preferably) by continuous infusion (0.5–2.0 μg/kg/min), can treat myocardial ischemia
- β-blockers by bolus or infusion ↓ HR and myocardial contractility and can prevent and treat ischemia
- RBCs to maintain Hct ≥ 28%

Postoperative Period

- 2nd and 3rd postop days are most common time for MI in noncardiac surgical patients; ischemia intraoperatively, designate as "high risk" in postoperative period
- Maintain good analgesia to ↓ stress response
- Maintain cardiac medications (esp β-blockers)
- Consider use of aspirin or other medications to ↓ coronary thrombosis in high-risk noncardiac surgical patients

CORONARY ARTERY SPASM (CAS)

Robert G. Merin, M.D.

RISK

• Incidence of pure disease is very low, but CAS may complicate atherosclerotic CAD.
• Difficult to differentiate from transient microthrombotic episodes
• More common in females, diabetics, and hypertensives

PERIOPERATIVE RISKS

• Low (classical): Dx based on ST-segment or wall motion evidence for myocardial ischemia without concurrent changes in determinates of myocardial oxygen balance (non–hemodynamically related [NHR]) may occur after CABG
• High (new view of cause of thrombosis in CAD): Not related to structural tight stenoses, but to humoral/endocardial factors that can also precipitate thrombosis

WORRY ABOUT

• Consequences of ischemia such as arrhythmia, ventricular failure, MI

OVERVIEW

• Classical: Diagnosed by normal coronary angiogram during chest pain and ST-segment depression and exaggerated coronary vasoconstriction to ergonovine

Two Distinct Syndromes

• Prinzmetal's (variant) angina (syndrome A): Demonstrable coronary vasospasm in epicardial vessels on coronary angiogram; regional, usually at site of small nonobstructing atheroma; can be demonstrated in patients with hypercholesterolemia without coronary atherosclerosis; often occurs at rest; no gender predominance; without concurrent CAD, prognosis is excellent. With concurrent CAD can lead to infarction.
• Syndrome X (microvascular angina): No demonstrable coronary vasospasm on coronary angiogram; rarely associated with CAD; limited coronary vascular reserve ($\uparrow$ coronary BF with dipyridamole or papaverine); sometimes chest pain at rest, but accentuated by exercise; predominantly female (70:30); prognosis usually excellent.

ICD-9-CM Code: 413.1 (Prinzmetal)

See also Coronary Artery Disease in Diseases section

ETIOLOGY

• Vascular endothelial dysfunction with decreased release of nitric oxide (or increased degradation by oxygen free radicals)
• Same risk factors as for CAD but cigarette smoking even more prevalent
• Predominantly vascular smooth muscle dysfunction; present in peripheral vessels as well; diabetes and Htn special risk factors.

USUAL TREATMENT

• Medical therapy: Calcium-channel blocking drugs and nitroglycerin are Rx for both syndromes; also potassium-channel agonists
• Angioplasty for discrete single proximal lesions in syndrome A

ASSESSMENT POINTS

SYSTEM	EFFECT	ASSESSMENT BY HX	PE	TEST
CV	Chest pain Myocardial ischemia Htn	Chest pain at rest NHR ischemia relieved by Ca^{2+}-channel blockers		ECG Coronary angio with ergonovine testing
RESP	Chest pain	May be caused by hyperventilation		
MS	Syndrome X ischemia	Claudication	Decreased or absent peripheral pulses	Angiography or Doppler

Key Reference: Maseri A, Davies G, Hackett D, Kaski JC: Coronary artery spasm and vasoconstriction: The case for distinction. Circulation 1990; 81:1983–1991.

PERIOPERATIVE IMPLICATIONS

Preoperative Preparation

• Continue Ca^{2+}-channel blockers and nitrates. Consider IV nitroglycerin and nicardipine.

Monitoring

• ST-segment analysis
• Consider intra-arterial BP
• Consider TEE if available

Airway

• None

Preinduction/Induction

• Control HR and BP

Maintenance

• Careful HR, BP, and temp control
• Consider thoracic epidural anesthesia

Extubation

• May be increased risk for vasospasm

Postoperative Period

• Adequate pain treatment
• Consider continuous epidural

Adjuvants

• Ca^{2+}-channel blockers, nitroglycerin

ANTICIPATED PROBLEMS/CONCERNS

• Differentiate coronary vasospasm from microemboli because treatment is different; untreated, either may lead to arrhythmias, CHF, MI

CRANIOSYNOSTOSIS

Yvon F. Bryan, M.D.

RISK

- May be isolated defect or part of malformation syndrome; isolated in 6 in 10,000 births
- Apert's syndrome occurs in 1 in every 10,000
- Several different mechanisms responsible for defect

PERIOPERATIVE RISKS

- Difficult airway
- Massive blood loss
- Increased intracranial pressure (ICP)

WORRY ABOUT

- Difficulty due to craniofacial anomalies
- Treatment of increased ICP
- Potential for massive fluid and blood replacement
- Venous air embolism if extensive bones work

OVERVIEW

- Premature closure of cranial sutures
- Degree of deformity depends on the number of sutures and time when fused
- May be isolated or part of a syndrome
- If only one suture involved usually sagittal and deformity repaired for cosmetic reasons
- With more than one suture, the infant may need repair to assess ↑ ICP
- Multiple sutures associated with syndromes, such as Apert's and Crouzon's, that affect cranium, cranial base, and face
- Crouzon's associated with strabismus and malignant hyperthermia

ICD-9-CM Code: 756.0

ETIOLOGY

- Congenital anomaly in which one or more of the cranial sutures close prematurely
- Sagittal sinus most commonly involved in ~57%
- Coronal synostosis is between 18 and 29%

- May be classified by 58 different syndromes
- Monogenic syndromes that are autosomal dominant, autosomal recessive, X-linked, or with an unknown inheritance pattern
- Other syndromes are chromosomal, environmental induced, or of unknown causes
- Teratogens that cause craniosynostosis are diphenylhydantoin, aminopterin, methotrexate, retinoic acid, oxymetazoline, and valproic acid
- Can also be due to metabolic and hematologic disorders

USUAL TREATMENT

- Operate between the ages of 2 to 6 mo
- May need to treat elevated ICP if present
- Manage associated problems involved with the rare syndromes
- May need airway management techniques that are different from the usual, including possible tracheotomy

ASSESSMENT POINTS

SYSTEM	EFFECT	ASSESSMENT BY HX	PE	TEST
HEENT	Difficult airway, maxillary hypoplasia, ocular proptosis, dental malocclusion	Hx of difficult intubation	Large tongue, micrognathia, short neck	Neck x-rays if indicated
CV	Congenital heart disease	Atrial septal defects, tetrology of Fallot, patent ductus arteriosus, etc.	Murmurs, irregular rhythms	ECG, ECHO, cardiac catheterization
RESP	Tracheal stenosis, tracheobronchomalacia, obstructive sleep apnea		Tachypnea, sternal retractions, accessory muscles	ABGs, room air saturation
METAB	Electrolyte abnormalities			Electrolytes
NEURO	↑ ICP, hydrocephalus, seizure disorders, mental retardation	Vomiting, lethargy, seizures		

Key Reference: Gregory G (ed): Pediatric Anesthesia, 3rd ed. New York, Churchill Livingstone, 1994, pp 394–395 and 702–704.

PERIOPERATIVE IMPLICATIONS

Preoperative Preparation
- Obtain Hx as to whether a single suture involved for cosmetic reasons as opposed to multiple sutures in a patient with congenital syndromes and increased ICP
- Assess potential of difficult airway by Hx, physical exam, or risk secondary to syndrome

Monitoring
- Single suture in healthy infant need only one IV (20 or 22 G); multiple sutures requires large-bore IVs, arterial line, central venous line, urinary catheter, precordial Doppler

Airway
- Plan to have surgeon for possible tracheotomy if know difficult and previous attempts at intubation were unsuccessful
- Awake fiberoptic intubation a possibility
- Numerous laryngoscope blades, airways, and masks available
- A reinforced endotracheal tube

Induction
- Normal airway in healthy child—an inhalational induction with either halothane or sevoflurane in nitrous oxide and oxygen
- Increased ICP may need intravenous induction without ketamine
- Need to modify induction depending on the syndrome involved

Maintenance
- Blood loss can be >150% of blood volume, requiring massive transfusions
- Coagulopathies, electrolyte abnormalities, acidosis, and inadvertent extubation are possible
- Warming devices necessary

Extubation
- A short procedure (one suture) with minimal blood loss can be extubated in OR
- Numerous suture involvement associated with significant blood loss may be extubated if warm, hemodynamics as preop
- For the difficult airway plan to have necessary equipment

- For procedures below the orbital ridge, may need to leave intubated until edema resolves

Adjuvants
- Obtain the blood products, equipment necessary for operation and transfer to the PACU or ICU

Postoperative Period
- Major concerns are the airway and problems with oxygenation and ventilation
- If remain intubated, the need to sedate and ventilate and to decide when and how to extubate can be discussed by the surgeons, anesthesiologists, and intensivists
- Bleeding and metabolic abnormalities may occur in the postop period

ANTICIPATED PROBLEMS/CONCERNS

- Airway difficulties
- Communication between the teams involved
- Adequate blood and fluid resuscitation

CREST SYNDROME

Valerie Sera, M.D.
Michael Faulkner, M.D.

RISK

- Incidence of all forms of scleroderma 20/1 million/y
- Rarely seen before age 25
- Women > men

PERIOPERATIVE RISKS

- Severe hypotension 2° to hypovolemia
- Hypoxia 2° to pulmonary Htn and restrictive disease
- Failed intubation

WORRY ABOUT

- GI reflux
- Obliterative vasculopathy leading to pulmonary Htn
- Restrictive lung disease
- Renal crises
- Mucosal tears

OVERVIEW

- CREST (calcinosis, Raynaud's phenomenon, esophageal dysmotility, sclerodactyly, and telangiectasia)
- CREST syndrome, otherwise known as limited cutaneous systemic sclerosis, describes the features seen in patients who have one form of systemic sclerosis
  - Must have 3 of 5 signs present
- Prominent feature in patients with CREST syndrome is telangiectases, particularly affecting the hands and face, but may also be seen late in the course of diffuse systemic sclerosis
- Calcinosis refers to cutaneous and subcutaneous deposits of calcium and is a manifestation of limited cutaneous systemic sclerosis. Calcinosis will typically occur on pressure points of the arms (extensor surfaces), buttocks, and finger pads.
- CREST syndrome should not be considered a disease entity separate from scleroderma (systemic sclerosis), but it is usually more benign

ICD-9-CM Code: 710.1 (Scleroderma)

ETIOLOGY

- Autoimmunity, genetics, hormones, environmental factors may all play role
- Autoantibodies: anticentromere

USUAL TREATMENT

- Begin during early inflammatory stage, strategies are target organ–specific
- Includes antifibrinolytic agents, anti-inflammatory drugs, immunosuppressive therapy, vascular drugs

ASSESSMENT POINTS

SYSTEM	EFFECT	ASSESSMENT OF HISTORY	PE	TEST
HEENT	Cutaneous fibrosis Mucosal telangiectases		Masked facies Small oral aperture Atrophy of gums Hyperpigmentation	Direct visualization of airway
CV	Pericardial disease Myocardial fibrosis Conduction abnormalities	DOE CHF Arrhythmia Syncope	Rales	ECHO ECG, Holter
RESP	Fibrosing alveolitis Obliterative vasculopathy Pulmonary Htn	Dyspnea Nonproductive cough		CXR PFTs Bronchoalveolar lavage ECHO
GI	Esophageal fibrosis/colonic dysmotility	Difficulty chewing Dysphagia Bloating Diarrhea	Weight loss	UGI/endoscopy
RENAL	Intrinsic renal vessel disease		Malignant Htn	Proteinuria Hematuria ↑ Renin Cr
DERM	Cutaneous fibrosis Calcinosis at pressure points		Fibrosis of limbs, ↓ sweating Atrophy and contractures Telangiectases	
MS	Raynaud's phenomenon	Excessive cold sensitivity Pain	Cyanosis of digits	

Key Reference: Pronk LC, Swaak AJ: Pulmonary hypertension in connective tissue disease. Report of three cases and review of the literature. Rheumatol Int 1991; 11:83–86.

PERIOPERATIVE IMPLICATIONS

Preoperative Preparation

- Proton pump inhibitors to reduce gastric acid
- Consider metoclopramide for early disease
  - Less effective for late disease

Monitoring

- Invasive arterial monitoring relatively contraindicated in patients with Raynaud's disease because of risk of digit ischemia, but ABGs may be indicated
- Blood pressure may be difficult because of reduced forearm blood flow
- Consider PA catheter if pulmonary Htn
- Skin temperature may be significantly lower (1.5°C) than core

Anesthetic Technique

- Regional anesthesia may be preferable, considering pulmonary problems
- Regional technique may be associated with prolonged block in the presence of epinephrine because of severe vasoconstriction
- May see vasomotor instability

Airway

- Patient may have severe decrease in oral aperture
- Direct visualization of the nasal and oropharynx with a flexible fiberoptic bronchoscope may be necessary to prevent tearing of telangiectases

Preinduction/Induction

- Extra attention should be paid to ensuring adequate padding during positioning intraoperatively
- Patient may be hypovolemic due to vasoconstriction
- Consider volume expansion
- May initially observe Htn followed by vasodilation and hypotension

Maintenance

- Usually require mechanical ventilation because of restrictive lung disease
- Intraoperative hypoxemia may develop 2° to pulm Htn

Extubation

- May require postop ventilation if significant pulmonary compromise
- Pain control important for pulmonary status

ANTICIPATED PROBLEMS/CONCERNS

- Difficult airway
- Hypoxemia
- Hypotension

CRI DU CHAT SYNDROME (5p SYNDROME) Barbara W. Palmisano, M.D.

RISK

- 1/50,000 births

PERIOPERATIVE RISKS

- Difficult airway management due to micrognathia
- Congenital heart disease

WORRY ABOUT

- Difficult mask ventilation
- Inability to visualize larynx
- Behavioral problems due to profound retardation

OVERVIEW

- Chromosomal abnormality
- Microcephaly with profound mental retardation and somatic growth failure
- Characteristic facies including micrognathia and facial asymmetry
- Characteristic high shrill cry in infancy that is central in origin, although laryngeal malformations occasionally reported (narrow diamond-shaped larynx, laryngomalacia; long, floppy epiglottis, hypoplastic epiglottis)
- Congenital heart disease common (30–50%)
- Occasional malformations of CNS, GI tract, kidneys, MS system

ICD-9-CM Code: 758.3

ETIOLOGY

- Partial deletion of short arm of chromosome 5 occurring sporadically (85%) or as an unbalanced translocation inherited from a carrier parent (15%)
- Characteristic high-pitched, catlike cry localized to 5p15.3; other clinical features localized to 5p15.2
- Milder forms have only deletion of distal critical region (5p15.3)

USUAL TREATMENT

- None for primary chromosomal abnormality

ASSESSMENT POINTS

SYSTEM	EFFECT	ASSESSMENT BY HX	PE	TEST
HEENT	Micrognathia Malocclusion High, vaulted palate Cleft lip/palate Asymmetric face	Feeding and swallowing difficulty	Receding mandible; reduced thyromental distance	
CV	Various congenital heart defects	Shortness of breath Night sweats	Murmur/gallop Dyspnea Tachycardia	ECHO ECG
RESP	Chronic aspiration Frequent URI with otitis media		Dyspnea Rales/rhonchi Wheezing	CXR
CNS	Retardation Seizures		Hypotonia in infancy Spasticity later	
MS	Scoliosis Various limb anomalies			

Key Reference: Tullu MS, Muranjan MN, Sharma SV, Sahu DR, Swami SR, Desmukh CT, Bharucha, BA: Cri-du-chat syndrome: clinical profile and prenatal diagnosis. J Postgrad Med 1998; 44:101–104.

PERIOPERATIVE IMPLICATIONS

Preoperative Preparation

- Develop strategies for difficult airway management

Monitoring

- Routine

Airway

- Laryngeal mask airway or fiberoptic bronchoscopy to facilitate endotracheal intubation

Preinduction/Induction

- Careful preop sedation in monitored setting for uncooperative patient

Maintenance

- Keep ectomorphic patients warm (warm room temperature, radiant warming and body covering during induction, heated and humidified inspired gases, warm intravenous fluids)

Extubation

- Awake extubation for patients with difficult airway management

Adjuvants

- No specific concerns

ANTICIPATED PROBLEMS/CONCERNS

- Intraoperative airway management may be difficult
- Postoperative airway obstruction secondary to anatomic factors and neurologic dysfunction
- Associated malformations, especially congenital heart disease

CROHN'S DISEASE

Kelvin Yee, M.D.

RISK

- Incidence of 2 cases per 100,000/y: prevalence of 20 to 40 per 100,000
- Race: Caucasians > African-Americans
- Increased incidence 3- to 6-fold in Jews compared with non-Jews
- Peak occurrence: between ages 15 and 35 y

PERIOPERATIVE RISKS

- Risk of exacerbation of underlying liver disease

WORRY ABOUT

- Intravascular fluid volume and electrolyte status
- Nutritional status and adverse effects associated with hyperalimentation
- Colonic and extracolonic complications (anemia, liver disease, arthritis)
- Corticosteroids supplementation if chronically receiving steroids to maintain fluid and electrolyte balance, and vascular reactivity

OVERVIEW

- Anemia may be due to chronic disease, iron deficiency, chronic hemorrhage, or folate or vitamin B_{12} deficiency
- Decreased intravascular fluid volume due to malnutrition and hypoalbuminemia
- Electrolyte abnormalities, especially hypokalemia due to diarrhea
- Potential for malignancy and intestinal obstruction/perforation/toxic megacolon
- Rectocutaneous fistulas, rectal fissures, or perirectal abscesses with Crohn's disease

ICD-9-CM Code: 555.9

ETIOLOGY

- Unknown
- Features of the disease have suggested a relationship with familial or genetic, infectious, immunologic, and psychologic factors
  – Susceptibility mapped to chromosome 16

USUAL TREATMENT

- Pharmacologic: anti-inflammatory agents (mesalamine [Pentasa], a 5-ASA agent), sulfasalazine, corticosteroids, antibiotics, and immunosuppressive therapy (azathioprine and cyclosporine)
- Surgical: surgery for symptomatic obstruction, fistula, abscesses, or perforation

ASSESSMENT POINTS

SYSTEM	EFFECT	ASSESSMENT BY HX	PE	TEST
CV	Dehydration, anemia	Bloody diarrhea, loss of weight	Postural hypotension, tachycardia	Hct, BUN/Cr, K^+, Mg^{2+}
GI	Fatty liver infiltration	Jaundice	Hepatomegaly	Alkaline phosphatase
	Pericholangitis			
	Cirrhosis			LFTs
	Toxic megacolon	Fever	Rebound tenderness	Abdominal series
	Intestinal perforation	Abdominal pain		
	Proctitis/rectal abscess	Bleeding/tenesmus		WBC
	Malabsorption		Cachexia, weight loss	Albumin, B_{12}, folate
RENAL	Secondary amyloidosis			Proteinuria
	Renal stones	Flank pain		
MS	Ankylosing arthritis	Joint mobility	↓ Joint ROM	

Key Reference: Stenson WF: Inflammatory bowel disease. *In* Goldman L, Smith LH Jr, Bennett JC (eds): Cecil Textbook of Medicine, 21st ed. Philadelphia, WB Saunders, 2000, pp 722–729.

PERIOPERATIVE IMPLICATIONS

Preoperative Preparation

- Assess volume status and ensure normality
- Hyperalimentation: if given preoperatively, need to maintain intraoperatively; assess glucose, PO_4^{2-}
- Assess concurrent steroid use and need for supplementation

Monitoring

- Routine

Airway

- None

Preinduction and Induction

- Rapid-sequence induction in patients with gastric outlet or duodenal obstruction

Maintenance

- Consider avoiding nitrous oxide if bowel distention/obstruction
- Potential adverse effects of hyperalimentation must be noted, with serum glucose checked regularly

Extubation

- Awake extubation for "full stomach"

Postoperative Period

- Monitor volume status, as third space losses and fluid mobilization will ensue

Adjuvants

- With underlying liver disease consider avoiding halothane, and for muscle relaxants dependent on hepatic elimination, reduced plasma clearance necessitates smaller than normal maintenance doses

- Hypoalbuminemia results in diminished protein binding, higher free drug levels, and increased volume of distribution, thus enhancing effects and clearance of highly protein bound drugs while reducing effects of other drugs

ANTICIPATED PROBLEMS/CONCERNS

- Nutritional deficiency, often severe, particularly with small bowel involvement or with short-bowel syndrome from extensive resection; may require supplementation of electrolytes, minerals, and vitamins
- Often marked hypovolemia and anemia exacerbated by third space losses; may need aggressive fluid hydration

CROUP (LARYNGOTRACHEOBRONCHITIS)

Maurice S. Zwass, M.D.

RISK

• Children between 6 mo and 6 y are at risk, (6 mo–3 y at greatest risk)
• Children with underlying airway abnormalities (e.g., subglottic stenosis) or difficult intubations (e.g., micrognathia) and symptoms are at increased risk and require particular planning

PERIOPERATIVE RISKS

• Difficulty with intubation because of very narrowed subglottic region
• Obstruction of the small tracheal tube because of airway secretions

WORRY ABOUT

• Risk of rebound tracheal edema several hours after racemic epinephrine treatment
• Cardiorespiratory crisis in progressive or severe Sx, agitation, younger patients, difficulties with oxygenation or ventilation, failure to oxygenate
• Bacterial superinfection of airway

OVERVIEW

• Common childhood ailment with prodromal illness accompanied by a characteristic cough (often sounds like seal barking)
• Sx and respiratory compromise from progressive swelling of subglottic region tracheal mucosa
• Frequently present when inspiratory stridor and respiratory distress develop
• Radiographs of neck often demonstrate gradual progressive tracheal narrowing, most narrow just below level of vocal cords (referred to as "steeple sign"); upper glottis on lateral neck radiograph is normal
• When obtained, evaluation of CBC is consistent with viral illness

ICD-9-CM Codes: 464.4 (Croup); 464.2 (Laryngotracheitis)

ETIOLOGY

• Viral agents are usual etiologies and include parainfluenza viruses (most common); adenoviruses, influenza virus, respiratory syncytial virus (RSV), and measles virus also associated

USUAL TREATMENT

• Cool mist often greatly improves Sx; supplemental O_2
• If symptoms more severe, aerosolized racemic epinephrine can dramatically reduce airway swelling (rebound tracheal edema risk several hours after administration necessitates observation in hospital)
• Steroid administration controversial; may ↓ severity of disease and ↓ need for tracheal intubation or hasten improvement in first 24 h of illness
• Small percentage with this disease need tracheal intubation
• Parenteral steroids (dexamethasone) and inhaled (budesonide) have been used
• Breathing helium-oxygen mixtures has been reported as helpful in some cases (lower density and viscosity)

ASSESSMENT POINTS

Differential points between croup (laryngotracheobronchitis) and epiglottitis

	CROUP	EPIGLOTTITIS
AGE	3 mo–3 y	1–7 y
ONSET	Gradual	More rapid (usually <24 h)
FEVER	Low grade	High
COUGH	Characteristic barking	None
SORE THROAT	Occasional	Frequently severe
POSTURE	Any	Frequently sitting forward, mouth open, drooling
AIRWAY SOUND	Inspiratory stridor	Inspiratory stridor
VOICE	Normal	Muffled
APPEARANCE	Nontoxic	Toxic
SEASONALITY	Peak winter, epidemic	Year-round

Key References: DeSoto H: Epiglottitis and croup in airway obstruction in children. Anesthesiol Clin North Am 1998; 16:853–868; Malhorta A, Krilov LR: Viral croup. Pediatr Rev 2001; 22:5–12.

PERIOPERATIVE IMPLICATIONS

Airway

• Airway support with good mask fit and positive pressure ventilation can generally overcome obstruction from swelling of airway
• Identification of larynx generally routine, but tracheal tube 0.5–1.0 mm diameter smaller than usual may necessitate having available extra-long or microlaryngeal tracheal tubes

• Tracheotomy rarely needed as therapy for these patients with current management and reserved only for unusual cases

Induction

• Induction common with IV access already obtained

ANTICIPATED PROBLEMS/CONCERNS

• Symptomatic patients who require intubation of trachea need tube 0.5–1.0 mm smaller in diameter than equivalent in children without croup.

• Patient who requires tracheal intubation usually requires sedative management to tolerate ventilation; often followed for development of leak around tracheal tube as a sign of improvement of edema; most patients improve within 2–4 days; when leak is present at 20–25 cm H_2O of pressure, extubation can be considered; complicated cases and patients with prolonged courses may benefit from examination of airway in operating room at time of extubation
• Although viral illness, some patients may acquire bacterial superinfection of airway and require antibiotic therapy

CRYPTOCOCCUS INFECTION

David H. Wong, Pharm.D., M.D.

RISK

- 0.15% incidence in general population
- 7% incidence in AIDS patients
- 80–90% of infections occur in patients with AIDS as risk factor

PERIOPERATIVE RISKS

- Possible respiratory insufficiency

WORRY ABOUT

- Underlying disease

OVERVIEW

- Encapsulated yeast that reproduces by budding
- Polysaccharide capsule prevents phagocytosis by PMNs
- Infection usually associated with defect in cell-mediated immunity
- Serum tests for diagnosis may be unreliable
- Pulmonary cryptococcosis Dx made by bronchoscopy or biopsy
- Cryptococcal meningitis—Dx usually made by CSF stain and culture
- Pulmonary cryptococcosis may spread systematically in 17% of patients or more
- If pulmonary cryptococcosis present, look for disseminated cryptococcosis (do blood, urine, CSF cultures; consider bone marrow cultures)
- Mortality of disseminated disease may be as high as 50%
- Relapses are common, particularly in AIDS patients
- Not contagious from human to human

ICD-9-CM Code: 117.5

ETIOLOGY

- Organism present in soil, and particularly in pigeon feces
- Usually enters body via inhalation, then spreads hematogenously
- Associated with chemotherapy, corticosteroid therapy, immunosuppressive therapy (i.e., organ transplant recipients), hemopoietic cancer, AIDS

USUAL TREATMENT

- Meningitis or disseminated cryptococcosis—IV amphotericin, IV fluorocytosine
- Lipid-based IV amphotericin may have less nephrotoxicity than IV amphotericin
- Meningitis may need intrathecal amphotericin
- Isolated pulmonary cryptococcosis—IV/PO fluconazole
- Surgical drainage of abcesses as indicated
- Taper corticosteroids if possible

ASSESSMENT POINTS

SYSTEM	EFFECT	ASSESSMENT BY HX	PE	TEST
RESP	Pulm infection	Cough, sputum production, dyspnea	Wheezes or signs of infection	CXR, sputum culture, bronchoscopy if necessary
RENAL				Azotemia or decreased renal function
CNS	Meningitis	Headache, nausea, vomiting, seizures	Mental status	CSF culture, India ink stain, Gram stain

Key Reference: Nunez M, Peacock J, Chin R: Pulmonary cryptococcosis in the immunocompetent host. Chest 2000; 118:527–534.

PERIOPERATIVE IMPLICATIONS

Preoperative Preparation

- Consider respiratory isolation circuit for anesthesia machine (for possible concomitant respiratory infections)
- Preop mental status may be depressed; may affect choice of anesthetic and need for airway protection

Monitoring

- Routine
- Pay particular attention to respiratory variables

Airway

- None

Preinduction/Induction

- None

Maintenance

- Administration of amphotericin B: if an anaphylactoid reaction occurs, may complicate interpretation of changes in vital signs or other physical signs

Extubation

- Consider if can adequately protect airway

Adjuvants

- None

Postoperative Period

- Pay particular attention to respiratory variables

ANTICIPATED PROBLEMS/CONCERNS

- Amphotericin B therapy associated with anaphylactoid reactions, hypotension, fever, chills, bronchospasm, nausea and vomiting. Chronic treatment can result in hypokalemia, hypomagnesemia, anemia, azotemia, renal tubular necrosis, and hepatic toxicity
- 5-Fluorocytosine therapy associated with thrombocytopenia, pancytopenia, and hepatitis

CUSHING'S SYNDROME

George H. Lampe, M.D.

RISK

- 10 million/y in USA treated with gluco-corticoids
- Those treated for >21 days are at risk for Cushing's syndrome
- 7500 cases/y due to increased endogenous production

PERIOPERATIVE RISKS

- Acute adrenal insufficiency (addisonian crisis) if replacement is not provided
- Hyperglycemia, gastric ulceration, increased risk of infection with replacement

WORRY ABOUT

- Adequate gluco/mineralocorticoid replacement

OVERVIEW

- A constellation of physical signs caused by glucocorticoid excess (Cushing's disease specifically refers to pituitary excess resulting in Cushing's syndrome)
- Exogenous administration of glucocorticoids for more than 3 wk may suppress adrenal function for up to 1 y
- Epidural depot corticosteroid administration can cause adrenal suppression
- Acute adrenal insufficiency is rare but life threatening, prompting the guideline "When in doubt, treat"

ICD-9-CM Code: 255.0
Includes all causes except for congenital adrenal hyperplasia (255.2)

ETIOLOGY

- Exogenous administration prescribed by physicians—very common
- Pituitary ACTH overproduction (Cushing's disease)—rare
- Adrenal overproduction—rare

USUAL TREATMENT

- Rx must include gluco/mineralocorticoid activity (hydrocortisone is the gold standard)
- Physiologic (low-dose) replacement 25 mg of hydrocortisone IV q8h
- Supraphysiologic (extreme stress) doses 100 mg of hydrocortisone q12h

ASSESSMENT POINTS

SYSTEM	EFFECT	ASSESSMENT BY HX	PE	TEST
HEENT	Breathing difficult owing to fat or enlargement	Snoring	Uvula visible Neck and mandible ROM	
CV	Htn	Continue antihypertensives	BP CV exam for CHF S_3 gallop CHF with basilar rales	ECG CXR (if indicated)
GI	Gastric ulceration	Epigastric pain or black stools		Hgb Stool Hemoccult (if indicated)
METAB/ ENDO	Adrenal suppression	Extended steroid exposure during last year	Centripetal fat, moon facies, cushingoid	ACTH stimulation test (rarely indicated) Glucose Na^+ and K^+ and electrolytes
	Hyperglycemia with Rx Electrolyte abnormalities with metabolic alkalosis Overweight			
CNS	Personality changes	Euphoria	Affect	
MS	Osteoporosis Delicate skin Muscle wasting	Pain Easy bruisability	Ecchymoses Thin extremities	X-rays (if indicated)

Key Reference: Acosta E, Pantoja JP, Gamino R, Rull JA, Herrera ME: Laparascopic versus open adrenalectomy in Cushing's syndrome and disease. Surgery 1999; 126:1111–1116.

PERIOPERATIVE IMPLICATIONS

Preoperative Preparation

- Steroid Rx in physiologic doses (25 mg q8h) for minor surgery; consider high dose (100 mg q12h) of hydrocortisone hemisuccinate for major surgery

Airway

- Assume difficult airway due to moon facies and delicate mucosa that is easily traumatized

Induction

- Etomidate may further suppress adrenal function—might avoid in patients at risk
- Careful positioning to prevent stress fractures and skin trauma

Extubation

- Use great care when removing tape to avoid skin avulsion and bruising

Postoperative Care

- Monitor lytes and glucose
- Monitor hemodynamics
- Monitor for occult GI blood loss
- Taper steroids daily over 3 days

ANTICIPATED PROBLEMS/CONCERNS

- Hypotensive without supplementation
- Need for ulcer prophylaxis and attention to infection, immune compromise, and potential for CHF supplementation given

CYANIDE POISONING

Peter H. Breen, M.D., F.R.C.P.C.

RISK

- Potent and rapid-onset toxin, especially inhalation of hydrogen cyanide (CN)
- CN ingestion → slower onset
- Diffuses rapidly through body with high intracellular fixation to cytochrome aa_3 in cellular mitochondria to paralyze aerobic metabolism

PERIOPERATIVE RISKS

- Main target organs: CNS and heart
- Animal experiments: apnea precedes cardiac collapse

WORRY ABOUT

- If CN toxicity resulted from fire or smoke exposure, consider also carbon monoxide (CO) and other toxins
- $1/3$ of patients from domestic fires with CO toxicity also have ↑ CN
- Be alert for CN poisoning in donor for organ transplantation

OVERVIEW

- Major route of CN detoxification: conversion to thiocyanate, which requires sulfane sulfur donor (e.g., thiosulfate) and enzyme (e.g., rhodanase); without renal excretion, ↑ thiocyanate can cause CNS abnormalities
- Minor route: hydroxocobalamin (one form of vitamin B_{12}) chelates CN to form cyanocobalamin
- Methemoglobin (metHb) ferric ion has high affinity for CN

ICD-9-CM Code: 989.0

ETIOLOGY

- Combustion product of natural and synthetic polymers
- Industrial chemistry (e.g., metals and plastics preparation)
- Plants: may contain cyanogenic glycosides
- Na nitroprusside: overtreatment (> 0.5 mg/kg/h within 24 h)
- Abuse (e.g., suicide, Chicago CN-laced–Tylenol murders [1982])

USUAL TREATMENT

- Intubation and ventilation with 100% O_2 (hyperbaric O_2, effective experimentally, is not practical)
- Na thiosulfate (25%) 150 mg/kg IV (minimal side effects but thiocyanate requires renal excretion or hemodialysis)
- Gastric decontamination (if necessary)
- Hydroxocobalamin, 4 g IV, safe and rapid but not yet available in USA
- Methemoglobinemia induction (metHb, 30%) with 10% sodium nitrite (5–10 mg/kg IV) slow and unpredictable; can be hazardous in presence of carboxyhemoglobin (from CO toxicity) because neither metHb nor COHb carries O_2; can be fatal in G6PD deficiency
- Dicobalt EDTA (ethylenediaminetetraacetate), 300–600 mg IV, followed by glucose infusion; potent and rapid but unsafe (esp arrhythmias, hypotension, and allergic reactions)

ASSESSMENT POINTS

SYSTEM	EFFECT	ASSESSMENT BY HX	PE	TEST
HEENT	↓ CNS → ↓ airway maintenance/protection	Concomitant smoke inhalation injury	Perioral burns Airway edema	Laryngoscopy/ bronchoscopy
CV	Stimulation at low CN conc Depression at high CN conc	Hypertension, tachycardia Hypotension, bradycardia	↑ Cardiac output ↓ Cardiac output Arrhythmias	ECG: arrhythmias, esp ↓ conduction, VTach, VFIB
RESP	Aerobic cellular respiration paralyzed Thermal/toxic airway and parenchymal injury	Concomitant smoke inhalation injury	Bronchoconstriction and pulm edema	↑ Blood PvO_2 and ↑ SvO_2 ↓ VO_2 ↓ $\dot{V}CO_2$ ↓ $PETCO_2$ Chest x-ray Bronchoscopy
METAB	Cellular aerobic metabolism disabled	Combination of ↑ SvO_2 and lactic acidosis suggests CN		Lactic metabolic acidosis Whole blood CN levels (Not available in all labs)
CNS	Stimulation at low CN conc	↑ Inhalatory CN intake Anxiety, dyspnea, headache Auditory/visual disturbances	↑ Resp rate Confusion	
	Depression at high CN conc		Apnea, convulsions, coma	Funduscopy: red retinal veins (↑ SvO_2)

Key Reference: Breen PH, Isserles SA, Tabac E, Roizen MF, Taitelman UZ: Protective effect of stroma-free metHb during cyanide poisoning in dogs. Anesthesiology 1996; 85:558–564.

PERIOPERATIVE IMPLICATIONS

Preoperative Preparation

- Continuous 100% O_2

Monitoring

- SpO_2 unreliable in presence of metHb
- Mixed venous continuous SO_2 or blood PO_2 (SvO_2, PvO_2)
- $PETCO_2$
- Measure of $\dot{V}O_2$ or $\dot{V}CO_2$ helpful

Airway

- Protect and maintain airway

Induction

- Avoid CV depressant agents

Maintenance

- 100% O_2 (no N_2O)

Extubation

- Ensure CNS status permits natural airway maintenance and protection

Adjuvants

- Consider treatment for concomitant CO poisoning (see Carbon Monoxide Poisoning in Diseases section)

Postoperative Period

- Maintain 100% O_2 breathing

ANTICIPATED PROBLEMS/CONCERNS

- Heart and brain are target organs
- Prompt CPR (ventilation with O_2) determines outcome
- Follow CNS function
- Seek concomitant smoke inhalation injury and CO toxicity

CYSTIC FIBROSIS

Theodore W. Striker, M.D.

RISK

- Prevalence 1:2500 births
- Incidence 20,000/y
- Race with highest prevalence: Caucasian

PERIOPERATIVE RISKS

- Increased risk of pulmonary problems:
  - Pneumothorax
  - V/Q abnormalities
  - Hypoxemia
  - Obstructive pattern of ventilation

WORRY ABOUT

- Hypoxemia
- Pneumothorax
- Copious secretions with inspissation
- Cor pulmonale

OVERVIEW

- Multisystem disease of exocrine secretory glands involving salivary, sweat, digestive, and pulmonary secretions
- Frequent associated bronchiectasis, hemoptysis
- Recurrent pulmonary infection—frequently antibiotic resistant

ICD-9-CM Code: 277.00

ETIOLOGY

- Recessive inherited disorder—both parents must carry gene to inherit
- Mucus-secreting glands secrete abnormally—precipitation in ducts of secretory glands

USUAL TREATMENT

- Pulmonary therapy—antibiotics for infection, humidity, bronchodilators, chest physiotherapy
- Sweat electrolyte changes—adequate electrolyte intake. Diet: nutrition and enzyme replacement.
- Gene therapy still experimental

ASSESSMENT POINTS

SYSTEM	EFFECT	ASSESSMENT BY HX	PE	TEST
HEENT	Frequent nasal polyps	Nasal obstruction Difficulty sleeping	Polyps of nose	
	Sinusitis	Fever, headaches	Sinus drainage	Sinus x-ray, culture
CV	Cor pulmonale	Dyspnea Cough Orthopnea Cyanosis	Tachypnea Rales, rhonchi, wheezing Clubbing of fingers Cyanosis	ECG (if indicated) CXR (if indicated)
RESP	Bronchiectasis Atelectasis Pneumonitis Bronchospasm	Dyspnea Poor exercise tolerance Orthopnea	Hyperinflation of chest Poor ventilation Cyanosis Clubbing Rales and rhonchi Cough, wheezing	CXR PFTs A-a gradient (if indicated)
GI	Cholelithiasis	Abdominal pain—may be asymptomatic	Jaundice	US (if indicated) Cholangiography (if indicated)
	Pancreatic insufficiency	Poor fat absorption Glucose intolerance		Glucose
	Hepatic fibrosis Intestinal obstruction	Abdominal pain	Abdominal rigidity	LFTs GI x-rays (if indicated)
MS	Poor muscle development	Hx of poor nutrition Muscle weakness	Cachexia	

Key Reference: Boat TF, Boucher RC: Cystic fibrosis. *In* Murray JF, Nadel JA (eds): Textbook of Respiratory Medicine, 2nd ed. Philadelphia, WB Saunders, 1994, pp 1418–1450.

PERIOPERATIVE IMPLICATIONS

Preoperative Preparation

- Pulmonary function studies close to time of anesthesia
- CXR
- Blood gases, serum electrolytes, blood glucose
- Bronchodilators, antibiotics, cardiotonic drugs
- Chest physical therapy

Monitoring

- Routine
- CVP if procedure and CV condition warrant
- Blood glucose—at frequent intervals

Airway

- Early oropharyngeal airway especially with nasal polyps
- Chest or esophageal stethoscope valuable if thorax not badly distorted

Induction

- Parenteral induction faster and more reliable than inhalation induction
- Avoid substances irritating to upper and lower respiratory tract

Maintenance

- High FIO$_2$
- Ventilatory assistance for severe obstructive airway and reactive airway disease
- Humidification of gases
- Regional techniques helpful for postanesthetic pain management. No evidence that patient is better served by regional instead of general anesthesia.

Extubation

- Should be delayed until adequacy of ventilation has reached preanesthetic levels
- May be accompanied by chest physical therapy, endotracheal suction, and reinflation

Adjuvants

- Bronchodilators
- Digitalis and diuretics in presence of cor pulmonale

Postoperative Period

- Pain management (may include narcotics) to encourage coughing and deep breathing
- Chest physical therapy
- Early activity

ANTICIPATED PROBLEMS/CONCERNS

- Pneumothorax
- Respiratory insufficiency
- Cor pulmonale
- Electrolyte disturbance (Na$^+$, Cl$^-$)

CYTOMEGALOVIRUS (CMV) INFECTION

Andrew D. Badley, M.D.
Carlos V. Paya, M.D., Ph.D.

RISK

- Seroprevalence in USA: <10 y—25%; 10–25 y—35%; 25–50 y—50%; >50 y—50+%
- Disease from CMV rare in immunocompetent individuals; can cause mononucleosis-like disease
- Disease from CMV in transplant recipients 10–40%
- Disease from CMV in HIV-positive patients 20–30% (increased risk with low CD4 count)
- Gender/race with highest prevalence: ?

PERIOPERATIVE RISKS

- Related to degree of CMV-induced organ dysfunction—pulmonary, CNS, hepatic, GI, cardiac, bone marrow, adrenal
- Risk of acquiring CMV from tissue or blood products of CMV-seropositive donor

WORRY ABOUT

- Giving CMV-seropositive blood products to a CMV-seronegative immunocompromised host. Alternatively, the use of filters that remove leukocytes from the blood can be used to prevent transmission of CMV if CMV-seropositive blood donors are used.
- Abnormal hepatic metabolism if CMV hepatitis
- Elevated ICP if CMV encephalitis/meningitis
- Abnormal oxygenation if CMV pneumonitis

- Myocardial dysfunction or arrhythmias if CMV myocarditis
- Perforated viscus 2° to colonic/gastric CMV
- Abnormal bleeding from thrombocytopenia
- Adrenal insufficiency due to CMV adrenalitis

OVERVIEW

- Double-stranded DNA virus; member of herpes family of viruses. Vast majority of North American adults have had prior exposures and are CMV seropositive.
- CMV disease if:
  - Perinatal infection
  - Intrauterine infection leading to congenital CMV disease
  - Infection of normal host is asymptomatic; rarely may cause a heterophile antibody–negative mononucleosis-like syndrome.
  - Infection in immunosuppressed individuals leading to symptomatic or asymptomatic viremia with or without organ involvement: retinitis, encephalitis, meningitis, myelitis, polyneuropathy, pneumonitis, esophagitis, gastritis, colitis, hepatitis, cholangitis, myocarditis, adrenalitis, vasculitis, bone marrow suppression

ICD-9-CM Code: 078.5

ETIOLOGY

- Double-stranded DNA virus
- Transmission through blood/blood products, sexually, perinatally, other contact (day care, ?medical facilities)

USUAL TREATMENT

- Medical treatment—ganciclovir (IV or oral maintenance), foscarnet (IV), occasionally IV immune globulin. Reduced immunosuppression.
- Surgical treatment—none

ASSESSMENT POINTS

SYSTEM	EFFECT	ASSESSMENT BY HX	PE	TEST
HEENT	Destruction of retina	Decreased visual acuity, blind spots	Funduscopy; white and red lesion	Ophthalmology evaluation
CV	Myocarditis; LV dysfunction	CHF symptoms, palpitations	Irregular rhythm, displaced PMI S_3	ECG, ECHO, heart biopsy
RESP	Pneumonitis; impaired gas exchange	Dyspnea, nonproductive cough	Wheezes, crackles	CXR, ABGs, bronchoscopy ± biopsy
GI	Viral infection of organ	Hepatitis/cholangitis: –Right upper quadrant pain –Jaundice, itching, acholic stools –Esophagitis: dysphagia, odynophagia –Colitis: diarrhea, abdominal pain –Gastritis: pyrosis, anorexia	Signs of hepatic failure, fetor hepaticus, asterixis, jaundice, bruising, painful liver, nonspecific abdominal pain	Liver function tests, ERCP, US, viral blood cultures ± biopsy
HEME	Bone marrow suppression	Rash, fatigue	Petechiae, pallor, tachycardia	CBC
CNS	Encephalitis	Motor or sensory abnormalities, altered mental status	Motor weakness, sensory abnormality, cerebellar ataxia, abnormal tests of cortical function	CT MRI Lumbar puncture

Key Reference: Barber L, Egan JJ, Lomax J, Haider Y, Yonan N, Woodcock AA, Turner AJ, Fox AJ: A prospective study of a quantitative PCR ELISA assay for the diagnosis of CMV pneumonia in lung and heart-transplant recipients. J Heart Lung Transplant 2000; 19:771–780.

PERIOPERATIVE IMPLICATIONS

Perioperative Preparation
- Evaluate for signs of cardiac/hepatic/CNS/bone marrow or adrenal dysfunction

Monitoring
- Routine

Airway
- May require high FIO_2 and PEEP

Preinduction/Induction
- Avoid tachycardia/hypotension

Maintenance
- Follow CO, PCWP, SaO_2, BP

Extubation
- No special concerns

Postoperative Period
- Monitor for clinical signs of disease progression

Adjuvants
- No special concerns

DEEP VEIN THROMBOSIS

Todd Dorman, M.D.

RISK

• 170,000 diagnosed new cases/y of deep vein thrombosis (DVT) in USA
• 90,000 recurrent cases/y
• True incidence (underdiagnosis) closer to 0.5 million cases/y
• Race with highest prevalence: ?
• Asthma ↑ with smoking, obesity, being bedridden, ↓ LVEF are predisposing factors
• Risk factors include age, previous DVT, paraplegia, spinal cord trauma, major orthopedic surgery, malignancy, hypercoagulable states
• Decreased risk with regional anesthesia vs. general

PERIOPERATIVE RISKS

• Without prophylaxis, DVT develops in close to 30% of general surgery cases
• Incidence of fatal pulmonary emboli: 0.1% (general)–5% (total knee replacement)

WORRY ABOUT

• Pulmonary embolism
• Cardiac arrest, electromechanical dissociation
• Hypoxemia and increased dead space potentially leading to respiratory acidosis in patient with controlled ventilation

OVERVIEW

• Clinical findings (e.g., Homans' sign) helpful less than 50% of the time
• Ascending phlebography (venography) is standard for comparison, but has 2–3% incidence of inducing peripheral thrombosis
• Impedance plethysmography (IP), which detects proximal veins, reasonable in symptomatic patients, but lacks sensitivity and specificity in asymptomatic patients
• Compression ultrasonography with Doppler flow imaging better than IP (proximal veins), yet sensitivity falls off in asymptomatic patients. If IP or Doppler-supplemented ultrasonography negative, patient needs serial exams to detect potential progression of distal disease.
• CT and MRI are reliable, yet are cumbersome, costly, and not routinely available

ICD-9-CM Code: 453.9 (Thrombosis, vein unspecified)

ETIOLOGY

• Stasis
• Activation of coagulation cascade by tissue trauma
• Hypercoagulability related to congenital or acquired antithrombin III, protein C, or protein S deficiency
• Hypercoagulability related to malignancy, smoking, sedentary lifestyle, ↑ physiologic age, ↓ LVEF
• Hyperviscosity states such as polycythemia vera

USUAL TREATMENT

• Heparin administration prior to warfarin to avoid acute decreases in endogenous anticoagulant protein C
• LMW heparin may be used
• Thrombolytics

ASSESSMENT POINTS

SYSTEM	EFFECT	ASSESSMENT BY HX	PE	TEST
CV			SVT RV strain	ECG
RESP	Pulmonary embolism	Chest pain Hemoptysis	Tachypnea Wheezing possible	ABGs End-tidal CO_2
HEME				PT, APTT Plt count Hgb
MS			Calf pain	Venography

Key Reference: Weinmann EE, Salzman EW: Medical progress: Deep-vein thrombosis. N Engl J Med 1994; 331:1630–1641.

PERIOPERATIVE IMPLICATIONS

Preoperative Preparation

• Sequential compression devices may decrease incidence by activating fibrinolytic system
• Anticoagulation needed for 6 mo after diagnosis and up to the time of procedure
• Consider preoperative placement of an IVC filter in high-risk patients

Monitoring

• Bleeding from residual anticoagulation or drug-induced thrombocytopenia

Airway

• None

Preinduction/Induction

• Regional anesthesia may reduce risk in some orthopedic and genitourinary procedures

Adjuvants

• Depends on etiology—examine specific etiology (e.g., Dilated Cardiomyopathy) in Diseases section
• Heparin, LMWH, warfarin tissue plasminogen activator, streptokinase/urokinase, anisoylated plasminogen-streptokinase activator complex all increase perioperative bleeding diathesis. Some effect of these agents on other drugs (verify specific drug effects in Drugs section).

Postoperative Period

• In high-risk patients consider full anticoagulation postoperatively as prophylaxis
• Continue sequential use of elastic stockings until patient ambulatory, but do not start in patients suspected of having DVT

ANTICIPATED PROBLEMS/CONCERNS

• Pulmonary embolism represents life-threatening complication of DVT

DEGENERATIVE DISK DISEASE

John E. Tetzlaff, M.D.

RISK

- Risk factors determined by spinal level
- Cervical spine—C3 and C4 most common, 10% of degenerative disk disease
- Thoracic—uncommon, can be related to trauma, tumor, 0.2–1.8% of disk disease
- Lumbar—very common, 85–90% of disk disease, third most common cause of chronic pain in USA

PERIOPERATIVE RISKS

- Difficult airway
- Spinal cord injury from airway manipulation or positioning
- Positioning injury from prone position
- Ischemic optic neuropathy

WORRY ABOUT

- Cervical spine instability or chronic subluxation
- Difficulty with intubation
- Injury to the spinal cord
- Pressure injuries or ventilatory difficulty with the prone position
- Optimum perfusion to the head. Ischemia or venous congestion may contribute to ischemic optic neuropathy.

OVERVIEW

- Pain from degeneration and herniation of an intervertebral disk is the third most common chronic disease in the USA and the most common indication for elective spine surgery
- Incidence varies among spinal segments, being absent in sacral area, most common in lumbar area, next in cervical region, and uncommon in thoracic region

ICD-9-CM Codes: 722.0 (Cervical); 722.11 (Thoracic); 722.10 (Lumbar)

ETIOLOGY

- Osteoarthritis
- Trauma
- Connective tissue diseases such as rheumatoid arthritis or ankylosing spondylitis

USUAL TREATMENT

- Conservative measures, such as rest, exercise, physical therapy, heat, and traction
- Symptoms are treated with analgesics and nonsteroidal anti-inflammatory drugs
- In acute phase, disk herniation can be treated with epidural steroid injection
- Surgery is performed to relieve compression on the spinal cord or specific nerve roots, and to expand the space for nerve root exit from the spinal column

ASSESSMENT POINTS

SYSTEM	EFFECT	ASSESSMENT BY HX	PE	TEST
HEENT	Difficult airway Visual acuity	Neck pain Patient report	Decreased ROM Patient report	Flexion/extension x-ray Eye examination
RESP	Lung tumor can mimic symptoms of thoracic disk disease	Chest pain	Abnormal pulmonary auscultation	CXR
GI	GI malignancy can mimic symptoms of thoracic or lumbar disk disease	Truncal pain, abdominal pain	Abdominal mass	CT, MRI
RENAL	Pyelonephritis, cancer of prostate can mimic symptoms of lumbar disk disease	Lumbar pain, muscle spasm, fever/chills	Costovertebral angle tenderness to percussion	Urinalysis, prostate-specific antigen, lumbar spine x-ray
CNS	Myelopathy, anterior spinal cord syndrome	Radiating pain, incontinence, sexual dysfunction, paraplegia	Long tract signs, abnormal reflexes, pathologic, Babinski reflex	X-ray, MRI
PNS	Radiculopathy, absent deep tendon reflexes, peripheral nerve deficits	Sciatica Numbess Weakness of the extremities	Sciatic pain with ROM Motor deficits Patches of decreased sensation	EMG
MS	Pain, decreased ROM, calcification	Pain, night pain, disability from work	Decreased ROM in spine	Spine x-ray, MRI

Key Reference: Rothman RA, Simeone FA: The Spine. Philadelphia, WB Saunders, 1989, Chapters 19–23.

PERIOPERATIVE IMPLICATIONS

Preoperative Assessment

- Evaluate coagulation if heavy NSAID use or symptoms of bleeding
- Airway assessment. If signs of cervical instability, flexion-extension x-ray of cervical spine.
- Antisialagogue if awake intubation
- Planned regional anesthesia may reduce minor complications, such as pain and nausea; intraop bleeding may be reduced

Monitoring

- Potential for air embolism, greater with sitting position for posterior approach to cervical spine
- Consider multilumen right atrial catheter, precordial Doppler

Airway

- If cervical spine not involved, then routine
- If abnormal, choices include awake intubation, inhalation induction, and intubation with induction drugs and muscle relaxants with the head maintained in a neutral position, possibly with traction

Induction

- If airway secured, induction dictated by other aspects of patient's health
- If regional anesthesia, technical difficulty with placement due to anatomic abnormality of the spine
- Consider paramedian dural puncture. Higher levels for dural puncture may result in a better block with spinal stenosis.

Maintenance

- Movement while prone with spinal cord exposed is dangerous. Avoid muscle relaxants after induction if spinal stimulation is used.
- If regional anesthesia, be prepared to re-inject block if duration of surgery exceeds duration of action of local anesthetic injected

Extubation

- Awake and supine are ideal
- Rapid-emergence agents (propofol, sevoflurane) may facilitate neuro exam in OR

Adjuvants

- Injury in the prone position to eyes, lips, teeth, tongue, chin, brachial plexus, ulnar nerves, genitalia, peroneal nerves, skin of the patella, and ankles
- Identify full neurologic function prior to extubation, since re-exploration for compressive hematoma could be indicated for major deficit

Postoperative Period

- Neurologic checks to identify deficits, pain control
- H_2-blocker therapy to prevent GI hemorrhage if large-dose steroid Rx chosen for nerve root swelling
- Evaluate visual acuity

ANTICIPATED PROBLEMS/CONCERNS

- Difficult airway if cervical involvement
- Air embolism—withdraw N_2O if any symptoms
- Transport bed availability and knowledge of how to remove frame, in case sudden transfer to supine position is necessary

DELIRIUM (POSTANESTHETIC)

David J. Cullen, M.D.

RISK

• Older patients (>70 y) and young patients
• Risk was 5.3% in 1961, although decreasing with newer drugs
• Premedication with barbiturates and/or scopolamine without opioids; phenothiazines; diphenhydramine
• Use of ketamine, Lomotil (atropine), meperidine
• Patients on high-dose steroids
• Withdrawal states—alcohol, barbiturates, meprobamate, or alprazolam
• Metabolic causes—hypoxia, hypercarbia, hyponatremia, hypochloremia, hyperosmolar states
• Incisional pain
• Gastric or urinary bladder distention, urethral irritation resulting from indwelling bladder catheter
• After major surgery (abdominal aortic and noncardiac thoracic surgery)
• Use of psychoactive medications
• Hypoalbuminemia

PERIOPERATIVE RISKS

• Attributing postanesthetic agitation, anxiety, or mental disturbances to drug effect when hypoxia and hypercarbia are the problem
• Patients can harm themselves and others

WORRY ABOUT

• Focusing on drug therapy while forgetting hypoxia and hypercarbia
• Damage to surgical site
• Violent behavior
• Residual hallucinations and nightmares (ketamine)
• Hyperthermia
• Augmenting resp depression from treatment with haloperidol or midazolam

OVERVIEW

• Rapid onset during early recovery from general anesthesia
• Specific cause that is usually reversible and diminishes with time
• Mental dysfunction: cognitive function impaired, emotional lability, inappropriate moods, agitation, belligerence, hallucinations, delusions, illusions, fluctuating state of consciousness

ICD-9-CM Code: 292.81 (Drug induced)

ETIOLOGY

• Most important: Establish a proper diagnosis. Hypoxia and hypercarbia must be ruled out. Treatment of delirium in presence of hypoxia and hypercarbia not only likely to fail but may accelerate resp depression and worsen hypoxia.
• Consider other metabolic disorders such as hypoglycemia, hyponatremia, hepatic encephalopathy, hyperpyrexia
• Anticholinergics (atropine and scopolamine)—parenteral or in eye drops. Delirium assoc with high serum levels of anticholinergics, though great variation in these levels in patients taking identical doses.
• Drugs with nonspecific CNS effects—phenothiazines, tricyclic antidepressants, sedatives, tranquilizers (diazepam, benzodiazepines, butyrophenones), barbiturates, meperidine, high-dose steroids
• Drug withdrawal from alcohol, barbiturates, benzodiazepines, opioids, or meprobamate
• Unrelieved pain, urinary retention, and gastric distention

USUAL TREATMENT

• Temporary physical restraint
• Nonspecific: opioids, tranquilizers, esp haloperidol in small IV doses
• Specific treatment: for anticholinergic-induced delirium, physostigmine, 0.5–2 mg IV

ASSESSMENT POINTS

SYSTEM	EFFECT	ASSESSMENT BY HX	PE	TEST
CNS	Postanesthetic delirium	Preop mental status, chronic drug therapy: Intraoperative anesthetic drugs, reversal drugs Oxygen status, ventilation, metabolic status, pain state	Anxiety, agitation, violent behavior, impaired cognition, emotional lability, agitation, hallucinations, fluctuating states of consciousness	O_2 saturation, ensurance of normal glucose and lyte status Response to physostigmine

Key Reference: Marcantonio ER, Goldman L, Orav EJ, Cook EF, Lee TH: The association of intraoperative factors with the development of postoperative delirium. Am J Med 1998; 105:380–384.

PERIOPERATIVE IMPLICATIONS

Preoperative Preparation
• Relieve anxiety by discussing anesthetic process with patient, answering all questions, providing assurances

Monitoring
• Routine

Airway
• Ensure clear airway, increase inspired oxygen concentration

Preinduction/Induction
• Avoid scopolamine without accompanying opioid

Maintenance
• Initiate analgesia coverage before ending anesthetic when appropriate

Extubation
• Evaluate for hypoxia and resp depression

Adjuvants
• Specific therapy: physostigmine 0.5–2 mg IV for anticholinergic-induced delirium
• Nonspecific drug–induced delirium:
  – Physostigmine 0.5–2 mg IV
  – Haloperidol 1–5 mg IV; wait 15–30 min to evaluate its effect and repeat or increase dose as needed
  – Midazolam 0.5–1 mg IV
• Assure a clear airway, monitor oxygen saturation, and increase inspired oxygen concentration

ANTICIPATED PROBLEMS/CONCERNS

• Use low-dose physostigmine 0.5–2 mg to avoid excess salivation and vomiting
• Prevention with physostigmine not as effective as treatment with physostigmine
• Opioid coverage during emergence helps limit incidence of delirium but may prolong awakening and promote resp depression
• Haloperidol is a potent antipsychotic with dopamine-blocking properties and relatively low anticholinergic effects and is available for IV use. Low doses of haloperidol are associated with few extrapyramidal side effects. Larger doses may be necessary but could compromise the airway unless the airway is properly protected.
• Always rule out hypoxia/hypercarbia before treating delirium with drugs or restraints

RISK

- People within USA: 4 million+
- Race with highest prevalence: unknown
- Affects 5–8% >65 y, 15–20% >75 y, and up to 50% of those >85 y.

PERIOPERATIVE RISKS

- Concomitant diseases in elderly patients include osteoarthritis, ASCVD, hypertension, renal disease, rheumatoid arthritis, and diabetes mellitus
- Risk increases with age and concomitant conditions

WORRY ABOUT

- Activities of other neurotransmitters (besides ACh) may be reduced: norepinephrine, serotonin, glutamate, and dopamine

OVERVIEW

- Dementia is a clinical diagnosis of progressive global intellectual impairment with 90% correlation at autopsy. Some rare forms of dementia, such as after head trauma, do not progress.
- Alzheimer's disease is thought most common cause of dementia; >50% of all cases in USA are Alzheimer's or vascular (including multi-infarct dementia)
- Another 10% due to alcohol abuse; multiple metabolic and other causes for the few secondary (reversible) dementias, most notably severe hypothyroidism
- Time from onset of symptoms until death, 2–15 y (average, 8 y)
- Dementia in young people may be due to HIV (more than 30% of all HIV cases)

ICD-9-CM Codes: 290.10 (Alzheimer's type); 290.40 (Multi-infarct dementia)

ETIOLOGY

- Histopathology shows senile neuritic plaques and neurofibrillary tangles containing cholinergic neurons, suggesting impaired cholinergic nerve transmission
- Extensive atrophy of cortical convolutions, especially in hippocampus and temporal lobes
- Changes normally seen in elderly brains, but markedly increased in Alzheimer's disease

USUAL TREATMENT

- Symptomatic treatment has been attempted with agents that affect cholinergic system, such as physostigmine, a centrally acting cholinesterase inhibitor; problems of short effect and high toxicity
- Tacrine (Cognex) and donepezil (Aricept) have been of some benefit in early Alzheimer's disease, but almost 50% of patients suffer serious side effects

ASSESSMENT POINTS

SYSTEM	EFFECT	PE	TEST
CV	~ 10% of those with dementia have CVD and generalized ASCVD	Hypertension	ECG
GI	Hepatic injury possible with alcohol abuse etiology		Liver enzymes
ENDO	Hypothyroidism can mimic or exacerbate dementia		T_3, T_4
CNS	Subdural hematoma and hydrocephalus possible causes		EEG, MRI, CT
PNS	Poor motor skills	Neurologic exam	
MS	Generalized stiffness and slowness; psychiatric disorders	Neurologic exam	

Key Reference: Goldstein MZ: Beyond morbidity and mortality: when older persons undergo anesthesia and elective surgery. Am J Geriatr Psychiatry 2000; 8:35–39.

PERIOPERATIVE IMPLICATIONS

Preoperative Preparation

- Patient most likely cannot give consent or a history; determine if guardian or surrogate identified
- Centrally acting anticholinergics (atropine, scopolamine) and sedatives best avoided; glycopyrrolate is acceptable

Monitoring

- Routine

Airway

- Cervical ROM may be limited by arthritis

Preinduction/Induction

- Propofol may offer most rapid recovery

Maintenance

- No one technique or agent best
- Avoid sedatives and narcotics with long half-lives

Extubation

- Extubate when awake; orientation postoperatively may be further impaired by drugs

Adjuvants

- Can see prolonged effect with sedatives, hypnotics, and narcotics

ANTICIPATED PROBLEMS/CONCERNS

- Poor candidates for regional anesthesia or for PCA in postop period
- Disorientation and delirium postoperatively common—provide familiar person and radio, written orientation material

DEPRESSION, UNIPOLAR

Barbara A. Dodson, M.D.

RISK

- 2–4% of adult population
- ~15% of patients with major depression commit suicide
- 4% of psychiatric admissions are for electro-convulsive therapy (ECT)

PERIOPERATIVE RISKS

- Risk of adverse drug interactions between antidepressants and anesthetic adjuncts resulting in cardiac arrhythmias and hypertensive crisis
- Cardiac arryhthmias, hypertension, ↑ cardiac output, and cerebral effects (↑ CMRO$_2$, ↑ CBF, ↑ ICP) 2° to ECT
- Potential systemic effects from deliberate drug overdoses

WORRY ABOUT

- Cardiac arrhythmias, hypotension, hypertension
- ↑ Cardiac output, ↑ BP, bradycardia, tachycardia, myocardial ischemia, and ↑ ICP from ECT
- Neuroleptic malignant syndrome
- Deliberate drug overdose

OVERVIEW

- Most common psychiatric disorder, distinguished from reactive grief and sadness by the severity and duration of the disturbances and presence of fatigue, anorexia, and insomnia
- Most problems are the result of interactions between antidepressants and anesthetic agents:
  – Tricyclics have antihistamine, anticholinergic, and sedating effects and can also interfere with AV conduction
  – MAO inhibitors ↑ norephinephrine stores, resulting in exaggerated responses to vasoactive agents
  – Selective serotonin reuptake inhibitors (SSRIs) can interact with MAO inhibitors, resulting in severe Htn, agitation, or coma
  – Patients frequently take over-the-counter and/or herbal drugs with potential drug-drug interactions
- ECT results in marked parasympathetic and sympathetic stimulation

See also Monoamine Oxidase Inhibitors; Reversible Inhibitors of Monoamine Oxidase in Drugs section and Electroconvulsive Therapy in Procedures section

ETIOLOGY

- Etiology is unknown
- ↓ Serotonin, dopamine, and norepinephrine levels in the CNS have been implicated
- Mechanisms underlying therapeutic effect of ECT remains unknown

USUAL TREATMENT

- Medical therapy—antidepressant drugs such as tricyclic and tetracyclic antidepressants, SSRIs, MAO inhibitors
- ECT used in patients who failed medical therapy or for whom antidepressants are contraindicated
- Supportive treatment of drug overdoses, with possible gastric lavage or hemodialysis

ASSESSMENT POINTS

SYSTEM	EFFECT	ASSESSMENT BY HX	PE	TEST
HEENT	Dry mouth, blurred vision	Glaucoma, retinal detachment	↓ Visual acuity	Funduscopic exam
CV	AV conduction delays, bradycardia, tachyarrhythmias, hypertensive crisis, hypotension	Angina, CHF symptoms, cardiac pacemaker, thrombophlebitis	Volume status, BP, S$_3$	ECG (± stress test) Echocardiography
RESP	Respiratory depression	CHF, severe pulmonary disease	S$_3$, rales, wheezing	CXR, ABGs
GI	Delayed gastric emptying	Reflux		
ENDO		Symptoms suggestive of pheochromocytoma	Unexplained severe hypertension	Vanillylmandelic acid levels
RENAL	Urinary retention	Difficulty urinating		
CNS	Neuroleptic malignant syndrome Seizures, coma	Recent CVA, intracranial surgery, intracranial mass lesion	Neurologic deficits, symptoms of ↑ ICP	CT, MRI, neurologic exam, toxicology screen
MS		Severe osteoporosis or major fractures	Fractures, limited joint mobility	Skeletal x-rays, MRI

Key Reference: Ghaemi SN, Boiman E, Goodwin FK: Insight and outcome in bipolar, unipolar, and anxiety disorders. Compr Psychiatry 2000; 41:167–171.

PERIOPERATIVE IMPLICATIONS

Preoperative Preparation
- Discontinuing MAO inhibitor 2 wk prior to surgery may not be necessary

Monitoring
- Consider arterial pressure monitoring

Airway
- Risk of gastric reflux
- Maintain cricoid pressure during induction

Maintenance
- Combination of pancuronium, halothane, and exogenous epinephrine can result in malignant tachyarrhythmias
- Meperidine is absolutely contraindicated in patients on an MAO inhibitor. Other opioids should be used with care.
- Indirect vasopressors should be avoided

- ECT results in marked parasympathetic, followed by sympathetic, stimulation

Extubation
- Risk of aspiration following extubation

Postoperative Period
- Potential problems with seizures or agitation
- May exhibit respiratory depression and delayed emergence from anesthesia

Adjuvants
- Esmolol for hypertensive crises. Atropine or glycopyrrolate for bradycardia.
- ECT usually performed using a short-acting IV anesthetic (e.g., propofol or methohexital) and a short-acting muscle relaxant

ANTICIPATED PROBLEMS/CONCERNS

- Tricyclic antidepressants have anticholinergic effects and can interfere with AV conduction
- MAO inhibitors ↑ norepinephrine stores, which can result in exaggerated responses to vasoactive substances
- Patients should be monitored for signs of neuroleptic malignant syndrome, such as hyperthermia, autonomic dysfunction, and muscle rigidity

DIABETES, TYPE I (INSULIN DEPENDENT)
Michael F. Roizen, M.D.

RISK

- People within USA: 1 million
- Race with highest prevalence: ↑ in Hispanics and Native Americans

PERIOPERATIVE RISKS

- Increased risk of CABG 5−10× if end-stage renal, CHF, or autonomic neuropathy; without renal, CHF, or autonomic dysfunction, risk is 1−1.5 × normal

WORRY ABOUT

- Autonomic neuropathy, gastroparesis, and sudden postop death
- Painless myocardial ischemia
- Atlanto-occipital joint immobility
- Tight glucose control might be indicated if pregnant, difficult weaning from bypass (ECC), or predictable global or focal CNS ischemia

OVERVIEW

- Endocrinopathy associated with end-stage renal, myocardial, and neuropathic disease
- Blood sugar control per se not associated with increased perioperative risk in absence of
  - Hypoglycemia
  - Hyperosmolar coma
  - Ketoacidosis
  - CNS ischemia
  - Pregnancy
  - Extracorporeal circulation
- Causes deranged autoregulation to CNS (blood sugar, 250 mg/dl), renal (blood sugar, 225 mg/dl), and cardiac (blood sugar, 100 mg/dl) vessels
- Need to control BP or blood sugar to decrease damage to these vessels and organs
- Check patient glucose log for degree of control
- Variable control may predict perioperative hypoglycemic episodes

ICD-9-CM Code: 850.09

See also Diabetic Ketoacidosis (DKA) in Diseases section

ETIOLOGY

- Genetic predisposition to autoimmune destruction of glucose transporter on islet cells → increased blood glucose—affects proteins via nonenzymatic glycosylations
- Swells cells (sorbitol is oncotically active)
- Increased viscous proteins (macroglobins), which impede blood flow
- Increased substrate for anaerobic metabolism
- Deranges autoregulation of blood flow

USUAL TREATMENT

- Insulin injections, diet, and exercise
- Pancreas transplant is option if renal disease is end stage
- Control of blood pressure

ASSESSMENT POINTS

SYSTEM	EFFECT	ASSESSMENT BY HX	PE	TEST
HEENT	Possible atlanto-occipital dislocation 2° to abnormal collagen glycosylation	Pain	Neck ROM Prayer sign	Usually not needed Neck x-rays in extension
CV	Angiopathy LV dysfunction (4−10× with hypertension) Ischemic PVD	Poor exercise tolerance Angina CHF symptoms	2-flight walk Chest exam for signs of CHF BP lying and standing	ECG CXR
RESP	↓ Lung elastance ↓ FEV; ↓ FVC	Poor exercise tolerance		Generally not needed
GI	Gastroparesis	Early satiety		
RENAL	Nephropathy, especially if hypertensive	N/V; impotence; orthostatic Sx Nonprotein foods		BUN/Cr
ENDO	↓ Insulin from islets			FBS, electrolytes
CNS	Autonomic dysfunction 2° to neuropathy	Early satiety; impotence; N/V; orthostatic symptoms		RR interval variation on ECG BP change on standing
PNS	Stocking-glove neuropathy → infections		PNS exam, especially if regional planned	
MS	Impaired joint mobility 2° to non-enzymatic glycosylation of collagen	Joint mobility	↓ ROM of joints	

Key Reference: Roizen MF: Miller Anesthesia, 4th ed. New York, Churchill Livingstone, 2000, pp 905−912.

PERIOPERATIVE IMPLICATIONS

Preoperative Preparation
- Metoclopramide (10 mg/70 kg) in patients with gastroparesis
- Assess myocardial and volume status

Monitoring
- Myocardial ischemia. Can have CHF if vol overload and LV dysfunction present.
- Blood sugar

Airway
- Atlanto-occipital dislocation possible—see HEENT—do prayer sign test; may have gastroparesis

Induction
- Osmotic diuresis can make hypovolemic; ANS and CV dysfunction make BP and HR fluctuate

Maintenance
- CV instability; volume status key to avoid renal and myocardial dysfunction with operation

Extubation
- CV and pulm drive insufficiencies common with neuropathies

Adjuvants
- Rx for tight control
- Regional: Diabetic nerves may be more prone to edema especially if epinephrine used. Reduce dose (e.g., lidocaine from 2.0% to 1.5%) for same effect.

Postoperative Period
- Sliding scale of insulin Rx based on q 1−3 h blood glucose determinations

ANTICIPATED PROBLEMS/CONCERNS

- Gastroparesis with presence of solid food 24 h after last meal if ANS dysfunction present. Consider Rx with metoclopramide 10 mg IM 1½ h prior to induction.
- ANS dysfunction associated with sudden death postop; can keep in ICU/PACU overnight; vested adult who can measure blood glucose and call 911 if sent home postop

DIABETES, TYPE II (NONINSULIN DEPENDENT)

Michael F. Roizen, M.D.
Stanley H. Rosenbaum, M.D.

RISK

- People within USA: 13–18 million
- Highest prevalence: Hispanics and Native Americans
- Gender predominance: none

PERIOPERATIVE RISKS

- Increased risk 5–10× if end-stage renal, CV, CHF, or autonomic neuropathy; without renal, CV, or autonomic dysfunction, risk is 1–1.5× normal
- Metabolic abnormalities increased with perioperative insulin Rx
- Unclear if same risks as for type I diabetes

WORRY ABOUT

- Autonomic neuropathy, gastroparesis, and sudden postop death
- Myocardial ischemia; CV instability
- Tight glucose control might be indicated in pregnancy (see under Diabetes, Type III), difficult weaning from bypass (ECC), predictable global or focal CNS ischemia
- Disordered autoregulation makes hypertensive BP fluctuations more dangerous
- Fluid and electrolyte imbalance

OVERVIEW

- Endocrinopathy that can cause same organ dysfunction as in diabetes type I: end-stage renal, myocardial, and neuropathic disease
- Associated with deranged blood flow autoregulation to CNS (at blood sugar 250 mg/dl), renal (at blood sugar 200 mg/dl), and cardiac (at blood sugar 100 mg/dl) vessels
- Ketosis is rare, since some endogenous insulin
- Primarily controlled by diet and/or oral agents, although insulin more frequently used
- Usually has high insulin levels for glucose level, but peripheral resistance to insulin effect. Can develop hyperosmolar nonketotic coma.
- Blood sugar control per se not associated with increased perioperative morbidity in absence of
  – Hypoglycemia
  – Hyperosmolar coma
  – CNS ischemia
  – Pregnancy
  – Extracorporeal circulation
- Check patient glucose log for degree of control

ICD-9-CM Codes: 250.00; 250.02 (Uncontrolled)

See also Diabetes, Type I, in Diseases section

ETIOLOGY

- Familial predisposition with very high concordance in identical twins
- Autosomal dominant with variable expression accentuated by conditions that increase peripheral insulin resistance (obesity, inactivity, certain changes, hormones), increase glucose production or metabolic demands (glucocorticoids, pregnancy), or decrease insulin secretion (certain β-adrenergic drugs)
- Increases nonenzymatic glycosylations
- Causes cell swelling
- Deranges autoregulation
- Increases viscous protein production
- Increases substrate for anaerobic metabolism

USUAL TREATMENT

- Hypoglycemic agents, diet, exercise, insulin
- BP control

ASSESSMENT POINTS

SYSTEM	EFFECT	ASSESSMENT BY HX	PE	TEST
HEENT	Possible atlanto-occipital dislocation	Pain	Neck ROM, prayer sign	
CV	Premature CAD Hypertension Peripheral vascular disease	Angina Claudication Symptoms of CHF	Peripheral pulses	ECG CAD-related tests as indicated
RESP	↓ Pulm elastance	Exercise tolerance		
GI	Gastroparesis	Early satiety		
ENDO	Hyperglycemia Osmotic diuretic–caused hypokalemia	Polyuria		Blood glucose, K^+
HEME	Infection from ↓ WBC phagocytic function		Site of infections	
RENAL	Nephropathy	Asymptomatic although often associated with neuropathy		BUN/Cr, UA for protein
CNS	Cerebrovascular disease Medication-induced hypoglycemia	TIAs, CVAs Long-acting oral hypoglycemic agents	CNS exam	
PNS	Distal neuropathy Postural hypotension	Impotence Foot infections	PNS exam, esp prior to regional anesthetic	
MS	Impaired joint mobility		ROM of joints	

Key Reference: Roizen MF: Miller's Anesthesia, 4th ed. New York, Churchill Livingstone, 2000, pp 905–912.

PERIOPERATIVE IMPLICATIONS

Preoperative Preparation
- Metoclopramide (10 mg/70 kg) if gastroparesis
- Assess myocardial and autonomic function and volume status, half-life of hypoglycemic agent(s) taken chronically

Monitoring
- Blood sugar (but ? tight control in type II diabetes and metabolic abnormalities)
- Painless myocardial ischemia can cause CHF if volume overload and LV dysfunction
- Peripheral vasculature and nerves vulnerable to pressure ischemia

Airway
- Atlanto-occipital dislocation possible—see HEENT, do prayer sign test

Induction
- Osmotic diuresis, autonomic nervous system, and CV dysfunction can make BP/HR fluctuate

Maintenance
- CV instability: volume status and avoidance of hypertension key to avoiding renal and myocardial dysfunction perioperatively

Extubation
- CV and pulmonary drive insufficiencies common with neuropathies

Adjuvants
- Regional: diabetic nerves may be more prone to edema, especially if epinephrine used. Reduce dose (e.g., lidocaine from 2.0% to 1.5%) for same effect.
- Oral hypoglycemics may ablate preconditioning

Postoperative Period
- Debate as to whether control to tighter than 60–250 ml/dl is of value in absence of hypertension

ANTICIPATED PROBLEMS/CONCERNS

- Autonomic nervous system dysfunction associated with sudden death postop; can monitor for resp function in ICU/PACU overnight; presence of adult at home who can measure blood glucose and call 911
- Infections and end-organ risk substantially increased with blood sugar >250 mg/dl. Hypoglycemic symptoms hidden by autonomic nervous system dysfunction, effects of regional, sedative-narcotic, and β-adrenergic blocking agents.

DIABETES, TYPE III (GESTATIONAL DIABETES MELLITUS) Richard B. Clark, M.D.

- Incidence of gestational diabetes mellitus (GDM) is 10 × higher than that of overt diabetes
- Increased in African-American and Hispanic women
- Risk factors are
  - Maternal age >25 y
  - Previous delivery of macrosomic infant
  - Previous unexplained fetal demise
  - Previous pregnancy with GDM
  - Strong immediate family history of NIDDM or GDM
  - Obesity (>90 kg)
  - Fasting glucose >140 mg/dl or random glucose >100 mg/dl

PERIOPERATIVE RISKS

- Unlikely renal, ocular, cardiac, neurologic, or orthopedic complications in GDM
- Hypoglycemia if insulin is used
- Fetal risk (if not controlled: polyhydramnios or macrosomia [6× normal])
- RDS (2–3 × normal); preeclampsia, neonatal hypoglycemia, prematurity

WORRY ABOUT

- Hyperglycemia and hypoglycemia

OVERVIEW

- GDM is defined as a carbohydrate intolerance that occurs (or is first recognized) during pregnancy.
- A glucose tolerance test is used to identify GDM. For details of the test, see the Key Reference.
- Maternal complications with GDM are few, but the fetus is at risk
- Complications, such as fetal polyhydramnios, macrosomia (6×), prematurity, birth trauma, RDS (2–3× normal rate), neonatal hypoglycemia, or morbidity, are as common with type III diabetes (GDM) as with type I diabetes (insulin-dependent)

ICD-9-CM Code: 648.8

See Pregnancy, Maternal Physiology; Diabetes, Type I; and Diabetes, Type II, in Diseases section

ETIOLOGY

- GDM occurs in genetically susceptible individuals
- Pregnancy, through secretion of substances from uterus, exerts diabetogenic effects

USUAL TREATMENT

- Use of insulin in GDM remains controversial. Diet has been used in management.
- Many clinicians obtain a single HbA_{1c} level at 6–12 wk gestation. In patients with mildly elevated plasma glucose levels and normal concentration of HbA_{1c}, dietary modification alone and a modest increase in exercise are often sufficient to normalize plasma glucose levels.
- If the fasting blood sugar exceeds 120 mg/dl, insulin may be required. Both regular and NPH insulin are used.

ASSESSMENT POINTS

SYSTEM	EFFECT	ASSESSMENT BY HX	PE	TEST
HEENT	Possible facial/pharyngeal edema	Snoring	Neck ROM Mallampati exam	
CV	CV changes of pregnancy—possible worse hypovolemia from osmotic diuresis		BP/HR with orthostatic maneuvers	
RESP	Resp changes of pregnancy, ↓ FRC, etc.			
GI	Gastroparesis of pregnancy	Early satiety		
ENDO	Neonatal hypoglycemia if maternal hyperglycemia Obesity			Blood sugar; glucose levels Acid-base status of fetus; HbA_{1c} in mother
HEME	Not present unless type I diabetes			
RENAL	↓ Renal function			BUN/Cr
CNS	ANS dysfunction	Gastroparesis, early satiety	Orthostatic BP	Tilt table test
PNS	Neuropathy not present unless type I diabetes			

Key Reference: Schwartz ML, Ray WN, Lubarsky SL: The diagnosis and classification of gestational diabetes mellitus: is it time to change our tune? Am J Obstet Gynecol 1999; 180:1560–1571.

PERIOPERATIVE IMPLICATIONS

Preoperative Preparation

- Full-stomach precautions: nonparticulate antacid administration usual

Monitoring

- Blood sugar in maternal and umbilical vein blood

Airway

- Examine for edema

Induction

- Regional anesthesia preferred to general anesthetic due to risks of aspiration and failed airway attainment if cesarean section is performed
- Osmotic diuresis can cause hypovolemia and increase BP and HR fluctuations

Maintenance

- CV instability: volume status is key to maintenance of uterine and other organ perfusion

Extubation

- Awake

Adjuvants

- Regional: diabetic nerves may be more prone to edema especially if epinephrine used. Reduced dose (e.g., lidocaine reduced from 1.5% to 1%) for same effect.

Postoperative Period

- Usually GDM cured by delivery

ANTICIPATED PROBLEMS/CONCERNS

- Fetal dysfunction, especially hypoglycemia and acidosis, if maternal hypoglycemia present
- Rapid changes in maternal blood glucose can accompany the pain/exertion of vaginal delivery of fetus and accompany the endocrine changes of uterine delivery

DIABETES INSIPIDUS
George J. Graf, M.D.

- Frequently occurs in childhood—early adulthood; males > females, males usually by sex-linked recessive transmission
- Nephrogenic diabetes insipidus (DI) rarely congenital; familial
- Racial predominance: none

PERIOPERATIVE RISKS

- Dehydration, hypernatremia, death
- Altered sensorium
- Hemodynamic instability
- Distended bladder, hydroureter

WORRY ABOUT

- Fluid and electrolyte imbalance during anesthesia
- New onset of central DI following serious head trauma
- Variable onset of central DI following pituitary surgery (1–6 days postop)
- Drug-induced renal tubular unresponsiveness to vasopressin (nephrogenic DI) (fluoride-related [or associated] toxicity, lithium, osmotic diuretics, etc.)

OVERVIEW

- Endocrinopathy associated with serum electrolyte and volume abnormalities
- Polyuria, excessive thirst, and polydipsia regularly present
- Dehydration unusual in awake patient
- Inadequate fluid replacement of excreted urine leads to hypernatremia and dehydration causing weakness, fever, altered sensorium, hemodynamic instability, and death
- Monitor urine output, serum osmolality, and electrolyte concentrations during perioperative period
- Ensure adequate fluid replacement

ICD-9-CM Code: 253.5

ETIOLOGY

- Inadequate production or release of vasopressin (ADH) from posterior pituitary
- Most frequently caused by neoplastic or infiltrative lesions of pituitary, pituitary surgery, severe head injury following cardiac resuscitation; may be idiopathic
- Renal tubular unresponsiveness to endogenous or exogenous vasopressin (ADH) usually acquired
  - Acute tubular necrosis
  - Renal transplantation
  - Drug-induced: lithium, amphotericin, osmotic diuretics, fluoride toxicity
  - Hypokalemia, chronic hypercalcemia
  - Systemic disorders: multiple myeloma, sickle cell disease

USUAL TREATMENT

- Hormone replacement: aqueous vasopressin, desmopressin
- Nonhormonal ADH stimulation: chlorpropamide
- Nephrogenic diabetes insipidus: hydrochlorothiazide, salt restriction

ASSESSMENT POINTS

SYSTEM	EFFECT	ASSESSMENT BY HX	PE	TEST
CV	Hypotension Tachycardia Myocardial ischemia	Orthostasis Reduced exercise tolerance	Orthostatic BP, HR	ECG
ENDO	Anterior pituitary dysfunction	Pituitary neoplasm or surgery	Multisystem effects 2° to multiple hormone deficiencies	Levels assess anterior pituitary function
RENAL	Polyuria 1° or 2° nephropathy	Frequent dilute urine	Urine volume	24-h urine; simultaneous measurement of plasma and urine osmolality
CNS	Visual disturbance Altered sensorium	Excessive thirst Polydipsia	Neurologic function	CT scan

Key Reference: Braunwald E (ed): Harrison's Principles of Internal Medicine, 13th ed. New York, McGraw-Hill, 1994, pp 1923–1928.

PERIOPERATIVE IMPLICATIONS

Preoperative Preparation

- Dx and appropriate Rx
- Assess electrolytes, serum osmolality, and volume status
- Rule out additional hormone deficiencies
- Discontinue provocative medications: lithium, mannitol

Monitoring

- Urine output with Foley catheter
- Serum electrolytes
- Intravascular volume

Airway

- Generally not affected

Induction

- Patient may be hypovolemic with BP and HR fluctuation, electrolyte abnormalities, and arrhythmias

Maintenance

- CV instability
- Fluid and electrolyte replacement dependent on multiple factors

Extubation

- Altered sensorium; unable to protect airway

Adjuvants

- Fluoride toxicity from prolonged enflurane or sevoflurane extremely rare as cause of renal tubular dysfunction

- Variable neuromuscular relaxant activity in presence of hypokalemia or hypercalcemia
- Chlorpropamide treatment for DI may cause hypoglycemia

ANTICIPATED PROBLEMS/CONCERNS

- Vasopressin therapy causes vasoconstriction, and acute treatment could precipitate myocardial ischemia in unstable patient with CAD
- Plasma osmolality affected by increases in BUN or glucose; urine osmolality below that of serum in severe cases of DI; urine osmolality will not increase following ADH therapy of nephrogenic origin

DIABETIC KETOACIDOSIS (DKA)

John R. Ammon, M.D.

RISK

- Patients with type I diabetes mellitus; rare in type II (see Diabetes, Type I in Diseases section)
- Diabetic with local or systemic septic process requiring surgery (e.g., appendicitis, perinephric abscess)

PERIOPERATIVE RISKS

- Cardiovascular collapse 2° to severe dehydration (diuresis, fluid deprivation, fever) and myocardial depression (severe acidosis)
- CNS injury 2° to cerebral edema with rapid correction of DKA
- Worsening of pre-existing end-organ dysfunction (e.g., nephropathy → ATN, CAD → perioperative MI)

WORRY ABOUT

- Fluid deficit of 3–8 L in established DKA
- Cardiac arrest or severe shock with onset of GA or regional anesthesia due to hypovolemia, acidosis
- Severe electrolyte derangements, esp total body potassium deficiency of several hundred milliequivalents
- Necessity of surgical therapy to treat etiology of DKA (abscess, gangrene)

OVERVIEW

- DKA is an acute metabolic emergency sometimes caused by a septic process requiring acute surgical care
- Absolute or relative deficiency of insulin and excess of glucagon causing severe hyperglycemia (250–600 mg/dl) with accompanying acidosis, dehydration, and organ dysfunction
- Perioperative approach as much hemodynamic as metabolic for favorable outcome

ICD-9-CM Code: 250.1

ETIOLOGY

- Type I diabetes with insulin deficiency caused by cessation of insulin therapy coupled with significant physical (infection, surgery) or emotional stress
- Glucagon, epinephrine, and cortisol operative in driving catabolic and ketogenic state
- Osmotic diuresis 2° to sustained hyperglycemia leads to volume depletion
- Metabolic acidosis a product of unrestrained free fatty acid release from adipose tissue and subsequent hepatic oxidation to ketone bodies from insulin lack and glucagon excess

USUAL TREATMENT

- Treat initiating cause
- Insulin, aggressive rehydration, correction of electrolyte derangements, hemodynamic support

ASSESSMENT POINTS

SYSTEM	EFFECT	ASSESSMENT BY HX	PE	TEST
CV	Hypovolemia	Duration of initiating event, postural symptoms	Tilt table test, BP HR, skin turgor Mucous membranes	CVP ABGs
RESP	Hyperventilation (Kussmaul's respiration)		Ventilatory rate and depth	ABGs
GI	Anorexia, N/V	Appetite, N/V		
RENAL	Diuresis	Urinary frequency, thirst		BUN/Cr
ENDO	Insulin deficiency, glucagon excess during severe catabolic stress	Type I diabetes		Blood glucose ABGs Potassium
CNS	Depression from lethargy to coma; late cerebral edema in children		Assess LOC Signs of ↑ ICP	

Key Reference: Skyler JS: Diabetes mellitus, types I and II. *In* Kelly's Textbook of Internal Medicine, 4th ed. Philadelphia, Lippincott Williams & Wilkins, 2000, pp 2751–2769.

PERIOPERATIVE IMPLICATIONS

Perioperative Preparation

- Vigorous isotonic saline infusion to restore hemodynamic stability (use 0.5 N saline if serum osmolality is >310 mOsm/L); CVP measurement appropriate in perioperative setting
- Insulin Rx usually begins with 0.1 U of reg insulin/kg IV with infusion of 0.1 U of reg insulin/kg/h

Monitoring

- Sequential glucose, pH, K+, serum K+ and Na+, chloride, urine output determinations during perioperative period; CVP catheter, possibly PA catheter if pre-existing myocardial dysfunction known; high incidence of occult CAD

Airway

- Potential stiff joint syndrome with difficult intubation; at risk for aspiration

Induction

- Hemodynamic instability likely if intravascular volume depletion not corrected; pre-existing autonomic neuropathy and CV dysfunction

Maintenance

- Protection of end-organs often compromised by diabetes mellitus, esp heart, CNS, renal

Extubation

- Awake

Adjuvants

- See under Diabetes in Diseases section

Postoperative Period

- Potential for hypoglycemic injury from rapid increase in insulin sensitivity when surgical cause of DKA corrected
- Medical management continued by physician with expertise in diabetes

ANTICIPATED PROBLEMS/CONCERNS

- Hemodynamic instability from combined volume deficiency, acidosis, and pre-existing CV disease
- CNS dysfunction from metabolic abnormalities, both early and late

DIAPHRAGMATIC HERNIA (CONGENITAL)
Joan M. Niehoff, M.D.

RISK

• Occurs in ~1/5000 births; 12–25% have associated anomalies

PERIOPERATIVE RISKS

• 30–60% mortality in live births
• Pulmonary hypoplasia and associated CNS and CV malformations affect mortality
• Timing of diagnosis associated with the prognosis (high-risk newborn presents with respiratory failure within first 6 h of life)

WORRY ABOUT

• Hypoxemia and acidosis
• Shock
• Tension pneumothorax

OVERVIEW

• Classified by site of herniation
• Posterolateral defects (Bochdalek) (90%), and left-sided defects occurring most frequently (80–90%); Morgagni hernias rare (5%); parasternal, less symptomatic, therefore, diagnosed at later age
• Degree of lung hypoplasia determined by time of defect during fetal development and amount of abdominal contents in chest, result in decreased numbers and function of alveoli; hypoplastic lung has high vascular resistance
• Ipsilateral lung most affected; both lungs abnormal
• Surgical treatment delayed for medical stabilization

ICD-9-CM Code: 756.6

INDICATIONS/USUAL TREATMENT

• Posterolateral defects require repair (does not resolve the pulmonary dysfunction)
• Small defects closed primarily; larger defects use artificial diaphragm, which contributes to postoperative respiratory failure
• ECMO indicated if severe pulmonary hypertension and/or hypercarbia despite maximal conventional management
• Fetal surgery still experimental

ASSESSMENT POINTS

SYSTEM	EFFECT	ASSESSMENT BY HX	PE	TEST
CV	Mediastinal shift Associated ASD, VSD, coarctation, tetralogy of Fallot (23%)	Displaced cardiac impulse	CV exam	ECHO
RESP	Respiratory distress, pulmonary hypertension	↓ Breath sounds on affected side Prominent ipsilateral chest	Pulmonary exam	CXR ABG
GI	Malrotation, atresia (20%)	Scaphoid abdomen	Abd exam	
GU	Hypospadias		Inspection	
CNS	Spina bifida, hydrocephalus, anencephaly (28%)		Inspection and neurologic exam	Ultrasound, CT scan
METAB	Acidosis, hypoxemia, hypercarbia			ABGs

Key Reference: Suda K, Bigras JL, Bohn D, Hornberger LK, McCrindle BW: Echocardiographic predictors of outcome in newborns with congenital diaphragmatic hernia. Pediatrics 2000; 105:1106–1109.

PERIOPERATIVE IMPLICATIONS

Perioperative Management

• ECMO provides temporary support until perinatal circulation matures and less sensitive to vasoconstrictive stimuli (1–2 wk)

Preoperative Preparation

• Avoid triggers for pulmonary vasoconstriction
• Goals include a $PaO_2 > 80$, $PaCO_2$ 25–30, normal or elevated pH, and normothermia
• Monitor pre- and postductal oxygenation
• NG tube
• Endotracheal intubation (unless small defect without respiratory distress)
• Sedation/analgesia/paralysis
• Watch for pneumothorax; consider prophylactic contralateral chest tube
• "Honeymoon" phase of adequate oxygenation after birth implies adequate alveolar surface

Anesthetic Technique

• Opioids well tolerated; inhaled halogenated anesthetics are not; avoid N_2O

Monitoring

• Routine and (preductal) arterial line

Surgical Stages

• Left subcostal incision usual; occasionally, thoracic approach used
• Reduction of herniated viscera by gentle traction, followed by excision of hernia sac
• Suture repair of defect; large defects may require flap or prosthetic material
• Small peritoneal cavity may limit closure (staged closure may be required)
• Ipsilateral chest tube usual before diaphragmatic closure and placed on water seal; prophylactic contralateral chest tube often used

POSTOPERATIVE CONSIDERATIONS

• If $A-aDO_2$ gradient >400 mmHg or if cardiopulmonary deterioration, continue respiratory assistance
• Persistent hypoxemia while on high FIO_2 suggests persistent pulmonary hypertension
• Minimize endotracheal suctioning, correct metabolic acidosis
• Deliver adequate nutrition
• Outlook dependent on pulmonary hypoplasia and bronchopulmonary dysplasia
• High degree of neurologic problems, whether or not infants placed on ECMO; seizures, developmental delay, and hearing loss in 20–30%

DIARRHEA, ACUTE AND CHRONIC

Michelle Braunfeld, M.D.

RISK

- Acute: 20% of population at sometime during year
- Chronic: 5% of population; ↑ with age
- Acute: male = female
- Chronic: female > male

PERIOPERATIVE RISKS

- Hypovolemia with hemodynamic instability
- Electrolyte abnormalities, especially hypokalemia
- Acid-base abnormalities: may be non–anion gap acidosis or alkalosis, depending on underlying cause

WORRY ABOUT

Chronic

- Underlying disease, especially iatrogenic (e.g., infection with antibiotic-induced diarrhea, end-stage liver disease with lactulose-induced diarrhea, or disaccharide [usually lactose] intolerance)
- Hormone-producing tumors (e.g., carcinoid, VIPomas, gastrinomas)
- Extraintestinal manifestations of inflammatory bowel disease (IBD) (e.g., deforming arthritis, cholangitis, vit K malabsorption with coagulopathy)
- Stress steroid therapy in IBD

- Psychological symptoms in up to 50% of patients with IBS; often alternates with constipation
- Postsurgical losses that may drain via ileostomy or fistula, or may be due to inadequate bowel absorption 2° to resection (short bowel syndrome)

Acute

- Viral, bacterial, or protozoan disease

OVERVIEW

- Acute: abrupt onset of loose stools in healthy individual: viral—self-limited, 1–3 days causing changes in small intestinal cells → shortened transit time; bacterial—tends to occur in groups of individuals (if within 12 h of a meal, usually due to preformed toxin); protozoan—prolonged watery diarrhea from contaminated water supply in endemic area
- Chronic: too-frequent passage of stools that are too loose for too long; >200 g/day of stool for >2–3 wk
- Multifactorial medical problem that requires supportive therapy and attention to the underlying etiology
- Only one in a spectrum of medical problems associated with an underlying disease or with treatment of disease. Supportive therapy includes fluid and electrolyte repletion and attention to acid-base balance.

- Toxic megacolon—extreme manifestation of inflammatory or infectious bowel disease is a surgical emergency. Patients often septic.

ICD-9-CM Code: 558.9

ETIOLOGY

Chronic

- Osmotic—laxatives, indigestible carbohydrates
- Secretory—hormone-producing tumors
- Exudative—inflammatory bowel disease, pseudomembranous colitis
- Decreased mucosal contact/mixing—short bowel syndrome, IBS

Acute

- Viral or bacterial (with or without toxin) or protozoan (see Overview)

USUAL TREATMENT

- Volume and electrolyte replacement
- Although acid-base correction often follows above, may occasionally need replacement
- Seek and treat underlying cause

ASSESSMENT POINTS

SYSTEM	EFFECT	ASSESSMENT BY HX	PE	TEST
CV	Hypovolemia	Postural symptoms, quantitation of bowel movements	Orthostatic changes Narrow pulse pressure Tachycardia Dry mucous membranes	
	Dysrhythmia 2° to electrolyte abnormalities			ECG
RESP	Compensatory hyperventilation			ABGs
METAB	Derangement dependent on underlying cause			Lab values include Ca^{2+}, Mg^{2+}, K^+, HCO_3^-; ECG
RENAL	Prerenal azotemia			BUN/Cr
CNS	Profound electrolyte abnormality Anemia—can be acute or chronic from acute GI losses or chronic disease state	Melena or hematochezia	Range from drowsiness to obtundation Stool guaiac	Hct

Key Reference: Cataldo R, Potash M: Atropine as a treatment of diarrhea after celiac plexus block. Anesth Analg 1996; 83:1131–1132.

PERIOPERATIVE IMPLICATIONS

Preoperative Preparation

- Assess volume status
- Repletion

Monitoring

- Consider arterial and central venous catheter (or some other fluid status monitor such as TEE) if significant hypovolemia and CV compromise present

Airway

- May require full-stomach precautions

Induction

- Hemodynamic instability and ↓ drug dosage if not repleted
- Sympatholytic drugs and sympathectomy with regional anesthesia can shorten transit time and increase diarrhea

Maintenance

- Tailor IV fluids to electrolyte and acid-base status (e.g., avoid normal saline if patient already has hyperchloremic acidosis)
- Continue electrolyte repletion if necessary

Extubation

- Routine, dependent on underlying condition

Adjustments

- Acid-base status and electrolytes may affect muscle relaxant duration and ability of antagonists to reverse block

ANTICIPATED PROBLEMS/CONCERNS

- Most operations do not affect underlying condition, but narcotics can make diarrhea less problematic, but use with caution in severe IBD as they may promote toxic megacolon
- Regional anesthesia that causes sympathectomy leaves parasympathetic system unopposed, which can cause shortened transit time and increase diarrhea

DILATED CARDIOMYOPATHIES (DCMs)   Frank W. Dupont, M.D.

RISK

• Prevalence varies from 8.3/100,000 to 36.5/100,000
• Higher mortality in elderly
• Racial predominance: African-American
• Gender predominance: male-to-female, 3:1
• 10,000 deaths from DCM reported annually in USA

PERIOPERATIVE RISKS

• Arrhythmias, CHF, autonomic instability, intracardiac thrombi, myocardial ischemia
• Smoking history, diabetes mellitus, and high diastolic blood pressure are reportedly predictors of mortality from idiopathic DCM (IDCM)

WORRY ABOUT

• Malignant arrhythmias, sudden death
• Worsening LV systolic and diastolic function, possibly RV dysfunction
• "Emboli," amiodarone- and implantable cardioverter-defibrillator (ICD)-related problems

OVERVIEW

• Disease characterized by dilatation of right, left, or both ventricles; increased EDV, ESV, and wall stress
• LV systolic ($\downarrow$ EF) and diastolic dysfunction (noncompliant ventricle), possibly AV valvular regurgitation
• Often tachyarrhythmias
• Intracardiac mural thrombi may be present
• High risk of sudden death

ICD-9-CM Code: 425.4 (Cardiomyopathy, idiopathic)

ETIOLOGY

• Primary (idiopathic) DCM: acquired with genetic predisposition, immunologic abnormality
• Secondary DCM: viral myocarditis (e.g., HIV), cytotoxic (ETOH, cocaine, doxorubicin), ischemic heart disease, metabolic (thyroid disease, diabetes mellitus), peripartum, neuromuscular disorders (muscular dystrophy [myotonic, Duchenne])

USUAL TREATMENT

• Medical treatment is primarily based on diuretics, digitalis, and vasodilators (ACE). Further, β-adrenergic receptor–blocking agents, immunosuppressives, anticoagulants, and antiarrhythmics (e.g., amiodarone, sotalol) or an ICD may be needed.
• Surgical treatment: cardiac transplantation, LVAD placement, cardiomyoplasty

ASSESSMENT POINTS

SYSTEM	EFFECT	ASSESSMENT BY HX	PE	TEST
CV	CHF	Dyspnea Orthopnea	Narrow pulse pressure, pulsus alternans Displaced PMI Systolic murmur (MR), S_3, S_4 JVD, ascites, pedal edema	CXR ECG ECHO Electrophysiologic testing Coronary angiography
	Myocardial ischemia Arrhythmias	Angina Palpitations		
RESP	CHF	Dyspnea Orthopnea	Rales Wheezing	CXR ABGs
GI		Anginal equivalent LUQ pain		See CV
HEME	Prolonged coagulation times	Bruising		PT/PTT
RENAL	Hypoperfusion	Nocturia		$\uparrow$ BUN/Cr ratio
CNS	Cerebral infarcts	Stroke	Focal neurologic deficits	CT scan
MS	Associated musculoskeletal disorders		Weakness	

Key Reference: Manolio TA, Baughman KL, Rodeheffer R, et al: Prevalence and etiology of idiopathic dilated cardiomyopathy (summary of a National Heart, Lung and Blood Institute workshop). Am J Cardiol 1992; 69:1458–1466.

PERIOPERATIVE IMPLICATIONS

Preoperative Preparation
• Optimization of cardiac condition for anesthesia (consider cardiology consultation)
• Checking of potassium, magnesium, and digoxin levels

Monitoring
• Consider ST-segment analysis
• Arterial line
• PA catheter if anticipation of large fluid shifts
• TEE is the monitor of choice for the assessment of biventricular function and AV valve regurgitation

Airway
• None

Preinduction/Induction
• Anesthetic principles based on afterload reduction, preload conservation, and prevention of myocardial depression
• Regional anesthesia techniques are not contraindicated provided hypotension is prevented
• ICD management precautions should be taken if applicable (see Implantable Cardioverter-Defibrillators [ICDs], Management, in Diseases section and Implantable Cardioverter-Defibrillators [ICDs], Implantation, in Procedures section)

Maintenance
• Potent inhalation agents often poorly tolerated; a narcotic-based anesthesia technique may be preferable, and N_2O should be used with caution
• Fluid management should be conservative to prevent fluid overload and acute CHF
• Inotropic support and FFP may be necessary

Extubation
• Beware of hypertension, arrhythmias, hypothermia

Adjuvants
• DCM predisposes to decreased blood flow to liver and kidney, which prolongs action of many agents; DCM also predisposes to increased volume of distribution of many drugs, thus often requiring increased initial dose and smaller and rarer subsequent doses (as with neuromuscular blocking agents, lidocaine, etc.); amiodarone-induced drug interactions (bradycardia, myocardial depression, hypotension)

ANTICIPATED PROBLEMS/CONCERNS

• Tachyarrhythmias, CHF, sudden death, emboli, hemodynamic instability, amiodarone interactions

DIPHTHERIA

Brian K. Bevacqua, M.D.

RISK

- People within USA: 5 cases/y (respiratory infections); 100 cases/y (cutaneous infections)
- Racial prevalence: none
- Age: children (age 15 y and younger) account for 25% of cases

PERIOPERATIVE RISKS

- Early (days after exposure): respiratory compromise; respiratory arrest; airway obstruction and hemorrhage; shock, coma, and death
- Late (2–6 wk after exposure): myocarditis; neuritis

WORRY ABOUT

- Early: progressive respiratory compromise caused by cervical and submandibular adenopathy, edema, and the characteristic "membrane" from the nasal pharynx to the bronchiolar level; systemic effects of exotoxin absorption (shock, coma, death)
- Late: myocarditis (10–20% of patients) characterized by tachycardia, S_3 gallop, dysrhythmias (atrial fibrillation, premature ventricular beats), and ECG changes (ST-segment changes, T-wave inversions, bundle branch block) that can lead to complete heart block CHF, cardiogenic shock, and myocardial fibrosis. Neuritis

(10%) involving both cranial (III, VI, VII, IX, and X) and peripheral nerves (motor > sensory); can resemble infectious polyneuritis.

OVERVIEW

- Infections and major complications are prevented by adequate levels of circulating antitoxic antibodies
- Requires complete primary immunization and periodic booster injections (every 10 y)
- Diagnosis of respiratory infections relies on recognition of the characteristic membrane
- Membrane begins as soft exudate patches that merge into a thin membrane, become thicker, and fuse to the underlying tissues
- Extent of membrane spread and exotoxin production determines degree of systemic involvement. The heart, kidneys, and nervous system are most likely to be involved.
- Myocarditis, the principal cause of death from diphtheria infections, begins as ST-segment and T-wave changes in the 2nd wk of illness
- Neuritis occurring 2–6 wk into the illness may involve cranial and peripheral nerves (motor > sensory) with compromise of speech, swallowing, and respiration

ICD-9-CM Codes: 032.0–032.9

ETIOLOGY

- Caused by *Corynebacterium diphtheriae*, a gram-positive rod with swellings at each end
- Encountered in patients who have never received complete primary immunization nor timely booster injections
- Can be spread from patients with respiratory or cutaneous infections (much more common than the respiratory form) or from chronic carriers

TREATMENT

- Early administration (within 48 h of onset) of equine antiserum essential
- Antibiotics (erythromycin or penicillin) should be given as soon as possible
- Immunize inadequately immunized individuals after exposure
- Isolation, bedrest, careful observation (for respiratory compromise)
- Symptomatic treatment (e.g., intubation or tracheostomy for respiratory distress)
- Pacemaker insertion for arrhythmia control

ASSESSMENT POINTS

SYSTEM	EFFECT	ASSESSMENT BY HX	PE	TEST
HEENT	"Membrane" spread and hemorrhage can cause airway obstruction	Altered speech, respiratory distress, croupy cough, hoarseness, chills, sore throat	Pharyngitis, fever, cervical and submandibular adenopathy and edema ("bullneck"); characteristic "membrane"	Gram stain and culture of "membrane," indirect laryngoscopy
CV	Conduction abnormalities, CHF, cardiogenic shock	Dyspnea with minimal exertion, symptoms of CHF, palpitations	Tachycardia, ectopic beats; atrial fibrillation, signs of CHF	ECG CXR
RESP	See HEENT	Tachypnea, dyspnea, presence of membrane	Progressive respiratory compromise	Indirect laryngoscopy
HEME/IMMUNO	Systems compromised dependent on amount of exotoxin			CBC; blood culture
GU	Proteinuria			UA
CNS	Interference with phonation, swallowing, respiration, resembles Guillain-Barré syndrome	Symptoms depend on involved nerves	Cranial nerves (most often III, VI, VII, X), peripheral nerves (motor > sensory)	

Key Reference: Southwick FS: Infections due to gram-positive bacilli. *In* Dale DC, Federman DD (eds): Scientific American Medicine. New York, Scientific American, Inc., 2000.

PERIOPERATIVE IMPLICATIONS

Preoperative Preparation

- Assessment of respiratory distress/airway compromise (with observation, indirect laryngoscopy, etc.)
- Assessment of immunization status and early intervention (within 48 h of symptoms) with antiserum and antibiotics
- Assessment of the immunization status of health care workers exposed to diphtheria and aggressive use of purified diphtheria toxoid as needed
- Assessment (late) of cardiac and neurologic involvement

Monitoring

- Consider pulmonary artery catheter or transesophageal echocardiography to assess degree of myocardial involvement

Airway

- Careful manipulation, as membrane will bleed if manipulated
- Aggressive use of endotracheal intubation/tracheostomy

Induction

- Compensate for problems of exotoxin shock (early) and possible CHF, cardiac arrhythmia (late)

Extubation

- Early: may need prolonged ventilation
- Late: cardiogenic shock/extensive polyneuritis may necessitate prolonged ventilatory support

Adjuvants

- Cardiac pacemaker for arrhythmia control/complete heart block

- Avoid digitalis preparations, as complete heart block is common and digoxin may worsen cardiac status
- Minimize use of sedative-hypnotics, as development of respiratory difficulties may be obscured

Postoperative Period

- Careful observation for respiratory (early), cardiac (late), and neurologic (late) compromise

ANTICIPATED PROBLEMS/CONCERNS

- Airway obstruction requiring tracheostomy/intubation
- Myocardial conduction problems that may necessitate pacemaker insertion
- Cardiogenic shock/CHF
- Neuritis that can present as a Guillain-Barré–like syndrome

DISSEMINATED INTRAVASCULAR COAGULATION (DIC)

Athos J. Rassias, M.D.
D. David Glass, M.D.

RISK

- Individuals at risk in USA: patients with sepsis, liver disease, shock, brain injury, tissue necrosis, leukemia, burns, fat embolism, retained placenta, amniotic fluid embolism, eclampsia, localized endothelial injury, disseminated malignancy, or intravascular hemolysis. In addition, certain toxins and immunologic disorders are associated with DIC.
- Gender/race predominance: none
- Mortality >50% in systemic DIC

PERIOPERATIVE RISKS

- Bleeding, poor coagulation
- Ischemic end-organ damage
- Concomitant problems (shock, hemolysis, obstetrical problems, etc.)

WORRY ABOUT

- Uncontrolled bleeding, from even minor sites of tissue trauma
- Usually occurs with other catastrophic problems, such as sepsis and major tissue damage
- End-organ damage from microthrombosis causing ischemic changes

OVERVIEW

- Syndrome consisting of activation of clotting cascade and fibrinolytic system
- Widespread formation of fibrin thrombi in microcirculation and resultant consumption of certain clotting factors and platelets
- Differential diagnosis: liver disease, massive transfusion, fibrinolysis, TTP, heparin overdose, dysfibrinogenemia/afibrinogenemia
- Dx: no specific laboratory finding pathognomonic for DIC. The laboratory findings must be correlated to the level of clinical suspicion given the presence of predisposing factors. If the patient has a clinical condition associated with DIC, the following laboratory findings are suggestive of DIC: platelet count <100,000/mm^3 or a rapid decline in the platelet count; prolongation of clotting times, such as PT and APTT; the presence of fibrin-degradation products (FDP); and low plasma levels of coagulation inhibitors, such as antithrombin III. D-Dimer, if positive, excludes primary fibrinogenolysis as a cause for a positive FDP.

ICD-9-CM Code: 286.6

ETIOLOGY

- Coagulation initiated and maintained by
  - Intrinsic processes that enzymatically activate procoagulant and protein
  - Release of inherent tissue factor by external factor, such as tissue trauma
- Risk of developing DIC increases with associated diseases and processes

USUAL TREATMENT

- Correction of underlying problem is most important goal, including aggressive general supportive measures, such as correcting hypoxemia, acidosis, and hypovolemia
- DIC warrants treatment only if significant bleeding, organ dysfunction, significant thrombosis, or treatment of underlying disease (e.g., acute promyelocytic leukemia) will worsen DIC
- Blood products:
  - PRBCs if significant hemorrhage
  - Cryoprecipitate for fibrinogen <50, aim to maintain at >100
  - Platelets, to maintain >20,000, and some recommend >50,000; FDPs impair platelet function; need liver function to clear FDPs
- FFP can be used if clotting factor deficiency
- Pharmacologic agents (controversial):
  - Heparin: used to turn off coagulation, allow coagulation factors to accumulate, and impede thrombus formation; amount given should not increase PTT
  - ϵ-Aminocaproic acid, an antifibrinolytic agent—can be effective in bleeding, but is generally not recommended as this may precipitate catastrophic thrombosis. May have a role in patients with 1e or 2e hyperfibrinolysis, such as those with acute promyelocytic leukemia or some patients with cancer. Note that the action of thrombin is usually greater than that of plasmin in DIC. Guideline for dosage in adults is to load with 3–4 g and maintain at 1 g/h.

ASSESSMENT POINTS

SYSTEM	EFFECT	ASSESSMENT BY HX	PE	TEST
HEENT	↑ Tendency for bleeding		Evidence of bleeding Engorged and friable mucous membranes	
CV	May have associated sepsis Microthrombi		Hypotension Signs of poor systemic perfusion	Invasive hemodynamic monitoring ECG ECHO
RESP	Bleeding Microthrombi	Dyspnea	Tachypnea	CXR ABGs
GI	Bleeding Microthrombi of liver			Nasogastric suctioning Stool heme testing LFTs
ENDO	Pituitary and adrenal microthrombi			ACTH-stimulation test
GU	Microthrombi			BUN/Cr
CNS	Bleeding Microthrombi			
MS	Petechiae			

Key Reference: Levi M, Ten Cate H: Disseminated intravascular coagulation. N Eng J Med 1999; 341:586–592.

PERIOPERATIVE IMPLICATIONS

Preoperative Preparation
- Correct disease process if feasible
- Blood products transfused as above
- Type and cross for PRBCs
- Regional anesthesia relatively contraindicated if significant coagulopathy present

Monitoring
- Routine
- Invasive monitors as indicated by condition
- Monitor coagulation

Airway
- Avoid tissue trauma

Induction
- Consider full stomach
- Septic patients likely hypovolemic and may have some degree of myocardial depression

Maintenance
- Coagulation monitoring frequently
- Transfusion of blood components according to clinical situation and coagulation status

Extubation
- Cardiovascular and pulmonary insufficiency may be present if acute DIC
- Consider postoperative mechanical ventilation

Adjuvants
- Muscle relaxants: may have concomitant hepatic and renal impairment, which alter metabolism of certain nondepolarizing muscle relaxants

ANTICIPATED PROBLEMS/CONCERNS

- Uncontrolled hemorrhage: patients may bleed from areas of even minor tissue trauma
- End-organ damage from microthrombosis
- Concomitant medical problems may present life-threatening situations

DIVERTICULOSIS

Stanley Deutsch, M.D., Ph.D.

RISK

• Age-dependent, ranging from 5% of the population by 40 y of age to 50% of the population after 80 y of age
• Common in the UK, North America, northern Europe, Australia, and New Zealand, but uncommon in southern Africa, the Middle East, the Far East, and the Pacific Islands

PERIOPERATIVE RISKS

• Because age-related, greater incidence of atherosclerotic heart disease, systemic atherosclerosis, and CHF, as well as reduced pulmonary and renal reserve

WORRY ABOUT

• Possibility of pelvic abscess, peritonitis, or bleeding

OVERVIEW

• A chronic condition, often asymptomatic, but in some patients, chronic pain with inflammation and flare-ups

ICD-9-CM Code: 562.1 (Colon)

ETIOLOGY

• A degenerative acquired disease related to low-residue diet with long transit time, as opposed to diets with high-fiber content with shorter transit time; an incidence of 96% in the sigmoid colon, with an incidence of 16% of disease in the entire colon
• With long transit times, intraluminal pressure ↑, colon becomes distended, followed by acute and then chronic inflammation of outpouches or diverticula

USUAL TREATMENT

• Anticholinergic antispasmodics, increased bulk by consuming a diet high in roughage (bran, fruit, and vegetables) to decrease transit time
• With severe abdominal pain, fever, and clinical signs of peritonitis, or pelvic abscess, exploratory laparotomy and antibiotics are indicated

ASSESSMENT POINTS

SYSTEM	EFFECT	ASSESSMENT BY HX	PE	TEST
CV	Hypotension Tachycardia Fever CAD	Angina	BP, HR Auscultation for rales, S_3	Pulmonary artery catheter Arterial line, ECG Urine output
RESP		Dyspnea with CHF	Rales with CHF	ECG CXR
GI	Abdominal pain, rigidity, pelvic mass on rectal exam, ileus			Free air under diaphragm if perforation Mass on CT scan
HEME	Anemia, leukocytosis, DIC with sepsis			Hgb, WBC, differential PT/PTT, FSP, plt count, fibrinogen
RENAL		May pass air with urine if perforation into urinary bladder		Urinalysis Urine output
CNS	Disorientation with sepsis			

Key Reference: Eijsbouts QA, de Haan J, Berends F, Siestes C, Cuesta MA: Laparoscopic elective treatment of diverticular disease: a comparison between laparoscopic-assisted and resection-facilitated techniques. Surg Endosc 2000; 14:726–730.

PERIOPERATIVE IMPLICATIONS

Monitoring

• Routine, including urine output
• With sepsis, monitor arterial pressure; pulmonary artery occlusion pressure might be considered

Maintenance

• Optimize intravascular volume, high oxygen content, and treat CHF

Postoperative Period

• Maintain intravascular volume, continued monitoring of CV variables, and urine volume

Adjuvants

• Antibiotics and potential interactions of antibiotics in prolonging muscle relaxation; interaction more bothersome if antibiotics have "washed" an inflamed peritoneum
• Volume expanders
• Component therapy if DIC develops
• Vasopressor support if required; no interactions

ANTICIPATED PROBLEMS/CONCERNS

• Pelvic abscess or peritonitis
• Cardiac or cerebral ischemia with infarction

DO NOT RESUSCITATE (DNR) ORDERS
David E. Lees, M.D.

RISK

- All facilities receiving federal funds (Medicare, Medicaid) must now inquire of the patient on admission as to the existence of an advance directive
- If the patient doesn't have one on admission, the hospital must inform the patient of the right to formulate such a document

PERIOPERATIVE RISKS

- Approximately 15% of patients with a DNR order come to surgery
- Almost 25% of USA population has recorded an advance directive

WORRY ABOUT

- Most commonly performed resuscitative procedures: vascular access, feeding gastrostomies, tracheostomies

OVERVIEW

- The DNR order is a limited expression of an advance directive, which is a legal instrument to ensure that a patient's wishes are carried out in the event of incapacitation
- Resuscitation is the usual response to sudden death; there is a presumed consent to resuscitation
- DNR orders arose because effectiveness of CPR is no longer categorically presumed, nor can the burden of a less-than-successful resuscitation be denied

ORIGIN

- In common law, unless contravened by statute or case law, the choices of a competent adult shall prevail
- US Supreme Court decision in the case of Nancy Cruzan affirmed that patients have the right to refuse treatment and that surrogates may act where patients have clearly and unequivocally made their views known
- Patient Self-Determination Act of 1991 and the JCAHO require that hospitals have written policies and procedures for dealing with advance directives under applicable state laws

TYPES/GOALS

- Several types of advance directives exist, including
  - DNR orders
  - Living wills
  - Health care proxies
  - Organ donation instructions
- Advance directives have 3 specific goals:
  - Give individual time to plan ahead
  - Provide someone to make surrogate decisions
  - Allow health care professionals and family members to make treatment plans in accord with patient's expressed wishes in event of incapacitation
- Web sites such as AdvanceDirectiveOnline.com provide online storage of advance directives and DNR orders. This site enables patients to store an advance directive on a secure Internet server, allowing health care facilities rapid access, should the need arise during a hospitalization.

Key Reference: Ethical Guidelines for the Anesthesia Care of Patients with Do Not Resuscitate Orders or Other Directives That Limit Care. Park Ridge, IL, American Society of Anesthesiologists, 1993; amended 1998.

PERIOPERATIVE IMPLICATIONS

- Remember, existence of a DNR order does not preclude surgery
- A DNR order should be reassessed whenever surgery is planned and should be either reaffirmed or suspended
- A thorough explanation of care to be provided to the patient must be given by the anesthesiologist; excluded procedures and temporal limits on any DNR suspension need to be established
- If personal views are in conflict with a patient's decision, all efforts need be made to find another anesthesiologist of comparable competence; an anesthesiologist does not have to surrender his or her own moral agency

- Anesthesiologists need be familiar with federal and state laws as well as local hospital policies
- When a patient with a DNR order is accepted for surgery, it must be remembered that a DNR order is not an excuse for suboptimal care
- Directives and policies should be frequently reviewed to determine the appropriateness of surgical and anesthetic care in such patients
- What is meant by *resuscitation*? Is treatment of hypotension on induction or correction of supraventricular dysrhythmia restricted in a DNR patient or is that part of total anesthetic care? Can only be answered by in-depth discussions with the patient.

- Did DNR status arise from unilateral consent? Was the DNR order instituted by a physician, claiming a resuscitation would be medically futile? Was this communicated to patient? Does patient agree?

ANTICIPATED PROBLEMS/CONCERNS

Anesthesiologists' Objections to DNR in OR

- Consent for anesthesia automatically presumes consent for resuscitation
- Fear of administrative harassment that may follow an intraoperative death
- Perceived responsibility for a patient's intraoperative death regardless of cause
- Fear of being sought out by terminal patients as "angel of death"

DOUBLE AORTIC ARCH

Carol L. Lake, M.D., M.B.A., M.P.H.

RISK

- Most common form of vascular ring; a very rare lesion, accounting for < 1% of congenital heart disease
- Race/gender predilection: none

PERIOPERATIVE RISKS

- Tracheal compression progressing to complete airway obstruction on induction and after neuromuscular blocking drugs

WORRY ABOUT

- Respiratory distress, wheezing, cyanosis
- Failure to thrive, poor growth, esophageal compression
- Associated cardiac disease such as transposition of the great arteries, tetralogy of Fallot, or VSD

OVERVIEW

- Double aortic arch produces a vascular ring around the trachea and esophagus, causing respiratory and esophageal obstruction of varying degrees
- Symptoms occur at birth or within the first 3 mo of life in most patients
- Surgical division of the extra arch breaks the compressing ring, but co-existent tracheomalacia may necessitate prolonged postop ventilation

ICD-9-CM Code: 747.21

ETIOLOGY

- Results from persistence of both arches during embryologic development instead of only the left arch. Ascending aorta divides into two arches passing on each side of the trachea and esophagus to join posteriorly to form the descending aorta. The left carotid and subclavian arteries arise from the smaller anterior arch, while the right carotid and subclavian arise from the dominant posterior arch.

USUAL TREATMENT

- Medical therapy: none
- Surgery: Via a left posterolateral thoracotomy, the smaller (anterior) arch is divided at its distal end just proximal to the junction with the larger posterior arch. The persistence of the carotid, temporal, and descending aortic pulses should be verified during temporary occlusion of the arch to be resected. Trachea and esophagus are freed above and below the point of obstruction, avoiding injury to the recurrent laryngeal nerve.

ASSESSMENT POINTS

SYSTEM	EFFECT	ASSESSMENT BY HX	PE	TEST
HEENT	Airway obstruction Esophageal obstruction	Dyspnea, apnea, intermittent cyanosis, dysphagia	Intercostal retractions, head hyperextended	CXR Barium esophagogram
CV	Depends on presence of associated heart disease; none if *only* double aortic arch present			
RESP	Recurrent respiratory infection	Coughing, wheezing		CXR (hyperinflated lung fields)

Key Reference: Lake CL: Pediatric Cardiac Anesthesia, 3rd ed. Norwalk, CT, McGraw-Hill, 1998, pp 368–370.

PERIOPERATIVE IMPLICATIONS

Preoperative Preparation

- Oxygen therapy if decreased arterial oxygen saturation present
- Antibiotics for bronchopneumonia

Monitoring

- Intra-arterial or central venous catheters with complex defects
- Doppler for persistent pulse presence

Airway

- Dynamic and static airway obstruction likely

Preinduction/Induction

- Inhalation induction without neuromuscular blockade until airway maintenance is documented by mask or tracheal tube is placed

- Secure IV access essential, as bleeding may occur during resection of anomalous arteries

Maintenance

- Depends on procedure
- Usually: GA with combination of narcotic and volatile agent

Extubation

- Extubation at end of case if tracheomalacia and stenosis absent

Postoperative Period

- Epidural analgesia delivered via caudal route provides good postop analgesia to minimize respiratory complications if early extubation possible

Adjuvants

- Anesthetic choices may be modified by co-existence of other cardiac lesions

ANTICIPATED PROBLEMS/CONCERNS

- Patients with double aortic arch may have mild to life-threatening respiratory obstruction and apnea

DOWN SYNDROME
James A. Greenberg, M.D.

RISK

- >300,000 individuals in the USA
- 80% of children with this condition survive beyond 1 y
- Number >50 y will ↑ by 200% by the year 2010
- Males > females 3:2
- No racial preponderance

PERIOPERATIVE RISKS

- Related to specific abnormalities in individual

WORRY ABOUT

- Congenital heart disease: 50% born with congenital heart disease (CHD), 8% with cyanotic CHD (usually tetralogy of Fallot)
  – May become profoundly hypoxic with R→L shunting; accidentally injected air bubbles may exit into systemic circulation (coronary and cerebral air emboli)
  – Adults less likely to have CAD
- Upper airway obstruction
  – Soft tissue obstruction of upper airway common immediately on induction of GA due to large tongue, small mandible, short neck
  – Subglottic stenosis is present in 20–25% and of particular concern in children
- Obstructive and central sleep apnea
- Cervical extension during intubation can cause neurologic symptoms (neck pain, arm pain, upper extremity weakness, torticollis)
- Generalized joint laxity; TMJ may sublux with jaw thrust
- Endocrine: hypothyroidism (4–6% in children; 15–20% in adults), hypothermia, obesity (difficult IV access)
- Mental retardation
  – May have overwhelming fears of unknown
  – Can become physically resistant to entering OR
  – Alzheimer's disease and other forms of mental illness (depression, psychosis) may co-exist

OVERVIEW

- Not a disease
- Incidence ↓ by prenatal screening and elective termination of pregnancy
- Wide variation in abilities and disabilities; neurologic development enhanced by external stimulation
- Institutionalized individuals have high incidence of seropositivity for hepatitis B
- More people living in group homes in community and becoming more self-sufficient in ADL

ICD-9-CM Code: 758.00

ETIOLOGY

- Genetic: trisomy 21
- Risk of parenting a Down syndrome fetus greatest in older (>35 y) parents (well characterized in mothers)

USUAL TREATMENT

- Depends on pathophysiology

ASSESSMENT POINTS

SYSTEM	EFFECT	ASSESSMENT BY HX	PE	TEST
HEENT	Large tongue Subglottic stenosis Hearing deficit in 66%	Hx of snoring Sleep apnea Intubation Hx		Audiology
CV	Tetralogy of Fallot in 4%	Sx of CHF "Tet spells"	Cyanosis Murmur	ECHO
ENDO	Hypothyroidism Obesity	Hypothermia	Obesity	
MS	Subluxation of C1/C2 Joint laxity			Cervical spine radiographs (controversy over whether these should be routine)

Key Reference: Mitchell V, Howard R, Facer E: Down's syndrome and anaesthesia. Paediatr Anaesth 1995; 5:379–384.

PERIOPERATIVE IMPLICATIONS

Monitoring

- Temperature (hypothermia)
- ECG (arrhythmias, ischemia); treat bradycardia from halothane or sevoflurane

Airway

- Have variety of alternative airway management devices available (e.g., oral and nasal airways, laryngeal mask, Bullard laryngoscope)
- Avoid neck extension during laryngoscopy if possible
- Smaller endotracheal tube may be necessary for narrowed subglottic space

Vascular Access

- Allow more time for IV placement
- Meticulously avoid injected air

Patient Management

- Soft, warm, kind, patient approach along with caregiver known to patient to help with initial management; warm, quiet OR

ANTICIPATED PROBLEMS/CONCERNS

- Hypoxia if R → L shunting develops
- Resistance to separation from caregiver
- Life-threatening upper airway obstruction with difficult vascular access
- Spinal cord ischemia with neurologic damage

DRUG ABUSE, LYSERGIC ACID DIETHYLAMIDE (LSD)

Michael J. Berrigan, M.D., Ph.D.
Herbert D. Weintraub, M.D.

RISK

• True prevalence of LSD use impossible to determine. In 1993, 13.2 million Americans over 12 y reported using LSD, an increase of 60% compared with 1985 data.
• LSD-related hospital visits remain low compared with those related to other major illicit drugs

PERIOPERATIVE RISKS

• LSD's sympathomimetic action may hinder evaluation of hemodynamics during surgery and anesthesia
• May prolong succinylcholine neuromuscular blockade and delay metabolism of ester local anesthetics (speculated inhibition of plasma cholinesterase)
• May potentiate analgesics

WORRY ABOUT

• CV: hypertension, tachycardia
• Psychiatric: visual illusions, labile mood, panic attacks
• GI: nausea
• Effects of concomitantly ingested drugs

OVERVIEW

• An odorless, tasteless, synthetic indolealkylamine that has been classified as a hallucinogen, although true hallucinations are rare. LSD commonly induces illusionary phenomena and synesthesia (blending of sensory modalities).
• Classified under Schedule I of the Controlled Substance Act
• Common route of ingestion is oral, and rapid GI absorption ensues. Distribution phase is rapid. LSD crosses the placenta.
• Tolerance rapidly develops, and no abstinence syndrome occurs
• Psychologic effects begin in 30–60 min and may last 8–12 h
• A very high therapeutic index. The human lethal dose is undetermined.
• Relatively inexpensive, with an average street unit costing $5. Currently, LSD dosages range from 20–80 μg, whereas the dosage range was 100–200 μg in the 1970s (DEA data).

ICD-9-CM Code: 305.3

ETIOLOGY

• Illicit drug use

USUAL TREATMENT

• Supportive reassurance
• Minimize external sensory stimuli
• Chlorpromazine, a phenothiazine, should be administered if it is certain no other hallucinogen has been ingested. If drug is given to a patient who has ingested STP (2,5-dimethoxy-4-methylamphetamine) or DMT (dimethyltryptamine), hypotension and shock may ensue.
• Benzodiazepines seem to be the most effective agents for treating "LSD psychosis" and visual disturbances

ASSESSMENT POINTS

SYSTEM	EFFECT	ASSESSMENT BY HX	PE
HEENT			Dilated, reactive pupils
CV	Sympathetic nervous system stimulation	Palpitations Sweating	Hypertension Tachycardia
RESP	No consistent changes		
ENDO	Hyperglycemia Mild hyperthermia		Elevated temperature
CNS	Euphoria Anxiety, labile mood Tremors Visual hallucinations and illusions Synesthesia Distorted sense of time	History of drug ingestion	Altered mental status

Key Reference: Micromedex—Drug Information Systems, Denver, CO, C.C.I.S. Expiration November 1998.

PERIOPERATIVE IMPLICATIONS

Preoperative Preparation
• Rule out associated traumatic injury
• Aspiration prophylaxis
• Sedation if agitation is severe

Monitoring
• Temperature
• Neuromuscular blockade

Airway
• None

Preinduction/Induction
• Exaggerated response to endogenous and exogenous catecholamines

Maintenance
• Maintain normothermia

Extubation
• At risk for aspiration
• Continue supportive reassurance

Adjuvants
• May have exaggerated response to sympathomimetic agents

• Theoretical potential for ester local anesthetic toxicity due to inhibition of plasma cholinesterase activity
• Theoretical potential for prolongation of succinylcholine neuromuscular blockade due to inhibition of plasma cholinesterase activity

ANTICIPATED PROBLEMS/CONCERNS

• Avoid injuries associated with agitation
• Possible concomitant drug/alcohol use by patient

DRUG OVERDOSE, RAT POISON (WARFARIN TOXICITY)

Michelle Braunfeld, M.D.

RISK

- Major risk is hemorrhage, esp CNS or GI
- Incidence: risk of hemorrhage in 2.4–8.1% of patients chronically anticoagulated. Risk is dose-related and proportional to PT prolongation. Thus, patients with a higher therapeutic INR (e.g., those with prosthetic valves) have higher risk. Age is associated with increased sensitivity to and increased incidence of bleeding complications. Patients >75 y may have >10× risk of CNS bleed than patients <65 y.
- Rx for DVT, cerebral vessel atherosclerosis, prosthetic heart valves, mitral stenosis, paroxysmal atrial fibrillation

PERIOPERATIVE RISKS

- Bleeding
- Drugs that potentiate anticoagulant effects: antibiotics (esp metronidazole, sulfonamides, cephalosporins), NSAIDs, phenytoin, cimetidine, barbiturates, alcohol

WORRY ABOUT

- Bleeding complications of invasive procedures
- Drug interactions
- Transient protein C deficiency preceding effect on procoagulant levels at initiation of warfarin therapy leading to thrombotic complications
- True poisoning with rodenticides ("super-warfarins") may result in prolonged clotting abnormality with abnormal PT values weeks to months post event

OVERVIEW/PHARMACOLOGY

- Vit K antagonist
- Cleared by hepatic and renal transformation and excretion. $T_{1/2}$ is ~40 h. Duration of action is 2–5 days.
- Onset of effect is delayed by 8–12 h because of time required to clear already synthesized clotting factors

ICD-9-CM Code: 286.9 (Coagulation defect)

DRUG CLASS/MECH OF ACTION/USUAL DOSE

- Blocks vit K–mediated carboxylation of factors II, VII, IX, X (procoagulants); protein C, protein S (anticoagulants)
- Carboxylation of coagulation factors oxidizes vit K. The vit K epoxide must be reduced to become active again. Coumarin anticoagulants block reduction of the epoxide. Thus, large and/or repeat doses of vit K are needed for large overdoses or for long-acting forms.
- Chronically taken for systemic anticoagulation for DVT, CVA, prosthetic valves, and atrial fibrillation either paroxysmal or associated with mitral stenosis
- Usual doses: loading regimen varies, but maintenance dose is 2.5–10 mg/d
- Alternatives: dicumarol, anisindione—while available, essentially never used. Neither shown to be superior to warfarin and both may have increased side effects.
- Phenprocoumin and acenocoumarol are prescribed in Europe. The former has a longer half-life than warfarin (5 days), the latter a shorter half-life (10–24 h).
- Heparin is drug of choice for acute anticoagulation, but must be given parenterally, usually as loading dose with an infusion

DRUG EFFECTS

SYSTEM	EFFECT	ASSESSMENT BY HX	PE	TEST
HEME	Abnormal levels of factor II, IV, IX, X, and protein C, protein S	Easy bruising, prolonged bleeding time	Ecchymoses	PT

Key Reference: Stoelting RK: Pharmacology & Physiology in Anesthetic Practice, 2nd ed. Philadelphia, JB Lippincott, 1991, pp 472–474.

POSSIBLE DRUG INTERACTIONS

Preoperative

Increased effect	Decreased effect
Antibiotics, NSAIDs	Methylxanthines
Oral hypoglycemics	Rifampin
Diazepam	Antihistamines
Cimetidine	Corticosteroids
Diuretics	Barbiturates
Phenytoin	

Adjuvants/Regional Anesthesia/Reversal

- Regional block—relatively contraindicated without reversal of anticoagulation
- Peripheral block—relatively contraindicated without reversal of anticoagulation

SPECIAL CONSIDERATIONS/CONCERNS

- Relatively minor surgical procedures may be performed without reversal of warfarin anticoagulation
- Major surgical procedures warrant discontinuation of drug 1–3 days preoperatively with a target PT within 20% of nml range. Alternatively, patient may be admitted 1–2 days prior to surgery. Warfarin is discontinued and heparin therapy instituted. Heparin is discontinued 6 h prior to surgery.
- In emergency surgery, patient may be given 10–20 ml/kg of FFP and 5–10 mg of vit K, with additional amounts of both given as needed
- Hypothermia will potentiate anticoagulant effect

DUCHENNE MUSCULAR DYSTROPHY
(PSEUDOHYPERTROPHIC MUSCULAR DYSTROPHY)

Richard I. Cook, M.D.

RISK

- Males (30/100,000 males); a few cases known in females
- Often undiagnosed until age 3–5 y
- Deterioration through puberty to death usually before age 25 y

PERIOPERATIVE RISKS

- Respiratory failure, prolonged mechanical ventilation
- Muscle weakness

WORRY ABOUT

- Poor cardiac function, cardiac arrhythmias, MVP (antibiotic prophylaxis)
- Poor respiratory function, pulmonary Htn from chronic sleep apnea, scoliosis
- Aspiration risk (delayed emptying)
- Hyperkalemic arrest with succinylcholine
- Association with malignant hyperthermia
- Consider supplemental steroids (if previous Rx with steroids)
- Poor long-term prognosis

OVERVIEW

- Most boys die from pneumonia but CHF is also seen in the later stages
- Gradual onset of the muscle wasting may go unnoticed for years after hyperkalemic response to depolarizing NM blockers develops. The infant may appear entirely normal. With age the body habitus may be normal or even athletic, but the muscle mass is gradually replaced by fat.
- ↑ Sensitivity to nondepolarizing NM blockers
- Use of Ca^{2+}-channel blocker (e.g., verapamil) may prolong or even cause NM blockade
- Up to ¼ of patients may have mitral valve prolapse
- Resting tachycardia common; cardiac involvement in 70% of cases, cardiac debilitation usually late
- ECG abnormal (increased RS in V_1, deep Q in precordial leads)

ICD-9-CM Code: 359.1

ETIOLOGY

- X-linked recessive disease; the muscles (including myocardium) are gradually replaced with fat and connective tissue. The defect is in the muscle cell membrane protein *dystrophin*.

USUAL TREATMENT

- At least 25 drugs have been tried without success; early trials of steroids have shown some promise
- Spinal rodding and fusion, often with AP approach, for the scoliosis that begins at 10–12 y can prolong comfort and ease of wheelchair use. Pulmonary deterioration continues, and life may be only minimally prolonged.
- Tendon releases for contractures
- Exploratory laparotomy for ileus

ASSESSMENT POINTS

SYSTEM	EFFECT	ASSESSMENT BY HX	PE	TEST
CV	Conduction	Tachycardia	Opening snap (MVP)	ECG, 24-h ambulatory ECG
	Contractile force	Difficult (Hx CHF Sx: orthopnea, DOE, PND)	CHF signs	ECHO, MUGA
RESP	↓ Volume and flows	Difficult	Unreliable	PFTs
	Sleep apnea/pulmonary Htn	Snoring, apneic spells	Unreliable	SaO_2?, sleep lab? ECHO?
GI	Dysmotility, gastric dilatation, paralytic ileus			
GU	Bladder paralysis, impotence			
CNS	↓ IQ		Mental status exam	
MS	Scoliosis, kyphosis Contractures			Spine films
	Muscle destruction	Progressive weakness		Abnormal myogram Elevated CK levels
	Macroglossia Poor IV access			

Key Reference: Frankowski GA, Johnson JO, Tobias JD: Rapacuronium administration to two children with Duchenne's muscular dystrophy. Anesth Analg 2000; 91:27–28.

PERIOPERATIVE IMPLICATIONS

Preoperative Preparation
- Avoid or limit sedation

Monitoring
- Consider PA catheter/TEE based on EF and surgical procedure
- Nerve stimulator

Induction
- Succinylcholine contraindicated because of hyperkalemia
- Avoid MH-triggering agents

- Consider avoiding depressants of cardiac contractility
- Consider long gastric emptying times, possible full stomach

Maintenance
- Variable response to NM blockers; titrate to effect
- Recommended to allow spontaneous recovery, as response to reversal agents varies

Emergence
- Potential for prolonged ventilator dependence when vital capacity <30% of predicted

- Late respiratory depression reported (cause unclear); may make outpatient surgery inadvisable

ANTICIPATED PROBLEMS/CONCERNS
- Respiratory failure
- Congestive failure
- Supraventricular tachydysrhythmias

WARNING
- The hyperkalemic response to succinylcholine (cardiac arrest) has been described in boys 4 mo old without clinical signs of Duchenne muscular dystrophy

DUODENAL ATRESIA

Lynne G. Maxwell, M.D.

RISK

- Incidence 1/10,000–40,000 live births
- M = F
- 20–30% have trisomy 21
- 45% are premature infants of pregnancy complicated by polyhydramnios
- Mortality 10%, due not to duodenal atresia but to associated congenital heart disease or prematurity

PERIOPERATIVE RISKS

- Hypoxemia associated with immature lungs
- Hypoxemia due to congenital heart disease, persistent fetal circulation

WORRY ABOUT

- Ventilation problems associated with prematurity
- Other associated anomalies in 50% of cases—esophageal atresia (7%), other intestinal atresias, renal anomalies (5%), malrotation of the gut (25%), volvulus, imperforate anus (3%), annular pancreas (25%)
- Congenital heart disease associated with trisomy 21 (ASD, VSD, AV canal)
- Aspiration on induction of anesthesia 2° to bowel obstruction
- May be associated with cystic fibrosis
- Late presentation can be associated with dehydration, hypovolemia, and hypochloremic alkalosis

OVERVIEW

- Frequently premature infant of pregnancy complicated by polyhydramnios
- Vomiting after birth: may be copious and bile stained
- Flat abdomen
- Diagnosis is made by "double bubble" on abdominal x-ray

ICD-9-CM Code: 751.1 (Atresia, small intestine)

ETIOLOGY

- Unknown in sporadic cases
- More common in trisomy 21

USUAL TREATMENT

- Surgical repair is curative

ASSESSMENT POINTS

SYSTEM	EFFECT	ASSESSMENT BY HX	PE	TEST
CV	Congenital heart disease—ASD, VSD, AV canal Persistent fetal circulation	Trisomy 21	Murmur Cyanosis	ECHO CXR Pulse oximetry
RESP	Respiratory distress syndrome of prematurity	Polyhydramnios Gestational age <36 wk	Tachypnea Retractions Flaring Grunting	CXR Pulse oximetry
GI	Duodenal obstruction Associated esophageal atresia	Bilious vomiting No gas in abdomen	Scaphoid abdomen	Abdominal x-ray Unable to pass OG tube
RENAL	Structural anomalies		Palpation of kidneys	Abdominal US

Key Reference: Murshed R, Nicholls G, Spitz L: Intrinsic duodenal obstruction: trends in management and outcome over 45 years (1951–1995) with relevance to prenatal counselling. Br J Obstet Gynaecol 1999; 106:1197–1199.

PERIOPERATIVE IMPLICATIONS

Preoperative Preparation
- OG tube to decompress stomach, reduce gastric contents
- Intravenous catheter placement with hydration (20 ml/kg NS) if diagnosis delayed beyond 24–48 h; correct electrolyte abnormalities
- Surfactant for premature infants with significant lung disease

Monitoring
- Arterial monitoring for ABGs, electrolyte, and Hgb determination only in premature infants with significant lung disease, those with congenital heart disease, or those with extreme dehydration due to protracted vomiting; otherwise NIBP sufficient as minimal blood loss expected
- Temperature
- Urinary catheter may be helpful in assessing adequacy of fluid resuscitation

Anesthetic Technique
- Suction OG tube prior to induction, intubation
- Awake intubation after preoxygenation only for actively vomiting, volume-depleted infants with abnormal airway anatomy
- Rapid-sequence induction after preoxygenation for normovolemic patients with normal airway anatomy

- Avoid N_2O to prevent intestinal distention; may be contraindicated in premature
- Nondepolarizing muscle relaxant helpful for surgical exposure
- Second peripheral IV after induction

Airway
- Precautions to prevent aspiration
- Abnormal airway anatomy unlikely

Preinduction/Induction
- Patient may be hypovolemic due to vomiting, poor feeding
- Correct dehydration, hypochloremic alkalosis (failure to do so can shift oxyhemoglobin dissociation curve to left and reduce oxygen delivery to tissues)
- De-bubble intravenous lines to prevent paradoxical air embolism
- Type-specific blood available for transfusion—rarely needed

Maintenance
- Mechanical ventilation with rate 15–20, PIP 20–25 to achieve adequate ventilation
- Air/oxygen mixture to achieve oxygen saturation 92–96%, although some use 100% oxygen to provide reserve; data on retinopathy of prematurity due to operative exposure to 100% oxygen is not conclusive, and surgical retraction may restrict ventilation and cause atelectasis, which can cause desaturation

- Surgical retraction/pressure on liver may decrease venous return and cause hypotension
- Fentanyl or remifentanil/pancuronium/isoflurane for premature infants
- In full-term infants who may be immediately extubatable, consider caudal catheter threaded to low thoracic position—dose with bupivacaine 0.25% with 1:200,000 epinephrine 0.5–0.75 ml/kg

Extubation
- May require postop ventilation if patient premature or has congenital heart disease
- Full-term infants with effective epidural anesthetic and no narcotic administration may be extubated

ANTICIPATED PROBLEMS/CONCERNS

- Prematurity/respiratory distress syndrome/apnea
- Congenital heart disease
- Risk of aspiration may continue postoperatively—leave OG or NG tube in place
- Later risk of GE reflux higher than normal (17%)
- Adequate fluid replacement
- Other associated anomalies

ECHINOCOCCOSIS

Anis S. Baraka, M.D., F.R.C.A.
Zuhayr A. Tabbarah, M.D.

RISK

- Common to endemic in sheep-raising countries worldwide (e.g., Mediterranean basin, Australia, Argentina, Far East) and in dog-eating populations
- Rare in USA except among immigrants from sheep-raising countries and residents of sheep-raising areas
- Racial predilection: none

PERIOPERATIVE RISKS

- Organ dysfunction, depending on site of hydatid cyst
- Sepsis
- Communication of cyst with biliary tree bronchopleural communications

WORRY ABOUT

- Spillage of hydatid fluid
  - Anaphylactic reactions
  - Dissemination of infestation
- Complications from scolicidal agents
  - Methemoglobinemia (with cetrimide); hypernatremia and sclerosing cholangitis (hypertonic saline, 15–20%); air embolism (hydrogen peroxide); ethanol intoxication (75–95%)

OVERVIEW

- Zoonosis caused by larval stage of *Echinococcus granulosus*, which produces unilocular cystic lesions; larvae burrow through mucosa of small intestine, enter portal circulation, and travel to liver
- Liver involved in >50% of cases, followed by lungs
- Cysts can involve any organ system including muscles, spleen, brain, spinal cord, kidneys, bones, and omentum; hydatid cysts grow slowly
- Sx related to mechanical pressure of cyst on surrounding structures
- Cyst may be infected and behave like abscess and/or acute cholangitis
- Spontaneous rupture/leak can occur, causing anaphylactic reactions and dissemination of infestation
- *Echinococcus* should be suspected when cystic mass is discovered in liver, lung, or other organs by ultrasound, CT scan, or CXR, with Hx of past exposure
- Dx can be confirmed by serologic studies (indirect hemagglutininemia, ELISA, others)

ICD-9-CM Code: 122.9

ETIOLOGY

- Caused by *E. granulosus;* adult worm lives in jejunum of canines (mainly dogs) for 5–20 mo; in addition to scolex and neck, it has 3 proglottides (1 immature, 1 mature, and 1 gravid); gravid segment splits before or after passage of stools and releases eggs that contaminate environment; intermediate hosts (sheep and occasionally humans) ingest food contaminated by *E. granulosus* eggs and develop cysts in liver, lungs, or other organs; life cycle of *E. granulosus* is complete when dogs consume infected viscera of sheep or other animals

USUAL TREATMENT

- Surgery, when feasible, principal definitive treatment; surgery may be conservative with use of scolicidal agent and evacuation of cyst or radical with pericystectomy or hepatic resection
- Laparoscopic approach to uncomplicated cysts of the liver and spleen is a safe and effective option. Also, video-assisted thoracoscopy may be used for pulmonary hydatid surgery.
- Puncture–aspiration–injection–reaspiration (PAIR) technique being used successfully in some countries
- Chemotherapy with albendazole is playing ↑ role as adjunct Rx to ↓ risk of dissemination and in nonoperable cases; usual dose, 10 mg/kg, to be started 1 mo–1 wk prior to surgery and for 1–6 mo postsurgery

ASSESSMENT POINTS

SYSTEM	EFFECT	ASSESSMENT BY HX	PE	TEST
CV	Hydatid cyst of heart Conduction defect Pericarditis	Chest pain		ECG ECHO Serology
RESP	Hydatid cyst of lung Rupture into bronchial tree	Cough, chest pain Hemoptysis		CXR Serology
GI	Hydatid cyst of liver, spleen, omentum	N/V Intermittent colic	Palpable mass Jaundice, fever	Ultrasound, CT scan Serology
RENAL	Hydatid cyst of kidney		Palpable mass	Ultrasound, CT scan, serology
CNS	Hydatid cyst of brain Space-occupying lesion, ↑ ICP Rupture into subarachnoid space	Headache	Signs of ↑ ICP Localizing signs	CT scan Serology
MS	Hydatid cyst mass of bones, muscles Pathologic fracture	Painless, localized swelling	Dull muscle ache on exertion	Ultrasound, CT scan, serology X-ray
SPINE	Mass effect	Weakness	Radicular distribution or paresis	X-ray CT scan

Key Reference: Craig PS: Current research in echinococcosis. Parasitology Today 1994; 10:209–211.

PERIOPERATIVE IMPLICATIONS

Preoperative Preparation

- Albendazole 10 mg/kg/d for 1 wk preoperatively (max 800 mg/d)
- LFTs, pulmonary function tests, depending on site of cyst
- Antihistamines part of premedication

Monitoring

- Routine monitors
- Other monitors depend on site of cyst

Airway

- Double-lumen tube for thoracotomy or thoracoscopy whenever hydatid cysts of lungs diagnosed

Induction

- Depends on site and function of organ involved

Maintenance

- 100% O$_2$ during one-lung ventilation for thoracotomy or thoracoscopy; cardiopulmonary bypass for cardiac hydatid cyst
- Avoidance of spillage of hydatid fluid
- Irrigation with scolicidal agents, such as cetrimide or hypertonic saline

Extubation

- Routine extubation, except in cardiac, pulmonary, or brain hydatid cysts, when extubation is tailored according to situation

Postoperative Period

- Routine except
  - Complications such as anaphylactic reactions, methemoglobinemia, or excessive bleeding
  - Specialized cases undergoing cardiopulmonary bypass, craniotomy, or thoracotomy complicated by bronchopleural fistula and/or excessive air leak

ANTICIPATED PROBLEMS/CONCERNS

- Anaphylactic reaction (2° to spillage); epinephrine first line of management
- Methemoglobinemia 2° to excessive cetrimide; methylene blue, 1–2 mg/kg, therapeutic

ECLAMPSIA

Therese K. Abboud, M.D.

RISK

- Preeclampsia: 6–8% of pregnant women
- Eclampsia: 0.2 to 0.67/1000 births
- Most often young primigravidas

PERIOPERATIVE RISKS

- Accounts for 20–40% of maternal mortality
- Severe hypertension, abruptio placentae, fetal distress, pulmonary edema
- Affects every organ system

WORRY ABOUT

- Hemodynamic variables and fluid changes
- Difficult airway
- Coagulopathy

OVERVIEW

- Preeclampsia Dx made if 2 or more of these criteria present: systolic BP >140 mmHg; diastolic BP >90 mmHg; proteinuria >2 g/24 h; and pedal edema
- Eclampsia implies seizures and may occur before, during, or after delivery; this worsens both maternal and fetal prognosis
- May manifest in virtually every organ system
- Disease process usually terminates 48 h after birth

ICD-9-CM Code: 624.4

ETIOLOGY

- Cause still speculative: genetic, immunologic, or simply ↓ in uterine blood flow
- Imbalance of thromboxane (↑) and prostacyclin (↓) with resultant ↑ vasoconstriction, platelet aggregation, uterine activity, and ↓ uteroplacental blood flow
- ↓ Placental perfusion releases fibronectin, which causes damage to tissues
- Seizures related to cerebral vasospasm, ischemia, edema, hemorrhage

USUAL TREATMENT

- Goal for eclampsia is stop convulsion, establish clear airway
- Definitive: delivery of fetus/placenta
- Magnesium: ↓ irritability of CNS and direct vasodilation (Rx range, 4–6 mEq/L)
- Antihypertensives: hydralazine, trimethaphan, labetalol, nitroglycerin, nitroprusside (caution, cyanide toxicity)
- Chronic aspirin Rx ↓ incidence

ASSESSMENT POINTS

SYSTEM	EFFECT	ASSESSMENT BY HX	PE	TEST
CV	Hypertension, CHF	Palpitations, fatigue, edema	High BP, edema, rales	ECG, ECHO
RESP	Pharyngolaryngeal edema, pulmonary edema	Cough, stridor, breathlessness, chest tightness	Tachypnea, dyspnea, rales, wheezing	CXR ABGs
HEME	Hypercoagulability, thrombocytopenia, platelet dysfunction, DIC, HELLP syndrome		Petechial oozing around IV puncture sites	Coagulation studies: platelet count PT, fibrin/fibrinogen
RENAL	Glomerulopathy, proteinuria, oliguria, ↑ Cr and BUN	↓ Urine output, edema	Rapid weight gain, edema	Urinalysis, 24-h urine protein, BUN/Cr
HEPATIC	↓ Hepatic blood flow, ↓ cholinesterase, periportal hepatic necrosis, subcapsular hemorrhage, abnormal LFTs	Epigastric and subcostal pain	Tenderness over liver area, hepatomegaly	Liver enzyme assay, ultrasound

Key Reference: Hood DD, Curry R: Spinal versus epidural anesthesia for cesarean section in severely preeclamptic patients: a retrospective survey. Anesthesiology 1999; 90:1276–1282.

PERIOPERATIVE IMPLICATIONS

Preoperative Preparation

- BP control
- Anticipate difficult airway
- Aspiration prophylaxis

Monitoring

- Routine
- Consider arterial catheter for severe cases
- PA catheter as indicated by oliguria, pulmonary edema, refractory hypertension, and persistent arterial desaturation

Airway

- Anticipate difficult intubation due to tissue swelling and airway bleeding

Labor/Delivery

- Epidural if no coagulation problems
- Avoid high-level block, prehydrate with caution

Cesarean Section

- Epidural if no coagulation defect
- General if bleeding abnormalities or in emergency
- Control BP with rapid-onset, short-acting antihypertensives
- MgSO₄ may potentiate muscle relaxant
- Avoid narcotics, sedatives, and high concentration of inhalation agents prior to delivery of fetus
- Extubate fully awake

Postpartum

- Eclamptic: observe in highly monitored situation
- Continue MgSO₄, hemodynamic control, and fluid balance concerns
- Adequate pain management: pain score, 2–5
- Observe for coagulopathy

Adjuvants

- Mannitol (cerebral edema), furosemide (pulmonary edema)
- Digitalis (CHF)
- Barbiturates, benzodiazepine to control seizures

ANTICIPATED PROBLEMS/CONCERNS

- Eclamptic seizures
- Pulmonary edema
- Hypertensive encephalopathy
- DIC

EISENMENGER'S SYNDROME

Michelle Burnett, M.D.
Theodore W. Striker, M.D.

RISK

- 3% of all congenital heart disease patients with atrial, ventricular, or aortopulmonary shunt
- VSD is most common lesion

PERIOPERATIVE RISKS

- Mortality rate of patients with ES carrying pregnancy to viability is 27–30%
- Fetal risks: ↑ risk of preterm labor, intrauterine growth retardation; fetal demise of 75%
- Cesarean section carries higher mortality: 70% vs. 30% for vaginal delivery
- Death most often occurs at delivery or post partum

WORRY ABOUT

- R → L shunt, pulmonary hypertension, right and left ventricular failure, hypoxemia, arrhythmias, paradoxical emboli, thromboembolic phenomena, hemoptysis
- ↓ Systemic vascular resistance of pregnancy worsens R → L shunt
- Inability to meet ↑ demand for O_2 with gestation and labor
- Thromboembolic disease (hypercoagulation of pregnancy, venous stasis, polycythemia with chronic hypoxia)

- Delivery produces autotransfusion with RV failure
- Excessive bleeding with previous heparinization
- Acute blood loss produces systemic hypotension, ↓ pulmonary blood flow, and hypoxia
- Postpartum increase in PVR

OVERVIEW

- Consists of pulmonary vascular occlusive disease with pulmonary hypertension with R → L shunt and right ventricular dysfunction
- Has poor prognosis; mean age at death, 25 y
- Hx of syncope, ↑ right-sided filling pressures, and systemic arterial desaturation below 85% indicate poor prognosis
- 50% of pregnant patients die in association with pregnancy; outcome is worst for patients with VSD (hemodynamic demands of pregnancy, labor, and delivery place excessive burdens)
- Some pulmonary vascular reactivity may exist in the pulmonary vasculature of pregnant women; may be due to systemic hormonal factors of pregnancy

ICD-9-CM Code: 745.4

ETIOLOGY

- Individuals with intracardiac shunts develop uncorrected L (systemic) → R (pulmonary) shunts

- Shunt occurs through ASD, VSD, patent ductus arteriosus, or aortopulmonary window
- L → R shunt overloads pulmonary vascular bed and RV
- Pulmonary vasculature becomes remodeled with relative fixed PVR
- ES follows with pulmonary hypertension, R → L or bidirectional shunt with peripheral cyanosis
- Pulmonary hypertension is fixed and not reversible by repair of intracardiac lesion

USUAL TREATMENT

- With expected high maternal mortality, pregnant patients with ES should initially be counseled to terminate pregnancy
- For the patient who wishes to continue with pregnancy:
  – Hospital admission early in 3rd trimester
  – Anticoagulation with heparin: SQ heparin 5000–10,000 U bid
  – Patients with O_2 sat <80% on room air should be fully anticoagulated
  – O_2 Rx
  – Monitor for preterm labor
  – Medical Rx: diuretics, antiarrhythmics, inotropes
- Long-term and postpartum: surgical treatment has been described: either heart and lung transplantation or lung transplantation with primary repair of congenital cardiac defects

ASSESSMENT POINTS

SYSTEM	EFFECT	ASSESSMENT BY HX	PE	TEST
CV	Right and left ventricular enlargement/failure	DOE, edema, orthopnea, anginal chest pain, syncope, fatigue	Elevated jugular venous pressure, increased intensity of S_2, split S_2 and S_3, rales Right ventricular heave	ECG CXR ECHO, angio
RESP	Pulmonary hypertension	Dyspnea, hemoptysis	Palpable pulmonary artery Cyanosis, clubbing	Pulse oximetry ABGs, Hct (polycythemia)

Key Reference: Smedstad KG, et al: Pulmonary hypertension and pregnancy: A series of eight cases. Can J Anaesth 1994; 41:502–512.

PERIOPERATIVE IMPLICATIONS

Preoperative Preparation
- Discontinuation of heparin; consider reversal with protamine
- Avoid aortocaval compression at all times
- Antibiotic coverage for subacute bacterial endocarditis

Monitoring
- Pulse oximetry
- With uncorrected patent ductus arteriosus, use simultaneous right hand (preductal) and foot (postductal) pulse oximetry to estimate changes in shunt fraction
- CVP line
- PA catheter use is controversial, may be relatively contraindicated, potential complications may outweigh benefits:
  – Difficult to position in PA
  – High risk of arrhythmias, thrombi, paradoxical emboli, PA hemorrhage
  – Misleading data: unreliable PCWP and measurement of CO with shunt

Airway
- Preoperative administration of Bicitra, metoclopramide, and ranitidine
- NPO for 8 h (if possible)

Preinduction/Induction
- For labor:
  – Provision of effective analgesia prevents ↑ release of catecholamines, which ↑ PVR
  – Coaxial technique: initial intrathecal dose of narcotic
- For cesarean section:
  – Regional: slow induction of epidural anesthesia; counteract sympathectomy with vasopressor and maintenance of preload
  – General anesthesia: avoid rapid-sequence with risk of precipitating ↑ in PVR or inducing myocardial depression; maintain cricoid pressure through induction; avoid ↑ in PVR, ↓ in SVR, hypoxia, hypercarbia, and myocardial depressants

Maintenance
- For labor:
  – Epidural infusion with low-dose local anesthetic/narcotic solution
  – Avoid Valsalva maneuver, pushing; delivery with vacuum or forceps
- For cesarean:
  – High-dose narcotic technique
  – Amnesia with benzodiazepine
  – Avoid halogenated agents: myocardial depression, ↓ SVR
  – Avoid nitrous oxide: ↑ PVR, higher FIO_2

Extubation
- High-dose narcotic technique neccessitates postop ventilation

Adjuvants
- Avoid N_2O
- Maintain SVR with dilute solution of phenylephrine
- Inotrope, vasodilator for treatment of failure
- Cautious use of oxytocin (systemic vasodilation)
- Avoid prostaglandin F (↑ in PVR)
- Resume anticoagulation in postpartum period

Postoperative Period
- Pain management is critical
- Death most often occurs at delivery or postpartum
- Possible hemodynamic changes:
  – Excessive blood loss; replace volume
  – Autotransfusion; treat with vasodilator, inotrope, judicious use of diuretic
  – Arrhythmias: sinus bradycardia, AV block, EMD
  – Pulmonary emboli
  – Postpartum ↑ in PVR; reason unknown

ANTICIPATED PROBLEMS/CONCERNS

- Unresponsive, ↑ PVR or ↓ SVR with loss of oxygenation
- CHF

EMPHYSEMA

William R. Furman, M.D.

RISK

- Prevalence, incidence, mortality ↑ with age
- Higher in males than females
- Higher in whites than nonwhites

PERIOPERATIVE RISKS

- Intraoperative bronchospasm
- N_2O expansion of bullae
- Postop respiratory failure
- Postop pulmonary infection

WORRY ABOUT

- Worsening of baseline pulmonary function, caused by
  - Bronchospasm
  - Acute bronchitis or pneumonia
  - Pulm embolism

OVERVIEW

- Anatomic: destruction of interalveolar septa and loss of pulmonary elastic recoil; leads to formation of bullae and development of irreversible expiratory airflow obstruction
- The prototypical "pink puffer" has dyspnea, hyperinflation, distant breath sounds, low diffusing capacity (↓ DLco to <60% predicted)
- Patients often have elements of chronic bronchitis and asthma
- Hypoxia, hypercarbia, cor pulmonale are late developments
- Mucociliary clearance is often worsened after inhalational anesthetics
- Diaphragmatic mechanics are impaired by anesthetics, sedatives, NM blockers, conduction blocks, supine positioning

ICD-9-CM Code: 492.8 (Resection of bullae)

ETIOLOGY

- According to the elastase-antielastase hypothesis, the lung is normally protected from injury to its elastic tissues by antielastases, including α_1 protease inhibitor (API), which is also called α_1 antitrypsin. According to this theory, emphysema may be acquired or genetic.
- Acquired: related to inhaled oxidants (cigarette smoke or other occupational exposures), which are believed to inactivate API, thus compromising lung matrix repair after injury
- Genetic: absent or abnormal API, also known as α_1 antitrypsin deficiency, which accounts for a small fraction of cases

USUAL TREATMENT

- Smoking cessation
- Relief of symptoms by treatment of bronchospasm and infection
- In advanced cases, if hypoxia and cor pulmonale have developed: oxygen
- Lung reduction surgery in cases of diaphragmatic dysfunction and disabling disease (experimental)

ASSESSMENT POINTS

SYSTEM	EFFECT	ASSESSMENT BY HX	PE	TEST
HEENT	Tumors 2° to smoking	Voice change	Hoarseness, stridor, inspiratory obstruction	
CV	Cor pulmonale (late)	Edema, severe dyspnea	Signs of pulm Htn Hepatosplenomegaly Pedal edema, cyanosis, pleural effusions, usually without pulmonary edema	CXR ABGs
	Pulmonary emboli	Episodic SOB Arrhythmias Hard to differentiate from course of underlying illness	May reveal DVT in legs	CXR V/Q scan Pulmonary angiogram
RESP	Bronchospasm	Recent ↑ in dyspnea or ↓ in exercise tolerance	↑ Resp rate ↑ Expiratory time ↑ Accessory muscle use	Spirometry pre- and post-bronchodilators
	Pneumonia	Fever, dyspnea, ↑ sputum	Signs of pulmonary consolidation	CXR

Key Reference: Seigne PW, Hartigras PM, Body SC: Anesthetic considerations for patients with severe emphasematous lung disease. Int Anesthesiol Clin 2000; 38:1–23.

PERIOPERATIVE IMPLICATIONS

Preoperative Preparation

- Optimize bronchodilation
- Eradicate any underlying bacterial infection
- Encourage smoking cessation

Monitoring

- Be cognizant of potential for increased gradient between $PETCO_2$ and $PaCO_2$

Airway

- None, unless tumor present in airway

Preinduction/Induction

- If patient has airway reactivity, consider issues related to asthma
- Usually best to avoid N_2O when expansion of bullae is a risk

Maintenance

- Recumbent positions impair chest wall muscle function, and abdominal muscle function usually needed for spontaneous ventilation
- Ventilator settings: long expiratory times may be required; try to avoid high positive pressures, especially if bullae are present

Extubation

- Residual anesthetics may compromise the ventilatory response to CO_2, increasing the risk of postop respiratory failure
- Unrelieved incisional pain, especially after abdominal or thoracic surgery, will impair breathing

- Patients may be semiconscious and combative owing to hypoxia and hypercarbia on emergence
- Evaluate whether postop ventilation may be the safest approach until the residual anesthetic effects have dissipated

Adjuvants

- β-Adrenergic agonists, theophylline, atropinic agents for airway reactivity
- Oral or inhaled steroids in selected patients

ANTICIPATED PROBLEMS/CONCERNS

- Postop respiratory failure
- Tension pneumothorax from ventilator-induced barotrauma
- Airway plugging from secretions

ENCEPHALITIS

Mary J. Njoku, M.D.
M. Jane Matjasko, M.D.

RISK

- Increased by exposure in endemic areas
- Increased during seasonal variation and epidemic outbreaks
- Associated with immunosuppression (HIV, transplant, oncology, chemotherapy)

PERIOPERATIVE RISKS

- Associated with mental status alteration, seizures, ↑ICP, SIADH
- Associated with increased sensitivity to sedative and amnestic effects of anesthetics and adjunct drugs
- Unrecognized, unexpected deterioration in mental status may occur perioperatively

WORRY ABOUT

- Delayed awakening
- Hyperkalemic response to succinylcholine
- Postop delirium
- Electrolyte abn 2° to SIADH

OVERVIEW

- Inflammation of parenchymal brain tissue
- May be primary manifestation of disease process or a component of another CNS or systemic illness
- Organisms enter CNS via blood stream, peripheral nerves, olfactory nerves
- Sx include fever, headache, photophobia, nuchal rigidity, vomiting, altered consciousness, behavioral changes, disorientation, lethargy, confusion, hallucinations, memory loss, seizures, coma, focal neurologic abnormalities
- Dx is established by symptoms, epidemiologic Hx (exposure, season, geographic location), CSF culture, CSF bacterial and viral antigens, brain biopsy, CT scan, MRI, ^{99m}Tc scan, EEG

ICD-9-CM Code: 064

ETIOLOGY

- Infectious
  - Viral
  - Nonviral—bacteria, protozoa, nematodes, fungi
- Noninfectious
  - Toxic, vascular, SLE, Behçet's disease

USUAL TREATMENT

- Acyclovir effective for herpes simplex encephalitis
- Other antimicrobial therapy should be given according to culture and sensitivity
- Supportive care
  - Intubate, ventilate, if dictated by mental status, airway reflexes
  - Hemodynamic support
  - Nutrition
  - DVT prophylaxis
  - GI prophylaxis
  - Physical therapy
  - Diagnosis and treatment of extracranial infections
- Management of complications: seizure, ↑ICP, SIADH, ventilatory failure

ASSESSMENT POINTS

SYSTEM	EFFECT	ASSESSMENT BY HX	PE	TEST
HEENT	Colonization of nasopharynx	Preceding URI		Nasopharyngeal culture
CV	Autonomic dysfunction		Labile BP, HR	
HEME	↑ or normal WBC			CBC, WBC differential, serum antibody titers
RENAL	SIADH	Water intoxication Anorexia N/V Personality disorders Neurologic abn	No evidence of volume depletion Normal skin turgor Normal BP Mental status changes from lethargy to coma	Serum Na$^+$ and osmolarity Urine Na$^+$ and osmolarity BUN, Cr
CNS	Focal, global neurologic disturbances	Fever Headache Seizure Personality change Memory loss Confusion Weakness	Focal neurologic deficits, altered mentation, papilledema; if spinal cord involvement: flaccid paraplegia, increased DTRs	CSF: cell count, protein, Gram stain, culture, antibodies, antigens, CT, MRI, ^{99m}Tc scan, EEG, brain biopsy

Key Reference: Irani DN, Hanley DF, Johnson RT: Acute viral encephalitis: Diagnosis and clinical management. *In* Tyler KL, Martin JB (eds): Infectious Diseases of the Central Nervous System. Philadelphia, FA Davis, 1993.

COMPLICATIONS

Preoperative Preparation

- Document neurologic exam
- Elicit Hx of ↑ICP or seizure
- If SIADH present, correct electrolyte and free water abn
  - Sodium administration or fluid restriction depending upon severity of hyponatremia
  - Beware of central pontine myelinolysis with rapid correction of hyponatremia

Monitoring

- Electrolytes
- Fluid I/O
- Consider ICP monitoring, EEG monitoring

Airway

- None

Induction

- Potential for hyperkalemic response to succinylcholine indicates preferred use of nondepolarizing NM blockers
- Autonomic instability

Maintenance

- If patient is receiving seizure prophylaxis, be aware of potentiation of sedative effects and alteration of hepatic metabolism of anesthetics and muscle relaxants

Extubation

- Delayed awakening
- Seizures on emergence

Postoperative Period

- Delirium
- Possible progressive deterioration

Adjuvants

- See interactions under Induction and Maintenance

ANTICIPATED PROBLEMS/CONCERNS

- Delayed awakening
- SIADH
- Hyperkalemic response to succinylcholine

RISK

- 1% of 60 million adult hypertensives
- 1.5–2.0 times greater in African-Americans than in remaining population
- Increased in unrecognized or undertreated hypertension

PERIOPERATIVE RISKS

- Increased risk of MI
- Cerebrovascular accident
- Renal failure

WORRY ABOUT

- Myocardial ischemia, failure
- Hemorrhagic CVA
- Neurologic deterioration postoperatively
- Aortic dissection
- Acute renal failure
- Microangiopathic hemolytic anemia

OVERVIEW

- Also called "hypertensive reversible posterior leukoencephalopathy"
- More common with hypertension, renal failure, eclampsia
- If untreated, follows rapid progress to severe injury or death
- Chronic hypertensives tolerate higher acute elevation in BP than those with recent onset of hypertension (e.g., eclampsia, renal failure)

ICD-9-CM Code: 437.2

ETIOLOGY

- Abrupt ↑ in BP in chronic hypertension
- Renovascular/renal parenchymal disease
- Pregnancy, eclampsia
- Endocrine: pheochromocytoma, Cushing's, renin-secreting tumors, mineralocorticoid hypertension
- Drugs: cocaine, sympathomimetics, tyramine with MAO inhibitors, erythropoietin, cyclosporine
- Autonomic hyperactivity; spinal cord lesions
- CNS disorders: head injury
- Thought to be caused by abrupt ↑ in SVR from circulating vasoconstrictors (e.g., ADH, angiotensin II), causing failure of the upper limit of cerebrovascular autoregulation

USUAL TREATMENT

- Rapidly reduce mean arterial pressure by 20–25% within 1 h
- Antihypertensives: nitroprusside, nitroglycerin, labetalol, ACE inhibitors, hydralazine, enalapril
- Anticonvulsants: phenytoin, benzodiazepines, barbiturates

ASSESSMENT POINTS

SYSTEM	EFFECT	ASSESSMENT BY HX	PE	TEST
CV	Hypertension (diastolic > 140 mmHg) CHF Myocardial ischemia	Past hypertension Angina Hx of CHF ↓ Exercise tolerance	S3 S4 gallop Rales	CXR ECG
RESP	↓ Lung elastance ↓ FEV, FVC	Exercise intolerance Cough Orthopnea	Rales	CXR O2 sat
GI	Aortic dissection Encephalopathy	Abdominal pain Back pain N/V	Abdominal mass	Ultrasound or arteriogram (if indicated)
RENAL	Renal failure	Anuria		UO, UA BUN/Cr
CNS	Severe headache Visual disturbances Paralysis Convulsions Stupor, coma	Mental status Examination	Retinal leak Arteriolar spasm Funduscopy	

Key Reference: Vaughan CJ, Delanty N: Hypertensive emergencies. Lancet 2000; 356(9227):411–417.

PERIOPERATIVE IMPLICATIONS

Preoperative Preparation

- Control BP: nitroprusside, nitroglycerin, hydralazine
- Treat CV failure, renal failure

Monitoring

- Invasive BP monitoring
- Invasive blood volume monitoring (CVP or pulmonary artery cath) or TEE

Airway

- Control BP during intubation

Induction

- Avoid ↑ in BP
- Control volume preinduction

Maintenance

- CV instability; volume status key to avoid fluctuations
- Control BP aggressively

Extubation

- Under BP control

Adjuvants

- Continued aggressive BP control

ANTICIPATED PROBLEMS/CONCERNS

- Labile BP
- Myocardial ischemia/failure
- CNS symptoms
- End-organ ischemia owing to angiopathic changes

Charles Weissman, M.D.

RISK

- 3.4–11% of medical ICU admissions
- 12–33% of multiple-organ dysfunction patients

PERIOPERATIVE RISKS

- With predisposing conditions, e.g., hepatic insufficiency, risk of developing or exacerbating metabolic encephalopathy
- Increasing severity of pre-existing encephalopathy

WORRY ABOUT

- Worsening hepatic insufficiency causing hepatic encephalopathy
- Diabetics' becoming hypoglycemic
- Postop hyponatremia
- Deteriorating renal insufficiency leading to uremic encephalopathy
- Pre-existing encephalopathy may be exacerbated by anesthetics, e.g., benzodiazepines, in hepatic encephalopathy
- Undiagnosed sepsis, hypothermia, high fever, CNS-acting drugs, including overdose
- CNS cause: brainstem CVA, meningitis, occult head trauma, encephalitis, brain tumor

OVERVIEW

- Altered sensorium, stupor, or coma without any other explanation in the setting of a metabolic disturbance
- Process affects global cortical function by altering brain biochemistry
- Distinguished from structural lesions by a nonfocal neurologic exam
- EEG shows diffuse background slowing, triphasic waves in hepatic encephalopathy
- Increased spontaneous motor activity—restlessness, asterixis, myoclonus, tremors, rigidity

ICD-9-CM Code: 348.3 (Unspecified encephalopathy)

ETIOLOGY

- Hypoglycemic encephalopathy—most commonly due to accidental or deliberate overdosing with insulin or oral hypoglycemic agents or prolonged ethanol intoxication
- Hepatic encephalopathy—acute or chronic hepatic insufficiency, Reye syndrome
- Uremic encephalopathy—renal failure. After dialysis "disequilibrium syndrome" caused by acute fluid and electrolyte shifts.

- Encephalopathy due to fluid and electrolyte abnormalities—hyperosmolar state, hyponatremia (acute decrease to <120 mEq/L), hypernatremia
- Pulmonary encephalopathy—combination of hypoxia and hypercarbia

USUAL TREATMENT

- Uremic encephalopathy—dialysis
- Hepatic encephalopathy—lactulose (oral or rectal), neomycin
- Hypoglycemic encephalopathy—intravenous glucose
- Septic encephalopathy—treatment of underlying infection
- Hyperosmolar/hyposmolar state—slow and careful restoration of electrolyte balance
- Pulmonary encephalopathy—quickly improve ventilation and oxygenation, mechanical ventilation

ASSESSMENT POINTS

SYSTEM	EFFECT	ASSESSMENT BY HX	PE	TEST
RESP	Sudden elevated $Paco_2$ (>65 mmHg)	COPD, drug overdose	Hypoventilation, papilledema	Pulse oximetry and end-tidal capnography, or ABGs
GI	Hepatic insufficiency	Liver disease, cirrhosis, alcoholism, portasystemic shunt	Asterixis, jaundice, ascites	SGOT, SGPT, bilirubin, ammonia PT
ENDO	Diabetes	Use of insulin or oral hypoglycemic agents		Blood glucose
	Apathy Thyrotoxicosis Hypothyroidism	Hyperthyroidism Hypothyroidism	Tachycardia Fever, sweating Hypothermia Pretibial edema	T_4, T_3 TSH
	Hypercalcemia	Hyperparathyroidism Malignancy		Serum Ca^{2+}
RENAL	Uremia Prerenal azotemia	Renal disease, ingestion of nephrotoxins, e.g., drugs	Asterixis	BUN/Cr, serum lytes Toxicology screen
CNS	Altered sensorium, stupor, coma, seizures		Nonfocal neurologic exam, altered mental status	EEG, CT Lumbar puncture
MS	Multifocal myoclonus, rigidity		Myoclonus	

Key Reference: Ravin PD: Metabolic encephalopathy. *In* Irwin RS, Cerra FB, Rippe JM (eds): Intensive Care Medicine, 4th ed. Philadelphia, Lippincott-Raven, 1999, pp 2078–2086.

PERIOPERATIVE IMPLICATIONS

Preoperative Preparation

- Assess and document preop mental status and neurologic function
- Uremic encephalopathy—preop dialysis, if possible

Monitoring

- Routine
- In hyperosmolar states, uremia and liver failure with ascites may need central monitoring

Preinduction/Induction

- Benzodiazepines should be avoided in hepatic encephalopathy.
- Increased potential for aspiration; consider rapid-sequence

Maintenance

- Carefully titrate anesthetics to avoid overdosing
- Careful attention should be paid to intravascular volume status, blood glucose, and lytes
- During and after TURP and hysteroscopy, sodium concentrations and volume status should be monitored

- In renal and hepatic failure, appropriate drugs and doses should be used. Long-acting drugs should be avoided.

Extubation

- Extubate only if patient is able to protect airway and maintain adequate ventilation

ANTICIPATED PROBLEMS/CONCERNS

- Poor mental status at the conclusion of surgery may require continued intubation
- Hyponatremia is a cause of postop metabolic encephalopathy

ENCEPHALOPATHY, POSTANOXIC

Charles Weissman, M.D.

RISK

• After successful prehospital cardiac resuscitation: 59–65% of patients remain comatose
• 0–5% of successful resuscitations result in chronic vegetative state

PERIOPERATIVE RISKS

• Worsening of neurologic status; blindness most common residuum
• Postpone surgery in all but emergency situations
• Do what is necessary to treat precipitating cause and to ↓ sequelae (e.g., ↓ ICP or edema by ↑ ventilation and slight ↑ in BP)

WORRY ABOUT

• Repeat of events that initially caused encephalopathy (e.g., arrhythmias leading to cardiac arrest)

OVERVIEW

• Definition: Brain injury resulting from "prolonged" period of insufficient cerebral oxygenation
• Clinical picture ranges from mild confusion to brain death
• Chances for acceptable neurologic recovery ~1% with continued coma after 24 h and lack of two of the following reflexes: pupillary, corneal, and oculovestibular
• Seizures occur in 25% of patients
• Anoxic damage may have been sustained by other organs (e.g., MI, shock liver, acute renal failure, stress ulcers, ARDS)
• Diabetes insipidus poor prognostic sign

ICD-9-CM Code: 348.1

ETIOLOGY

• Caused by inadequate O_2 delivery to CNS due to inadequate cardiac output, respiratory dysfunction, severe anemia, and/or ↑ICP
• Most often 2° to primary cardiac (MI or arrhythmia) or pulmonary (asthma, pulmonary embolism) event
• May also be result of carbon monoxide poisoning, suffocation, and cyanide poisoning

USUAL TREATMENT

• Prevent recurrence of inciting event
• Ventilatory and hemodynamic support, as needed
• Stress ulcer prophylaxis
• Treatment of seizures (with anticonvulsants, e.g., phenytoin) and myoclonus

ASSESSMENT POINTS

SYSTEM	EFFECT	ASSESSMENT BY HX	PE	TEST
CV	MI	Assess if cardiac disease was cause of arrest		ECG, other cardiac assessment CK, SGOT, LDH, troponins
RESP	ARDS	Assess if respiratory disease was cause of arrest Respiratory failure	Wheezing, stigmata of COPD	Pre-arrest PFTs ABGs
GI	Shock liver Stress ulceration	Hx of GI bleeding	Jaundice	SGOT, SGPT, bilirubin, alkaline phosphatase Hct NG output
RENAL	Renal failure	Assess if electrolyte abnormalities or acidosis caused initial event	Urine output	BUN/Cr
CNS	Altered mental status, diffuse and focal neurologic abnormalities	Changes in neurologic signs since hypoxic event	Neurologic and mental status exams, apnea test	CT scan EEG SSEP, BAER
MS	Myoclonus, posturing Contractures	Hx of abnormal movements, posturing Prolonged immobility	Decerebrate or decorticate postures Contractures	

Key Reference: Lippa CF, Moonis M: Generalized anoxia/ischemia of the nervous system. *In* Irwin RS, Cerra FB, Rippe JM (eds): Intensive Care Medicine, 4th ed. Philadelphia, Lippincott-Raven, 1999, pp 2086–2089.

PERIOPERATIVE IMPLICATIONS

Preoperative Preparation

• Assess and document neurologic function and mental status
• Review cause of anoxic event
• Assess damage to other organs

Monitoring

• If arrest was due to cardiac arrhythmias or MI/ischemia or if patient is hemodynamically unstable, may need specialized monitoring

Airway

• Assess potential for aspiration: gag reflex, ability to cough and clear secretions

Induction

• Avoid succinylcholine

Maintenance

• Must consider that patients may have pain perception and will require analgesia
• Do what is appropriate to ↓ sequelae (e.g., prevent cerebral edema, ↓ ICP with mild hyperventilation, and slight ↑ in BP)

Extubation

• If unable to maintain patent airway or sustain adequate minute ventilation, patient should remain intubated

Adjuvants

• Avoid long-acting anesthetics so that neurologic status can be assessed soon after surgery
• Avoid drugs that ↓ seizure threshold

ANTICIPATED PROBLEMS/CONCERNS

• Repeat of events (e.g., arrhythmias) that initially led to anoxic encephalopathy
• Worsening of neurologic condition during perioperative period
• Postpone all but emergency surgery if fluctuating neurologic deficits or acute encephalopathic condition exists

ENDOCARDIAL CUSHION DEFECT   Carol L. Lake, M.D., M.B.A., M.P.H.

RISK

- 2% of congenital heart disease is endocardial cushion defect (ECD)
- No gender predilection

PERIOPERATIVE RISKS

- Shunt reversal caused by anesthetic drugs, airway stimulation during light anesthesia, or airway obstruction
- Paradoxical embolism, particularly with shunt reversal
- Subacute bacterial endocarditis if antibiotic prophylaxis not given during "dirty" surgical procedures
- Pulmonary hypertensive crisis in patients with reactive pulmonary vasculature
- AV valve regurgitation, arrhythmias following surgical repair of ECD

WORRY ABOUT

- Development of pulmonary vascular obstructive disease and reversal of shunt
- Development of atrial arrhythmias

OVERVIEW

- ECD causes atrial and/or ventricular septal defects and clefts in anterior mitral and/or septal tricuspid valve leaflets
- Causes shunting at atrial or ventricular (or both) sites with or without associated AV valvular regurgitation
- Dx established by ECHO and cardiac catheterization
- ECD places patient at risk for development of shunt reversal leading to pulmonary vascular obstruction disease and Eisenmenger's syndrome

ICD-9-CM Code: 745.69

ETIOLOGY

- Atrioventricular canal defects result from failure of the endocardial cushions to grow and fuse with portions of the interatrial and interventricular septa in the 5–6-mm embryo

USUAL TREATMENT

- Medical: symptomatic therapy with digitalis and diuretics for heart failure
- Surgical: definitive therapy requires closure of the septal defects and repair of the clefts in the AV valves

ASSESSMENT POINTS

SYSTEM	EFFECT	ASSESSMENT BY HX	PE	TEST
HEENT	Feeding difficulties	Failure to thrive	< Normal wt/ht for age	Comparison of wt/ht to published values
CV	CHF Pulm Htn	Diaphoresis, coughing	Wheezing, rales, hepatosplenomegaly Worsening CHF	Cardiac catherization, ECG with RVH ECHO, cardiac catheterization
RESP	CHF	Dyspnea, tachypnea	Wheezing, rales	CXR
RENAL	Renal dysfunction due to heart failure			BUN, Cr
MS	Decreased exercise compared with peers			

Key Reference: Lake CL (ed): Pediatric Cardiac Anesthesia, 3rd ed. Norwalk, CT, Appleton & Lange, 1998, pp 290–291.

PERIOPERATIVE IMPLICATIONS

Preoperative Preparation

- Prophylactic antibiotics for subacute bacterial endocarditis
- Premedication to minimize anxiety and possible shunt reversal
- Diuretic if prone to CHF

Monitoring

- Intra-arterial catheter and central venous catheter if required by surgical procedure
- TEE if available and appropriate to anesthetic and surgical procedure

Airway

- May be difficult if associated congenital anomalies such as Down syndrome are present

Preinduction/Induction

- Meticulous air removal to avoid paradoxical embolism

- IV or inhalation induction depending on patient preference/cooperation. Choice of intravenous induction agent depends on severity of CHF and pulm Htn.

Maintenance

- Volatile agents that decrease systemic vascular resistance may worsen R → L shunting. Combinations of narcotic with low concentrations of volatile agents may be appropriate in patients with moderate disease.

Extubation

- At end of operation in patients without CHF or pulm Htn. If reactive pulm vasculature, may develop pulm hypertensive crisis requiring hyperventilation, ↑ FIO$_2$, sedation, or even nitric oxide or ECMO, which is more easily accomplished during mechanical ventilation.

Adjuvants

- Nitric oxide, nitroglycerin, prostaglandin to control pulm vascular tone. Inotropes for heart failure.

Postoperative Period

- Observe left and right atrial pressures, as LAP more than 6 mm >RAP suggests mitral valve incompetence/stenosis
- Residual shunting at atrial or ventricular level should be excluded by echocardiography.
- Heart block or other conduction defects may result from surgical repair
- Effective analgesia to minimize pulmonary hypertensive crisis, which may include epidural or spinal analgesia in some centers

ANTICIPATED PROBLEMS/CONCERNS

- Patients with partial or complete AV canal defects 2° to endocardial cushion defects who have CHF are likely to have moderate to severe AV valvular incompetence or pulm Htn following surgical repairs
- Significantly increased pulm blood flow 2° to L → R cardiac shunting increases the risk of developing pulm vascular obstructive disease and postop pulmonary hypertensive crisis

EPIDERMOLYSIS BULLOSA

RISK

- 1/17,000, 50% dystrophic form; equal racial distribution

PERIOPERATIVE RISKS

- Difficult IV access, airway, intraoperative positioning, reflux, steroid dependence, intraoperative hemorrhage, sepsis, iatrogenic corneal abrasion, blister formation, airway obstruction

WORRY ABOUT

- Difficult intubation (23%) 2° to microstomia
- Establishing monitoring, IV access
- Dehydration, malnutrition
- Anemia, hypoalbuminemia, electrolyte imbalance, thrombocytosis
- Septicemia
- Renal and adrenal dysfunction

OVERVIEW

- Characterized by epithelial blistering as a result of minor trauma by lateral shearing forces, not pressure
- 3 types: simplex (SEB), junctional (JEB), dystrophic (DEB)

- Associated conditions: growth retardation, pyloric stenosis, esophageal stricture, pseudosyndactyly, enamel hypoplasia, muscular dystrophy, squamous cell carcinoma, malignant melanoma
- SEB: Blisters are intraepidermal and are on soles and palms only in Weber-Cockayne form, are generalized in Kobner form, are generalized herpetiform in Dowling-Meara form, and are generalized in association with muscular dystrophy in MD form.
- JEB: Blisters are intralamina lucida and are in intertriginous areas in inversa form, are generalized with growth retardation in Herlitz form, are generalized without growth retardation in non-Herlitz form, and are generalized with pyloric atresia
- DEB: Blisters are sublamina densa and are in intertriginous areas in inversa form, are on ankles in pretibial form, are on arms and legs in pruriginous form, are generalized in non–Hallopeau-Siemens form, and are generalized with growth retardation and severe extracutaneous involvement in Hallopeau-Siemens form. Very aggressive squamous cell carcinomas are common.

ICD-9-CM Code: 757.39

ETIOLOGY

- SEB: Inherited autosomal, usually dominant, mutation producing abnormal keratin 5 or 14, abnormal plectin in MD form
- JEB: Inherited autosomal recessive mutation producing abnormal laminin 5, abnormal type XVII collagen, and abnormal $\alpha_6\beta_4$ integrin
- DEB: Inherited autosomal dominant or recessive mutation producing abnormal type VII collagen

USUAL TREATMENT

- No definitive treatment
- Trials using bioengineered skin, such as Apligraf
- Receive steroids and supportive treatment such as nutritional support, wound care, contracture release, esophageal dilation, oral surgery, and treatment of skin cancers

ASSESSMENT POINTS

SYSTEM	EFFECT	ASSESSMENT BY HX	PE	TEST
HEENT	Enamel hypoplasia: blisters, microstomia, ankyloglossia, supraglottic ulceration or narrowing	Delayed eruption, caries of teeth; painful peri- and intraoral lesions; hoarseness, respiratory obstruction; painful swallowing, spasm, food impaction	Poor oral hygiene, malocclusion; tongue atrophy; obliteration of vestibular sulci, stricture, webs, vocal cord lesions	Airway assessment, endoscopy
GI	Bullae Perianal blisters, poor absorption, diarrhea	Anal pain, tenesmus, constipation	Anal fissure or stricture	Endoscopy
GU	Blisters	Urinary diversion	Obstruction, sepsis	Renal function
MS	Contractures, growth retardation	Movement limitations, stature	Flexion contracture, pseudodactyly	
DERM	Blisters	Age at onset, Hx of remissions, infections	Scars, milia, nail dystrophy, cancer	Skin biopsy

Key Reference: Ames WA, Mayou BJ, Williams KN: Anesthetic management of epidermolysis bullosa. Br J Anaesthesia 1999; 82:746–751.

Web site: www.debra.com

PERIOPERATIVE IMPLICATIONS

Preoperative Preparation

- Careful planning of monitoring, IV placement, positioning in the OR, prevention of reflux, and airway management

Monitoring

- No contraindication to pulse oximeter use
- Pad automated BP cuff heavily, limit intervals
- Cut adhesive from ECG leads; hold in place with defibrillator jelly pads
- Suture invasive monitoring and IVs or wrap in place with petrolatum gauze
- Esophageal stethoscope may damage mucosa

Induction

- Regional anesthesia encouraged; use spray antiseptics or pour prep solutions; no intradermal local anesthetics
- No GA or muscle relaxant specifically contraindicated

Airway

- All airway management techniques reported successful
- Mask (or nasal mask) lubricated and padded with petrolatum gauze; pad chin under fingers; bullae occurred in 1 in 50
- LMA one size too small, heavily lubricated, cuff soft with audible leak, extubated deep to prevent trauma; lingual bulla occurred in 1 in 57
- Intubation less frequent; blind nasal, fiberoptic, and oral techniques; heavily lubricated small tube; lubricate laryngoscope heavily; cricoid pressure without lateral movement permissible; 66% class I or II view of larynx, 7–23% difficult airway incidence; soft lubricated gauze to prevent tube movement in mouth, no lateral forces on mouth corners by tube, no tape; trachea lined with columnar epithelium, so less likely to blister

Emergence

- Aim for a quiet emergence
- No suction on intraoral mucosa

ANTICIPATED PROBLEMS/CONCERNS

- Positioning: patient performs if possible; lateral shear forces from lifting cause blisters;
- Corneal abrasion: poor eyelid retraction; use ointment generously, protect eyes in prone position
- Treat hemorrhage with epinephrine or thrombin-soaked sponge
- Avoid sweating; warming devices, if unavoidable, no warmer than skin temperature
- Extremity tourniquets, IM or rectal medications, EMLA can be used
- Common procedures: release of syndactyly, dressing change, squamous cell carcinoma, esophageal dilatation, dental surgery

EPIGLOTTITIS

Maurice S. Zwass, M.D.

RISK

• Children 1–7 y, although epiglottitis (sometimes called supraglottitis) does occur in adults. (Decreasing incidence in children >3 y, related to vaccine against *Haemophilus influenzae* type B, but still found, particularly if not immunized.)

PERIOPERATIVE RISKS

• Acute deterioration of airway patency resulting in complete obstruction
• Difficulty in tracheal intubation due to severe edema of epiglottis and arytenoids

WORRY ABOUT

• Airway compromise in children who appear "toxic," with increasing distress, drooling, hypoxemia. The acute risks of airway compromise (of concern in small children) appear to be less critical in adults, most likely because of larger airway.
• Loss of airway control and aspiration

OVERVIEW

• An acute, potentially life-threatening cause of upper airway obstruction (etiologic agents may include bacteria other than *H. influenzae* type B)
• Produces inflammatory edema of epiglottis and other supraglottic structures
• Onset usually rapid; progression to severe obstruction can occur in several hours
• High fever, sore throat, and dysphagia frequently so severe that swallowing is inhibited and drooling results
• Differential diagnosis also includes retropharyngeal abscess (a bacterial infection), which can have same presentation. It can be differentiated from epiglottitis by presence of torticollis and trismus and with radiographic studies (contrast CT). Treatment is with antibiotics and surgical drainage.

ICD-9-CM Codes: 464.30; 464.31 (With obstruction); 478.24 (Retropharyngeal abscess)

ETIOLOGY

• *H. influenzae* type B is most often associated pathogen, though can be caused by β-hemolytic streptococci

USUAL TREATMENT

• Antibiotic therapy against bacterium (usually *H. influenzae*) and airway support, which generally requires tracheal intubation
• Because of high incidence of ampicillin-resistant strains, ampicillin plus a β-lactamase inhibitor (such as sulbactam) and/or chloramphenicol, cefuroxime, ceftazidime, or another penicillinase-resistant antibiotic as indicated by blood and epiglottis culture results
• Tracheal intubation classically performed in OR in a controlled fashion with surgical support for possible tracheotomy or cricothyrotomy present and gowned

ASSESSMENT POINTS

Differentiation between epiglottitis and croup (laryngotracheobronchitis):

	CROUP	EPIGLOTTITIS
AGE	3 mo–3 y	1–7 y
ONSET	Gradual	More rapid (usually <24 h)
FEVER	Low-grade	High-grade
COUGH	Characteristic barking	None
SORE THROAT	Occasional	Frequently severe
POSTURE	Any	Frequently sitting forward, mouth open, drooling
AIRWAY SOUND	Inspiratory stridor	Inspiratory stridor
VOICE	Normal	Muffled
APPERANCE	Nontoxic	Toxic
SEASONALITY	Peak winter, epidemic	Year-round

Radiographic studies may be helpful, because AP view of trachea appears normal but lateral neck view usually shows a markedly swollen, edematous epiglottis ("thumbprinting").

Key References: Benjamin B: Anesthesia for pediatric airway endoscopy. Otolaryngol Clin North Am 2000; 33:29–47; DeSoto H: Epiglottitis and croup in airway obstruction in children. Anesthesiol Clin North Am 1998; 16:853–868; Lee SS, Schwartz RH, Bahadori RS: Retropharyngeal abscess: epiglottitis of the new millennium. J Pediatr 2001; 138:435–437.

PERIOPERATIVE IMPLICATIONS

Preoperative Preparation

• With suspected epiglottitis, other personnel on patient care team can set up care (e.g., OR or ICU). Radiographs can be obtained, *but a team member capable of monitoring and securing the airway should be present.*
• Allow to remain in a position of comfort (often sitting with parent). Direct exam of oropharynx generally avoided, as are attempts to secure vascular access, because these may cause agitation leading to acute tracheal obstruction.
• Humidified oxygen should be delivered as tolerated.
• Aerosol therapy with racemic epinephrine may provide slight improvement of Sx, but not definitive. If Dx is confirmed, patient is taken to the location for intubation (most commonly OR).

Airway Management

• Anesthesia with sevoflurane or halothane and O₂, maintaining spontaneous ventilation
• IV catheter placed after induction of anesthesia, followed by direct laryngoscopy
• Large, swollen epiglottis can make identification of airway structures difficult, but once the epiglottis is identified, arytenoids and larynx are immediately below and tracheal tube can be inserted
• Because of upper airway swelling, a tracheal tube 0.5–1.0 mm smaller in diameter may be needed (tracheal tube of adequate length can be made available)
• Rarely is emergency tracheotomy necessary, but surgeons are "gloved" until airway secured
• Frequently orotracheal tube is changed to a nasotracheal tube for ease of securing and patient comfort

Post Airway Management Plans

• Once airway secured, cultures of blood and epiglottis are obtained, antibiotic therapy is initiated, and sedation plans are instituted

ANTICIPATED PROBLEMS/CONCERNS

• Resp support often for 24–72 h until swollen epiglottis returns to normal
• Usually require sedative management to facilitate tolerating mechanical ventilation
• Many patients (~25%) have associated pneumonia that requires treatment

FAMILIAL DYSAUTONOMIA
(RILEY-DAY SYNDROME)

Thomas J. Ebert, M.D., Ph.D.
William Hope, M.D., Ph.D.

RISK

• 1:10,000–20,000 in Jews originating from Eastern Europe (Ashkenazi)

PERIOPERATIVE RISKS

• Hemodynamic instability 2° to an erratic autonomic nervous system
• Pulmonary insufficiency 2° to a relative insensitivity to hypoxemia and hypercarbia

WORRY ABOUT

• Precipitation of a dysautonomic crisis characterized by intractable vomiting, Htn, tachycardia, and diaphoresis

OVERVIEW

• Rare, inherited disease of nervous system involving mainly peripheral sensory and sympathetic nerves
• Primarily a disease of children because mortality is high, particularly in early years; usually due to repeated aspiration pneumonias

ICD-9-CM Code: 742.8

ETIOLOGY

• Inheritance is autosomal recessive
• Symptoms due to diffuse sensory defect and an autonomic insufficiency with superimposed supersensitivity to acetylcholine and catecholamines

USUAL TREATMENT

• Symptoms are managed by conventional therapies

ASSESSMENT POINTS

SYSTEM	EFFECT	ASSESSMENT BY HX	PE	TEST
CV	Orthostatic hypotension	Dizziness, syncope	Supine and standing BP, HR	Autonomic function
RESP	Pneumonia Bronchiectasis	Pleuritic chest pain Secretions	Minimal	CXR
GI	Poor swallowing Aspiration pneumonia	Drooling Vomiting, Hx of "attacks"		Swallow study
GU	Dehydration	Emesis	Dry mucosa	Serum BUN, Cr
CNS	Seizure	Seizure		EEG

Key Reference: Axelrod FB, Donenfeld RF, Danziger F, Turndorf H: Anesthesia in familial dysautonomia. Anesthesiology 1988; 68:631–635.

PERIOPERATIVE IMPLICATIONS

Preoperative Preparation

• Difficulty swallowing: abundant secretions plus diminished laryngeal reflexes. Treat with antisialagogues.
• Avoid medications interacting with autonomic nervous system
• Vomiting crises: intractable vomiting associated with tachycardia, Htn, apprehension can be prevented by preop sedation with benzodiazepines
• H₂ blockers can decrease gastric volume and acidity
• Phenothiazines are associated with erratic hemodynamics at induction
• Treat chronic dehydration 2° to dysphagia and emesis
• Insensitivity to hypoxia, hypercarbia: minimize narcotics as premedication
• Insensitivity to superficial pain: lines placed without discomfort

Monitoring

• Routine
• Consider arterial line

Induction

• Consider rapid-sequence induction with etomidate because of poor airway reflexes and BP instability
• Use of nondepolarizing agents must be balanced against the risk of postop hypotonia and unpredictable effect of reversal agents on autonomic nervous system
• Lubricate eyes to avoid corneal abrasions

Maintenance

• Dysfunctional regulation can require exogenous treatment
• Aggressively treat blood loss, as hemodynamic instability exacerbated by ↓ intravascular volume
• Very sensitive to effects of exogenous catecholamines. If vasopressors required, use direct-acting agents.
• Consider controlled ventilation

Postoperative Care

• Although peripheral pain sensation is diminished, visceral pain sensation is usually intact and presents as anxiety, Htn, or tachycardia or can precipitate dysautonomic crisis. Treat pain with careful titration of narcotics and/or consider NSAIDs.

ANTICIPATED PROBLEMS/CONCERNS

• Respiratory function often compromised by aspiration, hypotonic musculature, and scoliosis, and abnormal response to hypoxemia and hypercarbia; some authors advocate endotracheal intubation until pain Rx no longer needed

140 DISEASES

FAMILIAL PERIODIC PARALYSIS (HYPERKALEMIC)

W. John Russell, M.B., F.R.C.A., F.A.N.Z.C.A., Ph.D.

RISK

- Rare, probably about 1/400,000
- Race appears to be exclusively Caucasian

PERIOPERATIVE RISKS

- No reported increase in mortality with any procedure, but severe myotonia could create respiratory difficulty
- Succinylcholine may not give relaxation, and therefore an unexpected difficult intubation may result
- Succinylcholine may also cause hyperkalemia and cardiac arrhythmia

WORRY ABOUT

- Cold can trigger an attack
- Hypoglycemia can trigger an attack; minimize fasting

OVERVIEW

- Intrinsic defect in muscle membrane allows depolarization of the muscle, but Na^+ channel does not close. Membrane thus remains inexcitable and a variable K^+ efflux continues.
- Patient may experience profound global stiffness and weakness after succinylcholine, exposure to cold, or spontaneously
- Dx by family Hx

ICD-9-CM Code: 359.3

ETIOLOGY

- Na^+ channel in skeletal muscle membrane has a defective α subunit
- Defect associated with chromosome 17 is substitution of a single base pair, usually methionine replacing threonine in fifth transmembrane segment of second domain
- An autosomal dominant condition; allows a persistent Na^+ influx with activation threshold ~ 10 mV more negative than normal
- Persistence of a Na^+ influx is associated with K^+ leak from cell
- Episodes of weakness associated with elevated serum K^+ levels

USUAL TREATMENT

- Avoid succinylcholine
- Avoid cooling during anesthesia
- Avoid hypoglycemia
- Do not give K^+-containing solutions
- Preop treatment with furosemide has been used
- Severe postop weakness may be alleviated with Ca^{2+}

ASSESSMENT POINTS

SYSTEM	EFFECT	ASSESSMENT BY HX	PE	TEST
MS	Weakness	Exercise, fatigue	Limb tone	Electromyography (discharges) K^+ load

Key Reference: Ashwood EM, Russell WJ, Burrows DD: Hyperkalaemic periodic paralysis and anesthesia. Anaesthesia 1992; 47:579–584.

PERIOPERATIVE IMPLICATIONS

Preoperative Preparation

- 24-h furosemide for K^+ depletion

Monitoring

- Temperature (esophageal) (keep warm)
- ECG (detection of hyperkalemia)
- Neuromuscular (minimize relaxant dose)

Airway

- No special difficulty, but may need support

Preinduction/Induction

- Avoid ketamine and succinylcholine
- Relaxation with nondepolarizing agents as indicated

Maintenance

- Keep warm
- Warm all IV fluid, use glucose 5% as maintenance

Extubation

- Normal reversal as indicated clinically
- Evidence of muscle weakness should be treated with IV calcium gluconate or chloride 10% 10 ml slowly over 5 min

Adjuvants

- Some experimental evidence suggests that condition, e.g., postoperative weakness, may be helped by phenytoin or by salbutamol
- Anticipate normal analgesic requirements for age and surgery
- Regional techniques are appropriate

ANTICIPATED PROBLEMS/CONCERNS

- Severe myotonia may create respiratory difficulty
- Succinylcholine may not give relaxation, and therefore intubation may be difficult
- Cold or hypoglycemia can trigger hyperkalemic attack
- Hyperkalemia can cause cardiac arrhythmia

FAMILIAL PERIODIC PARALYSIS (HYPOKALEMIC)

W. John Russell, M.B., F.R.C.A., F.A.N.Z.C.A., Ph.D.

RISK

- Rare, probably ~1000 people affected in USA
- Appears to occur in most races
- Presents usually in childhood or adolescence

PERIOPERATIVE RISKS

- Associated with supraventricular or conduction defect–type cardiac arrhythmias
- Treatment with lidocaine is contraindicated
- Weakness may be enhanced or precipitated by β-adrenergic blocking drugs
- Respiratory muscle weakness may occur postoperatively

WORRY ABOUT

- Attacks after glucose intake or insulin administration
- Cold triggers attacks
- Serum K^+ levels should be maintained above 4.0 mEq/L
- Cardiac dysrhythmias, especially bradycardias, during an attack

OVERVIEW

- Any severe hypokalemia may induce paralysis in susceptible persons even if they do not have familial disease. Limb weakness and paralysis have been reported after thyrotoxicosis, starvation, autoimmune and renal disease.
- Familial hypokalemic periodic paralysis is an autosomal dominant condition
- Usually the patient will be aware of the onset of weakness
- Prompt treatment with K^+ will usually abort an attack, although as much as 40 mEq of K^+ may be required hourly
- Attacks are most likely with anything that increases muscle activity; can be precipitated by exercise and also cold, presumably because of the increased muscle activity in shivering
- The symptoms in many patients can be controlled by regular K^+ supplements and acetazolamide

ICD-9-CM Code: 359.3

ETIOLOGY

- Intrinsic defect in muscle membrane appears to be associated with gene localized to 1q31–1q32 region near dihydropyridine receptor gene
- Unrelated to familial hyperkalemic disease
- Gene defect impairs voltage-sensitive Ca^{2+} channel, which may cause compensatory increase in the $Na^+/K^+/Cl^-$ cotransport and a reduced overall efflux in K^+

USUAL TREATMENT

- Avoid succinylcholine, cooling during anesthesia, hyperglycemia
- Give K^+-containing solutions
- Acetazolamide should be considered, if not already being given
- Severe postop weakness may be aggravated by Ca^{2+}
- Ventilation during anesthesia should be normocarbic to avoid K^+ shifts
- Maintenance by IPPV if evidence of weakness in postop phase

ASSESSMENT POINTS

SYSTEM	EFFECT	ASSESSMENT BY HX	PE	TEST
RESP	Inadequate	Noticeable SOB	Resp rate high	ABGs
MS	Weakness	Exercise, fatigue	Limb tone	Serum K^+ elevation < normal (normal = 0.8 ± 0.2 mEq/L) Glucose/insulin or ACTH infusion induces paralysis attack Plasma biochemistry after attack: elevated myoglobin, creatine kinase Muscle fiber conduction velocity may be slower than normal

Key Reference: Lema G, Urzua J, Moran S, Canessa R: Successful anesthetic management of a patient with hypokalemic familial periodic paralysis undergoing cardiac surgery. Anesthesiology 1991; 74:373–375.

PERIOPERATIVE IMPLICATIONS

Preoperative Preparation

- 24-h acetazolamide if not already given. Only glucose-free solutions IV. If Hx of frequent instability, prepare infusion with K^+.

Monitoring

- Temperature (esophageal) (keep warm)
- ECG (detection of hypokalemia may not be seen until late)
- Neuromuscular (minimize relaxant dose)

Airway

- No special difficulty, but may need support

Preinduction/Induction

- Regional techniques are appropriate

Induction

- Successful relaxation with succinylcholine and with atracurium has been reported

Maintenance

- Use warming blanket
- Warm all IV fluid, use glucose-free solutions as maintenance

Extubation

- Normal reversal as indicated clinically
- Evidence of muscle weakness should be treated with IV potassium chloride up to 40 mEq/h

Adjuvants

- Calcium-channel blockers do not appear to be contraindicated in patients with concomitant CV disease
- Anticipate usual analgesic requirements for age and surgery

ANTICIPATED PROBLEMS/CONCERNS

- May have associated supraventricular or conduction defect arrhythmias
- Respiratory muscle weakness may occur postoperatively
- Cold triggers attack
- Must maintain serum K^+ above 4.0 mEq/L

FAT EMBOLISM

Brian J. McGrath, M.D.

RISK

- Long bone fractures, pelvic fractures, multiple fractures
  - 80–100% fat embolism
  - 0.5–10% fat embolism syndrome (FES)
- Total hip, total knee replacement, intramedullary nailing:
  - 27–100% fat embolism
  - ?Incidence FES
- Unusual causes: liposuction, fat injection, bone marrow transplantation, cardiopulmonary bypass, CPR, burns, pancreatitis, hemoglobinopathies

PERIOPERATIVE RISKS

- FES: 5–20% mortality
- Pre-existing FES: respiratory failure/ARDS; RV dysfunction; coagulopathy; neurologic dysfunction
- Intraoperative fat embolism: shock; hypoxemia (severe)

WORRY ABOUT

- Pre-existing FES: hypoxemia; poor pulmonary compliance; pulmonary Htn; RV failure; abnormal CNS response to anesthetics; coagulopathy
- Intraoperative embolism: myocardial failure (right heart), hypoxemia (severe)

OVERVIEW

- Fat particles (globules of marrow fat) traveling into blood and lung
- Must distinguish fat embolism, which is common, from fat embolism syndrome, a much less common consequence of fat embolism
- FES can produce mild pulmonary dysfunction to severe ARDS
- Pulmonary Htn and acute right ventricular failure may occur in severe cases of FES
- Typically, there is delay in onset of signs and symptoms of up to 72 h following injury
- Occurs commonly during femoral reaming and cementing in hip arthroplasty

ICD-9-CM Codes: 958.1; 673.8 (Obstetric)

ETIOLOGY

- Usually occurs following orthopedic trauma with release of marrow fat into venous circulation
- Pathology produced by intravascular fat passing into the pulmonary and systemic arterial circulations and by production of endogenous inflammatory mediators

USUAL TREATMENT

- Early fracture fixation to ↓ embolization
- Use of noncemented prosthesis or venting of femoral shaft may reduce risk during hip arthroplasty
- O_2 therapy to maintain $SaO_2 > 90\%$
- Positive pressure ventilation with PEEP for ARDS
- Aggressive hemodynamic support with fluid and/or inotropes with shock
- Factor replacement for coagulopathy with bleeding
- Corticosteroids, heparin, ethanol, dextran: unproven benefit

ASSESSMENT POINTS

SYSTEM	EFFECT	ASSESSMENT BY HX	PE	TEST
CV	Intravascular fat	Fever		?Fat staining of blood
				?Bronchoalveolar lavage, macrophage staining
	Hypoperfusion	Syncope	Hypotension	PA catheter
	Pulm Htn	Obtundation	Tachycardia	
	RV failure		Oliguria	
			Vasoconstriction	
RESP	ARDS	Dyspnea	Tachypnea	CXR, ABGs, compliance measurement
	Hypoxemia		Cyanosis, rales	
HEME	Thrombocytopenia	Bleeding	Bleeding (rare)	CBC
	DIC			Platelets
	Anemia			PT, PTT
				D-Dimer
				Fibrinogen
DERM	Capillary fat embolism		Petechiae (60%)	
			• Axilla, chest	
			• Base of neck	
			• Conjunctiva	
			• Uvula	
CNS	Neurologic injury	Agitation	Delirium	
	Cerebral edema		Confusion	
			Focal deficits (rare)	
			Seizure (rare)	
			Coma (rare)	

Key Reference: Bulger EM, Smith DG, Maier RV, Jurkovich GJ: Fat embolism syndrome, a 10 year review. Arch Surg 1997; 132:435–439.

PERIOPERATIVE IMPLICATIONS

Preoperative Preparation

- Avoid sedatives/narcotics if patient is hypoxemic and not mechanically ventilated

Monitoring

- Arterial catheter; PA catheter may be helpful in severe cases

Airway

- May already be intubated and ventilated in severe cases
- Decreased FRC and oxygen "reserve" with ARDS

Induction

- Minimize myocardial depression

Maintenance

- CV: anticipate ↓ BP with femoral reaming/cementing: anesthetic reduction, fluid, vasopressors; patients with RV dysfunction may require longer-term inotropic support
- Resp: patients with ARDS may require increased FIO_2 and PEEP; avoid excessive airway pressures and tidal volumes
- Watch for embolism during femoral reaming, prosthesis cementing

Extubation

- Maintain intubation and mechanical ventilation in hemodynamically unstable patients and those requiring high FIO_2, high PEEP, or high minute ventilation
- Patients with CNS involvement may have a prolonged or exaggerated response to anesthetics and narcotics

ANTICIPATED PROBLEMS/CONCERNS

- Embolism during femoral reaming, prosthesis cementing
- Patients with ARDS may be difficult to ventilate and oxygenate

FOREIGN BODY ASPIRATION
Frederic Berry, M.D.

RISK

• Foreign body aspiration into the airway or esophagus is one of the most frequent and frightening pediatric surgical emergencies

PERIOPERATIVE RISKS

• Risk of aspiration is present but is very small. The danger period for vomiting or regurgitation with aspiration is primarily during the induction and recovery from anesthesia.

• Unless foreign body is immediate threat to survival, further consultation should be sought and, if necessary, the patient should be transfered to a specialized facility

OVERVIEW

• Acute presentation, with parent or caretaker observing the child swallowing or aspirating a foreign body and immediately developing respiratory distress or dysphagia; or chronic presentation after 1–2 wk of unexplained coughing, wheezing, or dysphagia; often with secondary infection behind the foreign body

ICD-9-CM Code: 934.0 (Trachea through orifice)

USUAL TREATMENT

• Bronchoscopy

ASSESSMENT POINTS

SYSTEM	EFFECT	PE	TEST
RESP	Main stem bronchus may have ball-valve effect	Involved lung cannot fully expire	Chest exam
	Pneumonia	Reactive airway with decreased breath sounds	CXR

Key Reference: Woods AM: Pediatric endoscopy. *In* Berry FA (ed): Anesthetic Management of Difficult and Routine Pediatric Patients, 2nd ed. New York, Churchill Livingstone, 1990, pp 199–242.

PERIOPERATIVE MANAGEMENT

• Divided into three time periods: preoperative, intraoperative, and postoperative

Perioperative Concerns

• NPO period: the stomach will not empty, so proceed expeditiously

• An IV should be started if possible and an anticholinergic agent administered. If the child has pneumonia, addition of antibiotics is indicated.

Induction

• Done in OR without presence of parents

• A technique of spontaneous ventilation usually with sevoflurane

• If IV present, small doses (1 mg/kg) of IV Pentothal or propofol to gently sedate and make inhalation induction smoother

Intraoperative Management

• If child is struggling to breathe or cyanotic, induction is with sevoflurane and O_2

• If only mild airway distress, nitrous oxide used for initial inhalation induction to facilitate administration of sevoflurane. Sevoflurane is the ideal induction agent, but there is controversy over whether to continue with sevoflurane or to use the more soluble anesthetic isoflurane. In addition, a propofol infusion may be added to stabilize the maintenance anesthetic. After initial inhalation induction, nitrous oxide is discontinued, sevoflurane increased, and ventilation gently assisted.

• Small amounts of PEEP (3–5 cm H_2O) useful for any degree of obstruction

• Topical anesthesia of larynx and cords with 4% solution of lidocaine, 5 mg/kg (4% lidocaine contains 40 mg lidocaine/ml) prior to laryngoscopy, so no response to introduction of ventilating bronchoscope

Monitoring

• End-tidal CO_2 (also the wave form) may be elevated into the 80s or 90s. As long as oxygen saturation remains in 85–95 range, the CO_2 is usually not a problem.

• Ventilating bronchoscope with a sidearm attachment for anesthesia circuit. Bronchoscope advanced through larynx into trachea and often into main stem bronchus. Desaturation may result from inadequate ventilation of contralateral lung. If this occurs consider administering PEEP until saturation can be returned to reasonable range.

• With pneumonia, saturations may not be able to be raised higher than the low 90s. Saturation of 85–90 is acceptable as long as it is stable. If rapidly falling oxygen saturation, bronchoscope must be withdrawn into trachea and ventilation assisted with PEEP.

• The surgeon grasps foreign body and starts to extract it from airway. If child starts to move or cough, management includes (1) releasing foreign body and re-anesthetizing; or (2) administering either muscle relaxant such as succinylcholine 1 mg/kg or propofol, lidocaine, or Pentothal (1–2 mg/kg) to deepen anesthesia.

Postoperative Management

• After trachea and bronchus rechecked with ventilating bronchoscope, trachea is intubated and awake extubation performed. If patient coughing but not sufficiently awake, lidocaine 1.5 mg/kg can be administered IV.

ANTICIPATED PROBLEMS/CONCERNS

• If PVCs develop because of elevated CO_2, can administer lidocaine 1.5 mg/kg, which can be repeated 2 times in 5 minutes, or switch anesthetic to isoflurane

FRIEDREICH'S ATAXIA

Mark Helfaer, M.D.

RISK

- Prevalence 2/100,000; 80–90% have cardiac involvement

WORRY ABOUT

- Cardiac involvement does not correlate with neurologic involvement

OVERVIEW

- Progressive degeneration of posterior columns and corticospinal and posterior spinocerebellar tracts
- Usual onset in childhood
- Proprioceptive sensory loss, areflexia, ataxia of limbs, Babinski's sign
- Pes cavus and scoliosis
- Cardiomyopathy

ICD-9-CM Code: 334.0

ETIOLOGY

- Inherited—usually autosomal recessive, but occasionally dominant
- Nucleotide has been mapped
- Fratoxin (mitochondrial iron content protein) deficiency

USUAL TREATMENT

- Usually untreatable and progressive
- Can be mistaken for metabolic disorders (hexosaminidase A deficiency, adrenomyeloneuropathy, vitamin E deficiency)

ASSESSMENT POINTS

SYSTEM	EFFECT	ASSESSMENT BY HX	TEST
CV	LV hypokinesia Concentric and asymmetric hypertrophy Cardiomyopathy	Severities of heart and neurologic manifestations are not proportional	ECG ECHO Endomyocardial biopsy
RESP	Severe scoliosis Neuromuscular impairment	Noncardiac dyspnea	Lung functions
MS	Pes cavus Scoliosis		

Key Reference: Mouloudi H, Katsanoulas C, Frantzeskos G: Requirements for muscle relaxation in Friedreich's ataxia. Anaesthesia 1998; 53:177–180.

PERIOPERATIVE IMPLICATIONS

Preoperative Preparation

- Usual premedication

Monitoring

- Train of four to monitor effects of neuromuscular blocking agent with unpredictable response due to NM disease

Airway

- None

Preinduction/Induction

- Case report of sensitivity to curare (0.06 mg/kg caused 90 min apnea)
- Possibility of hyperkalemia and cardiac arrhythmias after succinylcholine

Maintenance

- Case reports of successful spinal and epidural anesthesia
- Case reports of successful GA with cautious use of nondepolarizing agents
- Case report of successful use of hypotensive anesthesia with isoflurane
- Case report of marked decrease in cardiac output and supraventricular tachycardia with nitroprusside for hypotensive anesthesia
- Case report of successful use of epidural narcotic

Extubation

- If adequate strength from neuromuscular blocker and adequate pulmonary function, extubation is appropriate

Adjuvants

- See under Maintenance

Postoperative Period

- ECG monitoring for dysrhythmias

GASTRINOMA

RISK

- Annual incidence: 2–4/million
- More common in men than women: 3:2
- Predominantly diagnosed in patients 40–60 y
- 60% of gastrinomas are malignant

PERIOPERATIVE RISKS

- Risks associated with peptic ulcer disease
- Associated tumors (MEN type I)
- Risks associated with metastatic lesions (liver, bone, lungs)

WORRY ABOUT

- Likelihood of large gastric fluid volume
- Esophageal reflux (common)
- Electrolyte imbalance 2° to watery diarrhea
- Malnutrition 2° to chronic diarrhea and peptic ulcer disease
- 20–25% with other functioning endocrine adenomas (parathyroid, pituitary, thyroid, adrenal cortex)

OVERVIEW

- Gastroenteropancreatic neuroendocrine tumor arising from gastrin-secreting cells, occurring in pancreatic and extrapancreatic sites
- Secrete gastrin autonomously, leading to severe ulcer diathesis, abdominal pain, and diarrhea
- May occur sporadically or as part of the MEN I syndrome (benign or malignant cellular proliferation of at least two endocrine glands, mainly pancreatic islets, and parathyroid, pituitary, and adrenal glands)
- Constitutes part of the Zollinger-Ellison syndrome: gastric acid hypersecretion, intractable ulcer diathesis, and non–beta islet cell tumor of the pancreas

ICD-9-CM Code: 235.2

See also Multiple Endocrine Neoplasia (MEN) Types I and II in Diseases section

ETIOLOGY

- Often familial—may be inherited as autosomal dominant trait with a high but variable degree of penetrance

USUAL TREATMENT

- Correct gastric acid hypersecretion with H_2 blockers and proton pump inhibitors (omeprazole)
- Surgical exploration and resection

ASSESSMENT POINTS

SYSTEM	EFFECT	ASSESSMENT BY HX	PE	TEST
CV	Hypovolemia	Weakness, dizziness	Orthostatic BP	ECG
RESP[1]	Hypoxia	Dyspnea, decreased exercise tolerance	Breath sounds	CXR
GI	Gastric hyperacidity	Abdominal pain, esophageal reflux, diarrhea	Abdominal exam	Secretin stimulation test
ENDO[2]	Hyperparathyroidism	Multiple systems involved		Serum parathyroid hormone
RENAL[2]	Nephrolithiasis	Flank pain, hematuria	Costovertebral angle tenderness	Urinalysis
CNS[2]	Pituitary adenoma	Headaches, visual changes	Visual fields	MRI of sella turcica; prolactin levels
PNS[2]	Hypercalcemia	Somnolence, psychosis	Hyperreflexia	Ca^{2+} levels
MS[2]	Weakness, arthralgias	Proximal muscle weakness	Motor strength	Serum, urinary Ca^{2+}

[1] In the presence of pulmonary metastases.
[2] If gastrinoma presents as component of MEN I.

Key Reference: Dougherty TB, Cronau LH Jr: Anesthetic implications for surgical patients with endocrine tumors. Int Anesthesiol Clin 1998; 36:31–44.

PERIOPERATIVE IMPLICATIONS

Preoperative Preparation

- Assess electrolyte and volume status
- Control of gastric hypersecretion
- Consider other endocrinopathies of MEN syndrome

Monitoring

- Intravascular volume status. Can have significant volume shifts due to gastroduodenal pancreatic manipulations and resections. May need arterial line and central venous pressure monitoring. Measure urinary output with bladder catheter.

Airway

- Increased risk for aspiration and pneumonitis

Induction

- Rapid-sequence induction with cricoid pressure (awake intubation if extremely difficult airway by Hx or physical exam)
- May be hypovolemic from chronic diarrhea, abdominal pain

Extubation

- Careful assessment of pulm function and airway reflexes prior to extubation

Adjuvants

- Epidural catheter for postop pain control

Postoperative Period

- Possibility of continued acid hypersecretion
- Worry about pulmonary complications, e.g., decreased vital capacity and FRC—exacerbated by pain, ileus

ANTICIPATED PROBLEMS/CONCERNS

- 60% of gastrinomas are malignant and may metastasize to lymph nodes, liver, or lung, resulting in ↓ survival rate
- Lower cure rates after resection for patients with multiple gastrinomas

GASTROESOPHAGEAL REFLUX IN CHILDREN

Francine S. Yudkowitz, M.D.,F.A.A.P.

RISK

- Symptoms of gastroesophageal reflux (GER) persist past 6 wk of age in 1/500 infants
- 60% resolve by age 18 mo; 30% persist beyond age 4 y
- 5% develop esophageal stricture
- 5% die of complications of GER
- 10% of pyloric stenosis patients
- After esophageal atresia repair or gastrostomy
- Neurologically impaired or developmentally delayed children with spastic quadriplegia, hypoxic brain damage, or trisomy syndromes

PERIOPERATIVE RISKS

- Aspiration during induction of anesthesia
- Severe bronchospasm in patients with reactive airway disease (RAD)
- ↓ Pulmonary reserve 2° to chronic aspiration and pneumonitis

WORRY ABOUT

- Pulmonary complications from aspiration pneumonitis and RAD
- Anemia and malnutrition
- Steroid coverage for patients with RAD who are steroid dependent

OVERVIEW

- Patients may be relatively asymptomatic
- Presence of a hiatus hernia does not necessarily mean patient will have GER
- GER may result in regurgitation and vomiting
- Older children may complain of heartburn and chest pain
- Persistent regurgitation may result in failure to thrive
- Degree of reflux, duration of acid exposure in the esophagus, and ability of the esophagus to clear the reflux material determine extent of mucosal damage and degree of esophagitis
- Esophagitis may lead to bleeding, which may result in hematemesis, iron-deficiency anemia, and esophageal stricture
- GER may be a cause of neonatal apnea
- Diagnostic procedures include esophagography, esophagoscopy, and esophageal pH probe

ICD-9-CM Code: 530.81

ETIOLOGY

- Immature maturation of the lower esophageal sphincter
- Dyscoordination of swallowing mechanism in neurologically impaired patients

USUAL TREATMENT

- Medical:
  - Thickening of feeds
  - Maintaining the upright position after feeds
  - Antacids and/or H_2 blockers to ↓ gastric acidity
  - Metoclopramide to ↑ lower esophageal sphincter tone
  - Proton pump inhibitor, in older children
- Surgical:
  - Indicated when medical therapy fails or in the presence of life-threatening disease
  - Open or laparoscopic Nissen fundoplication. Success rate 95% in neurologically intact patients. Patients who are neurologically impaired have a greater morbidity and mortality with surgical repair.

ASSESSMENT POINTS

SYSTEM	EFFECT	ASSESSMENT BY HX	PE	TEST
RESP	Chronic aspiration	Cough, cyanotic episodes, apnea	Rales, rhonchi	CXR, ABGs (if indicated)
	RAD	Dyspnea, wheezing, cough	Wheezing ↓ BS, prolonged expiration	CXR, peak flow ABGs (if indicated)
HEME	Iron deficiency		Pallor	CBC
GENERAL	Malnutrition	Weight loss	↓ SQ tissue	Serum albumin

Key Reference: Holl JW: Anesthesia for abdominal surgery. *In* Gregory GA (ed): Pediatric Anesthesia, 3rd ed. New York, Churchill Livingstone, 1994.

PERIOPERATIVE IMPLICATIONS

Preoperative Preparation

- Assess the severity of pulmonary compromise
- Optimize respiratory status: treat pneumonia and control bronchospasm
- Correct anemia
- Improve nutritional status
- Confirm availability of blood
- Premedicate with a nonparticulate antacid and H_2 blocker

Monitoring

- Consider arterial line

Induction

- At risk for aspiration. Rapid-sequence induction with cricoid pressure.
- For patients with RAD, ensure adequate depth of anesthesia prior to instrumenting the airway

Maintenance

- No one anesthetic preferred
- Avoid N_2O in laparoscopic procedure
- Esophageal bougie may be required

- Watch for possible pneumothorax, trauma to viscera, hemorrhage, and vena cava compression or laceration. Air embolism may occur during laparoscopic procedures.
- During laparoscopic procedures, intra-abdominal pressures of ≤12 mmHg should be maintained

Extubation/Postoperative Period

- May be extubated after uncomplicated surgery
- Patients with severe respiratory compromise preoperatively or with neurologic impairment may require a period of postop ventilation
- Analgesic requirements will be less after laparoscopic procedures

SURGICAL PROCEDURE

- Fundus of the stomach is wrapped around the lower part of the esophagus. May be accomplished either open or laparoscopically.
- Pyloroplasty may be performed for associated delayed gastric emptying
- Pneumoperitoneum created during laparoscopic surgery will result in ↑ SVR, ↑ CVP, ↑ CO, and ↑ BP. Intra-abdominal pressures > 20 mmHg will ↓ venous return and ↓ CO, but the BP will remain unchanged due to ↑ SVR.

- Pneumoperitoneum will also elevate the diaphragm, which will ↓ lung volumes, ↓ FRC, ↓ compliance, ↑ airway resistance, and ↑ V/Q mismatch
- Pneumoperitoneum should not exceed 12 mmHg. Patients are placed in the reverse Trendelenburg position. This will help ameliorate both diaphragmatic elevation and the CVP elevation.
- Pneumoperitoneum is accomplished by the insufflation of CO_2, which may necessitate ↑ minute ventilation
- Laparoscopic procedures are associated with reduced rates of postop respiratory and wound complications and analgesic requirements, and shorter hospital stays

ANTICIPATED PROBLEMS/CONCERNS

- Respiratory compromise
- Unable to vomit postop and up to 3 mo after surgery. Therefore, intestinal obstruction in the postop period should be treated as a dire emergency.

GLAUCOMA, CLOSED-ANGLE

John V. Donlon, Jr., M.D.

- One tenth as common as open-angle glaucoma
- 200,000/prevalence in USA for angle-closure glaucoma (ACG)
- More common in white Northern Europeans
- No clear hereditary pattern

PERIOPERATIVE RISKS

- Acute ACG attack, optic nerve damage, visual loss

WORRY ABOUT

- Mydriasis precipitating acute attack of ACG
- Intraocular pressure (IOP) >30 mmHg
- Prolonged, stationary mid-dilation of the pupil at 3–6 mm

OVERVIEW

- Development of primary ACG a multifactorial phenomenon
- Usually associated with small eyes with flat anterior chambers but normal trabecular meshwork
- Attacks can be sudden and severe, with IOP reaching 60–70 mmHg within 1 h

ICD-9-CM Code: 365.20

ETIOLOGY

- Angle closure occurs when peripheral iris comes to rest against trabecular meshwork and covers it, preventing outflow of aqueous humor
- Relative pupillary block a common factor in most ACG episodes. Resistance of aqueous flow from posterior chamber increased owing to iris-lens apposition or synechia.

USUAL TREATMENT

- Acute episodes: promptly, pilocarpine 2% eye drops, a sympathomimetic used to cause miosis. Also consider topical β-blocker drops and acetazolamide 500 mg PO or IV. If IOP does not resolve to ≤30 mmHg, a peripheral or laser iridectomy can be performed.
- Chronic ACG: surgical iridotomy

ASSESSMENT POINTS

SYSTEM	EFFECT	ASSESSMENT BY HX	PE	TEST
HEENT	Increased IOP	Visual blurring	Red eye	IOP >30 mmHg
		Eye pain	Corneal edema	
		Nausea	Dilated pupil, fixed	Gonioscopy
		Vomiting	Narrow angle	
		Visual halos	Optic nerve edema	
			Shallow anterior chamber	

Key Reference: Campbell DG: Primary angle-closure glaucoma. *In* Albert DM, Jakobiec FA (eds): Principles and Practice of Ophthalmology, Vol 3. Philadelphia, WB Saunders, 1994, pp 1365–1388.

PERIOPERATIVE IMPLICATIONS

Preoperative Preparation

- Do not interrupt routine glaucoma medication regimen (except ecothiophate)
- Discontinue ecothiophate 2–3 wk before surgery
- Chronic acetazolamide therapy can cause modest Na^+ and bicarbonate diuresis and metabolic acidosis. Evaluate lytes.
- Avoid mydriasis
- Premedication with systemic antisialagogue such as glycopyrrolate or atropine has no significant effect on IOP

Induction

- Anesthetic agents tend to decrease IOP
- Succinylcholine may be used. (See Anticipated Problems/Concerns.)
- Laryngoscopy and intubation may cause a temporary, mild, clinically insignificant increase in IOP. Placement and removal of laryngeal mask airway disturb IOP less than endotracheal intubation.

Extubation

- Minimize cough and bucking
- Combinations of systemic neostigmine and atropine used to reverse effects of nondepolarizing muscle relaxants will not cause mydriasis or increase IOP

Postoperative Period

- Acute glaucoma attack presents as dull, periorbital headache. Eye will appear pale, dry, and firm. Treatment includes acetazolamide IV 5–7 mg/kg.

ANTICIPATED PROBLEMS/CONCERNS

- β-blocker eye drops such as timolol may have systemic effects: bradycardia, asthma. Selective β-blocker eye drops such as betaxolol are less likely to produce pulmonary effects.
- Ecothiophate eye drops rarely used today for treatment of glaucoma. Patients on ecothiophate therapy have decreased plasma cholinesterase activity. Succinylcholine may be safely used in these patients if titrated IV in small (5-mg) increments to a monitored train-of-four effect.

GLAUCOMA, OPEN-ANGLE

John V. Donlon, Jr., M.D.

- People within USA: 2 million
- African-Americans: Primary cause of blindness, 5× incidence of glaucoma among Caucasians
- Age: 10.5% prevalence in 70–79 y group

PERIOPERATIVE RISKS

- Optic nerve ischemia

WORRY ABOUT

- Mydriasis
- Sudden, significant increase in IOP
- Eye pain: dull, periorbital ache with a dry, pale, firm eye

OVERVIEW

- Primary open-angle glaucoma (POAG) is most common form
- Gradual, asymptomatic onset in midlife
- Bilateral disease with significant hereditary predisposition
- Untreated, leads to progressive optic nerve damage and blindness (4% of glaucoma patients in USA become blind)
- Chronic, incurable disease that requires lifetime control of IOP by medication or surgery

ICD-9-CM Code: 365.10

ETIOLOGY

- Pathogenesis unclear. Increased resistance to outflow of aqueous humor at videocorneal angle, probably in the cribriform layer of trabecular meshwork near canal of Schlemm.
- Multifactorial hereditary predisposition. Within families with Hx of POAG there is 6-fold prevalence for glaucoma.
- Risk factors for developing optic nerve damage include family Hx, age, African-American race, diabetes, and CV disease

USUAL TREATMENT

- Early detection, control IOP
- Topical eye drops: β-blocker such as timolol or, less often, ecothiophate, a long-acting anticholinesterase agent
- Laser trabeculoplasty
- Surgical intervention: iridectomy, Molteno valve, trabeculotomy, cyclodialysis, filtering procedures

ASSESSMENT POINTS

SYSTEM	EFFECT	ASSESSMENT BY HX	PE	TEST
HEENT	Increased IOP	Myopia	Asymmetric optic cups	IOP >23 mmHg
	Optic nerve damage	Family Hx of POAG	Firm, pale eyeball	Gonioscopy
		Dull eye pain		Slit lamp
		Visual changes		Visual fields

Key Reference: Sihota R, Gupta V, Agarwal HC, Pandey RM, Deepak KK: Comparison of symptomatic and asmptomatic, chronic, primary angle-closure glaucoma, open-angle glaucoma, and controls. J Glaucoma 2000; 9:208–213.

PERIOPERATIVE IMPLICATIONS

Preoperative Preparation

- Do not interrupt routine glaucoma medication regimen (except ecothiophate)
- Discontinue ecothiophate 2–3 wk before surgery
- Chronic acetazolamide therapy can cause modest Na^+ and bicarbonate diuresis and metabolic acidosis. Evaluate lytes.
- Avoid mydriasis
- Premedication with systemic antisialagogue such as glycopyrrolate or atropine has no significant effect on IOP

Induction

- Anesthetic agents tend to decrease IOP
- Succinylcholine may be used. (See Anticipated Problems/Concerns.)
- Laryngoscopy and intubation may cause a temporary, mild, clinically insignificant increase in IOP. Placement and removal of laryngeal mask airway disturb IOP less than endotracheal intubation.

Extubation

- Minimize cough and bucking
- Combinations of systemic neostigmine and atropine used to reverse effects of nondepolarizing muscle relaxants will not cause mydriasis or increase IOP

Postoperative Period

- Acute glaucoma attack presents as dull, periorbital headache. Eye will appear pale, dry, and firm. Treatment includes acetazolamide IV 5–7 mg/kg.

ANTICIPATED PROBLEMS/CONCERNS

- Ecothiophate eye drops rarely used today for treatment of glaucoma. Patients on ecothiophate therapy have decreased plasma cholinesterase activity. Succinylcholine may be safely used in these patients if titrated IV in small (5-mg) increments to a monitored train-of-four effect.
- β-blocker eye drops such as timolol may have systemic effects: bradycardia, asthma. Selective β-blocker eye drops such as betaxolol are less likely to produce pulmonary effects.

GLOMUS JUGULARE TUMORS

Ghaleb A. Ghani, M.D.

RISK

- 0.6% of head and neck tumors
- Slow-growing
- Can co-exist with other paragangliomas
- Histologically benign but can be malignant with metastases

PERIOPERATIVE RISKS

- Hypothermia
- Massive blood loss
- Venous air embolism
- Htn
- Bradycardia
- Hypotension, bronchospasm
- Tumor-part emboli

WORRY ABOUT

- Multiple locations, persistence of symptoms after resection of the tumor

OVERVIEW

- Tumors of neural crest at base of skull in jugular bulb area
- May extend into posterior fossa
- May damage lower cranial nerves (IX–XII)
- May secrete catecholamines
- May secrete serotonin, histamine
- May grow into lumen of jugular vein as far as the right atrium

ICD-9-CM Codes: 194.6 (Malignant); 227.6 (Benign)

ETIOLOGY

- Congenital (usually benign) hypertrophied arteriovenous anastomosis
- Epithelial cells with abundant capillary network common

USUAL TREATMENT

- Radiation
- Embolization, alone or preop
- Resection

ASSESSMENT POINTS

SYSTEM	EFFECT	ASSESSMENT BY HX	PE	TEST
HEENT	Cranial nerve injury	Hoarseness Dysphagia Tinnitus	Soft palate motion Gag reflex ↓ Hearing	Indirect laryngoscopy
CV	Htn Intravascular growth	Headaches	BP	Catecholamine level (if indicated) MRI/CT scans, angio (if indicated)
RESP	Aspiration	Cough Fever SOB	Rhonchi, wheezing	CXR
GI	Delayed gastric emptying	Heartburn Regurgitation		
GU		No different from normal		
CNS	Intracranial extension	Hearing loss Headaches Dizziness		CT scan (if indicated) MRI (if indicated) Paragangliomas in other locations

Key Reference: Jensen NF: Glomus tumors of the head and neck: anesthetic considerations. Anesth Analg 1994; 78:112–119.

PERIOPERATIVE IMPLICATIONS

Preoperative Preparation

- Control Htn (in cathecholamine-secreting tumors). Preparation is similar to pheochromocytoma (see under Pheochromocytoma in Diseases section)
- Treat pneumonia
- Metoclopramide for delayed gastric emptying
- Adequate venous access for rapid fluid infusion

Monitoring

- Consider A-line, CVP
- Monitor for venous air embolism (end-tidal CO_2, N_2; precordial Doppler)

Maintenance

- Watch out for
  - Massive blood loss
  - Htn
  - Hypotension
  - Bronchospasm
  - Venous air embolism
  - Bradycardia
  - Tumor-part emboli
- Provide controlled hypotension if needed
- Measure to ↓ the ICP for intracranial extension:
  - Mannitol
  - Hyperventilation
  - Optimize venous return from brain

Extubation

- Evaluate for cranial nerve (IX–XII) injury

Adjuvants

- Controlled ventilation
- Muscle relaxants to prevent spontaneous ventilation intraoperatively
- Controlled hypotension

ANTICIPATED PROBLEMS/CONCERNS

- Loss of upper airway reflexes
- Airway obstruction
- Aspiration
- Delayed gastric emptying
- Ileus
- CNS insult
- Intracranial hemorrhage

GLOSSOPHARYNGEAL NEURALGIA
Evelina Worwag, M.D.

RISK

- Patients with multiple sclerosis
- Age ≥40 y
- Increased in patients with carotid artery occlusive diseases, arachnoiditis, and extracranial tumors of larynx, pharynx, and tonsils
- M > F 2:3

PERIOPERATIVE RISKS

- Manipulation in throat can trigger pain and arrhythmia
- Profound bradycardia or even asystole can accompany attack of pain

WORRY ABOUT

- Cardiac arrhythmias, sudden death
- Chronic opioid use
- Signs of major depression and anxiety

OVERVIEW

- Involves episodic bursts of pain in distribution of cranial nerves IX and X
- Attacks can be precipitated by chewing, yawning, or swallowing
- Pain usually located in pharynx, tonsil, or ear (unilaterally)
- Bradycardia, tachycardia, syncope, hypotension, or seizures may accompany painful episodes
- Easily confused with sick sinus syndrome, carotid sinus syndrome, or atypical trigeminal neuralgia
- Pain and cardiac arrhythmia can be relieved by topical anesthesia to oropharynx
- Sick sinus syndrome can be ruled out by the absence of ECG changes (see under Sick Sinus Syndrome in Diseases section)
- Glossopharyngeal nerve block rules out trigeminal neuralgia

ICD-9-CM Code: 352.1

ETIOLOGY

- Usually idiopathic
- Can be caused by vascular compression in region of cerebellopontine angle, the entry zone of vagus and glossopharyngeal nerves, especially by cross-compression of the nerve
- Seen with vertebral and carotid artery occlusive disease, arachnoiditis, and extracranial tumors arising in area of pharynx, larynx, and tonsils

USUAL TREATMENT

- Anticonvulsants—Tegretol, Neurontin (gabapentin)
- Surgical exploration in posterior fossa (microvascular decompression of the nerve)
- Radiofrequency or cryoablation
- Local anesthetic block at the posterior tonsillar pillar—intraoral approach or extraoral at styloid process

ASSESSMENT POINTS

SYSTEM	EFFECT	ASSESSMENT BY HX	PE	TEST
CV	Bradycardia, tachycardia, syncope, hypotension	Syncope, palpitation, orthostatic symptoms	BP HR	ECG when pain triggered
CNS	Cranial nerves IX and X; seizures	Pain in cranial nerves IX and X distribution precipitated by chewing, yawning, or swallowing	Triggering of pain and pain relief	CT scan with infusion for microvessel localization and to rule out tumors

Key Reference: Minagar A, Sheremata WA: Glossopharyngeal neuralgia and MS. Neurology 2000; 54:1368–1370.

PERIOPERATIVE IMPLICATIONS

Preoperative Evaluation

- Adequate assessment of intravascular fluid volume and cardiac status with emphasis on ruling out treatable causes of syncope and bradycardia

Monitoring

- Consider arterial line and central venous line when need for pacemaker is possible

Airway

- Topical anesthesia to oropharynx before laryngoscopy
- Drying agent before induction
- Consider glossopharyngeal nerve block as premedication and prophylaxis

Maintenance

- Constant preparedness to treat cardiac arrhythmias, Htn

Extubation

- Worry about vocal cord paralysis

GONORRHEA

Jerry M. Calkins, M.D., Ph.D.

RISK

- Decreasing: 150 per 100,000
- Rate highest in teenagers, nonwhites, the poor, the poorly educated, urban people, unmarried people living alone
- Incidence higher among men, prevalence higher among women

WORRY ABOUT

- Universal blood and body fluid precautions

OVERVIEW

- Sexually transmitted disease
- Pathogenesis—initial attachment and mucosal colonization
- High incidence of co-existing chlamydial infections

Clinical Features

- Manifestation is a function of site of inoculation, duration of infection, virulence of strain, spread locally or systemically
- Disseminated gonococcal infection—myopericarditis, toxic hepatitis, docreased renal function, large number of skin lesions
- Mucosal infections—urethritis in men (incubation 2–5 days), urogenital tract disease in women, anorectal infection, pharyngeal infections, conjunctivitis in neonates and adults
- Invasive gonococcal disease—pelvic inflammatory disease (PID), perihepatitis (Fitz-Hugh–Curtis syndrome), disseminated gonococcal infection, septic arthritis, gonococcal endocarditis and meningitis

ICD-9-CM Code: 098

ETIOLOGY

- *Neisseria gonorrhoeae*
- Gram-negative intracellular diplococcus
- Humans only natural hosts for *N. gonorrhoeae*

USUAL TREATMENT

- Diagnosis "gold standard"—isolation of organism by culture, testing for antimicrobial resistance
- Serologic test for syphilis recommended
- Penicillin, ampicillin, amoxicillin, tetracyclines, and first-generation cephalosporins not recommended
- Uncomplicated infection—ceftriaxone, cefixime, ciprofloxacin, or ofloxacin; add doxycycline or azithromycin for co-existing chlamydial infections
- Symptoms may subside without treatment, leaving chronic asymptomatic carrier state
- Pharyngeal infection frequently asymptomatic, may clear spontaneously over several weeks, even without therapy
- Resolution of symptoms after treatment suggests cure; follow-up cultures are recommended

ASSESSMENT POINTS

SYSTEM	EFFECT	ASSESSMENT BY HX	PE	TEST
Mucosal				
HEENT	Conjunctivitis, ophthalmia neonatorum, adult gonococcal conjunctivitis Pharyngeal infection		Exudative tonsillitis	Cultures
GI	Anorectal infections Proctitis	Pain, pruritus	Purulent discharge, bloody diarrhea	Cultures
GU	*Women* Urogenital tract disease	Abnormal vaginal discharge, dysuria, urinary frequency, lower abdominal pain, labial pain, abnormal menstruation	Mucopurulent cervicitis	Cultures from urethra and vagina
	Men Acute epididymitis Prostatitis	Pain		
Invasive				
CV	Gonococcal endocarditis			
GI	Perihepatitis (Fitz-Hugh–Curtis syndrome)	RUQ tenderness		Liver enzyme elevation
GU	*Women* PID	Lower abdominal pain, vaginal discharge, fever, palpable adnexal mass		Endocervix cultures
	Men Urethritis	Dysuria	Purulent urethral discharge	Cultures from urethra
CNS	Gonococcal meningitis			
MS	Septic arthritis	Most common cause of septic arthritis in young adults Tends to involve single joints		

Key Reference: Holmes KK, Morse SA: Gonococcal Infections. *In* Harrison's Principles of Internal Medicine, 14th ed. New York, McGraw-Hill, 1998, pp 915–922.

PERIOPERATIVE IMPLICATIONS

Monitoring

- Awareness—Foley catheter placement; temperature

Airway

- Awareness if pharyngitis exists

Maintenance

- Awareness of extent of disease

Adjuvants

- Vary with hepatic involvement

ANTICIPATED PROBLEMS/CONCERNS

Measures to Control

- No vaccine available
- Follow-up cultures
- Effective antibiotics
- Testing isolates for antibiotic susceptibility
- Routine culturing of high-risk populations
- Diligent contact tracing and prompt referral; treatment of sexual partners
- Education targeted at high-risk groups
- Use of condoms and other barriers

RISK

- Prevalence: both sexes, all races, all ages but mostly affects young and middle-aged adults
- Worldwide illness, occurs all times of year
- Mortality rate 5–20%. Most patients eventually fully recover, 15% have significant residual weakness.

PERIOPERATIVE RISKS

- Respiratory failure 2° to polyneuropathy
- Autonomic dysfunction with profound CV instability

WORRY ABOUT

- Rapidity of symptoms—resp paralysis may occur within 24 h of onset
- Pulmonary complications

OVERVIEW

- Polyneuropathy most often encountered in critical care practice
  - Patients present initially with lower limb weakness that spreads
- Widespread, patchy, inflammatory demyelination of peripheral and autonomic nervous systems
- Dysautonomia from chromatolysis of anteromediolateral cell column and autonomic ganglia: fluctuating BP, Htn, hypotension, postural hypotension, tachycardia, arrhythmias
- CSF protein usually nml during first few days of illness, steadily rises and remains elevated for several months, even after recovery

ICD-9-CM Code: 357.0

ETIOLOGY

- Believed to be hypersensitivity reaction
- Cause unknown—slow virus, metabolic or autoimmune etiology speculated
- Antecedent illness within 4 wk of onset (resp or GI infection in 60–70% of cases)
- Other predisposing factors include surgery, pregnancy, malignancy, acute seroconversion to HIV
- Epidural anesthesia may be antecedent event or cause recurrence

USUAL TREATMENT

- Basis of treatment is symptomatic care
- Daily bedside evaluation of vital capacity and resp muscle strength; patients with ↓ resp reserve should be moved to ICU
- Elective tracheal intubation and mechanical ventilatory support when signs of resp distress are present *even before* $Paco_2$ rises or vital capacity falls
- Guidelines for ventilatory support:
  - Alveolar-arterial tension difference >300 mmHg with $FIO_2 = 1.0$
  - $Paco_2$ >50 mmHg
  - Maximum static inspiratory pressure <30 cm H_2O
  - Vital capacity <14 ml/kg
- Steroid therapy, immunosuppressants
- Plasmapheresis reduces hospital stay and time spent on ventilator if given to patients who do not improve or who worsen within first 7 days of onset of symptoms

ASSESSMENT POINTS

SYSTEM	EFFECT	ASSESSMENT BY HX	PE	TEST
HEENT	Inability to close eyes	Dry eyes	Dry eyes	
CV	Fluctuating hypo- and hypertension, postural hypotension, sinus tachycardia, arrhythmias	Orthostatic Sx Palpitations	BP/pulse	ECG
RESP	Respiratory failure 2° to weakness	Stamina—for breathing	↓ Strength on repeated ventilation	Macrophage-inhibiting factor
GI	Bowel obstruction	Inability to move bowels	Abdominal exam	Abdominal x-ray
CNS	Autonomic dysfunction	Early satiety Orthostatic hypotension Lack of sweating	BP lying and standing	ECG with R-R interval on deep breathing
MS	Weakness, joint fixation	Lack of stamina		

Key Reference: Asbury AK: New concepts of Guillain-Barré syndrome. J Child Neurol 2000; 15:183–191.

PERIOPERATIVE IMPLICATIONS

Preoperative Preparation

- Avoid rapid turning of patient—autonomic instability and postural hypotension may result
- Avoid head-up (reverse Trendelenburg) position—inability of patient to maintain CV stability with tilt
- Increased gastric acidity—treat with antacid and metoclopramide, 10 mg/70 kg
- Maintain appropriate environmental temperature

Monitoring

- Arterial line for continuous pressure monitoring started prior to anesthetic induction
- CVP or PA line to monitor for potential fluid shifts that result from positional changes and cardiac dysrhythmias
- Temperature—patients may become poikilothermic
- Neuromuscular monitoring

Airway

- Most patients have early tracheostomy; airway access should not be a problem; previous patients may have tracheal stenosis
- Fusion of TMJ—may make orotracheal intubation difficult

Induction

- Avoid barbiturates and phenothiazines, which may produce profound CV depression

Maintenance

- Local anesthesia preferred
- GA: nonsympatholytic technique such as nitrous oxide–oxygen supplemented by opioids or ketamine
- Sensitive to positive pressure ventilation and tracheal suction—may result in autonomic instability

Extubation

- Continue to ventilate postop if patient required ventilatory support preop
- Residual weakness from anesthetic agents and muscle relaxants may necessitate postop ventilation in patients not ventilated preop
- In ICU—wean from mechanical ventilation when vital capacity >10 ml/kg

Adjuvants

- Muscle relaxants
  - Avoid succinylcholine; can cause hyperkalemia with cardiac arrest
  - Patients have increased sensitivity to nondepolarizing muscle relaxants
  - May have residual muscle weakness after apparent full recovery from GA
- Volume
  - Maintain blood volume
  - Use colloid to maintain CVP >5 cm H_2O

ANTICIPATED PROBLEMS/CONCERNS

- Autonomic instability
- Respiratory failure

Special Problems

- Parturient: during third trimester, risk of exacerbation; for labor a regional anesthetic indicated to avoid exaggerated hemodynamic response to pain from autonomic dysfunction. Aspiration pneumonitis and respiratory failure may result in premature labor and maternal mortality. For C-section a regional anesthetic contraindicated even for patient with mild resp involvement.
- Fecal impaction
- Stress ulcers

HASHIMOTO'S THYROIDITIS
M. Lawrence Berman, M.D.

RISK
- People within USA: 100,000–400,000 new cases/y
- Most common cause of primary hypothyroidism in adults (10% over age 65)
- Race with highest prevalence: none known
- Gender predominance: F>M (8:1; age 30–50 y)

PERIOPERATIVE RISKS
- ↑ Risk of thyroid storm even if euthyroid preop
- Some risk of resp insufficiency and ↑ bleeding perioperatively

WORRY ABOUT
- Hyperthyroidism in perioperative period with thyroid storm (see under Hyperthyroidism in Diseases section)
- Chronic hyperthyroidism with its concomitants
- Co-existing autoimmune disease with adrenal failure

OVERVIEW
- Chronic inflammation of thyroid (painful or painless) with lymphocytic infiltration due to autoimmune factors
- Acute inflammation results in ↑ release of preformed hormone with hyperthyroidism
- Chronic inflammation results in ↓ thyroid gland function with resistant hypothyroidism

ICD-9-CM Code: 423.9

ETIOLOGY
- Autoimmune disease associated with other autoimmune diseases: Sjögren's syndrome, SLE, RA, pernicious anemia, autoimmune endocrinopathies, Addison's disease, hypoparathyroidism, diabetes mellitus, gonadal failure
- ↑ Incidence in patients with a family Hx and with chromosomal disorders—Turner's, Down, or Klinefelter's syndromes

USUAL TREATMENT
- Thyroid hormone replacement chronically in hypothyroidism
- NSAIDs in acute thyroiditis (painful) and propranolol to control symptoms of hyperthyroidism

ASSESSMENT POINTS

SYSTEM	EFFECT	ASSESSMENT BY HX	PE	TEST
HEENT	Swollen tender neck Enlarged tongue Tracheal compression	Neck pain, hoarseness	Examine airway and neck	Lateral neck x-rays or CT of neck
CV	Dehydration, tachy- or bradydysrhythmias	Orthostatic symptoms		Tilt table test ECG
RESP	↓ Resp muscle strength	SOB, DOE		
GI	Ileus Constipation			
ENDO	Acutely hyperthyroid Chronically hypothyroid	Shaking, anxiety, emotional lability	Reflex speed, HR Tremor, nervousness Mental status	Free T_4 estimate
	Other autoimmune dysfunction	Weakness	Inability to arise from chair without using hands	Serum K^+/Na^+
HEME	Anemia			Hgb, Hct
CNS	Cold intolerance Slow or fast movement, depending on stage	Cold intolerance	Reflexes, mental status exam	
MS		Arthralgias and myalgias		

Key Reference: Bennett-Guerrero E, Kramer DC, Schwinn DA: Effect of chronic and acute thyroid hormone reduction on perioperative outcome. Anesth Analg 1997; 85:30–36.

PERIOPERATIVE IMPLICATIONS

Preoperative Preparation
- Assess NPO status (poor gastric emptying)
- Cautious use of preop drugs (↑ sensitivity of CNS and resp system to depressants)
- Ensure that patient is euthyroid (to avoid thyroid storm)
- Assess fluid status
- Assess for co-morbidities (autoimmune/adrenal/pancreatic dysfunction)

Monitoring
- Temperature (consider placing cooling blanket on OR table as Rx for thyroid storm)
- Consider invasive monitoring if CV or resp compromise

Airway
- If normal preop, routine
- If displaced or distorted, consider awake fiberoptic and armored tube

Induction/Maintenance
- No data indicate one technique better than any other

Extubation
- Consider extubation in optimal situation for reintubation

Postoperative Concerns
- Routine + treatment of co-morbidities if co-existing autoimmune disease

Adjuvants
- Esmolol for acute hyperthyroidism
- Steroids sometimes needed for adrenal dysfunction
- Oral hypoglycemics (if chronic Rx) can cause hypoglycemia for longer duration and of greater severity in perioperative patient

ANTICIPATED PROBLEMS/CONCERNS
- Thyroid storm—clinical diagnosis of life-threatening illness if hyperthyroidism severely exacerbated by illness or operation—manifested by hyperpyrexia, tachycardia, alterations in consciousness
- Resp failure

Alan D. Kaye, M.D., Ph.D.
G.B. Racz, M.D.

RISK

- People within USA: >20 million
- Can start as early as 1 y of age, 10–20% of children by 20 y of age, male = female
- In adults, more frequent in women; declines after age 40 y
- Familial aggregation
- Can be associated with sinusitis; AVM; epilepsy; ischemic infarction; sensitivity to foods rich in tyramine, phenylethylamine, or octopamine (chocolate, wine, dairy products); electroencephelographic abnormalities

PERIOPERATIVE RISKS

- ↑ Incidence of Htn, stroke, CAD
- Gastric stasis
- Drug toxicity and side effects

WORRY ABOUT

- Toxic and side effects of antimigrainous preparations, adverse interaction with anesthetic drugs
- Associated intracranial disorders
- ↑ Aggregation of plts with ↑ risk of stroke and CAD

OVERVIEW

- Recurrent unilateral headache
- Typically, some or all of the following symptoms: recurrent abdominal pain with or without nausea or vomiting, unilateral throbbing cranial pain, sensory or motor aura, scalp tenderness, family history
- Diagnosis is history dependent
- Migrainous infarction with permanent neurologic damage is rare

ICD-9-CM Codes: 346.0 (Classic migraine); 346.1 (Common migraine. 5th digit subclassification: 0 without mention of intractable migraine, 1 with intractable migraine, so stated.)

ETIOLOGY

- Central or peripheral mechanisms incited by internal or external stimuli
- Lowering magnesium levels ↑ the affinity and release of serotonin at cerebrovascular and neuronal sites as well as NO production and activation of NMDA receptors
- Precipitated by trigger factors
- Cerebral and extracerebral arteries are most likely sources of pain
- Pain results from exaggerated pulsations in association with sensitization of nociceptors around blood vessels

USUAL TREATMENT

- No permanent cure
- Elimination of trigger factors, chronobiologic regulation
- Abortive therapy: sumatriptan; ergotamine, sphenopalatine ganglion block, nonopioid and opioid analgesics
- Prophylactic therapy: β-blocking agents, Ca^{2+}-channel blockers, anticonvulsants, antihistamines, antihypertensives, TCAs, and MAO inhibitors
- Behavioral treatment with biofeedback, self-hypnosis, relief by dark surroundings, sleep

ASSESSMENT POINTS

Mainly side effects and toxicity of antimigrainous therapy.

SYSTEM	EFFECT	ASSESSMENT BY HX	PE	TEST
CV	Ergotamine, sumatriptan –Worsening of Htn, ischemic heart disease, peripheral vascular disease, serotonin syndrome	Symptoms of angina and peripheral vascular insufficiency		ECG Stress ECG
	β-adrenergic receptor blocking agents and Ca^{2+}-channel blockers –Excessive depression of myocardial function	Symptoms of CHF	S_3 Rales	CXR
	Methysergide –Pericardial fibrosis, cardiac valvular fibrosis		↓ Heart sounds	CXR, ECHO
	TCAs and Ca^{2+}-channel blockers –Cardiac conduction abnormalities	Syncope		ECG
RESP	β-blockers –Worsening of COPD	Dyspnea	Expiratory wheezing	CXR ABGs
	Methysergide –Pleuropulmonary fibrosis	Dyspnea	Rapid shallow breathing	PFTs
GI	Gastroparesis	Early satiety		
CNS	Intracranial disorders TCAs, MAO inhibitors –Anticholinergic and CNS stimulation	Tachycardia, dry mouth, blurred vision, urinary retention, delayed gastric emptying	Focal deficit	Neuroimaging

Key Reference: Diamond ML, Solomon GD, Diamond S (eds): Diamond & Dalessio's the Practicing Physician's Approach to Headache, 6th ed. Philadelphia, WB Saunders, 1999.

PERIOPERATIVE IMPLICATIONS

Preoperative Preparation

- Detailed pharmacotherapy Hx
- Discontinue MAO inhibitors 14–21 days in advance, if possible (see Monoamine Oxidase Inhibitors in Drugs section)
- Gastroparesis: Metoclopramide (10 mg/70 kg patient)

Monitoring

- Routine, unless signs of ischemic heart disease

Airway

- None

Preinduction/Induction

- Patients receiving β-blockers and Ca^{2+}-channel blockers may develop reduced CO and hypotension

Maintenance

- Exaggerated response to indirect-acting vasopressors may occur with patients on ergotamine, sumatriptan, TCAs, and MAO inhibitors
- Hyperpyrexic coma reported after administration of narcotic to pts receiving MAO inhibitors

Extubation

- Increased risk of CNS stimulation with sumatriptan, ergotamine, TCAs, and MAO inhibitors

Postoperative Period

- Pain management may be critical
- Avoid withdrawal syndromes

ANTICIPATED PROBLEMS/CONCERNS

- Possible adverse interactions of anesthetic drugs and antimigrainous preparations
- No unique hazards of anesthesia administered to patients with migraine

HELLP SYNDROME

David J. Birnbach, M.D.

RISK

- If severe preeclampsia, 20% may exhibit HELLP syndrome
- Preeclampsia occurs in 5–10% of pregnancies

PERIOPERATIVE RISKS

- High maternal and fetal morbidity and mortality
- Increased C-section rate (up to 94%)
- Immediate delivery after diagnosis to prevent maternal and fetal death

WORRY ABOUT

- Confused with hepatitis, thrombotic thrombocytopenic purpura, gallbladder disease, and acute fatty liver of pregnancy
- Thrombocytopenia and coagulopathy increase risk of hematoma after regional anesthetic
- Upper airway and laryngeal edema leading to airway obstruction and difficult or failed intubation. Fluid management difficult; pulmonary edema may ensue.

OVERVIEW

- HELLP is an acronym for the findings that suggest hepatic involvement in preeclampsia patient: Hemolysis, Elevated Liver enzymes, Low Platelets
- Diagnostic criteria include hemolysis, defined by abnormal peripheral smear and ↑ bilirubin levels, elevated liver enzymes (SGOT >70 U/L, LDH >600 U/L), and thrombocytopenia (<100,000 / mm^3)
- Failure to treat may lead to eclampsia or death due to hepatic hematoma or rupture
- Not always associated with Htn

ICD-9-CM Code: 642.5 (Severe preeclampsia)

ETIOLOGY

- Poorly understood
- May be severe form of preeclampsia resulting from abnormal prostaglandin control, intravascular plt activation, and microvascular endothelial damage. Microangiopathic hemolytic anemia usual.

USUAL TREATMENT

- Definitive treatment is delivery as quickly as possible
- After delivery, many experience uneventful recovery, with plt counts returning to normal within 1 wk
- Glucocorticoids may accelerate fetal lung maturity and may also improve mother's plt count and reduce liver enzyme abnormalities
- Plts, FFP, and cryoprecipitate administered as needed
- Magnesium sulfate for CNS irritability and antihypertensives for Htn

ASSESSMENT POINTS

SYSTEM	EFFECT	ASSESSMENT BY HX	PE	TEST
HEENT	Upper airway edema	Dyspnea, voice change	Poor visualization on airway exam	Mallampati assessment
CV	LV failure	Dyspnea, desaturation	Adventitious sounds	CVP and/or PA pressures
RESP	Resp depression	Magnesium administration	↓ Reflexes	MgSO$_4$ level
GI	Liver swelling Subcapsular hematoma	Epigastric pain Nausea, vomiting		Elevated SGOT, SGPT
HEME	Thrombocytopenia Hemolytic anemia	Bruising Pallor, jaundice	Bleeding	Plt count LDH, bilirubin Peripheral smear
RENAL	Acute renal failure	Oliguria		Elevated uric acid, BUN, serum Cr
CNS	Eclampsia, cerebral edema	Seizures		

Key Reference: Haddad B, Barton JR, Livingston JC, et al: Risk factors for adverse maternal outcomes among women with HELLP syndrome. Am J Obstet Gynecol 2000; 183:444–448.

PERIOPERATIVE IMPLICATIONS

Preoperative Testing

- Obtain CBC, PT, PTT, fibrinogen, SGPT, SGOT, LDH, BUN, Cr
- Thromboelastography (TEG) may also be useful

Monitoring

- Consider arterial line if unstable
- Consider CVP or PA catheter if decreased UO or CHF

Airway

- Assess airway early and repeat airway exam periodically
- Laryngeal edema may preclude normal tracheal intubation in the event of emergency C-section
- Difficult intubation equipment might be readily available
- Consider preemptive epidural anesthetic

Induction

- Slow, controlled neuraxial anesthesia with incremental dosing, if not contraindicated due to coagulation abnormalities

- If general anesthesia is required, the hypertensive surge associated with endotracheal intubation can often be avoided by pretreatment with magnesium, antihypertensives, or opioids

Adjuvants

- If significant Htn, antihypertensive therapy prior to laryngeal intubation
- If receiving magnesium sulfate and needs GA, small doses of neuromuscular blocking agents with close monitoring

HEMOPHILIA
Vincent S. Cowell, M.D.

RISK

- Incidence: 1/10,000 male infants
- More than 15,000 people in the USA
- Hemophilia A, factor VIII (FVIII) deficiency, affects 80–85% of hemophiliacs; remainder have hemophilia B (Christmas disease) due to factor IX (FIX) deficiency
- Mode of inheritance and clinical features of hemophilias A and B are similar
- Females may be asymptomatic carriers of the hemophilia gene and may have partial deficiency of FVIII or FIX
- Hemophilia is without ethnic or geographic predilection

PERIOPERATIVE RISKS

- Prolonged and potentially fatal hemorrhage both during and after surgery
- Closed-space bleeding can lead to nerve injury or vascular or airway obstruction
- Surgery should not proceed without adequate supply of factor concentrate to support the procedure and postop course

WORRY ABOUT

- Spontaneous bleeding
- Postop hemorrhage despite optimal replacement therapy of deficient plasma coagulation factor

- Approximately 5–15% develop inhibitors, antibodies to FVIII or FIX (VIII much more often than IX)
- Factor replacement therapy risks exposure to viruses, including hepatitis and HIV

OVERVIEW

- Hemophiliacs can have severe deficiency (<1% of nml levels), moderate deficiency (1–5% of nml levels), or mild deficiency (5–30% of nml levels)
- Congenital disorder, inherited as an X-linked recessive trait, affecting males almost exclusively
- Acute and chronic complications often due to recurrent spontaneous bleeding (e.g., cycle of joint hemorrhage, inflammation, synovial proliferation, and erosion of cartilage, causing pain and disability)
- Treatment generally follows bleeding episodes
- New approaches to treatment involve the prophylactic use of clotting factors
- PTT is often elevated and used as a screening test for hemophilia; PTT and factor assays are used to monitor FVIII and FIX levels (PT and plt count are nml)

ICD-9-CM Code: 286.0

ETIOLOGY

- Hereditary disorder, X-linked recessive
- Dx made by abn plasma concentrations of FVIII or FIX
- About a third of all cases are the result of a new or spontaneous mutation

USUAL TREATMENT

- Plasma concentrations of deficient factors maintained at minimum of 40–70% throughout the perioperative period (2–7 days postop) for adequate hemostasis
- Hemophilia A: recombinant FVIII products
- Hemophilia B: recombinant FIX
- Desmopression (DDAVP injection or Stimate nasal spray) whenever possible for mild hemophilia
- Cryoprecipitate is no longer recommended as a treatment alternative except in life-threatening emergencies
- Recombinant factor VIIa (NovoSeven) for use in patients with inhibitors to FVIII or FIX
- FFP no longer used in routine treatment
- Gene insertion therapy is under investigation

ASSESSMENT POINTS

SYSTEM	EFFECT	ASSESSMENT BY HX	PE	TEST
HEENT	Pharyngeal bleeding	Often seen in children	Tongue and mouth lacerations	Examination
GI	GI bleeding not common	When it occurs, bleeding can be excessive	Stool exam, endoscopy	Hemoccult, angio
HEME	Anemia, hematoma formation, bruising	Lethargy, SOB, skin discoloration	Hematomas	PT/PTT FVIII and FIX assay, gene analysis
GU	Hematuria	Blood in urine		Urinalysis, cysto, IVP
CNS	Intracranial hemorrhage	Head trauma, headache, change in mental status	Any sign or symptom of head injury or trauma	Head CT
MS	Joint hemorrhage Joint deformities Muscle hemorrhage Compartment syndrome Chronic pain	Painful distention of the joint Bruising Restricted movement Narcotic dependence	Hemarthroses Limited ROM Tenderness	Physical exam X-ray

Key Reference: National Hemophilia Foundation. www.hemophilia.org

PERIOPERATIVE IMPLICATIONS

Preoperative Preparation
- Therapeutic levels (40–70%) of plasma FVIII or FIX before proceeding with surgery
- Avoid unnecessary IM injections

Monitoring
- Consider avoiding invasive monitoring unless absolutely essential

Airway
- Extra care to avoid trauma from instrumentation of airway

Induction
- No special considerations

Maintenance
- Risk of bleeding may outweigh the benefits of regional anesthetics

Extubation
- Be sensitive to extubating patients who have potential for bleeding in neck or pharynx that could compromise airway

Adjuvants
- When selecting anesthetic drugs, consider presence of co-existing liver disease due to hepatitis from previous transfusion

ANTICIPATED PROBLEMS/CONCERNS

- Transmission of blood-borne viruses (HIV, hepatitis viruses, and parvovirus) by clotting factor concentrates
- Universal precautions should be observed
- 20–33% of persons with hemophilia A develop inhibitors to FVIII
- Venous access can be challenging
- May want to avoid drugs that interfere with nml plt function such as aspirin and NSAIDs
- Chronic pain due to bleeding in joints or muscle tissue may lead to narcotic addiction

DISEASES **157**

HEPATIC ENCEPHALOPATHY

Jeffrey M. Baden, M.D.

RISK

- People in the USA: approximately 2000/y from fulminant liver failure and many more from chronic liver disease
- Race/gender with highest prevalence: unknown

PERIOPERATIVE RISKS

- Increased risk of CV depression, arrhythmias, sudden cardiac arrest
- Coagulopathy
- Cerebral edema, resp arrest, sepsis, renal failure, hypoglycemia, sodium abnormalities

WORRY ABOUT

- Deteriorating liver function
- Deteriorating renal function requiring hemodialysis
- Deteriorating CV and resp function

OVERVIEW

- Complex mental state associated with liver disease
- Key symptom is changed mental state ranging from confusion to coma
- Nature, extent, and complications of liver disease are main determinants of long-term survival

ICD-9-CM Code: 572.2

ETIOLOGY

- In $2/3$ of cases, failure of liver to remove ammonia and possibly other toxic substances before they enter systemic circulation
- Non-nitrogenous encephalopathy occurs in $1/3$ of cases and is often precipitated by drugs that depress consciousness
- Increased neuronal GABA activity

USUAL TREATMENT

- Most important measures:
  - Decrease dietary protein intake
  - Suppress ammoniagenic intestinal flora with oral neomycin
  - Stimulate ammonia fixation and removal with oral lactulose
  - Flumazenil and other benzodiazepine receptor antagonists

ASSESSMENT POINTS

SYSTEM	EFFECT	ASSESSMENT BY HX	PE	TEST
CV	CV depression Arrhythmias Sudden cardiac arrest		Low BP Abnormal pulse	ECG ECHO
RESP	Increased AV shunts Hypocapnia Lower O_2 consumption	Dyspnea	Cyanosis Hyperventilation	Pulse oximetry and capnography (if indicated) Blood gases
GI	Liver disease	Numerous causes, e.g., alcohol and viral hepatitis	Stigmata of liver disease Liver biopsy	Blood chemistry Viral hepatitis screens
HEME	Coagulation defects	Bleeds easily	Petechiae	CBC, prothrombin time
RENAL	Hepatorenal syndrome			Blood chemistries
CNS	Cerebral edema	Worsening mental state		EEG
METAB	Hypoglycemia Hypernatremia Hyponatremia			Blood chemistries

Key Reference: Mullen KD, Dasarathy S: Hepatic encephalopathy. *In* Schiff ER, Sorrell MF, Maddrey WC (eds): Schiff's Diseases of the Liver. Philadelphia, Lippincott-Raven, 1999, pp 545–581.

PERIOPERATIVE IMPLICATIONS

Preoperative Preparation

- Avoid opiates and sedatives

Monitoring

- Routine monitors
- ECG—sudden arrhythmias
- Consider intra-arterial and CVP monitoring—remember coagulopathy
- Frequent blood glucose and lyte analysis

Airway

- Bleeding of instrumented upper airway

Preinduction/Induction

- Avoid "fixed agents" when possible

Maintenance

- Volatile anesthetic of low arrhythmogenicity may be good choice

Extubation

- Remember hypoxia from disease itself

Adjuvants

- Use muscle relaxants sparingly and titrate carefully to effect
- Atracurium may be a good choice

ANTICIPATED PROBLEMS/CONCERNS

- Bleeding
- Prolongation of drug effects
- Cardiovascular depression and arrhythmias
- Tendency to hypoxia
- Sepsis
- Renal dysfunction
- Hypoglycemia

HEPATITIS, ALCOHOLIC
Johnathan L. Pregler, M.D.

RISK

- People within USA: 10% of men and 3–5% of women develop alcoholism, 10–15% of alcoholics will develop alcoholic hepatitis and cirrhosis

PERIOPERATIVE RISKS

- Mortality rate of 60–100% of patients undergoing surgery during active alcoholic hepatitis
- Poor prognosis when accompanied by ↑ bilirubin, ↑ Cr, PT >1.5× control, ascites, or encephalopathy
- Elective surgery should be postponed
- >10% develop DTs without prophylaxis

WORRY ABOUT

- Bleeding disorders and anemia
- Pulmonary shunting
- Altered mental status/encephalopathy/alcohol withdrawal with DTs
- Insulin resistance

OVERVIEW

- Acute inflammatory lesion of liver. As mild as nausea and vomiting or as severe as fulminant hepatic failure.
- In-hospital mortality 50% if elevated bilirubin, Cr, PT; ascites; and/or encephalopathy
- An intermediate stage between fatty liver and alcoholic cirrhosis
- May be preceded by period of heavy alcohol consumption

ICD-9-CM Code: 571.1

ETIOLOGY

- Daily consumption of a pint or more of alcohol or equivalent in wine/or beer for 10 or more years
- Amount and duration of consumption more important than type of alcohol or pattern of consumption
- Women at risk with lower consumption levels
- Inflammatory lesion with leukocytic infiltration. Progresses to hepatocellular necrosis and deposition of alcoholic hyaline.
- Repeated episodes precursor to cirrhosis after healing and scar tissue formation

USUAL TREATMENT

- Abstinence
- Recovery varies from several weeks to months
- Supportive care includes diet adjustment, multivitamin supplementation, lactulose, and neomycin if needed
- Steroid therapy is controversial, may be used for severe cases with encephalopathy

ASSESSMENT POINTS

SYSTEM	EFFECT	ASSESSMENT BY HX	PE	TEST
CV	High CO Low SVR Low CO (in advanced disease)	Exercise tolerance	Hyperdynamic cardiac exam	ECG ECHO
RESP	Pulmonary shunts Restrictive disease Pulmonary effusions Central hyperventilation	Orthodeoxia Ascites	Effusions on chest exam; ascites on abdominal exams	Respiratory alkalosis on ABG
GI/HEPATIC	Disrupted synthetic and metabolic function	Anorexia, N/V, malaise, wt loss, fever	Jaundice, ascites, tender hepatomegaly, splenomegaly	Elevated transaminases (SGOT/SGPT>2), PT, alk phos, bilirubin Decreased albumin
RENAL	Mg^{2+} and PO_4^{2-} wasting Free water retention		Ascites	Serum Mg^{2+} and PO_4^{2-} Hyponatremia
ENDO	Insulin resistance			Glucose
HEME	Anemia and thrombocytopenia GI blood loss Hypersplenism	Bruising/bleeding	Splenomegaly	Hgb/Hct, platelets
CNS	Decreased clearance of amines	Altered mental status	Neurologic exam	NH_3 levels

Key Reference: Gholson CF, Provena JM: Hepatologic considerations in patients with parenchymal liver disease undergoing surgery. Am Gastroenterol 1990; 85:487–496.

PERIOPERATIVE IMPLICATIONS

Preoperative Preparation

- Elective procedures should be postponed
- Extreme sensitivity to sedative medications
- Ascites may be treated by diuretics (spironolactone) or percutaneous drainage
- Hypokalemia and hyponatremia should be corrected slowly (over 24–36 h)
- Assess/correct coagulopathy by vit K administration and FFP, platelets if needed

Monitoring

- Glucose levels
- Large fluid shifts during abdominal procedures due to drainage of ascites may necessitate CVP or PA catheter

Airway

- At risk for aspiration if ascites and increased abdominal pressure

Induction

- Hypoalbuminemia may decrease V_d (Pentothal)
- H_2O-soluble drugs may have increased V_d owing to ascites
- Regional anesthesia well tolerated (if coagulation status permits)

Maintenance

- Maintain normocarbia
- Decreased clearance of hepatically metabolized drugs (meperidine, fentanyl, barbiturates)
- Conjugative metabolic pathways better preserved (morphine)
- Maintain hepatic blood flow (isoflurane is best inhalation agent) (no contraindication to N_2O)

Extubation

- Extubate when patient fully awake

Adjuvants

- MVI and vit K 10 mg SQ or IM

Postoperative Period

- Pain control ideally via regional to avoid sedative effects of systemic drug; however, must assess coagulation system
- Morphine metabolism is better preserved than other narcotics
- Monitor or treat for alcohol withdrawal

ANTICIPATED PROBLEMS/CONCERNS

- Poor regulation of glucose levels
- Need for prolonged airway protection because of altered mental status and pulmonary dysfunction
- Acute withdrawal from alcohol
- Multiple coagulation abnormalities due to synthetic dysfunction and hypersplenism

HEPATITIS, HALOTHANE

Aisling Conran, M.D.

RISK

• Greater if repeated exposures, obese, taking P450 inducing agent, middle age (>40 y, esp 50–60 y) female, genetic susceptibility
• Rare in infants and children: 1/10,000 to 1/40,000 halothane anesthetics

PREOPERATIVE RISKS

• Pre-existing liver disease; site, duration, or degree of surgery has NOT been shown to contribute to development

WORRY ABOUT

• Enzyme induction of hepatic cytochrome P450 system by other pharmacologic agents may predispose (esp INH)

OVERVIEW/PHARMACOLOGY

• Liver damage within 28 days of halothane exposure when other causes of liver dysfunction have been excluded
• Viral hepatitis, pre-existing liver disease, blood transfusion, sepsis, drug reactions, and intraop and postop hypoxia and hypotension must be excluded as causes of liver dysfunction
• In past, undiagnosed viral hepatitis, especially non-A, non-B hepatitis, confused clinical picture

• Clinical features include nausea, jaundice, fever, eosinophilia, rash and arthralgias, ↑ liver function test results, presence of autoantibodies

ICD-9-CM Code: 997.4 (Postoperative acute)

ETIOLOGY

• Hepatic hypoxia has been postulated as mechanism for development. While halothane, enflurane, and isoflurane decrease portal blood flow, both isoflurane and enflurane maintain hepatic blood flow better than halothane by increasing hepatic arterial flow. While persistent global hypoxia occurs rarely, local liver hypoxia may occur and contribute to the development of halothane hepatitis.
• Two forms: more common, mild form is associated with reductive metabolites of halothane metabolism. Fulminant form, occurring in approx 1:35,000 halothane anesthetics, is associated with a high mortality and is likely immune-mediated. This hypersensitivity hypothesis is supported by prevalence of eosinophilia, fever, Hx of previous or repeated exposures to halothane, Hx of drug allergy or atopy, and presence of IgG autoantibodies. IgG autoantibodies are found in 70%. The autoantibodies react with trifluoroacetic acid (TFA), a reactive metabolite that can bind to cellular components, changing "self" to "nonself." This new hapten provokes an immune hypersensitivity reaction in genetically susceptible individuals.
• Increased Ca^{2+} levels in cell may be final common pathway to cell destruction in liver. Halothane can inactivate endoplasmic reticulum's Ca^{2+} transport mechanism, resulting in an intracellular release of Ca^{2+}.

DRUG CLASS/METABOLISM

• Halothane is a nonflammable, halogenated alkene that is a potent volatile anesthetic agent. Undergoes biotransformation by the liver via two pathways, an oxidative and a reductive pathway. The oxidative pathway is favored in the presence of high oxygen tensions and the reductive pathway is more prevalent under both hypoxic conditions and in the presence of enzyme induction. Approximately 20% metabolism, a much higher rate than either enflurane (2.4%) or isoflurane (0.2%). TFA and bromide ion are the metabolites of the oxidative pathway and 2-chloro-1,1,1-trifluoroethane, 2-chloro-1,1-difluoroethylene, and fluoride ion are produced via the reductive pathway. None of the metabolites shown to be directly hepatotoxic. Binding of metabolites to hepatic cells is more likely under hypoxic conditions and therefore more likely to occur with the reductive pathway.

ASSESSMENT POINTS

SYSTEM	ASSESSMENT BY HX	PE	TEST
GI	Nausea	Jaundice (5th–6th day after exposure)	Eosinophilia Elevated LFTs Serum transaminases markedly increased Alkaline phosphatase may double Liver biopsy: centrilobular necrosis Antibody tests (still experimental but available)

Key Reference: Buchanan CC, Cameron RJ, Carpenter RD, Currie J, Spencer HT: Halothane and post–halothane exposure hepatitis. N Z Med J 1999; 112:19–20.

PREOPERATIVE IMPLICATIONS

• Assess patient for risk factors; review anesthetic records for possible prior halothane exposures

ANTICIPATED PROBLEMS/CONCERNS

• When evaluating a patient with postop liver dysfunction, many causes of postop jaundice need to be excluded, anesthesia records need to be reviewed, LFTs obtained and followed serially

• Hx of any contact with person with jaundice elicited, drug Hx and transfusion Hx obtained, serologies for viral hepatitis, antibody testing for volatile anesthetics, and liver biopsy obtained prior to making Dx

HEPATITIS A

Arnold J. Berry, M.D., M.P.H.

RISK

- Most common form of acute viral hepatitis in many parts of the world
- In USA, ~180,000 cases annually, representing about 50% of all clinically apparent cases of acute viral hepatitis
- Very common infection in economically developing countries of Africa, Asia, and Latin America; children are frequently sources for outbreaks in crowded households, day care centers, and institutions; ↑ risk of disease is associated with travel to developing countries, men who have sex with men, users of injection and noninjection drugs, persons with clotting-factor disorders
- Health care workers do not appear to be at ↑ risk for occupationally acquired infection
- Patients with chronic liver disease are at risk for fulminant hepatitis A

PERIOPERATIVE RISKS

- Elective surgery should not be performed on patients with acute hepatitis A virus (HAV) infection
- Worsening liver function

WORRY ABOUT

- With fulminant hepatitis A and coagulopathy, encephalopathy, cerebral edema, and multiple organ failure poss; mortality rate > 40%
- Maintenance of liver blood flow and oxygen delivery; metabolism of drugs with hepatic clearance; hypoglycemia; prolonged effect of sedatives

OVERVIEW

- In children <6 y of age, most HAV infections are asymptomatic, whereas among older children and adults, most infections are symptomatic, with jaundice occurring in >70%
- Symptoms do not occur until the viral load in the stool begins to decrease
- Chronic HAV infection does not occur; most acute infections resolve within 2 mo; 10–15% of symptomatic patients have prolonged disease lasting up to 6 mo
- Fulminant hepatitis with acute liver failure occurs in about 0.3% of pts with HAV infection; rate is 1.8% among adults >50 y of age; pts with chronic liver disease are at ↑ risk for fulminant hepatitis when infected with HAV

ICD-9-CM Code: 070.1

ETIOLOGY

- HAV is a 27-nm RNA, nonenveloped virus transmitted by the fecal-oral route by either person-to-person contact or ingestion of contaminated food or water; rarely, HAV has been transmitted by tranfusion of blood or blood products collected from donors during the viremic phase of infection
- Transmission by saliva has not been demonstrated
- HAV infection diagnosed by IgM anti-HAV in the acute phase and IgG anti-HAV occurs later; IgG anti-HAV persists and confers lifelong immunity

USUAL TREATMENT

- Immune globulin
- Hepatitis A vaccine
- Most patients treated at home unless dehydrated; complete recovery usually occurs within 3–6 mo
- Patients with acute liver failure require intensive support and may require liver transplantation

ASSESSMENT POINTS

(The following are for patients with acute hepatitis A or fulminant hepatitis A.)

SYSTEM	EFFECT	ASSESSMENT BY HX	PE	TEST
CV	Hypovolemia	Nausea, vomiting, GI bleed	Tachycardia, hypotension	Orthostatic BP changes; measure CO, SVR
RESP	Hypoxemia		Tachypnea	Oxygen saturation, ABG
GI	Bleeding	Hx of bleeding	Hemoccult + material	Hct, endoscopy
	Jaundice	Dark urine	Icteric sclerae	Bilirubin
	Nausea, vomiting	Nausea, vomiting		
	Hypoalbuminemia		Edema, ascites	Serum albumin
	Hepatitis		Abdominal pain	SGPT, SGOT
ENDO	Hypoglycemia	Altered consciousness		Blood glucose
HEME	Anemia	Tachycardia		Hct
	Thrombocytopenia	Easy bruising	Bruises	Plt count
	Immunosuppression	Infections		
	Coagulopathy	Abnormal bleeding	Bleeding in wounds	PT (low factor V, VII, IX, X, fibrinogen)
RENAL	Hepatorenal syndrome	Oliguria		Urinary Na⁺ low
	Hyponatremia	Altered consciousness, seizures		Serum Na⁺
CNS	Encephalopathy	Mental status exam	Level of consciousness	Serum ammonia level
	Cerebral edema		Level of consciousness	Measure ICP

Key Reference: Koff RS: Hepatitis A (seminar). Lancet 1998; 351:1643–1649.

PERIOPERATIVE IMPLICATIONS

(for patients with acute hepatitis A or fulminant hepatitis A)

Preoperative Preparation

- Elective surgery should be postponed in patients with acute hepatitis A
- Correction of clotting abnormalities with FFP, plts, cryoprecipitate as needed
- Administration of vit K to facilitate production of coagulation factors (prolonged PT), if time permits
- Premedicant depressive or sedative drugs should be avoided

Monitoring

- Arterial line for ABG, electrolytes, glucose, and BP
- Consider central venous or pulmonary artery catheter

Airway

- Consider rapid-sequence induction if nausea, vomiting, or upper GI bleeding exists

Preinduction/Induction

- Consider ketamine or etomidate in hypovolemic patients
- Acute liver failure is not likely to reduce plasma cholinesterase levels, so succinylcholine may be used if indicated
- Increased bioavailability of IV drugs if serum albumin concentration is decreased
- Limit sedative drugs

Maintenance

- Inhalation agent with high inspired oxygen concentration useful for maintaining hepatic blood flow and oxygen supply; should probably avoid halothane

- Effect of muscle relaxants with hepatic clearance may be prolonged
- Increased blood loss with coagulopathy

Extubation

- May need postop mechanical ventilation to ensure time for adequate metabolism of depressant drugs

Adjuvants

- Hypocalcemia may occur with citrate administration

ANTICIPATED PROBLEMS/CONCERNS

- Worsening of hepatic or renal function
- Delayed awakening from prolonged drug metabolism or encephalopathy
- Need to protect airway with reduced consciousness
- Hypoglycemia

HEPATITIS B

Arnold J. Berry, M.D., M.P.H.

RISK

- General population of USA: 3–5% have had the disease and 0.3–1.0% are carriers of hepatitis B virus (HBV)
- High-risk groups include immigrants from endemic areas, IV drug users, homosexual men, household contacts of HBV carriers, patients on hemodialysis, clients in mental institutions
- Before introduction of hepatitis B vaccine, about 20% of susceptible anesthesiologists had serologic evidence of prior hepatitis B infection

PERIOPERATIVE RISKS

- Depends on activity and stage of infection
- Worsening liver function, hepatic encephalopathy, coagulopathy

WORRY ABOUT

- With acute hepatic failure or end-stage liver disease: coagulation abnormalities, ↓ hepatic metabolism of drugs, ↓ levels of plasma cholinesterase, hypoxemia from pulmonary shunting, ascites and Na^+ overload, hepatic encephalopathy, impaired glucose metabolism, portal Htn and GI bleeding, hepatorenal syndrome
- Maintenance of liver BF and O_2 delivery

- Risk of disease transmission to susceptible anesthesia personnel associated with a hepatitis B surface antigen positive needlestick injury may be as great as 30%
- In addition to use of universal precautions by anesthesia personnel, use of sharp devices for invasive procedures should be minimized, and/or safety devices should replace standard sharp devices

OVERVIEW

- Hepatotropic viral infection: 90% have self-limiting acute hepatitis; 1% develop fulminant hepatitis; 10% become chronic HBV carriers with about half of those progressing to chronic active hepatitis, cirrhosis, or hepatocellular carcinoma
- 50% with acute infection asymptomatic whereas others have jaundice, malaise, nausea, abdominal pain
- HBV carriers are diagnosed by persistent positive serology for hepatitis B surface antigen (HBsAg)
- Hepatitis B surface antibody (anti-HBs) confers immunity (after resolution of infection or with immunization)

ICD-9-CM Codes: 070.30 (Acute); 070.32 (Chronic)

ETIOLOGY

- HBV (42-nm DNA virus) carried in and spread by blood and body fluid contact
- Transmitted to health care workers via parenteral or mucocutaneous exposure to HBV-infected blood or body fluids. One in four to one in five exposures causes disease in previously uninfected contact.

USUAL TREATMENT

- Prevention with hepatitis B vaccine
- Protocols should be in place for reporting and follow-up of percutaneous or permucosal exposures to blood or bloody body fluids
- Hepatitis B immune globulin for passive immunization after susceptible individual is exposed
- No specific Rx, bed rest for acute hepatitis B
- Orthotopic liver transplantation for liver failure

ASSESSMENT POINTS

(The following are for patients with fulminant hepatitis or cirrhosis from chronic hepatitis.)

SYSTEM	EFFECT	ASSESSMENT BY HX	PE	TEST
CV	Hyperdynamic circulation		Tachycardia Skin spiders	Measure CO, SVR
RESP	Hypoxemia		Tachypnea	SpO_2
GI	Bleeding Ascites Jaundice Hypoalbuminenia Hepatitis	Hx of bleeding Increasing abdominal girth Dark urine	Ascites, pedal edema Abdominal pain	Hct, endoscopy Bilirubin Serum albumin SGPT, SGOT
ENDO	Hypoglycemia	Altered consciousness		Blood glucose
HEME	Anemia Thrombocytopenia Immunosuppression Coagulopathy	Easy bruisability Infections Abn bleeding	Bruises	Hct Plt count PT (low factors V, VII, IX, X, fibrinogen)
RENAL	Hepatorenal syndrome Hyponatremia Hypokalemia	Altered consciousness, seizures Taking diuretics	Oliguria	Urinary Na^+ Serum Na^+ Serum K^+
CNS	Encephalopathy	Mental status exam	Level of consciousness Asterixis	

Key Reference: Koff RS: Viral hepatitis. *In* Schiff L, Schiff ER (eds): Diseases of the Liver, 7th ed. Philadelphia, JB Lippincott, 1993, pp 492–577.

PERIOPERATIVE IMPLICATIONS

(for patients with end-stage liver disease from hepatitis B)—emergency surgery only with acute infection

Preoperative Preparation

- Correction of clotting abnormalities with FFP, plt, cryoprecipitate as needed
- Administration of vit K to facilitate production of coagulation factors (prolonged PT), if time permits
- Paracentesis if resp compromise from massive ascites

Monitoring

- Arterial line for ABG and BP
- Consider need for central venous or pulmonary artery catheter

Airway

- Consider rapid-sequence induction if patient has ascites or upper GI bleeding

Preinduction/Induction

- Ketamine or etomidate in hypovolemic patients
- Duration of action of succinylcholine may be prolonged
- Increased bioavailability of IV drugs with low serum albumin
- Limit sedative drugs

Maintenance

- Inhalation agent with high FIO_2 useful for maintaining hepatic blood flow; should probably avoid halothane
- Choose muscle relaxants not dependent on liver metabolism
- Increased blood loss with coagulopathy

Extubation

- May need postop ventilation to ensure time for adequate metabolism of depressant drugs

Adjuvants

- Hypocalcemia may occur with citrate administration

ANTICIPATED PROBLEMS/CONCERNS

- Worsening of hepatic or renal function
- Fluid overload
- Delayed awakening from prolonged drug metabolism or encephalopathy
- Need to protect airway with reduced consciousness, esp with upper GI bleeding
- Hypoglycemia

HEPATITIS C

Arnold J. Berry, M.D., M.P.H.

RISK

- Hepatitis C virus (HCV) accounts for most cases of viral hepatitis in the USA with a prevalence of chronic HCV infection of 1.8%
- HCV is responsible for 80–90% of all cases of non-A, non-B hepatitis
- High-risk groups include IV drug users, sexual or household contacts of HCV carriers; transfusions account for 6% of new cases (90% of post-transfusion hepatitis is caused by HCV); increased prevalence in patients on hemodialysis
- About 2–3% of cases occur in health care workers

PERIOPERATIVE RISKS

- Worsening liver function, hepatic encephalopathy, coagulopathy
- Risk of transmission of HCV from carrier to anesthesia personnel is ~2% after percutaneous exposure

WORRY ABOUT

- With end-stage liver disease: coagulation abn, ↓ hepatic metabolism of drugs, ↓ levels of plasma cholinesterase, hypoxemia from pulm shunting, ascites and Na^+ overload, hepatic encephalopathy, glucose metabolism, portal Htn and GI bleeding, hepatorenal syndrome
- Maintenance of liver blood flow and O_2 delivery
- In addition to use of universal precautions by anesthesia personnel, use of sharp devices for invasive procedures should be minimized, and/or safety devices should replace standard sharp devices

OVERVIEW

- Hepatotropic insidious viral infection; fulminant acute hepatitis C rare
- After HCV infecion, 75–85% of patients develop chronic infection with active liver disease in 60–70%; cirrhosis develops in 10–20% of individuals with chronic hepatitis C and hepatocellular carcinoma in 1–5%

- Serologic testing with PCR can help detect anti-HCV in >99% of infected patients within 2 mo of initial infection, but anti-HCV does not correlate with resolution or confer immunity

ICD-9-CM Codes: 070.51 (Acute); 070.54 (Chronic)

ETIOLOGY

- HCV (30–60-nm RNA virus) carried in and transmitted by blood and body fluid contact

USUAL TREATMENT

- Type 1 interferon with or without ribavirin produces a sustained virologic response in up to 50% of infected patients
- Protocols should be in place for reporting and follow-up of percutaneous or permucosal exposures to blood or bloody body fluids; immune globulin and antiviral agents are not recommended for postexposure prophylaxis after occupational HCV exposure
- Orthotopic liver transplantation for liver failure

ASSESSMENT POINTS

(The following are for patients with end-stage liver disease from cirrhosis or chronic hepatitis.)

SYSTEM	EFFECT	ASSESSMENT BY HX	PE	TEST
CV	Hyperdynamic circulation		Tachycardia Telangiectases	Measure CO, SVR
RESP	Hypoxemia		Tachypnea	ABGs
GI	Bleeding Ascites Jaundice Hypoalbuminenia Hepatitis	Hx of bleeding Increasing abdominal girth Dark urine	Hemoccult+ material Fluid wave on abdominal exam Icteric sclerae Ascites, pedal edema Abdominal pain	Hct, endoscopy Bilirubin Serum albumin SGPT, SGOT
ENDO	Hypoglycemia	Altered consciousness		Blood sugar
HEME	Anemia Thrombocytopenia Immunosuppression Coagulopathy	Easy bruisability Infections Abn bleeding	Bruises	Hct Plt count PT (low factors V, VII, IX, X, fibrinogen)
RENAL	Hepatorenal syndrome Hyponatremia Hypokalemia	Altered consciousness, seizures Taking diuretics	Oliguria	Urinary Na^+ low Serum Na^+ Serum K^+
CNS	Encephalopathy	Mental status exam	Level of consciousness Asterixis	

Key Reference: Koff RS: Viral hepatitis. In Schiff L, Schiff ER (eds): Diseases of the Liver, 7th ed. Philadelphia, JB Lippincott, 1993, pp 492–577.

PERIOPERATIVE IMPLICATIONS
(for patients with end-stage liver disease from hepatitis C)

Preoperative Preparation

- Correction of clotting abnormalities with FFP, plt, cryoprecipitate as needed
- Administration of vit K to facilitate production of coagulation factors (prolonged PT), if time permits
- Paracentesis if resp compromise from massive ascites

Monitoring

- Arterial line for ABGs and BP
- Consider central venous or pulm artery catheter

Airway

- Consider rapid-sequence induction with ascites or upper GI bleeding

Preinduction/Induction

- Ketamine or etomidate in hypovolemic patients
- Duration of action of succinylcholine may be prolonged
- Increased bioavailability of IV drugs with low serum albumin
- Limit sedative drugs

Maintenance

- Inhalation agent with high FIO_2 useful for maintaining hepatic blood flow; should probably avoid halothane
- Choose muscle relaxants not dependent on liver metabolism

- Increased blood loss with coagulopathy

Extubation

- May need postop ventilation to ensure time for adequate metabolism of depressant drugs

Adjuvants

- Hypocalcemia may occur with citrate administration

ANTICIPATED PROBLEMS/CONCERNS

- Worsening of hepatic or renal function
- Fluid overload
- Delayed awakening from prolonged drug metabolism or encephalopathy
- Need to protect airway with reduced consciousness, especially with upper GI bleeding
- Hypoglycemia

HEREDITARY HEMORRHAGIC TELANGIECTASIA (OSLER-WEBER-RENDU DISEASE)

Kamla K. Prasad, M.D.

RISK

- Annual incidence in USA: 1/50,000
- Caucasians > other races
- No gender preponderance
- Autosomal dominant inheritance

PERIOPERATIVE RISKS

- Paradoxical air, bland, or septic embolism to brain (due to pulmonary AVMs in 20% of patients)

WORRY ABOUT

- Anemia 2° to hemorrhage, especially recurrent epistaxis
- High incidence of HIV, hepatitis B and C due to frequent transfusions (may exceed 100 units over a lifetime)

OVERVIEW

- A fibrovascular dysplasia
- Triad of telangiectases, AVMs, aneurysms distributed throughout body
- Great variability in severity of vascular lesions and organ dysfunction
- May present as frequent epistaxis, mucosal or GI bleeding, hypoxemia, central neurologic deficit, brain abscess, high-output CHF, or hepatic encephalopathy

ICD-9-CM Code: 448.0

ETIOLOGY

- Autosomal dominant disease with variable penetrance

USUAL TREATMENT

- High-dose progesterone and estrogen therapy (may increase risk of thromboembolism)
- Multiple transfusions

ASSESSMENT POINTS

SYSTEM	EFFECT	ASSESSMENT BY HX	PE	TEST
HEENT	Nasopharyngeal AVMs	Frequent epistaxis		
CV	High-output CHF Thromboembolism		Rales Neurologic deficit	CXR
RESP	AVMs/hypoxemia (R → L shunting)	Fatigue Exertional dyspnea Hemoptysis Hemothorax	Cyanosis Clubbing	ABGs CXR (rounded homogeneous masses of consistent density, rib notching)
HEPATIC	Hepatic failure (L → R shunting)	Bleeding Jaundice		PT, PTT LFTs
HEME	Anemia Coagulopathy	Recurrent epistaxis	Pallor	CBC Bleeding time (↓ plt aggregation) PT, PTT (factor XI deficiency, hepatic failure)
CNS	Paradoxical embolism	CVA Bacterial encephalitis Brain abscess	Neurologic deficits Fever	Brain CT Diagnostic lumbar puncture

Key Reference: Radu C, Reich DL, Tamman R: Anesthetic considerations in a cardiac surgical patient with Osler-Weber-Rendu disease. J Cardiothorac Vasc Anesth 1992; 6:461–464.

PERIOPERATIVE IMPLICATIONS

Preoperative Preparation

- Debubble IV lines to prevent paradoxical air embolism
- Meticulous aseptic line techniques to avoid septic embolism to brain

Monitoring

- Presence of esophageal varices or AVMs increase risk of esophageal stethoscope placement and gastric suctioning

Airway

- Risk of airway hemorrhage if oropharyngeal telangiectases
- Nasal intubation contraindicated if nasal telangiectases

Maintenance

- Risk of hepatic failure and high-output CHF modify anesthetic management

Postoperative Period

- Immobilization may predispose to CNS embolism

Adjuvants

- Precipitation of incompatible drugs in IV line or peripheral vein may send particulate matter to brain; avoid by careful technique and filter
- Prophylactic antibiotics to decrease risk of aerobic and anaerobic CNS infections
- NSAIDs, including ketorolac, may precipitate GI or mucosal bleeding
- Regional: AVMs may be present in epidural space

ANTICIPATED PROBLEMS/CONCERNS

- Anemia due to recurrent bleeding
- Transfusion is complicated: Low hematocrit may increase the risk of high-output CHF by increasing extent of arteriovenous shunting (↓ viscosity effect), but a high Hct may increase risk of thromboembolism
- Coagulopathy: Multiple hemostatic defects, including low-grade DIC, reduced plt aggregation, and factor XI deficiency, may aggravate bleeding caused by local vessel wall pathology
- Paradoxical embolism: Owing to pulmonary AVMs, peripheral microemboli (air, bland, or septic) bypass normal pulmonary capillary filtering and embolize, causing transient or permanent neurologic defects or brain abscess

HERNIATED NUCLEUS PULPOSUS Garfield B. Russell, M.D., F.R.C.P.C.

RISK

- Incidence: 1% of low back pain; cervical 1/1 million individuals
- Can be lumbar (most common), cervical, or thoracic (least common)
- 70% of adults experience low back pain; 40% experience sciatica
- 4–6% of the population experience clinically significant sciatica
- 20% of sciatica is caused by lumbar herniation
- Lumbar disks most prevalent ages 25–40 y
- Race with highest prevalence: none

PERIOPERATIVE RISKS

- Mortality rare: 0–0.5%
- Related to underlying conditions

WORRY ABOUT

- Associated psychologic problems if pain has been chronic; possible medications—narcotics, muscle relaxants, tranquilizers, antidepressants
- Potential litigious issues if injury is job- or accident-related

OVERVIEW

- Occurs in relatively healthy patients without increased risk for significant end-organ disease
- Injury risks of patient positioning:
  – Patients may be supine with arms tucked (cervical disks), prone on bolsters, prone on a Wilson frame, prone on an Andrew's table, in the Georgia-prone position (lumbar disks), in the lateral decubitus position (lumbar or anterior approaches to thoracic disks)
  – If supine, these include peripheral nerve injury (particularly ulnar) from poorly padded arm tucking, hyperextension injuries of the cervical spine, corneal abrasions
  – If prone, these include
    • Eyes—corneal abrasions, retinal artery or vein thrombosis from pressure, associated blindness, scleral edema
    • Nose—pressure necrosis
    • Mouth/pharynx—glossal edema, laryngeal edema, ETT kinking, pressure necrosis from poorly positioned oral airways.
    • Larynx/trachea—vocal cord paralysis 2° to recurrent laryngeal nerve pressure between retractor and ETT; mucosal injury from N$_2$O expanded ETT balloon H-retraction
    • CV— ↓ venous return and associated hypotension, particularly if in Georgia-prone position; venous air embolism—the free abdomen may generate pressure gradient in the IVC in relation to the surgical incision, allowing air to be entrained; the incidence is unknown
    • Resp—respiratory compromise if abdomen and diaphragm are not free and dependent. The ETT is at risk if not well secured.
  • GI—patients prone to reflux may experience passive regurgitation
- If substantial bone decompression is required with instrumentation for fusion, considerable blood loss is possible
- If bone fusion with a harvested bone graft, there is often postop discomfort from the site in excess of that from the diskectomy

ICD-9-CM Code: 722

ETIOLOGY

- Trauma
- Degenerative changes
- Risk factors include frequent lifting of objects >25 lb, exposure to whole-body vibration, cigarette smoking, narrow lumbar vertebral canals

USUAL TREATMENT

- Medical therapy with short period of rest, physical therapy, analgesics, muscle relaxants, and behavioral modification with a continued exercise program are usually successful
- Chemonucleolysis—much less frequently practiced because of anaphylactic reactions to chymopapain
- Traction
- Manipulation
- Surgical diskectomy

ASSESSMENT POINTS

SYSTEM	EFFECT	ASSESSMENT BY HX	PE	TEST
HEENT	↓ ROM, pain, difficult airway	Pain and limited ROM	Neck ROM	Cervical spine x-rays usually available for C-spine cases
CV	None primary	Predispositions: rheumatoid arthritis, obesity, family Hx	Murmurs Weight	None usually needed
CNS	None usual	Personality changes with pain or analgesic dependency	None	None usual
PNS	Pain ↓ Strength ↓ Sensation	New pain, paresthesias Impotence Bowel and urinary incontinence	Strength and sensory evaluation	None usual, possible EMG
MS	Muscle wasting Muscle spasm Limited motion Pain with activity	Strength changes Mobility	Spine ROM	None usual

Key Reference: Shapiro HM, Drummond JC: Miller's Anesthesia, 4th ed. New York, Churchill Livingstone, 1994, pp 1777–1779.

PERIOPERATIVE IMPLICATIONS

Preoperative Preparation
- Continued analgesia if necessary

Monitoring
- Routine
- Dermatomal somatosensory evoked potentials (dSSEP) have questionable clinical and practical applicability
- If spinal instrumentation with pedicle screw fixation used, free-run and triggered EMG monitor for bone cortex disruption and possible nerve root injury

Airway
- Associated with poor neck mobility and possible worsening with "sniffing" position
- Reinforced endotracheal tube
- Consider nasal endotracheal tubes for anterior cervical disks
- Fiberoptic intubation should be considered for patient with limited mobility, myelopathy, and associated stenosis of the spinal canal
- In particular, for anterior cervical diskectomy, ensure endotracheal balloon is not overfilled. Consider deflating and reinflating or decreasing air volume in balloon during cases, in particular if N$_2$O is administered.
- Light wand option to minimize flexion/extension

Induction
- Routine

Maintenance
- Simple lumbar diskectomies can be done with regional anesthesia (spinal preferable to epidural)

Extubation
- Prone positioning predisposes to significant upper airway edema
- Cervical disk patients may have a soft or hard neck collar in place

Adjuvants
- Some prefer no or limited NMB
- If neurophysiologic monitoring used: NMB can alter EMG, and many anesthetics, particularly volatile agents, interfere with dSSEP recording
- For anterior cervical diskectomies, esophageal stethoscope affords reliable landmark for the esophagus

Postoperative Period
- Analgesia requirements depend on surgical approach

ANTICIPATED PROBLEMS/CONCERNS

- Resolution of airway/facial/scleral edema for those positioned prone, particularly for longer cases
- Atelectasis after thoracic surgery
- Interference with swallowing by edema and discomfort from cervical surgery, particularly the anterior approach
- Possible postop stridor due to hematoma development after anterior cervical surgery

HERPES, TYPE 1

Eugene Y. Cheng, M.D., F.C.C.M.

RISK

- Rare in the immunocompetent host
- Frequency and severity markedly increased in patients with AIDS, hematologic and lymphoreticular malignancies, or recent organ transplantation

PERIOPERATIVE RISKS

- No evidence that surgery or anesthetics affect extent or duration of infection

WORRY ABOUT

- Transmitting infection to uninfected
- ↑ Risk of spreading HSV to other sites through examination or instrumentation
- Secondary infection of herpetic lesions with bacteria or fungi

OVERVIEW

- Transient viremia common; abnormal nonspecific and immune defenses unable to limit virus replication and spread, esp in immunosuppressed patients

- HSV-1 is often acquired during childhood and can cause gingivostomatitis, marked by fever and ulcers around the mouth and lips
- Recurrent infection slow to resolve and more likely to spread by contiguous extension
- Disseminated viral skin infection is usually self-limiting and resolves in 7–14 days
- Dx: Gold standard—viral culture; early in the course of infection, cultures are positive 80–90% of the time
- Rapid Dx:
  – Tzanck smear, positive approximately 50% of the time that a viral culture is positive
  – Direct fluorescent antibody testing, positive approximately 75% of the time that a viral culture is positive
  – Newer methods not widely used: enzyme immunoassay, PCR, DNA hybridization

ICD-9-CM Codes: 054.7 (Infection with specified complications); 054.8 (Infection with unspecified complications)

ETIOLOGY

- Ubiquitous human virus; HSV-1 responsible for 90% of infections above waist. Approx 80% of genital herpetic lesions caused by HSV-2 (genital herpes). In the family of Herpesviridae; other human herpesviruses are varicella-zoster (HHV-3), Epstein-Barr virus (HHV-4), cytomegalovirus (HHV-5), and human herpesvirus 6 (HHV-6).
- Humans the only natural reservoir; no vectors are involved with transmission
- Intact immune system will not prevent infection, but differences in immune system produce variations in pattern of disease (e.g., asymptomatic or disseminated)

USUAL TREATMENT

- Acyclovir for acute or recurrent infections; reduces viral shedding, lesion healing time, and symptoms
- Famciclovir and valaciclovir: mechanism of action is the same as acyclovir but offer improved oral bioavailability and more convenient dosing
- Foscarnet or vidarabine for acyclovir-resistant mutants

ASSESSMENT POINTS

SYSTEM	EFFECT	ASSESSMENT BY HX	PE	TEST
RESP	Pneumonitis	Aspiration of oral secretions; previous HSV esophagitis	Bilateral crackles	CXR—bilateral interstitial infiltrates
GI	Esophagitis	Odynophagia, dysphagia, substernal pain	Multiple shallow mucosal ulcers	
GU	Cystitis			
CNS	Encephalitis Meningitis	Headache, confusion, lethargy	Anosmia, memory loss, expressive aphasia, focal seizures	Brain biopsy
DERM	Cutaneous ulcers	Recurrent painful skin or mucosal ulcers	Multiple vesicular lesions on an erythematous base with subsequent ulceration	
	Stevens-Johnson syndrome	Extensive painful skin lesions	Deep bullous-erosive lesions	

Key References: Balfour HH: Antiviral drugs. N Engl J Med 1999; 340:1255–1268; Whitley RJ, Kimberlin DW, Roizman B: Herpes simplex viruses. Clin Infect Dis 1998; 26:541–555.

PERIOPERATIVE IMPLICATIONS

Preoperative Preparation

- Cover exposed herpetic lesions
- Strict adherence to universal precautions

Monitoring

- Avoid inserting catheters through any herpetic infected areas

Regional Anesthesia

- Contraindicated if needle must be inserted through herpetic infected area

Postoperative Period

- Thorough disinfection of any surface area that might have been in contact with oral secretions or herpetic lesions

ANTICIPATED PROBLEMS/CONCERNS

- No effective pre- or postexposure prophylaxis
- Most effective therapy is high-dose intravenous acyclovir for at least 10–14 days

HERPES, TYPE 2

Rosa M. Navarro, M.D.
Woo Chan Kim, M.D.

RISK

- People within USA: Estimated 40–60 million
- Highest prevalence in women, African-Americans, and lower socioeconomic groups
- Frequency and severity of infection increased in immunocompromised patients
- Incidence of neonatal HSV infection estimated at 1/2000–1/5000 deliveries

PERIOPERATIVE RISKS

- Vertical transmission from infected mother to fetus during vaginal birth
- Intrauterine fetal infection after rupture of membranes

WORRY ABOUT

- Transmission of infection to health care personnel resulting in herpetic whitlow via inoculation of virus into fingers
- Neonatal herpetic infection during vaginal births
- Viremia 2° to needle placement within infected area during regional anesthesia
- Extension of genital infection to adjacent areas during examination and instrumentation
- Secondary bacterial or fungal infection of herpetic lesions

OVERVIEW

- Causative primarily of infections below waist transmitted by sexual contact
- Maternal primary HSV-2 infection associated with spontaneous abortion
- Newborns infected with HSV-2 during vaginal delivery from the mother's genital infection (high neonatal mortality)
- Primary genital HSV-2 infection with highest incidence of systemic symptoms (malaise, fever, headache, myalgias)
- Latent infection remains dormant in sensory ganglia innervating infected area until reactivation
- Recurrent infection involves vesicular, ulcerative lesions in genital tract, labia, vulva, perineum, cervix, urethra
- Neuraxial opioid anesthesia does not reactivate or increase risk of recurrent genital HSV-2 infection
- Chronic recurrent HSV-2 infection associated with development of cervical cancer
- Diagnosis by viral culture most sensitive and specific (rapid Dx by Tzanck smear)

ICD-9-CM Codes: 054.9 (Infection); 771.2 (Congenital)

ETIOLOGY

- Double-stranded DNA virus in family of Herpesviridae
- Acquired genital infection primarily by sexual transmission of HSV-2
- Immunosuppression and increased number of sexual partners are risk factors for acquisition
- Diagnosed by multinucleated giant epithelial cells with intranuclear inclusion bodies on Giemsa stain smears (Tzanck preparation) taken from vesicle or tissue biopsy

USUAL TREATMENT

- IV acyclovir for neonatal HSV-2 infection
- Oral acyclovir and topical cream shorten duration of lesions for recurrent infections
- Most recommend that full-term parturients with visible genital lesions (especially primary infection) undergo abdominal delivery to decrease incidence of neonatal HSV infection

ASSESSMENT POINTS (PRIMARY AND RECURRENT)

SYSTEM	EFFECT	ASSESSMENT BY HX	PE	TEST
HEENT	Pharyngitis (primary)		Cervical adenopathy Mucosal ulceration	
GU (mucous membranes)	Cystitis (primary) Genital ulcers (recurrent)	Dysuria	Vaginal or urethral discharge Ulcerated lesions of penis or labia or cervix	Viral culture Tzanck smear; direct immunofluorescent assay Biopsy; intranuclear inclusion bodies
LYMPHATICS		Lymphadenopathy	Tender inguinal nodes	
SKIN	Herpetic whitlow (recurrent)	Painful vesicular or papular lesion	Pain	Tzanck smear
CNS	Aseptic meningitis (primary)	Headache	Cauda equina syndrome	
RECTAL	Herpes proctitis (primary)	Constipation Tenesmus Discharge		Proctosigmoidoscopy

Key Reference: Suligoi B, Cusan M, Santopadre P, Palu G, Catania S, Girelli G, Pala S, Vullo V: HSV-2 specific seroprevalance among various populations in Rome, Italy: the Italian Herpes Management Forum. Sex Transm Infect 2000; 76: 213–214.

PERIOPERATIVE IMPLICATIONS

Preoperative Preparation
- Universal precautions

Monitoring
- Routine

Regional Anesthesia
- Needle placement in infected area contraindicated 2° to risk of viremia and local extension into deep tissues
- Preferred in pregnant women with recurrent infection, no systemic symptoms, and no infection in area of block placement

Postoperative Period
- Universal precautions

ANTICIPATED PROBLEMS/CONCERNS

- Difficulty identifying asymptomatic carriers of HSV-2 with viral shedding
- No effective prophylaxis for newborns

HIRSCHSPRUNG'S DISEASE
Toni Anne Washington, M.D.

RISK
- Incidence: 1:5000 live births
- Male predominance 3.8:1
- Positive family history in 7%
- Associated with trisomy 21 (3–10%) and neural crest cell migrational disorders including congenital hypoventilation syndrome, Waardenburg's syndrome, and neuroblastoma

PERIOPERATIVE RISKS
- Intestinal obstruction with full stomach
- Hypovolemia
- Electrolyte abnormalities

WORRY ABOUT
- Abdominal distention/intestinal obstruction leading to regurgitation and aspiration
- Vomiting and diarrhea may result in electrolyte and fluid abnormalities
- Enterocolitis characterized by dehydration and septic shock (mortality 30%)
- Intestinal ischemia, perforation, and peritonitis leading to increases in third space losses

OVERVIEW
- Presentation variable from mild abdominal distention and stool retention to severe with toxic megacolon, enterocolitis, peritonitis, or perforation
- Diagnosis made 15% <1 mo, 64% <3 mo, 80% <1 y

ICD-9-CM Code: 751.3

ETIOLOGY
- Absence of ganglion cells in the bowel wall results in functional intestinal obstruction and distention of the normal proximal bowel
- Expression of inhibitory parasympathetic nerves is interrupted and relaxation of the bowel is inhibited, resulting in constant contraction of the aganglionic segment, internal anal sphincter, and anal canal
- Aganglionic region involves varying lengths of colon and is limited to the rectosigmoid region in 75% of cases; 8% of patients will have total colonic aganglionosis

USUAL TREATMENT
- Surgical resection of the aganglionic segment, operative mortality <1%
- Varying methods of staged repairs (Swenson, Duhamel, and Soave). Initial colostomy is created for decompression of the dilated proximal bowel. Resection of the aganglionic segment and colon pull-through with simultaneous or subsequent ostomy closure is performed 6–12 mo later.
- Newer techniques include laparoscopic-assisted endorectal pull-through. Colon and rectum are mobilized laparoscopically, and endorectal dissection is done through the anus. Primary single-stage transanal Soave without colostomy or intra-abdominal dissection is being performed in neonates with disease confined to the distal descending colon.
- Laparoscopic and single-stage procedures shorten postop recovery. On average, patients pass stool within the first 24 h, start feeds within 24–48 h, and are discharged in 3–4 days.

ASSESSMENT POINTS

SYSTEM	EFFECT	ASSESSMENT BY HX	PE	TEST
CV	Hypovolemia	UO IV replacement Extent of vomiting	Mucous membranes Orthostatic vital signs	BUN and Cr BUN/Cr ratio
GI	Intestinal obstruction	No meconium Diarrhea Vomiting Wasting	Mass in abdomen No feces in rectum Protruding abdomen	Abdominal films Barium enema

Key Reference: Motoyama EK, Davis PJ: Smith's Anesthesia for Infants and Children. St. Louis, CV Mosby, 1990, pp 598–599.

PERIOPERATIVE IMPLICATIONS

Preoperative Implications
- Assessment of volume status due to bowel preparation, vomiting, and diarrhea
- Consider other congenital anomalies

Monitoring
- Routine

Airway
- None other than those related to newborns or associated syndromes

Induction
- Consider need for rapid-sequence induction
- Monitor BP as anesthesia is deepened

Maintenance
- Prevent heat loss
- Need for muscle relaxation
- Premature infants: concern for retrolental fibroplasia and hyperoxia
- Consider combined general and regional anesthesia for profound relaxation of anal sphincter muscles and reduction of need for IV narcotics or muscle relaxation

Extubation
- Awake

Postoperative Period
- Concern regarding apnea in newborns receiving narcotics
- Association with congenital hypoventilation syndrome
- Postop pain management with continuous epidural anesthesia. Consider epidural catheter if concern exists with caudal catheters and fecal soiling.

Adjuvants
- Concern about apnea after opioids in newborns

ANTICIPATED PROBLEMS/CONCERNS
- Aspiration pneumonitis
- Postop surgical complications occur in 15–40% of cases and include disrupted anastomosis, fecal incontinence, constipation due to retained aganglionic segment, and enterocolitis
- Definitive treatment of complications may require operative management involving a redo pull-through procedure, fecal diversion, or anorectal myomectomy
- Postop enterocolitis carries a 30% mortality, with deaths occurring more than 2 y after uncomplicated surgical repair

HISTIOCYTOSIS
Hugh L. Preas II, M.D.

RISK

- Langerhans cell histiocytosis (LCH)
  - 3–4/million
  - Males:females, 2:1
  - Peak incidence at 1–3 y of age
- Hemophagocytic lymphohistiocytosis (HLH), primary or secondary
  - 1.2/million persons/y
  - Males = females
  - 1° HLH: 70% of cases present at <1 y of age
  - 2° HLH (infectious): 50% of cases present at <3 y of age
  - 2° HLH (malignancy): all ages

PERIOPERATIVE RISKS

- Depends on organ system involved and extent of dysfunction

WORRY ABOUT

- Specific organ dysfunction caused by infiltration with reactive histiocytes including hepatic, pulmonary, bone marrow, hypothalamic, and bone (lytic lesions, especially head and face, can include vertebrae and other bones)
- Treated with steroids and chemotherapy; may require perioperative steroid supplementation
- Diabetes insipidus due to infiltration of hypothalamus

OVERVIEW

- Clinical syndromes involving infiltration of organs with histiocytes or macrophages. Severity of clinical symptoms varies markedly. Can involve primarily skin and/or bone or liver, lung, or brain.
- Limited or progressive and fatal. Younger children with multiple or severe organ involvement have a high mortality.
- Clinical presentation in first decade of life

ICD-9-CM Codes: 277.8, (Acute chronic, subacute); 202.3 (Malignant)

ETIOLOGY

- LCH: Genetic pattern
- HLH: Genetic pattern (autosomal recessive) for 1° HLH, infectious or malignant etiology for 2° HLH

USUAL TREATMENT

- Chemotherapy (vinblastine, etoposide, mercaptopurine, doxorubicin, cyclophosphamide, methotrexate, others) and steroids
- Nonsteroidal agents for bone lesions
- Surgery required for biopsy and diagnosis, lytic bone lesions, and occasionally splenectomy
- Orthotopic liver or lung transplantation has been performed for end-stage disease
- Radiation therapy (bone lesions, pituitary disease)
- Bone marrow or stem cell transplant
- Immunomodulatory agents (cyclosporine A, antithymocyte globulin, FK-506, others)

ASSESSMENT POINTS

SYSTEM	EFFECT	ASSESSMENT BY HX	PE	TEST
HEENT	Soft tissue distortion of airway, loose teeth		Airway and dental evaluation	
RESP	Pneumothorax, reactive airways, infiltrates, fibrosis	Wheezing, dyspnea		CXR, ABGs, PFTs
GI	Ulceration, obstruction Hepatic dysfunction		Jaundice Hepatomegaly	Bilirubin SGOT, SGPT PT
CNS	Diabetes insipidus, neuropathy, exophthalmos	Polyuria, polydipsia	Neuro exam	Urine and serum Osm, electrolytes
HEME	Thrombocytopenia, anemia, leukopenia	Bruising or bleeding	Splenomegaly	CBC

Key Reference: Huang F, Arceci R: The histiocytoses of infancy. Semin Perinatol 1999; 23:319–331.

PERIOPERATIVE IMPLICATIONS

Preoperative Preparation
- Indicated by degree of organ dysfunction

Monitoring
- Routine

Airway
- Airway soft tissue or mandibular involvement may distort anatomy

Preinduction/Induction
- Usual precautions depending on severity of organ involvement

Maintenance
- Usual precautions depending on severity of organ involvement

Extubation
- If anatomy distorted and airway difficult, consider awake extubation

Adjuvants
- Vary depending on hepatic function

ANTICIPATED PROBLEMS/CONCERNS

- Organ dysfunction (hepatic, pulmonary, hematologic, hypothalamic, or bone)
- Diabetes insipidus
- Adrenal suppression due to chronic steroid therapy

HYDROCEPHALUS

Joseph R. Tobin, M.D.

RISK

- Newborns and children with anatomic CNS abnormalities (including myelomeningocele)
- Head trauma and intracranial hemorrhage patients
- CNS tumors
- Meningitis

PERIOPERATIVE RISKS

- Cerebral ischemia and neurologic sequelae
- Impaired airway reflexes, level of consciousness, gastric emptying
- Cardiorespiratory arrest

WORRY ABOUT

- Intracranial Htn
- Persistent nausea and vomiting
- Bradycardia
- Decreased level of consciousness

OVERVIEW

- Excess accumulation of CSF due to obstruction in normal CSF flow pattern from ventricular system to cortical surface (obstructive hydrocephalus); or from impaired reabsorption of CSF at arachnoid villi (communicating hydrocephalus)

- Slow progressive hydrocephalus well tolerated for weeks with slowly worsening symptoms (headache, nausea, papilledema)
- Acute hydrocephalus results in acute symptoms and may be life-threatening owing to herniation of brain with catastrophic ischemic injury; bradycardia, Htn, depressed level of consciousness, depressed airway reflexes and respiratory drive, and gastric atony

ICD-9-CM Codes: 331.4 (Obstructive); 331.3 (Communicating)

ETIOLOGY

Congenital

- Anatomic abnormalities: aqueductal stenosis, Arnold-Chiari malformation, Dandy-Walker syndrome

Posthemorrhagic/Post-traumatic

- Intraventricular hemorrhage (newborns or adults) with blood clot in ventricular system

Neoplastic

- Brain tumor obstructing normal CSF flow

Postinflammatory

- Meningitis, abscess, meningoencephalitis

USUAL TREATMENT

- Surgical correction of underlying cause or CSF diversion procedures (ventriculoperitoneal, ventriculoatrial, or lumboperitoneal shunts)
- Glucocorticoids are used acutely to diminish edema associated with neoplasm or abscess and may diminish associated intracranial Htn
- Acetazolamide to diminish CSF production
- Furosemide to acutely decrease cerebrovascular volume
- Mannitol to decrease ICP

ASSESSMENT POINTS

SYSTEM	EFFECT	ASSESSMENT BY HX	PE	TEST
CV	Bradycardia, Htn		Pulse, BP	
RESP	Impaired respiratory drive and airway reflexes		Cranial nerve exam, stridor Swallowing abnormalities	Pulse oximetry
GI	Nausea, vomiting, aspiration Abnormal feeding	Hx of progression of nausea/vomiting		
CNS	Depressed level of consciousness Increased ICP Headache	Timing of onset	Arousability and neurologic exam Tense fontanel, inferior eye deviation	CT scan

Key Reference: Cheek WR (ed): Pediatric Neurosurgery: Surgery of the Developing Nervous System. Philadelphia, WB Saunders, 1994.

PERIOPERATIVE IMPLICATIONS

Preoperative Preparation

- Assessment of urgency of presentation. Catastrophic increased ICP requires emergent intubation and hyperventilation. In young infants, direct neurosurgical needle puncture of a proximal lateral ventricle or previously inserted shunt may diminish ICP sufficiently to avoid a catastrophe.
- Secure IV access if possible

Monitoring

- Level of consciousness
- Routine

Airway

- Head up 10–20° and midline may diminish ICP
- Aspiration risk due to gastric atony

Preinduction/Induction

- Sedatives usually not indicated so that resp compromise or sedation does not increase ICP. Minimal sedation or use of local anesthetic to secure IV access without causing increased ICP due to pain, crying, or struggling.
- Rapid-sequence IV induction preferred (because of aspiration risk) unless in doubt of airway anatomy

- Debate over use of succinylcholine vs. rapid-onset nondepolarizing muscle relaxant (rocuronium or rapacuronium); thiopental, propofol, or etomidate IV agents preferred; avoid ketamine
- Mask induction may increase ICP by increasing cerebral blood volume. Sevoflurane may be the preferable agent for inhalation induction (well tolerated and minimal effects on cerebrovascular tone). Isoflurane and desflurane are associated with coughing and are not recommended for induction.
- Lidocaine 1–1.5 mg/kg IV may be useful adjunct to minimize increase in ICP due to laryngoscopy and endotracheal intubation

Maintenance

- Volatile anesthetic (most commonly sevoflurane or isoflurane) < 1 MAC, N_2O 0–70% (debatable), and opioid (i.e., fentanyl 2–5 μg/kg or equivalent)
- Maintain normothermia, cardiac output. Hyperventilation may be acutely helpful until CSF is diverted and ICP reduced.
- Normal saline at restricted or maintenance rate. Glucose support only for infants, and avoid hyperglycemia.

Extubation

- Ensure return of airway reflexes, level of consciousness, and respiratory drive
- Failure of achieving above criteria may require CT scan and/or ICU monitoring

Postoperative Period

- Usually unremarkable; depressed level of consciousness is concern for perioperative ischemic insult or hemorrhage
- EBL: minimal

Adjuvants

- Lidocaine, mannitol, furosemide, spontaneous hyperventilation by patient

ANTICIPATED PROBLEMS/CONCERNS

- Immediate postop neurologic exam should demonstrate improvement. If not improved, urgent CT scan and secure airway must be maintained. Postop ICU admission not required unless impaired neurologic status continues.

HYPERALDOSTERONISM (SECONDARY) Matthew K. Miller, M.D.

RISK

- Renovascular hypertension, found in 0.2–5% of the general population
- Malignant hypertension accompanied by intense secondary hyperaldosteronism
- Renin-producing tumors rare and usually found in young adults, producing severe hypertension and often severe hypokalemia
- Pregnancy is associated with a state of intense secondary aldosteronism
- ESRD results in some features of secondary hyperaldosteronism

PERIOPERATIVE RISKS

- Electrolyte disturbances (K^+, Na^+, Mg^{2+})
- Acid-base imbalance (metabolic alkalosis)
- Htn
- Volume disturbances ($\uparrow$ extracellular fluid volume, CHF, or hypovolemia, depending on etiology and preoperative therapy)

WORRY ABOUT

- Perioperative control of Htn and intravascular fluid volume
- Correction of hypokalemia and monitoring of acid-base balance
- Potential for $\downarrow$ BP when exposed to anesthetic, PPV, and changes in position
- Skeletal muscle weakness 2° to hypokalemia

OVERVIEW

- Secondary hyperaldosteronism occurs in states of low effective arterial blood volume, which activates the renin-angiotensin-aldosterone axis
- Renin acts as a proteolytic enzyme on angiotensinogen to yield angiotensin I
- Angiotensin I is converted to angiotensin II
- Angiotensin II acts on the adrenal gland to stimulate release of aldosterone
- Angiotensin II is a potent vasoconstrictor
- Aldosterone stimulates distal tubule reabsorption of Na^+ by the kidney to restore blood volume; $\uparrow$ H^+ and K^+ secretion
- In sustained states of hyperaldosteronism, the force for Na^+ reabsorption is transient and balanced by other factors, leaving only mild hypernatremia and volume excess; in contrast, the force for K^+ secretion and excretion remains elevated and may result in severe hypokalemia
- The ratio of plasma aldosterone (PA) to plasma renin activity (PRA) can differentiate between primary and secondary hyperaldosteronism; high (>50) PA/PRA ratio is associated with primary hyperaldosteronism, normal PA/PRA ratio is seen in secondary hyperaldosteronism

ICD-9-CM Code: 255.1

ETIOLOGY

- Associated with hypertension and edematous states (e.g., CHF, cirrhosis with ascites)
- Occurs in patients with dysfunctional kidneys that have areas of patchy ischemic kidney tissue in addition to areas of normal tissue
- Physiologically beneficial in pregnancy, ESRD
- Pathophysiologic in renovascular hypertension, malignant hypertension, and renin-producing tumors
- Iatrogenic in intestinal diversion (where GI structures are used for urinary diversion) and possibly in cyclosporine-induced hypertension
- All etiologies result in $\uparrow$ renin activity and ultimately $\uparrow$ aldosterone levels

USUAL TREATMENT

- As indicated: antihypertensive therapy, volume correction, K^+ replacement, and spironolactone
- Treatment of underlying disorder(s)

ASSESSMENT POINTS

SYSTEM	EFFECT	ASSESSMENT BY HX	PE	TEST
CV	Htn, fluid overload, overdiuresis	Dizziness, syncope	Edema, jugulovenous distention, diastolic Htn, S_3	ECG, CXR, invasive pressure monitoring
RESP	CHF	Dyspnea, orthopnea	Tachypnea, rales, wheezing	CXR, ABGs
GI	Associated with cirrhosis and ascites, urinary diversion to GI tract, excessive GI fluid loss	Liver disease, prior surgical Hx, severe vomiting or diarrhea, laxative or diuretic abuse	Ascites, postural hypotension, edema, spider angiomata	Na^+, K^+, HCO_3^-, Mg^{2+}
RENAL	Decreased glomerular filtration, severe K^+ depletion, renovascular Htn	Renal disease, Htn, muscle weakness	Edema, muscle wasting, severe Htn	Na^+, K^+, HCO_3^- ABG for acid-base status Consider Ca^{2+}, PO_4^-, Mg^{2+}, BUN/Cr, urine lytes Plasma aldosterone and plasma renin activity
MS	Muscle weakness, prolonged effects of NMB agents	Easy fatigability, muscle weakness	Muscle wasting, decreased muscle strength	Directed neurologic exam K^+

Key Reference: Corry DB, Tuck MF: Secondary aldosteronism. Endocr Metab Clin N Am 1995; 24:511–529.

PERIOPERATIVE IMPLICATIONS

Preoperative Preparation

- Assess and correct intravascular volume; if diuresis is needed consider spironolactone
- Assess and control BP
- Assess and correct electrolyte abnormalities, especially K^+, Mg^{2+}, Na^+, and HCO_3^-
- Determine etiology of hyperaldosteronism and correct underlying cause if possible

Monitoring

- Consider CVP or PA catheter for assessment of volume
- Consider arterial line if BP is labile
- Closely monitor neuromuscular blockade

Airway

- Routine, unless obesity or severe edema is present

Preinduction/Induction

- Consider volume status, BP, potential for K^+ shifts, and underlying disease state (e.g., CHF, hepatic insufficiency)

Maintenance

- Intravascular volume abnormalities can result in labile BP, especially with vasodilating effects of some anesthetic agents and PPV
- Hypokalemia may prolong NMB
- Hyperventilation and alkalosis may exacerbate hypokalemia
- Consider intraoperative ABGs
- In patients with intrinsic renal disease, consider avoiding enflurane and sevoflurane

Extubation

- Ensure return of neuromuscular function

Postoperative Period

- Continue monitoring of BP, volume, lytes

Adjuvants

- Hypokalemia may prolong and potentiate effects of NMB agents
- Altered distribution and clearance of some drugs secondary to abnormal intravascular fluid volume as well as hepatic and renal dysfunction secondary to underlying disease state(s)

ANTICIPATED PROBLEMS/CONCERNS

- Labile BP
- Exacerbation of end-organ hypoperfusion
- Poor myocardial performance in patients with underlying CHF

HYPERCALCEMIA

Michelle Braunfeld, M.D.

RISK

- Most often due to hyperparathyroidism in ambulatory outpatient—risk increased age >50 y
- Most often due to malignancy in hospitalized patient
- Female > male (2.5:1)
- 0.15%/y (1.5/1000 persons/y)

PERIOPERATIVE RISKS

- Hypovolemia and acid-base abnormalities
- Renal insufficiency
- Other electrolyte abnormalities, esp phosphorus, Mg^{2+}
- Full stomach and (in)ability to protect airway with altered mental status

WORRY ABOUT

- Volume status
- PUD associated with primary hyperparathyroidism
- Other manifestations of underlying disease, e.g., cardiopulmonary status in sarcoid, lytic bone lesions (esp in spine) in patient with malignancy with pathologic fractures
- Fluid overload and sodium retention with Rx
- Pancreatitis, esp with hyperparathyroidism

OVERVIEW

- Multifactorial medical problem that requires both supportive therapy and attention to underlying problem
- One in spectrum of problems associated with underlying disease or may be due to treatment of that disease (e.g., milk-alkali syndrome in PUD)
- Therapy includes volume replacement and possible further fluid/Lasix administration to induce Ca^{2+} excretion in exchange for Na^+

ICD-9-CM Code: 275.4

ETIOLOGY

- Increased GI absorption (e.g., milk-alkali syndrome), sarcoid
- Increased bone resorption (e.g., hyperparathyroidism) malignancy (8% renal cell carcinoma; 20% of squamous carcinomas including lung, female genital tract, head and neck; 8% of breast, lymphoma), Paget's, bone resorption, immobilization
- ↑ Renal reabsorption (e.g., thiazide diuretics, lithium)
- Less common causes are sarcoid, vit D intoxication, milk-alkali syndrome

USUAL TREATMENT

- <14 mg/dl in asymptomatic patient—no acute therapy more than hydration and diuresis aimed at lowering Ca^{2+} needed. Maintain good hydration and UO.
- >14 mg/dl or symptomatic patient <14 mg/dl—forced diuresis with saline (2–3 ml/kg/h) and Lasix (1–2 mg/kg/h). More potent agents (steroids, mithramycin, calcitonin, and bisphosphonates) needed if Ca^{2+} levels not reduced.
- Seek and treat underlying cause

ASSESSMENT POINTS

SYSTEM	EFFECT	ASSESSMENT BY HX	PE	TEST
HEENT	Band keratopathy			
CV	Hypovolemia	Postural symptoms	Orthostatic VS changes Narrowed pulse pressure Tachycardia	
	Conduction abnormalities, esp short QT_c interval Widened QRS			ECG Shortens QT_c interval—can follow in any one individual
GI		Nausea/vomiting		
ENDO	Excess PTH or production of PTH-related hormone			Radioimmunoassay of PTH or PTH-related peptides
CNS	Altered mental status Rarely, seizure	Confusion, obtundation, even coma		
MS		Bone pain		
RENAL	Calculi Renal insufficiency			Abd x-ray, IVP BUN/Cr

$QT_c = QT/\sqrt{RR}$; RR = RR interval.

Key Reference: Federman DD: Scientific American Medicine 1992, Endocrinology Section VI, pp 1–15.

PERIOPERATIVE IMPLICATIONS

Preoperative Preparation
- Assess volume, renal function
- Assess need to reduce serum calcium if level >14 mg/L
- Consider H_2-receptor antagonist metoclopramide

Monitoring
- UO—important to keep well hydrated
- Consider central venous catheter or other monitor of fluid status (such as TEE) if aggressive fluid therapy required and cardiovascularly compromised

Airway
- Full-stomach precautions
- Rule out lytic C-spine lesions

Induction
- Hypovolemia can lead to hemodynamic instability if usual dose of drugs given

Maintenance
- Hemodynamic instability if hypovolemic or myocardial contractility abnormalities
- Aggressive hydration—tailor IV fluids to lyte and acid-base status (avoid hypernatremia and acidosis from excessive N/S)
- Continue lyte replenishment if necessary (esp K^+, Mg^{2+})

Extubation
- Related to preop condition and underlying disease

Adjuvants
- May alter NMB duration and ability of antagonists to reverse block
- Associated acid-base and lyte derangements or renal insufficiency may affect duration of NMBs and ability to reverse block

ANTICIPATED PROBLEMS/CONCERNS

- Fluid and lyte overload from too aggressive hydration
- Bone fractures (pathologic)
- Lethargy, stupor, coma from high levels of Ca^{2+}

HYPERCHOLESTEROLEMIA

Uday Jain, M.D., Ph.D.

Uday Jain, M.D., Ph.D.

RISK

- People in USA: about 50 million
- Low-density lipoprotein (LDL) similar in African-Americans and Caucasians; high-density lipoprotein (HDL) higher in African-Americans. Death rate higher in African-Americans.
- Familial hypercholesterolemia (LDL > 260 mg/dl)—0.2% population
- Severe polygenic hypercholesterolemia (LDL > 220 mg/dl)—1% population
- Familial combined (multiple lipoprotein type) hyperlipidemia: elevated LDL and/or VLDL—1% population

PERIOPERATIVE RISKS

- Risk of myocardial ischemia and infarction
- Worsened CHF

WORRY ABOUT

- New-onset angina or increasing frequency or severity of angina
- Worsening or new-onset CHF
- TIAs of the CNS
- Peripheral atherosclerosis

OVERVIEW

- Normal total cholesterol < 200 mg/dl; 200–239 mg/dl borderline high; ≥ 240 mg/dl high
- HDL < 35 mg/dl low; ≥ 60 mg/dl high
- CAD: Keep LDL (total LDL–triglyceride/5) ≤ 100 mg/dl
- Lp(a) is a risk factor for CAD

ICD-9-CM Code: 272.0

See also Coronary Artery Disease, Atherosclerotic Disease, Lipidemias, Hypertriglyceridemia in Diseases section

ETIOLOGY

- Can be inherited or due to systemic illness such as diabetes, nephrotic syndrome, chronic renal failure, and hypothyroidism

USUAL TREATMENT

- Diet and exercise
- Cholestyramine and colestipol inhibit bile acid absorption
- Neomycin inhibits cholesterol absorption
- HMG CoA reductase inhibitors (lovastatin, pravastatin, simvastatin, atorvastatin) reduce cholesterol synthesis and are commonly used
- Thyroid hormone clears LDL
- Probucol reduces LDL but also HDL
- Nicotinic acid inhibits VLDL, LDL production
- Fibric acids clofibrate and gemfibrozil cause catabolism of triglyceride-rich lipoproteins
- Partial ileal bypass surgery

ASSESSMENT POINTS

SYSTEM	EFFECT	ASSESSMENT BY HX	PE	TEST
CV	Myocardial ischemia and infarction LV dysfunction	Angina or its equivalents Dyspnea, edema, exercise intolerance	Displaced PMI S_3	ECG, CXR, stress testing, ECHO, coronary angio
RESP	CHF	Dyspnea, orthopnea, cough	Rales and rhonchi	CXR
DERM	Lipid deposits		Xanthelasma, xanthoma, arcus juvenilis	
RENAL	Impaired renal perfusion	Nighttime urinary frequency		Cr
CNS	Cerebrovascular atherosclerosis	TIAs	Carotid bruit	Carotid US and angio

Key Reference: Jacobson TA: "The lower the better" in hypercholesterolemia: a reliable clinical guideline. Ann Intern Med 2000; 133:549–554.

PERIOPERATIVE IMPLICATIONS

Preoperative Preparation

- Assess for CAD and peripheral vascular disease
- β-blockers and nitrates perioperatively, as tolerated

Monitoring

- Consider PA catheter, TEE, in presence of large fluid shifts, ischemic Hx, and high-risk surgery

Airway

- May be overweight and difficult to intubate

Induction

- Hypovolemia may lead to hypotension

Maintenance

- Maintain hemodynamic stability without hypothermia or anemia (ideal Hct may be > 27%)
- No anesthetic agent or technique proven superior
- Monitor for ischemia and failure

Extubation

- For noncardiac surgery, this is the period of greatest risk for ischemia

Postoperative Period

- High incidence of tachycardia, ischemia, and MI for several days after noncardiac surgery
- Treat pain, hemodynamic and biochemical abnormalities aggressively

Adjuvants

- Depends on end-organ disease

ANTICIPATED PROBLEMS/CONCERNS

- Problems are related to atherosclerosis

HYPERGLYCEMIA

William L. Lanier, M.D.

RISK

- People within USA: can occur in virtually any anesthetized or critically ill patient
- Race with the highest prevalence: none

PERIOPERATIVE RISKS

- Increased likelihood of neurologic injury following brain ischemia, and perhaps traumatic brain injury and spinal cord injury
- Dehydration resulting from osmotic diuresis

WORRY ABOUT

- Electrolyte abnormalities, particularly hypokalemia, while treating hyperglycemia
- Hypoglycemia following insulin, resulting in insult to the CV system and CNS
- Polyuria complicates assessment of fluid balance

OVERVIEW

- Is not a disease
- Typically produces adverse effects by two mechanisms: increases in plasma osmolality and increases in postischemic tissue lactic acidosis
- Dx made by measuring blood glucose concentrations
- In acute setting, blood glucose concentrations can be estimated using indicator impregnated strips; confirmation can be made by mechanized techniques

ICD-9-CM Code: 790.6

See also Diabetes, Diabetic Ketoacidosis, Hyperosmolar Nonketotic Coma, Cushing's Syndrome, Acromegaly, Pheochromocytoma, Morbid Obesity in Diseases section; see Steroids in Drugs section

ETIOLOGY

- Results from DM (both insulin-requiring and non–insulin-requiring), other endocrinopathies (Cushing's syndrome, acromegaly, obesity, pheochromocytoma), physiologic stress, drug administration (particularly corticosteroids), and glucose-containing fluid infusions

USUAL TREATMENT

- Insulin
- Isotonic intravenous crystalloid solutions to treat hypovolemia and dilute existing blood glucose
- If possible, treat underlying cause (e.g., discontinue infusion of glucose-containing solutions, discontinue corticosteroids, reduce physiologic stress to patient)

ASSESSMENT POINTS

SYSTEM	EFFECT	ASSESSMENT BY HX	PE	TEST
HEENT	Dehydration in extreme cases		Dry mucosa in extreme cases	
CV	Mild inotropic effect with mild hyperglycemia Dehydration		Tachycardia, orthostatic hypotension	
GI		Polydipsia in extreme cases		
RENAL	Osmotically induced diuresis	Polyuria, urinary frequency		Elevated urine glucose
ENDO		See under Etiology		Elevated blood glucose
HEME	Diminished WBC activity; changes in serum sodium concentrations			Serum sodium concentration decreases 1.6 mEq/L for each 100 mg/dl increase in glucose concentration
CNS			Altered consciousness, neurologic deficits	Plasma osmolality

Key Reference: Aouifi A, Neidecker J, Vedrinne C, Bompard D, Cherfa A, Laroux MC, Brule P, Champsaur G, Lehot JJ: Glucose versus lactated Ringer's solution during pediatric cardiac surgery. J Cardiothorac Vasc Anesth 1997; 11:411–414.

PERIOPERATIVE IMPLICATIONS

Preoperative Preparation

- Glucose reduction with insulin
- Hydration
- Normalization of lytes

Monitoring

- Blood glucose concentrations in all cases
- In severe cases, blood lytes, blood osmolality, urine output

Airway

- Abnormalities typically related to DM (↓ range of motion and abn atlanto-occipital contractions), acromegaly (distorted anatomy), or chronic corticosteroid use or Cushing's syndrome (cushingoid Sx, friable tissues)

Maintenance

- Maintain hydration
- Insulin therapy
- K+ replacement

Extubation

- No special considerations, other than those related to underlying disease

Adjuvants

- Limit attempted reduction of blood glucose concentration to ~75 mg/dl/h to avoid problems with osmotic injury to brain and lyte disturbances
- Monitor ECG during correction of profound hyperglycemia

Postoperative Period

- Variations in physiologic stress, fluid administration, and drug usage make postop blood glucose concentrations difficult to predict and control

ANTICIPATED PROBLEMS/CONCERNS

- Increases in blood glucose concentrations by a mere 40 mg/dl may worsen outcome following cerebral ischemic insult. In contrast, hypoglycemia resulting from excessive use of insulin may result in irreversible neurologic injury, independent of ischemic event.

HYPERKALEMIA

Irving Hirsch, M.D.

RISK

- Any patient with plasma K$^+$ concentration >5.5 mEq/L

PERIOPERATIVE RISKS

- Cardiac conduction system abnormalities
- VFIB
- Cardiac standstill in diastole

WORRY ABOUT

- Adverse effects are likely to accompany acute increases in K$^+$
- Depolarizing muscle relaxants, esp if given to patients with burns, spinal cord transection, catatonia with immobility, or muscle trauma
- Digitalis toxicity
- Acidosis

OVERVIEW

- Condition that can be due to ↑ total body K$^+$ content or alterations in distribution between intracellular and extracellular sites

ICD-9-CM Code: 276.7

ETIOLOGY

- Diminished renal excretion
  - Acute oliguric renal failure
  - Chronic renal failure
  - Addison's disease
  - Hyporeninemic hypoaldosteronism
  - Potassium-sparing diuretics
  - Ingestion of potassium-rich foods by patient with renal insufficiency
- Transcellular shifts
  - Acidosis
  - Cell destruction—trauma, burns, rhabdomyolysis, hemolysis, tumor lysis
  - Hyperkalemic periodic paralysis
  - Diabetic hyperglycemia
  - Depolarizing muscle relaxant causing K$^+$ release esp in patients with burns, spinal cord transection, catatonia with im-

mobility, muscle trauma, or denervating muscle
- Factitious hyperkalemia
  - Tourniquet method of drawing blood
  - Hemolysis of drawn blood due to delay in chemical determination

USUAL TREATMENT

- Promote transfer of K$^+$ from ECF to ICF
  - Glucose and insulin—25 g glucose with 10–15 U regular insulin/70 kg
  - Sodium bicarbonate—40–150 mEq/70 kg
  - Hyperventilation—with each pH change of 0.1, there is an inverse change in K$^+$ of 0.6 mEq/L
- Enhance K$^+$ elimination—diuretics, exchange resins (Kayexalate), dialysis
- Calcium gluconate—10–30 ml of a 10% solution over 10–20 min/70 kg counteracts cardiac effects

ASSESSMENT POINTS

SYSTEM	EFFECT	ASSESSMENT BY HX	PE	TEST
CV	Tall peak T waves ↓ Amplitude R wave Widened QRS complex Decreased and eventual disappearance of P wave QRS blends into T wave—"sine wave of hyperkalemia"			ECG
	Ventricular arrhythmia	Possible hemodynamic instability		ECG
	Cardiac arrest	CV collapse		ECG
NM	Weakness Paralysis			
ENDO	↑ Aldosterone Insulin release ↑ Glucagon Epinephrine release	 ↑ BP, HR		K$^+$, renin, aldosterone, glucose

Key References: Cooper RC, Baumann PL, McDonald WM: An unexpected hyperkalemic response to succinylcholine during electroconvulsive therapy for catatonic schizophrenia. Anesthesiology 1999; 91:574–575; Kokko JP: Disorders of fluid volume, electrolyte, and acid-base balance. *In* Bennett JC, Plum F (eds): Cecil Textbook of Medicine, 20th ed. Philadelphia, WB Saunders, 1996, pp 525–551.

PERIOPERATIVE IMPLICATIONS

Preoperative Preparation

- Normal K$^+$ levels before elective surgery
- Avoid sedatives (↓ ventilation) prior to K$^+$ normalization

Monitoring

- ECG
- Plasma K$^+$ levels
- ABG concentration
- Peripheral nerve stimulator

Maintenance

- Adequate ventilation to avoid respiratory acidosis
- Avoid metabolic acidosis—arterial hypoxemia or excessive depths of anesthesia
- IV fluids—avoid lactated Ringer's or others containing K$^+$

Adjuvants

- Muscle relaxants—avoid depolarizing agents; increase K$^+$ 0.3–0.5 mEq/L with succinylcholine
- Dose of nondepolarizing relaxants required is unclear—may need diminished dose

ANTICIPATED PROBLEMS/CONCERNS

- Acute increases in K$^+$ leading to acute ECG changes or adverse cardiac effects. Rx: see Usual Treatment.
- Avoid use of depolarizing muscle relaxants in patients with burns, neuropathies, para- or quadriplegia, muscle trauma, or catatonia with immobility

DISEASES 175

HYPERMAGNESEMIA
David R. Gambling, M.B., B.S., F.R.C.P.C.

RISK

- Patients with renal insufficiency, especially those receiving Mg^{2+}-containing cathartics or antacids
- Parturients on $MgSO_4$ therapy
- "Runaway" infusion of Mg^{2+} during transportation to the OR can cause acute, life-threatening hypermagnesemia. Risk of developing very high serum Mg^{2+} levels in such cases can be reduced by always using a small volume Buretrol device in patients receiving IV Mg^{2+} therapy.

PERIOPERATIVE RISKS

- Potentiates nondepolarizing neuromuscular blocking agents
- May increase risk of modest hypotension during administration of regional anesthesia
- Potentiates hypotension associated with use of volatile anesthetics, Ca^{2+}-channel blockers, and butyrophenones
- Can exacerbate local anesthetic toxicity
- Hypermagnesemia may be associated with ↑ in bleeding time and TEG changes, although no clinically significant coagulopathies have been attributed to Mg^{2+}

WORRY ABOUT

- Intraoperative hypotension
- Muscle weakness (esp respiratory)
- Excessive sedation
- Myocardial depression and cardiorespiratory arrest with very high levels

OVERVIEW

- Defined as an elevated Mg^{2+} concentration in plasma, in excess of 1.1 mmol/L
- Equivalent Mg^{2+} concentrations in the three unit systems in common use: mg/dl, mEq/L, mmol/L
  - Normal serum level 1.8–2.4 mg/dl, 1.5–2.0 mEq/L, 0.75–1.0 mmol/L
  - Therapeutic level 4.8–8.4 mg/dl, 4–7 mEq/L, 2–3.5 mmol/L
  - Neuromuscular toxic level >12 mg/dl, >10 mEq/L, >5 mmol/L
- Mg^{2+} elimination is dependent on GFR; with GFR <30 ml/min, patients are at significant risk
- Sx vary with plasma concentration and become more serious as the plasma concentration increases >4 mmol/L
- CV, resp, MS systems are predominantly affected

ICD-9-CM Code: 275.2

ETIOLOGY

- Patients with chronic renal failure who are receiving Mg^{2+}-containing antacids or laxatives
- Often iatrogenic, e.g., excessive administration of $MgSO_4$ infusion to parturient pt with preterm labor or pregnancy-induced Htn
- Rarely Addison's disease, myxedema, or lithium therapy

USUAL TREATMENT

- Discontinue Mg^{2+} therapy and delay nonessential surgery
- Fluid load and diuretic therapy
- Adults—IV calcium gluconate 1 g (temporary but effective). Neonates—IV calcium gluconate 100–200 mg/kg over 5 min and continuous infusion 100–300 mg/kg/d.
- Peritoneal dialysis or hemodialysis for persistent or life-threatening hypermagnesemia
- Assist ventilation/protect airway if necessary

ASSESSMENT POINTS

The side effects of hypermagnesemia are more serious as the serum level of magnesium increases.

SYSTEM	SIGNS AND SYMPTOMS	SERUM Mg^{2+} CONCENTRATION
GENERAL	Normal	0.7–1.1 mmol/L (normal range)
CV	Warmth, flushing, headache, nausea, dizziness	2–3 mmol/L (range during parenteral treatment)
	Decreased AV and intraventricular conduction	>2.5 mmol/L
	ECG—prolonged PQ and widening of QRS	
	Possible hypotension	
	Cardiac arrest in diastole*	>12.5 mmol/L
CNS	Sedation	2–3 mmol/L
MS	Absent deep tendon reflexes	4–5 mmol/L
	Progressive muscle weakness and resp arrest	6–7.5 mmol/L

Patients with chronic renal failure frequently have Mg^{2+} levels up to 3 mmol/L but are seldom symptomatic.
Acidemia will decrease serum level at which side effects occur; e.g., in presence of acidemia, cardiac arrest can occur at a serum level of 8–10 mmol/L.
*The ability of this degree of hypermagnesemia to cause cardiac arrest is uncertain if ventilatory support and normal acid-base balance are maintained.

Key Reference: Koinig H, Wallner T, Marhofer P, et al: Magnesium sulphate reduces intra- and postoperative analgesic requirements. Anesth Analg 1998; 87:206–210.

PERIOPERATIVE IMPLICATIONS

Preoperative Preparation

- Discontinue $MgSO_4$ unless being used to treat seizures or ventricular dysrhythmias
- Check serum level
- ECG, Cr, lytes

Monitoring

- Routine

Airway

- Use full dose of succinylcholine for intubation
- Reduce dose of nondepolarizing neuromuscular blocking drugs (NMBs) by $1/3$–$1/2$

Preinduction/Induction

- Avoid sedative premedications
- Ensure full denitrogenation of lungs
- Avoid precurarization or priming dose of NMB

Maintenance

- May decrease requirement for anesthetics owing to decreased neurotransmitter release

Extubation

- Ensure full return of train-of-four, ability to sustain head lift and vital capacity >10 ml/kg
- Ensure patient responsiveness

Adjuvants

- Hypermagnesemia may exacerbate hypotension associated with hypovolemia, Ca^{2+}-channel blockers, volatile inhalation anesthetics, butyrophenones, lumbar epidural, or subarachnoid anesthesia
- Treat with IV calcium gluconate 1 g and fluid load and diuretics

Postoperative Period

- Beware of excessive sedation, weakness, hypoventilation, cardiac arrest
- May cause or aggravate neonatal hypotonia and hypotension
- May reduce postop analgesic requirements by antagonism of N-methyl-D-aspartate

ANTICIPATED PROBLEMS/CONCERNS

- Hypermagnesemia potentiates action of nondepolarizing NMBs by inhibiting release of acetylcholine from motor nerve terminal, decreasing sensitivity of postjunctional membrane, and reducing excitability of muscle fibers
- Many common anesthestic drugs exacerbate weakness and sedation associated with hypermagnesemia
- Potentiates local anesthetic toxicity
- Excessively high plasma Mg^{2+} concentrations can cause cardiorespiratory arrest

HYPERNATREMIA

John K. Hayes, Ph.D.
Kuang C. Wong, M.D., Ph.D.

RISK

- People with chronic liver disease treated with certain drugs (lactulose, mannitol, fructose)
- Patients with altered mental status, intubated patients, infants and elderly persons
- Elderly and pediatric populations with decreased H_2O acquiring skills

PERIOPERATIVE RISKS

- Brain shrinkage from hypernatremia can cause vascular rupture with cerebral bleeding, subarachnoid hemorrhage, coma, and death
- Mortality rate ranges from 16–60%

WORRY ABOUT

- Development of hypertonic encephalopathy
- High mortality rate associated with hypernatremia; of those recovering >40% may develop neurologic sequelae

OVERVIEW

- Serum sodium concentration and serum osmolality are closely controlled by water homeostasis, which is mediated by thirst, vasopressin, and the kidneys
- Physiologic or iatrogenic hypernatremia is defined by serum sodium concentration >145 mmol/L with serum osmolality >290 mOsm/L
- Hypernatremia can result in hypovolemia, euvolemia, and hypervolemia
- Cellular dehydration results from transmembrane fluid shift from cells to extracellular space

ICD-9-CM Code: 276.0

ETIOLOGY

- Impaired thirst
- Excessive water loss
  – Renal: nephrogenic diabetes insipidus (DI) (tubular damage)
  – Pituitary: pituitary diabetes insipidus (PDI)
  – Extrarenal: sweating, solute diuresis from glucose (diabetic ketoacidosis, nonketotic hyperosmolar coma) or mannitol or glycerol administration, kidney dialysis
- Brain tumors, head trauma, cranial surgery can cause DI states
- Infants or children: diarrhea
- Elderly: reduced water intake, ingestion of sodium bicarbonate

USUAL TREATMENT

- Adequate water intake/administration
- Fluid volume supplement:
  – To lower the serum Na^+ conc by ~0.5 mmol/L/h and to replace no more than half of the H_2O deficit in the first 24 h
  – To calculate the H_2O deficit where total body water in kg is 60% of lean body mass in men and 50% in women. H_2O deficit = total body water (serum $[Na^+] + 140 - 1$).
  – Circulatory collapse: give rapid plasma or blood substitutes to correct shock; then give normal saline (N/S)
- Acute hypernatremia without circulatory collapse: give 5% glucose at slow infusion rates
- Drug therapy (PDI)
  – Desmopressin (nasal spray, 5–10 μg)
  – Chlorpropamide (oral, 250–750 mg/d)

ASSESSMENT POINTS

SYSTEM	EFFECT	ASSESSMENT BY HX	PE	TEST
HEENT	Dry mouth Swollen tongue		Exam of mouth	
CV	Tachycardia Hypotension Possible circulatory collapse	BP on arising	HR BP	ECG
METAB	Fever			Temperature
CNS	Restlessness Weakness Maniacal behavior Delirium		CNS exam	
DERM	Flushed		Skin exam	
RENAL	Polyuria Hyposthenuria	Urinary frequency and color		Na^+, K^+, and Osm both urine and serum

Key References: Adrogue HJ, Madias NE: Hypernatremia. N Engl J Med 2000; 342:1493–1499; Reeves WB, Andreoli TE: The posterior pituitary and water metabolism. *In* Wilson JD, Foster DW (eds): Textbook of Endocrinology, 8th ed. Philadelphia, WB Saunders, 1992, pp 332–356.

PERIOPERATIVE IMPLICATIONS

Monitoring

- Blood electrolytes (esp Na^+ and K^+), serum and urinary osmolality, temperature

Airway

- None unless patient is unconscious

Maintenance

- Give adequate fluids (see under Usual Treatment)
- Sustain blood electrolytes and temperature in physiologic ranges

Extubation

- Dependent on neurologic function

ANTICIPATED PROBLEMS/CONCERNS

- Development of neurologic dysfunction/coma
- Enhanced mortality and morbidity with higher incidence in children

HYPEROSMOLAR NONKETOTIC COMA

(SEE ALSO UNDER DIABETES, TYPE II)

John R. Ammon, M.D.

RISK

- Elderly and pts with underlying medical problems, esp cardiac and renal
- Occurrence of perioperative catabolic stress state in type II diabetic
- Elderly diabetic with stroke or gram-negative infection, esp pneumonia

PERIOPERATIVE RISKS

- Hypotension, shock due to extreme osmotic diuresis from elevated glucose
- End-organ injury from deranged volume status and hemodynamic instability (renal, myocardial, in situ thrombosis) and hyperosmolarity (CNS)

WORRY ABOUT

- Underlying cause of hyperosmolar crisis, e.g., infection, CVA, loss of metabolic control perioperatively
- Hypovolemia
- CNS dysfunction and/or injury, e.g., hallucinations, focal neurologic deficits

OVERVIEW

- A grave metabolic emergency with mortality > 50%
- Characterized by extreme hyperglycemia, serum osmolality > 350 mOsm/L, profound fluid depletion
- Prevented perioperatively by appropriate metabolic monitoring and support

ICD-9-CM Code: 250.2

ETIOLOGY

- Type II diabetic in severe catabolic state resulting from infection, CVA, or uncontrolled perioperative metabolic stress
- Inadequate insulin present to prevent extreme hyperglycemia but enough to prevent or suppress diabetic ketoacidosis (DKA)

USUAL TREATMENT

- Urgent volume resuscitation for an average fluid deficit of 10 L; must treat circulation and improve renal perfusion and urine flow (oliguria or anuria in late stages)
- 0.9% Saline, then 0.45% saline; add 5% dextrose as blood sugar approaches normal
- Insulin usually required, although patients more sensitive than those in DKA
- Sodium bicarbonate only if significant lactic acidosis present from poor tissue perfusion

ASSESSMENT POINTS

SYSTEM	EFFECT	ASSESSMENT BY HX	PE	TEST
CV	Severe volume contraction and acidosis, shock in extreme cases		Vital signs	ABGs CVP, PAP ECG
RESP	Inadequate ventilation due to brainstem hypoperfusion		Ventilatory rate and depth	ABGs
ENDO	Inadequate insulin during severe catabolic stress	Type II diabetes Recent CVA, infection, or surgical procedure		Blood glucose
RENAL	Profound diuresis → oliguria, → anuria			UO BUN/Cr ratio
CNS	Clouded sensorium to coma; seizure; delayed anesthesia emergence	Altered CNS status over hours to days	Level of consciousness	Serum Osm, CSF culture

Key Reference: Skyler JS: Diabetes mellitus, types I and II. *In* Kelly's Textbook of Internal Medicine, 4th ed. Philadelphia, Lippincott Williams & Wilkins, 2000, pp 2751–2769.

PERIOPERATIVE IMPLICATIONS

Monitoring

- Sequential glucose determinations during surgical period in type II diabetic, esp when catabolic stress severe, e.g., CABG, trauma, major vascular surgery

Airway

- Airway protection lost by depressed CNS function

Induction

- If surgical procedure necessary (unlikely), volume resuscitation key step before induction; usual concerns for diabetic end-organ dysfunction (see under Diabetes, Type II, in Diseases section)

Maintenance

- Ongoing treatment of metabolism (blood glucose, insulin) and volume status; end-organ support

Extubation

- Intact CNS function and airway reflexes for airway and ventilatory adequacy

Postoperative Period

- Risk of hyperosmolar coma continues after surgery with ongoing catabolism and potential for inadequate insulin, extreme hyperglycemia

ANTICIPATED PROBLEMS/CONCERNS

- High mortality and severe morbidity due to CNS and myocardial ischemia, shock, ATN, widespread arterial and venous thromboses

HYPERPARATHYROIDISM

Michael L. Nahrwold, M.D.
Srinivas Mantha, M.D.

RISK

- People within USA: 50,000 patients/y
- Race with highest prevalence: none
- Male/female: 1:2
- Prevalence: 50–100/100,000 (increases with age)
- 0.8% in pregnancy

PERIOPERATIVE RISKS

- Hypovolemia and lyte abn
- ↑ Risk of cardiac dysrhythmias 2° to hypercalcemia
- Aspiration from full stomach
- Postoperative hypocalcemia

WORRY ABOUT

- Signs of hypercalcemia and other lyte irregularities
- Intravascular volume changes
- Fluid overload and Na^+ retention in CV fragile patients
- Renal, cardiac, and CNS abnormalities
- Pancreatitis secondary to hypercalcemia

OVERVIEW

- Endocrinopathy associated with elevation in parathyroid hormone (PTH) levels
- Primary problem is hypercalcemia
- Dx supported by ↑ PTH level associated with hypercalcemia
- Most patients with primary hyperparathyroidism are hypercalcemic but asymptomatic
- Hyperparathyroidism in pregnancy is associated with high (50%) maternal and fetal morbidity and can lead to neonatal hypocalcemia and tetany

ICD-9-CM Code: 252.0

See also Parathyroidectomy in Procedures section and Hypercalcemia in Diseases section

ETIOLOGY

- Primary hyperparathyroidism usually due to benign parathyroid adenoma (80–90%), hyperplasia (15%), or parathyroid carcinoma (uncommon)
- May be manifestation of MEN II, which includes pheochromocytoma, hyperparathyroidism, and medullary thyroid carcinoma
- Secondary hyperparathyroidism is usual in chronic renal failure patients undergoing dialysis

USUAL TREATMENT

- Surgically with parathyroidectomy
- Medically with saline hydration and furosemide in emergency situations to restore serum Ca^{2+} to a safe level (<14 mg/dl)
- Recent advances and techniques such as nuclear imaging for correct localization of parathyroid tumors; endoscopic, radiologically guided, or video-assisted surgical techniques for surgery; and quick hormone assays are allowing minimally invasive parathyroidectomy under local/regional anesthesia
- Mithramycin (for more resistant Ca^{2+} elevators), calcitonin, and steroids (for hypercalcemia associated with hyperphosphatemia)
- IV phosphates, indomethacin
- Pregnant women with primary hyperparathyroidism should be treated with parathyroidectomy ideally in the 2nd trimester

ASSESSMENT POINTS

SYSTEM	EFFECT	ASSESSMENT BY HX	PE	TEST
CV	Htn, dysrhythmias	Palpitation, headache	Abn pulse rate and/or rhythm, ↑ BP	ECG, lytes, total and ionized Ca^{2+} QT_c* interval
RESP	↓ Bronchial clearance of secretions	Cough	Adventitious sounds	
GI	Peptic ulcers, pancreatitis	Constipation, anorexia, nausea and vomiting, epigastric pain		
RENAL	Nephrocalcinosis, nephrolithiasis → renal dysfunction	Polyuria, hematuria		BUN, Cr
CNS	EEG abn, seizures	Depression, personality change, psychomotor retardation, memory impairment	Psychosis, disorientation, obtundation, coma	
MS	Hyporeflexia, osteopenia, osteitis fibrosa cystica	Weakness, bone pain	Muscular atrophy, arthritis, pathologic fractures	

*$QT_c = \dfrac{QT}{\sqrt{R\text{-}R}}$; R-R = R-R interval.

Key Reference: Udelsman R, Donovan PI, Sokoll LJ: One hundred consecutive minimally invasive parathyroid explorations. Ann Surg 2000; 232:331–339.

PERIOPERATIVE IMPLICATIONS

Preoperative Preparation
- Assess total and ionized Ca^{2+} levels
- Reduce serum total calcium to <14 mg/dl
- No intervention for Ca^{2+} level ≤12 mg/dl
- For higher levels use saline hydration and furosemide (rapid action), mithramycin (acts in 6–12 h), calcitonin (acts in 1–2 h), or glucocorticoids (cover intraoperatively with stress dose); reduce Ca^{2+} to <14 mg/dl
- Consider H_2 receptor antagonists and metoclopramide

Monitoring
- Routine; pay attention to changes in QT_c interval (QT_c by itself poorly correlated with ionized Ca^{2+}, but changes correlate)*

Airway
- Possibility of pathologic fractures requires careful positioning for laryngoscopy

Preinduction/Induction
- No preferred agents or techniques
- Hypovolemia can lead to hemodynamic instability if usual dose of drugs is given
- Minimally invasive procedures can be performed using local anesthesia or sedation

Maintenance
- No preferred agents or techniques. Possibility of pathologic fractures requires careful positioning and padding of pressure points.

Extubation
- Swelling of or bleeding into the neck or recurrent laryngeal nerve injury during surgery may cause airway compromise

Adjuvants
- Response to NM blockers may be unpredictable if Ca^{2+} level elevated

ANTICIPATED PROBLEMS/CONCERNS

- Cardiac arrhythmias due to hypercalcemia
- Postop airway compromise 2° to bleeding or recurrent laryngeal nerve injury
- Pneumothorax 2° to surgical procedure
- Fluid and lyte overload from too aggressive hydration

HYPERTENSION

Simon J. Howell, M.D.
Pierre Foëx, M.D.

RISK

• Prevalence in the USA population: 4% aged 18–29 y; 75% aged ≥ 80 y
• Ideal pressure of 115/76 or less present in only 4% of adult USA population

PERIOPERATIVE RISKS

• No evidence to suggest that BPs consistent with stage 1 or 2 Htn (i.e., systolic 140–180 mmHg or diastolic 90–110 mmHg) at the time of admission for surgery confer ↑ perioperative risk. However, being a known hypertensive even on antihypertensive medication is associated with an ↑ risk of perioperative complications. This increased risk appears to be a consequence of the sequelae of Htn, such as CAD and renal impairment.
• Associated with perioperative Htn, bradycardia, myocardial ischemia

WORRY ABOUT

• Stages 3 and 4 hypertension (> 180/110 mmHg)
• Evidence of end-organ damage (see Assessment Points)

OVERVIEW

• Hypertension can be essential or secondary
• Increased risk of coronary heart disease, stroke, CHF, renal insufficiency

ICD-9-CM Code: 401

ETIOLOGY

• Essential hypertension not fully understood: many putative factors: genetic factors (linkage to angiotensin gene), race, age, lifestyle (exercise), obesity, sodium intake, alcohol intake, childhood influences (birth weight, BP tracking), socioeconomic status
• Secondary hypertension uncommon; 5% of all Htn. Possible causes include renal artery stenosis, Cushing's syndrome, pheochromocytoma, Conn's syndrome.

USUAL TREATMENT

• Nonpharmacologic treatment: weight loss, reduction of alcohol intake, salt restriction, exercise, behavior modification
• Pharmacologic treatment: diuretic, β-blockers, Ca^{2+}-channel blocking drugs, ACE inhibitors, α-blockers

ASSESSMENT POINTS

SYSTEM	EFFECT	ASSESSMENT BY HX	PE	TEST
CV	CAD	MI, angina		ECG Exercise ECG Radionuclide scintigraphy Coronary angio
	LVH/LVF	Dyspnea, orthopnea	Displaced apex beat S_3, basal crepitations Rales	CXR ECHO Radionuclide angio
	Peripheral vascular/aortic disease	Claudication	Peripheral pulses Brachial-ankle BP ratio	Doppler Angio
RENAL	Renal impairment			Cr
CNS	TIA/CVA	Hx of TIA/CVA	Neurologic signs Carotid bruit	CT scan Doppler Angio

Key Reference: Howell SJ, Sear YM, Yeates D, et al: Risk factors for cardiovascular death after elective surgery under general anaesthesia. Br J Anaesth 1998; 80:14–19.

PERIOPERATIVE IMPLICATIONS

Preoperative Preparation

• Continue and/or increase antihypertensive medicine
• Short-acting vasodilator prepared
• Assess myocardial and volume status

Monitoring

• Consider direct arterial monitoring
• Volume status monitoring depending on LV function (e.g., PA cath, CVP, or TEE)

Induction

• Preintubation narcotics to prevent exacerbation of Htn
• Generous induction dose of IV agent
• Volume repletion prior to induction
• Consider short-acting β-blockers to prevent tachycardia

Maintenance

• CV stability best maintained by careful volume control and anticipation of noxious stimuli

Extubation

• Adequate pain relief prior to termination of anesthesia
• Short-acting vasodilator and/or β-blockers to prevent Htn and tachycardia

Adjuvants

• Regional: may prevent severe increases in BP, since intubation not needed. Severe dehydration may be present, resulting in profound hypotension.
• Continuous infusions of nitroglycerin, nitroprusside, or esmolol
• Severe hypotension may not respond to usual doses of vasoconstrictor due to prior drug treatment

Postoperative Period

• Restart antihypertensive medication ASAP in postop period
• Patch therapy for some drugs must start 12 h prior to anticipated need due to slow absorption from skin

ANTICIPATED PROBLEMS/CONCERNS

• Watch for Sx of CNS, renal, or myocardial dysfunction
• Preop period affords opportunity to educate patient about importance for complying with antihypertensive therapy

HYPERTENSION, UNCONTROLLED, WITH CARDIOMYOPATHY

Edward D. Miller, Jr., M.D.

Edward D. Miller, Jr., M.D.

RISK

- People within USA: 1 million
- Race with highest prevalence: African-American
- Male = female

PERIOPERATIVE RISKS

- Increased risk of myocardial ischemia and/or infarction
- Increased risk of stroke
- Increased risk of renal failure

WORRY ABOUT

- Tachycardia
- Severe elevations or depressions in BP

OVERVIEW

- Severe volume depletion may be present
- Silent myocardial ischemia may occur from supply-demand mismatches even in absence of CAD
- May be forerunner of renal failure and/or stroke
- CHF may be presenting sign
- May develop left ventricular hypertrophy (LVH) ± strain pattern on ECG
- May require >6 wk of treatment for regression of LVH

ICD-9-CM Code: 402

ETIOLOGY

- Genetic predisposition
- Secondary forms related to abnormalities of kidney or adrenal glands
- High peripheral resistance is accelerated with time

USUAL TREATMENT

- Variety of antihypertensive agents to decrease BP
- Surgical correction of secondary forms of Htn

ASSESSMENT POINTS

SYSTEM	EFFECT	ASSESSMENT BY HX	PE	TEST
CV	LV function LVH	Exercise tolerance	2-flight walk	ECG, CXR ECHO, MUGA Stress thallium
RESP	Pulm edema	Orthopnea Dyspnea	Rales	CXR
CNS	Stroke	Blackouts	Carotid bruit	Carotid study
RENAL	Nephropathy		Edema	BUN/Cr

Key Reference: Roizen MF: Patients with comorbidities. *In* Miller RD (ed): Anesthesia, 5th ed. New York, Churchill Livingstone, 2000, pp 933–937.

PERIOPERATIVE IMPLICATIONS

Preoperative Preparation

- Continue and/or increase antihypertensive medicine
- Short-acting vasodilator prepared
- Assess myocardial and volume status

Monitoring

- Consider direct arterial monitoring
- Volume status monitoring depending on LV function (e.g., PA cath, CVP, or TEE)

Induction

- Preintubation narcotics to prevent exacerbation of Htn
- Generous induction dose of IV agent
- Volume repletion prior to induction
- Consider short-acting β-blockers to prevent tachycardia

Maintenance

- CV stability best maintained by careful volume control and anticipation of noxious stimuli

Extubation

- Adequate pain relief prior to termination of anesthesia
- Short-acting vasodilator and/or β-blockers to prevent Htn and tachycardia

Adjuvants

- Regional: may prevent severe increases in BP, since intubation not needed. Severe dehydration may be present, resulting in profound hypotension.
- Continuous infusions of nitroglycerin, nitroprusside, or esmolol
- Severe hypotension may not respond to usual doses of vasoconstrictor due to prior drug treatment

Postoperative Period

- Restart antihypertensive medication ASAP in postop period
- Patch therapy for some drugs must start 12 h prior to anticipated need due to slow absorption from skin

ANTICIPATED PROBLEMS/CONCERNS

- Watch for Sx of CNS, renal, or myocardial dysfunction
- Preop period affords opportunity to educate patient about importance of complying with antihypertensive therapy
- Hypotension if therapy is continued, esp angiotensin receptor blocking drugs and receptor inhibitors; or if pt is untreated and volume depleted
- Htn if medications are discontinued

HYPERTHYROIDISM

Michael F. Roizen, M.D.

RISK

- People within USA: 400,000/y develop hyperthyroidism plus 5% of pregnant females (highest prevalence in 2nd trimester); 1/1000 females; 1/3000 males
- Race with highest prevalence: unknown

PERIOPERATIVE RISKS

- Risk related to occurrence of thyroid storm; ↑ risk of storm, even if made euthyroid prior to surgery
- Some increased risk of respiratory insufficiency
- Progressive increased risk of hypothyroidism after surgery on thyroid, radioactive Rx of hyperthyroidism, and thyroiditis

WORRY ABOUT

- Assessing that patient is euthyroid
- Securing airway in patient with large goiter or displaced trachea
- Postop risks of nerve injury (immediate stridor requires immediate reintubation), surreptitious bleeding (examine wound—can drain externally—prior to PACU discharge), and thyroid storm (uncommon without another acute illness or after 3 days postop)

OVERVIEW

- Endocrinopathy with CV disease—tachycardia (commonly idiopathic if no prior Dx of hyperthyroidism has been made), CHF, dysrhythmias (AFIB) as major manifestation
- Other target: resp and CNS (decreases drive to breathe; worsens anxiety, psychoses) and metabolic (hypermetabolism and increased protein turnover resulting in weakened muscles and malnourishment)
- If euthyroid prior to operation, risk of storm and of periop CV problems diminished by >90%
- If not euthyroid, try to delay operation until euthyroid
- If emergency (life-threatening trauma, ruptured viscus), use β-blocking agents and iodides to ↓ periop effects and ↓ further synthesis and release of thyroid hormones; keep in ICU until risk of storm has passed

ICD-9-CM Codes: 242.9 (Hyperthyroidism [thyrotoxicosis]); 242.0 (Graves' disease); 245 (Thyroiditis); 193 (Malignant thyroid disease); 198.89 (Metastatic malignant thyroid disease)

ETIOLOGY

- Multinodular diffuse enlargement (Graves' disease); almost never malignant, soft large gland, thought autoimmune (thyroid-stimulating IgGs that bind to TSH receptors on thyroid associated with goiter and ophthalmopathy)
- Pregnancy (ectopic TSH-like substance)
- Thyroiditis (autoimmune)
- Thyroid adenoma—toxic multinodular goiter (firm gland) later in life and rarely (almost never) malignant; unilateral solitary nodule with autonomous function earlier in life, also almost always benign
- Choriocarcinoma
- TSH-secreting pituitary adenoma
- Surreptitious ingestion of T_4 or T_3

USUAL TREATMENT

- Antithyroid drugs for 2–6 mo; if recurs, retreat; if recurs again, consider surgery or radioiodine Rx

ASSESSMENT POINTS

SYSTEM	EFFECT	ASSESSMENT BY HX	PE	TEST
HEENT	Weakened tracheal rings, distorted/displaced trachea Ophthalmopathy	Snoring, hoarseness, neck pain	Ask to vocalize "e"; examine airway and neck Look at eyes; test for diplopia	Check CXR (PA and lateral) lat neck films; CT scan of neck
CV	Dysrhythmias, AFIB, sinus tachycardia, mitral valve prolapse CHF, cardiomyopathies	Palpitations; ↑ HR during sleep DOE, orthostatic SOB	Standard exam	Rhythm strip or full ECG CV system is involved in either Hx or PE
GI	Weight loss, diarrhea, dehydration	Dizziness on arising; Hx of diarrhea, constipation	Skin turgor; other measures of volume status such as orthostatic vital signs	Increased serum alkaline phosphatase
HEME	Mild anemia, thrombocytopenia; agranulocytosis 2° to propylthiouracil or methimazole		Skin/mucous membranes for infection/petechiae	CBC with plt count and differential
CNS		Shaking, anxiety, emotional lability	Reflex speed, tremor, nervousness, mental status	
METAB	Need to assess if euthyroid Malnourished	Refer to all other systems, esp reflex speed, tremor, heat intolerance; fatigue; weakness; weight loss; anorexia, increased appetite	Reflex speed; HR	Free T_4 estimate

Key Reference: Roizen MF: Anesthetic implications of concurrent diseases. *In* Miller RD (ed): Anesthesia, 4th ed. New York, Churchill Livingstone, 2000, pp 927–930.

PERIOPERATIVE IMPLICATIONS

(See also under thyroidectomy, subtotal)

Preoperative Preparation
- Assess if euthyroid
- Assess for associated autoimmune diseases

Preinduction/Induction
- Prehydrate liberally if CV status will tolerate
- Check and protect eyes

Anesthetic Technique
- No one technique has proved superior
- Hyperthyroidism is associated risk factor for halothane hepatitis

Monitoring
- Temp (also place cooling blanket on OR table to treat thyroid storm if it occurs)
- Consider invasive monitoring if patient has dilated cardiomyopathy/thyroid storm/severe dysrhythmia

- If head-up position is utilized, consider air embolus monitoring and therapy

Airway
- Consider awake fiberoptic intubation if questions about adequacy of airway or distortion/involvement of trachea present
- Consider armored tube or equivalent if tracheal rings are affected

Induction/Maintenance
- Routine

Adjuvants
- Usually no requirement for muscle relaxants

ANTICIPATED PROBLEMS/CONCERNS

- Thyroid storm is life-threatening illness if hyperthyroidism has been severely exacerbated by illness or operation. Manifested by hyperpyrexia, tachycardia, striking alterations in consciousness. Early signs include delirium, confusion, mania, excitement. Differential Dx: malignant hyperthermia, pheochromocytoma crisis, NMS.
- Rx includes supportive care, propylthiouracil followed in 1 h by iodides and propranolol, decrease conversion of the less active T_3 to the more active T_4
- Surreptitious bleeding behind neck bandages can suddenly compromise airway function
- Recurrent laryngeal nerve injuries post thyroidectomy usually result in damage to abductor fibers, which results in hoarseness
- Bullous glottic edema can require immediate reintubation
- Occasionally late tetany (usually 2–3 days post thyroidectomy) can occur from accidental removal of or damage to parathyroid glands

HYPERTRIGLYCERIDEMIA

Uday Jain, M.D., Ph.D.

RISK

- People within USA: Combined with hypercholesterolemia in up to 20% of population
- Racial predilection: none

PERIOPERATIVE RISKS

- Some causes such as dysbetalipoproteinemia can cause atherosclerosis
- Primary chylomicronemia not atherogenic
- Acute pancreatitis and its complications (fatal hemorrhagic pancreatitis, pseudocyst, pancreatic exocrine insufficiency, and impaired insulinogenesis)

WORRY ABOUT

- Myocardial ischemia and infarction
- Acute pancreatitis when triglycerides >1000 mg/dl
- Serum electrolytes, hydrophilic species underestimated in laboratory
- Transient eruptive cutaneous xanthomas

OVERVIEW

- Not independent risk factor for CAD in absence of hypercholesterolemia
- Triglyceride is glycerol esterified by 3 fatty acid molecules of variable chain length and degree of saturation
- Chylomicrons and very low density lipoproteins (VLDLs) are lipoproteins primarily containing triglycerides
- Normal value of triglycerides <200 mg/dl; values >1000 mg/dl associated with ↑ risk of pancreatitis
- Spinal or epidural anesthesia and β-blockers reduce FFA levels
- Sympathetic stimulation, stress, insulin, increase FFA levels
- Heparin releases lipoprotein lipase inhibited by protamine and hepatic lipase resistant to protamine

ICD-9-CM Code: 272.1–3

See also Hypercholesterolemia, Lipidemias, Coronary Artery Disease, Atherosclerotic Disease in Diseases section

ETIOLOGY

- Primary hypertriglyceridemia or chylomicronemia; primary hyperprebetalipoproteinemia and mixed lipemias caused by several genetic disorders; combined hyperlipidemia and multiple lipoprotein type hyperlipidemia (excess of VLDLs and/or LDLs); familial dysbetalipoproteinemia (broad β disease, type III hyperlipoproteinemia)
- Due to diabetes, nephrotic syndrome, renal failure, rare dysproteinemias, oral contraceptives, thiazide diuretics, and β-blockers

USUAL TREATMENT

- Diet and exercise
- Nicotinic acid inhibits production of VLDLs and LDLs
- Fibric acids clofibrate and gemfibrozil may cause abdominal discomfort, cholesterol gallstones, or myalgias accompanied by high serum creatine phosphokinase

ASSESSMENT POINTS

SYSTEM	EFFECT	ASSESSMENT BY HX	PE	TEST
CV	Coronary and peripheral atherosclerosis (not without ↑ cholesterol) LV dysfunction	Hx of CAD—angina, CHF, MI Exercise tolerance	2-flight walk Displaced PMI S_3	ECG, CXR, ECHO, stress testing, angio
RESP		Exercise tolerance		Generally not needed
GI	Acute pancreatitis	Epigastric pain, obesity		
ENDO	Caused by poorly controlled DM	Ketoacidosis Hyperosmolar coma		Blood glucose level
DERM	Markedly elevated VLDLs may lead to transient eruptive xanthomas		Xanthomas occur on extensor surfaces such as elbows, knees, buttocks	
RENAL	Caused by nephrotic syndrome, renal insufficiency	Urinary problems		BUN, Cr
CNS	Lipemia retinalis when triglycerides > 3000 mg/dl		Whitish cast of venous vascular bed of retina	

Key Reference: Miller M: Current perspectives on the management of hypertriglyceridemia. Am Heart J 2000; 140:232–240.

PERIOPERATIVE IMPLICATIONS

Preoperative Preparation

- If serum triglycerides high, lytes may be underestimated. Cholesterol and glucose may be high while thyroid hormone may be low.
- Assess CV system and abdomen

Monitoring

- Routine

Preinduction/Induction

- FFAs are competitive inhibitors of barbiturates and other acidic drugs binding to albumin
- FFAs increase the likelihood of ventricular arrhythmias

Maintenance

- No agent or technique superior
- Negative inotropic properties of anesthetics may be enhanced
- Blood-gas partition coefficient of inhalational anesthetics is increased in hyperlipemia, slowing their uptake

Extubation

- Period of greatest risk for developing myocardial ischemia
- Epigastric pain may be felt if acute pancreatitis

Adjuvants

- Depends on etiology and end-organ diseases
- Lipid stores of anesthetic agents may alter awakening and return of psychomotor normality

ANTICIPATED PROBLEMS/CONCERNS

- Complications of CAD
- Acute pancreatitis

HYPOKALEMIA

Irving A. Hirsch, M.D.

RISK

- Any patient with plasma K$^+$ <3.5 mEq/L
- Patients on diuretic therapy for Htn or other conditions
- Htn affects 60 million people
  – Higher prevalence in African-Americans than in Caucasians
  – Increased with age in all groups
  – Increased in men vs. women <50 y
  – Increased in women vs. men >50 y

PERIOPERATIVE RISKS

- Cardiac arrhythmias—atrial and ventricular premature beats
- Muscle weakness
- Autonomic insufficiency

WORRY ABOUT

- Recent evidence suggests that cardiac arrhythmogenicity is dependent on acuteness or chronicity of hypokalemia
- Acute alkalosis
- β_2-adrenergic agonists may shift K$^+$ intracellularly, worsening hypokalemia
- Potential for prolonged response to nondepolarizing muscle relaxants

OVERVIEW

- Serum K$^+$ and its extracellular to intracellular ratio important for electrical excitation of excitable cells, including heart, skeletal muscles, nerves
- Acute shifts, in face of chronic hypokalemia, are more likely to produce life-threatening complications
- Chronic condition less dangerous because ratio of intracellular to extracellular K$^+$ is maintained

ICD-9-CM Code: 276.8

ETIOLOGY

- Inadequate intake: diet; alcoholism; anorexia nervosa; geophagia
- Excess renal loss: mineralocorticoid excess; primary or secondary hyperaldosteronism; Cushing's syndrome; chronic licorice ingestion; Bartter's syndrome; diuretics: pre–late distal tubule locus of action (such as hydrochlorothiazide and furosemide [Lasix]), osmotic diuretics, carbonic anhydrase inhibitors (acetazolamide); chronic metabolic alkalosis; antibiotics: carbenicillin, gentamicin, amphotericin B; renal tubular acidosis; Liddle's syndrome; acute leukemia; uretero-sigmoidostomy
- Gastrointestinal losses: vomiting; diarrhea; nasogastric suctioning; villous adenoma
- Etiology of acute hypercalemia
  – Acute alkalosis
  – Hypokalemic periodic paralysis
  – Barium ingestion
  – Insulin therapy
  – Vitamin B$_{12}$ therapy
  – Thyrotoxicosis (rarely)

USUAL TREATMENT

- Plasma K$^+$ decrease from 4 to 3 mEq/L = 100–200 mEq deficit
- Plasma K$^+$ <3 mEq/L = 200–400 mEq deficit
- Replacement:
  – Oral—potassium gluconate or citrate
  – IV—potassium chloride 10–20 mEq/h, larger amounts only under adequate monitoring of cardiac electrophysiology

ASSESSMENT POINTS

SYSTEM	EFFECT	ASSESSMENT BY HX	PE	TEST
CV	Arrhythmias ECG changes	PACs, PVCs	Prolonged P-R and QT intervals Flattened T waves, V waves ST-segment depression	ECG
ENDO	↓ Aldosterone ↓ Insulin release			Aldosterone Glucose
NM	Weakness Areflexic paralysis Ileus, abdominal pain Autonomic insufficiency Rhabdomyolysis	Muscle pain	Respiratory insufficiency Absence of bowel sounds Orthostatic hypotension	ABGs (rarely needed) BP CK
RENAL	K$^+$ conservation Polyuria Polydipsia ↑ Renal ammonia Edema and sodium retention	Frequent urination Frequent drinking		Urine K$^+$ Urine ammonia Urine sodium

Key Reference: Reddy VG: Potassium and anesthesia. Singapore Med J 1998; 39:511–516.

PERIOPERATIVE IMPLICATIONS

Preoperative Preparation

- K$^+$ levels (>2.7 and <5.8 mEq/L) before elective surgery
- Determine if hypokalemia is acute or chronic in onset

Monitoring

- ECG
- Plasma K$^+$ levels
- ABGs
- Peripheral nerve stimulator

Maintenance

- Adequate ventilation to avoid respiratory alkalosis (avoid hyperventilation)
- Avoid hyperglycemia—IV fluids with glucose
- Avoid epinephrine or other β_2-agonist, which may shift K$^+$ intracellularly

ANTICIPATED PROBLEMS/CONCERNS

- Decision to proceed with elective surgery depends on level and acuteness or chronicity of hypokalemia
- Hypokalemia may lead to arrhythmias, esp with catecholamines, digitalis, calcium, or hyperventilation
- Hypokalemia due to diuretics may cause or be associated with volume depletion
- Hypokalemic patients may be sensitive to vasodilators or cardiac-depressant effects of volatile anesthetics

184 DISEASES

HYPOMAGNESEMIA

James M. Feld, M.D.

James M. Feld, M.D.

RISK

- 60% of all patients admitted to either a surgical or medical ICU were hypomagnesemic

PERIOPERATIVE RISKS

- ↑ Risk for arrhythmias (atrial and ventricular)
- ↑ Risk for worsening ischemia/CHF
- ↑ Susceptibility to seizures, bronchoconstriction, vasospasm
- ↑ Mortality from endotoxin challenge

WORRY ABOUT

- Giving $MgSO_4$ too fast may cause burning at IV site, overall sense of warmth (has been used for postop shivering), mild transient hypotension

- As long as renal function is intact, excessive levels will be cleared over several hours
- Prolongation of neuromuscular blockade with all nondepolarizing drugs

OVERVIEW

- Common deficiency from multiple causes that results in decreased stability of excitable cells, decreased contractility and ↑ SVR
- Safe to give even if levels are high—may not truly reflect intracellular levels
- Must replete Mg^{2+} levels before correcting K^+ and Ca^{2+} deficiencies
- Primary concern is increasing susceptibility to worsening myocardial ischemia

ICD-9-CM Code: 275.2

ETIOLOGY

- Poor nutrition, diuretic therapy, aminoglycosides, digitalis, prolonged IV therapy, diabetes mellitus, large blood transfusions, increased alcoholic intake

USUAL TREATMENT

- Acute administration of 2 g $MgSO_4$ over 20–30 min
- 1 g $MgSO_4$ with every 20 mEq of KCl
- Give at beginning of case, as it may interfere with neuromuscular blockade reversal
- Keep in mind usual preeclamptic doses are 4–6 g bolus and 1–2 g/h; monitoring levels between 6 and 8 mg/dl

ASSESSMENT POINTS

SYSTEM	EFFECT	PE	TEST
CV	Myocardial ischemia		
	Htn		ECG
	Arrhythmias		BP
RESP	Bronchospasm	Wheezing	
		Airway pressure	
NEURO	Seizures (more marked in presence of cocaine)		
	Vasospasm		
OB	Htn of preeclampsia, eclampsia	Seizures	
MS	Weakness	Difficulty weaning	

Key References: James M: Clinical use of magnesium infusions in anesthesia. Anesth Analg 1992; 74:129–136; Seelig MS, Elin RJ, Antman EM: Magnesium in acute myocardial infarction: still an open question. Can J Cardiol 1998; 14:745–749.

PERIOPERATIVE IMPLICATIONS

Preoperative Preparation

- In patients susceptible to hypomagnesemia, give 2–5 g $MgSO_4$ over the first 1–2 h of surgery
- Initial 2 g will alter the catecholamine response to intubation and may contribute some analgesic effect

Intraoperative Period

- Give more Mg^{2+} only if patient is to be kept intubated postop and if UO is adequate, as reversibility of neuromuscular blockade may not be complete
- Mg^{2+} will potentiate vasodilators and slowing effect of digitalis in supraventricular arrhythmias.

Postoperative Period

- Rarely measure blood levels in routine case unless patient with heart disease is going to ICU and is on vasoactive drugs or requiring large amounts IV fluids
- 1–2 g $MgSO_4$ slow push in PACU may attenuate postop shivering

ANTICIPATED PROBLEMS/CONCERNS

- Levels above 8–10 mg/dl cause diaphragmatic weakness and are rarely reached with above recommendations
- Other than potentiating neuromuscular weakness, Mg^{2+} administration is safe
- In suspected MIs it should be given as early as possible

HYPONATREMIA

Kuang C. Wong, M.D., Ph.D.
John K. Hayes, Ph.D.

RISK

- Patients, especially the elderly, with adrenocortical insufficiency (Addison's disease) or syndrome of inappropriate antidiuretic hormone secretion (SIADH)
- Up to 25% of elderly males subjected to transurethral resection of the prostate (TURP), from irrigating fluid absorption
- Females subjected to endoscopic gynecologic surgery with excessively absorbed irrigating fluid
- Infants/children receiving multiple tap-water enemas

(See Addison's Disease and SIADH in Diseases section, and Transurethral Resection of Prostate in Procedures section)

PERIOPERATIVE RISKS

- Adrenocortical insufficiency associated with ↑ risk of inability to cope with stress and of CV collapse
- Iatrogenic dilution associated with CNS, cardiopulmonary, and skeletal muscle abnormalities

WORRY ABOUT

- Intraoperative TURP syndrome with iatrogenic hyponatremia
  - Water intoxication (cerebral and/or pulmonary edema)
  - Cardiac dysrhythmias
  - Visual or motor disturbance attributed to ammonia intoxication when glycine is the irrigation solution
  - Hypothermia

OVERVIEW

- Can occur in isotonic, hypertonic, and hypotonic forms—excretion of renal water impaired despite intake of dilute fluid(s)
- Serum sodium and intra- to extracellular ratio is important in maintaining cellular integrity and electrical activity of excitable cells. Low serum sodium from inadequate dietary intake, too vigorous diuresis, or absorption of sodium-free irrigating solutions.
- Dilutional hyponatremia is inevitable during TURP, so pre-existing conditions should be optimally stabilized before coming to the OR (e.g., lyte disturbance, cardiac ischemia, chronic pulmonary disease)

ICD-9-CM Code: 276.1

ETIOLOGY

- Dilutional hyponatremia results from absorption of sodium-free irrigating fluid
- SIADH can be caused by CNS or pulmonary tumors or dysfunction
- Impaired renal water excretion capacity
  - ↑ Plasma concentration of arginine vasopressin
  - Depletion of K^+ → imbalance in the ratio of exchangeable Na^+ to K^+ ions
  - Thiazide diuretics

USUAL TREATMENT

- Restricting free water administration (rate of rise of Na^+ to be < 1 mEq/L/h lest central pontine myelinolysis occur)
- Combined IV hypertonic saline (with IV diuretic) at sufficient pace and magnitude to reverse hyponatremia (CAUTION: reversal too fast may cause osmotic demyelination)
- Decrease symptomatic organ dysfunction (CHF Rx with diuresis, vasodilation)

ASSESSMENT POINTS

SYSTEM	EFFECT	ASSESSMENT BY HX	PE	TEST
CV	Dysrhythmias	Palpitations		ECG
	CHF	Orthopnea, DOE	S_3, rales	CXR
RESP	Pulm edema		S_3, rales	CXR
CNS	Confusion			Usually serum
	Restlessness			Na^+ < 123 mEq/L
	Visual disturbances			
	Seizure, coma			
MS	Hyporeflexia	Cramps, weakness	Weakness	Reflexes
	Cramps, weakness			
RENAL				Serum Na^+
				Serum and urine osmolality

Key Reference: Adrogue HJ, Madias NE: Hyponatremia. N Engl J Med 2000; 342:1581−1589; Liu WS, Wong KC: Anesthesia for genitourinary surgery. *In* Barash PG, Cullen BF, Stoelting RK (eds): Clinical Anesthesia. Philadelphia, JB Lippincott, 1992, pp 1160−1164.

PERIOPERATIVE IMPLICATIONS

Monitoring
- Blood lytes and serum osmolality
- ECG
- Body temperature
- EEG if patient receives GA

Airway
- Respiratory support in patients with ammonia-induced toxicity with hemodialysis if renal impairment

Maintenance
- Ensure optimal general or regional anesthesia
- Prevent hypothermia by using warmed irrigating and IV fluid

Extubation
- Cardiopulmonary problems should be stabilized following hyponatremia and water intoxication

Postoperative Period
- Pain management
- Restore lyte balance
- Replace blood loss if necessary (hypovolemia, tachycardia, hypoxemia)

ANTICIPATED PROBLEMS/CONCERNS

- Dilutional hyponatremia is generally related to the skill of the resectionist and the duration of resection
- Patient with pre-existing cardiopulmonary problems should be optimally stabilized
- ASA class 1 and class 2 patients will tolerate hyponatremia and water load better than classes 3 and 4 patients; chronic hyponatremia tolerated better than acute hyponatremia
- Risk of central pontine myelinolysis if hypertonic saline is administered

HYPOPHOSPHATEMIA

Alan S. Tonnesen, M.D.

RISK

- 0.3–1.5% of "healthy" adults; 5–20% of hospitalized patients
- Alcoholism, ketoacidosis, osmotic diuresis, acidosis, catabolism, acute burn injury
- Depressed intake: starvation, malabsorption, familial hypophosphatemia, hemodialysis, binding within gut, vitamin D deficiency
- Increased urinary losses: hyperparathyroidism, osmotic diuresis, acute volume expansion, acetazolamide, diuretic phase ATN, renal transplantation, acidosis
- Redistribution: glucose-insulin infusion, β-adrenergic agonists, resp alkalosis, recovery from malnutrition, alcohol withdrawal, theophylline overdose

PERIOPERATIVE RISKS

- Acute resp or cardiac failure, unclear etiology

WORRY ABOUT

- Postop resp or cardiac failure
- Hypocalcemia and vascular calcification if PO_4 administered too rapidly

OVERVIEW (P_i mol wt = 31)

- Need 10 mmol/1000 kCal; 1 mmol/kg/d
- 60–70% absorbed in duodenum and jejunum, stimulated by vitamin D, from dairy products, meat, eggs

- Excretion
  – Kidney: filtered, reabsorbed proximally (inhibited by PTH, cortisol, glucagon, calcitonin, osmotic diuresis, high dietary PO_4 intake); 10% absorbed distally
  – Gut: secreted, then reabsorbed; may be trapped by aluminum antacids, Ca^{2+}, sucralfate: may be lost by diarrhea or drainage via ostomies or fistulas
- Distribution
  – Total body content about 15 g/kg; volume of distribution about 400 ml/kg. Bone contains 85% of total.
  – Intracellular: 50–75 mmol/L, bound organic form, as high-energy phosphates, phosphorylated proteins, metabolic intermediates
- Factors favoring intracellular movement include glucose, fructose, alkalosis (especially resp), insulin, β-adrenergic stimulation, anabolism (rapid tumor growth, refeeding), osteoblastic metastases
- Extracellular fluid volume (ECFV): 1 mmol/L: 10% protein bound, 5% chelated. Normal P_i is 3.5–5.0 mg/dl (1.1–1.6 mmol/L); falls by 30% after carbohydrate ingestion; higher in females, children, postmenopausal women; lower in AM than PM; elevated after PO_4 ingestion; serum concentration is not closely related to body stores. Body stores assessed better by measuring excretion of PO_4, $FePO_4$, tubular reabsorption of PO_4/GFR.

- Functions
  – Buffer: binds 1, 2, or 3 hydrogen ions/mole, depending on pH. Store and release energy. Structure of proteins, cell membrane lipids, and bone; enzyme phosphorylation for activation. Carbohydrate metabolism: phosphorylate glucose during cellular entry; glycerol-PO_4 serves as gluconeogenic precursor.

ICD-9-CM Code: 275.3

ETIOLOGY

- Depressed intake, increased loss, redistribution

USUAL TREATMENT

- Measure Ca^{2+}, Mg^{2+}, and K^+. Administer 10–15 mmol/1000 calories, 20–30 mmol/d in critically ill. Dietary supplement may be limited by diarrhea.
- For severe hypophosphatemia (<1 mg/dl): Na or K phosphate, intravenously or enterally: multiply volume of distribution by the desired change in $[P_i]$; rate of administration not >0.04 mmol/kg/h to avoid hypocalcemia and tissue precipitation

ASSESSMENT POINTS

SYSTEM	EFFECT	RESULT
CV	Depressed ATP generation	Heart failure
	Impaired pressor response to norepinephrine and angiotensin	
HEME		
WBC	Impaired phagocytosis, bactericidal and migration functions	
Platelets		Thrombocytopenia, defective aggregation, megakaryocytosis
		Impaired clot retraction
RBC	Reduced RBC 2,3-DPG level	Increased HbO_2 affinity
	Spherocytosis, splenic sequestration	Hemolytic anemia (<0.2 mg/dl)
ENDO	Insulin resistance, impaired insulin secretion	Hyperglycemia
RENAL	Reduced GFR	
	Hypercalciuria	
	Hypermagnesuria	Hypomagnesemia
	Hypophosphaturia	
	↓ Proximal Na^+ reabsorption	
	↓ Tm for bicarbonate, reduced titratable acid excretion	
	↓ Tm for glucose	Bicarbonaturia, metabolic acidosis
CALCIUM	Inhibits PTH secretion	Hypercalcemia
CNS	Neurologic depression	Irritability, paresthesia, dysarthria
		Anisocoria, hyperreflexia
MS	Weakness	Proximal > distal
	Resp failure	Rhabdomyolysis
		CPK
		Myoglobinuria
		Aldolase
	Increased osteoclast activity	Bone pain
		Pseudofractures

Key Reference: Fisher M, Simpser E, Schneider M: Hypophosphatemia secondary to oral refeeding in anorexia nervosa. Int J Eating Disord 2000; 28:181–187.

PERIOPERATIVE IMPLICATIONS

- Severe hypophosphatemia corrected slowly over hours to days to fully replete body stores and avoid hypocalcemia and vascular and interstitial calcium precipitation

HYPOPITUITARISM

Johnathan L. Pregler, M.D.

RISK

• Pituitary tumor most common cause, with incidence of 0.2–2.8/100,000/y; prevalence of 8.9/100,000 for total of ~22,500 people in USA
• 30% of pituitary macroadenomas (>10 mm) cause one or more hormone deficiencies
• 50% of patients after pituitary radiation therapy by 4.2 y have hypopituitarism.

PERIOPERATIVE RISKS

• In patient with adequate hormone replacement, surgery presents no increased risk
• If due to secreting tumor, then ↑ risk of Cushing's disease, acromegaly, SIADH, or hyperthyroidism

WORRY ABOUT

• Hypoglycemia
• Airway abnormalities if due to GH-secreting adenoma

• Altered volume status due to ↑ urinary losses
• Adequacy of adrenal function
• ↑ Risk of CV disease

OVERVIEW

• Partial or complete disruption of pituitary gland secretion. Symptoms result from end-organ hypofunction or dysfunction. Organs affected include adrenals, thyroid, reproductive system, liver (glucose production), and kidneys.
• May manifest cortisol deficiency, hypothyroidism, amenorrhea, infertility, insulin-induced hypoglycemia, diabetes insipidus
• Pituitary apoplexy is sudden loss of pituitary function with hypotension, eye pain, blindness, ophthalmoplegia

ICD-9-CM Codes: 253.2 or 253.7 (if due to radiotherapy, post ablative, post hypophysectomy, or secondary to hormone therapy)

ETIOLOGY

• Common causes include pituitary adenoma, pituitary surgery, pituitary radiation therapy, pituitary apoplexy from hemorrhage or infarction
• Other causes: empty sella syndrome, head trauma, infiltrative disease, and internal carotid artery aneurysms
• Mechanical compression of normal pituitary cells by mass effect, impaired blood flow, and interference with hypothalamic regulatory hormone delivery may all be causes of dysfunction

USUAL TREATMENT

• Surgical resection of adenoma with appropriate hormonal replacement therapy includes for ACTH: prednisone or cortisone PO; for TSH: thyroxine PO; for LH and FSH: women: estrogen and progesterone PO; men: testosterone esters IM; for ADH: desmopressin intranasal

ASSESSMENT POINTS

SYSTEM	EFFECT	ASSESSMENT BY HX	PE	TEST
HEENT	Mandibular and oral soft tissue hyperplasia in acromegalics		Airway exam Check ring size	
CV	Hypovolemia Catecholamine resistance		Orthostatic hypotension	Give cortisol and observe BP effect
GI	Hypoaldosteronism	Anorexia, N/V, weight loss, abdominal pain		Hyperkalemia, hyponatremia, hypovolemia
ENDO	Decreased ACTH	Fatigue, fever, stress-induced hypotension, and hyponatremia	Fever, hypotension, weight loss, mental status	AM cortisol level, rapid ACTH stimulation test, insulin tolerance test
	Decreased LH, FSH	Decreased libido and sexual function Amenorrhea	Regression of secondary sexual characteristics	FSH, LH serum levels Serum estradiol and testosterone
	Decreased GH	Fatigue		Insulin-induced hypoglycemia Serum IGF-I
	Decreased TSH	Weight gain, cold intolerance, depression, constipation, hair loss	Myxedema, hyporeflexia	TSH, T_4
	Increased prolactin	Lactation, amenorrhea	Galactorrhea	Serum prolactin
MS	Increased GH in acromegalics		Large hands, feet, mandible, tongue	
RENAL	↑ Vasopressin ↓ Vasopressin	Excessive thirst Increased UO and thirst	Hypovolemia Hypotension	Hyponatremia Hypernatremia Dilute urine

Key Reference: Smith M, Hirsch NP: Pituitary disease and anaesthesia. Br J Anaesth 2000; 85:3–14.

PERIOPERATIVE IMPLICATIONS

Preoperative Preparation
• Ensure adequacy of hormone replacement therapy
• Check serum Na^+ and K^+ and correct if necessary
• Determine volume status and adequacy of fluid replacement
• In acromegalics: careful airway assessment
• Steroid supplementation considerations (hydrocortisone 100 mg/70 kg/d)

Monitoring
• Consider central venous pressures if indicated by co-existing CV abnormalities or inadequate preop correction of fluid status

• Frequent monitoring of electrolytes if hypo- or hypernatremia is not corrected preop
• Consider glucose monitoring

Airway
• Acromegalics with normal airway exam may be difficult to intubate. Have fiberoptic available.

Induction
• Little risk of ↑ ICP with pituitary adenomas
• No special technique if hormone replacement and volume status are adequate

Maintenance
• Maintain normocarbia for pituitary surgery

Extubation
• Routine (for nonpituitary surgery)

Adjuvants
• Intraoperative diabetes insipidus treated with vasopressin 5–10 IU SQ or IM q 4–6 h

Postoperative Period
• Polyuria and polydipsia with dilute urine may indicate development of diabetes insipidus
• Postop hypopituitarism may require steroid replacement therapy

ANTICIPATED PROBLEMS/CONCERNS

• Acromegalic should be treated as a difficult airway with possible awake fiberoptic intubation and extubation only when fully awake
• Patient with GH deficiency may manifest hypoglycemia

HYPOTHERMIA, MILD (CORE TEMPERATURE 34–36°C)

Daniel I. Sessler, M.D.

RISK

- Greater in infants and children
- Greater in longer, larger operations
- Similar in regional and GA

PERIOPERATIVE RISKS

- Myocardial ischemia
- Surgical wound infections
- Coagulopathy
- Altered drug kinetics
- Shivering and thermal discomfort

PERIOPERATIVE BENEFITS

- Resistance to cerebral ischemia
- Decreases triggering and severity of malignant hyperthermia

OVERVIEW

- Core temperature normally protected by responses including sweating, vasoconstriction, shivering
- Typical doses of general anesthetics ↑ the sweating threshold ~1°C and ↓ vasoconstriction and shivering thresholds 2–4°C, thus increasing the range of temp not triggering protective responses from ~0.2°C to ~4°C
- Regional anesthesia inhibits thermoregulatory control by preventing peripheral responses (such as vasoconstriction) and centrally by altering afferent input

ICD-9-CM Code: 991.6 (Accidental)

ETIOLOGY

- Initial 0.5–1.5°C decrease in core temp from core-to-peripheral redistribution of body heat

- Subsequently, slow, linear decrease in core temperature from heat loss exceeding heat production
- Finally, a core-temp plateau results when thermoregulatory vasoconstriction decreases cutaneous heat loss and constrains metabolic heat to core thermal compartment

USUAL TREATMENT

- Forced-air and resistive heating (electric blankets) are the most effective noninvasive warming methods, typically increasing mean body temp 1.5°C/h
- Fluids administered can be warmed. 1 L of crystalloid at 20°C or 1 U of blood at 4°C decreases mean body temp ~0.25°C in adults.
- Passive insulation (e.g., surgical drapes, cotton blankets) decreases heat loss only 30%
- Circulating-water mattresses less effective and may cause burns. Airway heating and humidification are ineffective.

ASSESSMENT POINTS

SYSTEM	EFFECT	DX	TREATMENT
CNS	Ischemia protection Thermal discomfort	None Visual Analogue Scale	Maintain hypothermia Active cutaneous warming
CARDIAC	Myocardial ischemia (usually postop)	ST-segment depression ECHO	Active cutaneous warming
VASC	Precapillary dilation; reduced SVR Arteriovenous shunt constriction; ↑ BP, ↓ HR	Associated with sweating Fingers feel cold	Active or passive cooling Active cutaneous warming
MS (shivering)	2–3-fold ↑ metabolic rate Patient discomfort Interference with monitoring	Visual inspection Oxygen consumption	Prevent hypothermia Meperidine 10–25 mg IV Clonidine 75 μg IV Active cutaneous warming
IMMUNO	Incidence of infections increases 2–3-fold	Clinical infections	Prevent hypothermia
HEME	10% ↑/°C in blood loss	Bleeding time PT/PTT falsely normal	Prevent hypothermia Defect probably not reversed by FFP and plt transfusions
METAB (increased drug action)	MAC decreases ~5%/°C ↓ Drug metabolism	Monitor drug action (rather than dose)	Titrate drug administration to desired end point Monitor twitch depression

Key Reference: Sessler DI: Perioperative heat balance. Anesthesiology 2000; 92:578–596.

PERIOPERATIVE IMPLICATIONS

Preoperative Preparation

- Active "prewarming" for 30–60 min usually minimizes hypothermia

Monitoring

- Four core temp sites are accurate: pulmonary artery, distal esophagus, tympanic membrane, nasopharynx
- Four additional sites suitable except during cardiopulmonary bypass: mouth, axilla, rectum, bladder

Intraoperative

- Maintain normothermia (core temp >36°C) unless otherwise indicated
- Sufficient passive or active reduction of heat loss will prevent hypothermia. Active warming often required.
- Once triggered, thermoregulatory vasoconstriction effective in preventing further core hypothermia

Postoperative

- Hypothermic patients can be aggressively rewarmed

- Shivering and thermal discomfort can be specifically treated
- Postop warming not a routine substitute for maintaining intraoperative normothermia

ANTICIPATED PROBLEMS/CONCERNS

- Thermal discomfort is not life-threatening, but many patients consider it the worst part of surgery

HYPOTHYROIDISM

John Butterworth, M.D.

RISK

• Subclinical hypothyroidism may be present in as many as 8–10% of adult women and 1–2% of adult men; overt hypothyroidism occurs in 0.5–1.5% of adult women and about 0.05–0.15% of adult men

PERIOPERATIVE RISKS

• Potential increased risk for hypothermia, hypotension, cardiac failure, and perioperative gastrointestinal dysfunction
• Perioperative mortality rate not increased unless overtly hypothyroid

WORRY ABOUT

• Predisposition to hypothermia
• Neuromuscular weakness may impair weaning from mechanical ventilation

OVERVIEW

• A common condition, particularly in adult women
• Elevated thyrotropin (TSH) concentration in blood is hallmark laboratory finding and may be present months to years before decrease in T_4
• Adequacy of treatment defined by normal TSH concentrations
• Total and free thyroxine (T_4) (and usually triiodothyronine [T_3]) concentration usually reduced

• Patients presenting with severe, untreated hypothyroidism or myxedema coma may also demonstrate hypothermia, hypoventilation, hyponatremia, hypotension, heart failure, bowel obstruction, and hypoglycemia

ICD-9-CM Code: 244.9

ETIOLOGY

• Hypothyroidism (decreased thyroid hormone secretion) may result from disease of thyroid or pituitary glands, or hypothalamus or generalized tissue resistance to thyroid hormone
• Most (95%) of cases result from primary disease of gland, most commonly autoimmune thyroiditis; previous ^{131}I treatment for hyperthyroidism and previous total thyroidectomy are also relatively common causes of hypothyroidism
• Patients with critical illness often have reduced total T_4 and reduced total and free T_3 with normal TSH concentrations ("euthyroid sick syndrome") but usually do not require thyroid hormone replacement
• Primary TSH deficiency may result from pituitary tumors and cysts or their treatment (either surgery or radiation), pituitary infiltration, necrosis, or infarction; secondary TSH deficiency may result from con-

genital deficiency of thyrotropin-releasing hormone (TRH), radiation therapy, infections, or tumors or cysts impinging on the hypothalamic–pituitary portal circulation

USUAL TREATMENT

• Maintenance outpatient therapy for adults consists of oral thyroxine 0.1–0.2 mg (1–3 μg/kg) daily
• Delay of up to 4 weeks for TSH to stabilize after T_4 dosage adjustment
• Long $T_{1/2}$ of T_4 (about a week) permits oral T_4 to be withheld safely for several NPO days
• Chronic rifampin and phenytoin increase metabolism of T_4 and increase T_4 dosage requirements
• 20% of patients with chronic angina will have increased symptoms with full T_4 replacement
• Myxedema coma may require use of intravenous T_3 (liothyronine) 0.15–0.3 μg/kg every 6 h and IV hydrocortisone 0.5–1 mg/kg every 8 h to cover for possible hypothyroid-impaired adrenal response to stress
• Intravenous liothyronine may also be indicated in other circumstances when peripheral conversion of T_4 to T_3 is impaired (e.g., hypothermic cardiopulmonary bypass)

ASSESSMENT POINTS

SYSTEM	EFFECT	ASSESSMENT BY HX	PE	TEST
HEENT	Enlarged tongue	Snoring	Enlarged tongue	
CV	↓ Heart rate, ↓ BP, heart failure	Palpitations, myocardial ischemia, arrhythmias, peripheral edema	Bradycardia, tachycardia	TSH, T_4 (or T_3) concentrations, ECG
RESP	Hypoventilation			Arterial P_{CO_2}; or HCO_3^-/ serum electrolytes
GI	Ileus	Constipation	↓ Bowel sounds	
RENAL	Decreased free water clearance	Fluid retention, edema	Edema	Serum Na^+ concentration
CNS	Obtundation, muscular weakness	Lethargy, weakness, mental slowness	Decreased deep tendon reflexes, impaired mental status examination	TSH, T_4 (or T_3) concentrations

Key Reference: Woeber KA: Update on management of hyperthyroidism and hypothyroidism. Arch Fam Med 2000; 9:743–747.

PERIOPERATIVE IMPLICATIONS

Preoperative Preparation
• Chronic thyroid replacement to maintain clinically euthyroid state

Monitoring
• Temperature (particularly in those who have not received full T_4 replacement)
• Routine

Airway
• Usually no abnormalities, but may have large tongue

Maintenance
• No significant effect of hypothyroidism on MAC for inhaled anesthetics

• Keep the patient warm
• Possible increased risk of perioperative heart failure, hypotension, and GI dysfunction (controversial)

Extubation
• Keep the patient warm
• Weaning from mechanical ventilation may be impaired

Adjuvants
• None (except in cases of myxedema coma, in which IV liothyronine and hydrocortisone may be indicated)

ANTICIPATED PROBLEMS/CONCERNS

• Only patients who have been inadequately treated with T_4 carry risks; those chronically receiving an appropriate dose of T_4 probably have (at most) minimally increased risks compared with other patients
• Inadequately treated hypothyroidism can lead to lethargy and fatigue, dementia, heart failure, resp weakness, fluid retention and edema, hyponatremia, clotting abnormalities, and generalized weakness

HYPOXEMIA

Ted J. Sanford, Jr., M.D.

RISK

- All patients undergoing anesthesia and surgery (7–35% in large series have Pa_{O_2} < 60 mmHg in OR or PACU)
- Patients with pre-existing pulmonary disease

PERIOPERATIVE RISKS

- Hypoxemia may lead to hypoxia and eventual severe neurologic/cardiac sequelae or death

WORRY ABOUT

- Inadequate delivery of O_2 to blood—greatest concern to the anesthesiologist is inadequate delivery of O_2 to patient
- Concern that inadequate delivery of O_2 to blood will lead to inadequate delivery of O_2 to tissues
- Misinterpretation of clinical manifestations of hypoxemia

OVERVIEW

- Hypoxemia—denotes low Po_2 in blood (vs. hypoxia, which denotes inadequate delivery of O_2 to tissues)
- Hypoxemia defined as (1) resting Po_2 > 2 SD below normal for age and FIO_2, (2) SaO_2 < 90%, (3) Pao_2 < 60 mmHg on room air, (4) a fall in SaO_2 > 5%
- Multiple clues in vital signs and patient symptoms that should be assumed to be due to hypoxemia

ICD-9-CM Code: 799.0 (Hypoxia)

ETIOLOGY

- Decreased FIO_2—failure to provide adequate inspired O_2 (e.g., O_2 supply failure, gas machine disconnect, airway disconnect, patients at higher altitude)
- Inadequate alveolar ventilation or alveolar hypoventilation: venous admixture accounts for majority of causes
  – V/Q mismatch—asthma, COPD, pulm embolism, pulm vascular disease, passive atelectasis due to pneumonia. Resorption atelectasis is most common when O_2 is taken up from an obstructed area of tracheobronchial tree; adhesive atelectasis seen with decreased surfactant; alveoli filled with blood, vomitus; FRC > closing capacity.
  – R → L cardiac shunts—ASD, VSD (*Note:* will not respond to increased FIO_2)
  – Diffusion problems—very rare cause

USUAL TREATMENT

- Determine cause of decreased O_2 delivery and treat
- Increase FIO_2—this will help in all situations of hypoxemia except those due to R → L shunts

ASSESSMENT POINTS

- Subjective signs
  – Anxiety, confusion, altered mental status, diaphoresis, seizures, cyanosis (both central and peripheral)
- Objective signs
  – Tachypnea—increased ventilation due to stimulation of carotid body chemoreceptors, lactic acidosis. May not occur in patients with severe lung disease or history of bilateral carotid endarterectomies.
  – Tachycardia—early signs due to sympathetic stimulation, not to be ignored as just light anesthesia or patient anxiety
  – Hypertension
  – Arrhythmia—due to myocardial ischemia
  – Hypotension
  – **BRADYCARDIA—LATE SIGN! ! !**
- Pulse oximeter—decreased or decreasing saturation. May be interpreted as artifacts or problems with machine. Be wary of pulse oximeter readings of 85% (equal saturated). May have many false positive results because of movements, cautery, or peripheral circulation problems.
- Arterial and venous blood gases—decreased Pa_{O_2}
- Alveolar-arterial oxygen difference—$P(A-a)O_2$ will be normal if hypoxemia is due to decreased Pao_2, increased if hypoxemia due to venous admixture problems
- CXR—look for areas of atelectasis, lung collapse, or evidence of aspiration

Key Reference: Greif R, Laciny S, Rapf B, Hickle RS, Sessler DI: Supplemental oxygen reduces the incidence of postoperative nausea and vomiting. Anesthesiology 1999; 91:1246–1252.

PERIOPERATIVE IMPLICATIONS

Monitoring

- Routine
- ABGs

Airway

- Must ensure patency and intact circuit at all times

Maintenance

- Adequate FIO_2 and alveolar ventilation

ANTICIPATE PROBLEMS/CONCERNS

- Must have a high index of suspicion whenever SaO_2 decreases or any of the clinical subjective or objective signs and symptoms are present. Always assume the decreased SaO_2 does not reflect a problem with the pulse oximeter but signifies a real problem.

IgA DEFICIENCY

David Bui, M.D.
Paul R. Knight III, M.D., Ph.D.

David Bui, M.D.
Paul R. Knight III, M.D., Ph.D.

RISK

- The most common immunodeficiency disorder
- Incidence has been estimated to be 1/300 to 1/600
- More prevalent among European descendants
- Most patients are clinically normal
- Increased risk of allergies and anaphylaxis
- Increased risk of malignancies

PERIOPERATIVE RISKS

- Increased incidence of pulmonary complications, atopic disorders, and postoperative infections

WORRY ABOUT

- Recurrent sinopulmonary infections leading to decreased pulmonary reserve
- Associated autoimmune disorders (e.g., lupus)
- Associated GI disorders leading to volume depletion
- Anaphylactic reactions from transfusion of blood products containing IgA

OVERVIEW

- An immunodeficiency syndrome with increased susceptibility to nosocomial infection
- Cell-mediated immunity is usually normal
- Co-existing diseases may include atopy, recurrent sinopulmonary infection, GI disease, and autoimmune disease
- Decreased synthesis or secretion of IgA

ICD-9-CM Code: 279.01

ETIOLOGY

- Absence of IgA on mucosal surface
- Decreased IgA "blocking" antibodies against environmental antigens
- Associated with histocompatibility groups HLA-A1, -B8, and -Dw3
- There have been several reported cases of acquired IgA deficiency
- Usually decreased rather than absent lymphocyte IgA secretion
- Expression of clinical sequelae may relate to changes in IgG subclass and/or compensatory IgM secretion

USUAL TREATMENT

- Should not treat with gamma globulin
- Increased suspicion of infections and aggressive antibiotic therapy
- Therapy directed toward specific co-existing diseases

ASSESSMENT POINTS

SYSTEM	EFFECT	ASSESSMENT BY HX	PE	TEST
CV	Decreased reserve, hypovolemia	Dypnea or exertion	Tachycardia, orthostatic hypotension	ECG, ECHO
RESP	Recurrent sinopulmonary infection, hemosiderosis, asthma	↓ Exercise tolerance	Wheezing, rales	CXR, PFTs Sinus x-rays
GI	Chronic gastroenteritis, malnutrition, malabsorption	Chronic diarrhea	Cachexia	Electrolytes, BUN, serum albumin
HEME	Nonspecific	Depends on the extent of co-existing diseases		Serum IgA, anti-IgA antibody, Coombs' test
RENAL	Nonspecific	Varies in severity depending on the extent of co-existing diseases		BUN, Cr
CNS	Degenerative, demyelinating	Mental retardation associated with ataxia-telangiectasia		MRI

Key References: Knight PR: In Lema MI (ed): Problems in Anesthesia. Philadelphia, JB Lippincott, 1993, pp 375–391.

PERIOPERATIVE IMPLICATIONS

Preoperative Preparation

- Consider antibiotic therapy
- Work up any indication of infection
- Optimize any underlying organ dysfunction and volume status

Monitoring

- Consider invasive hemodynamic monitoring in debilitated patients

Airway

- Strict aseptic technique
- Universal precautions
- May encounter difficult intubation in patients with associated rheumatoid arthritis

Induction

- Hypotension secondary to hypovolemia and/or decreased cardiac reserve
- Wheezing allergies relatively resistant to conventional therapy

Maintenance

- May require high inspired O_2
- Regional anesthesia and careful titration of anesthetic agents due to potential underlying cardiovascular and pulmonary diseases
- Use only "thoroughly" washed RBC transfusions

Extubation

- Careful assessment of neuromuscular function due to potential drug-drug interaction

Adjuvants

- Depend on organ dysfunction

Postoperative Period

- May require intensive pulmonary therapy
- Maintain strict antiseptic precaution
- Increased suspicion of bacterial infection

ANTICIPATED PROBLEMS/CONCERNS

- Anaphylactic reaction from transfusions of blood or blood products containing IgA to individual with IgA antibodies
- Asthmatic patient with IgA deficiency is relatively resistant to treatment
- Increased risk of nosocomial infection

IMMUNE SUPPRESSION

Paul R. Knight III, M.D., Ph.D.

RISK

• 0.25 to 1.5% of USA population have HIV or other cause of immune suppression
• Major risk factors: neutropenia, yeast overgrowth, and/or nosocomial colonization of skin and mucosa

PERIOPERATIVE RISKS

• 22.2% 30-day mortality in one study of AIDS patients undergoing intra-abdominal surgery
• Mortality greatest at the extremes of age
• Greatest source of morbidity and mortality is 2° to infection
• Pneumonia accounts for ~40% of all deaths
• Increased incidence of postoperative pneumonia, wound infection, postoperative sepsis, respiratory insufficiency, SIRS, and hypotension due to cardiovascular instability
• Increased healing time

WORRY ABOUT

• Nosocomial transmission of infection
• Transmission of pathogenic drug-resistant strains of microbial agents to medical personnel (e.g., new strains of TB)
• ↓ Pulm reserve due to repeated infections
• Decreased myocardial reserve 2° to underlying disease and generalized poor health
• Translocation of intestinal bacteria due to severe mucositis

OVERVIEW

• Immune suppression can arise from multiple causes
• Intraoperatively, surgical trauma, anesthetic agents, blood transfusion with/without severe hemorrhage decreases the immune response

ICD-9-CM Code: 279.3 (Immune deficiency)

ETIOLOGY

• Drugs, cancer, infections (HIV), massive burns, or trauma
• Primary immune deficiency
• Very young have immature immune systems
• Aged develop decreased cellular immune responses
• Smoking decreases respiratory defense mechanisms

USUAL TREATMENT

• Selective use of antibiotic prophylaxis, antivirals (e.g., acyclovir), antifungal agents (e.g., fluconazole), or immune enhancement (e.g., immune globulin)
• Strict sterile procedures and universal precautions
• Fastidious personal hygiene

ASSESSMENT POINTS

SYSTEM	EFFECT	ASSESSMENT BY HX	PE	TEST
HEME	Anemia, neutropenia, lymphocytopenia, hypoglobulinemia, recurrent bacteremia	Easy fatigue, recurrent fever, sweats, and chills	Pale, petechiae	Hct/Hgb, WBC, platelets, plasma proteins, special lymphocyte counts (e.g., CD4$^+$ cells)
CV	SBE, decreased cardiovascular reserve, hypovolemia, drug-induced injury (e.g., arabinomycin), mycotic aneurysms	Decreased exercise tolerance	Murmurs, orthostatic hypotension, abnormal HR	ECG, ECHO
RESP	Recurrent pulm infections, pulm fibrosis	Decreased exercise tolerance		CXR, spirometry
GI	Chronic gastroenteritis, chronic malnutrition, severe mucositis	Severe "cramping" diarrhea, fever, and chills	Cachexia	Electrolytes, albumin Blood cultures
RENAL	Chronic pyelonephritis, bladder infections, chronic cystitis, drug-induced injury (e.g., cyclosporine)	Recurrent urinary tract infections, frequency		BUN, Cr, pyelogram
CNS	Mycotic infarcts	Minor strokes	Focal lesions	Brain scan
MS	Osteomyelitis	Deep pain located over involved area	Point tenderness	X-ray

Key Reference: Knight PR: *In* Lema MJ (ed): Problems in Anesthesia. Philadelphia, JB Lippincott, 1993, pp 375–391.

PERIOPERATIVE IMPLICATIONS

Preoperative Preparation
• Continue or initiate antibiotic therapy and immune therapy
• Optimize underlying organ system dysfunction.
• Assess volume status
• Assess timing of administration of immune suppressive drug(s)

Monitoring
• Consider arterial line, PA line, or other invasive hemodynamic monitors in severely debilitated patients

Airway
• Strict aseptic technique and universal precautions when handling the airway

Induction
• Chronic respiratory injury may cause increased tendency to desaturate

• Hypotension due to decreased myocardial reserve and/or relative hypovolemia
• Decreased drug requirements 2° to decreased plasma proteins

Maintenance
• Increased inspired O_2 may be required due to chronic lung infections
• Decreased myocardial reserve may require careful selection and titration of anesthetic agents or local or regional anesthesia for peripheral procedures
• Preemptive pain management may protect against additional immune suppression

Extubation
• Due to weakness and drug-drug interactions, return of strength should be carefully evaluated

Adjuvants
• Transplantation and anticancer drug interactions need to be considered (e.g., cyclosporine and barbiturates, narcotics, and

muscle relaxants); bleomycin and O_2 administration

Postoperative Period
• Resp adequacy should be carefully followed and may require intensive care monitoring
• Maintain careful antisepsis procedures for extended periods

ANTICIPATED PROBLEMS/CONCERNS

• The greatest intraoperative risk to these patients is infection; therefore, strict hygienic practices are required
• The general state of nutrition, recurrent infections, and the underlying cause of the immune suppression all tend to generally decrease respiratory reserve and cardiovascular stability
• Risk of transmission of drug-resistant pathogenic microbial agents to medical personnel via blood products

IMPLANTABLE CARDIOVERTER-DEFIBRILLATORS (ICDS), MANAGEMENT

Paul D. Eckenbrecht, M.D.

RISK

• 400,000 Americans annually suffer sudden cardiac death (SCD)
• 200,000 Americans have ICDs, and 50,000 ICDs are implanted annually
• 76% of ICD patients are male, < 1% are pediatric patients

PERIOPERATIVE RISKS

• Presence of ICD is not a risk in itself
• Associated diseases: spontaneous dysrhythmias (VTach/VFIB)—100%; CAD—65%; cardiomyopathy—19%; LV dysfunction with mean LVEF—35 ± 10%; valvular disease—8%; MVP—4%; hypertrophic cardiomyopathy—1%; tetralogy, transposition, long QT syndrome—1%
• ↑ Risk of perioperative ventricular dysrhythmias, myocardial ischemia, and LV dysfunction with hypotension and CHF.

WORRY ABOUT

• Electromagnetic interference (EMI) can cause ICD malfunctions
• Strong, continuous EMI can (1) inhibit therapy because the system can no longer sense the intrinsic rhythm, (2) activate or deactivate any CPI Ventak series device when magnet and antitachycardia modes are enabled, (3) temporarily suspend both VTach and VFIB detection and therapy capability of most Medtronic and Ventritex devices as well as Ventak devices when the magnet mode is enabled and the antitachycardia mode is disabled
• EMI may cause inappropriate sensing and delivery of therapy, as well as inhibit antibradycardia pacing
• Transthoracic countershocks should be administered perpendicular to a line between epicardial patch electrodes or perpendicular to the ICD-transvenous lead system

OVERVIEW

• All ICDs have two interrelated functions: dysrhythmia detection and dysrhythmia therapy
• Dysrhythmia detection may be based on morphology (electrogram shape) or rate
• All devices implanted since 1993 have programmable, tiered therapy options: single-chamber, dual-chamber, or rate-responsive pacing for bradycardia; antitachycardia pacing (ATP) and low-energy cardioversion for VTach; and high-energy defibrillation for VFIB
• Before 1993, epicardial patch leads
• Since 1993, multiple percutaneous transvenous or subpectoral sense/pace and defibrillating leads are usually implanted

ICD-9-CM Codes: 427.1 (VTach); 427.41 (VFIB)

ETIOLOGY

• SCD is multifactorial: a structural cardiac abnormality interacts with an acute trigger and results in VTach/VFIB
• Myocardial damage is the primary dysrhythmic substrate
• Low LVEF (≤ 35%) is a strong, independent predictor for SCD
• Acute triggers include myocardial ischemia, sympathetic stimulation, lyte abn (K^+, Mg^{2+}), prodysrhythmic drug effects

USUAL TREATMENT

• Survivors of cardiac arrest due to VTach/VFIB not associated with acute MI and/or sustained VTach who at EP study are noninducible, nonsuppressed by drug or surgical therapy, or intolerant of drugs
• Nonsustained VTach with CAD, prior MI, LV dysfunction, and inducible VFIB or sustained VTach at EPS that is not suppressible by a class I antiarrhythmic
• First-line therapy for poorly tolerated VTach in association with impaired LV function, or VTach in patients who are not inducible at EPS
• 80% with an ICD receive concomitant antiarrhythmic therapy to reduce required device interventions

ASSESSMENT POINTS

SYSTEM	EFFECT	ASSESSMENT BY HX	PE	TEST
CV	Myocardial ischemia LV dysfunction	Angina symptoms Exercise tolerance DOE, anginal equivalent	S_3, rales	ECG, thallium exercise stress test ECHO, MUGA, Ventriculography
RESP	Amiodarone toxicity CHF	Exercise tolerance, DOE PND, orthopnea	S_3, rales	CXR, PFTs, ABGs CXR
NEURO	CV disease	Stroke, TIAs	Bruits	Carotid duplex
RENAL	Renal insufficiency		Edema	BUN, Cr
LYTES	Reversible VTach/VFIB	Diuretic Rx		Serum K^+ and Mg^{2+}

Key Reference: Singer I, Barold SS, Camm AJ (eds): Nonpharmacological Therapy of Arrhythmias for the 21st Century: The State of the Art. Armonk, NY, Futura Publishing Co, 1998.

PERIOPERATIVE IMPLICATIONS

Preoperative Preparation

• All ICD dysrhythmia detection and therapy functions turned (programmed) off preoperatively leaves antibradycardia pacing intact
• An external magnet will temporarily suspend both VTach and VFIB detection and therapy of most ICDs (done under emergent conditions when a programmer is unavailable), but *magnet behavior can be unpredictable*, so consultation with the manufacturer and interrogation with a programmer are the only means to determine magnet response
• CPI Ventak series devices can be permanently disabled by magnet placement when the magnet and tachy modes are enabled: with a magnet, R-wave synchronized tones will occur, 30 sec after which a continuous tone indicates device deactivation. Magnet reapplication until intermittent tones return indicates device reactivation.
• Transthoracic countershock becomes necessary for VTach and VFIB while the ICD is turned off. Transthoracic paddles should be positioned perpendicular to a line between epicardial patch electrodes, or perpendicular to the implanted ICD and transvenous lead.
• After anesthesia, all ICDs should be reinterrogated and re-enabled

Monitoring

• When PACs are removed they may dislodge defibrillating leads positioned in SVC
• Dislodgment of transvenous sense/pace and defibrillating leads placed in the RV apex is less likely, especially in those > 6 wk of age
• TEE a reasonable alternative to a PAC if hardware dislodgment is serious concern

Airway

• Tracheal intubation may cause sympathetic stimulation and myocardial ischemia, triggers of VTach/VFIB in patients at risk for SCD

Preinduction/Induction

• None

Maintenance

• Maintain normothermia and Hct ≥ 28 with CAD and LV dysfunction
• ↑ Incidence of intraoperative conduction defects atropine-resistant bradycardia, CHB, pacemaker and inotropic dependency, α-blockade with low SVR, and hepatic, thyroid, and pulmonary dysfunction in patients taking chronic, preop amiodarone

Extubation

• Same concern as intubation

Postoperative Period

• Reactivate ICD postop after electrocautery no longer needed.

ANTICIPATED PROBLEMS/CONCERNS

• ECG monitoring if ICD is disabled
• Energy requirements for defibrillation increase with antiarrhythmics (classes IA, B, C including lidocaine, propranolol, amiodarone, verapamil), halogenated hydrocarbons, hypothermia, myocardial ischemia, acidosis
• Bretylium has little effect and sotatol ↓ defibrillation threshold
• Skin potential produced by ICD discharge not harmful to caregivers in contact with patient
• ICD manufacturers: Biotronik (800-547-0391); CPI and Intermedics (800-227-3422); Medical (800-352-6466); Medtronic (800-328-2518); Ventritex, Pacesetter, and Telectronics (800-722-3774).

INFRATENTORIAL TUMORS
Marie L. Young, M.D.

RISK
- ~$\frac{2}{3}$ of intracranial tumors in children are in the posterior fossa
- Primary intra-axial lesions are generally malignant; extra-axial lesions are typically benign

PERIOPERATIVE RISKS
- Signs, symptoms of brainstem compression

WORRY ABOUT
- ↑ ICP, hydrocephalus
- Impaired protective airway reflexes, aspiration
- Irregular respiration due to brainstem compression, swelling
- Impaired level of consciousness

OVERVIEW
- Prognosis is poor with glioblastoma, infiltrating brainstem glioma
- Pediatric cystic cerebellar astrocytoma is associated with 80% survival at 20 years
- Benign lesions such as meningioma, acoustic neuroma have low morbidity, mortality, but may recur if resection is incomplete
- Degree of head elevation influences incidence, severity of air embolism (sitting > prone > park bench/lateral position)

ICD-9-CM Codes: 191.6; 191.7; 225.1; 225.2

ETIOLOGY
- Astrocytoma, medulloblastoma, brainstem glioma are the most common posterior fossa tumors in children
- Acoustic neuroma, metastases, meningioma are the most common posterior fossa tumors in adults

USUAL TREATMENT
- Surgical removal or debulking
- Primary or adjuvant radiotherapy
- CSF diversion (ventriculostomy or shunt)
- Steroids to ↓ peritumor edema

ASSESSMENT POINTS

SYSTEM	EFFECT	ASSESSMENT BY HX	PE	TEST
HEENT	Tonsillar herniation Cranial nerve VII compression	Dysphagia, change in voice Tinnitus, ipsilateral hearing impairment	Gag dysfunction	Indirect laryngoscopy Hearing exam
CV	Progressive brainstem compression Ischemic cardiomyopathy		Bradycardia Hypertension S_3 gallop, CHF	ECG
RESP	Progressive tonsillar herniation		Hyperventilation Irregular respiration Apnea	CT exam MRI
GI	↑ ICP	Nausea Vomiting		CT scan MRI
CNS	↑ ICP	Listlessness, headache, nausea, drowsiness, diplopia	Papilledema	CT scan MRI
MS	Lesion in cerebellar midline Lesion in cerebellar hemisphere	Truncal ataxia	Nystagmus Hypotonia, limb ataxia Intention tremor	Extraocular movement abnormalities

Key Reference: Wen DY, Haines SJ, Young ML: In Cottrell JE, Smith DS (eds): Anesthesia and Neurosurgery, 3rd ed. St. Louis, Mosby–Year Book, 1994, pp 323–363.

PERIOPERATIVE IMPLICATIONS

Preoperative Preparation
- Individualize to physical status, presence of ↑ ICP, anxiety level
- Avoid narcotic premedication if risk of ↑ ICP
- Oral benzodiazepines effective in reducing anxiety

Monitoring
- Goals are maintenance of adequate CNS perfusion and cardiorespiratory stability, detection/treatment of air embolism, and surgical brainstem compression
- Capnography, precordial Doppler ultrasound, right atrial catheter for air embolism detection/retrieval (TEE if available)
- Brainstem auditory evoked responses and cranial nerve VII stimulation may reduce morbidity from surgical manipulation

Airway
- Verify appropriate endotracheal tube position after final positioning; avoid large bite blocks and oral airways to minimize tongue and soft tissue compression, postoperative airway swelling

Induction
- Hypotension on induction can be offset by preinduction IV hydration

Maintenance
- Preserve autonomic reflexes; avoid long-acting vasodilators
- Monitor for changes in electrolyte balance due to loop and osmotic diuretics
- Avoid severe hypothermia (<32°C), hyperglycemia
- Controlled positive pressure ventilation, adequate hydration decrease risk of air embolism

Extubation
- Patient should be awake, following commands, and showing return of protective airway reflexes

Adjuvants
- Short-acting vasopressors or vasodilators for maintenance of cardiovascular stability

Postoperative Period
- Suspect brainstem compression or hematoma if postoperative hypertension or profound bradycardia persists in previously normotensive patient
- Avoid potent narcotic analgesic drugs that may produce hypercarbia, decreased intracranial compliance

ANTICIPATED PROBLEMS/CONCERNS
- Patients with higher-grade malignancy have greater likelihood of postoperative brain swelling

INSULINOMA

Jesse J. Muir, M.D.

RISK

- Rare tumors
- Clinically important hyperfunctional islet cell tumors have an incidence of <1/100,000

PERIOPERATIVE RISKS

- Hypoglycemia

WORRY ABOUT

- Intraoperative hypoglycemia
- Possibility of multiple endocrine neoplasia syndrome type I (MEN I), i.e., pituitary tumors, parathyroid tumors, islet cell tumors (often multiple)
- Multiple insulinomas are possible, even in absence of MEN I

OVERVIEW

- Hypoglycemia has many causes; extensive endocrine evaluation is needed to make diagnosis
- Diagnosis strongly suggested by Whipple's triad: (1) symptoms of hypoglycemia provoked by fasting; (2) blood glucose levels <50 mg/dl; and (3) relief of symptoms with glucose
- Diagnosis made by showing circulating insulin level is inappropriately high for existing blood glucose level; esp at time of hypoglycemia, two types of measurement can be made: during fasting (up to 72 h) and after provocative testing
- In normals, the ratio of plasma insulin (μU/ml) to blood glucose (mg/dl) is <0.4. A higher ratio suggests inappropriately high insulin levels for existing blood glucose.
- Tumor(s) localization vital if blind pancreatic resection is to be avoided

ICD-9-CM Code: 211.7 (Benign)

ETIOLOGY

- Unknown: most are solitary adenomas
- MEN I syndrome present in 4% of patients with insulinomas

USUAL TREATMENT

- Surgery
- Octreotide revolutionized preop management as it normalizes glucose levels, but uncertain if it hinders periop diagnosis, as no large trial is available that includes long-term follow-up
- Diazoxide if surgery fails or if patient not a surgical candidate and if octreotide fails

ASSESSMENT POINTS

SYSTEM	EFFECT	ASSESSMENT BY HX	PE	TEST
RENAL	May have renal stone if MEN I	Renal colic	Flank pain	Serum Ca^{2+}
ENDO	MEN I, possible hyperparathyroid Pituitary tumors	Renal colic Vision changes	Flank pain Look for signs of pituitary dysfunction	Serum Ca^{2+} Skull x-rays Appropriate endocrine testing
	Insulinoma	Seizures or "spells"	Mental status evaluation	Fasting blood glucose and insulin levels
CNS	Seizures or abnormal behavior secondary to hypoglycemia	Hx of seizure or spells Frequent meals to avoid "spells"	Mental status evaluation	Blood glucose

Key Reference: Tanaka Y, Funahashi H, Imai T, Naruse T, Suzumura K, Oda Y: The effectiveness of administering a minimal dose of octreotide long-term prior to surgery for insulinoma: report of a case. Surg Today 2000; 30:541−543.

PERIOPERATIVE IMPLICATIONS

Preoperative Preparation

- Monitor mental status for hypoglycemia
- Rule out MEN I
- Consider octreotide Rx perioperatively

Monitoring

- Measure plasma glucose every 10–15 min
- Intermittent sampling is safe as long as plasma glucose is kept above 60 mg/dl
- Consider arterial line or CVP to facilitate sampling ease

Airway

- None

Induction

- None

Maintenance

- Tend to be long procedures; careful attention to fluid status
- Have dextrose solutions available to Rx hypoglycemia

Extubation

- None

ANTICIPATED PROBLEMS/CONCERNS

- It has been proposed that glucose solutions be avoided intraoperatively so that hyperglycemic rebound can be used to confirm tumor removal; less than half of patients will have this "rebound" in first 30 min following tumor removal
- Hyperglycemic rebound cannot be used as proof of complete tumor removal; some patients who have hyperglycemia rebound continue to have hypoglycemic episodes
- Thorough pancreatic exploration combined with intraoperative sonography has been reported to be technique of choice to identify insulinoma intraoperatively
- Although patients may appear to have had successful tumor removal, they must be monitored for hypoglycemia in the postoperative period.

INTRACRANIAL HYPERTENSION (ICH)

Joseph Dooley, M.D.
Kevin J. Gingrich, M.D.

RISK

• People within USA: >50% of patients presenting with head trauma or other intracranial pathology (>600,000/y)
• Gender predominance: depends on etiology

PERIOPERATIVE RISKS

• ↑ Risk of brain ischemia and herniation leading to brain infarction, disability, coma, and death
• ↑ Risk of permanent CNS dysfunction

WORRY ABOUT

• Controlling intracranial pressure and preventing brain ischemia/herniation
• CV and resp instability
• Co-existing injuries in trauma patients (occult cervical spine and intra-abdominal injuries)

OVERVIEW

• Intracranial compartment has fixed volume with three components (brain = 85%, CSF = 10%, cerebral blood volume [CBV] = 5%)
• Increased volume of one component (e.g., tumor, hydrocephalus, or hemorrhage) elevates ICP, causing intracranial Htn (ICH: ICP >20 mmHg)
• ICH reduces cerebral perfusion pressure (CPP = MAP − ICP), causing brain ischemia/infarction
• ICH causes intracranial pressure gradients that may extrude brain parenchyma through dural or bony passages, resulting in herniation
• Some anesthetic agents, Htn, hypercapnia, and hypoxemia increase cerebral blood flow (CBF), increasing CBV and ICP

ICD-9-CM Code: 348.2 (Benign)

ETIOLOGY

• Usually a secondary process accompanying other pathology (e.g., head injuries, hemorrhage, hydrocephalus, abscess, primary and metastatic brain tumors, cerebral infarcts, hypertensive and metabolic encephalopathies, venous thrombosis, infection, burns, near-drowning, and status epilepticus) that increases brain, CSF, or cerebral blood volumes

USUAL TREATMENT

• Treatment of primary disease (e.g., removal of tumor, hematoma, or abscess)
• Avoid hypercapnia/hypoxemia and deliver moderate hyperventilation acutely
• Establish stable hemodynamics
• Head elevation (head above heart) and neutral neck position to promote cerebral venous return
• Osmotic therapy (mannitol) to decrease neuronal size
• Corticosteroids (neoplasm or abscess)
• CSF drainage
• Sedation and NMB in responsive patients

ASSESSMENT POINTS

SYSTEM	EFFECT	ASSESSMENT BY HX	PE	TEST
CV	Dysrhythmias, unstable vital signs Inferior wall myocardial ischemia		BP Pulse S$_3$ gallop	Tachycardia, bradycardia, prolonged QT interval, ECG, ECHO
RESP	Irregular breathing		Resp rate and pattern	
GI	Reduced gut motility	Vomiting		
RENAL	SIADH Central diabetes insipidus		Oliguria Polyuria	Urinalysis, serum electrolytes
CNS	Altered function	Headache, vomiting, unconsciousness	Neurologic deficits, papilledema	Direct ICP measurement (ventriculostomy, intracranial bolt, etc.)

Key Reference: Bekker AY, Mistry A, Ritter AA, Wolk SC, Turndorf H: Computer simulation of intracranial pressure changes during induction of anesthesia: comparison of thiopental, propofol, and etomidate. J Neurosurg Anesthesiol 1999; 11:69–80.

PERIOPERATIVE IMPLICATIONS

Preoperative Preparation

• Judicious or no preop sedation because of risk of hypoventilation
• Assess volume status

Monitoring

• Consider arterial catheter for BP monitoring and for serial ABGs to properly manage mechanical ventilation
• Consider ICP monitor and CVP line
• Glucose

Airway

• Neutral cervical spine position for tracheal intubation if possible traumatic injury
• Possible aspiration risk (emergency procedure or severe ICH)

Preinduction/Induction

• Neutral neck position and head elevation
• If patient cooperative, establish voluntary hyperventilation; otherwise hyperventilate as soon as possible
• Induction technique should maintain CV stability and not ↑ CBF (e.g., fentanyl, thiopental, nondepolarizing NM blocker; avoid succinylcholine unless airway concerns override)

Maintenance

• O$_2$, N$_2$O (controversial) or hypnotic (thiopental or propofol) infusion, and narcotic infusion with 0.25% isoflurane or equivalent sevoflurane. Up to 1.2% isoflurane without narcotic infusion. Avoid halothane and enflurane.
• Moderate hyperventilation (Paco$_2$ to ~30 mmHg) and avoid PEEP
• Maintain mean arterial pressure such that estimated CPP >60 mmHg

Extubation

• Maintain tracheal intubation if concerns about postop resp function; otherwise, prompt extubation for early neurologic evaluation

Adjuvants

• Benzodiazepines, β-blockers, antihypertensives

Postoperative Period

• If ICH persists, adequate ventilation/oxygenation, pain control, sedation essential

ANTICIPATED PROBLEMS/CONCERNS

• Use isotonic crystalloid or colloid IV solutions to minimize brain water and cerebral edema. Avoid dextrose since it may exacerbate effects of brain ischemia.
• Renal dysfunction and severe hypovolemia are possible from preop osmotic therapy

INTRAOPERATIVE RECALL
Randall C. Cork, M.D., Ph.D.

RISK
- People within USA: 2.5 million
- Gender/race prevalence: none

PERIOPERATIVE RISK
- 0.2–2.0% of all GA
- Incidence of recall is increased in obstetrics (7–28%), major trauma (11–43%), cardiopulmonary bypass (up to 23%), and bronchoscopy (8%), all associated with a "light level" of anesthesia

WORRY ABOUT
- Posttraumatic stress syndrome (PTSS)
- 7% of closed claims from intraoperative recall
- Poor postop recovery

OVERVIEW
- Explicit recall is conscious, deliberate recollection of events
- Implicit recall is change in behavior attributable to intraoperative event
- Both can lead to PTSS
- Underdiagnosed because of inadequate questioning by anesthesiologist and denial by patient

ETIOLOGY
- 70% due to technique, e.g., accidental or purposefully light anesthesia
- 20% due to equipment, e.g., empty vaporizer or faulty ventilator/circuit
- 10% unknown

USUAL TREATMENT
- Discuss the memories/feelings with patient
- Consult with psychologist or psychiatrist for treatment of PTSS

ASSESSMENT POINTS

SYSTEM	EFFECT	TEST
CV	Htn	BP
	Tachycardia	ECG
RESP	Tachypnea	Resp rate
	Sighing	Ventilatory compliance
	Breath holding	Observation
	Bronchospasm	
	↑ Peak inspiratory pressure for same volume	
CNS	Increased autonomic activity	ECG
	Htn	BP
	Tachycardia	Observation
	Diaphoresis	Bispectral index
	Lacrimation	Processed EEG
	Anesthetic depth	
MS	Spontaneous movement	Ventilatory compliance
	Increased tone	Observation

Key Reference: Hameroff SR, Polsoa JS, Watt RC: Monitoring anesthetic depth. *In* Blitt C, Hines R (eds): Monitoring in Anesthesia and Critical Care Medicine, 3rd ed. New York, Churchill Livingstone, 1995, pp 491–507.

PERIOPERATIVE IMPLICATIONS

Preoperative Preparation
- Inform patient about risk of explicit and implicit memory and assure that you will be there at all times
- Perhaps allow patient option of earplugs, music, or tape to listen to during operation (certainly for patients with this problem after prior operations/anesthetics)
- Use an amnesiac agent as part of preop medication

Monitoring
- If using muscle relaxants, use twitch monitor to maintain at least one twitch
- Use bispectral index or processed EEG as an indication of depth of anesthesia

Airway
- Delaying endotracheal intubation beyond the normal period after a short-acting induction agent may result in recall

Induction
- Use excess induction agent if possible, and supplement if more time is required to control airway
- Use an amnesiac agent

Maintenance
- Use spontaneous ventilation, if possible
- Supplement with volatile agent, and monitor end-tidal concentration
- Monitor twitch, and maintain one visible
- Apply earplugs or play audio tapes to patient

Extubation
- Reverse muscle relaxation well before decreasing anesthetic

Adjuvants (to decrease incidence)
- Amnesiac agents
- Volatile anesthetics

Postoperative Period
- Always ask
  - Last thing remembered before?
  - First thing remembered after?
  - Anything in between?
  - Dream?
- If evidence of recall, discuss memories/feelings with patient and consult a psychologist or psychiatrist to treat for PTSS

ANTICIPATED PROBLEMS/CONCERNS
- PTSS
- Talkative OR personnel

JAUNDICE

William T. Merritt, M.D., M.B.A.

RISK

- Chronic liver disease consistently 9th most common cause of death in USA
- Male:female 2:1
- African-American:Caucasian 2:1

PERIOPERATIVE RISKS

- Jaundice per se poses no special risks
- Risks associated with co-existing or underlying conditions

WORRY ABOUT

- Esophageal varices (incompetent lower esophageal sphincter)
- Ascites
- Low systemic vascular resistance
- Bleeding
- Inability to extubate at end of surgery

OVERVIEW

- Mostly unconjugated
  - Excess production
- Hemolytic anemias (e.g., sickle cell anemia; B-thalassemia major)
- Extravascular hemolysis (tissue infarction; hemorrhage into tissue, "postoperative jaundice")
- Ineffective erythropoiesis
  - ↓ Hepatic uptake
- Drugs (e.g., flavaspidic acid, novobiocin, some cholecystographic dyes)
- Severe, prolonged fasting
  - ↓ Conjugation
- Neonate: physiologic jaundice of the newborn; "breast milk" jaundice; hypothyroidism; galactosemia
- Sepsis
- Acquired transferase deficiency: drug inhibition (e.g., pregnanediol, chloramphenicol); hepatocellular disease (cirrhosis, hepatitis)
- Gilbert's disease: ↓ glucuronyl transferase
- Crigler-Najjar I (absent) and II (partial decrease) in glucuronyl transferase
- Mostly conjugated
  - ↓ Hepatic excretion
- Hereditary/familial: Dubin-Johnson, Rotor syndromes; recurrent intrahepatic cholestasis, benign; gestational cholestatic jaundice—($\sim$1:13,000 deliveries; 3rd trimester; preeclampsia, nulliparity; twin; ↓ plt)
- Acquired: sepsis; hepatocellular disease (drug- and viral-induced hepatitis); postoperative jaundice (pigment overload [transfusions, resorption of hematomas, hemolysis]; hepatocellular damage [drugs, including halothane; shock]; benign postoperative jaundice); drug-induced cholestasis (e.g., oral contraceptives, methyltestosterone)
  - Extrahepatic biliary obstruction (e.g., mechanical, from stones, stricture, tumor)
- Pseudojaundice
  - Dietary carotenoids (primarily infants; excessive intake of vegetables, such as carrots, tomatoes); TPN-associated liver dysfunction
  - Poisoning (picric acid)

ICD-9-CM Code: 782.4 (Jaundice, unspecified, non-newborn)

USUAL TREATMENT

- No specific treatment outside of newborn period
- For neonates: fluids, phototherapy, exchange transfusion, albumin, tin mesoporphyrin and IV immunoglobulin Rx have been shown to decrease the level of unconjugated bilirubin below levels regarded to be toxic to the neonatal brain
- The smaller and sicker the premature infant, the more aggressive the therapy needed

ASSESSMENT POINTS

SYSTEM	EFFECT	ASSESSMENT BY HX	PE	TEST
HEENT		Duration	Yellow sclerae	
CV	Hyperdynamic Poss ↓ SVR	General Sx	↑ HR; ↓ BP	
RESP	Cirrhotics have 6× increase in pulm Htn	Severe dyspnea, hypoxia, clubbing	Clubbing Cyanosis	ECHO; right-sided heart catheterization if indicated
GI	Severe dysfunction Prolonged effects of most anesthesia drugs	General Sx, reflux, ascites, varices, edema	Signs of chronic liver disease	LFTs Coagulation time Hgb, plt
ENDO/ METAB	↓ Synthetic function ↑ Enzymes, ↓ albumin, ↓ hepatic coag factors; ↓ clearance of toxins	General malaise Sx Easy bruising/ bleeding	Jaundice Ecchymoses Hematoma Ascites	LFTs Coagulation time NH_3
HEME	↓ Plt	Easy bruising/bleeding	Ecchymoses, hematoma	
DERM		Duration; evidence of bleeding	Yellow color	
RENAL	↓ Function		Edema	BUN, Cr; Cr may be spuriously lower with high bilirubin
CNS	Recurrent encephalopathy in cirrhosis Cerebral edema in fulminant hepatic failure Autonomic dysfunction	Mental status: Duration of illness Abnormal autonomic function	Normal to encephalopathy/ Comatose Orthostatic BP changes	Bilirubin interferes with cerebral near-infrared oximetry

Key Reference: LaMont JT, Isselbacher KJ: Postoperative jaundice. N Engl J Med 1973; 288:305–307.

PERIOPERATIVE IMPLICATIONS

- Drug: ↓ protein production leads to ↓ albumin binding, more active drug
  - Cimetidine/ranitidine—clearance reduced, esp in patients with ascites, hypoproteinemia, encephalopathy
  - Benzodiazepines—clearance of oxidative pathway markedly ↓ ; glucuronidation path (e.g., lorazepam) not greatly altered. Excessive sedation in severe liver disease.
  - Narcotics—meperidine clearance is severely affected; succinylcholine activity may be prolonged somewhat because of ↓ levels of pseudocholinesterase
  - Miscellaneous—phenobarbital and lidocaine have reduced clearance; diuretics may have reduced natriuretic efficacy
  - Halogenated agents—halothane should be avoided; association of enflurane with hepatic toxicity is less clear; isoflurane, seroflurane are preferred agents in setting of liver disease and best preserves liver hemodynamics
  - Pregnancy—jaundice may signal the HELLP syndrome and pregnancy-induced Htn
  - Cardiac surgery—jaundice occurs in about 20% post-CPB patients; risk factor for mortality

Preoperative Preparation

- Hydration should be adequate; if chronic liver failure, may be total body fluid ↑, but intravascularly ↓

Monitoring

- NMB—dose muscle relaxants to effect and consider path of elimination

Airway

- May have bleeding disorder

Induction

- Avoid benzodiazepines
- Consider cricoid pressure if varices present

Maintenance

- Be mindful of metabolic clearance paths
- When practical, use drugs cleared chiefly by nonhepatic paths

Extubation

- May have delay in awakening

ANTICIPATED PROBLEMS/CONCERNS

- Inability to extubate immediately postop due to prolonged action of NMB and sedative/hypnotic/narcotic medications

JEHOVAH'S WITNESS PATIENT

Meg A. Rosenblatt, M.D.

RISK

- Approximately 2 million members in USA, 4.9 million worldwide
- Headquartered in Brooklyn, New York

PERIOPERATIVE RISKS

- Mortality 2° to massive hemorrhage

WORRY ABOUT

- Understanding the rights and desires of patient vs. rights of physician prior to need to administer blood or blood products
- Problems arise in emergencies when little time is available for discussion of transfusion issues
- Competent adults are those who know the nature and consequences of their actions; such adults have the right to refuse specific therapies
- *Parens patriae,* the power of the state, represents the duty and interest of the state to preserve the health of minors

OVERVIEW

- Began as Bible study group in early 1800s; became Jehovah's Witnesses in 1931
- Strict interpretation of Bible passages, which forbid eating of blood, interpreted as prohibition of acceptance of blood products to sustain life
- Witnesses believe acceptance of blood products precludes achievement of eternal salvation

USUAL TREATMENT

- Discuss and document preoperatively the potential for life-threatening hemorrhage and therapies and interventions that would be acceptable to the patient
- Seek evidence of advance directive, an affidavit that confirms the patient's refusal to accept a transfusion (which forces discussion and releases physicians/hospitals of responsibility for outcome of the patient's decision)
- Optimize hematocrit, with erythropoietin, prior to elective procedures in which risk for transfusion is high
- Consider contacting a Jehovah's Witness Hospital Liaison Committee, which consists of a group of individuals trained to work as intermediaries in avoiding conflict between patients and physicians
- Contact legal counsel if patient is a minor, is unconscious, or is an incompetent adult

ASSESSMENT POINTS

SYSTEM	ASSESSMENT BY HX	TEST
HEME	Evaluate for treatable forms of anemia	Iron, folate, B$_{12}$ levels BUN/Cr

Key Reference: Dupuis JF, Nguyen DT: Anesthetic management of the patient who refuses blood transfusions. Int Anesthesiol Clin 1998; 36:117–131.

PERIOPERATIVE IMPLICATIONS

Preoperative Preparations

- Oral iron supplementation
- Consider erythropoietin, 75–100 U/kg SQ or IV, 3 times/wk for 3–4 wk
- Delay elective surgery until red cell mass is optimized

Monitoring

- Minimize phlebotomies/pediatric sampling tubes
- Consider oximetric pulmonary artery catheter if high possibility of hemorrhage

Therapeutic Options

- Hyper- or normovolemic hemodilution
- Hypotensive anesthetic techniques
- Colloid volume expanders: hydroxyethyl starch, dextrans
- Oxygen-carrying solutions: hemoglobin solutions (from recombinant hemoglobin), perflurocarbons
- Increase FIO$_2$
- Desmopressin
- Antifibrinolytic agents: aprotinin, tranexamic acid, ε-aminocaproic acid
- Hyperbaric oxygen

Surgical Options

- Meticulous surgical technique/experienced surgeons
- Laparoscopic/endovascular surgery
- Preoperative angiographic embolization
- Topical collagen

Adjuvants

- May accept use of red blood cell scavenging devices when the equipment is arranged in continuous series with patient's circulatory system
- May accept use of closed drainage systems that allow reinfusion of shed mediastinal or wound blood
- May accept use of "minor" blood fractions, such as albumin

Extubation

- Consider postoperative ventilation with neuromuscular blocking agents, sedation, and hypothermia for severe anemia; supplement with IV hyperalimentation, erythropoietin, iron dextran (which may add ~100 mg of iron per liter of TPN)

JEUNE SYNDROME (ASPHYXIATING THORACIC DYSTROPHY)   Anne Marie Lynn, M.D.

RISK

- Rare: 106 reported cases in literature
- Some cases in offspring of consanguineous parents
- Seen in families of Norwegian, African-American, and Japanese descent
- Four clinical forms: lethal, severe, mild, latent

PERIOPERATIVE RISKS

- 75% mortality in newborn period from restrictive lung disease
- Respiratory failure from small thoracic cage and hypoplastic lungs
- Affected individuals surviving infancy are reported to have progressive renal disease with cystic lesions
- Liver involvement with fibrosis, cysts, and pancreatic cysts also sometimes seen

WORRY ABOUT

- Respiratory failure with hypoxia and hypercapnia
- Barotrauma with positive pressure ventilation

- Renal failure may require careful fluid and electrolyte management and selection of nonrenally cleared muscle relaxants
- Liver involvement (rare cirrhosis) may affect drug handling

OVERVIEW

- Rare autosomal recessive form of dwarfism with a 75% mortality in the newborn period
- Respiratory failure from restrictive thorax and hypoplastic lungs
- If pulmonary involvement is milder, allowing survival, then changes in renal, hepatic, and pancreatic systems (often with cystic lesions and/or fibrosis) are reported
- Postaxial polydactyly is often seen, but nail dysplasia and facial changes are not, helping to separate this from Ellis–van Creveld syndrome
- Cardiac anomalies infrequent except for pulmonary hypertension
- Surgical enlargement of the thorax has been undertaken to increase pulmonary compliance; in some cases respiratory function improves with age, so long-term ventilatory support (months to years) has been attempted

- Larynx is reported to be small in affected children
- Renal transplantation has been reported in patients surviving infancy

ICD-9-CM Code: 756.4

ETIOLOGY

- Autosomal recessive inheritance
- Gene involved not identified but may reside on chromosome 12

USUAL TREATMENT

- Surgical thoracic enlargement requires long-term ventilation, which can be difficult and has a high incidence of barotrauma
- Older children require surgery related to renal failure (dialysis catheters, renal transplantation)

ASSESSMENT POINTS

SYSTEM	EFFECT	ASSESSMENT BY HX	PE	TEST
HEENT	Small larynx			
CV	Pulmonary hypertension	Syncope	↑ 2nd heart sound	ECG (RVH) ECHO
RESP	Stiff, small rib cage Hypoplastic lungs	Pneumonia/resp failure Assisted ventilation Asynchronous ventilation with agitation/crying	Small chest Horizontal ribs Cyanosis with crying	ABGs CXR Oximetry
GI	Hepatic fibrosis/cysts Pancreatic fibrosis/cysts	Failure to gain weight	Hepatomegaly	Abdominal US Bilirubin/LFTs
RENAL	Cysts Nephritis	Polyuria, polydipsia		BUN, Cr, lytes, Ca^{2+}, PO_4 Abdominal US
CNS	Occasional hydrocephalus Retinal degeneration			
MS	Short stature Short limbs Polydactyly of hands and feet			X-ray of thorax, pelvis

Key Reference: Baum VC, O'Flaherty JE: Jeune Syndrome in Anesthesia for Genetic, Metabolic, and Dysmorphic Syndromes of Childhood. Philadelphia, Lippincott Williams & Wilkins, 1999, pp 156–157.

PERIOPERATIVE IMPLICATIONS

Preoperative Preparation
- Assess ventilation
- Evaluate for possible pulmonary hypertension
- Evaluate renal function and consider liver function testing

Monitoring
- Consider arterial catheter

Airway
- Small larynx requires ↓ endotracheal tube size

Induction
- Agitation may make respiration asynchronous (chest/abdomen), causing hypoxemia

Maintenance
- Lung hypoplasia makes barotrauma high risk; consider with acute respiratory deterioration

Extubation
- Document adequate ventilation before extubation; postoperative ventilation may be needed for a prolonged period, especially after thoracoplasty

Adjuvants
- Renal function assessment guides selection of muscle relaxant and fluid management

ANTICIPATED PROBLEMS/CONCERNS

- Asynchronous ventilation during crying with hypoxia
- Barotrauma during assisted mechanical ventilation
- Renal failure
- Postoperative respiratory failure requiring ventilatory support
- Prolonged drug effect if hepatic cirrhosis (rare)

KARTAGENER'S SYNDROME

Russell C. Raphaely, M.D.
Maureen M. O'Rourke, M.D.

RISK

- In USA and Europe, prevalence of situs inversus varies from 1/6800 to 1/35,000
- ~20% of all persons with situs inversus have bronchiectasis and chronic paranasal sinusitis to complete syndrome described by Kartagener

PERIOPERATIVE RISKS

- Morbidity: Lung infection, pulm edema, atelectasis, sinusitis

WORRY ABOUT

- Airway obstruction due to ineffective clearance of secretions
- Bronchiectasis, which can lead to cor pulmonale and pulmonary edema
- Chronic disease with variable onset
- Chemical injury from aspiration in left lung, which is the larger lung in patients with Kartagener's syndrome

- Unintended bronchial intubation with single-lumen tracheal tube resulting in non-ventilation of right lung (in those with pulmonary inversion)
- Left-sided double-lumen tube may occlude orifice of left upper lobe
- Nasal catheters relatively contraindicated because of risk of paranasal sinusitis and ear infections

OVERVIEW

- Situs inversus (including dextrocardia)
- Primary ciliary dyskinesia resulting in chronic resp tract infections, bronchiectasis, sinusitis

ICD-9-CM Code: 759.3

ETIOLOGY

- Congenital defect in synthesis of various parts of cilia (dynein arms, radial spokes, nexin links); genetic-autosomal recessive
- 1/70 persons involved are heterozygous

USUAL TREATMENT

- Aerosol administration to reduce secretion viscosity
- Antimicrobial therapy for chronic respiratory tract infections, sinusitis
- Surgical intervention for pulm lobectomy
- Conventional and assisted airway clearance techniques (chest physical therapy, positive expiratory pressure [PEP mask], forced oscillation techniques, exercise programs, and physical activity)
- Nasal steroid sprays
- Inhaled bronchodilators and anti-inflammatory medications to treat bronchospasm
- Antimicrobial therapy for chronic respiratory tract infections, sinusitis

ASSESSMENT POINTS

SYSTEM	EFFECT	ASSESSMENT BY HX	PE	TEST
CV	Dextrocardia			CXR
				ECHO
RESP	Bronchiectasis	Dyspnea	Decreased	CXR
	Ciliary dyskinesia	Cough	breath sounds	Bronchoscopy
		Halitosis	Rhonchi	Spirometry
				Bronchography
IMMUNO	Chronic paranasal	Nasal drainage	Frontal and	Sinus films
		Morning sore throat	maxillary tenderness	(CT)
	Bronchitis	Cough	Rhonchi	Sputum and tracheal aspirate
		Mucus production		for culture and Gram stain
	Pneumonia	Cough	Rales	CXR
		Fever	Rhonchi	SpO_2
	Otitis media	Earache	Erythematous	Audiometry
			tympanic membrane	Tympanotomy

Key Reference: Ho AMH, Friedland MJ: Kartagener's syndrome: anesthetic considerations. Anesthesiology 1992; 77:386–388.

PREOPERATIVE PREPARATION

- Consider omitting anticholinergics and cough suppressant from preanesthetic medication.

PERIOPERATIVE IMPLICATIONS

Monitoring

- In dextrocardia, position of ECG leads should be the mirror image of normal, as should that of paddles of external defibrillation, cardioversion, and pacing
- Since the great vessels and thoracic duct are likely to be reversed, consider cannulation of the internal jugular vein from the left

Airway

- Emphasize aseptic technique
- Humidify inspired gases
- Inhalation injury usually occurs in left lung, which is also larger lung

- Bronchial intubation with a single-lumen tracheal tube usually involves left side
- Right bronchial suctioning will be more difficult to perform with nonangulated suction catheters
- Left-sided double-lumen tube may occlude orifice of left upper lobe
- When lung isolation is needed, consider tracheal intubation first with a bronchial blocker in the appropriate bronchus
- If double-lumen tube is required, consider inserting the left-sided tube with the bronchial tube on the right; the endobronchial stylet and the upper part of tube must be bent 180° from original orientation prior to insertion such that the normal curvature of the oropharynx is still followed. The same principles apply to use of a right-sided tube.

Anesthetic Technique

- Employ regional techniques when possible

Extubation

- As soon as possible

Postoperative Considerations

- Consider nonnarcotic analgesia

ANTICIPATED PROBLEMS/CONCERNS

- Lung infection common as result of ciliary dyskinesia
- Fluid overload can precipitate cor pulmonale and pulm edema
- Avoid nasal catheters/airways to minimize chances of paranasal sinusitis

KEARNS-SAYRE SYNDROME
Jeremy M. Geiduschek, M.D.

RISK

- Less than 300 reported cases
- Same incidence in males and females
- Onset of symptoms before age 20 y

PERIOPERATIVE RISKS

- Cardiac conduction defects progress to complete heart block

WORRY ABOUT

- Cardiac rhythm
- Increasing demand for O_2 leading to lactic acidosis
- Decreased respiratory efficiency 2° to muscle weakness

OVERVIEW

- Triad of findings: chronic progressive external ophthalmoplegia, retinal pigmentary degeneration, and cardiac conduction block
- Other findings may include short stature, muscle weakness, developmental delay, dementia, cerebellar ataxia, epilepsy, hypoparathyroidism, diabetes, hypogonadism, nephropathy, hepatic dysfunction, asymmetric septal hypertrophy, cardiomyopathy, ↑ CSF protein, and ↑ serum lactate

ICD-9-CM Code: None listed; Use 759.89 (Congenital malformation affecting multiple systems not elsewhere classified)

ETIOLOGY

- Caused by rearrangement of mitochondrial DNA, KSS is part of spectrum of mitochondrial myopathies and encephalomyopathies
- Heterogeneous disorders that are still being defined
- Sporadic inheritance
- Diagnosis based on clinical findings and muscle biopsy that show abnormal accumulation of mitochondria ("ragged red fibers"); more sophisticated genetic analyses are able to demonstrate mitochondrial DNA deletions or insertions

USUAL TREATMENT

- Complete cardiac evaluation, including Holter monitor and echocardiogram; prophylactic pacemaker insertion for any evidence of AV block
- Treatment with steroids may precipitate hyperglycemia and severe metabolic acidosis
- Routine medical management of any associated findings

ASSESSMENT POINTS

SYSTEM	EFFECT	ASSESSMENT BY HX	PE	TEST
CV	Conduction defect Cardiomyopathy	↓ Exercise tolerance Sx CHF	Bradycardia	ECG, Holter ECHO Electrophysiology
RESP	CHF and muscle weakness may affect respiratory function	↓ Exercise tolerance		
RENAL	Nephropathy			BUN/Cr
ENDO	Hypoparathyroidism Diabetes		Tetany Chvostek's sign Weakness	Calcium FBS
CNS	Ophthalmoplegia Retinal pigment degeneration Hearing loss Cerebellar ataxia Elevated CSF protein	Visual disturbance ↓ Night vision ↓ Mobility	↓ ROM of ocular muscles ↓ Visual acuity "Salt and pepper" pigment changes of retina on funduscopy ↓ Hearing Dysdiadochokinesia Wide-based gait	MRI Lumbar puncture
PNS	Peripheral neuropathy	Weakness	↓ Strength	
MS	Variable muscle weakness	↓ Mobility	↓ Strength Impaired gait	Muscle biopsy

Key Reference: DeVivo DC: The expanding clinical spectrum of mitochondrial diseases. Brain Dev 1993; 15:1–22.

PERIOPERATIVE IMPLICATIONS

Preoperative Preparation

- Be prepared to provide cardiac pacing
- Have magnet if pacemaker already present
- Assess cardiac status

Monitoring

- Routine, assuming no cardiomyopathy or CHF present

Airway

- Routine

Induction

- Consider regional or local anesthesia if applicable

- Avoid administration of muscle relaxant; if needed, use reduced dose

Maintenance

- No specific technique proven superior

Extubation

- Muscle weakness may delay extubation

Adjuvants

- Sedatives carefully titrated

Postoperative Period

- Watch for respiratory failure 2° to muscle weakness
- Continuous cardiac monitoring

ANTICIPATED PROBLEMS/CONCERNS

- Progression to complete heart block; consider pacemaker insertion with any degree of AV block; have ability to provide cardiac pacing (e.g., transcutaneous pacer)
- So far, mitochondrial myopathies have not been associated with malignant hyperthermia
- Not known if KSS or other mitochondrial myopathies create risk for severe hyperkalemia following succinylcholine administration

KLIPPEL-FEIL SYNDROME

Eric Weissend, M.D.
Ronald S. Litman, D.O.

RISK

- Incidence estimated at 1:40,000 live births (probably underestimate, as milder cases go unrecognized)
- Slight female predilection (63%)

PERIOPERATIVE RISKS

- Cervical spine instability and cardiopulmonary complications

WORRY ABOUT

- Exacerbation of cervical spine instability during airway maneuvers, endotracheal intubation, and subsequent positioning

OVERVIEW

- Not a disease
- Congenital abnormality consisting of the following triad of findings: (1) fusion of two or more cervical vertebrae; (2) low posterior hairline; (3) cervical immobility
- Severity ranges from mild (often not recognized until late in life) to severe (recognized at birth because of obvious deformity)
- Careful preoperative assessment of cervical spine anatomy and degree of instability
- Review of systems for other congenital abnormalities (many reported; see below)

ICD-9-CM Code: 756.16

ETIOLOGY

- Unknown

USUAL TREATMENT

- None

ASSESSMENT POINTS

SYSTEM	EFFECT	ASSESSMENT BY HX	PE	TEST
HEENT	Head and neck immobility		ROM of cervical spine, facial asymmetry, cleft palate, torticollis, vocal cord dysfunction	Flexion/extension radiographs of cervical spine Consider MRI of cervical spine
CV	Bradyarrhythmias and AV conduction pathway abnormalities (due to CNS malformations) Cardiac defects (most commonly VSD)	Syncope	Murmurs	ECG ECHO
RESP	Central alveolar hypoventilation Pulmonary agenesis or hypoplasia Restrictive lung disease (due to severe scoliosis)	Sleep apnea, snoring, difficulty breathing		ABGs CXR (if symptomatic)
RENAL	Urinary tract abnormalities Renal agenesis, ureteral duplication			BUN, Cr if indicated Renal US
CNS	Hindbrain abnormalities (e.g., syringomyelia, Arnold-Chiari malformation) Mental retardation Deafness, strabismus	Peripheral neurologic dysfunction (e.g., weakness, paresthesias, paraplegia, quadriplegia)	Neurologic exam	
MS	Scoliosis, Sprengel's deformity (scapular elevation) Hypermobility of C-spine, spondylosis/decreased mobility of C-spine		Exam of spine and shoulders	Radiographs if indicated

Key Reference: Smith B, Griffin C: Klippel-Feil syndrome. Ann Emerg Med 1992; 21:876–879.

PERIOPERATIVE IMPLICATIONS

Preoperative Preparation

- Careful and complete evaluation of cervical spine anatomy and instability and of other major organ system abnormalities

Monitoring

- Depends on patient's physical condition

Airway

- If indicated, awake intubation using maneuvers to stabilize cervical spine; complete immobility with use of fiberoptic intubating bronchoscope ideal

Preinduction/Induction

- Depends on patient's physical condition

Maintenance

- Careful positioning of head and neck with maintenance in neutral position

Extubation

- Depends on extent of cervical spine pathology and respiratory compromise

Adjuvants

- No special considerations

ANTICIPATED PROBLEMS/CONCERNS

- Exacerbation of pre-existing cervical spine instability leading to neurologic deterioration

LATEX ALLERGY

Mary A. Keyes, M.D.

RISK

- Myelomeningocele (25–30%)
- Congenital urologic anomalies
- Health care workers (5–10%)

PERIOPERATIVE RISKS

- Type I immediate hypersensitivity reactions involve IgE-specific latex proteins. Cutaneous contact may result in pruritus and urticaria. Airborne exposure may lead to sneezing and rhinitis. Systemic reactions including bronchospasm, hypotension, and vascular collapse are life-threatening manifestations.
- Type IV hypersensitivity or contact dermatitis occurs 24–48 h after exposure and is confined to cutaneous manifestations

WORRY ABOUT

- Life-threatening anaphylactic reactions from intraoperative exposure. Latex is a ubiquitous substance in the medical environment.

OVERVIEW

- Institution of universal precautions and recognition of latex allergy as a serious medical problem seem to have coincided. Billions of imported rubber gloves may be more allergenic due to more rapid production and more free latex particle aerosols.
- The combination of atopy and frequent exposure increases the risk in all groups. There is a spectrum of latex sensitivity from cutaneous manifestations to angioedema and anaphylaxis. Latex allergy should be suspected in any unexplained episode of intraoperative anaphylaxis.
- Radioallergosorbent (RAST) testing is specific but has variable sensitivity, 65–85%. Skin testing is more sensitive; however, there is a small but definite anaphylaxis risk.

ICD-9-CM Code: V15.07

ETIOLOGY

- Hypothesis that exposure early in life facilitates sensitization. Myelomeningocele group may represent a uniquely sensitive population, perhaps through intrathecal exposure during wound closure and ventriculoperitoneal shunting.

USUAL TREATMENT

- All patients with myelomeningocele can be treated in a *latex-free* environment from birth. Patients with congenital urologic anomalies could be considered for this precaution.
- Latex sensitivity is treated by meticulously preventing exposure. Pretreatment regimen of antihistamines and corticosteroids is often recommended, although there is no perfect evidence that pretreatment can prevent anaphylaxis.
- Anaphylaxis treatment: stop exposure, intravascular volume expansion, epinephrine as needed to support blood pressure and treat bronchospasm. Antihistamines and corticosteroids are secondary therapy.

ASSESSMENT POINTS

SYSTEM	ASSESSMENT BY HX	TEST
IMMUNO	Atopy, food allergies, asthma Hx of anaphylaxis	RAST, skin test

Key Reference: Landwehr LP, Boguniewicz M: Current perspectives on latex allergy. J Pediatr 1996; 128:305–312.

PERIOPERATIVE IMPLICATIONS

- Provide a latex-free environment. All hospitals and anesthesiology departments can have a handbook with latex-free materials listed. Since latex is an aeroallergen and present in the air for at least an hour after the use of latex gloves, patient can be scheduled as first case of the day. An Internet Web site is available to provide the most current information about safe products: *www.latexallergyhelp.com.*

ANTICIPATED PROBLEMS/CONCERNS

- Being aware of those at risk and providing a latex-free environment will eliminate most untoward events. However, be prepared to treat anaphylaxis.

LEIGH SYNDROME (SUBACUTE NECROTIZING ENCEPHALOPATHY)

Jeremy M. Geiduschek, M.D.

RISK

- Onset of symptoms usually in infancy
- Rare disorder

PERIOPERATIVE RISKS

- Respiratory failure after GA reported
- Other risks 2° to degree of symptoms and presence of cardiomyopathy and/or renal disease

WORRY ABOUT

- Abnormal regulation of respiration may lead to respiratory failure following sedation for procedures
- Decreased respiratory efficiency 2° to muscle weakness
- Metabolic acidosis

OVERVIEW

- Also called "subacute necrotizing encephalomyelopathy"
- Onset in infancy or early childhood
- Clinical features: failure to thrive, developmental delay, hypotonia, peripheral and optic neuropathy, ataxia, tremor, progressive respiratory dysfunction, aspiration pneumonias, brainstem dysfunction
- Occasional features: cardiomyopathy, renal disease
- Death usually within 2 y of onset of symptoms
- Laboratoy evaluation: elevated serum lactate and pyruvate, decreased CSF glucose
- Radiology findings (CT or MRI): lesions of the subcortex, midbrain, and brainstem (due to cysts, vascular proliferation, and demyelination)

ICD-9-CM Code: 330.8

ETIOLOGY

- Multiple modes of inheritance
- Due to a variety of mutations
- Enzyme defects causing severe deficiency of mitochondrial ATP production

USUAL TREATMENT

- Supportive measures
- Thiamine has improved status in some patients

ASSESSMENT POINTS

SYSTEM	EFFECT	ASSESSMENT BY HX	PE	TEST
HEENT	Swallowing difficulties		Sialorrhea	
CV	Cardiomyopathy	Sx CHF	Murmur, gallop, holosystolic murmur, pulm edema	ECG CXR ECHO
RESP	CNS disease will affect resp regulation Muscle weakness will affect resp regulation	Response to sedatives History of pneumonia		
GI	Chronic diarrhea	Episodes of dehydration	Hydration status	Electrolytes
ENDO/METAB	Lactic acidosis			Lactate
GU	Nephropathy			BUN/Cr
CNS	Ophthalmoplegia Optic atrophy Ataxia Seizures	Developmental history Loss of milestones	↓ ROM of ocular muscles ↓ Visual acuity Abnormal reflexes Wide-based gait	Cranial CT MRI
PNS	Peripheral neuropathy	Weakness	↓ Strength	
MS	Progressive hypotonia and weakness	↓ Mobility	↓ Strength	

Key Reference: Web site: Online Mendelian Inheritance in Man (OMIM). *http://www.ncbi.nlm.nlh.gov/Omim* (for Leigh Syndrome [MIM 256000]).

PERIOPERATIVE IMPLICATIONS

Preoperative Preparation

- Determine extent of cardiac involvement
- Give preoperative anticholinergic if oral secretions are copious
- Avoid prolonged fasting. Minor dehydration may worsen lactic acidosis.

Monitoring

- Routine, assuming no cardiomyopathy or CHF present

Airway

- Dependent on physical examination

Induction

- Consider nonlactated IV fluids
- No specific technique has been proven superior
- Succinylcholine avoided if peripheral neuropathy present

Maintenance

- No specific technique proven superior
- If NMB used, consider shorter acting agents with careful titration to desired end point

Extubation

- Muscle weakness may delay extubation

Adjuvants

- Sedatives carefully titrated due to ↓ consciousness and weakness

Postoperative Period

- Close monitoring of respiratory function

ANTICIPATED PROBLEMS/CONCERNS

- Not associated with malignant hyperthermia
- Not known if risk present for severe hyperkalemia following administration of succinylcholine (peripheral neuropathy would theoretically create risk)
- Fatal disorder, with death usually resulting from either progressive cardiac or pulmonary involvement

LESCH-NYHAN SYNDROME

Lawrence O. Larson, M.D.

RISK

- X-linked recessive disorder
- Incidence ~5.2 per million male births

PERIOPERATIVE RISKS

- Airway problems 2° to scarification from self-mutilation
- Impairment of renal function due to obstructive uropathy

WORRY ABOUT

- Aspiration pneumonia
- Drug metabolism and prolonged drug effects 2° to metabolic defect and impaired renal function

OVERVIEW

- Patients usually mentally subnormal
- Patients exhibit characteristic pattern of compulsive self-mutilation, spasticity, and choreoathetosis
- Primary biochemical defect is almost complete absence of hypoxanthine-guanine-phosphoribosyltransferase (HGPRT)
- Enzyme defect leads to excessive purine production and elevated uric acid concentrations

ICD-9-CM Code: 277.2

ETIOLOGY

- Genetic disease inherited as X-linked recessive trait

USUAL TREATMENT

- No specific treatment of enzyme deficiency
- Benzodiazepines frequently used to control self-mutilation and spasticity
- Gene therapy possibility
- Gabapentin

ASSESSMENT POINTS

SYSTEM	EFFECT	ASSESSMENT BY HX	PE	TEST
HEENT	Distortion of airway structures due to self-mutilation		Examine airway	
CV	Hypertension, CAD Adrenergic pressor response to stress is absent	Angina, angina-equivalent symptoms PND	Displaced PMI S_3	ECG Pharmacologic stress testing Coronary angiography and ECHO
RESP	Aspiration pneumonia	SOB following vomiting episode	Rales Wheezing	CXR
GI	Vomiting Athetoid dysphagia	Dysphagia		
RENAL	Decreased renal function due to obstructive uropathy			BUN Cr IVP
CNS	Retardation Seizure disorders Decreased MAO activity		Mental status questioning	EEG Mental function tests
MS	Spasticity Contractures		ROM	

Key Reference: Williams KS, Hankerson JG, Ernst M, Zametkin A: Use of propofol anesthesia during outpatient radiographic imaging studies in patients with Lesch-Nyhan syndrome. J Clin Anesth 1997; 9:61–65.

PERIOPERATIVE IMPLICATIONS

Preoperative Preparations

- Antacids
- H_2 blockers
- Metoclopramide
- IV access may be difficult

Monitoring

- Routine
- ST-segment analysis if CAD present

Airway

- Rapid-sequence induction
- Avoid succinylcholine
- Awake fiberoptic intubation

Preinduction/Induction

- Restraints
- Avoid agents with renal metabolism

Maintenance

- Avoid agents with renal toxicity
- No one agent or technique shown superior
- Administer exogenous catecholamines with caution

Extubation

- Awake to avoid aspiration

Adjuvants/Postoperative Period

- Restraints
- Benzodiazepines for spasticity

ANTICIPATED PROBLEMS/CONCERNS

- History unavailable or inaccurate because of retardation

LEKUEMIA

Subhash Jain, M.D.
Nolan Tzou, M.D.

RISK

- Incidence in USA: 2.8% all new cancers, 5/100,000 (acute) (children and adult)
  - ALL: 1/100,000
  - AML: 4/100,000
  - CLL: 2.5/100,000
  - CML: 1/100,000
- 15× greater incidence in patients with Down syndrome

PERIOPERATIVE RISKS

- Immunosuppression creates risk of both minor and major infections; sepsis, interstitial pneumonitis, encephalopathy
- Hematoma/bleeding 2° to thrombocytopenia and splenic sequestration of platelets

WORRY ABOUT

- Bone marrow suppression with nitrous oxide; no evidence that nitrous oxide adversely affects bone marrow engraftment
- Clinical case reports of patients with ALL who developed malignant hyperthermia
- Neuropathy related to chemotherapy
- Report of airway obstruction in all patients during central venous catheter insertion

OVERVIEW

- Hematologic malignancy with proliferation of cells may cause ↓ in amino acids, causing fatigue and metabolic starvation
- Invasion possible in all organ systems
- Usually outpatient treatment, but may require several procedures including bone marrow aspiration, central venous access placement, lumbar puncture, bronchoscopy, pericardiocentesis, external beam radiation

ICD-9-CM Codes: 208.0 (Undifferentiated, acute, blastic); 204.0 (Lymphoblastic)

ETIOLOGY

- Unknown
- Strong suspicion that leukemia and lymphoma are virus-induced

USUAL TREATMENT

- AML
  - Ara-C
  - Anthracyclines: daunorubicin, idarubicin
  - Vinca alkaloids: epipodophyllotoxin,vincristine/vinblastine
  - Bone marrow transplant
- CML
  - Busulfan
  - Hydroxyurea
  - Interferon alfa
  - Bone marrow transplant
- CLL
  - Cyclophosphamide
  - Corticosteroid
  - Fludarabine
  - Cytarabine

ASSESSMENT POINTS

SYSTEM	EFFECT	ASSESSMENT BY HX	PE	TEST
HEENT	Ulceration, oral lesions	Dysphagia	Airway assessment	
CV	Rare: Pericardial effusion, conduction defects, murmurs, CHF	Dyspnea, fatigue	Narrow pulse pressure, pericardial friction rub, cardiomegaly	CXR ECG ECHO
GI	Hepatosplenomegaly Nutritional support may be necessary to prevent hypoalbuminemia and loss of immunocompetence	Loss of appetite	Hepatosplenomegaly	Albumin
HEME	Anemia Leukostasis Thrombocytopenia	Weakness, fatigue	Pallor Ecchymoses Petechiae	CBC Bone marrow aspirate results
RENAL	Renal failure from tumor lysis syndrome (acute loss of tumor)	↓ Urine output	↓ Urine output	BUN/Cr ↑ Phosphate, ↑ or ↓ Ca^{2+} ↑ K^+
CNS	Cranial nerve infiltration (very rare) Meningeal leukemia (less common in adults) Vincristine neuropathy	Cranial nerve palsies, clouding of mental status Peripheral neuropathy	Weakness	EMG
MS	Infiltration of bony cortex and periosteum, synovial membranes	Bone pain	Bone swelling	X-ray CT scan

Key Reference: Fortney JT, Halperin EC, Hertz CM, Schulman SR: Anesthesia for pediatric external beam radiation therapy. Int J Radiat Oncol Biol Phys 1999; 44:587–591.

PERIOPERATIVE IMPLICATIONS

Preoperative Preparation

- Assess volume status, evidence of N/V, diarrhea, oral mucositis

Monitoring

- Routine

Airway

- Signs of dysphagia, ulcerations from chemotherapy and candidiasis
- Oral leukemia lesions can occur prior to or during therapy

Induction

- Brief heparinization and thrombocytopenia before bone marrow aspiration may influence choice of spinal or epidural

Maintenance/Extubation

- Based on clinical status of patient
- Usually very low postanesthetic complication rate, but include transient hypotension, dizziness, N/V, and temperature regulating

ANTICIPATED PROBLEMS/CONCERNS

- Risk of infection, aseptic technique with placement of all lines

Uday Jain, M.D., Ph.D.

RISK

- People within the USA: 10% of children, 25% of adult population
- Race with highest prevalence: none

PERIOPERATIVE RISKS

- Myocardial ischemia, infarction, CHF
- Stroke and TIAs
- Pancreatitis with hypertriglyceridemia

WORRY ABOUT

- New-onset angina, increasing frequency or severity of angina
- Worsening or new-onset CHF
- Transient ischemic attacks of CNS
- Peripheral atherosclerosis

OVERVIEW

- Hypertriglyceridemia, hypercholesterolemia (see separate sections)

- Hypolipidemia: Autosomal recessive Tangier disease (severe deficiency of HDL); familial hypoalphalipoproteinemia (HDL deficiency); LDL deficiency (autosomal recessive abetalipoproteinemia, autosomal dominant familial hypobetalipoproteinemia); normotriglyceridemic abetalipoproteinemia (LDL absent); 2° to cancer, myeloproliferative disorders, liver failure
- Lipodystrophy: Familial generalized lipodystrophy (Berardinelli-Seip syndrome: autosomal recessive, leads to macrosomia); Köbberling-Dunnigan syndrome (familial lipodystrophy of limbs and trunk, autosomal dominant, may lead to macrosomia)

ICD-9-CM Codes: 272.0–9

See also Coronary Artery Disease, Atherosclerotic Disease, Hypercholesterolemia, and Hypertriglyceridemia in Diseases section

ETIOLOGY

- Autosomal dominant or recessive inheritance
- Secondary to systemic illness

USUAL TREATMENT

- Diet and exercise
- Cholestyramine and colestipol inhibit absorption of bile acids derived from cholesterol
- Neomycin blocks cholesterol absorption
- HMG CoA reductase inhibitors (lovastatin, pravastatin, simvastatin, atorvastatin) reduce cholesterol synthesis and are commonly used
- Thyroid hormone clears LDL
- Probucol reduces LDL but also HDL
- Nicotinic acid inhibits VLDL, LDL production
- Fibric acids clofibrate and gemfibrozil cause catabolism of triglyceride-rich lipoproteins

ASSESSMENT POINTS

SYSTEM	EFFECT	ASSESSMENT BY HX	PE	TEST
HEENT	Tangier disease		Lobulated, bright orange-yellow tonsils	
CV	Myocardial ischemia and infarction LV dysfunction	Angina or its equivalents Dyspnea, edema, exercise intolerance, MI	Displaced PMI S_3 S_4	ECG, CXR, stress testing, ECHO, coronary angiography
RESP	CHF	Dyspnea, orthopnea, cough	Rales and rhonchi	CXR
RENAL	Impaired renal perfusion	Nighttime urinary frequency		BUN,Cr
CNS	Cerebrovascular atherosclerosis	TIAs	Carotid bruit	Carotid ultrasound and angiography

Key Reference: Ballantyne CM: Hyperlipidemia: diagnostic and therapeutic perspectives. J Clin Endocrinol Metab 2000; 85:2089–2112.

PERIOPERATIVE IMPLICATIONS

Preoperative Preparation

- Assess for CAD and peripheral vascular disease
- β-blockers and nitrates perioperatively, as tolerated

Monitoring

- Consider PA catheter, TEE in the presence of large fluid shifts, history of ischemia, and high-risk surgery

Airway

- Patients may be overweight, have large head and neck, be difficult to intubate

Maintenance

- Monitor for ischemia and cardiac failure
- Avoid hypothermia and anemia
- Heparin releases two triglyceride hydrolases: lipoprotein lipase inhibited by protamine and hepatic lipase resistant to protamine
- Insulin increases activity of lipoprotein lipase and releases free fatty acids (FFAs)
- Sympathetic stimulation, stress, and catecholamines release FFAs
- Spinal or epidural anesthesia and β-blockers reduce FFA levels

Extubation

- For noncardiac surgery, this may be period of greatest risk for ischemia

Adjuvants

- Depends on end-organ disease and lipid-drug binding

Postoperative Period

- High incidence of tachycardia, ischemia, and MI for several days after noncardiac surgery
- Treat pain, hemodynamic and biochemical abnormalities

ANTICIPATED PROBLEMS/CONCERNS

- Problems are related to atherosclerosis

LUDWIG'S ANGINA

John Penner, M.D.

RISKS

- About 70% have poor dentition, periodontal disease, and/or recent dental work. Other risks: sublingual lacerations, penetrating injuries to the floor of the mouth, sialadenitis, compound mandibular fractures, osteomyelitis of the mandible, otitis media, infected malignancy, and abscesses located under the thyrohyoid membrane.
- Associated with the following: acute glomerulonephritis, aplastic anemia, neutropenia, DM, immundeficiency states, dermatomyositis, and SLE

PERIOPERATIVE RISKS

- Potential for airway compromise to complete airway closure
- Spread of the infection along the deep cervical fascia can result in mediastinitis, mediastinal abscess, subphrenic abscess, jugular vein thrombosis, innominate artery rupture, pneumothorax, pericardial and/or pleural effusion, empyema, necrotizing fasciitis, and cervical or mandibular osteomyelitis

WORRY ABOUT

- Airway compromise
- The spread of infection remote to the site
- Mediastinitis, mediastinal abscess, subphrenic abscess, jugular vein thrombosis, innominate artery rupture, pneumothorax, pericardial effusion, pleural effusion, necrotizing fasciitis, or empyema

OVERVIEW

- Potentially lethal, rapidly spreading cellulitis involving the sublingual and submaxillary spaces
- Infection often starts as a periapical dental abscess of the 3rd or 4th mandibular molars, which have roots below the mylohyoid line of the mandible. Infection of the sublingual and submandibular spaces then follows.
- Accompanied by edema formation
- May present with tooth pain, swelling of the tongue and chin, fever, dysphagia, difficulty breathing, and inability to handle secretions

ICD-9-CM Code: 528.3

ETIOLOGY

- Results from bacterial infection; 50% are polymicrobial
- Most common isolates are streptococci and staphylococci. The most common anaerobe is bacteroides.

USUAL TREATMENT

- Treatment directed toward establishing a patent airway, treating the bacterial infection, and surgically decompressing the sublingual and submaxillary spaces

ASSESSMENT POINTS

SYSTEM	EFFECT	ASSESSMENT BY HX	PE	TEST
HEENT	Airway edema	Dysphagia Difficulty breathing Trismus	Drooling Stridor Retractions Cyanosis Sitting position Small oral aperture	CT/MRI of soft tissue
CV	Hypovolemia Pericardial effusion	Poor PO intake Hypotension	Orthostatic BP JVD Arrhythmia ↓ CO on PPV	Equalization of pressures across heart ECHO Pericardiocentesis
PULM	Pneumothorax Empyema Pleural effusion	Pleuritic pain Cough Dyspnea SOB SOB	Unequal breath sounds Tactile fremitus Ipsilateral hyperresonance	CXR CXR/thoracentesis CXR/thoracentesis

Key Reference: Spitalnic SJ, Sucov A: Ludwig's angina: case report and review. J Emerg Med 1995; 13:449–503.

PERIOPERATIVE PREPARATION

Preoperative Concerns

- High likelihood of difficult airway; tracheotomy tray available and a surgeon present
- Consider an antisialagogue to ↓ secretions and facilitate either direct or fiberoptic laryngoscopy.
- Review appropriate diagnostic tests for distant spread

Monitoring

- Routine; consider more if impending sepsis or significant co-morbidities exist
- If central access is desired, potential for jugular vein thombosis, which may make line placement difficult if not impossible

Airway Management

- Consider potential options for difficult airway
- After a deep enough level of anesthesia achieved, trismus may resolve
- Consider the potential for continued airway swelling after the oral ETT secured. One group recommends armored ETTs, as PVC nasotracheal tube may occlude 2° to continued pharyngeal swelling.

Induction

- Inhalation induction with spontaneous ventilation
- Consider the lateral position. Should obstruction occur, a nasal trumpet airway may be effective.

Maintenance

- Due to potential for pneumothorax, consider avoiding nitrous oxide

Extubation/Postoperative Period

- If extubated postop, consider a monitored setting

ANTICIPATED PROBLEMS/CONCERNS

- Consider postop intubation until swelling resolves
- If a nonarmored tube is chosen, consider possibility of tube occlusion 2° to airway swelling

LYME DISEASE

Sophia Socaris, M.D.
Philip D. Lumb, M.B., B.S., F.C.C.M.

RISK

- Most common arthropod-borne infection in USA
- Coastal areas in the east (3.7/100,000), from Maryland (6.1/100,000 [mid-Atlantic]) to Massachusetts; the Midwest in Wisconsin and Minnesota (0.7/100,000); and the far west, in northern California (0.6/100,000), southern Oregon (0.9/100,000), and western Nevada (0.6/100,000)
- Gender predilection: none
- Children < 15 y; adults 25–44 y

PERIOPERATIVE RISKS

- Increased risk of arrythmias and CHF in patients with cardiac involvement

WORRY ABOUT

- Fluid overload
- CHF
- AV block

OVERVIEW

- Stage 1—Early localized infection: erythema chronicum migrans (rash spreads centrifugally; lesion usually occurs at site of bite)
- Stage 2—Early disseminated infection: aseptic meningitis, cranial neuritis, and peripheral radiculoneuritis are neurologic manifestations
  - Carditis occurs in 4–8% of patients during this stage of disease
  - 2nd and 3rd degree AV block and myocarditis may be documented by ECG and heart failure; symptoms resolve in days to weeks
- Stage 3—Late persistent infection: intermittent episodes of asymmetric pain and swelling in a few large joints, especially the knees, over years; 62% of untreated patients develop frank arthritis a mean of 6 mo after

disease onset; 10% of untreated Americans with joint involvement develop chronic Lyme arthritis

ICD-9-CM Code: 088.81

ETIOLOGY

- Lyme disease is caused by the spirochete *Borrelia burgdorferi,* which is transmitted by the tick *Ixodes dammini*

USUAL TREATMENT

- Early doxycycline (within 24–48 h of bite) prevents infection in very high percentages
- Antibiotic therapy typically shortens stage 1 and generally aborts stages 2 and 3
- Vaccine available for adults

ASSESSMENT POINTS

SYSTEM	EFFECT	ASSESSMENT BY HX	PE	TEST
CV	AV node block CHF	Palpitations Fatigue Dyspnea Dizziness with exercise	Bradycardia Tachycardia	ECG
RESP		SOB	Rales	CXR
DERM	Erythema chronicum migrans	Erythematous annular lesions	Erythematous circular rash	
CNS	Meningitis Bell's palsy Radiculoneuritis	Headache Cognitive impairment Memory deficit	Cranial nerve facial palsy	Serology Lumbar puncture EMG
MS	Arthritis	Joint pain and swelling Musculoskeletal pain	Swelling of one or a few joints Erythema of joints	

Key Reference: Karsh R: Lyme disease. Rheum Dis Clin North Am 1993; 19:339–426.

PERIOPERATIVE IMPLICATIONS

Preoperative Concerns

- Ensure antibiotic Rx and cure of carditis prior to all but life-or-death emergency operations

Monitoring

- Routine

Airway

- Routine

Preinduction/Induction

- Avoid depolarizing muscle relaxants

Maintenance

- Routine

Extubation

- Routine

Adjuvants

- Avoid depolarizing muscle relaxants on induction, because of hyperkalemia

Postoperative Period

- Routine

ANTICIPATED PROBLEMS/CONCERNS

- Patients may develop arrhythmias

LYMPHOMAS

Alisa C. Thorne, M.D.

RISK

- Hodgkin's disease (HD) USA: 3/100,000 annually Dx
- Non-Hodgkin's lymphoma (NHL) USA: 13.7/100,000 annually Dx
- Race with highest prevalence of HD and NHL: Caucasian (90% of all cases)
- In past 15 y, 50% ↑ in incidence of NHL partly due to lymphoma in AIDS patients

PERIOPERATIVE RISKS

- Morbidity and mortality related to compression of organs and chemotherapy
- Mediastinal mass
- Superior vena cava syndrome; anthracycline cardiac toxic effects
- Bleomycin pulm toxic effects
- Pericardial effusion
- Radiation pneumonitis

WORRY ABOUT

- Tracheal or bronchial compression by large mediastinal mass

- Increased cardiac/pulm toxic effects with combination chemotherapy/radiation therapy (RT)

OVERVIEW

- Two major types of lymphoma: HD and NHL
- 7th most common cause of cancer-related death in USA
- 3rd most common childhood malignancy
- Average age at diagnosis: 42 y
- Often curable
- Accurate Dx and staging critical in determining Rx and prognosis

ICD-9-CM Codes: 200–202.8

ETIOLOGY

- HD: pathogenesis remains obscure, increased risk with inherited immunodeficiency syndromes, EBV, increased educational level

- NHL: pathogenesis involves clonal malignant expansion of B or T cells, increased risk with congenital and acquired immunodeficiency states, autoimmune disorders, infectious agents, phenoxyherbicides, organophosphates, ionizing radiation

USUAL TREATMENT

- Diagnostic laparoscopy or laparotomy
- RT
- Chemotherapy with multiple agents
- Combination RT and chemotherapy
- Chemotherapy commonly includes: bleomycin, doxorubicin, prednisone, nitrogen mustard, vincristine, procarbazine
- RT commonly includes neck, chest
- Both chemotherapy and RT have cardiac and pulmonary toxic effects
- Advanced or recurrent HD: treatment with biologics (e.g., radiolabeled immunoglobulin therapy, early reports show good response

ASSESSMENT POINTS

SYSTEM	EFFECT	ASSESSMENT BY HX	PE	TEST
HEENT	Bulky nodal disease Compression	SOB, DOE Tracheal deviation	Neck mass Wheeze, stridor	Indirect laryngoscopy CXR CT/MRI
CV	Mediastinal mass SVC syndrome (SVC obstruction)	SOB, DOE Cough, orthopnea Mental status change	Facial swelling, wheeze, may be asymptomatic Dilated veins upper half of body Edema of head, neck, and upper extremities, cyanosis	CXR, CT/MRI ECHO CT of airway
RESP	Pericardial effusion CHF due to anthracyclines Bronchial compression Obstructive pneumonia Pneumonitis due to bleomycin and/or RT	Frequently asymptomatic SOB, DOE Cough Wheeze Sx worse in supine position Fever, cough	↑ HR, ↓ BP, neck vein distention Rales, pedal edema	CXR, ECHO CT/MRI Flow-volume loop ABGs, PFTs, DLco
GI	Abdominal mass Upper/lower GI bleed Perforated viscus	Abdominal pain, GI bleeding	Palpable mass	CT/MRI
HEME	Bone marrow involvement			Alk phos, CBC, plts, bone marrow biopsy
CNS	Leptomeningeal disease or single or multiple mass lesions	Headache Cranial nerve abnormalities	Abnormal neuro exam	Spinal tap CT/MRI
RENAL	Ureteral compression			IVP, BUN/Cr

Key Reference: DeVita VT Jr, Hellman S, Rosenberg SA (eds): Cancer: Principles and Practice of Oncology, 5th ed. Philadelphia, Lippincott Williams & Wilkins, 1997, Ch 44.

PERIOPERATIVE IMPLICATIONS

Preoperative Preparation

- Assess extent bulky nodal disease causing upper or lower airway and/or cardiac compression
- Assess LV function after anthracyclines
- Assess pulmonary function after bleomycin, RT
- If large mediastinal mass, use local anesthetic if possible

Monitoring

- Routine

Airway

- Routine, unless large anterior mediastinal mass calls for awake fiberoptic intubation

- Use armored ETT
- Rigid ventilating bronchoscope on hand

Induction

- If large mediastinal mass: consider awake fiberoptic intubation, maintaining spontaneous ventilation, and semi-Fowler's position

Maintenance

- Spontaneous ventilation as above; avoid muscle relaxants
- Choose shortest acting agents for rapid wakeup
- After bleomycin use lowest FIO$_2$ possible

Extubation

- If mediastinal mass, extubate patient awake and breathing spontaneously and have rigid ventilation bronchoscope on hand

Adjuvants

- If asymptomatic with mediastinal mass, airway obstruction and/or cardiac compression may develop on induction

Postoperative Period

- Airway obstruction if mediastinal mass: observe longer in intensive nursing setting
- Monitor fluid status if significant LV dysfunction

ANTICIPATED PROBLEMS/CONCERNS

- If bulky nodal disease in neck and chest, at risk for SVC syndrome, difficult airway, and tracheobronchial compression on loss of spontaneous ventilation
- May have significant cardiac/pulmonary impairment due to combination chemotherapy/RT

MALIGNANT HYPERTHERMIA (MH) AND OTHER ANESTHETIC-INDUCED MYODYSTROPHIES (AIMs)

Henry Rosenberg, M.D.
John G. Shutack, D.O.

RISK

- Incidence of MH: 1/15,000–20,000 anesthetics in children; 1/50,000–100,000 in adults depending on use of trigger agents, gene pool
- Male > female

PERIOPERATIVE RISKS

- Mortality with MH in North America < 10%
- Mortality with other AIMs ~ 50%
- Masseter muscle rigidity (MMR)—10–20% of patients experiencing MMR develop clinical MH; generalized rigidity predicts clinical MH in > 60%
- Central core myopathy—very high risk for MH
- Hyperkalemia and cardiac arrest with Duchenne, Becker's dystrophy when succinylcholine used and sometimes with volatile agents only
- Certain forms of myotonia lead to risk for MH and/or hyperkalemia with succinylcholine

WORRY ABOUT

- Potent volatile anesthetics and succinylcholine contraindicated in MH and patients with AIM
- Availability of dantrolene
- Purge machine with 100% O_2 15–20 min prior to case
- Recrudescence of MH (about 25% of cases)
- Counseling family regarding risk and muscle biopsy testing

OVERVIEW

Malignant Hyperthermia

- Autosomal dominant myopathy
- Hypermetabolic disorder manifested by ↑ CO_2 production/O_2 consumption, acidosis, hyperkalemia, myoglobinuria/emia, tachycardia, tachypnea, increased end-tidal CO_2
- Untreated, mortality > 80%
- Dantrolene only specific treatment
- Dx by halothane/caffeine contracture test of biopsied muscle

ICD-9-CM Code: 995.89 (MH)

Other AIMs

- Patients with muscular dystrophy/myotonia may develop hyperkalemic arrest with succinylcholine and occasionally with potent volatiles only
- Signs of dystrophy subtle or not apparent in young children
- Obtain muscle specimens for dystrophin analysis, genetic testing if cardiac arrest
- Test for CK elevation in suspicious cases

ETIOLOGY

MH

- Defect in calcium release/control leads to ↑ intracellular calcium

- Heterogenetic predisposition
  - ? Ryanodine receptor, ? sodium channel, ? fatty acid production, ? inositol triphosphate system defect(s)
- Chromosomes 19, 17, 7, 3 linked in some cases

Other AIMs

- Muscular dystrophies—X-linked inheritance, several mutations
- Myotonia—genetic abnormality of sodium, chloride channels, or protein kinase, linked to chromosomes 19, 17, ? others
- Central core disease—in some families, linked to ryanodine receptor

USUAL TREATMENT

MH

- Discontinue triggers
- Hyperventilate patient with 100% O_2
- Dantrolene 2.5 mg/kg IV; may use more to treat acute episode
- Treat metabolic acidosis; actively cool
- Increase fluids $1\frac{1}{2}$ to 2 × maintenance
- No calcium-channel blockers
- Maintain UO 1–2 ml/kg, diuretics if necessary
- Assess for hyperkalemia and treat appropriately
- Coagulation profile, DIC a problem

Other AIMs

- Treat for hyperkalemia

ASSESSMENT POINTS

SYSTEM	EFFECT	ASSESSMENT BY HX AND PE	TEST
HEENT	Masseter muscle rigidity	Difficult intubation	ABGs/acidosis Hypercarbia Myoglobinuria
CV	MH: Tachycardia, arrhythmias AIM: Sudden bradycardia VFIB, asystole	Hyper/hypotension	Mixed venous and ABGs: ↑ End-tidal CO_2, myoglobinuria Hyperkalemia
RESP	Tachypnea	Tachypnea	↑ End-tidal CO_2
MS	Generalized rigidity	Developmental delay Muscle weakness	CK Muscle biopsy
RENAL	Renal failure	Low UO Dark urine	Myoglobinuria
SKIN	Vasoconstriction Heat	Mottled appearance (late) Hot skin Sweating	Core temperature

*The caffeine/halothane contracture test is used to assess MH susceptibility.

Key Reference: Rosenberg H, Fletcher JE, Brandone BW: Malignant hyperthermia and other pharmacogenetic disorders. *In* Barash P, Cullen B, Stoelting RK, (eds): Clinical Anesthesia, 4th ed. Philadelphia, JB Lippincott, 2000.

PERIOPERATIVE IMPLICATIONS

Perioperative Preparation for Known MH

- Avoid triggers (succinylcholine, all potent volatile agents)
- Use local anesthesia (amides and ester OK)
  - Regional anesthesia (epidural, spinal, regional block)
  - General—all following drugs are *not* triggers: pentothal (barbiturates), etomidate, ketamine, propofol, nitrous oxide, all nondepolarizing muscle relaxants, narcotics, benzodiazepines

- Anesthesia machine
  - Change circuit and bag
  - Remove and/or drain vaporizers
  - Oxygen flow at 10 L/min for 15–20 min prior to use
- Dantrolene prophylaxis not necessary
- Dantrolene and calcium-channel blockers together produce hyperkalemia

Monitoring

- Routine including end-tidal CO_2, core temperature

Perioperative Implications, Other AIMs

- Some, not all, patients with DMD and Becker's dystrophy will develop hyperkalemia with MH triggers
- Avoid succinylcholine in patients with myotonia

ANTICIPATED PROBLEMS/CONCERNS

- Sudden cardiac arrest in PACU
- Myoglobinuria, renal failure
- Rhabdomyolysis—follow CKs
- Hyperkalemia

DISEASES   213

MALNUTRITION

Srinivas Mantha, M.D.

RISK

- People within USA: generally 28% in surgical patients on admission to hospital
- For example, 39% in patients undergoing thoracic or abdominal surgery and 53% in patients with moderate to severe emphysema undergoing lung volume reduction surgery
- Race with highest prevalence: unknown

PERIOPERATIVE RISKS

- 18-fold increase for same operations compared with nonmalnourished
- Related to poor wound healing, infection, sepsis
- Presence of hypoalbuminemic malnutrition associated with poor outcome compared with protein-calorie malnutrition (PCM)
- 16.6% incidence of wound infections
- Prolonged respiratory support
- Prolonged length of hospital stay

WORRY ABOUT

- Respiratory muscle strength
- Impaired cellular immunity
- CHF

OVERVIEW

- Results from inadequate intake of macronutrients (carbohydrate, protein, fat); referred to as PCM
- There are two types of PCM:
  – Marasmic form (MF-PCM), which results in uniform loss of fat and muscle mass in all tissues and a concomitant loss of water in proportion to nonaqueous mass
  – Stress-induced hypoalbuminemic form of protein-calorie malnutrition (HAF-PCM), which results from neurohumoral modulation leading to depletion of visceral protein (in excess of muscle mass) and fat and is associated with an expansion of extracellular fluid compartment. Stress may be surgery, infection, inflammation, trauma, neoplasia.
  – In hospitalized patients, marasmic-kwashiorkor type (i.e., wasting of muscle and fat with hypoalbuminemia) is most common

ICD-9-CM Code: 261

ETIOLOGY

- Prolonged fasting and stress
- ↓ Dietary intake, ↑ metabolic demands and nutrient loss
- Surgical conditions associated with nausea and vomiting
- Malignant conditions involving GI tract. Tumors involving the neck. End-stage liver disease awaiting liver transplantation. Patients undergoing anterior and posterior spinal fusion.
- Common in ASA III and IV patients aged >60 years
- Burns
- Emphysema
- COPD: ↑ resting energy expenditure

USUAL TREATMENT

- If albumin level does not increase after 3–7 days of enteral or parenteral nutrition, mortality rate perioperatively exceedingly high

ASSESSMENT POINTS

SYSTEM	EFFECT	ASSESSMENT BY HX	TEST
CV	↓ Preload and stroke volume		ECHO
RESP	↓ FRC and diaphragmatic activity		CXR Expiratory spirogram
GI	↓ Gastric motility Gastric ulceration Gastric and intestinal atrophy	Anorexia, vomiting	Generally not needed
GENERAL	Malnutrition	Preadmission wt loss >10% of body wt in 6 mo or 5% in 1 mo, edema, anorexia, vomiting, diarrhea, ↓ food intake, chronic illness	BMI <20 kg/m^2 Voluntary hand-grip test Anthropometric measurements (midarm muscle circumference or triceps skinfold thickness: both <15th percentile of reference data)
IMMUNO	Impaired cell-mediated immunity Surgical wound infection and sepsis		Abnormally low lymphocyte count (<1500/mm^3) Anergy to a battery of 4 or 5 standard skin antigens
RENAL	↓ Mass ↓ Cr clearance and impaired ability to concentrate urine	↓ UO	Serum Cr/BUN
HEPATIC	↓ Protein synthesis		↓ Serum albumin (<3.5 mg/dl) and ↓ serum transferrin (<200 mg/dl)
PNS	↓ Peripheral nerve conduction and sensory abnormailities	Tingling and numbness in extremities	Generally not needed

Key Reference: Corish CA, Kennedy NP: Protein-energy undernutrition in hospital in-patients. Br J Nutr 2000; 83:575–591.

PERIOPERATIVE CONSIDERATIONS

Preinduction
- Consider prophylaxis for aspiration of gastric contents

Monitoring
- Routine

Induction
- None

Maintenance
- Patients receiving TPN must continue to receive it in intraop period. Alternatively, it may be replaced with 10% dextrose. TPN volume must be added to the total IV intake.
- Careful titration of volatile agents
- Hydration and UO

Extubation
- Resp muscle failure may preclude early extubation

Adjuvants
- Vecuronium metabolism impaired
- ↓ Binding (volume of distribution) of protein-bound drugs

ANTICIPATED PROBLEMS/CONCERNS

- Since edema is prominent feature of HAF-PCM, interpretation of anthropometric measurements may be difficult
- Perioperative nutritional support, if given for at least 10 days, reduces morbidity and mortality in patients with biochemical evidence of severe malnutrition, manifested as a low serum albumin (<3 mg/dl) and excessive weight loss
- Patients with end-stage chronic obstructive lung disease usually have malnutrition, and sudden refeeding perioperatively may precipitate acute respiratory failure

MARFAN'S SYNDROME

Laura Myers, M.D.
William J. Greeley, M.D.

RISK

- Prevalence is 2–3/10,000 population
- Inherited as autosomal dominant trait

PERIOPERATIVE RISKS

- Aortic arch dissection, MVP, mitral or aortic valve regurgitation, coronary artery abnormalities, cardiac arrhythmias, pneumothorax, restrictive lung disease

WORRY ABOUT

- Symptoms referable to progressive dilatation or rupture of ascending thoracic aortic aneurysm (e.g., chest pain radiating to interscapular region)
- Symptoms of mitral (midsystolic click) or aortic valvular insufficiency
- Myocardial ischemia (angina) due to medial necrosis of coronary arterioles
- Arrhythmias and conduction disturbances (palpitations)
- SOB (dyspnea) due to restrictive lung disease

OVERVIEW

- Familial disorder of connective tissue (CT) underlying defect of collagen synthesis decreases tensile strength and elasticity of CT. Involves skeleton, eye, and CV system, skin, fascia, lungs, skeletal muscle, CNS, and adipose tissue.
- Common causes of death are CV: aortic dilatation, dissection, or rupture; aortic or mitral valvular regurgitation; coronary artery insufficiency
- Skeletal features: increased length of long bones, joint laxity, scoliosis, pectus excavatum and carinatum, and possible laxity of cervical spine
- Pulm: spontaneous pneumothorax, restrictive lung disease with thoracic deformity, and obstructive problems during sleep due to laxity of soft tissue
- Ocular: lenticular subluxation or dislocation, cataracts, and glaucoma

ICD-9-CM Code: 759.82

ETIOLOGY

- Mutation in *FBNI,* the gene that encodes fibrillin-1, a major component of extracellular microfibrils (major components of elastic fibers, anchoring the dermis, epidermis, and ocular zonules)

USUAL TREATMENT

- No specific treatment
- Life expectancy can be normal

ASSESSMENT POINTS

SYSTEM	EFFECT	ASSESSMENT BY HX	PE	TEST
HEENT	Lens dislocation	Myopia	Retinal detachment	Ophthalmoscopy
CV	Aortic dissection Myocardial ischemia	Chest pain Angina		MRI, ECHO ECG Radionuclide studies Stress testing Angiography
	Arrhythmias	Palpitations	Pulse	Holter monitor Electrophysiology
RESP	Restrictive lung disease	Dyspnea	Pectus scoliosis	PFTs CXR
MS	Tall stature Joint hypermobility Recurrent dislocation Hernias			Arm span > height

Key Reference: Pyeritz RE: The Marfan syndrome. Annu Rev Med 2000; 51:481–510.

PERIOPERATIVE IMPLICATIONS

Preoperative Preparation

- Consider antibiotics for SBE prophylaxis
- Consider preoperative β-blockade Rx to mitigate increases in myocardial contractility and aortic wall tension (dP/dT)

Monitoring

- ST-segment analysis; consider TEE
- Invasive monitoring as appropriate for planned surgery

Airway

- High arched palate
- Potential cervical laxity/instability
- Potential for TMJ dislocation with direct laryngoscopy

Preinduction/Induction

- Avoid sudden increases in aortic wall tension
- Careful positioning to avoid dislocations

Maintenance

- No one technique has demonstrated superiority

Exubation

- Avoid sudden increases in CO, BP as this may increase dP/dT
- High risk for developing myocardial ischemia

Adjuvants

- Adequate pain management important
- May require ↑ doses of local anesthetic due to ↑ size and enlargement of the neural canal

ANTICIPATED PROBLEMS/CONCERNS

- CV: aortic dissection, MVP, mitral or aortic regurgitation, myocardial ischemia, cardiac arrhythmias
- Respiratory: pneumothorax, restrictive lung disease with thoracic deformity

MASTOCYTOSIS

Ron Yaniv, M.D.
Azriel Perel, M.D.

RISK

- People within USA; very rare
- Race/gender with highest prevalence: none

PERIOPERATIVE RISKS

- Increased risk of hypotension and bronchospasm as consequence of paroxysmal release of mast cell mediators
- Anesthetic drugs and procedure may induce mast cell degranulation
- Perioperative mortality rate—fatal cases reported

WORRY ABOUT

- Increased risk of hypotensive shock and bronchospasm
- Clotting factors may be disturbed as result of vitamin malabsorption, hepatic fibrosis, and massive heparin release from mast cells (uncommon)
- Profound cardiovascular collapse and death without signs of flushing or bronchospasm

OVERVIEW

- A spectrum of mast cell proliferative disorders (MPD): Common—indolent cutaneous MPD; Localized—solitary mastocytoma; Generalized—diffuse mastocytomas, urticaria pigmentosa (UP), telangiectasia macularis eruptiva perstans (TMEP)
- Initial manifestation is cutaneous eruption in many
- Episodic flushing, headaches, nausea, and vomiting
- Sometimes vascular collapse with syncope and palpitations, abdominal pain, wheezing
- Main concern—to avoid mast cell degranulators
- Rare—mast cell lymphoma/leukemia; rule out carcinoid syndrome as cause of symptoms (elevated urinary 5-HIAA)

ICD-9-CM Codes 202.6 (Mastocytosis); 238.5 (Mastocytoma); 757.33 (Mastocytosis syndrome)

ETIOLOGY

- Unknown
- MPD
- Also hypersensitive degranulation response of neoplastic mast cell

USUAL TREATMENT

- H_1 blockers—e.g., chlorpheniramine maleate, hydroxyzine, terfenadine; H_2 blockers—e.g., cimetidine, ranitidine followed by aspirin to block PGD_2 synthesis
- Disodium cromoglycate PO for GI symptoms
- Ketotifen
- Shock—IV epinephrine 2–10 μg/min and volume repletion
- EpiPen and epinephrine inhalers
- PUVA (psoralens plus ultraviolet A) for cutaneous manifestation
- Steroids—topical and systemic
- Anticholinergic agents
- Chemotherapy
- Splenectomy
- Protamine sulphate *rarely* necessary when endogenous heparin prolongs prothrombin time

ASSESSMENT POINTS

SYSTEM	EFFECT	ASSESSMENT BY HX	PE	TEST
HEENT	Rhinorrhea	Allergic rhinitis		
CV	Episodic vascular collapse			Episodic elevations of plasma histamine levels
RESP	Asthma	Wheezing		
GI	Malabsorption, GI bleeding Abdominal pain N/V; diarrhea		Hepatosplenomegealy	
HEME	Anemia, thrombocytopenia, leukopenia, mast cell leukemia			CBC Clotting studies Bone marrow biopsy
DERM	Mastocytoma UP TMEP	Pruritus Urticaria	Skin biopsy	(+ Giemsa)
PNS	Polyneuropathy		CNS exam	
MS	Bone pain			X-ray, ^{99m}Tc bone scan

Key Reference: Vaugh ST, Jones GN: Systemic mastocytosis presenting as profound cardiovascular collapse during anaesthesia. Anaesthesia 1998; 53:804–807.

PERIOPERATIVE IMPLICATIONS

Preoperative Preparation

- Refrain from ethanol, aspirin, NSAIDs
- Premedication with histamine-releasing drugs might be avoided
- Diazepam premedication—reported to be safe
- Start prophylactic H_1 and H_2 blockers
- Prophylactic disodium cromoglycate—yet to be confirmed (100 mg q6h)
- Predictive prick tests for drugs such as muscle relaxants—controversial

Monitoring

- Routine monitors
- Intra-arterial catheter (sudden BP changes)

Airway

- Intubation may be dangerous in the presence of mucosal lesions, as pressure can cause degranulation and bronchospasm or hypotension

Preinduction/Induction

- Avoiding atropine, scopolamine, and sodium thiopental has been recommended. Preinduction with H_1 blocker such as 25–50 mg diphenhydramine.
- Inhalational agents—safe (may even increase mast cell stability)

Maintenance

- Maintain normothermia
- Hypotension due to histamine release—IV epinephrine, 1–3 mg/kg
- Dopamine—not helpful
- Avoid dextran as colloidal solution

Extubation

- Should be smooth
- Keep patient warm

Adjuvants

- Blood transfusion—should be warmed and given only when essential

- Muscle relaxants: vecuronium recommended. Avoid potential histamine-releasing muscle relaxants in large doses, such as ditubocurarine, atracurium, gallamine.
- Regional: has been advocated but hypotension and bronchospasm reported to be even more common as well as urticaria and pruritus
- Antibiotics: avoid polymyxin B sulfate. Used safely: amikacin, cefazolin, metronidazole (± vancomycin).
- Miscellaneous drugs: avoid dipyridamole, papaverine, quinine, thiamine
- Radiologic contrast dyes can induce acute episode

Postoperative Period

- Continue with analgesics, H_1 and H_2 blockers

ANTICIPATED PROBLEMS/CONCERNS

- Hypotensive and bronchospastic crisis due to mast cell degranulation induced by anesthetic or surgical procedures

MEDIASTINAL MASSES
Jeffrey Rosenberg, M.D., Ph.D.

- Congenital lesion: 1/5000, M:F 1:1
- Thymoma, lymphoma, retrosternal goiter

PERIOPERATIVE RISKS
- Perioperative mortality rare
- Inability to ventilate or oxygenate
- Hypotension or tamponade

WORRY ABOUT
- Airway obstruction and inability to ventilate
- Vascular compression with hypoxia, hypotension, arrest
- Superior vena cava syndrome with airway edema and increased bleeding
- Recurrent laryngeal nerve injury
- Patients at risk with cough and pain, dyspnea and dysphagia, superior vena cava syndrome, tracheal deviation, Horner's syndrome, cyanosis, mediastinal widening, and hoarseness

OVERVIEW
- Severity of symptoms does not predict intra-operative course
- Airway obstruction or hemodynamic compromise has occurred with induction of GA, intubation, muscle relaxation, position change, and after extubation

ICD-9-CM Codes: 164.0 (Malignant thymoma); 201.9 (Hodgkin's lymphoma); 202.8 (Non-Hodgkin's lymphoma)

ETIOLOGY
- Adults: 97% malignant—80% metastatic bronchogenic carcinomas; 17% lymphomas (50% of lymphomas have mediastinal involvement); 20% thymomas (50% malignant; 35% association with myasthenia gravis)
- Pediatric: 87% malignant—16–36% of non-Hodgkin's lymphomas and 54–81% of Hodgkin's lymphomas, bronchial cysts, and teratomas

- Superior vena cava syndrome in 6–7% of lung cancer
- Others include parathyroid or thyroid tumors; lymphoid tumors; teratomas, aortic aneurysms, esophageal achalasia or diverticula, diaphragmatic hernia, bronchogenic or pericardial cysts, neurofibromas

USUAL TREATMENT
- For tissue diagnosis: biopsy under local
- If no tissue can be obtained or patient is uncooperative, approach is selective radiotherapy sparing some tumor for later diagnosis
  - If not diagnostic, then biopsy under GA
- Surgical resection for some tumors
- Cardiorespiratory complications during anesthesia are usually fewer after radiation

ASSESSMENT POINTS

SYSTEM	EFFECT	ASSESSMENT BY HX	PE	TEST
HEENT	Compression of trachea by mass	Cough Cyanosis Dyspnea Orthopnea	Wheezing Stridor	CXR Flow-volume loop CT scan
CV	Compression of PA or heart SVC syndrome	Fatigue, faintness Headache Dyspnea	Neck edema JVD Pulsus paradoxus ↓ BP	CXR ECHO supine and sitting
RESP	↓ Lung volume	Cough, cyanosis, dyspnea, orthopnea	↓ Breath sounds Wheezing; stridor	CXR, CT scan, PFTs
CNS	Compression of recurrent laryngeal nerve, sympathetic chain, spinal cord	Stridor Sympathetic instability Focal neuro Sx	BP changes with postural changes Paresthesias Focal weakness	Flow-volume loops Tilt table testing SSEP EMG

Key Reference: Pullerits J, Holzman R: Anaesthesia for patients with mediastinal masses. Can J Anaesth 1989; 36:681–688.

PERIOPERATIVE IMPLICATIONS

Preoperative Preparation
- Consider (including pediatric patients) an IV prior to induction (lower extremity if SVC syndrome)
- Those with PA or heart compression may need cardiopulmonary bypass (check availability prior to induction with cannulation sites prepped and draped)
- Consider light or no premedication except for anticholinergic

Monitoring
- Consider intra-arterial catheter, central venous, or pulm artery catheter
- If SVC syndrome, insert central venous access or PA catheter via femoral vein

Airway
- Tracheal or distal compression; may become obstructed with induction and muscle relaxation
- Maintain spontaneous ventilation throughout procedure unless ET tube is below obstruction
- Symptomatic patients in supine position are best maintained sitting or semi-sitting during induction

- Awake fiberoptic intubation not necessary if asymptomatic in supine position and CXR and/or CT scan do not reveal airway obstruction or compression
- If in doubt consider awake fiberoptic bronchoscopy to rule out obstruction or compression
- If compression seen in thoracic trachea, then consider a single-lumen armored ET tube with its tip distal to the compression
- If compression is at level of carina or distal, endobronchial intubation or a double-lumen endobronchial tube is recommended

Preinduction/Induction
- May develop airway obstruction with inability to ventilate
- May develop hypoxia from obstruction of pulm artery and blood flow to lungs

Maintenance
- Consider local anesthesia; otherwise keep patient breathing spontaneously
- If obstruction occurs consider altering patient's position, attempt rigid bronchoscopy, median sternotomy, or femorofemoral cardiopulmonary bypass

Extubation
- Deep extubation during spontaneous breathing recommended; try to minimize straining, coughing, or bucking with an increase in intrathoracic pressure
- Observe several hours after extubation to detect and treat delayed airway obstruction

ANTICIPATED PROBLEMS/CONCERNS
- Airway obstruction, hypotension, and hypoxia are major concerns
- Consider radiation and/or chemotherapy before GA
- If GA required, consider inspection of tracheobronchial tree with fiberoptic bronchoscopy
- If GA required, maintaining spontaneous ventilation preferable

MESOTHELIOMA

John R. Moyers, M.D.

RISK

- Diffuse mesothelioma: 15/1 million population
- Male:female 6–7:1
- 0.16% of all malignancies
- Localized mesothelioma extremely rare

PERIOPERATIVE RISKS

- Usually discovered in geriatric male undergoing lung biopsy
- Pleural effusion
- Previous needle biopsy of lung and thoracentesis make pneumothorax a concern
- General debilitation from malignancy

OVERVIEW

- Diffuse malignant mesothelioma is a sheetlike growth usually originating in lower part of chest cavity, invading diaphragm, and encasing lung and other mediastinal structures
- Peak incidence 20–40 y after asbestos exposure
- Usual onset of symptoms at age 55–70 y
- Median survival after onset of symptoms is 18 mo

ICD-9-CM Codes: 162.9 (Lung neoplasm); 199.1 (Mesothelioma, malignant site unspecified)

ETIOLOGY

- Diffuse mesothelioma related to asbestos exposure in 12–93% of cases
- Also associated with radiation therapy, erionite exposure, chronic inflammation and fibrosis, and other agents

USUAL TREATMENT

- Treatment has been controversial and largely ineffective
- Therapy has consisted of radiation to hemithorax, chemotherapy, and sometimes surgery (parietal pleurectomy and decortication or extrapleural pneumonectomy)

ASSESSMENT POINTS

SYSTEM	EFFECT	ASSESSMENT BY HX	PE	TEST
HEENT	Tracheal displacement			Lateral and AP CXR
CV				ECG
RESP	Pneumothorax	Cough, chest pain, increased SOB		ABGs, PFTs (rarely necessary) CXR (post biopsy; in expiration)
	Restrictive lung disease	Dyspnea, exercise	Percussion and auscultation of chest	
GI	Weight loss, debilitation, peritoneal tumors	Past body weights		CT scan of abdomen (not for perioperative care) Albumin (for degree of malnutrition) CBC (for malnutrition)
ENDO	Not associated with paraneoplastic syndromes			

Key Reference: Rusch VW: Diagnosis and treatment of pleural mesothelioma. Semin Surg Oncol 1990; 6:279–288.

PERIOPERATIVE IMPLICATIONS

Perioperative Preparation

- Usually come to surgery for lung biopsy via thoracoscopy or open-lung biopsy; some patients are scheduled for pleuropneumonectomy
- Assess pulmonary status; size of effusion, no pneumothorax
- Patient often had one or more recent needle biopsies of lung or thoracenteses
- Review CT scan for size and location of tumor

Monitoring

- Routine monitors
- Resp system via stethoscope, SpO$_2$, and PETCO$_2$
- Intra-arterial catheter for complex surgical procedures

Airway

- Look for tracheal and mediastinal displacement on CXR and CT scan

Induction

- Propensity for hypoxia, particularly from restrictive lung disease

Maintenance

- High FIO$_2$ may be necessary
- One-lung ventilation
- Lateral positioning

Extubation

- Ensure patient meets extubation criteria

Adjuvants

- Pain control after thoracoscopy or thoracotomy
- No special considerations for muscle relaxants, reversal agents, local anesthetics, or special drug interactions

Postoperative Period

- Monitor ventilation and oxygenation
- Pain relief; consider epidural or spinal analgesia after thoracotomies
- May have air leak postop

ANTICIPATED PROBLEMS/CONCERNS

- Anesthesia with one-lung ventilation for a geriatric patient with incurable malignancy
- Recent lung biopsy and thoracentesis prior to surgery and potential for complications from those procedures, including pneumothorax and dehydration
- Effective pain relief and monitoring of respiratory function postop
- Consider ICU stay for those undergoing complex procedures

METHEMOGLOBINEMIA

H. Michael Marsh, M.B., B.S., B.Sc.(Med)

RISK

- People within USA: rare
- Gender prevalence: none
- Socioeconomic/ethnic prevalence: none

PERIOPERATIVE RISKS

- Inadequate oxygen carriage and delivery to tissues
- Hemolysis may be induced by methylene blue, especially in patients with glucose-6-phosphate dehydrogenase (G6PD) deficiency

WORRY ABOUT

- % of methemoglobin or sulfhemoglobin. Acutely developing methemoglobinemia or sulfhemoglobinemia may become symptomatic at 1% with cyanosis; at 60%, acute CV collapse, coma, or death may occur.

OVERVIEW

- Present when >1% of circulating hemoglobin is oxidized to ferric form
- Two hereditary forms: (1) due to NADH-diaphorase (cytochrome b5 reductase) deficiency, inherited as an autosomal recessive trait; (2) due to abnormal globins, hemoglobin M, which are inherited as autosomal dominant traits
- Toxic methemoglobinemia occurs from exposure to agents that directly oxidize hemoglobin or facilitate its oxidation by molecular oxygen: nitrates ingested, nitroglycerin, isobutyl nitrite, and some local anesthetics

ICD-9-CM Code: 289.7

ETIOLOGY/PATHOGENESIS

- Fe^{2+} in hemoglobin is constantly oxidized in vivo, by NO and reactivity with O_2, to Fe^{3+}, methemoglobin. NADPH-diaphorase utilizes NADH generated by glyceraldehyde dehydrogenase, in the Embden-Meyerhof pathway, to reduce cytochrome b5, which in turn reduces Fe^{3+} in methemoglobin to Fe^{2+} in hemoglobin.

USUAL TREATMENT

- Medical therapy: ascorbic acid 300–600 mg/d in divided doses. Methylene blue 1 mg/kg IV, repeated once provided that patient is not G6PD-deficient, since hemolysis will occur in this case.
- Methylene blue may also be taken orally as 60 mg tid

ASSESSMENT POINTS

SYSTEM	EFFECT	ASSESSMENT BY HX	PE	TEST
RESP	SOB DOE	Hx of cyanosis if hereditary form	RR	Co-oximetry
HEME	Cyanosis if 1% methemoglobin is present or sulfhemoglobin seen	Cyanosed	Cyanosis	Spectrometry at 630 nm

Key Reference: Kern K, Langevin PB, Dunn BM: Methemoglobinemia after topical anesthesia with lidocaine and benzocaine for a difficult intubation. J Clin Anesth 2000; 12:167–172.

PERIOPERATIVE IMPLICATIONS

Preoperative Preparation

- Consider treatment if methemoglobin level is >1%. If sulfhemoglobin is present, may mean exchange transfusion.

Monitoring

- Use co-oximeter (IL282), since presence of methemoglobin will render pulse oximetry unreliable

Airway

- Routine

Induction

- Routine

Maintenance

- Routine

Extubation

- Routine

Adjuvants

- Avoid nitrates and local anesthetics that act as oxidizing agents

Postoperative Period

- See Monitoring

ANTICIPATED PROBLEMS/CONCERNS

- O_2 carriage is interfered with, proportional to concentration of altered hemoglobin present, and the interference with O_2 release and shift of tension-saturation curve from normal position
- Pulse oximetry overestimates SaO_2 in presence of methemoglobin. Methylene blue will decrease the SaO_2 for about 30 min after injection.

MITRAL REGURGITATION

Keith L. Stein, M.D.

RISK

- People within USA: 5–10% of population (if mitral valve prolapse included)
- Race with highest prevalence: unknown
- Female > male

PERIOPERATIVE RISKS

- Risk of atrial tachyarrhythmias, LV dysfunction, pulm edema, CHF, acute RV failure
- Bacterial endocarditis
- Acute mitral regurgitation (MR) associated with MI, CAD, and all associated risks (see Angina, Chronic Stable, in Diseases section)
- Low LV ejection fraction or severe symptoms associated with poor outcome

WORRY ABOUT

- Worsening symptoms of fatigue, DOE, nocturnal dyspnea, orthopnea, cachexia
- New-onset AFIB

OVERVIEW

- Evidence of right heart failure: hepatic congestion and hepatopathy, peripheral edema, jugular venous distention
- Disease of abnormal flow in heart, allowing some of systolic outflow to go back into left atrium
- Offloads LV by allowing low-pressure retrograde ejection
- Resulting hyperdynamic LV allows long period before symptoms; eventually, LV dilatation and hypertrophy progress to cardiac failure; left atrial distention leads to pulmonary Htn, pulmonary edema, and possible RV failure
- The more precipitous the onset, the more significant the acute heart failure
- Diagnosis made by Doppler, ECHO, cardiac catheterization

ICD-9-CM Code: 424.0

ETIOLOGY

- Chronic: degenerative (mitral prolapse, ruptured chordae), rheumatic, endocarditis, CAD, papillary muscle dysfunction, dilated LV, hypertrophic cardiomyopathy, SLE, rarely congenital (see also Mitral Valve Prolapse in Diseases section)
- Acute: ruptured chordae, endocarditis, MI with papillary muscle dysfunction, left atrial myxoma, trauma, prosthetic valve dysfunction
- May be accelerated by systemic Htn, ↓ left atrial compliance

USUAL TREATMENT

- Medical therapy: cardiac glycosides, angiotensin inhibitors, hydralazine, antibiotic endocarditis prophylaxis, CHF regimen (diuretics, nitrates)
- Surgical therapy (with symptoms of cardiomegaly): mitral valvuloplasty or mitral valve replacement

ASSESSMENT POINTS

SYSTEM	EFFECT	ASSESSMENT BY HX	PE	TEST
CV	Mitral regurgitation	Fatigue, exertional or nocturnal dyspnea	Pansystolic and late systolic murmur, rales	Doppler, ECHO Cardiac catheterization
	RV failure	Peripheral swelling RUQ pain, tenderness	Ankle edema Hepatomegaly Hepatojugular reflux	
	Cardiomegaly Left atrial enlargement		Displaced posterior MI	CXR
	AFIB	Palpitations	Irregular rhythm	ECG
RESP	CHF, pulm edema	Dyspnea, orthopnea	Gallop, rales	CXR
GI	Cachexia	Weight loss	Muscle wasting	Weight
	Congestive hepatopathy	Bleeding with minor trauma	Bruises	PT, PTT, LFTs
RENAL	↓ Perfusion	Oliguria		BUN, Cr
	Diuretic-induced ↓ in K^+, Mg^{2+}	Palpitations	Muscle weakness ↓ Reflexes	Serum K^+, Mg^{2+} ECG
MS	Cachexia		Muscle wasting	

Key Reference: Grewal KS, Malkowski MJ, Piracha AR, et al.: Effect of general anesthesia on the severity of mitral regurgitation by transesophageal echocardiography. Am J Cardiol 2000; 85:199–203.

PERIOPERATIVE IMPLICATIONS

Preoperative Preparation

- Continue chronic medications for AFIB rate control, CHF, afterload reduction
- Avoid hypoxemia, hypercarbia to limit increase in PVR and resultant risk of RV failure
- Consider antibiotic prophylaxis

Monitoring

- Consider PA catheter or TEE if LV dysfunction, aortic operations, or procedures with large fluid shifts or BP variations

Airway

- None

Preinduction/Induction

- Avoid bradycardia or acceleration of AFIB ventricular response
- Maintain preload, reduce afterload (full, fast, and vasodilated)
- Avoid myocardial depression

Maintenance

- Any technique that avoids ↑ afterload or myocardial depression, both of which manifest as cardiac failure
- Regional anesthetic technique may help ↓ afterload
- Maintain normovolemia, normocarbia, normotension, normal SaO_2
- Avoid excessive PEEP
- Follow CO, utilize IV vasodilators and vasodilating inotropes as needed

Extubation

- ↑ Risk of Htn inducing MR and CHF
- ↑ Risk of hypoventilation and hypoxemia inducing RV dysfunction

Adjuvants

- No known drug interaction problems unless CHF develops and ↓ liver or renal perfusion

Postoperative Period

- Maintain afterload reduction, digoxin levels, fluid balance
- Pain management may be critical to avoid Htn
- PCA, epidural analgesia potentially beneficial

ANTICIPATED PROBLEMS/CONCERNS

- Depressed LV ejection fraction, severe pulmonary Htn, and RV dysfunction may be best predictors of high perioperative risk
- ↑ LV afterload (Htn) rapidly worsens MR and induces pulm edema and CHF

MITRAL STENOSIS

Albert T. Cheung, M.D.

RISK

- Bimodal age distribution: 20–39 y and 50–60 y patients
- Most common among USA immigrants from regions where rheumatic fever is prevalent (e.g., Middle East, Asia, Latin America)

PERIOPERATIVE RISKS

- ↑ Risk of perioperative cardiac complications that include infectious endocarditis, pulm edema, heart failure, new-onset AFIB or atrial flutter, embolic stroke of cardiac origin

WORRY ABOUT

- Fluid status
- Paroxysmal AFIB or flutter
- Limited ability to increase cardiac output in response to ↑ metabolic demands
- Cardiomyopathy, pulm Htn, RV failure, hepatic dysfunction, tricuspid regurgitation, and associated aortic valve disease
- Pulmonary edema

OVERVIEW

- Diastolic emptying of blood from the left atrium into the left ventricle is impaired critically when the mitral valve area is < 1 cm^2
- Transmitral pressure gradient varies directly with cardiac output; acute increases in cardiac output and venous return to heart cause acute increases in pulm venous pressure. Pulm edema occurs when the pulm venous pressure > pulm capillary oncotic pressure.
- Left atrial dilation, AFIB, left atrial thrombosis, pulm Htn, RV failure, tricuspid regurgitation may develop
- Symptoms of mitral stenosis can be elicited by conditions (fluid overload, exercise, pregnancy, sepsis, operation) that demand an ↑ in cardiac output or diastolic blood flow (MR)
- Deformity of the mitral valve apparatus may cause both mitral stenosis and mitral regurgitation

ICD-9-CM Code: 394.0

ETIOLOGY

- Congenital heart disease (rare)
- Acquired mitral stenosis is sequela of rheumatic carditis developing after group A streptococcal pharyngitis
- Rheumatic carditis produces exudative and inflammatory lesions that lead to fibrosis, calcification, thickening, and fusion of the mitral valve leaflets

USUAL TREATMENT

- Anticoagulation to ↓ risk of thromboembolic events
- Digoxin or other antiarrhythmic agents to control ventricular rate in patients with AFIB
- Diuretic therapy for symptomatic pulm edema
- Percutaneous balloon valvotomy or open valvotomy in patients without extensive valve calcification or mitral regurgitation
- Mitral valve replacement or reconstruction

ASSESSMENT POINTS

SYSTEM	EFFECT	ASSESSMENT BY HX	PE	TEST
CV	Mitral stenosis	DOE Chest pain or tightness	Diastolic murmur	ECHO Cardiac cath
	AFIB Pulm Htn	Palpitations DOE	Irregular pulse Sternal heave Prominent S$_2$	ECG
RESP	Pulm edema	DOE Orthopnea Paroxysmal nocturnal dyspnea Hemoptysis	Tachypnea Rales Wheezes	CXR
GI	CHF		Hepatomegaly	Liver function tests
RENAL	Fluid retention Diuretic therapy	Dependent edema	Pedal edema	Serum lytes
CNS	Embolic stroke	Neurologic deficits TIAs	Focal neurologic deficits	Head CT scan TEE
HEME	Bleeding	Anticoagulation therapy	Ecchymosis	INR, PT, PTT

Key Reference: Savino JS, Cheung AT: Rheumatic mitral stenosis. *In* Oka Y, Konstadt S (eds): Transesophageal Echocardiography: A Problem Oriented Approach. Philadelphia, Lippincott-Raven, 1996.

PERIOPERATIVE IMPLICATIONS

Preoperative Preparation

- Optimize fluid status of patients in CHF
- Control ventricular rate in patients with AFIB
- Replete K$^+$ in patients with hypokalemia on digoxin therapy
- Antibiotic prophylaxis for infectious endocarditis
- Keep patient calm using reassurance, anxiolytics, and analgesics
- Assess the risk of bleeding in anticoagulated patients and correct the prolonged PT (INR) with FFP if necessary

Monitoring

- ECG to detect paroxysmal AFIB or flutter

- Consider arterial catheter for continuous BP monitoring and ABG sampling
- Consider PA catheter or TEE to guide intravascular volume status when large fluid shifts are anticipated.

Preinduction/Induction

- Cautious administration of drugs that decrease myocardial contractility, or cause arterial dilation or tachycardia
- Vasoconstrictors may worsen pulm Htn
- Hypoventilation and hypoxia may worsen pulm Htn
- Positive inotropic agents may precipitate pulmonary edema

Maintenance

- Control fluid administration

Extubation/Postoperative Period

- Provide adequate analgesia
- ↑ Risk of postop resp failure

Adjuvants

- Consider regional anesthesia or perioperative epidural anesthesia and analgesia

ANTICIPATED PROBLEMS/CONCERNS

- Patients have a limited ability to increase their cardiac output
- Acute pulm edema is precipitated by ↑ cardiac output, ↑ HR, pregnancy, anxiety, fluid overload, exercise, and postop mobilization of sequestered (third space) interstitial and extracellular fluid
- Bleeding in anticoagulated patients

MITRAL VALVE PROLAPSE
Albert T. Cheung, M.D.

RISK

- Believed to be most common form of valvular heart disease, with incidence of 5–10% of population and disproportionate frequency among young women
- ECHO indicates incidence in unselected general ambulatory population is only 2.4% with no predilection for gender or age using strict criteria
- Severity of the disease in patients with clinically significant MVP caused by structural abnormalities of the mitral valve apparatus increases with age

PERIOPERATIVE RISKS

- Infectious endocarditis
- Heart failure as a consequence of acute or chronic MR
- Embolic stroke
- Cardiac dysrhythmias

WORRY ABOUT

- Severity of MR
- Evidence of structural or pathologic abnormalities of the mitral valve apparatus such as leaflet thickening, myxomatous degeneration (leaflet redundancy), and chordal elongation by ECHO
- Clinical symptoms of MR or history of CHF, AFIB, infective endocarditis, or embolic stroke

- Associated conditions: Marfan's syndrome; Ehlers-Danlos syndrome, pseudoxanthoma elasticum, sudden cardiac death, pectus excavatum, scoliosis, hyperadrenergic state, anxiety disorders

OVERVIEW

- Severity of disease in patients labeled with the syndrome of MVP varies widely based on clinical and ECHO criteria used to establish the diagnosis
- Frequency of heart failure, AFIB, CVD, syncope, chest pain, dyspnea, and ECHO abnormalities has not been shown to be increased in patients with the mildest form of the disease, defined by isolated prolapse of the mitral valve leaflets >2 mm beyond the mitral valve annulus into the left atrium during systole
- If clinically significant MR by ECHO: risk of HF, infective endocarditis, AFIB, embolic stroke, and progression of disease
- Structural abnormalities or weakness of the valve apparatus causes displacement or prolapse of the leaflets beyond the mitral valve annulus into the left atrium during ventricular systole
- Progressive annular dilation, elongation of chordae tendineae, and stretching of valve leaflets impairs leaflet coaptation and leads to the development and worsening of MR

- Rupture of weakened chordae produces acute MR
- Surface abnormalities on valve apparatus ↑ the risk of infectious endocarditis and embolic stroke
- Chronic MR and left atrial dilation are associated with AFIB and risk of embolic stroke

ICD-9-CM Code: 424.0

ETIOLOGY

- Inherited connective tissue disorders
- Myxomatous degeneration (replacement of collagen and elastin by mucopolysaccharide)

USUAL TREATMENT

- No treatment in asymptomatic patients
- ACE inhibitors, β-blockers, and diuretics in patients with significant MR or CHF
- Antiarrhythmic agents and anticoagulation therapy in patients with AFIB
- Mitral valve replacement or repair in patients with severe MR

ASSESSMENT POINTS

SYSTEM	EFFECT	ASSESSMENT BY HX	PE	TEST
CV	Mitral valve prolapse	Atypical chest pain DOE	Mid- and late-apical nonejection systolic clicks	ECHO
	Mitral regurgitation	DOE CHF	Mid- to late-apical systolic murmur	ECHO
	Dysrhythmias	Palpitations Syncope	Abn pulse	ECG Holter
	Infectious endocarditis	Fever, chills	Embolic phenomena	TEE, blood culture
CNS	Stroke	Neurologic deficits TIAs	Focal neurologic signs	Head CT scan ECHO
MS	Skeletal deformities		Pectus excavatum Scoliosis	CXR

Key Reference: Freed LA, Levy D, Levine RA, Larson MG, Evans JC, Fuller DL, Lehman B, Benjamin EJ: Prevalence and clinical outcome of mitral-valve prolapse. N Engl J Med 1999; 341:1–7.

PERIOPERATIVE IMPLICATIONS

Preoperative Preparation

- Assess existence and severity of MR
- Antibiotic prophylaxis for infectious endocarditis in patients with MR detected by ECHO

Monitoring

- Routine

Preinduction/Induction/Maintenance

- Avoid Htn and acute increases in sympathetic tone
- Consider regional anesthesia

Adjuvants

- Therapeutic interventions that ↑ BP, myocardial contractility, preload, or sympathetic tone may ↑ severity of MVP, MR, or the risk of chordal rupture
- Antihypertensives and afterload reducing agents are effective for ↑ cardiac output in patients with significant MR

Extubation/Postoperative Period

- Avoid Htn and acute increases in sympathetic tone

ANTICIPATED PROBLEMS/CONCERNS

- Htn and positive inotropic stimulation may increase severity of MVP, the regurgitant LV ejection fraction when MR is present, and risk of acute rupture of chordae tendineae
- Presence of severe MR or associated connective tissue disorders may alter routine management of patients with isolated MVP (see Mitral Regurgitation and individual connective tissue disorders in Diseases section)

MOBITZ I (SECOND DEGREE ATRIOVENTRICULAR BLOCK)

James R. Zaidan, M.D.

RISK

• Occurs after inferior myocardial infarction, or occasionally in trained athletes or in normal, sleeping people

PERIOPERATIVE RISKS

• Without associated heart disease and without symptoms, should not present undue risk during anesthesia
• If occurs secondary to inferior myocardial infarction, the perioperative risk depends on extent of ischemic area

WORRY ABOUT

• Advancing to a higher degree block if ischemic zone extends to anterior wall
• Papillary muscle dysfunction may occur

OVERVIEW

• Found usually in presence of CAD
• Block generally occurs in AV node, resulting in normal QRS complexes
• ECG reveals progressive lengthening P-R intervals at decreasing increments and progressively shortening R-R intervals
• Bradycardia usually responds to atropine

ICD-9-CM Code: 426.13 (Mobitz I)

ETIOLOGY

• Acquired, usually with MI
• Increased resting parasympathetic tone relative to resting sympathetic tone (i.e., may be some parasympathetic and decreased sympathetic tone)

USUAL TREATMENT

• Specific therapy in absence of heart disease not necessary unless patient is symptomatic
• Treatment of an infarction-related Mobitz I block includes observation and medical therapy with atropine
• Temporary pacing is necessary only if medically unresponsive patient is symptomatic
• Permanent pacing seldom required and considered only in persistently blocked, symptomatic patients

ASSESSMENT POINTS

SYSTEM	EFFECT	ASSESSMENT BY HX	PE	TEST
CV	Commonly no Sx Bradycardia on occasion	Exercise tolerance Angina SOB	Signs of CHF and ↓ perfusion	ECG CXR
RENAL	Likely normal			Renal function testing?
CNS	No effect or ↓ perfusion of CNS	No Sx or only mild Sx: fainting, dizziness	Normal Bruits	PE Carotid US

Key Reference: Hung KC, Lin FC, Chern MS, Chang HJ, Hsieh IC, Wu D: Mechanisms and clinical significance of transient atrioventricular block during dobutamine stress echocardiography. J Am Coll Cardiol 1999; 34:998–1004.

PERIOPERATIVE IMPLICATIONS

Preoperative Preparation
• Consider availability of transcutaneous pacing

Monitoring
• Based upon co-existing disease
• Observe for and prepare to treat third degree block when positioning PA catheter in patient with Mobitz I block

Airway
• None

Induction/Maintenance
• Regional or general
• No contraindications to any standard anesthetic drugs
• Intraoperative processes and drugs that increase atrial rate could decrease ventricular rate

Extubation
• None

Adjuvants
• Cautious use of drugs that slow AV conduction

ANTICIPATED PROBLEMS/CONCERNS

• Extension of infarcted area with higher degree block and CHF

MOBITZ II (SECOND DEGREE ATRIOVENTRICULAR BLOCK)

James R. Zaidan, M.D.

RISK

• Occurs after anterior infarction and can quickly proceed to a third degree heart block

PERIOPERATIVE RISKS

• Risk of developing third degree block

WORRY ABOUT

• Rapid development into a third degree block, which requires temporary transvenous pacing

OVERVIEW

• Block is located in bundle of His or bundle branches, resulting in lengthening QRS duration
• P-P and R-R intervals are constant, and P-R intervals are constant prior to the dropped QRS complex

ICD-9-CM Code: Mobitz II: 426.12

ETIOLOGY

• Acquired, usually associated with MI

USUAL TREATMENT

• Temporary pacemaker insertion should be considered soon after onset of this block, because third degree block commonly occurs
• Pacing does not improve survival
• Atropine usually does not improve conduction

ASSESSMENT POINTS

SYSTEM	EFFECT	ASSESSMENT BY HX	PE	TEST
CV	Bradycardia	Exercise tolerance Angina SOB	Signs of CHF and ↓ perfusion	ECG CXR Other tests as indicated
GU	Likely normal			Renal function testing?
CNS	↓ Perfusion of CNS	Fainting, dizziness	Normal? Bruits	PE Carotid US

Key Reference: Hung KC, Lin FC, Chern MS, Chang, HJ, Hsieh IC, Wu D: Mechanisms and clinical significance of transient atrioventricular block during dobutamine stress echocardiography. J Am Coll Cardiol 1999; 34:998–1004.

PERIOPERATIVE IMPLICATIONS

Preoperative Preparation

• Evaluation of CAD important
• Likely a transvenous pacemaker will be in place
• Transcutaneous pacing should be available if temporary transvenous pacing was not established prior to induction of anesthesia

Monitoring

• Based on severity of heart disease and extent of infarcted area
• Prepare to treat third degree block when positioning a PA catheter

Airway

• None

Induction/Maintenance

• No contraindications to any standard anesthetic drugs
• Any intraoperative process or drug increasing atrial rate could worsen block and decrease ventricular rate

Adjuvants

• Cautiously use drugs that slow conduction through AV node unless they also slow SA nodal rate and allow 1:1 AV conduction and ↑ ventricular rate
• First degree AV block will persist if 1:1 conduction occurs

MORBID OBESITY

Susan L. Polk, M.D., M.S.Ed.

RISK
- About 5% of Americans

PERIOPERATIVE RISKS
- Morbidity or mortality twice normal, owing to associated CV and resp abnormalities, hypercoagulability

WORRY ABOUT
- Technically difficult procedures: intubation, establishing IV lines
- Restrictive ventilatory dysfunction and hypoxemia
- Associated sleep apnea (may be associated with problematic narcotic epidural analgesia)
- Systemic and pulm Htn
- LV and RV failure
- Hypercoagulability
- ↑ Gastric emptying time and hiatus hernia
- Liver disease
- Psychologic disorders

OVERVIEW
- Defined as twice ideal body weight [ideal body weight (kg) = height (cm) − 100] or body mass index >35 [BMI = weight (kg)/height^2 (meters)]
- CV and resp dysfunction due to increased body mass to be perfused and oxygenated. Increased demand for O_2 and CO_2 excretion from metabolic demand of increased tissue mass. Increased work of breathing due to decreased chest wall compliance.
- Obstructive and/or central sleep apnea due to increased upper airway soft tissue mass relaxing during sleep. Patients extremely sensitive to resp depressant effects of sedatives and hypnotics.
- Psychologic dysfunction may interfere with postop stir-up routine and contribute to pulm and thromboembolic phenomena

ICD-9-CM Code: 278.0

ETIOLOGY
- Unknown. Presumed genetic predisposition but an acquired disease.

USUAL TREATMENT
- Dietary intervention with exercise and behavioral modification
- Surgical: Gastric stapling or bypass, or intestinal bypass

ASSESSMENT POINTS

SYSTEM	EFFECT	ASSESSMENT BY HX	PE	TEST
CV	Htn	Dyspnea, pounding	BP Cardiomegaly	ECG, CXR, BUN
	Pulm Htn	Dyspnea at rest and on exertion, orthopnea	Rales	CXR, ECG
	Ventricular dysfunction	Dyspnea Orthopnea, poor exercise tolerance	Venous engorgement Rales, S_3 and S_4 Cardiomegaly	CXR, ECG, ECHO
	CAD	Angina, poor exercise tolerance		Stress ECHO, ECG, angio
RESP	Restrictive dysfunction	Dyspnea at rest or on exertion Orthopnea	Rapid resp rate Shallow breathing, ruddy color	ABGs, PFTs, Hct, CXR (pulm Htn) Pulse oximetry on room air while supine
	Sleep apnea	Snoring, frequent sleep interruptions Daytime somnolence	Upper airway tissue, ruddy color	ABGs, Hct, polysomnogram
GI, METAB	Hepatic dysfunction	Jaundice Bleeding disorders Ascites	Hepatomegaly, ascites, spider angiomas, jaundice	LFTs, PT, PTT BUN and Cr
	Full stomach NIDDM	Heartburn, hiatus hernia Polydipsia, polyuria		Fasting glucose Urinalysis, GTT
DIFFICULT AIRWAY		Snoring	Visualization of uvula and tonsillar pillars	Lateral neck x-ray may be helpful

Key Reference: Michaloudis D, Fraidakis O, Petrou A, et al: Continuous spinal anesthesia/analgesia for perioperative management of morbidly obese patients undergoing laparotomy for gastroplastic surgery. Obes Surg 2000; 10:220−229.

PERIOPERATIVE IMPLICATIONS

Preoperative Preparation
- Metoclopramide 10 mg, cimetidine 300 mg PO the night before and IV preoperatively
- Assess myocardial and volume status

Monitoring
- Routine monitors plus consider arterial line if BP cuff does not fit well or takes too long to inflate
- Frequent ABGs
- UO
- Possible CVP or PA catheter if volume status likely to be significantly altered

Airway
- Awake intubation may be indicated if difficulty anticipated on basis of examination
- Elevation of shoulders and head on a bolster facilitates insertion of laryngoscope

Induction
- Patient may need to remain semisitting if SaO_2 drops when supine
- Preoxygenation should be complete

Maintenance
- Volume status can change precipitously, esp with position change
- Oxygenation may deteriorate with upper abdominal surgery or increased intra-abdominal pressure
- All agents tapered at the end to minimize postop sedation

Extubation
- As soon as adequate to maintain normocapnia and patient is responsive to command

Adjuvants
- Initial dose of induction agent and narcotics calculated on a mg/kg basis and muscle relaxants calculated on estimated lean body mass

- Subsequent doses of sedatives, hypnotics, relaxants, narcotics calculated on estimated lean body mass. Regional anesthesia if physically possible and if patient can use accessory muscles to help with breathing.

Postoperative Period
- Pain control necessary to facilitate early stir-up routine. PCA acceptable in sleep apnea, but not in continuous mode. Some think epidural narcotic infusions are contraindicated unless continuously monitored for resp depression.

ANTICIPATED PROBLEMS/CONCERNS
- Resp insufficiency and pneumonia postop avoided by minimal sedation, appropriate pain control, early ambulation
- Postop thromboembolic phenomena also avoided by above
- Poor motivation, resulting in poor ambulation, avoided by intensive preop teaching and postop coaching

MOYAMOYA

Francine S. Yudkowitz, M.D., F.A.A.P.

RISK

- Occurs in both children and adults
- Occurs predominantly in children
- More frequent in females

PERIOPERATIVE RISKS

- Stroke

WORRY ABOUT

- Hypocarbia and hypercarbia
- Adequate cerebral blood flow
- Hypotension
- Hypothermia

OVERVIEW

- Progressive occlusive cerebrovascular disorder—narrowing of internal carotid and basilar arteries leads to proliferation of arteries, particularly at the base of the brain
- Adults present with intracerebral/intraventricular hemorrhages
- Children present with TIAs and strokes that lead to neurologic deficits. Symptoms may start from birth to age 5 y, with rapid deterioration in neurologic function over the next 2–3 y.
- Symptoms in children are precipitated by activities that involve hyperventilation, which results in hypocarbia. Changes in body temperature may also precipitate attacks.
- Abnormal vessels have intimal thickening or deficiency of the internal elastic lamina

ICD-9-CM Code: 437.5

ETIOLOGY

- Not clearly defined
- Congenital—both cerebral and systemic vasculature involved
- Acquired—results from meningitis, neurofibromatosis, connective tissue disease, and chronic inflammation in the neck region
- Childhood moyamoya may be associated with optic glioma, neurofibromatosis, congenital heart disease, Down syndrome, basal brain tumors, and prior RT

USUAL TREATMENT

- Medical
  - Antiplatelet agents
- Surgical
  - EDAS (encephalodural arteriosynangiosis). The scalp artery or temporal artery is placed onto the arachnoid surface of the brain. Collaterals to ischemic brain occur over time.

ASSESSMENT POINTS

SYSTEM	EFFECT	ASSESSMENT BY HX	PE	TEST
CV	Congenital heart disease	Exercise tolerance, cyanosis	Auscultation	ECG, ECHO, CXR
CNS	Decreased CBF	TIAs, strokes	Neuro deficits	
	Seizures			EEG

Key Reference: Soriano SG, Sethna NF, Scott RM: Anesthetic management of children with moyamoya syndrome. Anesth Analg 1993; 77:1066–1070.

PERIOPERATIVE IMPLICATIONS

Preoperative Preparation

- Assess for associated abnormalities
- Avoid sedatives and narcotics that would result in hypercarbia

Monitoring

- Arterial line for blood pressure monitoring and blood gas analysis

Induction/Maintenance

- No one anesthetic technique is best. Maintaining cerebral and systemic hemodynamics is more important.
- Minimize increases in $CMRO_2$ with adequate levels of anesthesia during painful stimuli
- Ensure adequate CBF by avoiding hypotension, hypocarbia, and hypercarbia
- Maintain normal temperature with warming blanket if needed

Postoperative Period

- Monitor for hypoventilation to avoid hypercarbia-induced neurologic symptoms
- Provide adequate analgesia

ANTICIPATED PROBLEMS/CONCERN

- Stroke

MUCOPOLYSACCHARIDOSES

James J. Fehr, M.D.

RISK

- Only males affected in Hunter syndrome (X-linked)
- People within USA: incidence estimated to be 1/30,000

PERIOPERATIVE RISKS

- Estimated perioperative mortality: 20%
- Difficult intubation (25%), failed intubation (8%)

WORRY ABOUT

- Difficult airway, cardiac lesions, poor IV access, resp failure

OVERVIEW

- Child may appear normal at birth; by age 1 y often shows signs of both growth and mental retardation. Dx made by characteristic physical findings and ↑ urinary mucopolysaccharides (MPs).

- Hurler syndrome, considered prototype, is characterized by involvement of heart, liver, and bones. Most severe form and also associated with corneal clouding, developmental delay, frequent respiratory infections, stiff joints, abnormal airway.
- Scheie syndrome is milder form of Hurler syndrome; patients have normal intelligence and life expectancy but may have stiff joints and aortic regurgitation
- Hunter syndrome has diffuse joint limitations, short neck, short stature, ischemic cardiomyopathy
- Morquio syndrome has severe kyphoscoliosis, possible cervical subluxation and aortic regurgitation
- Maroteaux-Lamy syndrome has kyphoscoliosis, cardiac involvement, mild joint stiffness
- Recurrent hernias often occur in mucopolysaccharidoses

ICD-9-CM Code: 277.5

ETIOLOGY

- Hereditary, progressive disorders of lysosomal enzymes responsible for metabolism of MPs resulting in intracellular accumulation of incompletely metabolized MPs in tissues throughout body. Leads to progressive alteration of cellular structure and function. Death often results from cardiac or pulmonary failure.
- All forms are autosomal recessive except for Hunter syndrome, which is X-linked recessive

USUAL TREATMENT

- None at present; prenatal diagnosis is available

ASSESSMENT POINTS

SYSTEM	EFFECT	ASSESSMENT BY HX	PE	TEST
HEENT	Large tongue, small mouth, micrognathia Difficult airway anticipated Atlantoaxial subluxation possible		Neck ROM	X-ray
CV	Difficult IV access Frequent valvular lesions Compliance often reduced Possible ischemic disease (even at a young age)	Exercise tolerance Angina Hx		ECG CXR ECHO
RESP	Propensity to develop pneumonia Obstructive apnea Bronchospasm			
GI	Frequent hepatomegaly Hepatic function usually normal			
CNS	Mental retardation, deafness are frequent Cervical myelopathy in Morquio syndrome Hydrocephalus in Hurler and Hunter syndromes			
MS	Short neck, severe skeletal abnormalities Anticipate difficulty in positioning			

Key Reference: Butler MG: Specific genetic diseases at risk for sedation/anesthesia complications. Anesth Analg 2000; 91:837–855.

PERIOPERATIVE IMPLICATIONS

Preoperative Preparation

- May be resistant to sedative premedications
- Anticipate possible airway obstruction/cardiopulmonary difficulties
- Antisialagogue, e.g., glycopyrrolate
- Antibiotic prophylaxis for cardiac lesions

Monitoring

- Routine

Airway

- Abnormal airway and short neck predispose to complicated airway management, including difficulty in performing a tracheotomy

- Consider fiberoptic bronchoscopy
- LMA may be useful

Preinduction/Induction

- IV placement before induction
- Padding and positioning

Maintenance

- Avoid myocardial ischemia

Extubation

- Conscious with intact airway reflexes prior to extubation

Adjuvants

- Utilize local anesthetics and regional techniques when appropriate

Postoperative Period

- Delayed emergence
- Respiratory complications including pneumonia, bronchospasm, and apnea

ANTICIPATED PROBLEMS/CONCERNS

- Airway is likely to be difficult to manage
- Cardiac and pulmonary systems frequently affected

MULTIPLE ENDOCRINE NEOPLASIA (MEN) TYPES I AND II

Burnell R. Brown, Jr., M.D., Ph.D.*
Edward J. Frink, Jr., M.D.

RISK

- People within USA: 1/15,000 (?)
- Racial predominance: unknown
- Usually transmitted in autosomal dominant pattern but may have variable penetrance

PERIOPERATIVE RISKS

- See specific syndrome

OVERVIEW

- MEN I (Werner's syndrome), IIa (Sipple's syndrome), and IIb (also called MEN type III) are a group of familial diseases involving hyperplasia and/or malignancies of several endocrine organs
- MEN I: characterized by parathyroid, pancreas, and pituitary tumors. 90% have hyperparathyroidism (hyperplasia); 20–40% have peptic ulcers (hypergastrinemia); 80% have islet cell tumors (Zollinger-Ellison syndrome); 25% have acromegaly.

- MEN IIa: characterized by medullary carcinoma of thyroid; pheochromocytoma (50%); hyperparathyroidism (25% incidence, primarily adenomas)
- MEN IIb: Characterized by medullary thyroid carcinoma, pheochromocytoma, marfanoid habitus, and multiple mucosal neuromas

ICD-9-CM Code: 258.0

ETIOLOGY

- Both are genetic diseases inherited in autosomal dominant fashion

USUAL TREATMENT

- MEN I: parathyroid disease treated by subtotal parathyroidectomy. Pancreatectomy (partial or total) may be required for control of hyperinsulinism (hypoglycemia). Diazoxide and streptozocin may be helpful for hypoglycemia. Therapy for gastrin-secreting tumors is total gastrectomy.
- MEN IIa: excision of pheochromocytoma if present is lifesaving (usual site is adrenal glands). Subtotal parathyroidectomy for hyperparathyroidism. All patients with either pheochromocytoma or hyperparathyroidism (hypercalcemia) should have total thyroidectomy.
- MEN IIb: excision of pheochromocytoma. Medullary thyroid carcinoma (as with IIa) is of calcitonin-producing cells. Therapy is surgical excision and follow-up for metastases.

ASSESSMENT POINTS

DISEASE	EFFECT	ASSESSMENT BY HX	PE	TEST
MEN I	Parathyroid hyperplasia	Family Hx essential	Acromegaly possible (usual tumor is a benign chromophobe adenoma)	Glucose Ca^{2+}
	Nephrolithiasis; nephrocalcinosis			
	Pancreatic tumors, severe hypoglycemia			CT scan of sella;
	Pituitary tumors, acromegaly			CT scan of abdomen; growth hormone level
MEN IIa & b	Pheochromocytoma	Family Hx Sweating; tachycardia	Htn (paroxysmal)	CT scan Urinary catecholamines
	Medullary cancer of thyroid	Metastatic disease	Thyroid gland	Calcitonin levels
	Parathyroid adenoma	Family Hx Hx urinary stones		Ca^{2+} Cr BUN Pelvic x-rays

Key Reference: Dougherty TB, Cronau LH: Anesthetic implications for surgical patients with endocrine tumors. Int Anesthesiol Clin 1998; 36:31–44.

PERIOPERATIVE IMPLICATIONS: MEN I

Monitoring
- Cardiac arrhythmias, prolonged QT interval (hypercalcemia)
- UO
- CNS monitoring for pituitary adenomas
- Blood glucose

Airway
- Acromegalics very difficult to intubate

Maintenance
- Monitor blood glucose
- Maintain renal function, NaCl infusion (high-output diuretics such as furosemide)
- Usual neurosurgical precautions for operations for adenomas of pituitary

PERIOPERATIVE IMPLICATIONS: MEN II

Monitoring
- Usual monitoring for pheochromocytoma removal (intra-arterial line, PA cath); ECG
- UO
- Venous pressure
- Thyroidectomy (possible air embolism)

Airway
- Usually no problem. Post thyroidectomy may precipitate problem (severed recurrent laryngeal nerve, tracheomalacia).

Maintenance
- Keep BP at acceptable levels (volatile anesthetics, nitroprusside, phentolamine)
- Carefully monitor volume status
- Be prepared to treat hypercalcemic cardiac arrhythmias
- For thyroidectomy, metabolic maintenance

Adjuvants
- Pretreatment with phenoxybenzamine for pheochromocytoma
- Calcium-lowering drugs (mithramycin) preop, if necessary. Try fluid loading (saline) and furosemide first.

ANTICIPATED PROBLEMS/CONCERNS

- MEN I: hypoglycemia; hypercalcemia; postparathyroidectomy hypocalcemia with tetany
- MEN II: problems associated with pheochromocytoma (Htn, stroke, MI)

*Deceased

MULTIPLE MYELOMA
Kamla K. Prasad, M.D.

RISK

- Incidence in USA: 3/100,000/y
- 1% of all malignant disease
- African-American 2× > Caucasians
- Median age at diagnosis: 61 y; only 2% < 40 y
- Median survival 3 y; nearly 100% fatality rate

PERIOPERATIVE RISKS

- ↑ Risk of acute renal failure and exacerbation of chronic renal failure
- ↑ Risk of neurologic sequelae

WORRY ABOUT

- ↑ Risk of infection from multifactorial causes
- Multifactorial coagulopathy

OVERVIEW

- Neoplastic proliferation of a single clone of plasma cells
  - Pathology by bone marrow invasion and excessive monoclonal Ig production
- Potentially severe adverse renal, neurologic, hemostatic, immunologic, pulmonary consequences perioperatively

ICD-9-CM Code: 203.0

See also Waldenström's Macroglobulinemia in Diseases section

ETIOLOGY

- Unknown, with possible genetic predisposition
- Massive production of monoclonal Ig's causes derangements in most organ systems and overwhelms host

USUAL TREATMENT

- Alkylating chemotherapeutic agents
- Glucocorticoids (high dose)
- Interferon alfa-2b
- Localized irradiation

ASSESSMENT POINTS

SYSTEM	EFFECT	ASSESSMENT BY HX	PE	TEST
HEENT	Instability of axial spine	Vertebral bone pain	Neurologic deficits	Neck radiographs
CV	Hyperviscosity syndrome (microvascular sludging)	Angina, fatigue, CHF, blurred vision	Venous thrombosis, oronasal bleeding	Serum viscosity > 5 cP (nml: ≤ 1.8 cP)
RESP	Pneumonia Resp insufficiency	Recurrent infections Rib/thoracic spine pain	Pathologic rib fractures	CXR Thoracic spine x-ray
ENDO	Malnutrition	Cachexia		Albumin
HEME	Abnormal plt function Thrombocytopenia Factor I, II, XI inhibition Normochromic, normocytic anemia	Easy bruisability Prolonged bleeding		Bleeding time PT, PTT CBC
RENAL	Glomerular and tubular failure (due to precipitated Ig's, hypercalcemia, hyperuricemia)			Bence Jones proteinuria BUN/Cr Serum Ca^{2+} Uric acid
CNS	Spinal cord compression	Radicular pain	Neurologic deficits	X-rays (vertebral collapse, lytic lesions)
PNS	Peripheral nerve compression	Carpal tunnel syndrome	Neurologic deficits	
METAB	Hypercalcemia ↑ Infection susceptibility	Lethargy; weakness Recurrent infections		ECG (QT, P-R) WBC
MS	Pathologic fractures	Bone pain	Pathologic fractures	X-rays: fractures, punched-out bony lesions

Key Reference: Kyle RA: Maintenance therapy and supportive care for patients with multiple myeloma. Semin Oncol 1999; 26(suppl 13):35–42.

PERIOPERATIVE IMPLICATIONS

Preoperative Preparation
- Recombinant erythropoietin to ↓ transfusion requirements
- Positioning to prevent pathologic fractures
- Antibiotic and γ-globulin prophylaxis

Monitoring
- UO: maintain to prevent hypercalcemia and renal failure
- Temp: maintain normothermia to prevent microvascular sludging

Airway
- Axial spine fractures/cord compression may be present
- Macroglossia if amyloidosis

Maintenance
- Adequate hydration to minimize renal failure, hypercalcemia, hyperviscosity syndrome

Extubation
- Pulm insufficiency due to rib and vertebral fractures and pneumonia

Adjuvants
- All protein-bound drugs: unpredictable pharmacokinetics due to alterations of relative proportions of globulins and albumin in plasma
- Regional: relatively contraindicated owing to multifactorial coagulopathy, pre-existing neurologic deficits, and extensive pathologic bone lesions

Postoperative Period
- ↑ Pulm complications: venous thrombosis (hyperviscosity) and pneumonia (presence of rib fractures)—adequate hydration/aggressive pulm toilet mandated
- Encourage early ambulation to prevent hypercalcemia and venous thrombosis
- ↑ Infection risk due to functional hypogammaglobulinemia/neutropenia
- Plasmapheresis to treat hyperviscosity syndrome

ANTICIPATED PROBLEMS/CONCERNS

- Transfusion to treat anemia may precipitate hyperviscosity syndrome; plasmapheresis may be indicated before transfusion
- Treat hypercalcemia with hydration, prednisone, furosemide—consider biphosphonates (pamidronate), calcitonin (see Hypercalcemia in Diseases section)

MULTIPLE SCLEROSIS

Armin Schubert, M.D.

RISK

- Prevalence: 10–80/100,000 in North America
- Occurs primarily in temperate climates
- Female predominance 8:1
- Onset usually in 3rd decade of life
- Racial predominance: Caucasian 6× incidence of all other races

PERIOPERATIVE RISKS

- Exacerbation of Sx with temp elevation, stress of surgery, infection, emotional trauma, postpartum state
- Risk of positioning injury (muscle wasting), hyperkalemia with succinylcholine, DVT
- Steroid therapy predisposes to adrenal suppression, gastric ulceration

WORRY ABOUT

- Advisability of major conduction block; greater neurotoxicity of local anesthetics due to demyelination
- Presence of transverse myelitis and other major motor neuron disease (risk of hyperkalemia with depolarizing NMB)
- Cranial nerve involvement with loss of airway integrity
- Temp increase: as little as 0.5° can aggravate symptoms
- Autonomic dysfunction

OVERVIEW

- Demyelinating disease of brain and spinal cord (peripheral nerves are not affected), with chronically remitting and relapsing or progressive course
- Associated conditions include seizures and uveitis; CNS components involved are cortex (cognitive dysfunction, memory loss, personality change, emotional lability)
- Chronic dysesthetic pain and spasticity contribute to disability

- Paroxysmal Sx may mimic cerebral ischemia, spinal cord compression, tic douloureux

ICD-9-CM Code: 340

ETIOLOGY

- Cause unknown
- Autoimmune, genetic, environmental factors thought to combine to attack CNS myelin

USUAL TREATMENT

- No treatment curative
- Steroids, ACTH, azathioprine, cyclophosphamide ameliorate relapses
- Carbamazepine used for paroxysmal Sx (including pain), baclofen, and, occasionally, surgery for spasticity (thalamotomy)
- Interferon-β now thought to shorten attacks, prolong time between attacks, delay onset of disability

ASSESSMENT POINTS

SYSTEM	EFFECT	ASSESSMENT BY HX	PE	TEST
HEENT	Pseudobulbar palsy	Hx of swallowing difficulty	Cranial nerves IX, X	
RESP	May have aspirated from bulbar dysfunction, seizure	Review with family	Auscultation	CXR, oximetry
GI	GI effects of steroids	Hx of pain, bleeding		
CNS	Cognitive dysfunction, optic neuritis, seizures, dysesthesias, ophthalmoplegia, autonomic dysfunction Monoplegia, transverse myelitis, quadriplegia	Hx of memory loss, emotional lability, "dropping" things, visual problems Lhermitte's sign (electric shock to legs); check with family for description of seizures	Mental status exam Neurologic exam (esp motor and sensory) Orthostatic vital sign changes	CSF electrophoresis (elevated IgG and myelin basic protein); MRI (plaques); evoked potentials; EEG

PERIOPERATIVE IMPLICATIONS

Preoperative Preparation

- Consider steroid supplementation; avoid anticholinergics
- May need benzodiazepine premedication
- Carefully document preop neurologic status
- Adequate volume status

Monitoring

- Routine

Airway

- None

Preinduction/Induction

- Spinal anesthesia implicated in aggravating MS symptoms and considered contraindicated

- Caution with epidural anesthesia: (1) need clear indication, such as in obstetrics, (2) patient informed of possible symptom exacerbation, (3) use lower concentrations of local anesthetics, (4) epidural opioids OK to use
- Peripheral nerve blocks OK
- Succinylcholine may precipitate hyperkalemia
- Avoid elevation of body temp
- Avoid proconvulsant anesthetics

Maintenance

- Avoid large temp swings, esp hyperthermia
- Continue steroid stress coverage
- Careful titration of nondepolarizing NMBs

Extubation

- Patients with brainstem involvement should be extubated awake
- Spasticity may diminish maximal inspiratory effort

Adjuvants

- Duration of most NMBs shortened by phenytoin and carbamazepine

Postoperative Period

- Be aware of exacerbation of MS symptoms; perform neuro exam
- Continue supplemental steroid coverage
- Unknown risk-benefit from interferon-β prophylaxis
- Treat hyperthermia
- Spasticity may interfere with pulmonary toilet

ANTICIPATED PROBLEMS/CONCERNS

- Unpredictable appearance of new neurologic deficits perioperatively
- Exacerbation of MS symptoms with hyperthermia
- Hyperkalemia with succinylcholine
- Emotional lability and need for sedative premedication

MULTISYSTEM ORGAN FAILURE, LUNG DYSFUNCTION IN

Lisa M. Weavind, M.B., B.Ch.
Thomas W. Feeley, M.D.

RISK

- Lung dysfunction in multisystem organ failure (MSOF) occurs in 150,000 people/y in USA
- Multiple risk factors include systemic sepsis, pulm contusion, inhalation of toxic substances, near-drowning, long-bone fractures, severe pancreatitis, diffuse pneumonia, DIC
- Risk of developing lung dysfunction (acute respiratory distress syndrome—ARDS) in MSOF is additive based on number of risk factors involved.
- Age not an important risk factor, although COPD is

PERIOPERATIVE RISKS

- Hypoxemia
- ↓Venous return and preload 2° to PEEP and ↑intrathoracic pressure
- Pulm Htn with RV dysfunction
- Pneumothorax
- Acute inability to ventilate 2° to alveolar derecruitment
- Mortality perioperatively 10–90% determined by ability to oxygenate and cause of MSOF

WORRY ABOUT

- Ventilator-associated lung injury (VALI) and oxygen toxicity
- Mechanical device malfunction
- Unsuspected auto-PEEP
- Death from primary cause of MSOF
- Deteriorating resp function during transition from ICU to anesthesia ventilator

OVERVIEW

- MSOF results when multiple disease processes often have a common pathologic pulm end point, ARDS. Pathogenesis of lung dysfunction involves uncontrolled inflammatory response to massive insult, leading to vascular endothelial damage and allowing pulm edema to occur.
- Lung dysfunction in MSOF consists of hypoxemia, ↓ FRC, ↓ compliance, ↑ intrapulmonary shunt and pulm interstitial infiltrates
- Long-term resp function good for survivors

ICD-9-CM Code: 518.4 (Lung edema, not of cardiac etiology)

ETIOLOGY

- Pulm and systemic infections, esp gram-negative septic shock, have high association with lung dysfunction of MSOF with mortality as high as 90%
- MSOF from DIC caused by systemic agent
- The lung itself may initiate MSOF secondary to initiation of SIRS by alveolar recruitment/derecruitment injury

USUAL TREATMENT

- Treatment of underlying cause and supportive
- Reversal of life-threatening hypoxemia of utmost importance
  – Administration of supplemental O_2
  – Intubation and mechanical ventilation employing PEEP (see Acute Respiratory Distress Syndrome in Diseases section)
  – Avoid VALI by limiting alveolar overdistention, using small tidal volume ventilation and avoiding alveolar recruitment/derecruitment injury by optimizing PEEP

ASSESSMENT POINTS

SYSTEM	EFFECT	ASSESSMENT BY HX	PE	TEST
CV	Hypovolemia ↓ CO RV dysfunction	Hypotension	Gallops S_3 Dysrhythmias	ECG PA catheterization
RESP	Hypoxemia Noncompliant lungs Pulm Htn Pulm edema	Tachypnea Dyspnea	Crackles ↑ P_2	Oximetry, ABGs PA catheterization CXR Peak pressures
GI	Ileus Distention Hemorrhage	Abdominal discomfort Nausea/vomiting Hemorrhage	↓ Bowel sounds Guaiac + stool	KUB, endoscopy
HEME	Anemia (↓ Hct) Thrombocytopenia DIC		Pallor Bleeding	CBC with plt count PT/PTT Fibrinogen level, FSPs
RENAL	Renal failure	Oliguria	Edema	BUN/Cr
CNS	Cerebral hypoxia	Altered mental status		

Key Reference: Ware LB, Matthay MA: The acute respiratory distress syndrome. N Engl J Med 2000; 342:1334–1349.

PERIOPERATIVE IMPLICATIONS

Preoperative Preparation

- Demonstrate stable oxygenation with standard Ambu bag and PEEP valve. Check ventilator settings and verify lack of movement of ETT during transport.
- Consider transport to OR on transport ventilator to avoid alveolar derecruitment
- Re-evaluate least PEEP

Monitoring

- Routine and consider PA catheter and airway pressure to follow changes in compliance and reduce barotrauma
- Consider TEE or PA catheter and arterial catheter to follow blood gases and filling volumes

Airway

- Ensure airway is secure

Preinduction/Induction

- Hypoxemia and hypercarbia may exacerbate pulm Htn leading to RV dysfunction
- Reduced FRC neg impact on shunt and V/Q

Maintenance

- PEEP is mainstay in supportive Rx of lung dysfunction in MSOF by restoring FRC, decreasing shunt, and improving V/Q mismatch.
- Administer fluids to maintain adequate pulm capillary wedge pressure and cardiac index
- Administer blood and inotropes as needed to optimize O_2 delivery
- Underlying cause (sepsis/bleeding/DIC) can be made much worse by surgical trespass
- Consider continuous ventilation on transport ventilator and total intravenous anesthesia to maintain gas exchange

Extubation

- Usually left intubated on ventilatory support until improvement in lung function
- Prevent ↑ in O_2 consumption, e.g., shivering

Adjuvants

- Unconventional modes of ventilation, artificial gas exchange, specific therapies targeted at pathogenic pathways, and more recently nitric oxide, prostacyclins, thrombolytics, and surfactant

Postoperative Period

- Close monitoring of volume status, PEEP
- Reduce FIO_2 to nontoxic level ASAP

ANTICIPATED PROBLEMS/CONCERNS

- Significant complications of supportive therapy for lung dysfunction in ARDS are pulm infections and pulm barotrauma, including pneumothorax, pneumomediastinum, pneumopericardium, and venous or arterial air embolism
- Adequate oxygenation on a nontoxic FIO_2 requires vigilant and creative attention to volume

MYASTHENIA GRAVIS

Cecil O. Borel, M.D.

RISK

- Individuals within USA: 10,000–15,000
- Affects all races
- Females: males 2:1

PERIOPERATIVE RISKS

- Postop neuromuscular ventilatory failure
- Postop pneumonia due to poor cough and secretion clearance

WORRY ABOUT

- Preop optimization of muscle strength
- Anticholinesterase medications, steroids, plasmapheresis

OVERVIEW

- Characterized by weakness and fatigability of skeletal muscles:
  - Inspiratory muscle weakness from residual paralysis from nondepolarizing neuromuscular blocking agents
  - Exacerbation of underlying bulbar (airway) musculature
  - ↑ Sensitivity to hypoventilation with narcotic analgesics
- Muscle strength improves similarly in both myasthenia gravis and nondepolarizing blockade after administration of anticholinesterase drugs

ICD-9-CM Code: 358.0

ETIOLOGY

- Autoimmune disease of neuromuscular junction mediated by reduction in number of acetylcholine receptors at neuromuscular junction

USUAL TREATMENT

- Anticholinesterase medications (pyridostigmine, Mestinon)
- Immunosuppression: steroids, azathioprine, IV immunoglobulin
- Plasmapheresis
- Thymectomy

ASSESSMENT POINTS

SYSTEM	EFFECT	ASSESSMENT BY HX	PE	TEST
NM	Peripheral muscle weakness	Easy fatigability	Arm adduction times < 1 min	Repetitive nerve stimulation
RESP				
Airway	Bulbar weakness	Difficulty swallowing	Head lift < 5 sec	Formal swallowing evaluation
Ventilation	Inspiratory muscle weakness	Orthopnea, breathlessness	Paradoxical inspiratory motion	NIF < 30 cm H_2O FVC < 1000 ml
Ventilatory drive	CO_2 retention	Morning headache		ABGs
Secretion clearance	Weak cough	Recurrent pneumonia	↓ Ventilation of bases	CXR

Key Reference: Borel CO, Hanley DF: Muscular paralysis—myasthenia gravis and polyneuritis. *In* Parrillo JE, Bone RC (eds): Critical Care Medicine: Principles of Diagnosis and Management. Philadelphia, Mosby–Year Book, 1994, pp 1193–1215.

PERIOPERATIVE IMPLICATIONS

Preoperative Preparation

- Anticholinesterase medications: hold 2–4 h preop, then start IV neostigmine 1 h before emergence at 1/30–1/60 daily pyridostigmine dose, infuse over 24 h
- Steroid maintenance

Monitoring

- Routine
- Train-of-four twitch monitor if short-active nondepolarizers used

Induction/Intubation

- Consider breathe-down techniques
- Intubation without muscle relaxation in severe disease

Maintenance

- Minimize or avoid use of muscle relaxants

Extubation

- Check NIF (> 30 cm H_2O), head lift, cough, gag, ensure full return of twitch

Adjuvants

- Avoid or minimize use of nondepolarizing muscle relaxants
- Depolarizing relaxants may have ↑ or ↓ efficacy
- Consider epidural analgesic, particularly for thymectomy

ANTICIPATED PROBLEMS/CONCERNS

- Postop ventilatory failure, pneumonia, aspiration

MYCOPLASMA PNEUMONIAE INFECTION

Bobby Su-Pen Chang, M.D.
Scott C. Streckenbach, M.D.

RISK

- Infections in the USA population: 60/1000/y
  - Asymptomatic infections—12/1000/y
  - Tracheobronchitis, pharyngitis: 46/1000/y
  - Pneumonia: 2/1000/y (2 million cases annually)
- Ages 5–20 y common; all ages possible
- Virulent in neonates
- Closed populations such as military camps and schools
- Epidemic outbreaks during fall and early winter in temperate climates
- Patients with Down syndrome, sickle cell disease (functional asplenism), and immuno-compromised hosts may manifest more severe disease

PERIOPERATIVE RISKS

- No perioperative risk data; ↑ hemagglutination and hemolysis with hypothermia during CPB

WORRY ABOUT

- Progression or unmasking of pulmonary and extrapulmonary disease

OVERVIEW

- Atypical pneumonia: differential Dx includes influenza, adenovirus, RSV, CMV, *Chlamydia,* and *Legionella*
- Clinical disease
  - Incubation period 2–3 wk
  - Insidious onset—fever (101–102°F), malaise, headache, scratchy throat, nonproductive cough
  - 5–10% progress to pneumonia
- Diagnosis
  - Hx and clinical picture
  - CXR—bronchopneumonia, plate-like atelectasis, nodular infiltration, hilar adenopathy
  - Gram stain—polymorphonuclear leukocytosis only. Organism does not stain because of absence of cell wall.
  - Culture—gold standard; organism may take 5–20 days to culture

- Serology—complement fixation test (single titer >1:32 or 4-fold ↑ over 2–3 wk)
- Cold agglutinins—IgM antibodies directed to I-antigen on RBC membranes; a titer >1:32 during acute stage is presumptive evidence of *M. pneumoniae*
- Rapid diagnostic tests—enzyme immunoassay (IgM), polymerase chain reaction (DNA)

ICD-9-CM Code: 483.0

ETIOLOGY

- Transmitted by respiratory droplets

USUAL TREATMENT

- Antimicrobial therapy is not necessary for most cases of *Mycoplasma* upper respiratory infections
- Antibiotics (erythromycin, ciprofloxacin, tetracycline) will shorten course of pneumonia

ASSESSMENT POINTS

SYSTEM	EFFECT	ASSESSMENT BY HX	PE	TEST
HEENT	Pharyngitis, sinusitis, myringitis, conjunctivitis			
CV	Pericardial effuson Pericarditis Myocarditis	Reported incidence as high as 10%; ↑ incidence with advanced age	Distant heart sounds S_3, JVD Pericardial rub	ECG ECHO Effusion tap
RESP	Tracheobronchitis Pneumonia Pleural effusion Bullous disease ARDS Hemoptysis	See above	Rhonchi, wheeze, ↓ breath sounds, egophony, substernal pain	CXR Sputum
HEME	Hemagglutination and hemolysis due to cold agglutinins Anemia Thrombocytopenia TTP	Effect of cold agglutinins occurs when surface or core temp falls below critical temp Peak cold agglutinin titer occurs ~4 wk into illness	Physical signs rare at room temp except for peripheral cyanosis	Cold agglutinins Blood smear CBC Free Hgb UA Direct Coombs'
DERM	Rash Stevens-Johnson syndrome	Most patients with rash have associated pneumonia	Erythematous maculopapular and vesicular exanthems	
CNS	Aseptic meningitis Meningoencephalitis Transverse myelitis Guillain-Barré dysfunction Peripheral neuropathy	0.1% of infections have CNS involvement 7% of patients with pneumonia have CNS involvement	Meningeal signs Focal or generalized neurologic deficits	CSF Blood culture MRI

Key Reference: Keegan BM, Lowry NJ, Yager JY: *Mycoplasma pneumoniae*: a cause of coma in the absence of meningoencephalitis. Pediatr Neurol 1999; 21:822–825.

PERIOPERATIVE IMPLICATIONS

Preoperative Evaluation
Hypothermic procedures:
- Routine screen
- If screen reveals presence of cold agglutinins (CA), determination of thermal range of reactivity (cold screen) and titer recommended.
- If significant CA with high thermal range (>20°C), consider postponing case. CA may persist up to 2–3 mo. Plasmapheresis can help.
- If emergent procedure: Keep pt temp above thermal range of CA by warming pt, fluids, blood, room, and gases; use normothermic technique if need CPB

Monitoring
- Consider invasive monitoring if cardiac disease suspected

Airway
- Rapid desaturation 2° to reduced FRC
- Hyperreactive airway 2° to inflammation

Maintenance
- Warm all fluids and blood products, humidified inspired gases
- If hemolysis suspected, maintain UO with maintenance of intravascular volume, osmotic and/or loop diuretics, alkalinization of urine

Extubation
- Clear sensorium and adequate analgesia to participate in postop mechanical toilet

ANTICIPATED PROBLEMS/CONCERNS

- Cold agglutinins
  - Hemagglutination
  - Hemolysis
- Cold agglutinins and CPB
  - Inadequate myocardial protection
  - CPB circuit obstruction
- Hyperreactive airway
- Impaired oxygenation if lung involved

MYOCARDIAL CONTUSION

Andrew L. Rosenberg, M.D.

RISK (BLUNT CHEST TRAUMA)
- 2 Million motor vehicle accidents/y with ~40% involving closed chest injury
- 20–70% incidence by clinical criteria
- 16–20% incidence by autopsy
- Motor vehicle > falls > crush injuries
- Males > females (5:1)

PERIOPERATIVE RISKS
- Abnormal ECG
- Nonspecific ST-T wave changes (70%) in trauma patients
- Ventricular arrhythmias most common in contusion
- Q wave and ST elevation
- 7–17% false negative
- 60% false positive
- Other cardiac conditions: thrombosed, lacerated coronary arteries in spasm; ventricular hypofunction; pericardial effusion/tamponade; pericarditis; valvular insufficiency, left-sided > right-sided; ventricular wall rupture

- Possible ↑ risk of cardiac complications (arrhythmias, hypotension) with ↑ CK-MB troponins, and abnormal ECHO
- No evidence of ↑ mortality associated with GA

WORRY ABOUT
- Malignant ventricular arrhythmia
- Cardiac conduction blocks
- Volume status
- Acute hypotension
- Associated injuries: pulmonary contusion–hypoxemia, thoracic aorta injuries, flail chest

OVERVIEW
- Traumatic injury with hemorrhagic, well-circumscribed lesions of partial or full thickness from myocardial contusion
- Usually of RV but can be multichambered
- Frequently in severe blunt chest trauma and after CPR, precordial thumps, but difficult to definitively diagnose

- Incorporation of clinical suspicion, anginal chest pain unrelieved by nitrates, ECG—especially ventricular dysrhythmia, troponin I and T levels, 2-D ECHO for Dx
- Amount of malignant arrhythmias may be proportional to severity of myocardial contusion

ICD-9-CM Code: 861.01

See also under Trauma in the index

ETIOLOGY
- Mechanical contusion of myocardium from posterior sternum
- "Ram effect" from ↑ transdiaphragmatic pressure
- Automobile accident = 15%
- Falls ~10%
- Crash, sports-related assaults ~15%

USUAL TREATMENT
- Supportive
- Adequate volume replacement

ASSESSMENT POINTS

SYSTEM	EFFECT	ASSESSMENT BY HX	PE	TEST
CV	Ventricular contusion	Angina-like chest pain unrelieved by nitrates Dyspnea	Chest wall, sternal tenderness Hypotension with severe dysfunction S_3 Rales	ECG, serial CK-MB, troponin I and T ECHO SPECT
	Arrhythmia	Palpitations, dizziness, syncope	Pulse	ECG monitoring
	Valvular disruptions	Dyspnea	Auscultatory murmurs	ECG
	Coronary artery injury: thrombosis, laceration, spasm	Chest pain		Angio
	Effusion/tamponade			TEE
		Chest pain	Pericardial friction Diminished heart sounds Distended neck veins	2-D cardiography PA catheter
RESP	CHF Pulm contusion	Dyspnea Orthopnea Chest tightness	S_3 Rales Wheezing Tachypnea	CXR Oxygen saturation

Key References: Capan L, et al: Management of thoracoabdominal injuries. *In* Caplan LM, Miller SM, Turndorf H (eds): Trauma, Anesthesia and Intensive Care. Philadelphia, JB Lippincott, 1991, pp 492–495; Rudusky BM: Cardiac troponin in the diagnosis of myocardial contusion. Chest 1996; 109:413–414.

PERIOPERATIVE IMPLICATIONS

Preoperative Preparation
- 2-D ECHO or TEE abnormalities predict perioperative hypotension
- Assess and ensure adequate volume replacement
- Assess and treat associated concurrent injuries
- No evidence for benefit of prophylactic antiarrhythmic agents

Monitoring
- Continuous ECG for arrhythmias
- PA catheter for large fluid shift operations or patients with signs of LV dysfunction
- ↑ Risk of perioperative arrhythmias without ↑ mortality

Airway
- Evaluation for associated airway injury

Preinduction/Induction
- Adequate volume replacement
- Hypotension more likely with large contusions
- Extra attention to avoid hypoxia, hypovolemia

Maintenance
- No one agent or technique shown superior
- Avoid known pulm vasoconstrictors: catecholamine, hypoxia, acidosis, histamine-releasing agents ($MgSO_4$, mivacurium)
- Consider high inspired oxygen if contusion
- Nitrous oxide can aggravate pulm Htn
- Elevations in PVR may unmask RV failure
- ↑ LV filling pressures and ↓ cardiac output often reflect hypovolemia or are 2° to RV failure, not LV failure

Extubation
- May leave intubated if concerns for resp failure and hypoxia present

Adjuvants
- Combination of appropriate intravascular volume replenishment and vasodilators (nitroglycerin) for pulmonary Htn

Postoperative Period
- Delayed hypoxia from pulmonary injury common and can cause pulmonary Htn leading to hypotension if RV severely contused

ANTICIPATED PROBLEMS/CONCERNS
- Variable diagnostic criteria, total CK-MB >50 U/L and ≥5% total CK.
- Possible higher risk of cardiac complications with ↑ CK-MB
- Almost any arrhythmia reported, especially conduction delays; more severe contusion associated with ↑ malignant ventricular arrhythmia
- Watch for RV failure leading to ↑ LV pressure but ↓ LV diastolic filling.

MYOCARDIAL ISCHEMIA (MIsch)

Dennis T. Mangano, M.D., Ph.D.
Michael F. Roizen, M.D.

RISK

- People within USA:
  - 1.5 million/y develop acute myocardial infarction (MI)
  - 8 million have $\geq 70\%$ narrowing of 1 or more coronary arteries
- European and African-American heritage > Japanese, but environment of North America equalizes risks
- Highest in patients with known other atherosclerotic disease (including prior MI): smokers (3.5-fold ↑); hypertensives (3-fold ↑); diabetics (4-fold ↑); hypercoagulable or chronic inflammatory diseases (3-fold ↑); stressed, divorced, or unstable marriage (2.5-fold ↑); with weight gain since age 20 y (1.5-fold ↑ for each 5 kg ↑); ↑ LDL cholesterol in those who do not exercise (1.4–3.4-fold ↑); who do not drink or take folate or aspirin; whose parent died of CAD at < age 40 y.

PERIOPERATIVE RISKS

- Increases risk 9-fold of perioperative CV complication (MI, CHF, arrhythmia requiring Rx)
- 2-y survival: rate in high-risk patient with perioperative MIsch is 25%, vs. 85% for those without periop MIsch

- Inadequate coronary perfusion (1.5 to 6% reinfarction rate with general surgery; higher with vascular/thoracic/upper abdominal surgery); lower with cataract/prostate/peripheral surgery with 1-limb anesthesia only
- Can lead to ↑ LV or RV compliance and CHF and dysrhythmias
- Can lead to inadequate perfusion of other organs and their insufficient function (brain/kidney/liver/gut)

WORRY ABOUT

- Postop period if stressed by perturbations that increase demand (pain, sepsis, fever, hyper- and hypovolemia, and tachycardia), or limit supply (thrombosis, hyperviscosity states, diseases limiting pulm function and gas exchange [restrictive, obstructive, parenchymal], hematocrit < 28%)

OVERVIEW

- Condition of inadequate supply of O_2 and nutrients to myocardial cells relative to need associated with the ↑ stress of perioperative period
- Treatment and prophylaxis of this and related disorders consumes 5–20% of total health expenditures. Perioperative CV complications increased onefold with MIsch, with 3-fold reduction in 2-y survival and survival and 3-fold increase in perioperative costs for major surgery
- Major focus of clinical and basic studies to decrease incidence of and risks from concern

over risk-benefit ratio and cost-effectiveness, identifying high-risk patients prior to surgery and segregating them for prior therapy (smoking cessation, control of Htn, hypercholesterol states, hypercoagulable states, PTCA, CABG) or increased perioperative vigilance and care (PA lines, TEE, ICU care, prophylactic pain therapy)

ICD-9-CM Code: 410.09

ETIOLOGY

- Known atherosclerotic risks (genetic predisposition, smoking, Htn, diabetes, divorced or unstable marriage, inflammation, hypercoagulable states, ↑ LDL cholesterol, weight gain)
- Known conditions that increase perioperative demands on heart (tachycardia, 2-fold greater for HR > 90; 11-fold greater for HR > 110); or limit supply (vasospastic states; $PaCO_2$ < 25; Hct < 28%; hyperviscosity and hypercoagulable states; inadequate O_2 exchange)

USUAL TREATMENT

- Decrease atherogenic risk factors
- Decrease perioperative demands on heart
- Consider preop segregation for β-blocker and nitrate therapies, antispasm and sympatholytic therapies, PTCA or CABG considerations, or stepped-up postop care of increased monitoring, intensive normalization of hemodynamics, greater prophylactic pain therapies

ASSESSMENT POINTS

SYSTEM	EFFECT	ASSESSMENT BY HX	PE	TEST
HEENT	Plaques in other areas	Risk factor search: smoking stain; hypercholesterolemic lesions	McArdle's earlobe	
CV	↓ LV or RV compliance ↓ Pump function arrhythmias Autonomic pain	SOB, DOE Angina ↓ Exercise tolerance Palpitations PND	HR/BP prior to and after 2-stair climb; S_3; rales; JVD; use character and rhythm	ECG, CXR, stress ECHO or dipyridamole thallium or ambulatory Holter
RESP		Nocturnal cough, orthopnea		
RENAL	Perfusion insufficiency	Nocturia		BUN/Cr
CNS	Autonomic pain syndromes Other atherosclerotic syndromes	Pain in neck or left arm Stroke/TIA Hx	CNS and cranial nerve exam	Carotid Doppler Autonomic NS testing

Key Reference: Sorrentino MJ, Roizen MF: Secondary prevention of coronary artery disease: duplications for the peripheral vascular disease patient. Problems Anesth 1998; 11:157–166.

PERIOPERATIVE IMPLICATIONS

Preoperative Preparation

- Consider segregation procedures and prophylactic regimens (see under Usual Treatment)

Monitoring

- ST-T waves of area of myocardium identified as at risk (or II and V_5) (II esp for CNS surgery); ST-segment trend analysis
- Consider PA line or TEE and arterial line and approaches to intensively normalize hemodynamics

Airway

- Routine

Induction

- Without hemodynamic disturbance and especially with HR control

Maintenance

- Tachycardia or hypovolemia and Hct <28 can precipitate ischemia
- No agent with demonstrated outcome superiority
- Intensively normalize hemodynamics and HR

Extubation

- In nonstressful fashion for patient without compromising supply of O_2 to myocardium
- Aggressive stepped pain therapy recommended

Adjuvants

- CHF decreases liver blood flow and clearance of drugs requiring hepatic metabolism (such as lidocaine)
- β-adrenergic receptor antagonists and nitrates can be associated with profound hemodynamic disturbances if drug interactions or sudden preload/afterload/or contractility perturbations (such as rapid onset of spinal anesthesia) occur

ANTICIPATED PROBLEMS/CONCERNS

- Pre- and postoperative periods at least as great a cause of morbidity as intraoperative period
- Consider compassionate anxiety-relieving yet aggressive preop consultation and intensive stepped pain prophylaxis consultations postop

MYOTONIA DYSTROPHICA (MYOTONIC DYSTROPHY, STEINERT'S DISEASE)   Arthur J. Klowden, M.D.

RISK

• 2.4–5.5/100,000 births

PERIOPERATIVE RISKS

• Operative/anesthetic and postop morbidity/mortality are increased
• High incidence of cardiopulmonary complications, including sudden death, cardiac failure, cardiomyopathy

WORRY ABOUT

• Increasing frequency of symptoms
• Signs of resp or cardiac decompensation

OVERVIEW

• Degenerative disease of skeletal muscles. Progressive distal muscle wasting. Triad of characteristic features described as frontal baldness, cataracts, and mental retardation.
• Onset of symptoms in 2nd and 3rd decades of life. Death frequently in 5th or 6th decade of life, usually due to cardiopulmonary complications.
• Persistent contracture after cessation of stimulation or voluntary contraction of the muscle. This inability of the skeletal muscle to relax is diagnostic. EMG is corroborative and pathognomonic, showing continuous low-voltage activity with high-voltage, fibrillation-like potential bursts.
• Intrinsic disorder of skeletal muscle linked to myotonin-protein kinase gene on chromosome 19q13.2. Defect in Na^+ and Cl^- channel function produces electrical instability of the muscle membrane and self-sustaining runs of depolarization. May also have abnormal CA^{2+} metabolism.

ICD-9-CM Code: 359.2

ETIOLOGY

• Inherited autosomal dominant trait

USUAL TREATMENT

• Quinine, procainamide, phenytoin, tocainide, mexiletine (depress Na^+ influx)

ASSESSMENT POINTS

SYSTEM	EFFECT	ASSESSMENT BY HX	PE	TEST
HEENT	Visual disturbance		Presenile cataract, ptosis, strabismus	Exam by ophthalmologist
	Speech/swallowing impaired		Generalized weakness of pharyngeal, mandibular (and thoracic) musculature Dysarthria, facial weakness Expressionless facies	
CV	Dysrhythmias Cardiomyopathy	CHF uncommon but may occur with pregnancy	Delayed intraventricular conduction Heart block Up to 20% with mitral valve prolapse	ECG ECHO, Holter Cardiology consult
RESP	Restrictive lung disease	Weak cough Dyspnea Hx of pneumonias	Wasting of sternocleidomastoid muscles; resp muscle weakness Lungs intrinsically normal; ↓ VC, ERV	PFTs ABGs
GI	High aspiration potential Delayed esophageal and gastric emptying Gastric dilation/atony ↑ Incidence of cholelithiasis	Weak swallowing ability		
ENDO	Gonadal atrophy Diabetes mellitus ↓ Thyroid function Adrenal insufficiency Frontal balding ?Malignant hyperthermia		Thyroid nodules	Blood/urine glucose tests Thyroid function tests
CNS	Mental retardation Associated with central sleep apnea and hypersomnolence Emotional abn		Myotonic handgrip (delayed, incomplete release), ↑ CK in serum Myotonia can be initiated or worsened by exercise or cold temp	EMG CK
GYN	Pregnant patient is a challenge. Resp function threatened by ↓ FRC and myotonic weakness, which may be exacerbated by pregnancy. Seems to be added risk for uterine hemorrhage at delivery due to uterine atony and retained placenta. C-section may be safer.			

Key Reference: Aldredge LM: Anaesthetic problems in myotonic dystrophy. A case report and review of the Aberdeen experience comprising 48 general anesthetics in a further 16 patients. Br J Anaesth 1985; 57:1119–1130.

PERIOPERATIVE IMPLICATIONS

Preoperative Preparation
• Ensuring NPO status
• No preop analgesics or sedatives
• Warm ambient room air in OR may ↓ incidence and severity of myotonia

Monitoring
• Routine

Airway
• Propensity for frequent jaw dislocation
• Potential inability to secure airway because of jaw muscle spasm

Preinduction/Induction
• Risk for aspiration of gastric contents
• Succinylcholine-induced skeletal muscle contraction may be so severe and prolonged (2–5 min) as to make adequate ventilation difficult

• May be hard to differentiate from onset of MH

Maintenance
• Myotonia may be precipitated by drugs (propofol, succinylcholine, anticholinesterases, halothane, etc.), physical factors (cold, shivering), surgical manipulation, or electrocautery
• Regional or local anesthesia acceptable, but will not block myotonic response
• IV regional may be preferable when suitable

Extubation
• Beware airway obstruction because of jaw muscle weakness
• Delayed recovery from anesthetic common

Adjuvants
• ↑ Sensitivity to ventilatory depressant effects of all premedicants, sedatives, opioids

• Reversal agents can theoretically precipitate skeletal muscle contraction by facilitating depolarization of NMJ, but adverse responses do not predictably occur

Postoperative Period
• ↑ Sensitivity to respiratory depressant effects of opioids or sedatives, including epidural opioids
• Pulm complications due to poor cough possible

ANTICIPATED PROBLEMS/CONCERNS

• If myotonia develops intraoperatively, neither general or regional anesthesia, nor NMBs will attenuate it. Local infiltration of involved muscles may help. Even asymptomatic patients may have some degree of cardiomyopathy. Beware premature extubation, consider postop ventilation.

MYXOMA

Solomon Aronson, M.D.

RISK

- Although primary cardiac tumors are rare (< 0.01%) this is the most common (50%)
- 75% develop in left atrium
- Rarely develop in ventricle
- More common in females (70%)

PERIOPERATIVE RISKS

- May be friable and embolize
- Risk of LV or RV inflow obstruction
- May simulate pulm Htn and/or constrictive pericarditis

WORRY ABOUT

- Hypotension due to obstruction of ventricular inflow and/or incompetence of tricuspid (right) or mitral (left) valve
- Tumor "flips" on stalk across valves, causing stenotic or incompetent symptoms
- RV hypertrophy due to long-standing left inflow obstruction
- Rare pulm or systemic embolization

OVERVIEW

- Is a true neoplasm and distinct from a thrombus
- Usually polypoid with 1–2 cm stalk projecting into cavity, round with smooth margins
- Typically grows very slowly before symptomatic (10–20 y)

ICD-9-CM Code: 215.4 (Thorax myxoma)

ETIOLOGY

- Polyhedral cells with small nuclei are separated by an afibrillar, eosinophilic myxomatous stroma that is predominantly a mucopolysaccharide
- Rarely extends deeper than endocardium
- Although "benign," this tumor can undergo malignant degeneration

USUAL TREATMENT

- Surgical
- Cardiopulmonary bypass required
- Atriotomy with transseptal approach through fossa ovalis

ASSESSMENT POINTS

SYSTEM	EFFECT	ASSESSMENT BY HX	PE	TEST
CV	Mitral stenosis or insufficiency syndromes	Edema, CHF	Left atrial enlargement Systolic murmur (MI) Diastolic murmur (mitral stenosis)	ECHO ECG CXR
RESP	Pulm emboli (right)	DOE, cough	Rales, wheezing, ↑ P_2	ECHO, CXR, ECG
GI		CHF	Hepatic enlargement	Hepatic enzymes (if Sx of CHF)
RENAL	Emboli (left)			Urinalysis Cr clearance
CNS	Stroke (left)	CNS dysfunction	CNS dysfunction	ECHO
GENERAL	Constitutional symptoms	Fever, malaise	Weight loss	

Key Reference: Larsson S, Lepore V, Kennergren C: Atrial myxomas: results of 25 years experience and review of the literature. Surgery 1989; 105:695.

PERIOPERATIVE IMPLICATIONS

Preoperative Preparation

- Differential Dx includes mitral stenosis/insufficiency (left), tricuspid stenosis/insufficiency (right), constrictive pericarditis, pulm Htn, subacute bacterial endocarditis
- Mitral stenosis: hemodynamic aim is to keep in normal sinus rhythm with adequate preload and high normal afterload (see Mitral Stenosis in Diseases section).
- Mitral insufficiency (regurgitation): hemodynamic aim is to keep HR normal or fast and vasodilate
- Hemodynamics can mimic any or all of above depending on load-dependent variables prevailing in the cardiac cycle at the time (e.g., preload, afterload, HR)

Monitoring

- Routine monitors otherwise needed for cardiopulmonary bypass (e.g., temp, ECG, coagulation, Foley)
- Intra-arterial catheters

- Beware of central line with right-sided atrial myxoma (may cause dislodgment of friable debris as pulm emboli)
- TEE most sensitive way to guide hemodynamic management and assess therapeutic approach

Airway

- Routine

Preinduction/Induction

- May develop hypotension if preload ↓ or HR ↑
- Avoid insertion of central venous or PA monitoring catheters or cannula with right-sided tumor
- Intraop TTE helpful diagnostic (prior to induction): concern about right inflow obstruction exacerbated by PPV

Maintenance

- May dislodge pieces during CPB venous cannulation; direct assessment of anatomy, physiology; and even placement of cannula should be guided by TEE
- If pedunculated, tumor may obstruct inflow track and hemodynamics may present as low BP, low CO; ↑ CVP (right) or ↑ PCWP (left)

Extubation

- Expect excellent recovery from primary myxomatous lesion and ventricular function
- Criteria should be based on myocardial protection techniques and post-CPB bleeding risk
- Early extubation consideration is reasonable

Postoperative Period

- Beware residual ASD (as tumors typically originate in atrial septum in region of fossa ovalis)
- Beware conduction, dysrhythmia disturbance (especially in pediatric population)
- Symptoms of pulm Htn usually regress quickly

ANTICIPATED PROBLEMS/CONCERNS

- Hypotension with inadequate preload when lesion obstructs inflow dynamics

DISEASES   237

NARCOLEPSY

Douglas Martz, M.D.

RISK

- Prevalance: 1/4000
- Race with highest prevalence: none

PERIOPERATIVE RISKS

- Risks related to treatment medications
- ↑ Sensitivity to anesthetic agents
- ↑ Incidence of delayed emergence and postop hypersomnia after GA

WORRY ABOUT

- Tricyclic drugs increase incidence of perioperative hypotension
- Tricyclic drugs blunt pressor response to indirect-acting sympathomimetic agents (e.g., ephedrine) and exaggerate pressor response to direct-acting sympathomimetic agents (e.g., phenylephrine)
- ↑ Incidence of postop apneic episodes
- Possible ↑ sensitivity to anesthetic agents

OVERVIEW

- Lifelong disease that usually develops in childhood/adolescence
- Initial symptom is excessive daytime sleepiness with irresistible sleep attacks
- Secondary symptoms of cataplexy, hypnagogic hallucinations, disrupted nocturnal sleep, and automatic behavior have variable incidence and occur later in the disease
- Sleep attacks appear as clinically normal sleep lasting from seconds to minutes. Can be easily awakened by auditory or tactile stimulation.
- 80% incidence of cataplexy (sudden brief loss of voluntary muscle control). Usually precipitated by strong emotional response (e.g., laughter, anger, surprise). Patient remains conscious. Majority of patients develop a flat affect to suppress the emotional trigger.
- Diagnostic work-up includes nocturnal polysomnogram (documents adequacy of sleep and rules out obstructive sleep apnea) followed by a Multiple Sleep Latency Test

(MSLT) to document hypersomnolence and REM onset sleep. Patients with narcolepsy fall asleep quickly (usually < 5 min) and have early onset of sleep.
- Often confused with obstructive sleep apnea syndrome

ICD-9-CM Code: 347

ETIOLOGY

- Association with HLA-DR15 and DQ6 antigens

USUAL TREATMENT

- Psychosocial support, therapeutic naps, medications
- Sleep attacks most commonly treated with indirect sympathomimetic drugs such as pemoline, mazindol, methylphenidate, and amphetamines
- Cataplexy and other secondary symptoms treated with tricyclic antidepressants and/or serotonin reuptake inhibitors

ASSESSMENT POINTS

SYSTEM	EFFECT	ASSESSMENT BY HX	TEST
HEENT		Obstructive symptoms (rare)	
CV	Conduction abnormalities due to tricyclics		ECG
CNS	Flat affect Fatigue	Daytime sleep attacks	

Key Reference: Mesa A, Diaz A, Froth M: Narcolepsy and anesthesia. Anesthesiology 2000; 92:1194–1196.

PERIOPERATIVE IMPLICATIONS

Preoperative Preparation

- Avoid sedative premedication
- Continue medical therapy on day of surgery
- If antisialagogue needed use non–central acting agent

Monitoring

- May have conduction abnormalities on ECG
- Patients with a history of chronic amphetamine therapy may benefit from direct arterial pressure monitoring

Induction

- May have exaggerated hypotension if taking tricyclics
- Hydrate prior to induction

Maintenance

- ↑ Sensitivity to anesthetic agents. Consider use of propofol, desflurane, sevoflurane, and N_2O instead of longer acting intravenous/inhalation agents.
- Exaggerated pressor response to direct-acting sympathomimetics (e.g., phenylephrine) if taking tricyclics. Use small doses if clinically indicated.
- Blunted/unpredictable pressor response to indirect-acting sympathomimetics if taking tricyclics. Probably best to avoid.

Adjuvants

- Muscle relaxants: life-threatening arrhythmias have been reported with the use of pancuronium in patients on tricyclics
- Anesthetic agents: life-threatening arrhythmias have been reported with the use of halothane in patients on tricyclics

Postoperative Period

- May be prone to postoperative apneic episodes especially with use of intravenous and/or neuraxial narcotics for postop analgesia

ANTICIPATED PROBLEMS/CONCERNS

- Patients often on tricyclic therapy and CNS stimulant therapy. Will often be sensitive to anesthetic agents. If on tricyclics need to be concerned about exaggerated pressor responses with direct-acting sympathomimetics. Indirect-acting sympathomimetics have a blunted pressor response and probably should be avoided. Postop apnea is of theoretical concern. Postop obstruction symptoms are extremely rare.

238   DISEASES

NECROTIZING ENTEROCOLITIS

Robert M. Insoft, M.D.
I. David Todres, M.D.

RISK

- Most common life-threatening intestinal surgical emergency in the newborn
- Occurs predominantly in premature infants, with 75% in infants < 1500 g
- Increasing incidence in term and near-term neonates as well

PERIOPERATIVE RISKS

- Cardiovascular instability, acidosis, shock, bowel ischemia, bacteremia, patent ductus arteriosus, polycythemia

WORRY ABOUT

- Persistent metabolic acidosis and intestinal perforation are ominous signs

OVERVIEW

- Presents commonly with generalized signs of sepsis, including glucose instability, hypothermia, apnea, feeding intolerance, and metabolic acidosis
- Terminal ileum most commonly involved, followed by the distal small bowel and ascending colon. Bowel ischemia may lead to gangrene of bowel with perforation as well as peritonitis, CV and respiratory collapse, shock, and death.
- Multisystem failure is commonly associated involving the respiratory, CV, renal, and hepatic systems. Abnormally elevated inflammatory mediators, such as TNF, IL-6, and PAF, are associated.
- In severe cases, abdominal wall may be erythematous, signifying intestinal perforation and peritonitis

- Pneumatosis intestinalis is evident as a linear collection of air and hydrogen gas in the wall of dilated loop of bowel; may extend into portal venous circulation

ICD-9-CM Code: 777.5

ETIOLOGY

- Associated with bowel ischemia, enteral feeds, infection, and prematurity. Clearest link is with prematurity, leading to the theory that an underlying developmental immaturity of bowel is potentially the initiating problem leading to this life-threatening condition.

ASSESSMENT POINTS

SYSTEM	EFFECT	ASSESSMENT BY HX	PE	TEST
CV	Shock PDA	Pulm edema, RDS, shock	Murmur BP/HR	ABGs, BP UO
RESP	RDS	Apnea or tachypnea		ABGs CXR
ID	Sepsis	Bacteremia Peritonitis	Abd wall cellulitis, peritonitis	Blood and peritoneal fluid cultures
GI	Peritonitis, bloody stools, malabsorption	Large feeding residuals, bilious emesis	Residuals, guaiac stools	Lytes, bowel sounds, KUB Temp instability
RENAL	Prerenal failure		UO, BP	BUN, Cr
HEME	DIC Polycythemia	Bleeding		Hct, plt count, Fibrinogen PT/PTT

Key Reference: Kanto WP: Recognition and medical management of necrotizing enterocolitis. Clin Perinatol 1994; 21:335–346.

PERIOPERATIVE MANAGEMENT

Preoperative Preparation

- Most neonates may be treated medically with fluid resuscitation, antibiotics, ventilatory support, and hyperalimentation
- Surgery indicated for pneumoperitoneum from intestinal wall perforation, intestinal gangrene (detected by abdominal paracentesis), and presence of portal vein gas. Other indications include clinical deterioration, abdominal wall erythema, and an unresolved ileus.
- Discontinue enteral feeds and insert nasogastric tube connected to suction for intestinal decompression
- Therapeutic goals include normalization of vital signs, ensuring adequate oxygenation and ventilation (e.g., tracheal intubation, mechanical ventilation, adequate perfusion)

- Vigorous fluid resuscitation to keep up with third space losses from peritonitis and sepsis
- Correct metabolic acidosis—achieved through fluid resuscitation
- Inotropic agents such as dopamine and dobutamine may be required to optimize cardiac output
- Correct coagulopathy with FFP, plts, and packed RBCs
- Administer broad-spectrum antibiotics, with anaerobic coverage highly considered as well

Monitoring

- Routine plus glucose and electrolytes

Induction/Maintenance

- Potent anesthetic agents are poorly tolerated
- Carefully titrated narcotic and muscle relaxant technique is satisfactory
- N_2O is usually avoided because of its potential for causing bowel distention

- Fluid resuscitation (lactated Ringer's, 5% albumin, and sometimes packed RBCs) is actively carried out during surgical procedure

Postoperative Period

- Closely monitor in NICU for ongoing fluid requirements as third space loss continues
- Prolonged TPN is often required
- Stricture formation leading to partial or total bowel obstruction is a common complication in both medically and surgically treated neonates
- Short-bowel syndrome can occur, leading to long-term complications

ANTICIPATED PROBLEMS/CONCERNS

- Hypovolemia and bowel ischemia
- Acidosis, shock, and death

NECROTIZING FASCIITIS

Avery Tung, M.D.

RISK

- Rare: 5000 in USA
- No race or gender preference
- Risk factors include diabetes (20–50% of cases), atherosclerosis (20–30%), CV or renal disease, alcoholism, malnutrition

PERIOPERATIVE RISKS

- Highly lethal condition with 30–60% mortality depending on speed of Dx and spread of infection
- Death by septic shock and associated multiorgan system failure
- Need for surgery often emergent
- Associated chronic medical conditions complicate anesthetic care

WORRY ABOUT

- Incomplete initial fluid and pressor resuscitation
- Associated CV, renal, liver disease
- Metabolic derangements: acidosis, hypocalcemia, DIC

OVERVIEW

- Progressive, usually polymicrobial, soft tissue infection involving subcutaneous tissue and spreading along fascial planes
- Can progress rapidly to severe systemic toxicity with septic shock, pulm and renal dysfunction, and extreme third space sequestration of fluid
- Extensive surgical debridement usually performed. Hyperkalemic responses to succinylcholine usually not a concern, as necrotizing infection spares muscle.
- Use of N_2O not a concern if gaseous pockets exist, as surrounding tissue is avascular and necrotic

ICD-9-CM Code: 729.4

ETIOLOGY

- Minor trauma, wounds, or decubiti in patients with diabetes, alcoholism, chronic CV and renal disease, or poor nutrition. Subsequent bacterial seeding event.
- Can also occur in young, otherwise healthy patients following surgery or cuts/abrasions
- Spread of necrotic infection along fascial planes with sparing of skin
- Onset of severe systemic toxicity, septic shock, end-organ dysfunction, death
- Malignant bacterial species

USUAL TREATMENT

- Antibiotics
- Wide, often repeated surgical debridement
- Hemodynamic, resp, nutritional support perioperatively

ASSESSMENT POINTS

SYSTEM	EFFECT	ASSESSMENT BY HX	PE	TEST
HEENT	Possible infection	Edema complicating intubation	Airway exam	
CV	↓ SVR ↑ CO	↓ Mentation	Orthostatic hypotension	Invasive monitoring
RESP	ARDS Pulm edema	SOB Dyspnea	Rales	ABGs CXR
ENDO	Metabolic abn			ABGs, electrolytes PT/PTT, Hct
RENAL	↓ Renal function	↓ UO		BUN/Cr
CNS	Disoriented 2° to sepsis		Neuro exam	

Key Reference: Conly J: Necrotizing fasciitis. *In* Hall JB, Schmidt GA, Wood LDH (eds): Principles of Critical Care, 2nd ed. New York, McGraw-Hill, 1998, pp 406–408.

PERIOPERATIVE IMPLICATIONS

Preoperative Preparation

- Surgery often emergent
- Verify adequacy of initial resuscitation including volume status
- Patient may not be on NPO status

Monitoring

- Often persistently hypotensive, tachycardic, with septic physiology
- Consider invasive monitoring including arterial line, CVP or PA catheter, or transesophageal ECHO to manage intraoperative volume status

Airway

- Spread of fascial infection can be clinically silent
- Can cause airway edema if infectious spread to neck or face

Induction

- May be severely septic and hypotensive with massive fluid requirements
- Relative hypovolemia may accentuate hypotensive response to anesthetic induction

Maintenance

- Hemodynamic instability. Monitor volume status and adequacy of cardiac output.

Extubation

- Often need repeat exploration within 24 h if sepsis and hemodynamic instability continue postop. Consider postop intubation and ICU management between debridements.

Adjuvants

- No contraindication to N_2O
- Efficacy of hyperbaric oxygen therapy for anaerobic infection unproven but felt worthwhile by some

Postoperative Period

- Consider ICU care
- Will likely need repeat debridement within 24 h
- Prognosis worst with perineal/truncal infection, extensive spread, associated diabetes/CV disease

ANTICIPATED PROBLEMS/CONCERNS

- Need for emergent surgery in potentially unstable patient
- Massive fluid requirements 2° to edema formation and septic physiology
- Associated metabolic abnormalities

NEUROFIBROMATOSIS

Zeev N. Kain, M.D.

RISK

- Prevalence: 1/3000 people

PERIOPERATIVE RISKS

- Risk depends upon tumor and location

WORRY ABOUT

- Difficult intubation
- Intraoperative Htn and tachycardia

OVERVIEW

- Genetic disorder in which multiple organs, such as skin and nervous system, are site of tumors and hamartomas
- Hallmark is café-au-lait spots (more than 6 that are >1.5 cm in diameter) and multiple neurofibromas
- Laryngeal and tracheal compression may occur 2° to associated tumors
- Surgery may be indicated for patients with NF-1, esp for removal of tumors (e.g., neurofibromas, pheochromocytoma), skeletal dysplasia (e.g., tibial pseudoarthrosis), scoliosis, and renovascular Htn

ICD-9-CM Codes: 237.7; 171.# (Malignant)

ETIOLOGY

- Autosomal dominant, although about 50% of cases represent new mutations. The gene for NF-1 appears to reside on the long arm of chromosome 17.

USUAL TREATMENT

- Radiation and surgical treatment for various tumors involved

ASSESSMENT POINTS

SYSTEM	EFFECT	ASSESSMENT BY HX	PE	TEST
HEENT*	Pharyngeal compression Laryngeal compression Airway obstruction	Dyspnea, dysphonia	Evaluation of airway	X-ray CT of neck
CV	Renovascular Htn Pheochromocytoma	Headache, perspiration		BP/HR Urinary catecholamines
RESP*	Restrictive lung disease Cor pulmonale Interstitial lung disease Hypoxemia	Exercise tolerance	Cyanosis Clubbing	CXR ECG ABGs PFTs (rare)
GU*	Obstruction and uremia			
CNS	Mental retardation Seizures Neurofibromas			
MS*	Kyphoscoliosis Macrocephaly Craniofacial/vertebral dysplasia			

*In severe cases

Key Reference: Richardson MG, Setty GK; Rawoof SA: Responses to nondepolarizing neuromuscular blockers and succinylcholine in von Recklinghausen neurofibromatosis. Anesth Analg 1996; 82:382–385.

PERIOPERATIVE IMPLICATIONS

Preoperative Preparation

- Evaluation of airway for possible laryngeal and pharyngeal tumors
- Asymptomatic intraspinal neurofibromas can make identification and entry into epidural and subarachnoid spaces very difficult. A careful examination of the back is indicated before any regional technique is considered.

Monitoring

- Routine
- Consider arterial line depending on resp status and presence of pheochromocytoma

Airway

- Consider awake fiberoptic intubation or tracheotomy if laryngeal and pharyngeal involvement

Preinduction/Induction

- No particular anesthetic drug or technique recommended
- Consider potential for spinal cord neurofibromas if regional considered
- Consider potential for increased ICP
- Consider potential of pheochromocytoma (see Pheochromocytoma in Diseases section)
- Although some thought abnormal response to NMBs, recent evidence suggests no or minimal effect

Maintenance

- CV instability if pheochromocytoma present
- Several reported cases of prolonged NMB in response to administration of succinylcholine, pancuronium, d-tubocurarine

Extubation

- Routine considerations

Postoperative Period

- Pain management may be critical

Adjuvants

- Prolonged response or resistance to NMBs

ANTICIPATED PROBLEMS/CONCERNS

- Presence of pheochromocytoma
- Potential for increased ICP if expanding intracranial tumor

OCCLUSIVE CEREBROVASCULAR DISEASE

Ian A. Herrick, M.D., F.R.C.P.C.

RISK

• People within USA: stroke incidence = 0.1%/y (all causes)
• Races with highest prevalence: Japanese/Eastern European (incidence 0.3%/y)

PERIOPERATIVE RISKS

• Stroke
  – Major general surgery at age >50 y = 0.4%; at age >80 y = 2.5%
  – Major peripheral vascular reconstruction = 1%
  – CABG = 1–5%, carotid endarterectomy (CEA) = 3% or less

WORRY ABOUT

• Cerebral ischemia
• Myocardial ischemia (CAD, leading cause of morbidity following CEA)
• Control of co-existing CAD, DM, Htn

OVERVIEW

• Two main clinical presentations
  – Patients with known occlusive CVD undergoing CEA or carotid angioplasty. Risk factors include CAD/CHF; stroke in evolution, frequent TIAs; severe Htn; carotid siphon stenosis; COPD; poor cerebral collateral flow; age >70 y; intraluminal thrombus. Criteria for patient selection and acceptable perioperative morbidity and mortality rates are now well established for CEA.
  – Patients with known or possible CVD presenting for other surgery. Risk factors are poorly defined. Most perioperative strokes occur postop and do not correlate with presence of CVD. Highest risk with CABG.
• Asymptomatic carotid bruits are inconsistent predictors of CVD but predict poor CVD survival

ICD-9-CM Code: 434.9

ETIOLOGY

• Vasculopathy 2° to advanced atherosclerosis
• Risk factors include age, Htn, diabetes mellitus, smoking
• High incidence of concomitant CAD and peripheral vascular disease

USUAL TREATMENT

• Antiplatelet drugs (esp ASA); CEA
• Carotid angioplasty with or without stent placement undergoing evaluation as an alternative treatment to CEA in some patients

ASSESSMENT POINTS

SYSTEM	EFFECT	ASSESSMENT BY HX	PE	TEST
HEENT	Possible positional cerebral ischemia	Sx of cerebral ischemia with head movements	Neck ROM	
CV	Htn Vasculopathy LV dysfunction, CHF	Exercise tolerance Angina, MI, CHF Claudication	Arterial BP S_3 Peripheral pulses	ECG, CXR ECHO Stress test
RESP	COPD due to smoking Irritable airway	Dyspnea Chronic cough Smoker	Wheezing Accessory muscles	CXR ?ABGs ?PFTs
ENDO	Possible diabetes			Glucose
RENAL	Possible nephropathy	Diabetes, Htn		Cr, urea
CNS	Cerebral ischemia	TIA, stroke	Neurologic deficits	Cerebral angio prior to CEA

Key Reference: Lownie SP, Pelz DM: Carotid angioplasty and stenting: current status. Can Med Assoc J 2000; 162:1451–1454.

PERIOPERATIVE IMPLICATIONS

Preoperative Preparation
• Neurologic assessment
• Optimize control of co-existing Htn, CAD, diabetes, COPD
• Evaluate normal BP range

Monitoring
• Arterial catheter and ST-segment monitoring
• For CEA, consider neurologic monitor: EEG or regional anesthetic with awake patient (if practical)
• Carotid angioplasty usually performed with the patient awake

Induction/Maintenance
• Have surgeon block carotid sinus nerve if bradycardic
• Maintain hemodynamic stability based on preop BP range
• Maintain normocapnia based on preop pH and $PaCO_2$
• Light IV sedation often administered during angioplasty
• Embolic stroke or severe, vagal-mediated, bradycardia can accompany carotid dilation during angioplasty

Extubation
• Be prepared to manage hemodynamic instability following CEA
• Avoid straining on ET tube with fresh arteriotomy following CEA

Postoperative Period
• Hemodynamic instability due to baroreceptor dysfunction following CEA
• Adequate analgesia, supplemental O_2
• Awake patient allows early and frequent neurologic evaluation

ANTICIPATED PROBLEMS/CONCERNS

• Most patients with CVD also at high risk for CAD. Consistent approach to management of both problems includes hemodynamic stability, adequate oxygenation, normocapnia, adequate analgesia, normoglycemia.
• Caution regarding use of succinylcholine in patients with previous paretic CVA
• Angioplasty is not associated with substantial discomfort. Only minimal sedation is typically needed for comfort.

OPITZ-FRIAS SYNDROME (THE G SYNDROME) Bruno Bissonnette, M.D.

RISK

- Overall incidence not reported
- Very rare congenital disorder

PREOPERATIVE RISKS

- Very high risk of recurrent pulmonary aspiration; hypoplasia of both pulmonary and vascular components of one lung
- High mortality rate in infancy

WORRY ABOUT

- Neuromuscular dysfunction of laryngo-esophageal apparatus
- Laryngotracheoesophageal cleft or fistula
- Difficult tracheal intubation due to craniofacial deformity
- Associated congenital anomalies

OVERVIEW

- Known also as the hypospadias-dysphagia syndrome
- Emergency presentations are for cardio-pulmonary resuscitation, upper resp obstruction, severe resp stridor, regurgitation, aspiration
- Presence of one hypoplastic lung
- Laryngeal hypoplasia
- Laryngotracheoesophageal cleft or fistula
- Anticipate very difficult tracheal intubation
- Any male infant presenting for TEF with genital defect should be suspected
- Classically—weak, hoarse cry

ICD-9-CM Code: 759.9 (Congenital anomaly, unspecified)

ETIOLOGY

- X-linked recessive inheritance
- Autosomal dominant inheritance or new mutation
- Partial male sex limitation
- Autosomal recessive inheritance, high parenteral consanguinity
- Females can be equally or nearly as severely affected as males

USUAL TREATMENT

- Prophylactic gastrostomy
- Feeding jejunostomy
- Cervical esophagostomy if unable to swallow
- Prophylactic antibodies (pulm infection)

ASSESSMENT POINTS

SYSTEM	EFFECT	ASSESSMENT BY HX	PE	TESTS (IF INDICATED)
HEENT	Cleft lip–palate (35%) Ankyloglossia Micrognathia	Feeding difficulties Speech anomalies	Short lingual frenulum	
CNS	Dolichocephaly (20%) Large metopic sagittal suture and anterior fontanel	Mental dysfunction Prominent forehead	"Cone-head" Palpation	CT (if indicated)
FACIES	Hypertelorism/telecanthus (90%) Mongoloid palpebral fissures Strabismus	Mother-related disease	Large nasal bridge downslanting	Face x-ray
CV	Congenital heart defects (40%) (ASD, VSD, PDA, coarctation of aorta)	Failure to thrive	Auscultation	ECG TEE, ABGs
RESP	Agenesis, hypoplasia of one lung Tracheoesophageal cleft, fissure Hypoplasia of vocal cord Tracheomalacia Short trachea, high carina	Polyhydramnios on delivery Coughing, choking, cyanosis Hoarse, weak cry Stridorous resp	Auscultation Tracheal stenosis	CXR Bronchogram Esophagogram
GI	Achalasia of the cardia (70%) Neuromuscular dysfunction of esophagus	Dysphagia		Esophagogram (if indicated) Cinefluoroscopy of swallowing (if indicated)
GU	Hypospadias with descended testis Ureteral stenosis or duplication		Perineal or penoscrotal	Nephrogram

Key Reference: Conlon BD, O'Dwyer T: The G syndrome/Opitz ocular-genital-laryngeal syndrome/Opitz BBB/G syndrome/Opitz-Frias syndrome. J Laryngol Otol 1995; 108:244–246.

PERIOPERATIVE IMPLICATIONS

Preoperative Preparation

- Evacuation of the stomach with NG tube
- Feeding: clear water or apple juice
- Consider H_2 blocker
- No atropine IM or metoclopramide
- Give sodium citrate through NG tube
- IV access 24 h before surgery to reduce stomach content

Monitoring

- All standard monitors
- Invasive arterial pressure if unstable

Airway

- Tubes smaller than normal 2° to laryngeal hypoplasia

Preinduction

- Warm OR
- Decompress stomach with suction
- Atropine and succinylcholine backup

Induction

- Maintain spontaneous respiration
- Danger of regurgitation and aspiration requires careful inhalation induction
- Cricoid pressure should be applied

- Atropine 20 μg/kg of induction to prevent bradycardia during intubation

Maintenence

- Hand ventilation (low PPV)
- Avoid hypothermia

Extubation

- Based on patient's lung condition

Adjuvants

- All medications can be used

ANTICIPATED PROBLEMS

- Regurgitation and pulm aspiration. Difficult tracheal intubation. ↑ Incidence of pneumothorax. High mortality rate in infancy.

OSTEOARTHRITIS

Denise J. Wedel, M.D.

RISK

• Osteoarthritis (OA) most common cause of impairment in the elderly
 – 63–85% of Americans >65 y have radiographic signs
 – 35–50% have pain, stiffness, or limitation of movement
 – 9–12% are significantly disabled
 – 46 million doctor visits and 68 million work days lost per annum
• Risk factors differ across joints: knee—obesity, injury; hand—repetitive use; hip—congenital or developmental abn, male preponderance

PERIOPERATIVE RISKS

• Often associated with obesity
• Common analgesics include NSAIDs and intra-articular steroid injections
• Rarely affects neck or jaw
• Reported association with diabetes, hypothyroidism, hyperparathyroidism, gout

WORRY ABOUT

• Anesthetic problems with associated obesity
• Positioning may be difficult owing to joint pain and stiffness
• Possible associated metabolic conditions
• Effect of medications on plt function and frequent steroid injections

OVERVIEW

• OA is age-related but not caused by aging
• Early radiographic findings include joint space narrowing, osteophytes, subchondral stenosis
• With progression, osteophytes, subchondral cysts, intra-articular osseous bodies seen
• Subchondral bone collapse is a late finding
• Knees most common joint affected (41%), followed by hands (30%) and hips (19%)
• Risk factors for symptoms are obesity (knees) and severe radiographic findings

ICD-9-CM Code: 715.0 (Generalized)

ETIOLOGY

• Cartilage shows ↑ water with softened cartilage and depletion of keratan sulfate
• Age-related decreases in blood supply, followed by changes in distribution of forces causing damage to cartilage nutrition
• Repetitive use or previous injury may cause subchondral microfractures over time with strain on overlying cartilage
• Autosomal dominant in some with co-segregation of OA with a mutation in type II procollagen gene

USUAL TREATMENT

• Conservative therapy: weight loss, physical therapy to maintain function and mobility, analgesics (aspirin, acetaminophen, NSAIDs), steroid injections
• Surgical replacement

ASSESSMENT POINTS

SYSTEM	EFFECT	ASSESSMENT BY HX	PE	TEST
HEENT	Rare C-spine involvement	Pain	Neck ROM	Usually not needed C-spine x-rays
CV	Age-related changes	Exercise tolerance may be limited by joint changes	HR and tolerance to 2-flight stair climb	ECG CXR
RESP	Nonspecific	Exercise tolerance		CXR
GI	Sensitivity to NSAIDs	Gastric upset		
ENDO	Associated diabetes			Fasting blood sugar
CNS	Age-related changes	TIAs or stroke		
MS	Multiple joint involvement	Joint pain	Joint ROM	
RENAL	Age-related changes			Cr

Key References: Carr AJ: Beyond disability: measuring the social and personal consequences of osteoarthritis (review). Osteoarthritis Cartilage 1999; 7:230–238; Slagbool PE, Heijmans BT, Beekman M, Westendorg RG, Meulenbelt I: Genetics of human aging: the research for genes contributing to human longevity and diseases of the old (review). Ann N Y Acad Sci 2000; 908:50–63.

PERIOPERATIVE IMPLICATIONS

Preoperative Preparation

• Assess joint involvement and ROM
• Question patient regarding nonprescription analgesics
• Consider regional anesthetic techniques
• Evaluate for steroid need

Monitoring

• Routine

Airway

• Assess neck ROM

Induction

• Age-related considerations: elderly patients may have slow circulation times, CV disease, fluctuations in BP

Maintenance

• Position with consideration of other joint involvement

Extubation

• No special considerations

Adjuvants

• Elderly patients may be more sensitive to narcotics

Postoperative Period

• Consider continuous regional technique with local anesthetic and/or narcotic for pain management

ANTICIPATED PROBLEMS/CONCERNS

• Usually neck and airway normal
• Concomitant risk factors—esp obesity
• Often several joints involved with pain and decreased ROM
• Regional anesthesia well suited

OSTEOPOROSIS

David B. Albert, M.D.

RISK

- All elderly patients of European descent considered at risk
- Female > male 3:1
- Postmenopausal female, small frame, low wt
- Risk factors: positive family history, nulliparity, long-term glucocorticoid fracture, long-term anticonvulsant fracture, thyrotoxicosis, hyperparathyroidism, smoking, heavy alcohol use

PERIOPERATIVE RISKS

- Concomitant medical conditions in elderly
- Pneumonia
- Co-existing metabolic or endocrine disorders
- Fractures

WORRY ABOUT

- Positioning because of increased risk of bone fractures
- Vertebral fractures
- Pulm function/restrictive disease, esp if kyphosis present

OVERVIEW

- Imbalance between bone resorption and formation causes loss of bone substance, resulting in bone fractures
- Most common fracture sites: vertebral body, neck of femur, distal radius, proximal humerus, pelvis
- Severe kyphosis common
- Type I (postmenopausal) osteoporosis: women 15–20 years after menopause; vertebral and Colles' fractures most common
- Type II (age-related) osteoporosis: men and women ≥70 y. Hip and vertebral fractures most common. Also pelvis, humerus, femur.
- Biphasic pattern of bone loss
  – Slow phase occurs in both sexes beginning at age 40 y; 0.6–1%/y, cortical and trabecular bone
  – Accelerated phase in women after menopause: 2–3%/y cortical bone; 4–6%/y trabecular bone

ICD-9-CM Code: 733.00

ETIOLOGY

- Insufficient accumulation of bone mass during skeletal growth
- Age-related factors: decreased bone formation at cellular level begins in 4th decade and becomes more severe with age. Age-related ↑ in parathyroid function with age-related ↓ in calcium absorption.
- Menopause: accelerated phase of bone loss is the result of estrogen deficiency
- Sporadic factors: twofold increased risk with cigarettes and high alcohol consumption

TREATMENT

- Calcium and vitamin D; estrogen (newer nonestrogen bone matrix–enhancing drugs); calcitonin; discontinuation of glucocorticoid if due to chronic use; sodium fluoride; surgical stabilization of fractures

ASSESSMENT POINTS

SYSTEM	EFFECT	ASSESSMENT BY HX	PE	TEST
HEENT	Osteoporosis of skull Vertebral fractures	Pain		Skull x-ray Neck x-ray
RESP	Kyphosis	Dyspnea	Dowager's hump	Flow-volume loop ABGs
ENDO	Parathyroid function ↓ in Type I ↑ in Type II Calcium absorption ↓ Metabolic disorders of vitamin D			Ca^{2+}
MS	Back pain Loss of height Spinal deformity Fractures	Acute back pain Remittance and recurrence until chronic	Dowager's hump ↓ Height Multiple fractures	X-ray Vertebral bone density

Key Reference: Riggs BL: Osteoporosis. *In* Wyngaarden JB, Smith LH (eds): Cecil Textbook of Medicine, 18th ed. Philadelphia, WB Saunders, 1988, pp 1510–1515.

PERIOPERATIVE IMPLICATIONS

Preoperative Preparation
- Move and position carefully owing to risk of bone fractures

Monitoring
- Routine
- Consider ABGs if pulm disease or pneumonia present

Airway
- Cervical fractures may require neck stabilization and fiberoptic intubation
- Acromegaly may occur with osteoporosis

Musculoskeletal
- Vertebral collapse may make spinal/epidural anesthesia more difficult

ANTICIPATED PROBLEMS/CONCERNS

- Susceptible to fracture with routine positioning and moving

OTITIS MEDIA

Yvon F. Bryan, M.D.
Toni Anne Washington, M.D.

RISK

- Most common infectious disease in children, after respiratory tract
- By age 3, 80% of children have had at least one episode of otitis media
- 10% develop persistent effusion after 3 mo of initial episode
- Winter months have higher rates

PERIOPERATIVE RISKS

- Peak prevalence 6–36 mo of age; risk of anesthetic complications high in this age group, esp under 1 y of age
- Children may have concurrent URI
- Abnormal eustachian tube function
- Patients may fail antimicrobial therapy
- History of recurrent otitis media with effusion or persistent effusion
- May have upper airway obstruction 2° to adenoids

WORRY ABOUT

- URI
- Large adenoids/tonsils causing airway obstruction

USUAL TREATMENT

- Antibiotics, usually ampicillin and gentamicin (IM/IV) if patient < 1 mo of age
- For older children other medications may be used and be administered PO
- Do not treat with ear drops
- Myringotomy and tubes if persistent effusions, recurrent infection, or in specific cases
- Adenoidectomy may be indicated in selected patients

OVERVIEW

- A common infectious disease treated with antibiotics that usually resolves
- Patients who present for surgery either are young (< 6 mo of age) or have COM with effusion or multiple infections

- Specific indication for surgery (myringotomy) in sick patients or those ventilated who have otitis media

ICD-9-CM Code: 382.9

ETIOLOGY

- Abnormal function of eustachian tube
- Reflux or aspiration of secretions of nasopharyngeal bacteria
- Most common pathogens obtained by needle tympanocentesis were *Streptococcus pneumonia* and *Haemophilus influenzae*
- URI for a few days followed by classic triad of fever, hearing loss, and otalgia

ASSESSMENT POINTS

SYSTEM	EFFECT	ASSESSMENT BY HX	PE	TEST
HEENT	Adenoid hypertrophy Serous effusion	Ear pain, tugging at ear Fever Airway obstruction	Purulent otorrhea Inflamed tympanic membrane	Otoscopy Temperature
RESP	URI	Preceded OM	Auscultation	Pulse oximetry CXR
CNS	Complications of COM if left untreated Depending on extra- or intracranial pathology	Irritability Anorexia		

Key Reference: Oski FA: Principles and Practice of Pediatrics. Philadelphia, JB Lippincott, 1994, pp 974–976.

PERIOPERATIVE IMPLICATIONS

- Patients with CHD or susceptible to MH may require IV placement for sedation to avoid use of inhalational agents

Monitoring
- Pulse oximeter
- Temperature

Airway
- Enlarged adenoids may cause airway obstruction

Maintenance
- Inhalational anesthetic using either sevoflurane or halothane for induction/maintenance in a healthy child and no IV placed

Extubation
- Patients are usually not intubated unless problems occur during procedure

Adjuvants
- May want to administer PO, PR, or intranasal analgesics either preop or intraop for pain relief

Postoperative Concerns
- Minimal, unless pain not relieved or patient in discomfort from being NPO

PROBLEMS/CONCERNS

- If intraop problems occur such as a need to intubate, may need to have a longer period of recovery prior to discharge

PACEMAKERS

Mark F. Trankina, M.D.

RISK

- People within USA: 0.5 million
- >115,000 permanent pacemakers implanted/y

PERIOPERATIVE RISKS

- No proven increase in risk due to pacemaker itself
- Risk related to associated medical problems

WORRY ABOUT

- Perioperative loss of capture due to electromechanical interference (EMI)—underlying rhythm
- Magnet should be placed on generator only if (1) response to magnet is absolutely known in that patient or (2) patient has become hemodynamically unstable owing to pacemaker failure and failure of other measures
- Newer designs (rate-adaptive) may alter rate by perioperative hemodynamic/respiratory manipulations and have very unpredictable responses to magnet placement

OVERVIEW

- While pacemaker is indication of cardiac disease, it can be considered adjunct to successful anesthetic management and not a problem in itself
- Indications (permanent): symptomatic brady-dysrhythmias, asymptomatic Mobitz II or greater, sinus node dysfunction, some types of SVT or VTach, orthotopic heart transplantation, hypertrophic and ?dilated cardiomyopathy, ?long QT syndrome
- Indications (temporary): following cardiac surgery, treatment of drug toxicity resulting in dysrhythmias, certain dysrhythmias complicating MI
- Codes: 1st letter refers to the chamber paced, 2nd to the chamber sensed, and 3rd to response to sensed event. Final 2 letters refer to programmability and antitachycardia (AICD) functions. In 1st position A refers to atrium, V to ventricle; D implies that both atrium and ventricle are paced. For 2nd position the same letters are utilized for chamber or chambers sensed. O indicates that no chamber is sensed. In 3rd position I refers to inhibition, T to triggering, D to double (atrium-triggered, ventricle-inhibited), O to none. A newer class of pacemakers, designated by R (rate-adaptive) in 4th position (i.e., DDDR), is designed to deliver more physiologic response by changing rate in response to exercise.

ICD-9-CM Code: V45.0 (Pacemaker status postsurgical)

ETIOLOGY

- Congenital
- Acquired: CAD, MI, Htn, post cardiac surgery, post evoked potential study, dilated and infiltrative cardiomyopathy, inflammatory, infectious, neoplastic, radiation, neuromuscular, idiopathic, neurally mediated

USUAL TREATMENT

- Possible electrophysiology study
- Permanent pacemaker placement followed by regular telephone evaluations

ASSESSMENT POINTS

SYSTEM	EFFECT	ASSESSMENT BY HX	PE	TEST
CV	Dysrhythmia Pacemaker 50% significant CAD 20% Htn	Pacemaker indication, syncope Review recent phone checks Exercise tolerance, angina, Sx CHF BP control	ECG/pulse 2-flight walk	ECG ?programming; CXR (leads)
ENDO	10% insulin-dependent diabetes			
CNS	Other causes of syncope	TIA, CVA	Bruits	
MS		PNS exam if regional planned		

Code	Indication	Function	Perioperative Management
VVI	Bradycardia without need for preserved AV conduction	Demand ventricular pacing	Magnet utilization may be helpful and converts to asynchronous pacing, usually at 72 bpm
VVIR	Bradycardia without need for preserved AV conduction, chronotropic incompetence	Allows somewhat physiologic response to exercise	Pacemaker may sense perioperative changes (e.g., temp and respiratory rate) as related to exercise, unpredictable response to magnet placement
DDD	Bradycardia when AV synchrony can be preserved	Provides more physiologic response, maintains AV concordance	Unpredictable response to magnet placement
DDDR	Patients requiring physiologic response of heart rate, i.e., chronotropic incompetence	Allows somewhat physiologic response to exercise, maintains AV concordance	Pacemaker may sense perioperative changes (e.g., temp and respiratory rate) as related to exercise, unpredictable response to magnet placement

Key Reference: Trankina MF: Pacemakers and antitachycardia devices: perioperative management. *In* Atlee JH (ed): Complications in Anesthesia. Philadelphia, WB Saunders, 1999, pp. 375–379.

PERIOPERATIVE IMPLICATIONS

Preoperative Preparation

- Magnet available
- Alternate pacing modality (e.g., esophageal, transcutaneous)
- IV chronotropes (isoproterenol, ephedrine)
- Discuss cautery precautions with surgeon
- Regional offers CNS perfusion monitoring
- ?Cardiology consult—probably not needed if patient asymptomatic and recent evaluations of generator OK. Generator programming check always advisable if feasible.

Monitoring

- ECG/pulse relationship, especially during cautery (consider arterial catheter)

Induction

- Succinylcholine may cause pacemaker inhibition with myopotentials in older pacemakers

Maintenance

- Vigilant ECG/pulse monitoring
- Electrocautery, which emits radiofrequency energy, has potential to cause transient or permanent changes in pacemaker function. Most common problem is inhibition of pacemaker. In one study, 21% of patients exposed to electrocautery during surgery had pacemaker reprogram to the backup mode. Grounding plate away from operative site (circuit should not go through generator/leads), bipolar if possible, short bursts, lowest current. X-rays OK, MRI not advisable.
- Magnet: should be applied only if effect known or if pacemaker dysfunction has caused hemodynamic compromise. Once placed, removed only with pacemaker programmer's presence

Extubation

- ECG/pulse, recheck generator status before proceeding

Adjuvants

- K+ rapid fluctuations could affect capture

Postoperative Period

- Programming recheck advisable, especially after cardioversion/defibrillation or if magnet has been placed

ANTICIPATED PROBLEMS/CONCERNS

- Intraoperative reprogramming, loss of pacing capture
- Postop generator failure, loss of pacing capture
- Risks related to associated medical problems

PANCREATITIS, ACUTE

Jeffrey J. Schwartz, M.D.

RISK

• Incidence of 100–200/1 million in larger cities
• No gender/racial predilection

PERIOPERATIVE RISKS

• Most mortality occurs with surgery for complications of acute pancreatitis: 10–40%
• Risk of nonpancreatic surgery probably dependent on severity of attack

WORRY ABOUT

• Severe hypovolemia 2° to sequestration of fluid in retroperitoneal space
• Electrolyte abn, including hypocalcemia, hyperglycemia, acidosis
• Systemic complications such as alcohol withdrawal, ARDS, acute renal failure, DIC, multisystem organ failure, sepsis (see these topics in Diseases section)

OVERVIEW

• Intense inflammatory response caused by release of activated pancreatic enzymes with resultant tissue destruction, fluid and electrolyte loss
• Most commonly a mild self-limited disease diagnosed by abdominal pain radiating to the back, elevated serum amylase, CT imaging
• Occasionally severe with renal, pulm, coagulation, septic complications

ICD-9-CM Code: 577.0

ETIOLOGY

• Many diverse causes
• Most commonly alcohol, gallstones, trauma, CPB, medications, hypertriglyceridemia, infection
• 10% of cases idiopathic

USUAL TREATMENT

• In most cases, nonspecific and supportive only
• Adequate volume replacement and correction of electrolyte abn
• Intensive care of organ system failures
• Parenteral analgesia; meperidine preferred to morphine
• Rarely, judiciously timed surgery to drain abscesses or debride necrotic tissue

ASSESSMENT POINTS

SYSTEM	EFFECT	ASSESSMENT BY HX	PE	TEST
CV	Hypovolemia	Orthostatic dizziness Cold	Lying and sitting BP and HR Hypotension Oliguria	BUN/Cr
RESP	ARDS	Dyspnea Tachypnea	Chest exam may be nonspecific	ABGs CXR
GI	Ileus GI bleed	Nausea, vomiting Hematemesis		
ENDO	Hyperglycemia			Serum glucose
HEME	DIC		Bleeding	PT/PTT, plt FSP, fibrinogen Hct
RENAL	Acute renal failure Hypocalcemia		Tetany	BUN/Cr Serum Ca^{2+}
CNS	Psychosis Encephalopathy		Mental status	

Key Reference: Steinberg W, Tenner S: Medical progress: acute pancreatitis. N Engl J Med 1994; 330:1198–1210.

PERIOPERATIVE IMPLICATIONS

Preoperative Preparation

• Assess and correct volume status, hypocalcemia, hyperglycemia, acidosis

Monitoring

• Consider arterial catheter if need for blood draws or hypovolemia
• Consider CVP or PA catheter for monitoring of volume status

Airway

• Routine

Induction

• Peritoneal irritation frequently leads to ileus and ↑ risk of aspiration
• Anticipate hypovolemia

Maintenance

• CV instability due to massive sequestration of fluid; depending on severity >10 L of isotonic fluid may be required over 24 h

Extubation

• Will likely require postop mechanical ventilation

Adjuvants

• Multiple interaction of protein-bound drugs, esp if patient malnourished or undergoing alcohol withdrawal (see Malnutrition in Diseases section and Alcohol Abuse in Diseases section)

ANTICIPATED PROBLEMS/CONCERNS

• Patients with pancreatitis presenting for abdominal surgery are typically critically ill and require postop intensive care to manage hypovolemia, ARDS, DIC, acute renal failure, sepsis
• Hypoglycemia, hyperglycemia are life-threatening risks after pancreatectomy
• Alcohol withdrawal can be life-threatening
• ECG may show signs of inferior (II, III, aVF) current of injury

PANCREATITIS, CHRONIC

Jeffrey J. Schwartz, M.D.

RISK

- Unknown

PERIOPERATIVE RISKS

- Perioperative mortality directly related to chronic pancreatitis (rare)
- Associated malnutrition may lead to difficulty with wound healing and infection
- Endocrine insufficiency leads to glucose intolerance, but ketosis, coma, and chronic diabetic complications are rare

WORRY ABOUT

- Management of pain and narcotics if patient is addicted owing to chronic administration

OVERVIEW

- A nonlethal condition characterized by fibrosis, inflammation, loss of exocrine pancreatic tissue
- Characterized by severe persistent or episodic abdominal pain
- Malabsorption and diabetes mellitus are consequences of loss of pancreatic tissue
- Endocrine insufficiency occurs later than exocrine insufficiency

ICD-9-CM Code: 577.1

ETIOLOGY

- Most commonly chronic alcohol use leads to proteinaceous plugs in the ducts and atrophy of acinar tissue with fibrosis
- Other causes are pancreatic duct obstruction, cystic fibrosis, protein-calorie malnutrition
- Acute pancreatitis does not lead to chronic pancreatitis
- 30–40% of cases are idiopathic

USUAL TREATMENT

- Strict avoidance of alcohol
- Pancreatic enzyme supplements for exocrine insufficiency
- Insulin for glucose intolerance
- Selected patients may occasionally achieve pain relief with surgery

ASSESSMENT POINTS

SYSTEM	EFFECT	ASSESSMENT BY HX	PE	TEST
GI	Malabsorption	Diarrhea	Orthostatic hypotension	BUN/Cr Albumin
ENDO	Glucose intolerance	Polyuria, polydipsia		Serum glucose

Key Reference: Steer ML, Waxman I, Freedman S: Medical progress: chronic pancreatitis. N Engl J Med 1995; 332(22):1482–1490.

PERIOPERATIVE IMPLICATIONS

Preoperative Preparation
- If patient is receiving chronic narcotics, the usual dose should be given on the day of surgery
- Glucose/insulin management

Monitoring
- Routine

Airway
- Routine

Induction
- Consider full stomach if abdominal pain

Maintenance
- Consideration of narcotic tolerance must be incorporated in plan

Extubation
- Routine

Adjuvants
- Multiple interventions and adjustments needed for protein-bound drugs if patient is malnourished (see Malnutrition in Diseases section)

ANTICIPATED PROBLEMS/CONCERNS

- Difficulty managing pain and narcotics in patients on large doses of narcotics for chronic pain
- Pancreatic endocrine insufficiency may lead to impaired glucose intolerance without chronic sequelae of diabetes mellitus

PARKINSON'S DISEASE (PARALYSIS AGITANS)

Michael D. Sharpe, M.D., F.R.C.P.C.
William Zimmermann, M.D.

RISK

- Prevalence rate: 347/100,000 population >40y
- Gender with higher prevalence: males; 40–60 y (1.4:1)

PERIOPERATIVE RISKS

- Associated with ↑ incidence of arteriosclerosis and obstructive lung disease

WORRY ABOUT

- Increased sensitivity to anesthetic agents
- Laryngospasm/diaphragmatic spasms
- Visual and tactile hallucinations
- Reduced VC leading to pulm complications
- Violent tremors
- Muscle tremors mimicking VFIB
- Postop delirium/psychiatric disturbances
- Side effects of L-dopa therapy

OVERVIEW

- Degenerative disease of extrapyramidal system characterized by bradykinesia, rigidity, tremor
- Dementia in up to 50% of patients
- Symptoms may worsen on emergence from GA
- Classic signs: (1) poverty of movement (bradykinesia), (2) muscular rigidity, (3) resting tremor, (4) postural instability

ICD-9-CM Code: 332.0

ETIOLOGY

- Parkinsonism or Parkinson's disease
  - Unknown
  - Some clusters related to 1927 influenza epidemic

- Secondary parkinsonism
  - Postencephalitis, CO poisoning, manganese poisoning, n-MPTP poisoning, chronic ingestion of dopamine-inhibiting antipsychotic drugs

USUAL TREATMENT

- Levodopa (L-dopa) in combination with α-methylhydrazine (carbidopa) (Sinemet)
- Bromocriptine and lergotrile: provide direct stimulation of dopaminergic receptors; use in combination with Sinemet
- Amantadine: reduces symptoms via presumed anticholinergic and enhanced dopamine effect
- Anticholinergics (benztropine): cholinergic side effects limit use; cholinergic crisis precipitated by acute withdrawal of chronic therapy
- Stereotaxic surgery more commonplace
- Experimental treatment with fetal adrenal implantation

ASSESSMENT POINTS

SYSTEM	EFFECT	ASSESSMENT BY HX	PE	TEST
HEENT	Laryngospasm Cervical/facial muscle rigidity		Mouth opening Neck ROM	
CV	Orthostatic hypotension Hypovolemia Htn Autonomic dysfunction Dysrhythmias	Fainting Sx		BP drop with postural change ECG
RESP	Aspiration pneumonitis Obstructive lung disease	Exercise tolerance, chest tightness, cough	Rales, wheezing Fever Assess cough, ability to take deep breath	CXR O_2 sat PFTs ABGs
	↓ Vital capacity	Difficulty with coughing, deep breathing exercises, resp infection Sx		
GI	Gastroparesis, N/V, dysphagia, poor nutrition	Early satiety		Albumin/transferrin
CNS	Agitation, confusion, depression, dementia Visual/tactile hallucinations			
MS	Impaired joint mobility due to rigidity Violent skeletal muscle tremors	Joint mobility		ROM of joints Tremor severity
RENAL	Urinary retention	Frequency, incontinence, suprapubic pain	Bladder distention	Residual urine volume

Key Reference: Furuya R, Hirai H, Andoh T, Kudoh I, Okumura F: Successful perioperative management of a paitent with Parkinson's disease by enteral levodopa administration under propofol anesthesia. Anesthesiology 1998; 89:261–263.

PERIOPERATIVE IMPLICATIONS

Preoperative Preparation

- Administer anti-Parkinson's therapy up to time of surgery; benefits last 6–12 h
- Avoid phenothiazines, butyrophenones, and metoclopramide—exacerbate extrapyramidal Sx
- Avoid meperidine and selegiline combination
- Assess intravascular volume status
- Preop instruction of deep breathing/incentive spirometry

Monitoring

- Close attention to ECG in presence of arrhythmogenic anti-Parkinson's agents (e.g., L-dopa)

Airway

- Muscle rigidity may impede airway manipulation and impair ventilation
- Increased risk of aspiration

Induction

- Intravascular volume depletion and inadequate response to hypotension (due to ↓ renin release and depletion of noradrenaline stores 2° to L-dopa therapy) make BP and HR fluctuate
- Ketamine may cause exaggerated sympathetic response
- Potential hyperkalemic response to succinylcholine

Maintenance

- Normal response to nondepolarizing muscle relaxants
- Use agents that have rapid recovery

Extubation

- Ensure full recovery of NMB
- Laryngospasm and impaired ventilation 2° to muscle rigidity
- Violent tremors/hallucinations on emergence

Adjuvants

- Avoid indirect-acting sympathomimetics if patient is on deprenyl
- Regional: preferred over GA owing to emergence problems
- N/V and ileus following GA may prevent reinstitution of oral anti-Parkinson's therapy
- Muscle relaxants eliminate rigidity

Postoperative Period

- Close attention to respiratory status (e.g., physiotherapy, incentive spirometry)
- Close attention to CNS state—potential for delirium and other psychotic disturbances
- Begin anti-Parkinson's therapy immediately postop

ANTICIPATED PROBLEMS/CONCERNS

- Skeletal muscle tremor may mimic VFIB on ECG monitor

PAROXYSMAL ATRIAL TACHYCARDIA

Jeffrey R. Balser, M.D., Ph.D.
Michael J. Breslow, M.D.

RISK

- Common in surgical ICU patients
- Incidence in USA population estimated at 1.9%
- No racial prevalence
- Commonly with mitral valve prolapse

PERIOPERATIVE RISKS

- Rapid heart rate impairs LV filling and may adversely affect LV function in patients with LV failure, LV hypertrophy, aortic stenosis, or mitral stenosis

WORRY ABOUT

- Hypotension—esp in patients with systolic or diastolic dysfunction
- Ischemia—patients with CAD
- VFIB—in Wolff-Parkinson-White (WPW) patients who develop AFIB

OVERVIEW

- Paroxysmal atrial tachycardia (PAT), aka paroxysmal supraventricular tachycardia (PSVT), describes supraventricular arrhythmias other than AFIB and atrial flutter
- Usually seen postop in critically ill patients, most commonly after major vascular surgery, pneumonectomy, cardiac procedures; also in patients who develop postop infectious complications
- Causes poorly defined, probably multifactorial, and may include catecholamine excess and pericardial inflammation
- Common types of PAT
  - Re-entrant rhythms: AV nodal re-entrant tachycardia; AV reciprocating tachycardia through accessory pathway
  - Unifocal or ectopic atrial tachycardia
  - Multifocal atrial tachycardia

ICD-9-CM Code: 427.0

ETIOLOGY

- Re-entrant rhythms
  - AV nodal re-entry: re-entrant pathway within AV node. Most common form of PAT; seldom associated with organic heart disease.
  - Accessory pathway mediated: re-entrant rhythm that involves an accessory pathway from atrium to ventricle. In sinus rhythm, the bypass tract may cause a pre-excitation pattern on ECG (WPW syndrome: short P-R interval and δ wave on ECG) or may not be apparent.
- Unifocal atrial tachycardia: arising from a single atrial muscle site other than SA node. Associated with catecholamine excess states (light anesthesia) or digitalis toxicity (triggered activity with 2:1 or 3:1 AV block).
- Multifocal atrial tachycardia: arising from multiple atrial sites, usually seen in patients with pulm disease or CHF

USUAL TREATMENT

- Initial therapy: vagal maneuvers or adenosine to terminate the arrhythmia. Adenosine 6 mg/70 kg IV over 1–3 sec; if unresponsive in 1–2 min (and no hypotension) may administer 12 mg/70 kg. Avoid carotid sinus massage in patients with known carotid artery disease. Adenosine may provoke bronchospasm in patients with reactive airway disease, or excessive (prolonged) bradycardia in patients taking carbamazepine or in denervated heart transplant patients. Adenosine may be ineffective in patients taking methylxanthines (i.e., theophylline).
- The goal of second-line therapy is to achieve ventricular rate control and possible conversion when PAT does not respond, or

rapidly recurs, after adenosine. When LV function is preserved: IV Ca^{2+}-channel blockers (diltiazem or verapamil) or β-blockers are preferred; IV digoxin is much slower in onset and less potent. With LV dysfunction (EF < 0.4): caution is warranted in administering AV nodal blockers due to negative inotropic effects, and digitalis and diltiazem are preferred IV agents.
- When AV nodal block is unsuccessful, electrical cardioversion is considered. If infeasible or unsuccessful, antiarrhythmic agents may also be used. When LV function is preserved, IV options include procainamide and amiodarone. The proarrhythmic potential of these agents makes them less desirable than AV nodal blockade. In patients with poor LV function, IV amiodarone is preferred.
- Patients with accessory pathway re-entrant rhythms who develop AFIB are at risk for VFIB, and this scenario is exacerbated by agents that reduce the accessory bundle refractory period (digoxin, Ca^{2+}-channel blockers, β-blockers, and adenosine). Hence, WPW patients who experience AFIB should not receive AV nodal blockers, and IV procainamide and amiodarone are preferred agents for slowing the rate and to achieve conversion.
- Multifocal and unifocal PAT: Correct underlying abn (hypoxia, lytes). Therapy: Electrical cardioversion and procainamide are not effective. Effective IV agents available for use include AV nodal blockers (Ca^{2+}-channel blockers, β-blockers) and amiodarone. While digoxin slows the ventricular rate, toxicity may provoke automatic atrial tachycardia.

ASSESSMENT POINTS

SYSTEM	EFFECT	ASSESSMENT BY HX	PE	TEST
CV	WPW AV nodal re-entry Symptomatic unifocal atrial tachycardia	Palpitations Diaphoresis	Prominent jugular venous pulsations	ECG Electrophysiologic studies

Key Reference: Guidelines for cardiopulmonary resuscitation and emergency cardiovascular care. Circulation 2000; 102(suppl 8):I-112–I-128.

PERIOPERATIVE IMPLICATIONS

Preoperative Preparation

- If possible, continue Ca^{2+}-channel blockers and β-blockers perioperatively to avoid withdrawal-associated arrhythmias

Monitoring

- Continuous intraoperative ECG monitoring and postop ECG monitoring in high-risk patients

Induction/Maintenance/Extubation

- Avoid tachycardia, light anesthesia, hypoxia, and lyte abn
- Aim for effective postop analgesia
- Consider β-blockers in hyperadrenergic postop patients with adequate cardiac output

Adjuvants

- Limit use of vagolytic agents such as pancuronium and atropine

ANTICIPATED PROBLEMS/CONCERNS

- Transient side effects with adenosine include flushing, dyspnea, and chest pain. Adenosine may provoke hypotension, especially in patients with borderline hemodynamic status.
- Wide complex rhythms: adenosine may be used if the rhythm is confirmed by other means to be supraventricular in origin. The use of adenosine to discriminate VTach from SVT is now discouraged due to vasodilatory side effects (worsened hypotension) in patients with VTach.

PATENT DUCTUS ARTERIOSUS
George A. Gregory, M.D.

RISK
- People within USA: 20,000–30,000/y
- Highest in preterm infants
- Racial predilection: none

PERIOPERATIVE RISKS
- Hemorrhage: <2%
- Hypoxia with collapsing lung for surgery
- Hypotension due to hypovolemia and preop dehydration

WORRY ABOUT
- Hypovolemia due to fluid restriction
- Chronic lung disease
- CHF

OVERVIEW
- PDA primarily occurs in preterm infants
- Present in ~70% of neonates with birth wt <1250 g
- CHF in 10–20% of patients
- Onset 1–10 days of age as lung function improves
- ↑ Pulmonary blood flow—85% of cardiac output may flow through lungs

ICD-9-CM Code: 747.0

ETIOLOGY
- Prematurity
- Prostaglandin
- Inadequate innervation of ductus arteriosus
- Inadequate muscle in ductus arteriosus

USUAL TREATMENT
- Restrict fluid intake to 120 ml/kg/d
- Indomethacin (0.1–0.25 mg/kg) IV q12 h × 3 (modify based on age)
- Mechanical ventilation
- Ligation of ductus arteriosus

ASSESSMENT POINTS

SYSTEM	EFFECT	ASSESSMENT BY HX	PE	TEST
CV	Pulmonary edema	↑ O$_2$ and myocardial ventilation requirement ↑ O$_2$ desaturation	Palmar pulses Hypotension Low diastolic pressure Bounding pulses and precordium	ECHO
RESP	CHF	↑ Myocardial ventilation requirement, worsening oxygenation	Rales; ↓ breath sounds	CXR
GI	Necrotizing enterocolitis	Abdominal distention Poor feeding Blood in stool Free air in peritoneum	Distended tense abdomen Edema of abdominal wall Tender abdomen	Abdominal x-ray
RENAL	Oliguria	↓ UO due to ↓ renal blood flow		Volume of urine
CNS	CNS hemorrhage	↑ Fontanel pressure ↓ Hct	↑ Fontanel size and tension	Head sonogram

Key Reference: Radtke MD: Current therapy of the patent ductus arteriosus. Curr Opin Cardiol 1998; 13:59–65.

PERIOPERATIVE IMPLICATIONS

Preoperative Preparation
- Stabilize ventilation
- Replenish intravascular volume
- Optimize vasopressors

Preinduction/Induction
- Mechanical ventilation
- Consider inducing anesthesia with fentanyl (10–50 μg/kg) or other opioid

Monitoring
- Intra-arterial pressure (continuous)
- SaO$_2$ right arm (preductal); end-tidal CO$_2$; CVP if available
- Airway pressure
- Blood gases, pH

Airway
- Routine

Maintenance
- Support arterial pressure with fluid (Ringer's lactate, 5% albumin or blood) and vasopressors
- Ensure adequacy of blood gases; keep SaO$_2$ 87–92% to reduce risk of retinopathy of prematurity
- Provide adequate anesthesia to prevent Htn

Extubation
- Continue mechanical ventilation postop
- Maintain normal blood gases

Adjuvants
- None

Postoperative Period
- Provide adequate pain relief
- Maintain normal blood gases and pH

ANTICIPATED PROBLEMS/CONCERNS
- Patients may develop necrotizing enterocolitis due to low gut blood flow
- Intracranial hemorrhage may occur if BP increases with ligation of PDA

PEMPHIGUS

James M. Sonner, M.D.
Jeffrey A. Katz, M.D.

RISK

- Incidence in USA: 0.1–0.5/100,000/y for pemphigus vulgaris (the most common form of pemphigus)
- Age: most common from age 30–60 y; can occur in children or elderly
- Most common in people of Mediterranean descent

PERIOPERATIVE RISKS

- Infection
- Electrolyte abn with extensive lesions

WORRY ABOUT

- Pharyngeal blisters, sloughing of mucosa, bleeding produced by airway manipulations
- Consequences of steroid treatment (e.g., Htn, hyperglycemia, gastric or duodenal ulceration, myopathy, infection, psychic disturbances, osteoporosis) or immunosuppressive therapy (bone marrow suppression)

OVERVIEW

- Autoimmune, intraepidermal blistering disease of skin and mucous membranes. Oral lesions most common. Blisters rupture easily, heal slowly, usually do not scar.
- Four types: vulgaris (most common and severe form), vegetans, foliaceus, erythematosus
- 5-y mortality 5–15% for treated pemphigus vulgaris. Most common cause of death is infection, usually with *Staphylococcus aureus*.
- Occasionally co-exists with other autoimmune diseases, thymoma (with or without myasthenia gravis), or malignancies

ICD-9-CM Code: 694.4

ETIOLOGY

- Autoimmune disease in which autoantibodies are produced to cell adhesion molecules (desmosomal glycoproteins) on keratinocytes. More common in patients with certain HLA haplotypes. Immune response leads to acantholysis and blistering.
- Uncommonly, pemphigus is drug induced.
- Rarely, may occur in association with malignancy (paraneoplastic pemphigus)
- Endemic pemphigus foliaceus (South America) possibly caused by an infectious agent

USUAL TREATMENT

- Corticosteroids
- Adjuvant therapy
  – Immunosuppressive agents (e.g., azathioprine, methotrexate, cyclosporine)
  – Oral gold, dapsone, or mycophenolate mofetil occasionally used
  – Plasmapheresis or photopheresis occasionally used to decrease antibody titer in refractory disease

ASSESSMENT POINTS

SYSTEM	EFFECT	ASSESSMENT BY HX	PE	TEST
HEENT	Oral and pharyngeal erosions and blisters	Painful oral lesions ↑ Salivation Painful swallowing	Oral lesions	
CV	Htn (due to steroids)		BP	
RESP	At risk for pneumonia	Fever, cough, sputum	Diminished breath sounds, Dullness to percussion	CXR
GI	Gastric or duodenal ulcer (due to steroids)	Epigastric pain Dark stools		
MS	Myopathy (due to steroids)	Fatigability, weakness		
DERM	Blisters Denuded areas Lyte abn	Blisters	Blisters Denuded or crusted areas of skin	Electrolytes

Key Reference: Korman NJ: New and emerging therapies in the treatment of blistering diseases. Dermatol Clin 2000; 18:127–137.

PERIOPERATIVE IMPLICATIONS

Preoperative Preparation

- Patients may require supplemental steroids
- Avoid tape on skin—it can generate new lesions
- Secure IV with loose cloth bandage or suture

Monitoring

- Consider monitors that do not adhere to skin. Consider removing adhesive from ECG pads and oximeter probes and securing with loose bandage. Place soft padding (e.g., Webril) under BP cuff.

Airway

- Patients may have oral erosions or blisters; new blisters may form from airway management. Risk is of airway obstruction or bleeding. Consider lubricating mask and laryngoscope blade to decrease friction, using small ET tube; minimal cuff inflation; and suture or hold tube in place. Avoid LMA owing to unquantified risk of pharyngeal trauma.

Preinduction/Induction

- Lubricate eyes—do not tape
- Allow patient to position self on well-padded OR table, to decrease risk of blister formation with positioning. Ensure all pressure points are padded once patient is on table.

Maintenance

- Neither general nor regional anesthesia clearly superior
- Local infiltration probably contraindicated owing to risk of blister formation

Extubation

- Minimize coughing during extubation

Postoperative Period

- New lesions of skin or mucous membranes may appear

Adjuvants

- Depends on agents and effects of agents used for chronic treatment
- Consider need for steroid supplementation

ANTICIPATED PROBLEMS/CONCERNS

- Minor frictional trauma to skin or mucosa may generate new lesions. Airway must be instrumented gently and tape avoided anywhere on the skin.
- Patients are at risk of infection and lyte abnormalities from pemphigus and of side effects of steroid and immunosuppressive therapy

PERICARDIAL EFFUSION

Bruce D. Spiess, M.D.

RISK

- Occurs rarely
- Postop open heart or PTCA: blood/serous
- Infection: viral, bacterial, fungal
- Neoplastic: lymphoma, leukemia
- Post acute MI (especially transmural)
- Gender predominance: male > female

PERIOPERATIVE RISKS

- If unknown, tamponade causing CV collapse possible with low probability of determining cause ante mortem
- If known, risk of CV collapse, especially with induction and institution of positive pressure ventilation

WORRY ABOUT

- Hypovolemia
- Limited filling of cardiac chambers

OVERVIEW

- Found in sac surrounding heart; if severe can restrict filling of heart
- Ventricular filling is depressed in both RV and LV
- Fluid bolus and inotropes do little to improve cardiac output
- Must have surgical drainage for proper treatment

ICD-9-CM Code: 423.9

ETIOLOGY

- Postsurgical and catheterization procedures
- During or after viral, bacterial, or fungal infection
- Postinflammatory process: acute transmural, SLE, rheumatoid arthritis
- Neoplastic

USUAL TREATMENT

- Drainage either percutaneous or open

ASSESSMENT POINTS

SYSTEM	EFFECTS	ASSESSMENT BY HX	PE	TEST
CV	Tamponade limiting CO Hypotension		Neck veins HR BP	Equalization of all pressures in heart ECG
	Arrhythmias			
RESP	↓ CO on institution of IPPB (mechanical ventilation)	Change in BP on institution of mechanical ventilation		Pulmonary artery, right atrial, left atrial pressures
METAB	Metabolic acidosis			ABGs

Key Reference: Sagrista-Sauleda J, Merce J, Permanyer-Miralda G, Soler-Soler J: Clinical clues to the causes of large pericardial effusions. Am J Med 2000; 109:95–101.

PERIOPERATIVE IMPLICATIONS

Preoperative Preparation

- Appropriate monitoring before induction
- Preoxygenation—not always effective
- Support hemodynamics-catecholamines, acid-base balance—keep "full and fast"
- Consider draining transthoracically if hemodynamic compromise severe
- Consider prep and drape prior to induction with surgeon ready
- Positive pressure ventilation may significantly worsen hypotension, resulting in shock and death
- Consider placing external defibrillator patches prior to anesthetic induction

Monitoring

- Arterial line indicated as BP may change suddenly; sampling of Hct for bleeding and acid-base status in low cardiac output state is useful
- Consider PA catheter—useful in making diagnosis and following surgical treatment. If pressures not relieved on surgical drainage, question original diagnosis.
- TEE—useful but less so than PA monitoring

Induction/Maintenance

- Do not decrease preload
- Avoid moderate to full dose barbiturates or propofol
- Monitor hemodynamics and use anesthetic, if tolerated, or etomidate
- Ketamine and pancuronium have been advocated for new tamponade situations
- Initiation of positive pressure ventilation may cause severe CV compromise due to ↓ filling of RV and LV

Subject Approach

- Post open heart surgery hemorrhage—reopening sternum to explore for sites of hemorrhage—usually relieved by first few sutures released
- Infections/neoplasia—subxyphoid pericardial window
- Small incision—open pericardium under direct vision; chest tube placed behind heart

Adjuvants

- Depends upon etiology

Extubation

- Consider awake extubation or postop mechanical ventilation, depending on etiology

ANTICIPATED PROBLEMS/CONCERNS

- Many different causes, all with different sequelae
- Hypotension on induction of anesthesia or positive pressure ventilation

PERICARDITIS, CONSTRICTIVE
Stephen N. Harris, M.D.

RISK

- 1/1000 people hospitalized have diagnosis of acute pericarditis (27,000/y in USA)
- Chronic constrictive pericarditis is a rare sequela of acute pericarditis (found in 2–6% of autopsies)
- Males > females
- Mean age at operation: 30–35 y with symptoms present for ≤ 2 y

PERIOPERATIVE RISKS

- 12–15% operative mortality; may be as high as 25% when due to hemothorax after CABG
- Hypotension from loss of preload during induction or intraoperative blood loss
- High incidence of arrhythmias during dissection

WORRY ABOUT

- For noncardiac surgery, extremely heart rate and preload dependent
- During pericardiectomy, arrhythmias and low-output syndrome following operation

OVERVIEW

- Occurs after initial episode of acute pericarditis with subsequent fibrin deposition leading to a pericardial effusion, which may be subclinical
- Large fibrotic thickened pericardium symmetrically encases and affects all four chambers to restrict diastolic filling with eventual equilibration of diastolic pressures and PCWP. Calcium contributes to stiffening.
- Early diastolic filling owing to rapid ↑ CVP. Late diastolic filling halted owing to ↑ intraventricular pressures. Prominent "y descent" on CVP.
- Intrathoracic pressures not transmitted to pericardial space and intracardiac chambers: venous and right-sided pressure ↑ during inspiration
- Severe cases—CVP ↑ with respiration (Kussmaul's). Systolic function depressed owing to myocardial atrophy, fibrosis, and compression of superficial coronary arteries.
- Approach for pericardiectomy through median sternotomy or left thoracotomy

- Differential diagnosis—suspect in patients with JVD, unexplained cardiomegaly, hepatomegaly, systemic edema, and ascites

ICD-9-CM Code: 423.2

ETIOLOGY

- Unknown; usually occurs after subclinical viral pericarditis
- In undeveloped countries, 25–50% of cases due to tuberculosis
- Can be a late result of mediastinal irradiation, chronic renal failure, RA, and SLE. Increasing in frequency owing to hemopericardium and after acute MI.

USUAL TREATMENT

- Early—diet and diuretics
- Late—with increasing symptoms, pericardiectomy

ASSESSMENT POINTS

SYSTEM	EFFECT	ASSESSMENT BY HX	PE	TEST
HEENT	May mimic SVC obstruction		↑ JVD, rapidly collapsing negative wave of diastolic "y descent"	
CV	Impaired ventricular filling	Cardiac cachexia	Diastolic pericardial knock, widened aortic and pulmonic heart sounds	ECHO; right and left heart catheterization
RESP	Pleural effusions, pulmonary venous congestion, left atrial enlargement	SOB	↓ Breath sounds, rales	CXR
GI	Hepatomegaly due to ↑ CVP Chronic passive congestion of liver		Pulsatile liver, ascites	↓ Albumin, ↑ globulin, ↑ conjugated and unconjugated bilirubin
HEME		Malaise		Normochromic and normocytic anemia
RENAL	↑ Venous pressure within kidney			Albuminuria and proteinuria consistent with nephrotic syndrome
MS	Venous congestion	Upper extremity wasting, gradual swelling of lower extremities	May be markedly edematous in severe cases	

Key Reference: Braunwald E (ed): Heart Disease: A Textbook of Cardiovascular Medicine, 4th ed. Philadelphia, WB Saunders, 1992, pp 1482–1489.

PERIOPERATIVE IMPLICATIONS

Preoperative Preparation
- Rehydrate to optimize filling pressures

Monitoring
- 2-lead ECG; consider arterial and CVP or PA catheters
- Consider transesophageal ECHO

Airway
- Significant venous congestion may make visualization difficult

Preinduction
- Avoid drugs and techniques that may cause bradycardia and ↓ venous return

Maintenance
- No specific agent or technique superior
- During excision of pericardium, arrhythmias and fluctuations in blood pressure common

Extubation
- Keep full; avoid anticholinesterase bradycardia

Postoperative Period
- Monitor for signs of myocardial depression due to epicardial myocardial stripping

ANTICIPATED PROBLEMS/CONCERNS

- Postop low-output syndrome seen in 14–28% of patients
- In-hospital mortality associated with preoperative NYHA class 3 or 4; severity of pericardial constriction and elevated RVEDP

PERIPHERAL VASCULAR DISEASE — Jacqueline M. Leung, M.D., M.P.H.

RISK

- 10–15% of those > age 50 y
- Long-term mortality increased 2–3 × in those with "overt" CAD, large vessel arterial disease, diabetes mellitus
- 5-y mortality rate 30–40%

PERIOPERATIVE RISKS

- High prevalence of co-existing CAD and carotid artery disease
- Presence of CAD increases operative mortality
- Pulmonary and renal insufficiency can cause prolonged recovery or morbidity

WORRY ABOUT

- Aortic clamping: may induce myocardial ischemia or ventricular failure; hypotension with declamping
- ↑ Risk of perioperative myocardial ischemia and cardiac complications
- Postop thrombosis in arterial grafts
- Postop delirium, esp if > 70 y or hypoxemic

OVERVIEW

- Vascular abnormalities involving extremities increase in frequency with age
- Co-existing diseases common (diabetes mellitus, COPD resulting from smoking, Htn, CAD)

ICD-9-CM Code: 443.9

ETIOLOGY

- Chronic arterial occlusive disease
- Less common: Takayasu's syndrome and thromboangiitis obliterans

USUAL TREATMENT

- Reconstitute pulsatile blood flow to distal vascular tree to allow healing of ulcerated or gangrenous tissue, relieve ischemic rest pain with the goal of salvaging a functional limb
- Most common surgical procedures are aortofemoral bypass, femoropopliteal bypass, femorotibial bypass
- Angiogenesis gene therapy now being combined with percutaneous angioplasty techniques in experimental protocols

ASSESSMENT POINTS

SYSTEM	EFFECT	ASSESSMENT BY HX	PE	TEST
CV	Htn Coronary artery stenoses MI	Usually asymptomatic Angina, may be asymptomatic	Normal if treated S_3 and/or S_4 Cardiomegaly	Vital signs ECG Exercise ECG Treadmill Pharmacologic stress test Coronary angiography
	Ventricular dysfunction	Exercise intolerance Sx of heart failure		ECHO Radionuclide studies
PERIPHERAL VASC EXAM	Occlusive lesions Abdominal aortic aneurysm may co-exist	Claudication Abdominal pain, may be asymptomatic	↓ Pulses Pulsatile abdominal mass	Angio Aortogram MRI
RESP	COPD (many are smokers)	DOE	↓ Breath sounds Prolonged expiration Wheezes	ABGs PFTs
ENDO	Diabetes mellitus and associated effects such as angiopathy, peripheral and autonomic neuropathy, nephropathy	Attention to CV, PNS for autonomic nervous system and other evaluation	Obesity (in DM type II) Cardiomegaly Foot ulcers	Fasting blood sugar
CNS	Ischemic CNS disease	Scotoma CNS and mental status evaluation Absence spells	CNS exam Search for carotid bruits	Doppler or angio (if indicated)

Key Reference: Leung J: Monitoring of patients during vascular surgery. Anesthesiol Clin North Am 1995; 13:67–81.

PERIOPERATIVE IMPLICATIONS

Preoperative Preparation

- Attention to and stabilization of concomitant medical conditions such as CAD, COPD, diabetes mellitus
- Identification of high-risk patients who may benefit from coronary angioplasty or CABG surgery prior to peripheral vascular operations
- Consider perioperative β-blockade to decrease myocardial ischemia

Monitoring

- ST trending if available
- In aortic surgery, consider placement of CVP or PA catheters or TEE for monitoring preload

- Use of transesophageal ECHO may elucidate the mechanism(s) of declamping hypotension (hypovolemia vs. ventricular dysfunction) and regional ventricular function (myocardial ischemia)

Airway

- None

Preinduction/Induction

- Prevent tachycardia (use of short-acting β-blockers desirable) and treat BP changes aggressively
- Epidural anesthesia combined with epidural analgesia shown to decrease incidence of reoperation and arterial thrombosis of graft as compared with GA

Maintenance

- See above

Extubation

- Same hemodynamic concerns as in induction
- Use of postop epidural analgesia decreases likelihood of arterial graft thrombosis

Adjuvants

- β-blockers and other antihypertensives useful in hyperdynamic situations
- Prophylactic nitroglycerin and Ca^{2+}-channel blockers to treat myocardial ischemia not conclusively proven efficacious

ANTICIPATED PROBLEMS/CONCERNS

- Perioperative myocardial ischemia and cardiac complications, thromboembolic events of grafts, CHF, renal failure

RISK

- Highest for children < age 5 y, adolescents, and adults
- Females > males
- 95–100% of unimmunized infants, children, adults
- Immunization 80% effective
- Mortality highest for infants < age 1 mo

PERIOPERATIVE RISKS

- Pneumonia (22%), seizures (3%), encephalopathy (1%) most common complications
- Erythromycin-treated children less than 6 wk of age at risk for hypertrophic pyloric stenosis

WORRY ABOUT

- Infectivity and contagion
- Hypoxemia and decreased pulmonary reserves
- Altered mucociliary function
- Subglottic swelling

OVERVIEW

- Humans are only known host for *Bordetella pertussis*
- 90% of nonimmune household contacts acquire disease
- 46% of cases found in adolescents and adults, 43% in children < 5 y

- Severe disease with 1.3% case-fatality rate for infants < age 1 mo and 0.3% case-fatality rate each for infants 2–5 mo and 6–11 mo
- Immunization in childhood has decreased but not eliminated incidence
- Acellular vaccines decreasing but not eliminating vaccine-related injuries
- Adolescents and adults display milder symptoms that may be indistinguishable from less serious causes of URI/LRI
- Catarrhal stage mimics less serious URI
- Paroxysmal stage associated with cough, cyanosis, apnea, vomiting, seizures
- Convalescent stage marked by persistent or episodic cough
- Infection of upper respiratory tree often accompanied by more severe symptoms (pneumonia, seizures) from gram-negative bacillus (*B. pertussis*)

ICD-9-CM Code: 033.0

ETIOLOGY

- *B. pertussis*, a fastidious, gram-negative, pleomorphic or rod bacillus
- Culture, isolated from nasopharyngeal mucus with Dacron or calcium alginate swab for plating on special medium
- 10–14 day incubation period
- Direct immunofluorescent assay (DFA) has variable sensitivity and low specificity

- Nucleic acid amplification methods hold promise for improving future diagnosis of *B. pertussis* and *Bordetella parapertussis*
- A whooping cough syndrome also caused by *B. parapertussis, Chlamydia trachomatis, Chlamydia pneumoniae, Bordetella bronchiseptica,* and many adenoviruses

TREATMENT

- Hospitalization, with intensive care in severe cases, to support nutrition, control cough, treat hypoxemia, monitor apnea, and treat severe sequelae such as pneumonia, seizures, and encephalopathy
- Erythromycin (40–50 mg/kg/d, orally, qid, for 14 day maximum erythromycin dose 2 g/d) ameliorates catarrhal stage and ↓ bacterial transmission in paroxysmal and convalescent stages
- Azithromycin (10–12 mg/kg/d, orally, in 1 dose) or clarithromycin (15–20 mg/kg/d, orally, in two divided doses, maximum one per day) for 5–7 days is of unproven efficacy
- TMP/SMX (8 mg/kg/d to 40 mg/kg/d, orally, bid) is unproven alternative when erythromycin not tolerated
- Corticosteroids and β_2-agonists have an unclear role in paroxysmal stage
- Transmission control is essential

ASSESSMENT POINTS

SYSTEM	EFFECT	ASSESSMENT BY HX	PE	TEST
HEENT	Upper airway obstruction	Difficulty feeding Difficulty breathing Immunization Hx	Rhinorrhea Lacrimation Conjunctivitis	Nasal culture DFA
CV	High O_2 consumption	Irritability	Tachycardia	ECG
RESP	Cough V/Q mismatch Pneumonia	Apnea, SOB Tachypnea, rales As above	Inspiratory whoop Cyanosis Rales	Culture + DFA Pulse oximetry CXR, ABGs
GI	Pyloric stenosis symptoms Poor oral intake Fatty liver Post-tussive emesis Cough-induced hernias	Treated infant <6 wk of age Dehydration Inability to retain food Inguinal hernias	Palpable pyloric olive Altered turgor Hepatomegaly Wt loss Reducible hernias	Abdominal US, contrast study Weigh on scale LFTs
RENAL		Oliguria		
CNS	Seizures Encephalopathy	Seizure type Immunization Hx Altered neuro status	Seizure type Neuro exam	EEG, CT, MRI LP, glucose

Key Reference: 2000 Red Book, Report of the Committee on Infectious Disease, American Academy of Pediatrics, 2000, pp 435–448.

PERIOPERATIVE IMPLICATIONS

Preoperative Preparation

- Maintain high index of suspicion for disease
- High infectivity requires isolation control precautions
- Uncomplicated disease resolves in 6–10 wk; optimize respiratory function and nutrition prior to surgery
- Postpone elective surgery minimum of 6 wk after resolution of symptoms. Consider D and T immunization 2 wk prior to surgery.
- Emergency surgery benefits must exceed risks
- Use disposable anesthesia circuit system

Monitoring

- Routine monitors
- Arterial catheter in emergency cases

Airway

- Nasal secretions may obstruct upper airway and increase risk of laryngospasm

- Upper and lower airway edema plus secretions ↑ risk of V/Q mismatch and hypoxemia
- Inspissated secretions may cause ETT blockage, contribute to postop pneumonia

Preinduction/Induction

- Consider regional anesthesia whenever possible
- Consider short-term topical nasal decongestant (e.g., xylometazoline) to clear upper airway
- Downsize ETT selection if tracheal intubation unavoidable
- Laryngeal mask airway of undetermined benefit
- Ensure adequate preoxygenation and prehydration
- Avoid respiratory depressant premedication

Maintenance

- Keep warm and hydrated
- Use disposable, humidified anesthesia delivery system
- PEEP as needed only to maintain oxygenation

- Suction ET tube prn, using saline to moisten secretions
- Control ventilation to minimize development of atelectasis

Extubation

- Expand atelectatic lungs prior to extubation
- Moisten and suction thickened secretions
- Bronchodilators as needed

Postoperative Period

- Caudal or epidural analgesia for pain relief
- Apnea monitoring and ICU observation as indicated
- Aggressive pulmonary toilet as tolerated

ANTICIPATED PROBLEMS/CONCERNS

- Risk of transmission of infection to all contacts, including OR personnel
- Development of severe respiratory insufficiency at bronchoalveolar level during perioperative period

PHEOCHROMOCYTOMA

Michael F. Roizen, M.D.

RISK

• People within USA: 0.03–0.04% (~80,000) by autopsy of nonselected individuals; 0.1–1% of individuals with sustained Htn have pheochromocytoma
• Race with highest prevalence: Caucasian

PERIOPERATIVE RISKS

• If emergency (life-threatening trauma, ruptured viscus), use α- and β-blockers and nitroprusside and keep in ICU until most painful time has passed or adrenergic control is attained
• ↑ Risk of hypertensive crisis with bleeding into myocardium, brain, or kidney or ischemia
• Mortality rate of 0–3% even if appropriately prepared for tumor resection and in "good" hands for adrenalectomy—may be higher for undiscovered case undergoing nonadrenal surgery
• 25–50% of those who die in hospitals of pheochromocytoma crisis do so during induction of anesthesia, during stressful perioperative periods, or during labor and delivery
• Associated with cholelithiasis and renal stones

WORRY ABOUT

• Pheochromocytoma (catecholamine excess) crisis with hemorrhage/infarcts in vital organs
• Major goal is to avoid pheochromocytoma crisis; pre- and intraoperative goals of management of extra-adrenal surgery are same as for adrenal surgery. If adrenergic blockade not present prior to surgery, try to delay operation until patient has appropriate degree of α-blocker. Judge appropriate blockade by
 – No BP readings > 165/90 mmHg for 48 h
 – Presence of orthostatic hypotension, but BP on standing should not be < 80/45 mmHg
 – ECG free of ST-T changes
 – Absence of other signs of catecholamine excess, and presence of signs of α-blocker

OVERVIEW

• Tumor of catecholamine-producing tissue (90% in adrenals). Painful (stressful) events cause exaggerated stress response if less than perfectly anesthetized or in daily living. Even small stresses can lead to blood catecholamine levels of 2000–20,000 pg/ml. However, infarction of tumor, with release of products onto retroperitoneal surfaces or pressure causing release of products, can result in blood levels of 200,000–1 million pg/ml—a situation that should be anticipated during tumor resection.
• Endocrinopathy associated with CV disease—tachycardia, CHF, dysrhythmias (AFIB)
• Need α-blocker prior to β-blocker lest vasoconstrictive effects of latter go unopposed, thereby increasing risk of dangerous Htn. β-blocker suggested if persistent arrhythmias or tachycardia not resolving with α-blocker or when aggravated by α-blocker.
• If α-blocker, appropriately, risk of crisis diminished by >90%

ICD-9-CM Code: 194.0

INDICATIONS AND USUAL TREATMENT

• 90% are spontaneously arising and 10% familial (autosomal dominant genetics involving chromosome 7 implicated)
• Associated with MEA IIA (medullary thyroid carcinoma; primary hyperparathyroidism) and IIB (medullary thyroid carcinoma and mucosal neuromas)
• Associated with neurofibromatosis, von Hippel–Lindau disease (retinal and cerebellar hemangioblastoma), ataxia-telangiectasia syndrome, Sturge-Weber syndrome

ASSESSMENT POINTS

SYSTEM	EFFECT	ASSESSMENT BY HX	PE	TEST
HEENT		Nasal stuffiness (from α-adrenergic blockade)		
CV	Htn; dysrhythmias; AFIB, sinus tachycardia, mitral valve prolapse; CHF, myocardial fibril necrosis or myocarditis	SOB, poor exercise tolerance, palpitations, Htn (50% sustained, 40% paroxysmal)	Standard exam + BP q 1 min in stressful environment + orthostatic maneuvers with BP/HR q 1 min	ECG, ECHO (if cardiomyopathy is suspected)
GI	90% of tumors adrenal or abdominal	Wt loss, diarrhea Dehydration	Palpating abdomen can trigger pheo crisis	No different from normal
HEME		Mild polycythemia, thrombocytopenia (2° to ↓ intravascular fluid)		Hgb (↓ polycythemia way to judge volume expansion by α-blocker)
GU	Renal stones from dehydration			
CNS	↑ Catecholamine effects	Headache, tremor, anxiety, ↓ pain threshold, fatigue		
METAB	Associated with hyperparathyroidism	Glucose intolerance from α-adrenergically induced gluconeogenesis and ↓ insulin secretion		Insulin Rx often before Dx made; Ca²⁺

Key References: Roizen MF: Pheochromocytoma. *In* Miller RD (ed): Anesthesia. New York, Churchill Livingstone, 2000, pp 924–927; Witteles RM, Kaplan EL, Roizen MF: Safe and cost-effective preoperative preparation of patients with pheochromocytoma. Anesth Analg 2000; 91:302–304.

PERIOPERATIVE IMPLICATIONS

Preoperative Preparation
• "Prehydrate" liberally over 6–60 days if CV status will tolerate; expand with high salt/fluid diet while increasing α-adrenergic blockade over 7–60 days

Monitoring
• Temp
• Art line placement prior to induction difficult and painful but desired because of variations in BP
• PA catheterization or TEE if CV system severely affected; CVP used in minority of cases

Anesthetic Technique
• No technique/group of agents associated with better outcome; use of droperidol controversial; agents that block reuptake (ketamine) or cause catecholamine release might be avoided

Induction/Maintenance
• Prehydrate liberally if CV status will tolerate
• Gentle induction with nitroprusside infusion plugged into IV line and running slowly
• Dopamine infusion in reserve for ready use
• Painful or stressful events often cause exaggerated response. Caused by release of catecholamines from nerve endings that are "loaded" by the reuptake process.

Postoperative Care
• See Adrenalectomy for Pheochromocytoma in Procedures section
• Postop: if catecholamine-producing tumor removed or if α-adrenergically blocked, do not chase or force high UO with large crystalloid infusions, as patients have tendency to CHF because they have been on endogenous inotrope for many years
• Early mobilization and deep breathing a must but fraught with difficulty owing to disturbed psyche that removal of catecholamines present for a long time often causes

Adjuvants
• Drug interactions possible with chronic antiadrenergic agents such as between verapamil or diltiazem and β-blockers in depressing AV nodal conduction if patient chronically or acutely receiving a β-blocker or decreased clearance of phenytoin, barbiturates, rifampicin, chlorpromazine, and cimetidine

ANTICIPATED PROBLEMS/CONCERNS
• Important to interview family members and perhaps advise them to inform their future anesthesiologists about potential for such familial disease

PHYSIOLOGIC ANEMIA AND THE ANEMIA OF PREMATURITY

Mary A. Keyes, M.D.

RISK

• Occurs in all infants but with variable severity

PERIOPERATIVE RISKS

• Well tolerated by healthy, term infant. In preterm infant, may be associated with episodes of apnea, bradycardia, tachycardia, lactic acidosis.

WORRY ABOUT

• Surgery requiring blood transfusion with physiologic anemia (9–12 wk of age)
• Episodes of apnea/bradycardia that are more severe the lower the hemoglobin in preterm infants

OVERVIEW

• Normal physiologic response to extrauterine life. Nadir at 9th–12th wk and is 9.5 to 11 g/dl.
• In preterm infant, nadir at 4–8 wk and may decrease to 8 g/dl

ICD-9-CM Code: 776.6 (Anemia, prematurity neonatal)

ETIOLOGY

• Hypoxic intrauterine environment ↑ erythropoietin levels. With the sudden rise in arterial O_2 saturation following birth, erythropoietin levels abruptly fall and do not rise for several weeks.
• Survival of neonate's erythrocytes is shorter than that of adult's
• Rapid increase in blood volume that accompanies rapid gain leads to hemodilution

USUAL TREATMENT

• No treatment necessary in term infant
• Preterm infants with episodes of apnea and bradycardia, tachycardia, lactic acidosis may benefit from RBC transfusion
• Trials of recombinant human erythropoietin in preterm infants may prove beneficial

ASSESSMENT POINTS (APPLY TO PRETERM INFANTS ONLY)

SYSTEM	EFFECT	ASSESSMENT BY HX	PE	TEST
CV	Tachycardia	None	Tachycardia	± ECG
RESP	Apnea/bradycardia	No. episodes/d		

Key Reference: O'Brien RT, Pearson HA: Physiologic anemia of the newborn infant. J Pediatr 1971; 79:132–138.

PERIOPERATIVE IMPLICATIONS

Preoperative Preparation
• Timing of elective blood-losing surgery depending on Hgb levels

Monitoring
• Routine

Airway
• None

Preinduction/Induction
• Routine

Extubation
• If apnea and bradycardia, extubation may be delayed until any drugs given during anesthesia are eliminated

Adjuvants
• Spinal anesthesia, when appropriate, may be beneficial in preterm infant

Postoperative Care
• Consider monitoring preterm infant for apnea and bradycardia for 24 h

ANTICIPATED PROBLEMS/CONCERNS

• Anemia is significant risk factor for postop apnea in preterm infant undergoing surgery and anesthesia

PICKWICKIAN SYNDROME
Susan L. Polk, M.D., M.S.Ed

RISK
- 5–10% of morbidly obese patients
- Usually associated with long-standing obesity

PERIOPERATIVE RISKS
- Much ↑ over that of normal patients
- 40% serious morbidity in intra-abdominal or intrathoracic procedures of >2 h duration

WORRY ABOUT
- Hypoventilation
- Hypercarbia
- Hypoxemia
- Polycythemia, thrombophlebitis, and subsequent pulm embolism
- Pulm Htn
- Hypersomnolence
- Biventricular cardiac failure

OVERVIEW
- Morbidly obese patients who hypoventilate because of sleep apnea and severe restrictive ventilatory disorder and have permanent pulm Htn, acidosis, and polycythemia because of their chronic hypoxemia and CO_2 retention
- Usually associated with systemic Htn and compensatory increased circulating blood volume, leading to right and left ventricular failure

ICD-9-CM Code: 278.8

ETIOLOGY
- Long-standing morbid obesity with sleep apnea, restrictive ventilatory disorder, hypercarbia, hypoxemia

USUAL TREATMENT
- Weight loss
- CPAP
- Uvulopalatopharyngoplasty

ASSESSMENT POINTS
(See under Morbid Obesity in Diseases section)

SYSTEM	EFFECT	ASSESSMENT BY HX	PE	TEST
HEENT	Difficult airway access	Snoring	Poor visualization	X-ray of neck may be helpful
CV	Biventricular failure	Dyspnea, poor exercise tolerance	Venous engorgement, S_3 and S_4, dyspnea	ECG, ECHO, CXR
	CAD	Angina, poor exercise tolerance		ECG, stress ECHO, angio
RESP	Hypoventilation	Dyspnea Sleeping upright Poor exercise tolerance	Rapid shallow breathing, cyanosis	ABGs, Hct, CXR

Key Reference: Suratt PM, Read B: The pickwickian syndrome revisited. New treatment for an old disease. Va Med Q 1996 Fall; 123:256–257.

PERIOPERATIVE IMPLICATIONS
(See also Morbid Obesity in Disease section)

Preoperative Preparation
- Consider pulm function tests with bronchodilator to determine if reversible restrictive component present
- Assess for bronchitis/pneumonia that can be improved with pulm toilet and antibiotic therapy
- Assess myocardial and volume status
- Consider maintaining semi-sitting position to avoid sudden shift of volume to central circulation and pulm edema (obesity sudden death syndrome)

Monitoring
- Frequent ABGs
- Resp volumes and pressures
- Consider PA catheter or transesophageal ECHO to monitor filling volumes and wall motion

Airway
- Awake intubation frequently required
- Shoulders and head elevated on bolster can sometimes facilitate entry to mouth

Induction
- Do not expect to ventilate patient adequately by mask. Establish airway first.

Maintenance
- May have to remain in reverse Trendelenburg position to allow adequate ventilation

Extubation
- In sitting position without residual sedation
- Ensure adequate volumes and preop levels of CO_2 retention

Adjuvants
- Regional anesthesia only if patient is able to maintain ventilation
- Residual sedation or narcosis may preclude early extubation

Postoperative Period
- Consider prophylaxis for thromboembolism—early stir-up and ambulation may minimize pulm and thromboembolic complications
- May be extremely sensitive to resp depressant effects of sedatives and narcotics

ANTICIPATED PROBLEMS/CONCERNS
- All those associated with morbid obesity apply to pickwickian patients
- Early stir-up and ambulation may minimize pulm and thromboembolic complications.
- Preparation of patient for possible prolonged postop mechanical ventilation, especially after upper abdominal procedures

PIERRE ROBIN SYNDROME
Charles B. Cauldwell, M.D., Ph.D.

- 1/8500 live births
- No known sex or race predilection

PERIOPERATIVE RISKS

- Associated congenital anomalies, e.g., cardiac

WORRY ABOUT

- PA Htn, cor pulmonale, or pulmonary edema secondary to chronic airway obstruction
- Acute resp failure due to exhaustion or aspiration
- Cachexia due to feeding difficulties

OVERVIEW

- An anomaly consisting of micrognathia and glossoptosis, often associated with cleft palate, leading to varying degrees of airway obstruction and feeding difficulties
- Airway obstruction can lead to hypoxia, brain damage, or CHF
- Feeding problems may cause aspiration or malnutrition
- Obstruction often improves by several months of age, secondary to mandibular growth, if hypoxia and malnutrition are avoided

ICD-9-CM Code: 756.0

ETIOLOGY

- Congenital, found either as isolated syndrome or as part of multiple defect syndromes

USUAL TREATMENT

- Prone positioning, lavage feeding
- Nasopharyngeal or oral airway, for short-term treatment
- Glossopexy or tracheotomy, if surgery necessary

ASSESSMENT POINTS

SYSTEM	EFFECT	ASSESSMENT BY HX	PE	TEST
HEENT	Airway obstruction	Sleep pattern		
CV	PA Htn Cor pulmonale			CXR
RESP	Pulm edema Aspiration pneumonitis			CXR
GI	Feeding problems	Failure to thrive	Percentile wt	
CNS	Hypoxia	Seizures Developmental delay		

Key Reference: Jones SE, Derrick GM: Difficult intubation in an infant with Pierre Robin Syndrome and concomitant tongue tie. Paediatr Anaesth 1998; 80:510–511.

PERIOPERATIVE IMPLICATIONS

Preoperative Preparation

- Avoid sedative premedication
- Consider antisialagogue

Monitoring

- Oximeter and precordial stethoscope particularly important

Airway

- May obstruct in supine position while awake or early during inhalation induction
- Consider oral or nasopharyngeal airway
- Intubation may be very difficult
- Consider awake intubation in neonates
- Have fiberoptic bronchoscope and experienced personnel available
- Have surgeon in OR capable of performing tracheotomy when induction begins

Preinduction/Induction

- See Airway

Extubation

- Child must be awake for extubation, may need to be prone to maintain patent airway

Adjuvants

- Do not use muscle relaxants unless absolutely sure patient can be intubated

ANTICIPATED PROBLEMS/CONCERNS

- Airway obstruction during all phases of anesthesia very common

PITUITARY TUMORS

Ira J. Rampil, M.D.

RISK

- People within USA: 7500/y
- Female:male 8:1

PERIOPERATIVE RISKS

- ↑ Risk due to secondary endocrine syndromes from secreting adenomas, e.g., acromegaly, Cushing's syndrome, diabetes mellitus, hyperthyroidism

WORRY ABOUT

- Angina, cardiomyopathy with evidence of CHF, lyte imbalance
- Difficult airway

OVERVIEW

- Symptoms due to hormonal dysregulation or local mass effect
- Microadenomas (secreting)
  – Prolactinoma (↑ PRL)
  – Cushing's disease (↑ ACTH)
  – Acromegaly (↑ GH)
- Macroadenoma (mass lesion)
  – Panhypopituitarism
  – ↑ ICP
  – Bitemporal hemianopsia

ICD-9-CM Code: 253.8

(See also Hypothyroidism in Diseases section)

ETIOLOGY

- Usually a nonmalignant clonal tumor derived from Rathke's pouch
- Incidence ↑ with age, up to 20% by 80 y (most asymptomatic)
- May occur as a component of MEN I, an autosomal dominant trait associated with deletion at q13 locus of chromosome 11

USUAL TREATMENT

- Incidental (asymptomatic) microadenoma: conservative
- Prolactin-secreting microadenoma: bromocriptine or cabergoline (dopaminergic agonists)
- Transsphenoidal resection is viewed as safe, and curative in ~90%

ASSESSMENT POINTS

SYSTEM	EFFECT	ASSESSMENT BY HX	PE	TEST
HEENT	Acromegaly: prognathism, lingular and laryngeal hyperplasia, mandibular enlargement		Mallampati class	Indirect laryngoscopy
CV	Cushing's disease: ↑ BP Acromegaly: ↑ BP, cardiomyopathy	Exercise tolerance	Volume status, BP	ECG (± stress test) ECHO
RESP		Sleep apnea		Usually not needed
ENDO	Acromegaly: diabetes mellitus Cushing's disease: hyperglycemia Prolactinoma: infertility, amenorrhea, galactorrhea, impotence (male) Macroadenoma (usually due to a glycoprotein-secreting adenoma leading to panhypopituitarism by compression/atrophy)		Truncal obesity, striae, moon facies	Serum cortisol; petrosal venous sampling of corticotropin; dexamethasone suppression test Serum GH and glucose suppression Serum prolactin, glycoprotein, TSH
CNS	Suprasellar compression of optic chiasm	Visual field cuts		Formal visual field testing
MS	Acromegaly: hypertrophy of facial bones and airway tissue Cushing's disease: osteoporosis, truncal obesity, skin fragility		Weakness	

Key Reference: Razis PA: Anesthesia for surgery of pituitary tumors. Int Anesthesiol Clin 1997; 35:23–34.

PERIOPERATIVE IMPLICATIONS

Preoperative Preparation

- Replacement therapy for panhypopituitarism

Monitoring

- Invasive arterial pressure monitoring usually required if intercurrent disease
- Continuous end-tidal CO_2 and N_2 to detect venous air embolism
- Consider CVP in severe acromegaly

Airway

- Have variety of laryngoscope blades and small ET tubes available
- Consider awake, oral fiberoptic intubation if macroglossia is present

Maintenance

- Htn frequently associated with epinephrine infiltration of nasal mucosa and hammering of nasal speculum. Anticipate and pretreat.

Extubation

- Despite pharyngeal packing and suctioning, pharynx and stomach may contain blood and irrigant. Patient should be fully awake and capable of protecting airway to prevent aspiration following extubation.

Postoperative Period

- UO should be followed to detect onset of diabetes insipidus

Adjuvants

- Esmolol and phentolamine (during epinephrine infiltration)

ANTICIPATED PROBLEMS/CONCERNS

- Patients with hypersecretion of ACTH or GH at ↑ risk of myocardial injury if tight hemodynamic control not maintained during the transient, intense stimulations associated with transsphenoidal surgery.

PLACENTA PREVIA

Paul W. Shabaz, M.D., Ph.D.
Karen S. Lindeman, M.D.

RISK

- Incidence: 1/345 to 1/53 deliveries
- Highest incidence: multiparous deliveries, repeat C-section, previous placenta previa

PERIOPERATIVE RISKS

- Maternal mortality: <1%
- Fetal mortality: ~20%
- Life-threatening hemorrhage of mother or fetus
- Fetal hypoxia

WORRY ABOUT

- Blood loss, hypovolemia
- Full-stomach considerations due to pregnancy or recent oral intake
- Placenta accreta, increta, and percreta possibly requiring hysterectomy
- Fetal compromise from inadequate intervillous blood flow
- Preterm labor

OVERVIEW

- Placental implantation in advance of fetal presenting part; mode of delivery depends on relationship between placenta and cervical os
- Often presents as painless vaginal bleeding
- Dx confirmed by US or exam of cervical os under "double setup" conditions
- Concomitant tocolytic therapy can alter hemodynamic responses to hemorrhage

ICD-9-CM Code: 641.1

ETIOLOGY

- Unknown

USUAL TREATMENT

- Expectant management
- Delivery by C-section for persistent hemorrhage or when fetus is mature in patient with total placenta previa

ASSESSMENT POINTS

SYSTEM	EFFECT	ASSESSMENT BY HX	PE	TEST
HEENT	Airway edema	Pregnancy	Mallampati class	
CV	Hypovolemia, anemia	Amount of bleeding	Tachycardia, hypotension	Hct
RESP	Reduced FRC	Pregnancy		
GI	Full stomach, decreased lower esophageal sphincter tone	Reflux symptoms		

Key Reference: Mayer DC, Spielman FJ: Antepartum and postpartum hemorrhage. *In* Chestnut DH (ed): Obstetric Anesthesia. St. Louis, Mosby, 1994, pp 699–721.

PERIOPERATIVE IMPLICATIONS

Preoperative Preparation

- Nonparticulate oral antacid premedication
- Assess volume status
- Crossmatch blood and consider transfusion
- Large-gauge IVs (2)
- Consider regional anesthesia if hemodynamically stable

Monitoring

- Routine monitors
- Consider arterial and/or central venous catheter if hemodynamically unstable

Airway

- Airway edema may make intubation more difficult
- Full stomach

Preinduction/Induction

- Preoxygenate with four vital capacity breaths of oxygen
- Consider awake or rapid-sequence induction
- Induction with thiopental or ketamine, depending on hemodynamics, plus succinylcholine

Maintenance

- Low-concentration inhalational agent 0.5–0.75 MAC before delivery
- Use of nitrous oxide before delivery of baby is controversial
- Can use nitrous oxide with IV opioid and consider benzodiazepine after delivery
- Restore intravascular volume

Extubation

- Extubate awake; greatest risk is pulmonary aspiration of gastric contents

Adjuvants

- Oxytocin, methylergonovine, prostaglandin $F_{2\alpha}$ to enhance uterine contraction and decrease bleeding after delivery

Postoperative Period

- None

ANTICIPATED PROBLEMS/CONCERNS

- Blood loss
- Full stomach
- Urgent induction of anesthesia
- Fetal distress

PNEUMOCYSTIS CARINII PNEUMONIA (PCP)

Neal H. Cohen, M.D., M.P.H.

RISK

- Respiratory infection in severely immuno-compromised patients
- Patients with acquired or congenital immunodeficiency syndromes
- Seen in all age groups
- >40% of all opportunistic infections in people with advanced AIDS, if no anti-*Pneumocystis* prophylaxis is provided

PERIOPERATIVE RISKS

- Resp failure necessitating mechanical ventilatory support
- Pneumothorax
- Hemodynamic instability associated with induction of anesthesia, positive pressure ventilation
- Persistent expiratory airflow reduction after resolution of acute infection

WORRY ABOUT

- Progressive respiratory failure
- Pneumothoraces, either spontaneous or associated with positive pressure ventilation
- Persistent pulm function abn after recovery
- Other causes of cough, dyspnea, fevers
- Associated with other opportunistic infections
- Toxicity from treatment, including methemoglobinemia, anemia, leukopenia, and severe skin rashes
- Emerging drug resistance

OVERVIEW

- Indolent disease that can progress to severe respiratory failure
- Associated with spontaneous pneumothoraces
- Extrapulmonary sites of infection rare since institution of aerosolized pentamidine prophylaxis
- Often associated with co-existing infections (tuberculosis, bacterial, viral, fungal) and malignancies (Kaposi's sarcoma, lymphoma) in immunosuppressed patients

ICD-9-CM Code: 136.3

ETIOLOGY

- *Pneumocystis carinii*, previously thought to be parasite, now classified as fungus
- Organisms reside in lungs, usually as latent infection; activated in immunosuppressed host
- High prevalence of antibodies to *Pneumocystis carinii* in nonimmunosuppressed humans, suggesting that most are infected early in life
- Person-to-person transmission has never been documented

USUAL TREATMENT

- TMP-SMX
- Pentamidine
- Primaquine
- Corticosteroids
- Prophylactic therapy with aerosolized pentamidine, oral TMP-SMX, or dapsone
- Supportive respiratory care

ASSESSMENT POINTS

SYSTEM	EFFECT	ASSESSMENT BY HX	PE	TEST
HEENT	Oropharyngeal lesions	Fever, chills, sweats	Circumoral, acral, and mucous membrane lesions	
CV	Intravascular volume deficits Myocardiopathy	Fluid intake, resp rate	Hemodynamic lability Neck veins distended Heart sounds	Orthostatic BP changes
RESP		Cough, usually nonproductive Progressive dyspnea Hemoptysis	Tachypnea Breath sounds Exam often normal	ABGs PFTs Transbronchial biopsy Gallium scan of lung LDH
GI	Hepatopathy Bowel lesions	Often associated with wt loss, other infections causing diarrhea, GI Sx	Hepatospleno-megaly	LFTs
HEME	Anemia, leukopenia Coagulopathy			CBC Clotting studies
RENAL	Nephropathy, oliguria	Oliguria		BUN, Cr
CNS	Encephalitis, meningitis	CNS changes	Abn mental status	

Key Reference: Mansharamani NG, Garland R, Delaney D, Koziel H: Management and outcome patterns for adult Pneumocystis carinii pneumonia, 1985 to 1995: comparison of HIV-associated cases to other immunocompromised states. Chest 2000; 118:704–711.

PERIOPERATIVE IMPLICATIONS

Preoperative Preparation

- Ensure adequacy of oxygenation, ventilation, acid-base balance
- Assess pulm function
- Review CXR for evidence of infiltrates, abscesses, cystic lesions or cavitations, bullae, pneumothorax, effusions

Monitoring

- Confirm presence or absence of methemoglobinemia
- Use pulse oximeter with caution, if metHb present; measure SaO$_2$ by co-oximeter

Airway

- Minimize airway pressures, tidal volume
- Increased airway reactivity

Induction

- Maintain adequate PaO$_2$
- Minimize airway pressures, risk of pneumothorax
- Hypotension associated with myocardial depressants, vasodilators, positive pressure ventilation
- Ensure adequate intravascular volume

Maintenance

- Ensure adequate oxygenation, ventilation
- Minimize airway pressures

Extubation

- May be delayed
- Prolonged ventilatory support often required

Postoperative Period

- Ensure adequate oxygenation, ventilation
- Maintain intravascular volume
- Continue anti-*Pneumocystis* therapy

ANTICIPATED PROBLEMS/CONCERNS

- Deterioration of respiratory status, prolonged respiratory failure
- Pneumothorax; may require surgical repair if tube thoracotomy unsuccessful
- Nosocomial infections
- Difficulty monitoring oxygenation with pulse oximeter, if patient treated with dapsone, primaquine
- Drug resistance

POST TRANSPLANT LYMPHOPROLIFERATIVE DISEASE

Tracy Koogler, M.D.

RISK
- 2% of all allograft organ transplants, with children affected more often
- Patients receiving cyclosporine, tacrolimus, and anti-T lymphocyte monoclonal antibodies (OKT3) have an increased incidence

PERIOPERATIVE RISKS
- Increased risk of obstructed airway or thoracic compression
- Increased risk of organ dysfunction

WORRY ABOUT
- Enlarged tonsils and cervical adenopathy increasing difficulty of airway
- Thoracic adenopathy complicating intubation, ventilation, and cardiac output
- Pulmonary involvement causing decreased oxygenation/ventilation
- Disease causing end-organ dysfunction, esp kidneys, liver
- Immunosuppression causing an increased rate of infection

OVERVIEW
- Can present as a mononucleosis-type picture with fever, pharyngitis, and cervical lymphadenopathy; usually presents early and occurs in younger patients with a more favorable prognosis
- Can present late in older patients as a localized tumor or mass in either the transplant organ or another site, such as lung, kidney, or prostate, with a poorer prognosis
- GI tract is a common location for multifocal distribution, which can lead to perforation and obstruction

ETIOLOGY
- Of all transplants, a 2% risk, greater in pediatric patients who are EBV seronegative at the time of transplant
- B lymphocytes are activated by EBV. These cells rapidly lymphoproliferate 2° to immunosuppression, and genetically change to malignant cells and lymphoid tumors.
- PTLD is thought a defect in the balance between cellular destruction and cellular proliferation

USUAL TREATMENT
- Change immunosuppressives and start antivirals such as acyclovir or ganciclovir.
- Surgery may be necessary to debulk large masses and relieve bowel obstructions
- Chemotherapy for disseminated unresponsive disease

ASSESSMENT POINTS

SYSTEM	EFFECT	ASSESSMENT BY HX	PE	TEST
HEENT	Cervical adenopathy Pharyngitis Enlarged tonsils with pseudomembranous appearance Otitis media Sinusitis Laryngeal edema	Difficulty swallowing Sore throat Headache Facial pain, ear pain Difficulty talking, breathing	Lymphadenopathy Tonsillar enlargement Spotty, erythematous tonsils Otitis media Tenderness over sinuses Drooling, tripod position	CT
RESP	Lung nodules Pleural effusions Hilar and mediastinal adenopathy	SOB Orthopnea	Decreased breath sounds Crackles, egophony	CXR CT
CV	Heart failure	SOB, tires easily Edema	New murmur, crackles Pitting edema	ECHO ECG
GI	Liver dysfunction Bowel obstruction Bowel perforation Tumors anywhere in GI tract	Nausea, vomiting Abdominal pain and discomfort Distention Swelling, tenderness over graft site	Jaundice Abdominal distention Tenderness over graft Rebound tenderness	LFTs Abd x-ray CT US
RENAL	Renal insufficiency or failure	Decreased urine output Swelling	Pitting edema Crackles	BUN, Cr, electrolytes
ID	Mononucleosis syndrome Generalized lymphadenopathy Sepsis	Fatigue, fever	Elevated temperature	
CNS	Brain tumors	Headache Loss of consciousness Seizure	Stupor, coma Seizure	CT, MRI

Key Reference: Nalesnik MA: Posttransplantation lymphoproliferative disorders (PTLD): current perspectives. Semin Thorac Cardiovasc Surg 1996; 8:139–148.

PERIOPERATIVE IMPLICATIONS

Preoperative Preparation
- Difficult airway techniques and consider GE reflux precautions
- Evaluate alternatives to GA if mediastinal mass or airway issues
- Consider stress dose steroids if receiving steroids

Monitoring
- Urine output for renal insufficiency
- Consider ICP monitor as indicated for CNS involvement

Airway
- Bag/mask technique may be difficult to maintain 2° to enlarged tonsils or airway edema or mediastinal masses
- Consider fiberoptic techniques if upper airway masses or edema or mediastinal masses

Preinduction/Induction
- Mediastinal mass can compress aorta and SVC, leading to significant hypotension if supine. Consider sitting induction.
- Consider lower extremity for volume resuscitation if a large mediastinal mass

Maintenance
- Avoid paralytics if a mediastinal mass
- If a mediastinal mass, keep in semi-Fowler's position and turn to lateral or prone position if hemodynamics become compromised

Extubation
- Risk of airway obstruction if manipulated during surgery

Postoperative Period
- Airway edema can become a problem
- Continue stress dose steroids

ANTICIPATE PROBLEMS/CONCERNS
- Airway issues

POSTOPERATIVE ENCEPHALOPATHY, METABOLIC

Steven Roth, M.D.

- Patients undergoing any surgical procedure are at risk. Especially of concern following brain or cardiac surgery, or patients with COPD, renal or hepatic failure, lyte abnormalities.
- No gender predominance

PERIOPERATIVE RISKS

- Aspiration, fluid and lyte imbalances, circulatory failure, hypoxia, insulin use

WORRY ABOUT

- Suspect in any patient who fails to awaken or awakens more slowly than expected following GA
- Evaluate for presence currently or earlier in perioperative period of severe hypotension, hypoxemia, fluid and lyte disorders, renal or liver dysfunction, thyroid abnormalities
- Seizures, ↑ intracranial pressure, persistent coma may result

OVERVIEW

- Altered state of consciousness that becomes apparent in perioperative period
- Patients may fail to awaken after GA for these reasons: (1) anesthetic-induced: narcotics, inhalational anesthetics, benzodiazepines, hypnotics may impair consciousness, (2) brain injury: direct surgical intervention (e.g., occlusion of major intracranial vessel, intracranial hemorrhage, edema) may result in impaired consciousness, or (3) embolization to a major artery may occur (e.g., during or after cardiac surgery)
- Metabolic abnormalities: circulatory failure, hypoxia, insulin use, hepatic and renal insufficiency, lyte abn can result in failure or slowness to awaken. In all cases, Dx should proceed quickly in order to treat underlying cause before severe brain injury results.

ICD-9-CM Code: 348.3 (Encephalopathy)

ETIOLOGY

- Anoxic-ischemic encephalopathy
- Hypercapnic encephalopathy ($PaCO_2$ >70 mmHg)
- Hypoglycemic encephalopathy (glucose ≤30 mg/dl)
- Hyperglycemic coma (glucose ≥450 mg/dl; Osm >319 mOsm/mm³)
- Acute hepatic encephalopathy: liver failure
- Uremic encephalopathy: renal failure
- Lyte imbalance: hypokalemia or hyponatremia, hypercalcemia
- Endocrine abn: thyrotoxicosis, hypothyroidism
- Drug/toxin exposure (search for drug/toxin exposure—drug/toxicology screen)

USUAL TREATMENT

- This depends upon the etiology—see Assessment Points

ASSESSMENT POINTS

ETIOLOGY	EXAMPLES	DIAGNOSIS	TREATMENT
ENDO	Hyperthyroid Hypothyroid	Thyrotoxicosis Myxedema	PTU Thyroid hormone replacement
ANOXIC-ISCHEMIC	Cardiac arrest Prolonged shock Hypoxemia	Obvious from clinical course	Reverse acute event Then, ↓ cerebral edema, maintain BP, ↓ temp??, prevent seizures
HYPERCAPNIC	Narcotic-induced Severe COPD Sleep apnea	↑ Heart rate and BP ↑ End-tidal or arterial PCO_2	Reverse narcotic Mechanical vent to ↓ PCO_2
HYPOGLYCEMIC	Insulin overdose Ethanol ingestion Neonatal (idiopathic)	No IVF or PO ingestion From Hx and alcohol level ↓ Blood glucose	IV glucose (D50)
HYPERGLYCEMIC	Hyperosmolar nonketotic coma Ketoacidosis	Suspect in known diabetic Ketones in blood, urine Acidosis	Insulin, correct acidosis and fluid volume deficit
ION DISTURBANCES	↓ Na^+ ↓ K^+	Serum Na^+ <125 mmol/L, e.g., SIADH Serum K^+ <2.5 mEq/L Severe muscle weakness	Hypertonic saline (caution) NaCl and diuretics K^+ replacement
RENAL	Renal failure		
HEPATIC	Hepatic encephalopathy		

Key Reference: Bozbora A, Coskun H, Erbil Y, Ozbey N, Orham Y: A rare complication of adjustable gastric banding: Wernicke's encephalopathy. Obes Surg 2000; 10:274–275.

PERIOPERATIVE IMPLICATIONS

- Correct ion and fluid disturbances
- Normalize blood glucose
- Optimize organ function (e.g., renal, hepatic)
- Adequate hormone replacement
- Search for drug/toxin exposure (glycine from fluid used for bladder irrigation; sedative/hypnotics; ethanol and its street substitutes such as ethylene)

PRADER-WILLI SYNDROME

Navil F. Sethna, M.B., Ch.B.

RISK

- Incidence 1/25,000 live births
- Gender predominance: none
- Highest prevalence (95%) in USA: Caucasians, persons of European descent

PERIOPERATIVE RISKS

- 65% of infants born prematurely. Initial marked hypotonia and failure to thrive with poor resp effort
- Morbid obesity; frequently develop kyphoscoliosis: resp embarrassment, hypoventilation, arterial desaturation with RV strain and eventually failure
- Risk of gastric content aspiration due to reduced tendency to vomit combined with rumination and obesity
- Potential difficult intubation due to craniofacial abnormalities and limited mouth opening (fish mouth)
- Diabetes mellitus
- Regional anesthesia: avoid technical difficulties due to obesity and lack of cooperation of an awake patient because of behavioral problems associated with mental retardation

WORRY ABOUT

- Difficult intubation and aspiration pneumonitis
- Cardiopulmonary insufficiency

OVERVIEW

- Dx: combined clinical criteria and molecular genetic data
- Clinical features: hypotonia, hypogonadism, obesity, developmental delay, dysmorphic facial features, thermoregulatory disturbance, ↓ sensitivity of skin, hyperphagia, short stature
- Age at Dx: infantile stage of hypotonia followed by childhood obese phase
- Prognosis: morbid obesity leading to death early in adulthood due to cardiopulmonary insufficiency

ICD-9-CM Code: 759.81

ETIOLOGY

- Inheritance: sporadic and autosomal recessive
- Genetic abnormality: 50% have normal chromosomes. A common abnormality is deletion of long arm of chromosome 15 between bands 15q11–15q13. Less commonly, chromosome 15 has balanced translocation, mosaicism, or marker chromosomes containing duplicated segments.

USUAL TREATMENT

- Strict dietary and behavior modification
- Diabetes mellitus type II usually responds to weight control

ASSESSMENT POINTS

SYSTEM	EFFECT	ASSESSMENT BY HX	PE	TEST
HEENT	Facial dysmorphia Poor mask fit Difficult intubation	Obstructive apnea	Small mouth (fish mouth) Micrognathia Short neck, limited cervical and mandibular mobility	
CV	Pulmonary Htn RV hypertrophy and failure Polycythemia	Orthopnea Arrhythmias Myocardial ischemia	Accentuated pulm component of S_2	CXR ECG ECHO Hct
RESP	Restrictive chest wall Hypoventilation	Orthopnea Sleep apnea	Tolerance of supine position	Sleep study
GI	Delayed gastric emptying Regurgitation	Rumination	Partially digested food in mouth	
ENDO	Nonketotic diabetes mellitus Central obesity Temp instability	Hypo-/hyperglycemia Hypo-/hyperthermia		Glucose tolerance test

Key Reference: Sloan TB, Kaye CI: Rumination risk of aspiration of gastric contents in the Prader-Willi syndrome. Anesth Analg 1991; 73:492–495.

PERIOPERATIVE IMPLICATIONS

Preoperative Preparation

- Only a well-supervised patient should be considered NPO

Monitoring

- Temp
- Evaluation of adequacy of oxygenation in presence of advanced obesity
- Right atrial catheter to monitor RV function (in the absence of LV dysfunction) and safety of IV fluid infusion during major surgery

Airway

- Small mouth opening, micrognathia, short neck, poor anesthetic mask fit, difficult intubation

Maintenance

- Maintain normal body temp
- Avoid long-acting hypnosedatives and opioids in presence of obesity-hypoventilation syndrome
- No specific drug or combination recommended in obese patients
- Maintain adequate depth of anesthesia during induction and maintenance to avoid elevation of pulm vascular resistance

Extubation

- Morbidly obese child frequently requires ventilatory support in immediate postop period, especially after major surgical procedure

Postoperative Period

- Pain management is important to avoid pulm complication
- Epidural/peripheral nerve block as adjunct to GA whenever possible to minimize opioid requirement

ANTICIPATED PROBLEMS/CONCERNS

- Facial and airway anomalies
- Uncontrolled nonketotic diabetes
- Hyperthermia/hypothermia
- Cor pulmonale
- Morbid obesity
- Rumination and aspiration pneumonitis

PREECLAMPSIA

Andrew M. Malinow, M.D.

RISK

- 2.5–7% of all pregnancies
- Young, nulliparous, or multiparous with previous preeclampsia/eclampsia Hx
- May be increased with Hx of other microangiopathy (e.g., chronic Htn, diabetes, renal disease)
- Lower socioeconomic status; malnutrition; no prenatal care

PERIOPERATIVE RISKS

- ↑ Risk of fetoplacental or maternal deterioration necessitating (often operative) delivery
- Preeclampsia and eclampsia account for 20% of maternal and perinatal deaths

WORRY ABOUT

- Hypertensive crisis leading to intracerebral bleed or LV failure
- ↑ Interstitial volume leading to edema
- Maternal hypotension producing placental hypoperfusion
- Thrombocytopenia may contraindicate regional anesthetic
- Eclampsia (or seizure in a severely preeclamptic patient) necessitating difficult tracheal intubation

OVERVIEW

- Marked by Htn, proteinuria, edema
- Maternal vasoconstriction: possibly leading to acute cardiorespiratory deterioration
- Proteinuria: sign of deteriorating renal function and widespread endothelial damage
- Edema: ↑ total body water, proteinuria, Htn lead to ↑ interstitial edema and ↓ intravascular volume
- Hematologic: widespread endothelial damage often leads to thrombocytopenia, a poor prognostic sign for fetoplacental well-being
- Epigastric pain an ominous sign of liver subcapsular edema and possible rupture. Delivery should be urgently effected. HELLP (Hemolysis, Elevated Liver enzymes, Low Platelet count) a poor fetoplacental prognostic sign.
- Headache: seizure may be impending

ICD-9-CM Codes: Preeclampsia: 642.4 (Mild), 642.5 (Severe); 642.7 (With preexisting hypertension); 760.0 (Affecting fetus or newborn)

ETIOLOGY

- Acquired disease of unknown etiology
- Imbalance in circulating mediators of vascular tone and response (e.g., thromboxane vs. prostacyclin)
- Pregnant patients who later manifest the disease have been shown to have demonstrated hyperdynamic CV response early in pregnancy compared with patients who do not go on to manifest disease
- Microangiopathy leading to endothelial change, platelet consumption, hemolysis

USUAL TREATMENT

- Prevention with daily low-dose aspirin beginning in 2nd trimester has had limited success
- Delivery becomes cure
- In hospital, therapy includes antihypertensives, seizure prophylaxis and support of maternal perfusion, with magnesium sulfate (therapeutic blood levels = 5–7 mg/dl), and intravascular rehydration
- Analgesia, esp epidural analgesia for labor, reduces catecholamine response to pain, increasing placental perfusion

ASSESSMENT POINTS

SYSTEM	EFFECT	ASSESSMENT BY HX	PE	TEST
HEENT	Edema		Airway exam	
CV	Systemic vasoconstriction ↓ Intravascular volume		Rales JVD BP	ECG CXR ECHO
RESP	Pulm edema	Dyspnea Chest discomfort	Rales/rhonchi Cyanosis	SaO_2 CXR ECHO
GI	Hepatic subcapsular edema	Epigastric pain	Enlarged liver edge	LFT
HEME	Thrombocytopenia	Easy bruising		Plt count
RENAL	↑ Capillary permeability	Wt gain	Nondependent edema	Urinary protein Cr clearance Serum uric acid
CNS	Seizure Intracerebral hemorrhage Cerebral edema	Headache Blurred vision Seizure	Retinal edema CNS exam	CT scan
OB	↓ Placental perfusion		FHR—lack of variability or bradycardia	FHR monitoring Doppler velocimetry

Key Reference: Gambling DR, Writer D: Hypertensive disorders. In Chestnut DH (ed): Obstetric Anesthesia Principles and Practice, 2nd ed. St. Louis, Mosby, 1999, pp 875–920.

PERIOPERATIVE IMPLICATIONS

Antepartum Management

- Optimize maternal perfusion while lowering systemic diastolic BP <110 mmHg
- Ensure therapeutic blood magnesium sulfate level
- Replenish intravascular volume

Monitoring

- Consider art catheter
- Consider CVP or PA catheter for oliguria or pulm edema
- Fetal heart monitoring

Airway

- Often difficult 2° to edema
- Prepare for emergent airway

Preinduction/Induction

- Epidural analgesia/anesthesia induces venodilation. Maintain maternal perfusion with judicious use of intravascular volume (and small increments of intravenous ephedrine, prn).
- Rapid-sequence induction of anesthesia, titrating infusions of intravenous antihypertensive drugs

Maintenance

- Hemorrhage at delivery may lead to dramatic hypotension
- Titrate antihypertensive agents

Extubation

- Extubate awake, control pressor response

Adjuvants

- Magnesium sulfate; IV antihypertensive

drugs (most often hydralazine, labetalol, nitroprusside, or trimetaphan antepartum); rarely (but esp in postpartum) dopamine to increase renal perfusion; finally, other inotropic support if demonstrable LV dysfunction

Postoperative Period

- Risk for developing pulm edema due to previous (appropriate) intravascular hydration
- Effective postcesarean analgesia beneficial in BP control

ANTICIPATED PROBLEMS/CONCERNS

- Maternal Htn causes maternal morbidity/mortality; maternal hypotension causes fetoplacental hypoperfusion
- Eclampsia (seizure in a severely preeclamptic patient) associated with CNS residua

RISK

- Implantation of fetus or blastocyst outside uterus
- Overall incidence, 1/90. More common in nonwhites and in 35–44 y age range than in 15–24 y.

PERIOPERATIVE RISKS

- Second leading cause of maternal mortality (leading cause in 1st trimester), accounting for 14.7% of all maternal deaths; nearly 2 times greater in nonwhites
- 85% of deaths due to hemorrhage, 5% due to infection, 2% due to anesthetic complications
- Highest mortality associated with intra-abdominal and interstitial tubal pregnancies 2° to larger size at time of diagnosis and therefore ↑ blood supply

WORRY ABOUT

- Hemorrhagic shock, ↓ intravascular volume
- Blood availability—may need type-specific or O neg blood
- Full-stomach/aspiration risk
- Consider physiologic changes of pregnancy if diagnosis made late in gestation, esp with intra-abdominal location (see Pregnancy, Intra-abdominal, in Diseases Section)
- If laparoscopic approach, consider effects of CO_2 insufflation, ventilation, and steep Trendelenburg position (see Laparoscopy, Gynecologic, in Procedures section)

OVERVIEW

- Primary concerns with ruptured ectopic are intravascular volume, airway management
- Differential Dx of abd pain: appendicitis, any intra-abdominal infection or process. Dx made by Hx and physical—95% have pelvic pain, 75% amenorrhea, 60–80% uterine bleeding.
- β-hCG—elevated in 100% of ectopics, US to rule out intrauterine pregnancy. Laparoscopy useful in Dx of acute pelvic pain and to rule out ectopic.

ICD-9-CM Code: 633

ETIOLOGY

- Mechanical factors: salpingitis, peritubal adhesions, previous ectopic, prior tubal surgery, multiple prior abortions
- Functional factors: external ovum migration, menstrual reflux, altered tubal motility

USUAL TREATMENT

- Surgical
  - 70% of ectopics diagnosed before rupture; an acutely ruptured ectopic is a surgical emergency
  - Salpingo-oophorectomy—advocated by some if other adnexa appear normal and future pregnancy desired
  - Salpingectomy—most common treatment
  - Salpingostomy used to salvage unruptured tube
  - Laparoscopy—diagnostic and can be used to remove small ectopic; associated with decreased morbidity and hospital stay
- Medical
  - Methotrexate used for unruptured small ectopics. Surgery avoided and possibly increased potential for future fertility
- Combined surgical/medical management—direct injection of methotrexate in fallopian tube
- Expectant management—primarily used for small ectopics following β-hCG
- Prognosis: 40% of patients will never conceive again. Of the 60% who do conceive, 12% will have repeat ectopics and 15–20% will spontaneously abort.

ASSESSMENT POINTS

SYSTEM	EFFECT	ASSESSMENT BY HX	PE	TEST
HEENT		Snoring/difficult airway	Airway exam	
CV	Hypovolemia 2° to hemorrhage	Orthostatic dizziness	Vitals, neck veins, orthostatic vital signs Weak, thready pulse Cold legs and arms of vasoconstriction	
HEME	Blood loss 2° to rupture Hemoperitoneum/vaginal bleeding	Vaginal bleeding Orthostatic dizziness	Orthostatic vital signs	Hct
CNS	Hypoperfusion causing mental status changes and decreased urine production	CNS Hx	CNS exam	BUN/Cr UA

Key Reference: Chestnut DH: Obstetric Anesthesia Principles and Practice. St. Louis, Mosby–Year Book, 1994, pp 259–262.

PERIOPERATIVE MANAGEMENT

Preoperative Preparation
- Assessment of volume status; 2 large-bore IVs
- Blood availability—at least O neg; type-specific preferable
- Consideration of full stomach

Anesthetic Technique
- GA: preferable in unstable patient with ruptured ectopic, if laparoscopy to be used or contraindication to regional
- Regional anesthesia: spinal or epidural T2–T4 level needed; consider in hemodynamically stable patients

Monitoring
- Routine; once ectopic bleeding stopped, fluid resuscitation for replacement only; too zealous replacement can lead to pulm edema

Airway
- If difficult airway, awake fiberoptic; otherwise rapid-sequence

Induction/Maintenance
- If unstable, consider etomidate or ketamine, maintenance with O_2, inhalational, and narcotic with muscle relaxants
  - Choice of drugs less important than anesthetic management

SURGICAL STAGES

Induction
- Possible CV instability 2° to uncorrected hypovolemia, as well as full-stomach/aspiration potential
- Skin incision
  - If laparotomy for rupture, hemoperitoneum and hypotension, and uncontrolled bleeding. Upon opening abdomen, a release of tamponade may result in ↓ BP.
  - Incision—Pfannenstiel or low midline
  - Laparoscopy—infraumbilical and 1–4 suprapubic incisions. Peritoneal insufflation: monitor end-tidal CO_2 and intraperitoneal pressures—should be <18 mmHg. Potential for CO_2 embolus or intra-abdominal injury during introduction of the Veres needle.
- Dissection: minimal to extensive depending on location of ectopic and degree of bleeding

Definitive Surgery
- Salpingectomy, ipsilateral oophorectomy—used for ruptured ectopic hysterectomy; may be necessary if interstitial implantation
- Salpingotomy
  - Technique of fallopian tube conservation
  - Can be performed via laparoscope; used to remove small ectopic <2 cm; preferred technique for unruptured ectopic

- Approximate duration: 1–2 h
- Fluid shifts can be large with ruptured ectopic
- Closure: minimal if laparoscopy; low midline or Pfannenstiel 15–20 min

Extubation
- Awake

Postoperative Period
- Blood loss may be extensive; check Hct
- Pain score: 4–6 laparoscopy, 5–8 laparotomy
- PCA or neuraxial narcotics; local anesthetics if regional ± neuraxial narcotics

ANTICIPATED PROBLEMS/CONCERNS

- CV: instability from massive hemorrhage from ruptured ectopic
- Potential for pulm edema, fluid overload in postop period due to massive crystalloid infusion and subsequent mobilization of third space fluid
- Postop shoulder and chest pain from unabsorbed gas and peritoneal irritation—30%
- Gastric dilation 3%, thrombophlebitis 3%, pulmonary embolism 2%, ureteral injury/stenosis 1% with laparotomy
- Postop infection, abscess

PREGNANCY, INTRA-ABDOMINAL

Richard J. Palahniuk, M.D.

RISK

- 11/100,000 live births in USA
- Higher incidence in African-Americans, Asians, and immigrant populations from Third World countries
- Higher incidence following in vitro fertilization procedures
- Maternal mortality 100× that of intrauterine pregnancy

PERIOPERATIVE RISKS

- Usually misdiagnosed at the time of laparoscopy or exploratory laparotomy
- Exsanguinating hemorrhage possible pre-, intra-, or postoperatively

WORRY ABOUT

- Hemorrhage

OVERVIEW

- Correct diagnosis is made preoperatively in only 10% of cases
- Differential diagnosis includes abruptio placentae, placenta previa, pelvic inflammatory disease, and bowel obstruction
- Patient usually has a normal early pregnancy and presents with midtrimester abdominal pain, nausea and vomiting, weakness, and vaginal bleeding
- Exsanguinating intra-abdominal bleeding can occur at any time
- Cases of twin fetuses, one intrauterine and one extrauterine, have been described

ICD-9-CM Code: 761.4

ETIOLOGY

- Intra-abdominal pregnancy always results from a missed ruptured tubal ectopic pregnancy
- Fertilized ovum may implant anywhere in the peritoneal cavity, including uterine surface, adnexa, and bowel

USUAL TREATMENT

- Volume resuscitation
- Emergency diagnostic laparoscopy or exploratory laparotomy with delivery of the fetus and excision of the placental implantation site

ASSESSMENT POINTS

SYSTEM	EFFECT	ASSESSMENT BY HX	PE	TEST
CV	Hemorrhage	Postural dizziness	Hypovolemia, hypotension	Hct
GI	Bowel obstruction GI bleed if bowel implantation	Nausea/vomiting	GI bleed	Abdominal x-ray, CT, MRI, abdominal ultrasound falsely negative
CNS			Decreased consciousness if massive hemorrhage	

Key Reference: Atrash HK, Friede A, Hogue CJ: Abdominal pregnancy in the United States: frequency and maternal mortality. Obstet Gynecol 1987; 69:333–337.

PERIOPERATIVE IMPLICATIONS

Preoperative Preparation
- Assess volume status
- Fluid/blood resuscitation

Monitoring
- Arterial and central venous lines valuable if diagnosis known

Airway
- Rapid-sequence induction

Induction
- Rapid-sequence using ketamine or etomidate
- Two or three large venous access lines prior to induction

Maintenance
- Ensure vascular stability

Extubation
- May need to delay extubation for postoperative care
- Extubate awake

Adjuvants
- None

Postoperative Period
- May require intensive care if large fluid shifts or perioperative severe hypotension/hypoxia

ANTICIPATED PROBLEMS/CONCERNS

- Hemorrhage

PREGNANCY, MATERNAL PHYSIOLOGY — Ronald P. Chavez, M.D.

RISK

- All pregnant females: ~3.8 million/y in USA deliver children

PERIOPERATIVE RISKS

- Maternal mortality: 1/14,000 live births for women 20–24 y; 1/2000 live births for women >40 y
- Perinatal mortality: 15.9/1000 live births. Higher in socioeconomically deprived and minorities.
- PT/PTT ↓; ↑ incidence of thrombotic complications during first 3–5 days post partum
- Risk of severe hypotension after pharmacologic sympathectomy 2° to dependence on sympathetic nervous system for maintaining hemodynamic stability

WORRY ABOUT

- Risk of aortocaval compression and impairment of uteroplacental perfusion
- Difficult airway due to wt gain, breast and capillary engorgement, swelling of nasal oral pharynx, larynx, trachea
- Hypoxia occurs more quickly owing to ↓ FRC and ↑ O_2 consumption
- ↑ Incidence of gastric reflux, silent regurgitation, active vomiting, aspiration

OVERVIEW

- Every body system affected by pregnancy
- ↑ Risk of hypoxia due to ↓ FRC, ↑ A-a gradient, ↑ O_2 consumption
- Airway management more challenging
- Incidence of failed ET intubation 1:280 vs. 1:2230 in nonpregnant patients
- Risk of aortocaval compression due to gravid uterus, which may result in signs of shock and ↓ uterine blood flow
- Pseudocholinesterase activity ↓, but recovery from succinylcholine usually not prolonged
- Concentrations of plasma proteins (e.g., albumin, α_1-acid glycoprotein) decreased, affecting pharmacokinetics
- ↑ Plt turnover, clotting, fibrinolysis
- Bile concentrates with slowing of gallbladder emptying predisposing to gallstones
- Increased GFR results in glucosuria, ↓ serum creatinine and BUN
- Blood glucose may be elevated 2° to a reduced tissue sensitivity to insulin
- Response to anesthetics different owing to ↓ MAC and ↓ FRC, which results in faster induction and risk of anesthetic overdose
- More rapid onset and longer duration of spinal anesthesia compared with nonpregnant females

ICD-9-CM Code: v22.2 (Pregnancy)

ETIOLOGY

- Fetal and maternal hormone production combined with size of the uterus

USUAL TREATMENT

- Delivery

ASSESSMENT POINTS

SYSTEM	EFFECT	ASSESSMENT BY HX	PE	TEST
HEENT	Capillary engorgement/swelling of nasal and oral pharynx, larynx, trachea	Epistaxis Voice changes Difficult nasal breathing	Exam of airway Temporomandibular distance Mallampati class	
CV	CO, SV, HR, ejection fraction ↑ SVR ↓, 3rd and 4th heart sounds, grade I–II midsystolic murmur		Auscultation of heart, pulse, pulse pressure	ECHO, ECG, PA catheter (all rarely needed)
RESP	Tidal volume ↑, FRC ↓ Minute and alveolar ventilation ↑, diaphragm excursion ↓	Dyspnea		PFTs (rarely needed)
GI	Reduction in tone of lower esophageal high pressure zone ↑ Gastric reflux ↑ Intragastric pressure	Heartburn Sx		
HEME	↑ Hgb, ↑ coag factors (I, VII, VIII, IX, X, XII), ↑ plt turnover, PMN function impaired	↑ Incidence of infection		Hgb, Hct, plt conc
GU	GFR ↑, Cr clearance ↑			

Key Reference: Chestnut DH: Obstetric Anesthesia Principles and Practice, 2nd ed. St. Louis, Mosby–Year Book, 1999, pp 17–42.

PERIOPERATIVE IMPLICATIONS

Preoperative Preparation

- Large-bore IV
- Nonparticulate antacid (e.g., Bicitra) administration within 1 h prior to surgery
- Transport patient in left uterine displacement
- Good oropharynx exam to determine if larynx difficult to visualize
- Preoxygenate if GA

Monitoring

- Routine

Airway

- Consider short-handled blade
- Have plan for management of difficult intubation
- Avoid manipulation of nasal airway

Preinduction/Induction

- If GA, preoxygenate with 100% O_2 high-flow rates, prevent aspiration with cricoid pressure and rapid sequence
- Maintain left uterine displacement
- Maintain normal maternal ventilation and oxygenation (hyperventilation may result in fetal hypoxemia and acidosis)

Maintenance

- If GA, maintain normal maternal ventilation and oxygenation; can use low-dose inhalational agent and nitrous oxide concentration of 50%
- Muscle relaxants titrated to effect

Extubation

- Awake without residual muscle relaxant blockade

ANTICIPATED PROBLEMS/CONCERNS

- Airway more challenging; incidence of failed intubation greater, and obvious anatomic features consistent with difficult intubation may not be present
- CV instability if regional or general anesthesia due to volume shifts (aortocaval compression, blood loss), usually increased cardiac output and HR
- Pain control desirable to maintain uterine perfusion

PREGNANCY-INDUCED HYPERTENSION
Susan K. Palmer, M.D.

RISK

- PIH incidence not known because diagnosis may not be made in hospital discharge summary unless it progresses to preeclampsia (PE)/eclampsia (EC)
- PE may occur in 5% of all pregnancies

PERIOPERATIVE RISKS

- 12.3% of maternal mortality related to Htn in pregnancy
- Progression to PE/EC is unpredictable and may occur up to 7 days postpartum

WORRY ABOUT

- ↓ Intravascular fluid (IVF) volume in patients with interstitial volume overload
- Hyperresponsive to endogenous and exogenous vasopressors
- Decreased uteroplacental perfusion despite ↑ maternal BP
- Edema in larynx and airway

OVERVIEW

- A blood-borne placental factor "activates" maternal vascular endothelium, which then directly affects vascular smooth muscle (VSM) tone/growth, causing Htn; endothelium also regulates the adherence and transmigration of WBCs (inflammation) and stimulates the aggregation of plts (coagulation cascade); endothelium controls access to the interstitium throughout the body (permeability, edema)
- PIH—BP >140/90 *after* 20 wk gestation in previously normotensive patient; BP must show this elevation at least twice >6 h apart and not associated with uterine contraction
- PE—above BP rise, plus evidence of other organ system involvement, e.g., proteinuria, nondependent edema, ↑ liver enzymes, ↓ plt count, CNS dysfunction
- Severe PE—*either* BP >160/110 *or* proteinuria >5 g/24h, *or* evidence of consumptive coagulopathy (DIC), *or* liver swelling/failure (epigastric or RUQ pain), *or* pulmonary edema (desaturation), *or* evidence of CNS edema (severe headache)

- Eclampsia—PIH/PE plus seizure; can occur up to 1 wk postpartum

ICD-9-CM Code: 642.11

See also Eclampsia in Diseases section and Preeclampsia in Diseases section

ETIOLOGY

- Causation unknown, no animal models. Placental factors initiate maternal endothelial malfunction, which causes failure of normal CV adjustments needed for successful pregnancy and normal fetal growth.

USUAL TREATMENT

- Control of BP, maintenance or improvement of uteroplacental perfusion, and prevention of seizures are primary goals
- Epidural analgesia may relieve vasospasm and improve uteroplacental perfusion
- Seizure prophylaxis can be accomplished with $MgSO_4$, benzodiazepine, barbiturate, or phenytoin
- Delivery of fetus and all of placenta usually, *but not always, followed by amelioration of symptoms*

ASSESSMENT POINTS

SYSTEM	EFFECT	ASSESSMENT BY HX	PE	TEST
CV	Vasospasm, ↑ CO (usually)	↓ Exercise tolerance		Consider PA catheter Measure CO, PVR
	↓ IVF	↓ UO	BP	UA, 24-h output BUN, uric acid, Cr
RESP	Swelling	"Hoarse" voice		Airway exam
HEME	↑ Hct, ↑ or ↓ plt ↓ Albumin ↑ BUN, Cr, uric acid			CBC Albumin, BUN, Cr
RENAL	Oliguria Proteinuria			UA, 24-h quantified proteinuria
HEPATIC	↑ Enzymes	RUQ pain, jaundice		Liver enzymes
CNS	Cerebral edema	Anxiety, headache Hyperreflexia (DTR) Optic disc edema		

Key Reference: Roberts J, Redman CWG: Pre-eclampsia: more than pregnancy-induced hypertension. Lancet 1993; 341:1447–1451.

PERIPARTUM IMPLICATIONS

Preoperative Preparation

- PIH can go directly to EC, especially if BP is much higher than nonpregnant baseline. Before delivery, control BP using mostly vasodilators, since large doses of β-blockers raise intrauterine pressure, compromising fetoplacental circulation.
- Rapid-onset regional or general anesthesia may cause severe hypotension due to intravascular fluid deficit

Monitoring

- Consider arterial line for BP management for severe PE or malignantly increasing BP
- Perioperative fluid challenge with plain balanced electrolyte solutions (with or without albumin) should increase renal output and improve fetal status. If no improvement, CVP/PA catheter may identify patients with low (<150% nonpregnant) cardiac output (CO) who need both vasodilation and cardiac contractility improvement.

- Mg^{2+} blood levels or repeated exam of DTRs necessary to prevent overdosage in patients who may develop renal failure during labor

Airway

- Edema may obscure normal structures, making rapid-sequence intubation difficult or impossible
- Mask ventilation may be difficult if face, lips, tongue also swollen
- Awake, surface anesthetized, fiberoptic endotracheal tube placement recommended if airway is swollen or looks difficult. Avoid unopposed α-agonist in nasal spray because of systemic Htn.

Maintenance

- Pregnancy lowers MAC by 30% for all inhalation agents
- All inhalation anesthetics cause uterine relaxation. May require greater than normal oxytocin infusion to contract uterus after delivery.

Extubation

- Extubate only when awake and strong, since half of maternal aspirations occur during emergence

Adjuvants

- Nerve stimulator can be used to monitor Mg^{2+}-potentiated effects of nondepolarizing muscle relaxants

Post Delivery

- Diuresis after delivery
- Still at risk for severe complications and may need intensive care for several days

PRETERM INFANT

David J Steward, M.B., B.S., F.R.C.P.C.

RISK

- < 37 wk gestation 10% of pregnancies in USA
- Very low birth weight (VLBW) (<1500 g) represented 1.4% of births in 1996 in USA, and these infants have over 93% survival rate
- Extremely low birth weight (ELBW) (1000–1500 g) have 85% survival rate
- Micropremie (50–750 g): 50% survival rate

PERIOPERATIVE RISKS

- Inadequate pain management
- Apnea and bradycardia
- Bleeding
- Hypovolemia or hypervolemia
- Cold stress and hypothermia
- Electrolyte disturbances
- Pneumothorax
- Infection and sepsis
- Intracerebral hemorrhage

WORRY ABOUT

- Respiratory status (? RDS or chronic sequelae)
- Volume status and/or presence of anemia
- Maintain body temp, avoid cold stress
- Blood glucose level (too low or too high)
- Serum sodium level (too high or too low)
- Coagulation status: thrombocytopenia, low factors V, VII, VIII
- Bilirubin level; kernicterus prone, esp with acidosis
- Retinopathy of prematurity (ROP)—safely limit inspired O_2
- Care with aseptic technique
- Postoperative apnea after minor surgery

OVERVIEW

- Immature organ systems, but many survive to adulthood
- Feel pain, which if inadequately treated causes adverse physiologic effects and outcomes
- RDS and intracerebral bleeding are major causes of morbidity and mortality in preterm infants. Chronic lung disease may follow RDS.
- Cerebral palsy (CP) is common in preterms, especially those <1500 g, and may be due to prenatal and neonatal factors
- The preterm has an immature immune system and is very prone to sepsis
- Preterms often require surgery; inguinal hernia is very common, some require anesthesia for retinal surgery. More major surgery is required for patent ductus arteriosis (PDA) ligation or necrotizing enterocolitis (NEC).

- In some cases preferable to perform surgery in NICU rather than transport to OR
- Postoperative apnea may occur in the first 24 h after minor surgery, whether general or regional analgesia is used. The incidence is inversely related to the gestational age at birth and the postconceptional age at surgery. Anemia increases the risk.

ICD-9-CM Code: 765.x (Premature infant)

ETIOLOGY

- Multiple risk factors include maternofetal endocrine activity, anatomic uterine factors, local or systemic inflammation, placental hemorrhage

USUAL TREATMENT

- Cared for in a neutral thermal environment
- Adequate calories for growth must be provided, often by parenteral route
- Early surfactant therapy; intensive respiratory care, using IPPV, PEEP, CPAP, as indicated
- Oxygen administration is limited to that required to achieve saturation of 90–95%
- Intracranial/intraventricular hemorrhage (IVH) is common and is the leading cause of morbidity and mortality

ASSESSMENT POINTS

SYSTEM	EFFECT	ASSESSMENT BY HX	PE	TEST
HEENT	Difficult airway Intracranial bleed ROP	Intracranial hemorrhage ROP or retinal examination Airway normal?	Fontanel Airway	Cranial ultrasound MRI or CT Ophthalmology report
RESP	RDS Respiratory failure Pneumonia Pneumothorax	RDS or history of RDS? History of apnea of prematurity Intubated and/or ventilated Pneumonia FIO_2 and SpO_2	Respiratory rate (>60 abnormal) Intercostal retractions Grunting Rales or rhonchi	Chest x-ray Blood gases
CVS	Hypovolemia Hypervolemia PDA CHF	Vital signs chart Weight chart Urine output Inotropes infusing	HR (120–160), murmur Bounding pulses (PDA) BP normal Liver enlarged (CHF) Edema: feet or eyelids	ECG, ECHO CXR
HEME	Anemia Sepsis Coagulopathy	Birth asphyxia (low factors) Vit K given Bleeding	CBC, WBC and differential Platelet count	
METAB	↑ or ↓ glu, ↓ T Hypocalcemia, hypomagnesemia Hyperbilirubinemia Na^+ or K^+ disturbance	Review charts and reports	Twitching Seizures Hypotension	Serum electrolytes, Ca^{2+}, Mg^{2+} Blood glucose, serum bilirubin

Key Reference: Henderson-Smart DJ, Steer P.: Postoperative caffeine for preventing apnea in preterm infants. Cochrane Database Syst Rev 2000, CD000048.

PERIOPERATIVE IMPLICATIONS

Preoperative Preparation

- Correct metabolic status
- Treat coagulopathy (Vit K, FFP, cryo, pH)
- Warm the OR, prepare Bair Hugger, etc.
- Ensure T maintained during transport
- 2-h fast for clear fluids, 4-h fast for breast milk/formula
- Reassess cardiopulmonary and volume status
- Ensure reliable IV line present (use EMLA)
- ICU bed may be used as an OR table

Monitoring

- Precordial or esophageal stethoscope
- Preductal SpO_2 (right upper limb or head), ECG, BP cuff, temperature
- End-tidal CO_2, art line for major procedures
- Make sure all monitors are secure

Airway

- Large tongue, small mouth may lead to difficulty
- Anesthetize prior to intubation to avoid, ↑ICP
- ETT must pass glottis and subglottic region easily and allow audible leak at 20 cm H_2O airway pressure
- Ensure that ETT cannot kink

Induction

- Use low concentrations of sevoflurane (<3%) and monitor BP carefully
- Alternatively, thiopental (1–2 mg/kg) plus fentanyl 5–10 μg/kg followed by relaxant
- In minor surgery: IV caffeine 10 mg/kg will reduce postop apnea

Maintenance

- Low concentrations; control ventilation but avoid hyperventilation
- Bradycardia usually indicates hypoxia

- BP is guide to volume replacement
- Infuse glucose at 4–6 mg/kg/min and monitor blood glucose levels with a glucometer
- Dilute saline solutions can lead to hyponatremia

Extubation

- After major surgery most benefit from continued respiratory support

Postoperative Period

- Ensure that monitoring is continued
- Minor surgery: patients <50 wk postconceptional age and a history of apnea or chronic pulmonary disease should be placed on an apnea monitor and observed for 24 h
- Anemic patients <60 weeks postconceptional age should be monitored as above.

ANTICIPATED PROBLEMS/CONCERNS

- Postoperative apnea
- Hypothermia

PROTEIN C DEFICIENCY

Charles Weissman, M.D.

RISK

• Congenital deficiency: heterozygote ~ 1/200–1/300
• Homozygote is estimated at 1/160,000–1/360,000
• Acquired deficiency also occurs

PERIOPERATIVE RISKS

• Patients with protein C deficiency are at risk for venous thrombosis and pulm embolism (immobility, endothelial damage, and ↓ blood flow during perioperative period may be triggers)

WORRY ABOUT

• Increased incidence of thrombophlebitis and pulm embolism
• Thrombosis of other vessels, such as intracerebral and coronary arteries, can occur

OVERVIEW

• Protein C is a vitamin K–dependent protein found in blood and synthesized in liver
• Inhibits blood coagulation by proteolytic inactivation of factors V and VIII
• Protein S is a cofactor of protein C
• Stimulates fibrinolysis possibly by neutralizing plasminogen activator inhibitors
• Deficiency causes hyperthrombotic state
• Skin necrosis can occur after warfarin therapy begun

ICD-9-CM Code: 286.9 (Coagulation factor deficiency)

ETIOLOGY

• Inherited—autosomal dominant with variable expressivity
• Homozygotes develop life-threatening visceral vessel thrombosis or purpura fulminans (massive cutaneous necrosis) in early neonatal period

• Heterozygotes may develop venous thrombosis and thromboembolism
• Acquired causes: hepatic dysfunction, vitamin K deficiency, DIC

USUAL TREATMENT

• Heterozygotes:
  – If acute thrombosis; start heparinization
  – Long-term anticoagulation with warfarin in patients with Hx of thrombosis. (Heparin therapy continued until warfarin is at therapeutic levels to prevent skin necrosis.)
  – With acute thrombosis may need transfusions of FFP to increase protein C levels
• Homozygotes:
  – Periodic FFP or purified protein C concentrate transfusions to provide protein C
• Acquired:
  – Vitamin K deficiency—parenteral vitamin K
  – DIC—treatment of underlying cause

ASSESSMENT POINTS

SYSTEM	EFFECT	ASSESSMENT BY HX	PE	TEST
HEENT	Retinal vein thrombosis	Hx of vision problems	Ophthalmoscopic examination	
CV	MI Angina Peripheral arterial disease	Hx of MI, angina Peripheral vascular thrombosis	Peripheral pulses	ECG
RESP	Pulm embolism	Hx of previous pulm embolism		
GI	Mesenteric thrombosis	Hx of bowel infarction		
HEME	Thrombophlebitis	Hx of thrombophlebitis, pulm embolism	Exam of veins in legs	
RENAL	Renal vein and artery thrombosis	Hx of renal problems		BUN/Cr Urine protein
DERM	Necrosis	Cutaneous necrosis after warfarin is begun	Cutaneous necrosis	
CNS	Intracerebral artery thrombosis	Hx of CVA, TIA	Neurologic exam	

Key Reference: Nachman RL, Silverstein R: Hypercoagulable states. Ann Intern Med 1993; 119:819–827.

PERIOPERATIVE IMPLICATIONS

Preoperative Preparation

• In homozygotes and symptomatic heterozygotes, FFP can be administered to increase protein C levels
• Warfarin can be stopped a few days before surgery to allow PT to return to normal range and heparin administered until surgery
• Intermittent pneumatic compression stocking can be placed prior to induction of anesthesia

Airway

• Some have suggested that the ET tube cuff not be inflated to prevent tracheal venous thrombosis
• In neonates, there should be an audible leak

Preinduction/Induction

• Regional anesthesia may be preferable, if possible

Maintenance

• Special attention can be paid to positioning to reduce venous and arterial stasis
• FFP should be given to patients with prior thrombotic manifestations and for prolonged operations

Adjuvants

• Intermittent pneumatic compression stockings can be used
• Postop heparinization should be started as soon as deemed safe

ANTICIPATED PROBLEMS/CONCERNS

• Increased risk of thrombosis, esp thrombophlebitis and pulm embolism
• When switching from heparin anticoagulation to warfarin, heparin can be continued until warfarin has achieved therapeutic effect to decrease risk of skin necrosis

PULMONARY ATRESIA

James F. Arens, M.D.

RISK

- 1.5% of normal births
- 0.5% of all congenital heart disease

PERIOPERATIVE RISKS

- RV failure
- Hypoxemia
- Metabolic acidosis
- Deterioration in 1st days of life

WORRY ABOUT

- Progressive metabolic acidosis
- Maintaining a patent ductus arteriosus
- RV hypoplasia: 50% incidence
- Maintaining prostaglandin infusion
- High risk: >50% do not survive 1st year

OVERVIEW

- Associated with other cardiac lesions, e.g., patent foramen ovale, patent ductus arteriosus, possible VSD
- High-risk infant
- Resuscitation—anesthetic technique

ICD-9-CM Code: 424.3

ETIOLOGY

- Congenital

USUAL TREATMENT

- Prostaglandin E$_1$ infusion
- Systemic to pulm shunt
- Infective endocarditis prophylaxis
- Palliative therapy

ASSESSMENT POINTS

SYSTEM	EFFECT	ASSESSMENT BY HX	PE	TEST
CV	RV failure Hypoxemia Metabolic acidosis Patent foramen ovale	SOB	Cyanosis Metabolic acidosis	ECG—right atrial enlargement CXR—left- or right-sided arch CXR— ↓ pulm vascular markings ABGs
RESP	↓ Pulm blood flow	SOB	Tachypnea	ECHO, cardiac catheter
SYSTEMIC	Signs of RV failure			

Key Reference: Kambaun J: Cardiac Anesthesia for Infants and Children. St. Louis, CV Mosby, 1994.

PERIOPERATIVE IMPLICATIONS

Preoperative Diagnosis

- Pulm atresia vs. pulm valve stenosis at cardiac cath; a Rashkind balloon septostomy was likely attempted

Preoperative Considerations

- Palliative surgery initially
- Type of shunt to be performed
- Which systemic artery is to be used for shunt? Don't stick it during CVP attempts.
- May surgically create a VSD
- Degree of hypoxemia, metabolic acidosis
- Right ventricle may be hypoplastic

Monitoring

- Routine
- A-Line
  - Umbilical artery if good trace
  - Radial artery—opposite side of shunt
  - Could clamp (partially) subclavian artery—same implication for pulse oximeter placement
- CVP for resuscitation drugs
- Temp

Airway

- Endotracheal

Preinduction/Induction

- Do not be rushed
- Prostaglandin infusion to keep baby alive (0.03–0.1 μg/kg/min)—patent ductus arteriosus needs to be open, as it may be keeping baby alive
- Intubation—smooth and quick by experienced individual
- Hypoxemia, bradycardia disastrous
- Avoid increased pulm vascular resistance:
  - Coughing, bucking; ↑ PEEP; ↑ CO$_2$; ↓ Po$_2$
  - ↓ Systemic vascular resistance
  - Air in all lines

Maintenance

- Hemodynamically stable anesthetic, e.g., ketamine plus low-dose narcotic or inhalational agent
- Normal heart rate—avoid bradycardia, tachycardia
- Normothermia
- Normal filling volumes
- Normal myocardial contractility
- Aiming for early extubation

Extubation

- As early as reasonably safe

Postoperative Care

- Provided in the area where the most physicians and nurses are thoroughly experienced in pediatric care
- Prostaglandin infusion maintained

ANTICIPATED PROBLEMS/CONCERNS

- Palliative surgery only
- Definitive procedure later, e.g., Fontan, Rastelli
- Hypoxemia progressing—inadequate shunt/ductus closing
- Tachypnea worsening—hypoxemia, laryngeal swelling, pneumothorax (small chest tube easily occluded)

PULMONARY EMBOLISM

Ronald G. Pearl, M.D., Ph.D.

RISK

- People within USA: 600,000/y
- No racial predilection
- Increased incidence in women

PERIOPERATIVE RISKS

- Risk for hypoxemia and right heart failure
- Perioperative mortality of ~90% for acute thromboendarterectomy, of ~10% for chronic thromboendarterectomy
- Postop pulm embolism in up to 1% of surgical patients

WORRY ABOUT

- Recurrent pulm embolism
- Right heart failure and CV collapse
- Hypoxemia
- Hemorrhage in patients on anticoagulants or thrombolytics

OVERVIEW

- Pulm embolism noticed in ~20% of autopsied patients
- Clinical presentation may range from asymptomatic to chest pain and hypoxemia to CV collapse
- Most patients have DVT
- Dx involves a combination of clinical suspicion, ventilation-perfusion lung scan, evaluation of the deep venous system of the legs, helical (spiral) lung CT scan, and pulm angiogram
- Negative D-dimer test excludes Dx in selected patients

ICD-9-CM Code: 415.1

ETIOLOGY

- Acquired disease
- Risk factors present in almost all patients: age >40 y, obesity, malignancy, recent surgery, trauma, pregnancy, immobilization, estrogen use, prior Hx of DVT, hypercoagulable state (factor V Leiden, deficiency of protein C, protein S, or antithrombin III)

USUAL TREATMENT

- Therapy decreases mortality from 35% to <5%
- Heparin (PTT 1.5–2.5 × normal) followed by warfarin sodium (INR 1–2) for most patients; LMWH at least as effective as dose-adjusted continuous intravenous unfractionated heparin
- Thrombolytic therapy for massive pulm embolism
- Vena caval filter if massive pulm embolism or if cannot receive anticoagulants
- Surgical thromboendarterectomy in selected cases

ASSESSMENT POINTS

SYSTEM	EFFECT	ASSESSMENT BY HX	PE	TEST
CV	RV failure	Syncope Dyspnea Palpitations	↑ JVP; RV heave Hypotension Tachycardia Hepatojugular reflux	ECG ECHO
RESP	Pulm infarction V/Q abn Pain from pleural irritation	Hemoptysis Chest pain Shoulder pain	Tachypnea	CXR, SaO$_2$ ABGs Lung V/Q scan Spiral CT scan Pulm angio
CNS	Syncope	Syncope		
MS	Phlebitis	Hx DVT Leg edema, pain	Leg edema Inflammation Palpable cord	Doppler US Impedance plethysmography Venography

Key Reference: Elliot CG, Goldhaber SZ, Visani L, Derosa M: Chest radiographs in acute pulmonary embolism. Results from the International Cooperative Pulmonary Embolism Registry. Chest 2000; 118:33–38.

PERIOPERATIVE IMPLICATIONS

Preoperative Preparation

- Preop Rx with heparin, warfarin, sequential compression devices decreases incidence of perioperative DVT and PE
- If active DVT, consider preop vena caval filter

Monitoring

- Consider PA catheter
- TEE may demonstrate RV dysfunction and PA thromboembolism

Airway

- None

Preinduction/Induction

- May develop hypotension due to RV failure

Maintenance

- Adequate preload essential to RV function

Extubation

- None

Adjuvants

- None

ANTICIPATED PROBLEMS/CONCERNS

- RV failure may be initial presentation of PE or may develop with recurrent PE

PURPURA, IMMUNE THROMBOCYTOPENIC (ITP)

Evan G. Pivalizza, M.B., Ch. B., F.F.A.S.A.

RISK

- Rare
  - Children, M:F 1:1
  - Adults, M:F 2–4:1 (pregnancy 1–2/1000 deliveries)

PERIOPERATIVE RISKS

- Hemorrhage
- Infection and thrombocytosis post splenectomy

WORRY ABOUT

- Preop corticosteroids, immunosuppressives
- Splenectomy
- Hemorrhage (clinically important bleeding rare if plts >10,000; growing surgical comfort with plts <50,000)

OVERVIEW

- Acute, intermittent, or chronic immune-mediated thrombocytopenia (accelerated destruction with appropriate megakaryocyte response) with dermal, mucosal, and CNS hemorrhage (most critical)
- Obstetric implications include risk of transient neonatal thrombocytopenia

ICD-9-CM Code: 287.3

ETIOLOGY

- "Immune" in title (previously "idiopathic") reflects presence of antiplatelet IgG autoantibody (majority plt-associated with some in plasma)
- Postulated action against plt membrane glycoproteins

USUAL TREATMENT

- Corticosteroids: initial therapy (1 mg/kg/d) with 30–60% response rates (up to 80% initially)
- IV immunoglobulin G (0.4–1 g/kg/d)
- Anti-D (if Rh$^+$ patient) cheaper, easier than IV IgG
- Splenectomy: defer as along as possible in children. Increasingly laparoscopic (requires disruption of spleen into bag before extraction to prevent splenosis). In chronic disease, indicated if steroids cannot be tapered or poor response to therapy. In acute disease, failed medical response and platelet transfusion.
- Other: azathioprine, vincristine, danazol
- Platelets: although have shorter survival, can temporarily elevate platelet count

ASSESSMENT POINTS

SYSTEM	EFFECT	ASSESSMENT BY HX	PE	TEST
HEENT	Airway manipulation—potential hemorrhage	Oral bleeding		
CVS	Vascular access			
HEME	Thrombocytopenia	Hemorrhage	Petechiae	Plts <20–80,000 × 10^3/mm^3 (depending on author), megakaryocytes, anti-platelet antibody
CNS	Hemorrhage in acute disease			Radiology if indicated
OB	Controversy predicting neonate at risk (10–15%) and mode of delivery			

Key Reference: Kelton JG, Bussel JB: Idiopathic immune thrombocytopenic purpura: an update. Semin Hematol 2000; 37:219–221.

PERIOPERATIVE IMPLICATIONS

Preoperative Preparation

- Consider preoperative steroids, IV IgG ± anti-D to raise platelet count
- Steroid supplement
- Premedication: avoid IM injections
- Pneumococcal, meningococcal vaccine (+ *Haemophilus* in children)

Monitoring

- Routine
- Protect pressure points and mucosal surfaces

Airway

- Avoid nasal ET intubation
- Careful instrumentation, esp with plt count <50,000 × 10^3/mm^3

Induction

- Avoid hypertensive response to ET intubation, esp with plt count <20,000 × 10^3/mm^3

Maintenance

- Theoretical disadvantage of volatile agents (see also Purpura, Thrombotic Thrombocytopenic [TTP] in Diseases section)

Fluids

- If plt required, transfuse after splenic pedicle ligation. Intraoperative thromboelastography and Sonoclot analysis of plt function may be useful guide to replacement therapy.

Extubation

- As above: care of mucous membranes and hemodynamic response

Adjuvants

- Individual analysis of risk-benefit for neuraxial technique, esp in parturient patient (report of thromboelastography and Sonoclot use in addition to BT in decision-making). If time, consider steroids, IV IgG ± anti-D to raise plt count.

Postoperative Period

- Risks of thrombocytosis not as crucial as in TTP, and initial reports of laparoscopic splenectomy herald decreased risk of postop pulm complications

ANTICIPATED PROBLEMS/CONCERNS

- Massive surgical hemorrhage
- CNS and airway hemorrhage

PURPURA, THROMBOTIC THROMBOCYTOPENIC (TTP)

Evan G. Pivalizza, M.B., Ch.B., F.F.A.S.A.

RISK

- Rare (1/1 million) but 20% fatality rate

PERIOPERATIVE RISKS

- Patient for splenectomy has not responded to medical therapy; hence, risks of microthrombi with CNS and renal dysfunction combined with thrombocytopenia

WORRY ABOUT

- Preop drugs and therapies
- CNS, renal dysfunction
- Thrombocytopenia (although usual quantitative plt triggers do not apply)

OVERVIEW

- Severe microvascular occlusive disease characterized by thrombocytopenia, microangiopathic hemolytic anemia, multisystem organ involvement (particularly CNS and kidney), often indistinguishable from hemolytic uremic syndrome

ICD-9-CM Code: 446.6

ETIOLOGY

- Combination of abnormal PAF, von Willebrand's factor multimers, and plt aggregation with suppression of prostacyclin production and endothelial damage, all leading to arteriole/capillary occlusion with microthrombi.
- Recent association with ticlopidine.

USUAL TREATMENT

- Parity of randomized, controlled studies, and usually combination of therapies:
  - Plasmapheresis of primary importance (plt-poor FFP) with rapid clinical response
  - Plt aggregator inhibitors: aspirin, dipyridamole, dextran
  - Immunosuppression: corticosteroids, vincristine (risk of neurotoxicity and abnormal ADH secretion), γ-globulin
  - Splenectomy: often in failed medical responses or to prevent relapses (laparoscopic)
  - Avoid plt transfusion

ASSESSMENT POINTS

SYSTEM	EFFECT	ASSESSMENT BY HX	PE	TEST
HEENT	Airway manipulation with potential hemorrhage			
CV	Rare conduction pathway involvement		Baseline MAP for perfusion of CNS/kidney Vascular access	ECG
RESP	Rare infiltrates causing hypoxemia			CXR
RENAL	Proteinuria, hematuria, with ARF less common than with HUS			BUN, serum Cr, urine sediment
HEME	Thrombocytopenia	Hemorrhage	Petechiae Jaundice	Plts 8000–44,000 × 10³/mm³; PT, PTT, fibrinogen usually normal Fragmented RBCs (Hgb 8–9 g/dl); ↑ LDH, bilirubin
CNS	Diagnostic fluctuating course	Spectrum—headache, seizures, coma		Lumbar puncture, EEG, neuroradiology studies rarely performed
OB	May precipitate episode or relapse	Differentiate from HELLP/PIH	Termination of pregnancy not as crucial	

Key Reference: George JN: How I treat patients with thrombocytopenic purpura–hemolytic uremic syndrome. Blood 2000; 96:1223–1229.

PERIOPERATIVE IMPLICATIONS

Preoperative Preparation

- Steroid supplement
- Premedication: not IM, caution with CNS involvement
- Pneumococcal, meningococcal (*Haemophilus* for children) if splenectomy

Monitoring

- Protect skin and mucous membrane (NIBP cuff, esophageal probe, pressure points)
- Usually have central access for plasma exchange. If CVP required, avoid subclavian (difficulty in compressing hematoma).
- Theoretical risk of radial arterial line with thrombotic process

Airway

- Avoid nasal ET tube. Careful instrumentation, especially if plt count <50,000 × 10³/mm³.

Induction

- Avoid sympathetic intubation response (risk of intracranial hematoma), but maintain MAP > CNS, renal autoregulatory thresholds (>50–60 mmHg)

Maintenance

- Theoretical advantage of inhibitory effect of volatile anesthetics on plt aggregation (halothane>isoflurane>enflurane)

Fluids

- Do not transfuse plts: reports of deterioration due to further plt thrombi
- Bleeding managed with RBCs (>48 h old to avoid active plts) and FFP (plt-poor)

Extubation

- As above: care of mucous membranes and hemodynamic response

Adjuvants

- Individual analysis of risk-benefit for neuraxial technique in thrombocytopenic patient (if in remission)

Postoperative Period

- Mobilize early because of precipitous increase in plt count and viscosity with risk of thrombotic events
- Risk of atelectasis from LUQ incision and dissection

ANTICIPATED PROBLEMS/CONCERNS

- Hemorrhage due to thrombocytopenia
- Microthrombi with CNS dysfunction

PYLORIC STENOSIS

John Peder Erickson, M.D.

RISK

- Incidence 1/300–1/1000 of all live births
- Children of affected parents have higher incidence (3–5%)
- Male predominance

PERIOPERATIVE RISKS

- Similar to other abdominal procedures in patients of same age
- Some association with other GU anomalies
- Some have elevated unconjugated bilirubin related to decreased glucuronyl transferase activity; returns to normal after correction of stenosis

WORRY ABOUT

- Potential of full stomach
- Dehydration from recurrent emesis leads to alkalosis

OVERVIEW

- Reduced size of gastric outlet impedes emptying of contents, which can cause abnormal nutrition, repeated vomiting, and dehydration
- Onset of symptoms 3–6 wk of age
- Usually surgically cured

ICD-9-CM Code: 750.5 (Congenital)

ETIOLOGY

- Almost exclusively genetic in infants
- Can be acquired in adults

USUAL TREATMENT

- Normalize fluid/electrolyte status: this is not a surgical emergency
- Surgical: pyloromyotomy can usually be undertaken within 2–24 h of admission (unless fluid derangements are severe)
- Short procedure (<1 h)

ASSESSMENT POINTS

SYSTEM	EFFECT	ASSESSMENT BY HX	PE	TEST
GI	Small bowel obstruction	Projectile emesis	Pyloric "olive" palpable in upper abdomen	Contrast study

Key Reference: Holl JW: Anesthesia for abdominal surgery. *In* Gregory GA (ed): Pediatric Anesthesia, 3d ed. New York, Churchill Livingstone, 1994, pp 549–570.

PERIOPERATIVE IMPLICATIONS

Preoperative Preparation
- Correct fluid and acid-base deficits
- Pyloric stenosis is not a surgical emergency

Monitoring
- Routine

Airway
- Potential for full stomach

Preinduction/Induction
- Some will pass orogastric/nasogastric tube to suction stomach (still does NOT guarantee empty stomach)
- Consider IV rapid-sequence induction

Maintenance
- No technique is absolutely contraindicated by pyloric stenosis alone

Extubation
- Potential of full stomach

Adjuvants
- Consider potential of associated liver and GU abnormalities

Postoperative Period
- Pain score: 2–5

ANTICIPATED PROBLEMS/CONCERNS

- Potential for full stomach
- Need to correct fluid/electrolyte imbalances preop

Q FEVER

Paul R. Knight III, M.D., Ph.D.
Thomas A. Russo, M.D., C.M.

RISK

- Greatest after direct or indirect exposure to infected cattle, sheep, or goats; particularly at parturition
- Less from a variety of other animals, rarely from blood products
- Abattoir workers, veterinarians, and other animal workers at greatest risk
- Immunocompromised state at higher risk (e.g., HIV, steroids)
- Mortality 2.4% overall, chronic infection ~16%

PERIOPERATIVE RISKS

- Decreased respiratory reserve 2° to pneumonia
- Decreased myocardial reserve 2° to endocarditis
- Increased hepatocellular damage in presence of liver involvement

WORRY ABOUT

- Respiratory complications
- Decreased myocardial performance and emboli with endocarditis
- Increased hepatic or neurologic injury

OVERVIEW

- Acute infection: asymptomatic (~50%) to moderate severity (2% hospitalized)
- Acute symptomatic disease presents as nonspecific febrile syndrome ± pneumonitis (?50%), hepatitis (80%+), pericarditis/myocarditis (<5%), neurologic disease (<5%)
- Chronic disease occurs in <1% of infections, usually without fever
- Chronic disease, primarily endocarditis (particularly abnormal or prosthetic valves) and occasionally bone

ETIOLOGY

- *Coxiella burnetii* is a fastidious, obligate, intracellular bacterium
- Spore stage can withstand harsh environmental conditions for prolonged periods, facilitating indirect transmission
- Highly infectious (1–10 organisms) primarily by inhalation, ? unpasteurized milk, ? tick bite
- Incubation period ~20 days (range, 3–40 days)
- Bacterium targets reticuloendothelial cells, resulting in granuloma

USUAL TREATMENT

- Diagnosis: epidemiologic circumstance and serology (positive in 2–4 wk)
- Acute disease: doxycycline or quinolones for 2–3 wk hastens resolution
- Chronic disease: doxycycline and rifampin for 1–3 y, ± valve replacement with endocarditis

ASSESSMENT POINTS

SYSTEM	EFFECT	ASSESSMENT BY HX	PE	TEST
CV	Endocarditis, Immune-complex vasculitis, Microthromboembolism	Rash, ↓ exercise tolerance	Clubbing, rash, murmurs, petechiae	ECHO, ECG, culture negative
RESP	Atypical pneumonia, asymptomatic pneumonia, rapidly progressive pneumonia, interstitial pulmonary fibrosis	Pleuritic chest pain, cough, dyspnea	Consolidation, rales, pleural effusions	CXR, Sputum cultures
GI	Acute hepatitis	N/V, fatigue, diarrhea, sweats and chills	Hepatomegaly or hepatosplenomegaly	SGOT, SGPT, bilirubin, granulomas on liver biopsy
HEME	Hyperglobulinemia, anemia, thrombocytosis-cytopenia	Easy fatigue, bleeding tendency	Pallor; purpuric eruptions	Sedimentation rate, Hct/Hgb, plt
OB	Immune-complex vasculitis			Microscopic hematuria
REPROD	Q fever complications 2° to reactivation of infection during pregnancy	↑ Spontaneous abortions		Isolation of *C. burnetii* from placenta
CNS	Meningoencephalitis, Optic neuritis	Weakness, seizures, meningismus, blurred vision, headache	Focal deficits, sensory loss	↑ Monocytes and protein in CSF; normal glucose
MS	Immune-complex vasculitis, vertebral osteomyelitis	Myalgia	Point tenderness	X-ray

Key Reference: Marrie TJ: *In* Mandell GL, Bennett JE, Dolin R (eds): Principles and Practice of Infectious Diseases, 5th ed. New York, Churchill Livingstone, 2000, pp 2043–2050.

PERIOPERATIVE IMPLICATIONS

Preoperative Preparation

- Continue or initiate antibiotic therapy and optimize any organ system dysfunction
- Only emergency surgery should be performed
- Assess respiratory and cardiac reserve and hepatic and neurologic status
- With chronic Q fever, subacute endocarditis prophylaxis may be appropriate

Monitoring

- Arterial line may be necessary if pneumonia present
- Myocardial valvular disease may require PA line or other invasive hemodynamic monitors
- Increased arterial line complications due to vasculitis (rare)

Airway

- None

Induction

- Pneumonia may cause rapid desaturation
- Hypotension and CV instability if cardiac valvular injury present

Maintenance

- If acute hepatitis, avoid drugs that require hepatic metabolism or decrease blood flow to liver

Extubation

- Respiratory status and CV stability need to be considered

Adjuvants

- Depends on hepatic/renal impairment

Postoperative Period

- Respiratory/myocardial status carefully followed and may require ICU monitoring
- Liver enzymes followed if hepatic involvement

ANTICIPATED PROBLEMS/CONCERNS

- Emergent surgical patients who present with an acute infection might require extended antibiotic therapy to prevent persistent *C. burnetii* infection

RAYNAUD'S PHENOMENON

Stephan J. Cohn, M.D.

RISK

- 1.9% of population (based on reporting of color changes on exposure to cold)
- Almost all with disease are ages 15–40 y; almost all with secondary phenomenon are over age 40 y
- Often associated with scleroderma, systemic lupus erythematosus, and/or primary pulm Htn

PERIOPERATIVE RISKS

- Rare morbidity

WORRY ABOUT

- Arterial thrombosis
- Low blood flow states (e.g., prolonged hypotension or use of tourniquet) can lead to gangrene of extremities

OVERVIEW

- Abnormal sensitivity of small arteries and arterioles to vasoconstrictive stimuli
- Often manifested in a bilateral symmetric pattern, with hands being affected more often than feet
- Patients exhibit triphasic color pattern in affected areas: pallor, then cyanosis due to small arterial occlusion, followed by erythema and edema as vessels suddenly reopen

ICD-9-CM Code: 443.0

ETIOLOGY

- Unknown
- Likely hypothesis: hyperactive sympathetic nervous system with excess neurotransmitter and/or little or no inactivation of norepinephrine

USUAL TREATMENT

- Prevention is most effective—avoid prolonged exposure to cold, avoid cigarette smoking
- IV regional blocks with lidocaine at regular intervals. Reserpine, bretylium, and guanethidine all used as additives to lidocaine in IV regional blocks.
- In severe cases, surgical sympathectomy an option but not always beneficial (see also Systemic Lupus Erythematosus in Diseases section)

ASSESSMENT POINTS

SYSTEM	EFFECT	ASSESSMENT BY HX	PE	TEST
RESP	Associated with primary pulmonary Htn	Chest discomfort DOE Weakness	JVD Pulmonic ejection click	CXR—right cardiomegaly Dilated pulmonary artery ECG—right atrial enlargement, renal vascular hypertension
MS	Impaired joint mobility due to pain or scleroderma	Joint mobility		
VASC	Small arterial occlusion	Triphasic color pattern	Often associated with numbness and diaphoresis	

Key Reference: Nay PG, O'Brien K: Acute vasospastic attack after extradural block in a patient with Raynaud's disease. Anesth Analg 2000; 90:1417–1418.

PERIOPERATIVE IMPLICATIONS

Preoperative Preparation

- Keep warm
- Assess for co-existing disease

Monitoring

- Assess risk-benefit ratio if considering arterial cannulation because of danger of thrombosis
- Monitor patient's temp and check pressure points and distal pulses frequently

Airway

- ↓ TMJ mobility if associated with scleroderma

Induction

- General or regional anesthetic options acceptable

Maintenance

- Use of tourniquet controversial

Adjuvants

- When using regional anesthetic, consider avoiding epinephrine

Postoperative Period

- Keep as warm as possible
- Check pulses in all extremities

REFLEX SYMPATHETIC DYSTROPHY
(COMPLEX PERIPHERAL PAIN SYNDROME)

Lloyd R. Saberski, M.D.
Jerry M. Calkins, M.D., Ph.D.

RISK
- People within USA: 1–6 million? (underestimated)
- 1.5% of total peripheral nerve injuries
- No racial predilection

PERIOPERATIVE RISKS
- Heightened postop pain if operation on involved extremity
- Frequently hypertensive, and with ↑ incidence of CAD

WORRY ABOUT
- Pain can be made worse by adrenergic agonists
- Avoid vascular access in involved extremities
- Position involved extremity carefully and document

OVERVIEW
- Neuropathic pain after injury, characterized as burning associated with severe allodynia, hyperpathia, and decreased range of motion
- Dx made on clinical basis from major criteria (burning pain, allodynia, hyperpathia, edema, temp changes) and minor criteria (nail and hair growth changes, skin changes)
- Considerable ambiguity as to who is afflicted
- Dx primarily of exclusion
- Regional sympathetic dysfunction may be present
- Operations upon involved extremities can lead to further postop neuropathic pain with significant sympathetic discharge
- No correlation between severity of injury and incidence, severity, and course of symptoms

ICD-9-CM Codes: 337.20 (Reflex sympathetic dystrophy—unspecified site); 337.21 (Reflex sympathetic dystrophy—upper limb); 337.22 (Reflex sympathetic dystrophy—lower limb); 337.29 (Reflex sympathetic dystrophy—other specified site)

ETIOLOGY
- Unknown, although involves altered peripheral and CNS response thresholds to afferent impulses
- Sympathetic dysfunction may be present. No specific diagnostic test available. (Triple phase bone scan, thermography, galvanic skin response helpful.)
- Associated with antecedent trauma, iatrogenic causes (amputation, tight casts), and visceral, neurologic, and musculoskeletal diseases

USUAL TREATMENT
- Early diagnosis—early treatment
- Some cases spontaneously subside
- Desensitization therapy
- Neuropathic pain medications
- Sympatholytic medication
- Sympatholytic blocks—document degree of success of blockade
- Spinal cord stimulation
- Sympathectomies (surgical) rarely indicated
- Multiple therapeutic regimens

ASSESSMENT POINTS

SYSTEM	EFFECT	ASSESSMENT BY HX	PE	TEST
GI	Slow peristalsis	Constipation	↓ Bowel sounds	
DERM	Dry, shiny skin Excessive sweating Vasomotor and sudomotor disturbances		Dry, shiny, moist, clammy, cool skin Nails brittle ↓ Hair growth	Abn galvanic skin response Thermography
PNS	Pain, allodynia Hyperalgesia Hyperesthesia	Pain to touch		
MS	Weakness, atrophy Trophic skin changes in skin, bones, joints	Weakness	Joints sclerosed	Triple phase bone scan

Key Reference: Loeser J: Bonica's Management of Pain. Philadelphia, Lea & Febiger, 2000.

PERIOPERATIVE IMPLICATIONS
- Avoid tourniquets, BP cuffs, and vascular punctures of involved extremity
- Carefully position patient and protect involved extremity
- Consider plexus infusion of local anesthetic 24–72 h before surgical procedure

Monitoring
- Routine

Induction
- Consider regional anesthetic infusion that can be continued postop; can be combined with GA (without succinylcholine)
- Consider avoiding sympathomimetic agents such as ketamine
- Pressors can aggravate sympathetic responsive pain and should be titrated incrementally
- Avoid Bier blocks since exsanguination and compression with tourniquet can be painful

Maintenance
- Consider combining conduction anesthetic with sedation or nonsympathomimetic GA
- Keep affected extremity warm

Adjuvants
- IV phentolamine can decrease sympathetic responsive pain
- Neuropathic medications such as lidocaine, phenytoin, and clonidine may decrease pain and anesthetic requirements

Postoperative Period
- Balanced analgesia: plexus infusion with local anesthetic, adjuvants, opioid

SPECIAL CONSIDERATIONS
- Conduction anesthetics along with neuropathic medication may decrease plasticity (wind-up) of CNS and decrease postop pain

RENAL FAILURE, ACUTE (ARF)

Robert N. Sladen, M.B., Ch.B., M.R.C.P., F.R.C.P.C.

RISK

- People within USA: 1% of all hospital admissions (community-acquired), 5% of all general hospital patients (hospital-acquired), 10–30% of ICU patients
- Population with highest prevalence: elderly (>65 y)

PERIOPERATIVE RISKS

- Overall mortality of perioperative ARF: 60–90%
- Acute pulm edema, electrolyte abn, arrhythmias
- Aspiration
- Bleeding (plt dysfunction)

WORRY ABOUT

- Difficult IV and arterial access
- Intolerance of hemodialysis
- GI symptoms
- Clinical signs of coagulopathy
- Hyperkalemia and arrhythmias

OVERVIEW

- Elective surgery is contraindicated with new-onset ARF; procedures are urgent or emergency
- Underlying disorder may still be present
- Repeated hemodynamic insults markedly impair renal recovery
- Dialysis partially controls thrombocytopathy and enteropathy, but does not decrease risk of sepsis and poor wound healing

ICD-9-CM Codes: 584 (Acute); 977.5 (Due to procedure)

ETIOLOGY

- ATN (ischemic, nephrotoxic)
  - Sepsis in 70% of all cases, multiple system failure in 80% of ICU patients
- Vascular injury (thromboembolism, occlusion, intra-abdominal Htn)
- Systemic disease (atherosclerosis, vasculitis, sickle cell)
- Acute interstitial nephritis, acute glomerulonephritis

USUAL TREATMENT

- Medical therapy
  - Fluid and electrolyte restriction, loop diuretics
  - Hyperkalemia: hyperventilation, bicarbonate, Ca^{2+}, insulin-glucose, Kayexalate enema
- Dialysis—peritoneal dialysis, intermittent hemodialysis, continuous arteriovenous or venovenous dialysis

ASSESSMENT POINTS

SYSTEM	EFFECT	ASSESSMENT BY HX	PE	TEST
HEENT	Edema		Airway edema	
	Coagulopathy	Epistaxis		See heme
CV	VTach, VFIB	Syncope, cardiac arrest		Serum K^+, Mg^{2+}
	Pericardial effusion	Dyspnea, pleuritic chest pain	Muffled heart sounds	ECG, CXR, ECHO
RESP	Pulm edema	Dyspnea, orthopnea	Rales	CXR
GI	Impaired motility	Reflux	Abdominal distention	NG, stool guaiac
	Ileus	GI bleeding	Tenderness, guarding	KUB series
	Serositis	Abdominal discomfort	Absent bowel sounds	Endoscopy
	Ulceration	Constipation, diarrhea		CT scan
HEME	Plt dysfunction	Excessive bleeding	Petechial hemorrhages	Bleeding time
RENAL	ARF	Oliguria, anuria	Edema	Urinalysis, BUN, Cr, Cr clearance Renal US, scintigraphy
CNS	Encephalopathy	Confusion, disorientation		EEG
		Coma		CT scan
MS	Rhabdomyolysis	Crush injury, limb ischemia	"Red urine"	Urine myoglobin Serum CK

Key Reference: Lote CJ, Harper L, Savage CO: Mechanism of acute renal failure. Br J Anaesth 1996; 77:82–89.

PERIOPERATIVE IMPLICATIONS

Preoperative Preparation

- Dialysis to control fluid overload, hyperkalemia, metabolic acidosis, acute uremia
- Consider metoclopramide, H_2-blocker to reduce reflux risk
- Consider DDAVP 0.3 μg/kg to enhance plt function (effective 8–12 h)
- Regional techniques may be contraindicated by coagulopathy
- DDAVP, insulin-glucose, Kayexalate can complicate perioperative care

Monitoring

- ECG for arrhythmia detection
- Consider PA catheter for large fluid shift operations with or without LV dysfunction
- Avoid arterial catheters and blood pressure cuffs in limbs with AV shunts

Airway

- Consider awake intubation with airway edema
- Avoid nasal intubation (epistaxis)

Preinduction/Induction

- Manage fluids as if renal function were normal (risk of hypovolemia)
- Treat as for full stomach: head up, cricoid pressure
- Succinylcholine is relatively contraindicated (avoid if K^+ conc $\geq$ 5.0 mEq/L)

Maintenance

- Restrict maintenance fluids, but replace losses appropriately guided by hemodynamic monitoring
- Avoid morphine, meperidine, pancuronium
- Increase minute ventilation to compensate for metabolic acidosis; sedative-hypnotic administration may lead to acidosis by decreasing resp rate in spontaneously breathing patient
- Anticipate increased volume of distribution but decreased clearance of most drugs
- Check ABGs, serum K^+

Extubation

- Anticipate delayed emergence
- Treat as for full stomach

Postoperative Period

- Careful assessment of CV, resp status: check ABGs, serum K^+
- Morphine, meperidine have active metabolites that are renally excreted: use with caution
- May require ultrafiltration for excess fluid removal in early postop period

ANTICIPATED PROBLEMS/CONCERNS

- Ventricular arrhythmias may occur without premonitory ECG signs. Rapid K^+ flux more ominous than high serum K^+ itself.
- Dialysis preferred 24 h preop to avoid disequilibrium during anesthesia

RENAL FAILURE, CHRONIC

Donald S. Prough, M.D.

RISK

• People within USA: >100 cases of end-stage renal disease (ESRD)/1 million population
• Racial prevalence: African-Americans ~200 cases/1 million; Hispanics ~100/1 million; Caucasians ~50/1 million

PERIOPERATIVE RISKS

• Overall perioperative mortality of patients with ESRD: 4%
• Overall perioperative morbidity of patients with ESRD: 50% (hyperkalemia, infections, hypotension/Htn, bleeding, dysrhythmias, clotted fistulas)

WORRY ABOUT

• Perioperative progression from chronic renal insufficiency (CRI), not requiring dialysis, to dialysis-dependent ESRD
• Hypovolemia and hypokalemia (esp if recently dialyzed)
• Hypervolemia, metabolic acidosis, and hyperkalemia (esp if not recently dialyzed)

• Autonomic dysfunction (excessive hypotensive responses)
• Exaggerated hypertensive responses to noxious stimuli
• Prolonged responses to renally excreted drugs and metabolites (e.g., vecuronium, pancuronium, narcotics)
• Impaired immune status

OVERVIEW

• ↓ Excretory and other functions of kidney related to long-standing disease—with dialysis, a disease that can persist for many years
• Associated with multiple complications of failed renal excretory function, including volume overload, accumulation of products of catabolism (e.g., potassium and hydrogen ions), plt dysfunction, and side effects of dialytic therapy, including hypovolemia
• Associated with complications of concurrent diseases (e.g., diabetes mellitus, Htn)
• Volume status and electrolyte balance related to recency of dialysis

ICD-9-CM Code: 585

ETIOLOGY

• Htn (15% Hispanics; 20% Caucasians; 40% African-Americans)
• Diabetes mellitus (20% Caucasians; 30% African-Americans; 37% Hispanics)
• Glomerulonephritis (12% African-Americans; 22% Hispanics; 25% Caucasians)
• Other causes: polycystic disease, collagen-vascular disease, pyelonephritis

USUAL TREATMENT

• CRI: fluid restriction, protein restriction, diuretics, antihypertensives
• Peritoneal dialysis or hemodialysis; continuous venovenous hemofiltration or continuous venovenous hemodialysis while hospitalized
• Renal transplantation (often combined with pancreatic transplantation in diabetics)

ASSESSMENT POINTS

SYSTEM	EFFECT	ASSESSMENT BY HX	PE	TEST
CV	CHF LVH Dysrhythmias	Exercise intolerance Htn Palpitations	Crackles; S_3, S_4 Pulse, auscultation	CXR ECG
GI	N/V, anorexia GI bleeding	N/V, anorexia Melena, rectal bleeding	Malnutrition	Positive occult blood
HEME	Plt dysfunction Anemia	Easy bruising Fatigability	Ecchymoses Pallor	Bleeding time Hgb
RENAL	↓ Concentrating ability (CRI)	Nocturia, frequency		Urine Osm BUN, Cr
CNS	Encephalopathy Autonomic dysfunction	↓ Mental acuity, disorientation Postural hypotension	Mental status Tilt table test: ↓ BP, ↑ HR when tilted	
PNS	Peripheral neuropathy	Paresthesias, burning, itching of lower extremities	Excoriations	

Key Reference: Sladen RN: Anesthetic considerations for the patient with renal failure. Anesthesiol Clin North Am 2000; 18:863–882..

PERIOPERATIVE IMPLICATIONS

Preoperative Preparation

• Assess adequacy of dialytic therapy, volume and acid-base status, Hgb concentration, CV status, serum K^+
• If not dialysis-dependent, assess renal reserve, CV status

Monitoring

• Temp, ECG (rhythm, rate, hyperkalemia)
• Pulse oximeter, capnometer, peripheral nerve stimulator
• Consider arterial catheter if chronically hypertensive; consider PA catheter for high-risk surgery in patients with cardiac dysfunction

Airway

• Gastroparesis precautions if diabetic

Preinduction/Induction

• Reduce dose of thiopental
• Exaggerated response to benzodiazepines
• Consider avoiding renally excreted neuromuscular blockers (vecuronium, pancuronium)
• Use narcotics cautiously
• If not dialysis-dependent, avoid sevoflurane and enflurane for prolonged cases
• Exaggerated BP swings with induction and intubation
• Reduce dose of local anesthetics if metabolic acidosis present or if sedatives will cause resp acidosis

Maintenance

• Precise volume management; titration of agents

Extubation

• Ensure adequate reversal of neuromuscular blockers
• Evaluate airway reflexes

Adjuvants

• Avoid renally excreted neuromuscular blockers

Postoperative Period

• Dialyze if necessary
• Monitor for frequent causes of postop morbidity (see above)

ANTICIPATED PROBLEMS/CONCERNS

• Hyperkalemia—treatment with $CaCl_2$, insulin/glucose, or $NaHCO_3$ may be necessary; intraoperative dialysis occasionally required
• Balancing intraoperative volume requirements with need for postop fluid removal
• Exaggerated drug effects

RESPIRATORY DISTRESS SYNDROME
T. James Gallagher, M.D.

RISK
- People within USA: up to 400,000/y
- Race/gender predominance: none

PERIOPERATIVE RISKS
- ↑ Risk in patients with generalized septic conditions including perforated colon and pancreatitis
- May develop following large-volume fluid resuscitation and blood replacement

WORRY ABOUT
- ↓ Oxygenation
- ↓ Pulm compliance

OVERVIEW
- Patients rarely die directly of respiratory distress syndrome
- Contributes to prolonged mechanical ventilation and increased stay in ICU
- May last from 3 days to several weeks
- Complicated by bacterial or yeast pneumonia
- Primarily results from generalized sepsis, which increases pulm vascular permeability

ICD-9-CM Code: 518.5 (Following trauma and surgery)

ETIOLOGY
- Represents a symptom or sign of generalized sepsis
- A vascular disease with altered permeability
- Alterations of permeability result from endotoxin release and stimulation of other cytokines, including TNF
- Lymphatic drainage usually overwhelmed, resulting in ↑ water accumulation in interstitial spaces
- ↑ Intravascular volume and ↓ colloid oncotic pressure can contribute to severity

USUAL TREATMENT
- Ventilatory support
- PEEP and CPAP to improve oxygenation
- Elimination of septic source
- Appropriate antibiotic therapy
- Inhaled nitric oxide may improve oxygenation or reduce need for mechanical ventilatory support

ASSESSMENT POINTS

SYSTEM	EFFECT	ASSESSMENT BY HX	PE	TEST
CV	Decreased O_2 delivery ↑ Intravascular volume	SOB ↓ Peripheral perfusion	Tachycardia S_3, S_4 Ischemia	ECG BP PCWP Cardiac output
RESP	↓ Oxygenation, CO_2 accumulation	Dyspnea Tachypnea	Rales Nasal flaring	CXR ABGs
CNS	Agitation Confusion	Disorientation		Level of consciousness

Key Reference: Esteban A, Alia I, Gordo F, de Pablo R, Suarez J, Gonzalez G, Blanco J: Prospective randomized trial comparing pressure-controlled ventilation and volume-controlled ventilation in ARDS. For the Spanish Lung Failure Collaborative Group. Chest 2000; 117:1690–1696.

PERIOPERATIVE IMPLICATIONS

Preoperative Preparation
- Avoid surgery if possible
- May require mechanical ventilator used in ICU rather than a standard anesthesia ventilator because of high airway pressures

Monitoring
- Oxygenation guided by pulse oximetry and blood gas analysis
- Peak inflation pressures
- PA catheter to judge fluid status, cardiac function frequently indicated

Airway
- Maintain intubation
- High FIO_2

Preinduction/Induction
- May develop hypoxemia
- Avoid agents requiring supplemental gases
- Anesthetic agents may blunt hypoxic PA vasoconstriction and reduce cardiac output

Maintenance
- ↓ Oxygenation may appear as a reduction in O_2 saturation or PaO_2
- ↓ Lung function may be evidenced by increase in peak inflation pressure or decrease in tidal volume
- Once the abdomen has been opened, compliance may improve; tidal volumes may become excessively high
- Closure of abdomen may result in extraordinarily high pressures and inability to ventilate

Extubation
- The patient should almost always remain intubated at end of procedure

Adjuvants
- Muscle relaxation may improve gas exchange
- It may be necessary to maintain paralysis in postop period

Postoperative Period
- Oxygenation and ventilation should be monitored in ICU in the postoperative period
- Ventilator changes should be based on x-ray and blood gas analysis
- If paralysis required, sedation also necessary

ANTICIPATED PROBLEMS/CONCERNS
- Oxygenation will almost always worsen following surgery
- If pulm parenchymal changes deteriorate or worsen, patients may have difficulty with CO_2 elimination

RETT SYNDROME
Catherine R. Bachman, M.D., F.R.C.P.C.

RISK

- Almost exclusively females
- Thought to be the second most common cause of profound mental retardation in females, after Down syndrome

PERIOPERATIVE RISKS

- Abnormal control of ventilation, with periods of apnea and hyperventilation
- May have GE reflux
- Multiple orthopedic and motor movement disorders

WORRY ABOUT

- Risk of perioperative apnea unknown
- Risk of succinylcholine-induced hyperkalemia unknown
- Aspiration due to GE reflux
- Intraoperative positioning because of spasticity and contractures

OVERVIEW

- Diagnosis based on consistent constellation of clinical features with absence of other causes of severe developmental delay
- Normal development for the first 5–6 mo of life followed by rapid loss of acquired cognitive, verbal, and motor skills with eventual severe impairment in all areas
- Abnormal EEG in virtually all patients (nonspecific)
- Pathognomonic stereotyped hand movements—tortuous hand-wringing or -washing or other bizarre hand automatisms
- Seizures of various types common
- Respiratory abnormalities when awake in 75% of patients—hyperventilation, breathholding, cyanotic spells, aerophagia with abdominal bloating. Respiratory pattern appears normal during sleep.
- Orthopedic and movement disorders such as spasticity, ataxia, scoliosis

- Vasomotor disturbances with cool mottled extremities
- Cachexia

ICD-9-CM Code: 330.8

ETIOLOGY

- Unknown
- No specific diagnostic test available
- A genetic basis considered likely—X-linked?
- Diagnosis made by history and clinical features (inclusion and exclusion criteria established)

USUAL TREATMENT

- Supportive only
- Aimed at improving quality of life, seizure control, nutrition, physical therapy, possible surgery for orthopedic problems
- Several therapeutic medication trials underway (L-carnitine, magnesium, melatonin)

ASSESSMENT POINTS

SYSTEM	EFFECT	ASSESSMENT BY HX	PE	TEST
HEENT	Nonspecific Spasticity may make airway difficult		Neck ROM Normal face	Neck x-rays if indicated
CV	No primary heart involvement Peripheral vasomotor disturbances	? Exercise tolerance (patients inactive) Extremities cool, trophic changes	Secondary cardiac changes only	As indicated by Hx and physical findings
RESP	Abn control of ventilation with hyperventilation, apnea, cyanosis, desaturation Lung changes due to scoliosis or aspiration	Hx of apnea, cyanosis Hx of scoliosis, aspiration	Observation Chest exam	O$_2$ saturation CXR PFTs unlikely (poor cooperation)
GI	GE reflux possible, swallowing difficulties, constipation Growth failure	Hx of GE reflux, feeding difficulties	Thin, small for age	X-ray studies for GE reflux
CNS	Severe developmental delay Seizures Ataxia Abn control of ventilation Abn sleep characteristics	Developmental level seizure activity Presence of apnea, cyanosis	Assessment of cognitive and movement disorders	EEG Resp studies, sleeping and awake
MS	Hypotonia (early); spasticity (late); ataxia Secondary orthopedic manifestations: scoliosis, joint contractures	Progress and extent of MS abnormalities	Chest exam for scoliosis Limb and joint positions	X-rays

Key Reference: Ellaway C, Christodoulou J: Rett syndrome: clinical update and review of recent genetic advances. J Paediatr Child Health 1999; 35:419–426.

PERIOPERATIVE IMPLICATIONS

Preoperative Preparation

- As for any patient with developmental delay
- Optimize respiratory status
- Assess respiratory control
- Minimize aspiration risk

Monitoring

- Routine
- More invasive depending upon procedure

Airway

- Normal face
- Spasticity may make positioning difficult

Preinduction/Induction

- Risk of hyperkalemia following succinylcholine unknown
- Possible aspiration risk due to GE reflux

Maintenance

- Respiratory control abnormal; unknown if spontaneous ventilation under anesthesia associated with significant apnea
- Attention to body temp because of thin body habitus and peripheral vasomotor disturbances

Extubation

- Possible aspiration risk
- Assess respiratory control

Postoperative Period

- Respiratory control abnormal
  - Effect of anesthetic agents
  - Duration of respiratory monitoring
  - Effect of narcotics vs. local anesthetics for pain control

Adjuvants

- None

ANTICIPATED PROBLEMS/CONCERNS

- Respiratory control abnormalities not well understood. Therefore, effect of anesthetic agents intra- and postoperatively on respiration not known. Need for postop monitoring for apnea unknown.

REYE'S SYNDROME

Mary A. Keyes, M.D.
Tracy Koogler, M.D.

RISK

- Incidence prior to 1990 was 0.3–0.6/100,000 <16 y
- During early 1980s, association between aspirin and Reye's syndrome was recognized and incidence dramatically declined

PERIOPERATIVE RISKS

- Surgery (all but life-and-death emergencies) contraindicated during Reye's syndrome. Following recovery, evaluate liver function tests.

WORRY ABOUT

- Recurrent liver dysfunction
- Permanent neuropsychologic deficits

OVERVIEW

- An acute encephalopathy with hepatic dysfunction predominantly in children; typically starts several days after unremarkable viral illness
- Encephalopathy heralded by protracted, severe vomiting, with abnormal behavior and combativeness that progress to coma
- Dx made by unexplained encephalopathy with one or more of following: serum transaminases elevated to at least 3× normal; blood ammonia levels at least 3× normal; or hepatic microvesicular fatty infiltration on liver biopsy. CSF is normal.
- Most children have moderate illness that does not progress to deep coma
- Prognosis depends on severity and duration of cerebral dysfunction. Severe disease may lead to subtle neuropsychologic defects.

ICD-9-CM Code: 331.81

ETIOLOGY

- Multifactorial; abnormal reaction to viral illness modified by exogenous toxin in susceptible host
- Most frequently linked with influenza A and B and varicella. Exogenous toxin is aspirin in majority of cases.

USUAL TREATMENT

- Early recognition of mild cases and control of ICP
- Management varies with severity of illness: fluids should be restricted in patients with cerebral edema. ICP monitoring aids in improving cerebral perfusion pressure and decreasing ICP.
- Mannitol to induce cerebral dehydration and barbiturates to decrease cerebral metabolic demand
- Coagulopathies treated with vitamin K and/or FFP

ASSESSMENT POINTS

SYSTEM	EFFECT	ASSESSMENT BY HX	PE	TEST
GI	Hepatic dysfunction	Severe vomiting	Hepatomegaly	Hepatic transaminases Ammonia levels Liver biopsy PT, PTT
CNS	Delirium Combative behavior Seizures Lethargy Coma	Alteration in mental status	No focal signs	CT scan ICP monitor

Key Reference: Sullivan KM, Belay ED, Durbin RE, Foster DA, Nordenberg DF: Epidemiology of Reye's syndrome, United States, 1991–1994: comparison of CDC surveillance and hospital admission data. Neuroepidemiology 2000; 19:338–344.

PERIOPERATIVE IMPLICATIONS

- Surgery not undertaken except in life-and-death emergencies

Adjuvants

- Early recognition of mild cases and control of ICP
- Management varies with severity of illness: fluids should be restricted in patients with cerebral edema. ICP monitoring aids in improving cerebral perfusion pressure and decreasing ICP.
- Mannitol to induce cerebral dehydration and barbiturates to reduce cerebral metabolic demand
- Coagulopathies treated with vitamin K and/or FFP

ANTICIPATED PROBLEMS/CONCERNS

- Hepatic dysfunction
- Encephalopathy

RHEUMATOID ARTHRITIS

Stephen F. Dierdorf, M.D.

- 1% of USA population
- Male:female 1:2−3

PERIOPERATIVE RISKS

- Increased risk for new neurologic disturbances 2° to occult cervical spine damage
- Myocardial damage insidious and may not be clinically evident
- Increased perioperative pulm complications 2° to pulm fibrosis and restrictive lung disease

WORRY ABOUT

- Laryngoscopy and tracheal intubation may be difficult 2° to rheumatoid damage to cervical spine
- Hx of previous tracheal intubation not predictive of current conditions
- Cervical cord damage during laryngoscopy and tracheal intubation

- Occult pericarditis and myocardial dysfunction
- Difficult to determine exercise tolerance because of limitation of movement 2° to joint dysfunction

OVERVIEW

- Chronic inflammatory disease affecting multiple joints and organ systems
- Systemic effects include anemia, pericarditis, cardiac tamponade, myocarditis, aortitis, peripheral nerve compression, and renal dysfunction
- Renal failure common cause of death

ICD-9-CM Code: 714

ETIOLOGY

- Autoimmune disorder triggered by an antigen in genetically susceptible individuals

- Variability in clinical course may be due to differences in triggering antigens and/or immune response
- Pathologic changes: cellular hyperplasia of synovium and synovial invasion by lymphocytes, plasma cells, and fibroblasts with ultimate destruction of cartilage and articular surfaces

USUAL TREATMENT

- First-line drugs include aspirin and NSAIDs: ibuprofen, indomethacin, naproxen, piroxicam, sulindac, and tolmetin
- Second-line drugs that alter immune response include hydroxychloroquine, methotrexate, sulfasalazine, azathioprine, penicillamine, and gold
- Significant side effects of long-term corticosteroid therapy; limit them to patients failing second-line response

ASSESSMENT POINTS

SYSTEM	EFFECT	ASSESSMENT BY HX	PE	TEST
HEENT	Edematous mucosa	Epistaxis	Friable mucosa	Direct laryngoscopy
	Arthritis of larynx	Hx of voice change	Voice, airway exam	
CV	LV dysfunction	Dyspnea	S$_3$	ECG
		Orthopnea	Rales	Stress ECG
		Reduced exercise		ECHO
	Aortitis	Reduced exercise	Diastolic murmur (AI)	ECHO
	Pericarditis	Dyspnea	Distant heart sounds	ECHO
			Friction rub	
RESP	Fibrosis	Dyspnea	Dry rales	CXR, PFTs
GI	Peptic ulcer	Epigastric pain, N/V		
RENAL	Renal dysfunction	Drug induced		Cr
CNS	Spinal cord compression	Neck pain	Sensory deficits	Radiography
	Neurologic dysfunction	Numbness	Motor deficits	MRI
			ROM of neck	
MS	Arthritis	Joint pain	Swelling	Radiography
			Pain with motion	
			Restricted motion	

Key Reference: Mackenzie CR, Sharrock NE: Perioperative medical considerations in patients with rheumatoid arthritis. Rheum Dis Clin North Am 1998; 24:1−17.

PERIOPERATIVE IMPLICATIONS

Preoperative Preparation

- Mobility of cervical spine and TMJ. Check cervical spine films and/or MRI if available; ROM of shoulders, elbows, wrists, hips, and knees.
- Review treatment drugs and their effects

Monitoring

- Routine for procedure and co-morbidities of patient

Airway

- Poor cervical spine mobility may necessitate awake tracheal intubation
- Smaller than predicted tracheal tube (laryngeal arthritis)

Preinduction/Induction

- No specific contraindications to common induction agents
- Greater decreases in BP 2° to myocardial dysfunction
- ↑ Risk of aspiration pneumonitis
- Careful positioning to avoid aggravation of major joint dysfunction

Maintenance

- Drug-induced hepatic dysfunction; potential for halothane hepatitis
- Exaggerated CV effects of volatile anesthetics

Extubation

- Postextubation laryngeal edema and stridor more common

Adjuvants

- Neuraxial anesthesia difficult because of spinal arthritis
- Drug interactions between anesthetics and antiarthritic drugs (see under drug in Drugs section, or in Goodman and Gilman)

ANTICIPATED PROBLEMS/CONCERNS

- Difficult tracheal intubation
- Increased neurologic deficits 2° to cervical spine degeneration
- May need perioperative corticosteroid supplementation

ROCKY MOUNTAIN SPOTTED FEVER

Paul R. Knight III, M.D., Ph.D.
Thomas A. Russo, M.D., C.M.

RISK

- All states in USA, most common southeast and south central, ~ 1000 cases/y
- Exposure to tick-infested terrain or dogs
- Severe infection, young and healthy at risk for death
- Mortality 20% untreated, 5% with treatment
- Mortality increases with delay in diagnosis, ↑ age, and male sex

PERIOPERATIVE RISKS

- Increased mortality 2° to CV instability and noncardiogenic pulmonary edema
- Increased risk of organ injury due to compounded insults
- Increased bleeding tendency

WORRY ABOUT

- Severe intravascular volume depletion leading to shock
- Electrolyte disturbances

- Cardiac arrhythmias
- Microvascular hemorrhage
- Consumptive coagulopathy
- Intraoperative respiratory and renal failure

OVERVIEW

- Uncommon but severe infection
- Pathophysiology primarily due to endothelial cell infection resulting in ↑ vascular permeability, edema, hypovolemia, and ischemia
- Initial symptoms in 1–3 days: nonspecific, mimicking a viral syndrome
- Rash appears in 3–5 days, initially as macules progressing to petechiae; usually centripetal progression; rash absent in 10%
- Disease progression (more likely with delay in treatment) results in multiorgan involvement: noncardiac pulmonary edema, CNS, myocarditis, hepatitis, bleeding (2° to thrombocytopenia and direct vessel damage), and renal failure

ETIOLOGY

- *Rickettsia rickettsii* transmitted in saliva of ticks after 6 h of attachment and feeding or by exposure to infected tick hemolymph
- Incubation period ~ 7 days (2–12 days)
- Obligatory intracellular bacterium that replicates in endothelial cells, causing direct cell injury with loss of vascular integrity

USUAL TREATMENT

- Dx difficult, primarily clinical and epidemiologic (potential tick exposure)
- Doxycycline, tetracycline, chloramphenicol (pregnant women)
- Correct hypovolemia, coagulation defects, thrombocytopenia
- Provide intensive, supportive care for various organ system failures

ASSESSMENT POINTS

SYSTEM	EFFECT	ASSESSMENT BY HX	PE	TEST
CV	Extensive microvascular leak; interstitial myocarditis	Rash, swelling	Rash, edema, arrhythmias	ECG, CXR Lytes, BP
RESP	Noncardiac pulm edema; interstitial pneumonitis	↓ Exercise tolerance, dypsnea	Rales by auscultation	CXR, spirometry
GI	Gastroenteritis; liver, spleen, and pancreatic microvascular hemorrhage and edema	N/V, pain, diarrhea	Abdominal tenderness Hepatosplenomegaly	SGOT, bilirubin
HEME	Thrombocytopenia, anemia	Easy bleeding, malaise	Rash	Hct/Hgb, plt/PT, PTT
RENAL	Microvascular hemorrhage and edema, interstitial nephritis, prerenal azotemia	Lumbar pain		BUN, Cr Lytes
CNS	Meningoencephalitis	Focal defects, deafness, meningismus, photophobia		CSF: ± ↑ WBC, ↑ protein
MS	Microvascular hemorrhage and edema	Myalgia	↓ ROM	

Key Reference: Walker DH, Raoult D: *In* Mandell GL, Bennett JE, Dolin R (eds): Principles and Practice of Infectious Diseases, 5th ed. New York, Churchill Livingstone, 2000, pp 2035–2039.

PERIOPERATIVE IMPLICATIONS

Preoperative Preparation

- Antibiotic therapy and correction of underlying organ system dysfunction
- Surgery only for emergency
- Assess volume, respiratory, renal status

Monitoring

- Consider PA catheter, arterial line, UO
- Intraoperative ABGs and lytes
- Plt and other coagulation variables

Airway

- Severe edema of oropharynx and ↑ bleeding tendency can lead to difficult intubation

Induction

- Hypovolemia can cause hypotension
- Microvascular leak in lung can cause rapid desaturation
- ↑ Cardiac arrhythmias

Maintenance

- Owing to CV instability, volume status is key
- Possibility of resp failure and constant volume resuscitation should be anticipated when selecting anesthetic technique

Extubation

- Oropharyngeal edema and ↑ bleeding tendency may make reintubation very difficult

Adjuvants

- Vasoactive drugs used in acute resuscitation should be readily available
- Lidocaine for treatment of cardiac arrhythmias

Postoperative Period

- Intravascular volume shifts; coagulation defects, respiratory failure, CV instability, renal failure

ANTICIPATED PROBLEMS/CONCERNS

- Owing to the possibility of multisystem failure, prolonged postop ICU management may be required
- Since early treatment with antibiotics is curative and highly successful in preventing complications, high index of suspicion, e.g., after tick exposure in endemic areas, is needed

SARCOIDOSIS

Andrew D. Rosenberg, M.D.

RISK

- Varies: $\leq 1-80/100,000$ with highest incidence in Sweden; in USA 30/100,000
- Presenting ages 20–40 y in USA
- More common in African-Americans than Caucasians in USA
- Females > males (2:1)

PERIOPERATIVE RISKS

- Severity depends on degree of airway, lung, cardiac, and CNS involvement

WORRY ABOUT

- Airway granulomas distorting and obstructing anatomy
- Degree of lung involvement and pulm fibrosis
- Cardiac involvement, heart block, arrhythmia, CHF
- CNS involvement

OVERVIEW

- Multisystem granulomatous disorder with widespread noncaseating epithelioid cell granulomas
- Lung most frequently affected organ
- Airway abnormality 2° to granulomas
- Local organ distortion can result in symptoms
- Mononuclear inflammatory cells: T-helper cells + mononuclear phagocytes lead to formation of granulomas

ICD-9-CM Code: 135.0

ETIOLOGY

- Unknown disease due to exaggerated cellular immune response involving mononuclear phagocytes and T lymphocytes

USUAL TREATMENT

- Steroids: prednisone 30–40 mg/d, tapered to 10–15 mg every other day; also chloroquine
- If steroids ineffective: methotrexate or immunosuppressive agents

ASSESSMENT POINTS

SYSTEM	EFFECT	ASSESSMENT BY HX	PE	TEST
HEENT	Involvement of nares, polyps with distorted anatomy; larynx granulomas, epiglottis, arytenoid involvement	Dyspnea Breathing difficulty	Nasal stuffiness, wheezing, hoarseness, stridor	Laryngoscopy
CV	Heart block Cor pulmonale 2° to RV enlargement	Palpitations	Arrhythmia Rales	ECG
RESP	Pulm granulomas, airway obstruction Bilateral hilar lymphadenopathy (eggshell calcifications of hilar nodes); pulm fibrosis; interstitial disease	Dyspnea Wheezing, cough	Dry rales Wheezes	CXR PFTs ($\downarrow$ vital and diffusing capacities) ABGs
GI	Liver involvement			$\uparrow$ LFTs; $\uparrow$ alkaline phosphatase
ENDO	Diabetes insipidus	Thirst		
RENAL	$\uparrow Ca^{2+}$ resorption			BUN/Cr
CNS	Nerve involvement Diabetes insipidus	Space-occupying lesions Seizures Psychiatric examination	Focal nerve deficits	

Key Reference: Newman LS, Rose CS, Maier LA: Sarcoidosis. N Engl J Med 1997; 336:1224–1234.

PERIOPERATIVE IMPLICATIONS

Preoperative Preparation
- Adequate steroid coverage

Airway
- Distortion or obstruction 2° to granulomas
- Hypoxia 2° to lung disease

Monitoring
- Observe for heart block
- Arrhythmia

ANTICIPATED PROBLEMS/CONCERNS

- Airway problems 2° to distorted anatomy
- Pulm problems 2° to lung involvement

SARCOMA

Stephan P. Nebbia, M.D.
Douglas R. Bacon, M.D.

RISK

- Osteosarcoma: 1:100,000; 2000 new cases/y in USA; 2nd decade (mean age 15)
- Soft tissue sarcoma: >20 types, 5500 new cases/y in USA, peak incidence in children and adults age 45–50 y
- Equal in male/female, all races

PERIOPERATIVE RISKS

- Morbidity and mortality related to surgical procedure
- Metastatic vital organ involvement, esp pulm, hepatic
- Mass effect, direct compression of organs, vascular structures

WORRY ABOUT

- Adriamycin-induced cardiotoxicity (global LV hypokinesis)
- Mitomycin-induced acute pulm toxicity, pulm fibrosis, ARDS with increased FIO_2
- Immunosuppression, hemorrhagic cystitis, renal failure induced by antineoplastic chemotherapeutic agents

OVERVIEW

- Malignant tumors derived from embryonic mesoderm
- Multiple types in connective tissue, muscle, fat, vasculature, neural and other tissues
- Spread aggressively by local invasion and early hematogenous spread, esp to lung

ICD-9-CM Code: 171 (depends on type)

ETIOLOGY

- Genetic factors, high-dose radiation, carcinogens (dibenzanthracene, methylcholanthrene), Maloney sarcoma virus may predispose to sarcoma
- von Recklinghausen's disease: 10–12% develop neurofibrosarcomas
- Paget's disease: 0.9% develop osteosarcoma
- Kaposi's sarcoma in AIDS patients and immunodeficient patients

USUAL TREATMENT

- Wide surgical resection
- Antineoplastic chemotherapeutic agents
- Radiation

ASSESSMENT POINTS

SYSTEM	EFFECT	ASSESSMENT BY HX	PE	TEST
CV	Atrial myxoma—ball-valve effect	Sx CHF, pulm edema	Rales S_3	CXR ECHO
	Vena caval obstruction	RV failure, CV collapse	Possible caput medusae, venous engorgement, edema	Angio
	SVC syndrome	Head, airway edema ↑ICP	Venous congestion of head and neck	Angio V/Q scan
RESP	Pulm embolus	Dyspnea		CXR, angio
GI	Gastroparesis	Early satiety		
	Bowel obstruction	Vomiting	Abdominal distention	Plain film of abdomen
	Hepatic metastases	Obstructive jaundice	Jaundice	EGD, bilirubin
	Sarcoma of ampulla of Vater	Hepatic dysfunction		
HEME	Hypercoagulable			PT/PTT
	Immunosuppressive chemotherapy	Alopecia		CBC
	Anemia, due to GI hemorrhage		Gross rectal bleeding	Guaiac
RENAL	Compression of ureters by retroperitoneal tumor	Sx uremia		BUN/Cr Renal US
CNS	CN compression	Various symptoms Dysphagia Loss of sensation, motor function	Neurologic exam	EMG
MS	Bone sarcomas	Hypercalcemia	Chvostek's	Blood Ca^{2+}
	Limb loss		sign	Albumin

Key Reference: Makela J, Kiviniemi H, Laitinen S: Prognostic factors predicting survival in the treatment of retroperitoneal sarcoma. Eur J Surg Oncol 2000; 26:552–555.

PERIOPERATIVE IMPLICATIONS

Preoperative Preparation
- Metoclopramide, sodium citrate, ranitidine in patients with gastroparesis
- Assess end-organ impairment 2° to antineoplastic chemotherapeutic agents

Monitoring
- Arterial line and CVP or PA catheter for resection of large tumors

Airway
- Risk of aspiration with large abdominal mass, or brainstem compression

Induction
- Cautious: with cardiac involvement, caval compression may have hemodynamic instability

Maintenance
- Potential CV instability

Extubation
- Awake, if at risk for aspiration

Adjuvants
- Altered pharmacokinetics with hepatic or renal involvement

Postoperative Period
- Pulm embolism, coagulopathy

ANTICIPATED PROBLEMS/CONCERNS

- Adverse effects of chemotherapeutic agents (see in Drugs section)
- Resp compromise due to pulm metastases
- Mass effect/organ compression and functional impairment
- Effects of prolonged anesthesia
- In prolonged abdominal cases; hypothermia, complications of massive transfusion

SCHIZOPHRENIA

Michael Ho, M.D.

RISK

- Incidence in USA: 2.5–4.75 million
- Estimated lifetime prevalence: 0.5–1.0%, constant worldwide
- Gender predominance: none
- First-degree biologic relative: 10× risk

PERIOPERATIVE RISKS

- Marked deterioration of function and self-care
- Surgery does not necessarily exacerbate, but rate of postop complications may be greater

WORRY ABOUT

- Uncooperative, combative, or catatonic patient
- Previously undiagnosed or poorly controlled co-existing disease
- Drug side effects and interactions

OVERVIEW

- DSM-IV: One of several psychotic disorders, all of which are delusional
- Dx based on strict criteria: hallucinations, disorganized speech, grossly disorganized or catatonic behavior, negative symptoms (decreases in affect, speech, action)
- No protection from systemic disease, including cancer, diabetes, allergies (except possibly arthritis)
- High lifetime mortality, primarily by accidents and suicide (10% of all schizophrenics complete suicide; 2–3% of all patients completing suicide are schizophrenic)
- Most devastating psychiatric illness

ICD-9-CM Code: 295.9

ETIOLOGY

- Functional hyperactivity of dopamine transmission, perhaps due to increase in D_2 receptors
  - Evidence: dopamine antagonists treat while agonists exacerbate disease
- Genetic vs. environmental factors controversial

USUAL TREATMENT

- First-line: dopamine antagonist antipsychotics (phenothiazines, butyrophenones, thioxanthenes, dihydroindolones, dibenzoxazepines)
- Side effects: extrapyramidal, anticholinergic, sedation, neuroleptic malignant syndrome (NMS)
- Prevent/Rx extrapyramidal side effects: anticholinergics, amantadine, bromocriptine, antihistamines, benzodiazepines, clonidine
- Clozapine: atypical antipsychotic (dibenzodiazepines); fewer extrapyramidal side effects, but agranulocytosis possible
- Adjuvants: benzodiazepines, lithium, antidepressants, propranolol

ASSESSMENT POINTS

SYSTEM	EFFECT	ASSESSMENT BY HX	PE	TEST
HEENT	Possible high-arched palate		Careful airway assessment	
CV	Orthostatic hypotension (α-blockade), dysrhythmias, and rare sudden death from antipsychotics	Dizziness Palpitations	Orthostasis Dysrhythmias	ECG: T-wave inversion, QT or P-R prolongation, ST-segment depression
GI	Elevation of LFTs from antipsychotics			LFTs
HEME	Leukopenia from antipsychotics			CBC
NEURO	Extrapyramidal side effects: 1. Parkinsonism 2. Acute dystonia 3. Akathisia 4. Tardive dyskinesia 5. Anticholinergic delirium 6. Sedation		1. Catatonia, rigidity, akinesia 2. Slow, sustained contractions of neck, jaw, tongue, extraocular muscles, larynx, face, body 3. Subjective discomfort leading to agitation, pacing, restlessness 4. Choreoathetoid movements of head, limbs, trunk 5. Confusion plus other anticholinergic symptoms	
GENERAL	NMS	Chronic antipsychotic use	Hyperthermia, autonomic lability, dysrhythmias Tachypnea, cyanosis, impaired consciousness	LFTs, WBC (leukocytosis), CK, UA (myoglobinuria)

Key Reference: Black DW, Andreasen NC: Schizophrenia, schizophreniform disorders, and delusional (paranoid) disorder. *In* Hales RE, Yudofsky SC, Talbott JA (eds): The American Psychiatric Press Textbook of Psychiatry. Washington, DC, American Psychiatric Press, 1994, pp 411–464.

PERIOPERATIVE IMPLICATIONS

Preoperative Preparation
- Hx may be unreliable, unobtainable
- Ensure adequate control of psychotic symptoms
- Address any tachycardia, dysrhythmias, or hemodynamic instability (rule out NMS, anticholinergic toxicity)
- Acute psychotic episode may be treated with haloperidol 2 mg IV or benzodiazepines
- Informed consent from legal guardian (unless emergency)

Monitoring
- Routine

Airway
- None

Preinduction/Induction
- No specific technique clearly superior

- Avoid drugs predisposing to tachycardia or dysrhythmias if pre-existing CV instability or dopamine antagonists (droperidol, metoclopramide)

Maintenance
- With chronic antipsychotic therapy, NMS and anticholinergic toxicity do not acutely occur intraoperatively
- Antipsychotics may alter temp regulation (predisposing to hyperthermia) and lower seizure threshold (theoretically, may want to avoid enflurane, etomidate, methohexital, ketamine)

Extubation
- Usual criteria

Adjuvants
- Rx NMS: discontinue antipsychotics, dantrolene, bromocriptine, ECT, benzodiazepines, anticholinergics

Postoperative Period
- Difficulty in assessing mental status and pain

- Discharge to home under supervision of responsible adult guardian

ANTICIPATED PROBLEMS/CONCERNS

- Anticholinergic side effects: blurred vision, mydriasis, dry mouth, mucous plugging, constipation, urinary retention, hot skin, delirium
  - Rx anticholinergic crisis: physostigmine 1–4 mg IV/IM (careful with angle-closure glaucoma, prostatic hypertrophy). Excess physostigmine risks cholinergic crisis (N/V, bradycardia, seizures), which can be treated by atropine.
- Symptoms of NMS similar to malignant hyperthermia, except onset of NMS more insidious (occurring over days) and extrapyramidal side effects present
- With antipsychotic-induced α-blockade, epinephrine may cause paradoxical hypotension due to unopposed β-mediated vasodilation

SCLERODERMA

Lee A. Fleisher, M.D.

RISK

- Incidence 20/1 million/y
- Prevalence 100–300/million
- Woman > men, 3–7:1, with higher mortality
- More severe in Native Americans and African-Americans
- 10-y survival: 60%

PERIOPERATIVE RISKS

- Severe hypotension 2° to hypovolemia
- Hypoxia 2° to pulmonary Htn and restrictive disease
- Failed intubation

WORRY ABOUT

- GI reflux
- Obliterative vasculopathy leading to pulmonary Htn
- Restrictive lung disease
- Renal crises

OVERVIEW

- Onset 35–50 y
- Chronic, systemic disease that targets skin, lungs, heart, GI, kidneys, and musculoskeletal system
- Three features: tissue fibrosis, small blood vessel vasculopathy, autoimmune response
- Two major classifications: limited and diffuse cutaneous scleroderma
- May have overlap syndromes with other rheumatic diseases

ICD-9-CM Code: 710.1 (Diffuse), 701.0 (Localized)

ETIOLOGY

- Autoimmunity, genetics, hormones, environmental factors may all play role
- Autoantibodies: antitopoisomerase in diffuse forms, anticentromere in limited form
- Twin studies suggest limited genetic role

USUAL TREATMENT

- Begin during early inflammatory stage, strategies are target-organ specific; include antifibrinolytic agents, anti-inflammatory drugs, immunosuppressive therapy, vascular drugs

ASSESSMENT POINTS

SYSTEM	EFFECT	ASSESSMENT BY HX	PE	TEST
HEENT	Cutaneous fibrosis		Masked facies Small oral aperture Atrophy of gums Hyperpigmentation	
CV	Pericardial disease Myocardial fibrosis Conduction abnormalities	DOE CHF Arrhythmia Syncope	Rales	ECHO ECG, Holter
RESP	Fibrosing alveolitis Obliterative vasculopathy Pulmonary Htn	Dyspnea Nonproductive cough		CXR PFT Bronchoalveolar lavage ECHO
GI	Esophageal fibrosis/colonic dysmotility	Difficulty chewing Dysphagia Bloating Diarrhea	Weight loss	UGI/endoscopy
RENAL	Intrinsic renal vessel disease		Malignant Htn	Proteinuria Hematuria BUN or Cr
DERM	Cutaneous fibrosis		Fibrosis of limbs Sweating Atrophy and contractures Telangiectasis	
MS	Raynaud's	Excessive cold sensitivity Pain	Cyanosis of digits	

Key Reference: Wilkes NJ, Peachey T, Beard C: Spinal anesthesia for Cesarean section in a patient with systemic sclerosis. Anaesthesia 1999; 54:1020–1026.

PERIOPERATIVE IMPLICATIONS

Preoperative Preparation

- Proton pump inhibitors to reduce gastric acid
- Consider metoclopramide for early disease
  - Less effective for late disease

Monitoring

- Invasive arterial monitoring relatively contraindicated in patients with Raynaud's disease because of risk of digit ischemia, but ABG may be indicated
- Blood pressure may be difficult because of reduced forearm blood flow
- Consider PA catheter if pulmonary Htn
- Skin temperature may be significantly lower (1.5°C) than core temperature

Anesthetic Technique

- Regional anesthesia may be preferable considering pulmonary problems
- Regional technique may be associated with prolonged block in the presence of epinephrine because of severe vasoconstriction
- May see vasomotor instability

Airway

- Pt may have severe decrease in oral aperture
- Consider awake FOB intubation
- May require nasal intubation

Preinduction/Induction

- Pt may be hypovolemic due to vasoconstriction
- Consider volume expansion
- May initially observe Htn followed by vasodilation and hypotension

Maintenance

- Usually requires mechanical ventilation because of restrictive lung disease
- Intraoperative hypoxemia may develop secondary to pulm Htn

Extubation

- May require postoperative ventilation if significant pulmonary compromise
- Pain control important for pulmonary status

ANTICIPATED PROBLEMS/CONCERNS

- Difficult airway
- Hypoxemia
- Hypotension

SCOLIOSIS AND KYPHOSIS

Ralph L. Bernstein, M.D.

RISK

- Idiopathic scoliotic curves of $>10°$ occur in 2–3% of children <16 y
- Overall female:male prevalence 3.6:1
- In severe curves (30° or greater) female:male 10:1

PERIOPERATIVE RISKS

- Neurologic damage
- Massive blood loss
- Atelectasis, pneumonia
- Ileus

WORRY ABOUT

- Neurologic damage from direct trauma or from spinal cord injury during corrections as result of interference with blood supply to spinal cord, or during positioning intubation in surgery unrelated to correction
- Adequate blood and fluid replacement
- Pulmonary insufficiency

OVERVIEW

- Curves measured by Cobb method (which draws a line from superior surface of superior end vertebra of curve and a line along the inferior surface of inferior end vertebra). Intersecting perpendicular lines are drawn from these lines to give angle of curve.

- Kyphosis—abnormal dorsal curvature of spine, flexible or rigid, treated with AP correction. Angular acute may be congenital, post-traumatic, or postinfection; may develop neurologic impairment. Treated by decompression and fusion in situ.
- In idiopathic scoliosis with curves diagnosed before age 10 y there is high risk (88%) of progression
- Progression related to growth potential, onset of menarche in girls, and skeletal age
- In patients with neuromuscular scoliosis (cerebral palsy, Friedreich's ataxia, poliomyelitis, muscular dystrophy) there are problems with swallowing, aspiration, pulm infection, poor cough, CV disease (muscular dystrophy), poor nutrition
- Progression of scoliosis may lead to cardiorespiratory problems and painful back in adulthood
- Neuromuscular patients may not be able to sit because of pelvic obliquity

ICD-9-CM Code: 737.39

See Scoliosis and Kyphosis Surgery in Procedures section

ETIOLOGY

- Idiopathic scoliosis from upper and lower motor neuron diseases and from myopathic causes
- Kyphosis (Scheuermann's type) may be metabolic, with different types of collagen in affected end-plates, and may result from juvenile osteoporosis

USUAL TREATMENT

- Bracing for mild curves
- Surgery for progressive curves involving fusion instrumentation, correction of curve, and fusion with bone grafts
- In some instances anterior (thoracolumbar) correction and fusion combined with posterior instrumentation and fusion
- In kyphosis, pain treated first with bracing, then surgery if needed
- AP fusion, acute angular decompression, and fusion in situ

ASSESSMENT POINTS

SYSTEM	EFFECT	ASSESSMENT BY HX	TEST
HEENT	Pharyngeal dysfunction Swallowing problems Poor cough in neuromuscular patients	Regurgitation on feeding, spitting Choking	
CV	Cardiomyopathy in muscular dystrophy	Dilated cardiomyopathy	ECG, ECHO, CXR ECG—abn ECG, tall R: right precordial leads Deep Q: left precordial lead
RESP	Frequent pneumonias from aspiration		CXR, PFTs in neuromuscular dystrophy
GI	Poor nutrition Underweight	Poor feeding	Serum protein, albumin measurements
HEME	Antiepileptic medication can interfere with coagulation (especially valproic acid)	Prolonged bleeding time	Bleeding time Change medication to control seizure prior to surgery

Key Reference: Bernstein RL, Rosenberg AD: Scoliosis. *In* Manual of Orthopedic Anesthesia and Related Pain Syndromes. New York, Churchill Livingstone, 1994.

PERIOPERATIVE IMPLICATIONS

Preoperative Preparation

- Idiopathic scoliosis
  - Predonation of autologous blood
- Neuromuscular scoliosis
  - Nutritional preparation—may need gastrostomy feedings to establish adequate serum protein levels. Treat resp problems. If vital capacity <30–35% of predicted, may need ventilatory assistance postop.

Monitoring

- Somatosensory evoked potentials (SSEPs), motor evoked potentials

Airway

- May need fiberoptic scope

Maintenance

- Position patient so that chest and abdomen are free from pressure, and no tension on spine

Extubation

- In patients with idiopathic scoliosis, extubation when extubation criteria met
- In patients with neuromuscular scoliosis, ventilatory support may be needed
- Weaning important as soon as possible to avoid prolonged ventilatory support—this may lead to further muscle weakness. Check neurologic status immediately.

Adjuvants

- Valproic acid may interfere with coagulation

SEIZURES, EPILEPTIC

W. Andrew Kofke, M.D.

RISK

- Incidence of epilepsy 0.5–2%; 25–30% of epileptics have seizures more often than 1/mo
- 300,000 people have medically uncontrolled epilepsy

PERIOPERATIVE RISKS

- Many rare syndromes are associated with epilepsy, which can involve disturbances in major organ systems
- Various psychiatric disorders
- Sudden death syndrome reported with epilepsy, but incidence unknown

WORRY ABOUT

- Proconvulsant and anticonvulsant properties of anesthetics
- Antiepileptic drug therapy–induced resistance to NMBs and fentanyl
- Anticonvulsant-induced blood dyscrasia and hepatitis

OVERVIEW

- Poorly controlled epilepsy results in inability to maintain normal lifestyle. Intellectual and social deficits can result from brain-damaging effect of uncontrolled recurrent seizures, negative attitudes of society, or side effects of antiepileptic drug therapy.
- Seizures are categorized as partial (simple, complex, or with generalization) or generalized (inhibitory, excitatory), pseudoseizures, or unclassified

ICD-9-CM Code: 345

ETIOLOGY

- *Congenital* often associated with other syndromes such as tuberous sclerosis, neurofibromatosis, multiple endocrine adenomatosis, Jervell–Lange-Nielsen syndrome
- *Acquired* often associated with trauma, stroke, or idiopathic causes

USUAL TREATMENT

- Antiepileptic drugs such as phenytoin, phenobarbital, clonazepam, carbamazepine, and many others
- 13% of epileptic patients are thought to be candidates for epilepsy surgery, but only about 1% actually undergo surgery

ASSESSMENT POINTS

SYSTEM	EFFECT	ASSESSMENT BY HX	PE	TEST
HEENT	Gingival hyperplasia	Phenytoin use		
CV	Cardiac tumors with tuberous sclerosis ↑ Incidence of sudden death with epilepsy (anesthetic implications unknown)	Tuberous sclerosis	Murmur possible	ECHO
RESP	Pulm involvement with neurofibromatosis	Neurofibromatosis Exercise tolerance	Cor pulmonale	CXR ECG
GI	Anticonvulsant-induced hepatitis	Anticonvulsant use	Icterus Tender RUQ	LFTs if symptomatic
ENDO	Hyponatremia	Carbamazepine use (rare)		Na^+
CNS	Tolerance to fentanyl Psychiatric disturbances	Anticonvulsant use		Assess effects of preop sedatives
MS	Tolerance to NMBs	Anticonvulsant use		Train-of-four monitoring in OR

Key Reference: Kofke WA, Tempelhoff R, Dasheiff RM: Anesthetic implications of epilepsy, status epilepticus, and epilepsy surgery. J Neurosurg Anesth 1997; 9:349–372, 1997.

PERIOPERATIVE IMPLICATIONS

Preoperative Preparation
- Assess neuropsychiatric status
- Determine antiepileptic drug history
- Assess for murmur suggestive of myocardial tumor (tuberous sclerosis) or stigmata of neurofibromatosis

Monitoring
- For seizure surgery EEG may be placed intraoperatively

Airway
- Routine considerations

Preinduction/Induction (For Epilepsy Surgery)
- GA ultrafast-acting thiobarbiturate such as thiopental. If intraoperative EEG, etomidate or methohexital suitable alternative.
- For conscious analgesia craniotomy: position determined with protection of pressure points. O$_2$ delivered by nasal prongs with capnography and impedance resp monitor. Fentanyl 0.5–0.75 μg/kg and droperidol 0.15 mg/kg. Local anesthetic injected before surgical incision.

Maintenance
- If intraoperative EEG not planned, use an anticonvulsant anesthetic maintenance regimen such as isoflurane with or without nitrous oxide or moderate-dose opioid
- For GA with intraoperative EEG, N$_2$O-narcotic techniques with avoidance of both isoflurane and halothane. Enflurane produces high-voltage spikes on EEG; has been used to synchronize and activate epileptogenic foci. Methohexital, 25–50 mg, alfentanil, 50–100 μg, and remifentanil, 2.5 μg/kg, have been used as activating agents.
- For conscious analgesia continued titrated sedation during painful parts of procedure anticipated with fentanyl

Extubation
- NMB agents and narcotics may not last as long as expected, with unanticipated coughing as procedure comes to close

Adjuvants
- Muscle relaxants: ↓ effect with antiepileptic drugs

- Opioids: tolerance with antiepileptic drug therapy
- Most anesthetics have potential to precipitate seizures during or *after* surgery
- Antiepileptic drug levels can be significantly affected by anesthetics, changes in body physiology, and prolonged NPO status

Postoperative Period
- Blood levels of antiepileptic drugs can be unpredictable, and parenteral antiepileptic drugs such as phenytoin or phenobarbital may be required
- Numerous case reports of postop seizures with a variety of anesthetics suggest concern for this possibility

ANTICIPATED PROBLEMS/CONCERNS

- Blood levels of antiepileptic drugs can be significantly affected by anesthetics, changes in physiology, and prolonged NPO status
- Opioid tolerance may result in increased need for pain medication

SEIZURES, GRAND MAL (TONIC-CLONIC)

Marek A. Mirski, M.D., Ph.D.

RISK

- 500,000–1,000,000 in USA with recurrent tonic-clonic seizures
- 10–20 million at risk to have one tonic-clonic seizure 2° to alcohol withdrawal, febrile convulsions (in children), CNS pathology, metabolic disturbances

PERIOPERATIVE RISKS

- Intraoperative and postop seizures
- Status epilepticus (unrecognized intraoperatively)
- Delayed awakening
- Todd's paralysis
- Pulmonary aspiration
- Transient hypoxemia, tachycardia, Htn
- ↑ ICP

WORRY ABOUT

- Check serum anticonvulsant levels preop, consider free vs. total serum phenytoin levels in nutritionally depleted patients. May be best to normalize low serum levels preop.
- Caution with intraoperative IV phenytoin (hypotension, 50 μg/min limit) or phenobarbital (somnolence)

- Prudent to avoid drugs that may lower seizure threshold: tricyclics, ?etomidate, ketamine

OVERVIEW

- Although typically a benign event, trauma to head or extremities is common if precautions not taken (padded hospital bed). May lead to status epilepticus, a life-threatening condition requiring active and immediate intervention to terminate attack before cerebral injury results (30–60 min). Subtherapeutic anticonvulsant serum levels and alcohol withdrawal most commonly provoke status epilepticus.
- During seizures and postictally, airway reflexes are typically preserved—intubation *not* indicated unless aspiration is strongly suspected
- Postictally, enhancement of previous neurologic motor deficit is common (Todd's paralysis) for hours after seizure

ICD-9-CM Code: 345.3

ETIOLOGY

- Leading cause (30%) is idiopathic; undetermined fraction have genetic predisposition
- Acquired—2° to congenital defects, perinatal asphyxia, trauma, CNS infection, drug withdrawal (alcohol most common), metabolic pathology resulting in low Na^+, Ca^{2+}, or Mg^{2+} or ↑ BUN

USUAL TREATMENT

- For one seizure, no therapy required. Check serum anticonvulsant levels.
- For recurrent or prolonged seizures: IV midazolam 1–3 mg, diazepam 5–10 mg. Alternatively, thiopental 50–100 mg/70 kg, propofol 1 mg/kg. Ventilatory assistance should be available for greater dosage requirements.
- To prevent recurrence, IV phenytoin should be considered to reach serum target level of 10–20 μg/dl (15–20 mg/kg load in patient not currently taking phenytoin)

ASSESSMENT POINTS

SYSTEM	EFFECT	ASSESSMENT BY HX	PE	TEST
HEENT	Gingival hyperplasia (phenytoin) Seizure-induced oral trauma		Oral exam	
CV	Drug-induced SIADH (carbamazepine) Thrombocytopenia (several drugs)			CBC, electrolytes
RESP	Aspiration pneumonia	SOB, fever, supplemental O_2	Auscultation	CXR, O_2 sat ABGs, sputum culture
GI	Poor absorption of anticonvulsant Drug-induced increase of hepatic P450 Drug-induced transaminase elevation	Low serum levels Increase dosage requirement of various drugs		Drug levels
CNS	Postictal somnolence Possible multiple CNS abnormalities	Developmental Hx	Cognitive, motor	
MS	Seizure-induced focal injury			

Key Reference: Kofke WA, Tempelhoff R, Dasheiff RM: Anesthetic implications of epilepsy, status epilepticus, and epilepsy surgery. J Neurosurg Anesthesiol 1997; 9:349–372.

PERIOPERATIVE IMPLICATIONS

Preoperative Preparation

- Ensure therapeutic anticonvulsant levels
- Provide protection from injury should seizure occur

Monitoring

- Routine
- EEG postop if poor emergence observed

Airway

- Evaluate for past seizure-induced oral trauma
- Gingival hyperplasia (phenytoin)

Induction

- Standard induction drugs provide anticonvulsant action
- Benzodiazepines useful adjunct

Maintenance

- CV changes may be indicative of seizure

Extubation

- Extubate awake if possible
- Delayed emergence could signal postictal state or status epilepticus—EEG suggested

Adjuvants

- Anticonvulsants for acute seizure: IV benzodiazepines, propofol, barbiturates
- Load with phenytoin or barbiturate; oral drugs less reliable absorption
- Muscle relaxant doses altered by some anticonvulsants

Postoperative Period

- Check serum anticonvulsant levels
- EEG indicated if postop level of arousal not as expected

ANTICIPATED PROBLEMS/CONCERNS

- Clinical seizure preinduction—injury and aspiration risk if sedative drugs given
- Intraoperative seizure with consequent delayed emergence
- Subclinical or convulsive status epilepticus

SEIZURES, INTRACTABLE

René Tempelhoff, M.D.

RISK

- People within USA: 600,000 epileptics/y have uncontrolled seizures
- Racial predominance: none

PERIOPERATIVE RISKS

- Sudden death
- Status epilepticus
- Seizure-mediated cardiac dysrhythmias

WORRY ABOUT

- Liver toxicity from anticonvulsants
- Perioperative trauma from convulsions
- Sudden death
- Status epilepticus postoperatively
- Altered pharmacologic responses due to chronic drug therapy

OVERVIEW

- Neurologic disease associated with birth, congenital malformation, trauma, CNS pathology, idiopathic
- Perioperative risks increased for acquired seizure disorder, but furthermore some epilepsy/congenital malformations carry their own anesthetic risks
- Check type of seizures, clinical manifestations, duration, frequency
- Anticonvulsant therapy and side effects (liver function, level of consciousness)

ICD-9-CM Code: 780.3 (Seizure, recurrent)

ETIOLOGY

- Congenital (e.g., tuberous sclerosis/infantile seizure)
- Idiopathic
- CNS pathology: trauma, tumor, hemorrhage

USUAL TREATMENT

- Anticonvulsant and diet
- Surgery for ablation of foci
- GA regarded as a last resort for seizure that is unresponsive to sedative-hypnotics and resulting in decrease in consciousness or significant (< 7.28) metabolic acidosis

ASSESSMENT POINTS

SYSTEM	EFFECT	ASSESSMENT BY HX	PE	TEST
HEENT	Tongue biting/swallowing		Airway assessment	
CV	Cardiac dysrhythmias	Syncope Tachycardia		ECG ECHO Holter
RESP	Hyperventilation due to metabolic acidosis			ABGs
GI	Altered liver function Anticonvulsant toxicity Tuberous sclerosis		Jaundice	LFTs Anticonvulsant levels
ENDO	Associated multiple endocrine adenomatosis			Glucose Ca^{2+}, thyroid function tests
RENAL	Renal dysfunction Tuberous sclerosis			Cr
CNS	Psychiatric problems CNS pathology			
MS	Occult trauma from seizures		Check joints, bones Examine tongue	

Key Reference: Kofke WA, Tempelhoff R, Dasheiff RM: Anesthesia for epileptic patients and epileptic surgery. *In* Anesthesia and Neurosurgery, 3rd ed. St. Louis, CV Mosby, 1994, pp 495–520.

PERIOPERATIVE IMPLICATIONS

Preoperative Preparation

- Usual anticonvulsant regimen

Monitoring

- Routine monitors
- End-tidal CO_2: increase in CO_2 production could be indirect sign of seizure
- Consider EEG monitoring

Induction

- Have sodium thiopental and/or benzodiazepines to treat possible seizures
- Significantly higher requirement for nondepolarizing muscle relaxants and narcotics

Maintenance

- Avoid proconvulsants (ketamine, etomidate, enflurane, and probably sevoflurane)
- Continue scheduled anticonvulsants
- GA is sometimes used as treatment for status epilepticus

Extubation

- To be delayed in case of doubt or situation such as:
  – High end-tidal CO_2 despite adequate ventilation can be a sign of active seizure
    – Patient nonresponsive
    – Obvious convulsions
- Consider adding anticonvulsant (benzodiazepines) and ordering EEG

Adjuvants

- See specific anticonvulsant used

Postoperative Period

- Watch end-tidal CO_2 on awakening, as high production may indicate seizure activity
- Resume anticonvulsants
- Treat seizures ad lib

ANTICIPATED PROBLEMS/CONCERNS

- Seizures on induction and awakening are treated with first-line benzodiazepine Rx (e.g., lorazepam) rather than long-acting drugs (e.g., phenytoin)
- Evolution to status epilepticus: GA?
- Sudden death (ventricular arrhythmias?)

SEIZURES, PETIT MAL (ABSENCE)

Marek A. Mirski, M.D., Ph.D.

- Approximately 75,000–100,000 in USA
- Pure cases almost exclusively a risk in children, with age at onset 4–10 y

PERIOPERATIVE RISKS

- Few. Risk of transition of petit mal absence seizures into tonic-clonic seizures or status epilepticus is exceedingly low.

WORRY ABOUT

- Maintenance of serum anticonvulsant levels
- Inducing seizures with hyperventilation

OVERVIEW

- Relatively common seizure of childhood
- Seizure typified by brief absence (5–20 sec) with impairment of consciousness, 3/sec spike-wave EEG, mild facial motor manifestations
- Attacks may be few or occur > 100/d
- Hyperventilation and bright flickering lights are common triggers
- "Atypical absence" seizures may have more motor features and be of longer duration
- Trauma from seizures rare, axial posture almost never affected
- No postictal sequelae; EEG and level of awareness return immediately
- Spontaneous resolution frequent in adolescence (25–30%); ~ 50% go on to develop tonic-clonic seizures

ICD-9-CM Code: 345.2

ETIOLOGY

- Strong genetic predisposition in otherwise normal children
- Structural lesions in adults

USUAL TREATMENT

- Valproic acid (VPA) or ethosuximide (ESM) is drug of choice
- No emergent therapy required unless other seizure type present

ASSESSMENT POINTS

SYSTEM	EFFECT	ASSESSMENT BY HX	PE	TEST
CV	Mild thrombocytopenia (VPA) Pancytopenia (ESM)			CBC with platelet count
RESP	Hyperventilation may induce seizure			
GI	↑ Liver enzymes (ESM, VPA) GI upset (VPA) Hepatotoxicity (VPA—rare > age 2 y)	GI Sx		SGPT, SGOT
CNS	EEG typically normal between seizures Normal development is rule			EEG
MS	Mild myoclonic movements		Movements	

Key Reference: Kofke WA, Tempelhoff R, Dasheiff RM: Anesthetic implications of epilepsy, status epilepticus, and epilepsy surgery. J Neurosurg Anesthesiol 1997; 9:349–372.

PERIOPERATIVE IMPLICATIONS

Preoperative Preparation

- Continue anticonvulsant therapy
- Verify adequate anticonvulsant levels: ESM 40–100 μg/ml, VPA >50 μg/ml (variable)

Monitoring

- No issues

Airway

- No issues

Preinduction/Induction

- Avoid bright flashing lights and hyperventilation

Maintenance

- Normocarbia unless otherwise indicated

Extubation

- Normocarbia

Adjuvants

- Muscle relaxant action is affected by some agents used to treat petit mal seizures

Postoperative Period

- Pain management beneficial if it results in avoidance of stress-induced hyperventilation

ANTICIPATED PROBLEMS/CONCERNS

- Major perioperative morbidity rare
- Major concern is to document if other seizure types, such as tonic-clonic seizures, occur, which *would* affect perioperative risk

SEPTIC HYPERDYNAMIC SHOCK; SYSTEMIC INFLAMMATORY RESPONSE SYNDROME (SIRS)

Myer H. Rosenthal, M.D.

RISK

- Incidence in USA: unknown
- All ages; more frequent and less well tolerated in elderly
- Males = females

PERIOPERATIVE RISKS

- Splanchnic circulatory insufficiency leading to increased bowel permeability and reticuloendothelial dysfunction with endotoxemia
- Organ hypoperfusion and release of variety of cytokines causing ARDS and MODS

WORRY ABOUT

- Worsening hypotension, vital organ hypoperfusion, and metabolic acidosis
- Development of ARDS or MODS from release of cytokines leads to capillary permeability, intravascular hypovolemia, and cell death; ATN and hepatic, myocardial, and cerebral insufficiency 2° to free radical destruction

OVERVIEW

- Failure of heart to pump blood into aorta in sufficient quantity and under sufficient pressure to maintain adequate tissue perfusion
- Initiating pathophysiologic response is reduction in SVR, often accompanied by compensatory rise in cardiac index, in an attempt to maintain satisfactory systemic perfusion
- Initial reduction in SVR complicated by impaired preload (hypovolemia), due to vasodilation, ↑ vascular permeability, and hypocontractility (cardiac failure), due to coronary hypoperfusion, β-adrenergic receptor hyporesponsiveness, direct negative inotropic effect of bacterial toxins and humoral mediators

ICD-9-CM Code: 785.59

ETIOLOGY

- Any microorganism may initiate sepsis
- SIRS produced by septic process with liberation of a variety of vasoactive humoral factors
- Common with splanchnic circulatory insufficiency that can accompany major abdominal, vascular, or bowel surgery or pathology. Failure of bowel or hepatic perfusion and low oxygen tension in bowel wall lead to ↑ bowel permeability and reticuloendothelial dysfunction with resultant endotoxemia. Pathophysiologic changes similar to those seen with hyperdynamic shock—decrease SVR.

ASSESSMENT POINTS

SYSTEM	EFFECT	ASSESSMENT BY HX	PE	TEST
CV	Vasodilation ↑ Capillary permeability Hypoperfusion, hypovolemia, hypocontractility	Edematous, yet signs of organ hypoperfusion, cold extremities, infection	BP lying and standing Degree of vasoconstriction, HR, obtundation, tachypnea	PAOP, CVP, CO, SVR ECHO Lactate, ABGs
GI	Hepatic/GI insufficiency Vomiting Diarrhea	Bowel habits		Gastric mucosal pH, temperature
HEME	Infection; hemodilution; hemolysis; thrombocytopenia; DIC	Immunocompromised bleeding, febrile	Warm, full pulses; petechiae; bleeding	WBC with differential, Hct, cultures, coagulation studies
RENAL	ATN, oliguria, anuria	UO		↑ BUN, Cr, inactive excretion of Na$^+$
METAB	Acidosis 2° to inadequate tissue perfusion		Tachypnea Mottled extremities	ABGs Lactate
RESP	Tachypnea, hypoxemia, increased work of breathing		Cyanosis Tachypnea Fatigue	ABGs
CNS	Hypoperfusion Acidosis Obtundation	Level of consciousness	Somnolent Obtunded Confused, comatose	

Key Reference: Muret J, Marie C, Payen D, Cavaillon JM: Ex vivo T-lymphocyte derived cytokine production in SIRS patients is influenced by experimental procedures. Shock 2000; 13:169–174.

PERIOPERATIVE IMPLICATIONS

Preoperative Preparations
- Ensure optimal perfusion to organs—possible within context of removing infective agent
- Aggressive invasive hemodynamic monitoring
- Optimize preload
- Evaluate and optimize oxygenation
- Verify ventilator settings and line positions

Monitoring
- Consider need to assess preload, SVR, and CO (PA catheter or TEE) and arterial (± mixed venous) blood gas tensions
- Consider Foley catheter

Airway
- No special considerations

Induction
- If MAP < 65 mmHg, consider fluids if PAOP < 15 mmHg, or inotropes if PAOP > 15 mmHg, or vasoconstrictor if CI > 4.50 L/min/m^2

Maintenance
- Selection of optimal inotropic therapy controversial with support for dopamine (DA), epinephrine (EPI) and dobutamine (DOB)
- Factors including ↓ enzymatic conversion of DA to EPI, β-receptor hyporesponsiveness, and pre-existing vasodilation favor a predictable potent β-adrenergic agonist without vasodilator properties, namely EPI at a dose range 20–175 ng/kg/min. Routine therapy to produce supranormal values for oxygen delivery and CI based on anecdotal reports. However, inconsistent results with one report using DOB resulting in ↑ mortality compared with controls not treated to supranormal levels. Adequate oxygen delivery must guide therapy.
- Consider avoiding agents with vasodilator and negative inotropic properties
- If using agents with α_1 vasoconstrictor effect, consider dopamine at 2–3 µg/kg/min to avoid renal hypoperfusion

Extubation/Postoperative Period
- Consider hemodynamic and acid-base status
- Verify infusion rates/ventilator/lines prior to and after transport

Adjuvants
- Consider renal status before administering drug dependent on kidney for excretion

ANTICIPATED PROBLEMS/CONCERNS
- Necessity for aggressive surgical drainage of infected foci may require anesthetic administration to a patient with hyperdynamic shock

SHY-DRAGER DISEASE

Lisa A. Caramico, M.D.

Lisa A. Caramico, M.D.

RISK

- More common in men than women
- Symptoms begin in 5th–7th decades

PERIOPERATIVE RISKS

- Autonomic dysfunction with CV collapse
- Aspiration risk

WORRY ABOUT

- Orthostatic hypotension
- Obstructive sleep apnea—found in advanced stages
- Vocal cord paralysis—found in advanced stages

OVERVIEW

- A parkinsonism-plus syndrome
- Clinical manifestations include orthostatic hypotension, parkinsonian symptoms, urinary and bowel dysfunction, impaired potency and libido, and decreased sweating
- Pathologic changes include widespread degeneration of CNS
- Irreversible progressive neurodegenerative disease primarily with autonomic failure
- Death often occurs 7–8 y after onset of symptoms
- Difficult to treat the parkinsonian symptoms as dopaminergic drugs may exacerbate orthostatic hypotension

ICD-9-CM Code: 333.0

ETIOLOGY

- Unknown

USUAL TREATMENT

- Symptomatic relief of orthostatic hypotension
- Liberal salt intake
- Fludrocortisone
- Elastic stockings
- Midodrine—peripheral α-adrenergic agonist
- Sympathomimetics—ephedrine
- Prostaglandin inhibitors—indomethacin, ibuprofen
- MAO inhibitors
- Common to also receive antiparkinsonian drugs

ASSESSMENT POINTS

SYSTEM	EFFECT	ASSESSMENT BY HX	PE	TEST
HEENT	Vocal cord paralysis Obstructive sleep apnea	Obstruction; apnea episodes; stridor; snoring; dysphonia; dysarthria	Bilateral abductor paralysis	Direct laryngoscopy Nasoendoscopy
CV	Orthostatic hypotension Fixed HR	Syncope; dizziness	Postural changes in BP	Tilt table test ECG
RESP	Irregular resp			
GI	Gastroparesis Fecal incontinence, diarrhea, constipation, sodium loss	Early satiety, dysphagia	Loss of rectal sphincter tone	Electrolytes
GU	Urinary incontinence	Nocturia Sexual impotence Atonic bladder		
CNS	Parkinsonian symptoms Anhidrosis Heat intolerance		Cogwheel rigidity Shuffling gait Anisocoria Horner's syndrome	
MS	Osteoporosis and aseptic necrosis (may be associated with autonomic dysfunction)		Muscle atrophy Fasciculations	

Key Reference: Niquille M, Van Gessel E, Gamulin Z: Continuous spinal anesthesia for hip surgery in a patient with Shy-Drager syndrome. Anesth Analg 1998; 87:396–399.

PERIOPERATIVE IMPLICATIONS

Preoperative Preparation

- Reduce venous pooling; increase peripheral vascular resistance; increase plasma volume. Care must by taken using these techniques in the attempt to decrease postural hypotension, as fluid overload can occur.

Monitoring

- Arterial and central venous catheters if fluid shifts likely to guide fluid replacement
- Temp—reduced sweating may lead to elevations in temp

Airway

- Vocal cord paralysis and dysautonomia with gastroparesis may make awake intubation the more desirable choice

Preinduction/Induction

- Consider steroid supplementation if on fludrocortisone
- Consider effects of MAO inhibitors
- Avoid agents that may cause a decrease in cardiac output, decrease in HR, or vasodilatation, as profound hypotension may occur

Maintenance

- IPPV may cause a decrease in venous return and exaggerate hypotension
- Norepinephrine stores at the nerve endings may be reduced. Therefore, the response to adrenergic drugs may be reduced or exaggerated: Use direct-acting drugs in small doses titrated to effect.
- Atropine may not increase the HR owing to parasympathetic deficiency

Extubation

- Awake

Postoperative Period

- Autonomic dysfunction

ANTICIPATED PROBLEMS/CONCERNS

- Autonomic dysfunction with CV collapse
- Aspiration risk

SICK SINUS SYNDROME (SSS)

John L. Atlee, M.D.

RISK

- Acquired condition resulting from aging in association with CAD or cardiomyopathies
- Incidence unknown. More common indication for permanent pacing than AV heart block.
- Gender or racial predominance: none
- Usually develops in 6th–7th decades but can occur sooner

PERIOPERATIVE RISKS

- Circulatory insufficiency 2° to sinus bradycardia, escape rhythms, or bradycardia with SA or AV heart block
- Association of sinus node dysfunction with paroxysmal atrial tachyarrhythmias (bradycardia-tachycardia syndrome), esp AFLT/AFIB, but also atrial tachycardia and re-entrant SVT

WORRY ABOUT

- Associated coronary heart disease or cardiomyopathy in >1/2 of patients with SSS
- Thromboembolism and stroke in patients with SSS and AFLT/AFIB

OVERVIEW

- In symptomatic patients with SSS, lightheadedness, dizziness, and syncope (when due to arrhythmias) are usually caused by bradyarrhythmias. Palpitations are usually produced by tachyarrhythmias and suggest the presence of the bradycardia-tachycardia syndrome. Patients may also complain of angina or have symptoms suggestive of heart failure.
- Antiarrhythmic drugs used to control tachyarrhythmias may aggravate bradycardia or ↑ asystolic sinus pauses following spontaneous termination of tachycardia

ICD-9-CM Code: 427.81

ETIOLOGY

- Atrophy or fibrous degeneration of the sinus node and extensive lesions, including fatty infiltration, of the approaches to the SA and AV nodes. Inflammatory or degenerative changes of the nerves and ganglia surrounding the SA node.
- Extrinsic causes for SA node dysfunction include autonomic reflexes, hypothermia, and effects of drugs. In the absence of intrinsic SA node dysfunction, anesthetics should not cause severe bradycardia.

USUAL TREATMENT

- Chronotropes (atropine, ephedrine, isoproterenol) to increase sinus rate
- Temporary or permanent pacing for bradycardia and to suppress tachyarrhythmias
- Systemic anticoagulation for patients with chronic AFLT/AFIB

ASSESSMENT POINTS

SYSTEM	EFFECT	ASSESSMENT BY HX	PE	TEST
CV	Arrhythmias	Palpitations, dizziness, syncope, fatigue, lethargy	Pulse too slow, fast, or irregular	ECG, Holter monitoring Electrophysiologic studies
	Structural HD	Exercise intolerance, dyspnea, fatigue, angina	S_3, rales, wheezes	ECHO Reperfusion scintigraphy Coronary angio
	Implanted pacemaker	Sx suggesting device malfunction	Suppressed pacemaker	Pacing system analyzer, programmer, or vagal maneuvers to ascertain function
RESP	CHF, COPD	Dyspnea, orthopnea, cough	S_3, rales, wheezes	CXR
GI	Hypoperfusion	GI distress, diarrhea		
RENAL	Hypoperfusion	Polyuria		BUN/Cr
CNS	Ischemia/stroke	Syncope episodes, paralysis, dementia	Neurologic or mental deficits	See CV assessment

Key Reference: Kastor JA: Arrhythmias, 2nd ed. Philadelphia, WB Saunders, 2000, pp 566–591.

PERIOPERATIVE IMPLICATIONS

Preoperative Preparation

- Consider temporary pacing for patient without pacemaker and symptomatic bradycardia
- Patient with a pacemaker: deactivate adaptive-rate pacing feature; reprogram to an asynchronous mode if electrocautery or other electromagnetic interference likely to alter device function. Have device function checked after surgery.
- If acute onset AFIB/AFLT (≤3 days), consider cardioversion and anticoagulation

Monitoring

- ECG with ST-T trending; strip-chart recorder
- Consider direct arterial pressure and PA catheter monitoring with significant ventricular dysfunction
- For patient with pacemaker, monitor pulse waveform to detect device inhibition

Induction

- AFLT/AFIB or severe bradycardia with significant ventricular dysfunction ↑ risk of untoward circulatory dynamics
- Caution with agents such as thiopental or propofol
- Desflurane, ketamine, and pancuronium may accelerate ventricular rate with AFLT/AFIB
- Expect ↑ circulatory lability due to bradycardia or paroxysmal tachycardia

Maintenance

- With associated ventricular dysfunction, less tolerance of large fluid shifts or blood loss
- No anesthetics especially contraindicated, but caution with drugs that slow sinus rate
- Hyperdynamic circulation in response to catecholamine surge (surgical stress, airway stimulation) may ↑ risk for paroxysmal tachyarrhythmias and thromboembolic phenomenon

Adjuvants

- Do not rely on atropine to increase sinus rate; direct-acting β-adrenergic agonists are more reliable
- Use Ca^{2+}-channel blocker or β-blocker, not digitalis, for ventricular rate reduction with AFLT/AFIB

Postoperative Period

- Susceptibility to bradycardia and escape rhythms or paroxysmal tachyarrhythmias does not decrease

ANTICIPATED PROBLEMS/CONCERNS

- Chronotropes used to treat bradycardia may be ineffective or cause paroxysmal tachyarrhythmias
- Perioperative pacemaker malfunction in patients with permanent pacemakers

SICKLE CELL DISEASE

William A. McDade, M.D., Ph.D.

RISK

- Affects persons with ancestors from areas endemic for falciparum malaria: Greeks, Turks, Italians, Arabs, Asian Indians, Africans
- In USA, 1/500 African-Americans (0.2%) have sickle cell anemia
- Early mortality—median age of death in men is 42 y and in women is 48 y

PERIOPERATIVE RISKS

- Patients have 30% overall complication rate; risk decreases with increased levels of fetal Hgb
- Complications include anemia, stroke, acute chest syndrome, myonecrosis, heart failure, MI, hepatic or splenic sequestration, retinal hemorrhage, hematuria, renal failure, atelectasis and pneumonia, new-onset tonic-clonic seizure, intraoperative stasis and hypotension, wound infection, urinary tract infection, unexplained death

WORRY ABOUT

- Degree of anemia, dehydration, sepsis, stress, acid-base status, hypoxemia
- Percentage of HbSS-containing cells
- Postop atelectasis and pneumonia
- Previous renal or heart failure

- Precipitation of vaso-occlusive crisis
- Risk of hemolytic transfusion reaction due to alloimmunization

OVERVIEW

- Lifelong cause of painful vaso-occlusive episodes
- Average rate of painful episodes per patient-year is 0.8
- 5.2% of patients with 3–10 episodes/y account for 33% of all episodes
- Mortality positively correlates with increased pain rate in adults
- Only Hct and percentage of fetal Hgb have predictive value in defining risk of painful crisis
- End-organ damage due to vaso-occlusion causes morbidity and mortality. Key conditions are pregnancy, heart failure, MI, CVA, acute chest syndrome, sequestration crisis, and severe anemia.
- Enhanced O_2 delivery by sickle Hgb causes rightward shift (P50 = 31 mmHg) of oxyhemoglobin dissociation curve
- Inherited hemoglobinopathy permits deoxygenated Hgb molecules to polymerize into rigid insoluble intraerythrocytic fibers, resulting in sickled cells

- Organ damage is due to vaso-occlusive ischemia, which occurs because the sickled cells are unable to traverse narrow capillary beds, leading to distal blood flow impairment. Also, there is an enhanced tendency for sickle cells to adhere to the endothelium and cause release of vasoactive substances.

ICD-9-CM Code: 282.60

See also Sickle Cell Trait in Diseases section

ETIOLOGY

- Molecular lesion is on β-chain of Hgb at position 6 glu → val
- Sickle erythrocytes are more fragile with shortened life span, which leads to chronic hemolysis and anemia

USUAL TREATMENT

- Vaccines against pneumococcus and *Haemophilus influenzae* type b, and prophylactic penicillin therapy effective in autosplenectomized patients
- Palliative care for painful crisis
- Simple and exchange transfusions
- Hydroxyurea to increase fetal Hgb

ASSESSMENT POINTS

SYSTEM	EFFECT	ASSESSMENT BY HX	PE	TEST
HEENT	Hypoxemia due to sleep apnea	Snoring or sleep apnea Hx	Tonsillar hypertrophy	ABGs
CV	MI; LV and RV dysfunction; CHF	Angina Sx; poor exercise tolerance; dyspnea	Displaced PMI S_3, S_4	ECG, exercise ECG; ECHO, Hct
RESP	Acute chest syndrome; lung and rib infarction; pneumonia	Previous acute chest syndrome; dyspnea	Point tenderness over rib; rales; crackles	CXR
GI	Gallstones; sickle girdle syndrome (mesenteric ischemia); hepatic sequestration crisis	RUQ pain; abdominal pain	Jaundice; RUQ tenderness	Bilirubin
HEME	Sickle pain crisis; asplenia or splenic sequestration crisis; anemia; infection	Pain in affected areas; fatigue; sepsis	Pallor; splenic enlargement; flank tenderness; fever	Hgb, Hct, WBC, % HbSS Electrophoresis
RENAL	Renal failure and insufficiency	Hematuria; hemodialysis Hx		UA, BUN, Serum Cr
REPROD	Preterm labor and delivery; perinatal mortality; placenta previa; abruptio placentae	Vaginal bleeding		US
CNS	Stroke; intracranial hemorrhage; pneumococcal meningitis; retinopathy and hyphema; seizure	Previous CNS Sx (weakness, TIA, or neurologic dysfunction); headache; vomiting or altered mental status	Focal deficits, stupor or coma; nuchal rigidity	Head CT; EEG
MS	Leg ulcers; myonecrosis; myofibrosis; infant hand-foot syndrome; shoulder or hip avascular necrosis; osteomyelitis	Pain in affected areas	ROM; skin changes; fever	WBC, UA, x-ray

Key Reference: Vichinsky EP, Haberkern CM, Neumayr L, et al: A comparison of conservative and aggressive transfusion regimens in the perioperative management of sickle cell disease. N Engl J Med 1995; 333:206–213.

PERIOPERATIVE IMPLICATIONS

Preoperative Preparation

- Latest data suggest there is no benefit in exchange transfusion preop. Rather, transfuse to a Hgb of 10 g/dl, independent of HbSS percent, with HbAA erythrocytes using extended matched transfusions (minor group E, K, C, Fya).
- Alkalinization has no benefit
- Autotransfusion—predonated units and Hgb-based O_2 carriers remain of unestablished efficacy
- Venous access may be difficult and a central line or implantable reservoir is useful
- Preop hydration for 12 h preceding surgery

Monitoring

- Routine
- If PA catheter indicated due to co-morbidity and surgical setting, an oximetric catheter is

useful in providing continuous mixed venous blood Po_2 sat for assessment of oxygen utilization and delivery

Airway

- None

Induction

- Avoid oversedation, which may decrease respiration and lead to hypoxemia
- Avoid hypovolemia
- Retrobulbar blocks appear safe
- No differences in morbidity or mortality shown among various anesthetic agents or between regional and GA techniques

Maintenance

- Cardiopulmonary bypass presents special problems causing dilutional anemia, mechanical hemolysis, hypothermia, low-flow state, and plt activation

- Tourniquet use is relatively contraindicated, but unproven to show ↑ risk for sickle patients

Extubation

- Analgesic-induced resp depression at extubation may contribute to atelectasis, pulm infections, and hypoxemia

Postoperative Period

- Adequate hydration; analgesia; pulmonary toilet, including incentive spirometry; supplemental oxygen therapy for 12–48 h postop

ANTICIPATED PROBLEMS/CONCERNS

- All blood transfusions in these patients carry high risk for hemolytic reaction due to previous exposure
- Avoid all situations leading to hypoxemia, hypovolemia, or stasis

SICKLE CELL TRAIT

Michael F. Roizen, M.D.

ICD-9-CM Code: 282.5

RISK

- People within USA: 2.5 million
- Race with highest prevalence: African-Americans

PERIOPERATIVE RISKS

- Increased risk of complications following CABG
- Perioperative mortality rate in published cases of SA trait is 0.8%
- Some increased risk of CVA and pulmonary infection but not well quantified

WORRY ABOUT

- Increased risk of vaso-occlusive phenomenon with hypoxia and stress

OVERVIEW

- Is not a disease
- Is not a cause of abnormalities in blood count
- Does not produce vaso-occlusive symptoms under physiologic conditions—painful crisis not a hallmark or concomitant of condition
- Does not adversely affect individual's life expectancy
- Dx established by Hgb electrophoresis

ICD-9-CM Code: 282.5

See also Sickle Cell Disease in Diseases section

ETIOLOGY

- Heterozygous in which individual has one beta S and beta A globin gene (SA disease)

USUAL TREATMENT

- None, except iron supplementation (debated)

ASSESSMENT POINTS

SYSTEM	EFFECT	ASSESSMENT BY HX	TEST
RESP	Pulm embolism		
HEME	Hgb level usually 13–15 g/dl	Hx SOB: poor exercise tolerance 10–40% of Hgb S—same cells as Hgb A	Hgb
GU	Painless hematuria and bacteriuria; pyelonephritis (especially with pregnancy)		UA (culture if prosthesis planned)
CNS	Stroke	Migraine headache	

Key Reference: Djaiani GN, Cheng DC, Carroll JA, Yudin M, Karski JM: Fast track cardiac anesthesia in patients with sickle cell abnormalities. Anesth Analg 1999; 89:598–603.

PERIOPERATIVE IMPLICATIONS

Preoperative Preparation
- Warm room
- Consider prehydration

Monitoring
- Temperature

Airway
- Occasionally distorted anatomy 2° to extramedullary erythropoiesis
- Sinusitis possible
- Prehydrate liberally if CV status will tolerate

Induction
- Routine

Maintenance
- Keep warm
- Keep vasodilated
- Keep without stasis
- High O_2 content

Extubation
- Keep warm

Adjuvants
- Vary if hepatic or renal insufficiency exists

Postoperative Period
- Aggressively prevent pain, hypovolemia, and hypothermia

ANTICIPATED PROBLEMS/CONCERNS

- Stroke and/or pulm emboli or infection have been reported after CPB. Five of 544 patients in literature of sickle trait disease died perioperatively.

SILICOSIS

Karen B. Domino, M.D., M.P.H.

RISK

- Occupational exposure to respirable dust containing crystalline free silica or crystalline quartz
- Males >> females
- No racial predominance
- Potential number of exposed workers: 1.2 to 3 million people, but with use of protection devices, disease is rare

PERIOPERATIVE RISKS

- Increased risk of hypoxemia, bronchospasm, pneumothorax, atelectasis, chronic bronchitis, pneumonia, mycobacterial and fungal pulm infection, and perioperative resp failure
- Pulmonary Htn and cor pulmonale

WORRY ABOUT

- Resp failure and increased risk of pulm infection, especially after abdominal and thoracic surgery
- Cor pulmonale

OVERVIEW

- Pulm fibrosis (silicosis) develops after chronic occupational exposure
- Primarily restrictive changes in pulm function (stiff lungs with reduction in lung volumes); obstructive changes may be present. In late stages, ventilatory failure, pulmonary Htn, and cor pulmonale develop.
- Increased risk of postop resp failure, especially following thoracic and abdominal procedures

ICD-9-CM Codes: 502 (Nodular); 503 (Non-nodular)

ETIOLOGY

- Major occupational exposures include mining, stone cutting, abrasive industries, foundry work, packing silica flour, and quarrying, particularly of granite, causing dose-related pulm fibrosis
- Progressive pulm fibrosis (silicosis) occurs after many (15–20) years of exposure

- In some cases of intense exposure (e.g., sand blasting), acute silicosis may occur after <1 y of exposure
- Pathogenesis involves phagocytosis of silica by macrophages, rupture of phagolysosomes, cellular lysis, collagen production, and interstitial fibrosis
- Initial lesions are pulm nodules containing silica dust. Massive fibrosis results when nodules coalesce. Bleb and bulla formation and distortion of airways and vascular bed by these nodules complicate advanced disease.

USUAL TREATMENT

- Discontinue occupational exposure
- Supportive therapy
- Prophylaxis for complicating infections (pneumococcal and influenza vaccines, tuberculosis)
- Sometimes corticosteroids used

ASSESSMENT POINTS

SYSTEM	EFFECT	ASSESSMENT BY HX	PE	TEST
CV	Pulm Htn Cor pulmonale	Dyspnea Exercise tolerance Leg swelling	S_3 Peripheral edema Distended neck veins	ECG CXR
RESP	Pulm fibrosis Bulla/bleb formation	Cough Sputum production Dyspnea Exercise tolerance	Rales, rhonchi, wheezing Cyanosis Use of accessory muscles of resp Resp rate	CXR ABGs PFTs Inspiratory force Diffusing capacity Lung biopsy
GI	Weight loss			
MS	Generalized weakness			
IMMUNO	Hilar adenopathy (eggshell calcification) ↑ Susceptibility to infection, especially pulm	Cough Fever Sputum production		CXR Sputum culture and sensitivity

Key Reference: Weill H, Jones RN: Occupational pulmonary diseases. *In* Fishman AP (ed): Pulmonary Diseases and Disorders, 2nd ed. New York, McGraw-Hill, 1988, pp 819–860.

PERIOPERATIVE IMPLICATIONS

Preoperative Preparation

- Treat bronchitis and pulmonary infection
- Treat bronchospasm if obstructive component present

Monitoring

- Consider repetitive ABGs and lung mechanics (forced vital capacity, tidal volume, inspiratory force, resp rate) especially postop
- Consider PA catheter if pulm Htn and fluid shifts expected

Airway

- Routine

Preinduction/Induction

- Caution with IV agents that depress ventilation and regional techniques that affect accessory muscles of respiration (e.g., high subarachnoid block, interscalene block)
- Maintain adequate preload and cardiac output. Avoid hypoxemia, hypercapnia, and metabolic acidosis, as these may increase PA pressures and worsen cor pulmonale.

Maintenance

- Controlled ventilation preferred during GA
- Ventilation may require increased airway pressures because of poor lung compliance
- Observe for spontaneous pneumothorax, especially in severe disease

Extubation

- Consider temporary postop mechanical ventilation, especially after upper abdominal and thoracic surgery, until stringent criteria met

Postoperative Period

- Pain management critical to avoid ↑ pulm Htn

Adjuvants

- Bronchodilators, supplemental O_2, incentive spirometry may improve ability to wean

ANTICIPATED PROBLEMS/CONCERNS

- Increased risk of resp failure and complications especially after upper abdominal and thoracic surgery
- Patients with cor pulmonale at increased risk for cardiac complications

SINGLE (INCLUDING COMMON) VENTRICLE

Daniel Nyhan, M.D.
Laura A. Hastings, M.D.

RISK

- Hypoplastic left heart syndrome (HLHS) is most common congenital heart malformation involving a single ventricle
- HLHS accounts for 7.5% of those with CHDs
- Slight male predominance for HLHS

PERIOPERATIVE RISKS

- Risk of complications of chronic hypoxemia— hyperviscosity, ↓ coagulation factors and platelets
- Risk of surgical shunts—narrowing of vessels anastomosed, obstructed shunts
- Risk of infective endocarditis
- Risk of paradoxical emboli
- Additional risk proportional to specific anatomy

WORRY ABOUT

- Diastolic dysfunction
- Elevated PVR, PAP
- PA distortion
- AV valve regurgitation
- Systolic dysfunction

OVERVIEW

- Wide variety of lesions usually associated with atresia of the ipsilateral AV or semilunar valve result in single ventricle physiology
  - Tricuspid atresia (TA) is the prototypic single left ventricle. See Tricuspid Atresia in Diseases section.
  - HLHS is the prototypic single right ventricle
- Some patients with biventricular hearts have specific anatomy that precludes a "2-ventricle" repair
- Initial lesion requires complete, unobstructed mixing of the systemic and pulmonary

venous return at the atrial or ventricular level. The single ventricular output is then divided between the pulmonary and systemic circulations.
- Balance of blood flow in each circulation (Qp:Qs) is determined by the relative resistance to flow. Resistance to flow in the pulmonary circulation is determined by pulmonary valve obstruction, arteriolar resistance, and pulmonary venous and LA pressure. Resistance to flow in the systemic circulation is determined by anatomic obstructions (coarctation, arch hypoplasia) and systemic vascular resistance.
- Goal throughout all stages is to balance the Qp:Qs at ~1:1
  - With complete mixing, this results in saturations of 75–80%
- FIO_2, CO_2, and pH management can be used to manipulate the Qp:Qs
- Qp:Qs >> 1 results in pulmonary overcirculation/pulmonary vascular congestion
- Qp:Qs << 1 results in hypoxemia

ICD-9-CM Code: 746.7 (HLHS)

ETIOLOGY

- Specific to the exact lesion
- Usually isolated

USUAL TREATMENT

- Once identified as a single ventricle repair, a series of palliative repairs ensues
- First, stable blood flow is established to the PA in the newborn period
  - For TA, a BT shunt is placed
  - For HLHS, a stage I Norwood procedure is performed

- Complete intracardiac mixing of blood is imperative
- Stage I Norwood consists of creating a neoaorta utilizing native PA tissue and homograft/patch as necessary to connect the single ventricle to the aortic arch and appropriately augment the hypoplastic component of the arch. A BT shunt is placed to supply pulmonary blood flow since the PA has been disconnected to create the neoaorta. An atrial septectomy is performed for complete intracardiac mixing of systemic and pulmonary venous blood. See also Blalock-Taussig (BT) Shunt in Procedures section.
- The eventual goal is to separate the circulations in order to provide normal (or near-normal) oxygen saturations and to reduce the volume workload on the single ventricle. Thus, the next stage consists of a cavopulmonary or atriopulmonary connection. This is commonly done around 6 mo of age. Venous flow from the SVC is directed to the PAs and IVC blood is directed to the single ventricle. Low PVR is necessary to promote pulmonary blood flow.
- The final stage is a completion Fontan. The IVC blood is directed, either intracardiac or extracardic, to the PAs. This effectively separates the circulations. Frequently a fenestration, or small hole from the conduit to the atrium, allows decompression of the "right" side if the PA pressures are elevated. This maintains cardiac output but at the expense of decreased oxygen saturations. The fenestration creates a right-to-left shunt.

ASSESSMENT POINTS

SYSTEM	EFFECT	ASSESSMENT BY HX	PE	TEST
CV	CHF	Dyspnea, tachypnea, feeding difficulties	S_3, rales, wheeze, metabolic acidosis	CXR, pulse oximeter, ABGs
	Hypoxia	Dyspnea, tachypnea, feeding difficulties cyanosis	Cyanosis	CXR, pulse oximeter, ABGs
HEME	Polycythemia	See above	See above	Hgb, Hct

Key Reference: Kawahito S, Kitahata H, Tanaka K, Nosaki J, Oshita S: Intraoperative evaluation of pulmonary artery flow during the Fontan procedure by transesophageal Doppler echocardiography. Anesth Analg 2000; 91:1375–1380.

PERIOPERATIVE IMPLICATIONS

Preoperative Preparation
- Depending on the stage of the palliative process (Norwood stage I, Glenn/hemi-Fontan, completion Fontan), hemodynamics are best optimized preoperatively
- Higher oxygen saturation can ↓ O_2 delivery to the tissues by facilitating overcirculation to the lungs

Monitoring
- Arterial blood pressure monitoring
- CVP is controversial due to the risk of clot in the SVC and the profound implications for subsequent staging, which requires patency of these vessels
- Consider TEE

Preinduction/Induction
- Dependent on exact anatomy and stage of palliation

Airway
- PPV affects the PVR and can have profound effects on the hemodynamic stability. Heavy sedation also leads to hypoxia and hypercarbia, which increase PVR.

Maintenance
- Frequently IV based

Extubation
- After stage I Norwood, patient ventilated overnight or longer
- After stage II (Glenn or hemi-Fontan) or the completion Fontan, early extubation is recommended to facilitate pulmonary blood flow.

High intrathoracic pressure from PPV impedes the venous flow to the pulmonary circulation, while negative intrathoracic pressure (spontaneous respiration) enhances flow.

ANTICIPATED PROBLEMS/CONCERNS

- Low cardiac output syndrome
- Arrhythmias
- Overcirculation
- Hypoxemia
- Pleural and pericardial effusions

SLEEP APNEA, CENTRAL AND MIXED
Andreas M. Ostermeier, M.D.
Michael F. Roizen, M.D.

RISK

- People in USA: 4% of middle-aged adults; M:F ratio, 2:1; obstructive or mixed
- Risk increases with male sex, old age, obesity, Hx of snoring with impaired daytime performance
- In elderly, risk is 2× higher for African-Americans

PERIOPERATIVE RISKS

- Increased risk of central and mixed (central and obstructive) apnea. In mixed SAS, obstructive apnea component can mask central apnea.
- Risk for respiratory depression also in intubated, tracheotomized, and awake patients
- Increased risk with sedative-hypnotic narcotics, postoperatively with any form of pain relief

WORRY ABOUT

- See medical records for previous problems
- Look for related medical disorders (e.g., cor pulmonale, cardiac arrhythmias, erythrocytosis)

- Apnea even several hours postoperatively possible, especially after epidural anesthesia
- When administering O_2, think of possible dependence of ventilation on hypoxic drive

OVERVIEW

- Central implies failure of resp rhythmogenesis. In SAS patients, at least 30 periods of apnea, defined as cessation of airflow for ≥10 sec, are found during normal nocturnal sleep.
- Obstructive sleep apnea relates to a failed or inadequate respiratory activation of upper airway muscles, resulting in lack of airflow
- In central apnea, hypoventilation persists despite relief of obstruction
- Central apnea is unaccompanied by any respiratory effort, in contrast to obstructive sleep apnea
- Related to central alveolar hypoventilation syndrome (CAHS), also known as Ondine's curse

ICD-9-CM Code: 306.1 (Psychogenic apnea)

ETIOLOGY

- Central: familial basis is evident in some cases, possible relation to neurologic disorders (e.g., encephalitis in childhood, damaged respiratory centers, autonomic neuropathy in diabetes)
- Mixed: has obstructive component. Upper airway narrowing superimposed on co-existent abnormality of neurologic control or function of upper airway muscle tone or ventilatory control.
- Associated with obesity, nasal obstruction (polyps, rhinitis, deviated septum, acromegaly, hypothyroidism, Htn)

USUAL TREATMENT

- Continuous positive airway pressure (CPAP)
- Tracheotomy and mechanical vent at night
- Diaphragmatic pacing, especially at night
- Surgery to remove obstruction
- For central/mixed apnea, additional medical treatment with protriptyline, progesterone
- For mixed apnea, also wt loss and physical aids
- Avoid narcotics, benzodiazepines, alcohol

ASSESSMENT POINTS

SYSTEM	EFFECT	ASSESSMENT BY HX	PE	TEST
HEENT	Obstructive apnea	Snoring, partner gives Hx of patient's awakening at night with grunts	Visualization of uvula and tonsillar pillars	
CV	Htn	Dyspnea at rest, DOE Poor exercise tolerance, angina	Cardiomegaly S_3/S_4 murmur	ECG, ECHO
RESP	Right-sided heart dysfunction, snoring, resp dysfunction, DOE	Awakening at night with grunts	Venous engorgement Rapid resp rate Cardiomegaly	SaO_2 supine ECG, CXR, ABGs, Hct Polysomnogram
GI	Hepatic dysfunction Full stomach NIDDM	Jaundice, bleeding disorders, ascites, heartburn, hiatus hernia, polydipsia, polyuria	Hepatomegaly, ascites, spider nevi, jaundice	LFTs, PT, PTT Fasting glucose
ENDO	Obesity Hypothyroidism Acromegaly		Mental function reflexes BMI	Free T_4 estimate TSH, GH levels
HEME	Polycythemia		Plethora, clubbing, cyanosis	O_2 sat, Hct
CNS	Disturbed sleep, impaired daytime performance, morning headache, memory problems, irritability	Daytime sleepiness, complaints of disrupted sleep Ask for encephalitis, autonomic neuropathy, brainstem damage		Polysomnogram

Key Reference: Ostermeier AM, Roizen MF, Hautkappe M, Klock PA, Klafta JM: Three sudden postoperative arrests associated with epidural opioids in patients with sleep apnea. Anesth Analg 1997; 85:452–460.

PERIOPERATIVE IMPLICATIONS

Preoperative Preparation
- Take sleep Hx, if possible from bed partner
- Avoid preop sedation with benzodiazepines and narcotics
- Examine airway carefully
- Consider metoclopramide 10 mg, cimetidine 300 mg PO the night before and IV preop
- Assess myocardial and volume status
- Initiate CPAP therapy over periop period

Monitoring
- Routine; consider arterial line
- UO, possible CVP or PA catheter if volume status likely to be significantly altered

Airway
- Airway control necessary if prominent central component and sedation mandatory
- Awake, sitting, fiberoptic intubation may be indicated if difficulty anticipated

Induction
- Patient may need to remain semi-sitting if SaO_2 drops when supine. Preoxygenation should be complete.

Maintenance
- Oxygenation may deteriorate with upper abdominal surgery or increased intra-abdominal pressure
- Consider the use of short-acting substances (e.g., propofol, remifentanil)
- Minimize postop sedation

Extubation
- Extubate as soon as patient maintains normocapnia and responds to command
- Consider close monitoring after extubation

Adjuvants
- Initial dose of induction agent and narcotics calculated on a mg/kg basis and muscle relaxants calculated on estimated lean body mass
- Subsequent doses of sedatives, hypnotics, relaxants, and narcotics calculated on estimated lean body mass
- Regional anesthesia if physically possible and if patient can use accessory muscles to help with breathing

Postoperative Period
- Pain control with opioids only when NSAIDs and/or regional anesthesia is contraindicated and/or insufficient, as (sudden) complete pain relief may increase risk of respiratory arrest
- Some think epidural or narcotic indicated and others think relatively contraindicated
- Extended respiratory monitoring
- Stabilize ABGs to adequate levels
- Pain control necessary. PCA acceptable in sleep apnea, but not in continuous mode.

ANTICIPATED PROBLEMS/CONCERNS

- Resp insufficiency and pneumonia postop
- Postop thromboembolic phenomena
- If problems occur, inform patient before discharge with written instructions, especially for further anesthetic interventions

SLEEP APNEA, OBSTRUCTIVE

Charles Ahere, M.D.
Claude Brunson, M.D.
Michael F. Roizen, M.D.

RISK

- People in USA: 0.5–3% of whole population
- Gender predominance: males > females, 2:1
- Race with highest prevalence: unknown

PERIOPERATIVE RISKS

- Increased risk of pulm Htn, RV failure, systemic Htn
- Some patients may be polycythemic and have an increased risk of CVA
- Complications associated with obesity
- Increased risk in supine position of sudden arrest postop

WORRY ABOUT

- Airway obstruction with sedating drugs: need for awake, sitting intubation without sedation if obstructs when supine
- Increased sensitivity to sedating drugs
- Difficult airway management: mask ventilation and intubation
- Aspiration risk in morbidly obese
- Postop airway obstruction or resp depression
- Nasal obstruction from NG tubes, e.g., may lead to resp compromise

OVERVIEW

- Apnea refers to cessation of airflow at the mouth for >10 sec
- Sleep apnea: repetitive episodes of upper airway occlusion during sleep, often with oxygen desaturation to 85%, nearly always associated with loud snoring. Episodes of apnea often terminate with a snort or gasp.
- Upper airway obstruction from relaxation of muscles of oropharynx
- Frequent periods of apnea lead to hypoxia and hypercarbia, which could lead to cor pulmonale
- Polycythemia may result from chronic hypoxia
- Nocturnal cardiac arrhythmias are common
- Monitoring of depth and quality of sleep along with cardiopulmonary variables in those with severe symptoms
- Other name is pickwickian syndrome associated with morbid obesity (see also Morbid Obesity in Diseases section)

ICD-9-CM Codes: 780.57, 278.0 (Morbid obesity)

ETIOLOGY

- Cessation of airflow due to complete obstruction of upper airway
- Narrowing due to enlarged tonsils, adenoids, uvula, low soft palate, or craniofacial abn superimposed on co-existent abnormalities of upper airway muscle tone and/or neurologic control
- Obesity exacerbates upper airway obstruction
- Structural abn such as tonsillar hypertrophy, enlarged tongue, and micrognathia may contribute to airway obstruction

USUAL TREATMENT

- Weight loss in overweight patients
- Avoidance of alcohol and sedatives before sleep
- Nasal CPAP
- Physical aids such as devices to detect and prevent snoring, keep patient off back while sleeping (e.g., tennis ball sewn on nightshirt)
- Nasopharyngeal or oropharyngeal airway
- Uvulopalatopharyngoplasty
- Tracheotomy in extreme cases
- Electrophrenic pacing for central sleep apnea

ASSESSMENT POINTS

SYSTEM	EFFECT	ASSESSMENT BY HX	PE	TEST
HEENT	Obstructive apnea	Snoring; partner gives Hx of patient's awakening with grunts at night	Visualization of uvula and tonsillar pillars	
CV	Htn	Dyspnea at rest and on exertion Poor exercise tolerance	Rapid respiratory rate ↑ BP, cardiomegaly	ECG; ECHO
RESP	Right-sided heart dysfunction Restrictive dysfunction	Snoring; partner gives Hx of patient's awakening with grunts at night DOE	Venous engorgement, rales, S_3 and S_4, cardiomegaly	Pulse oximetry on room air while supine ECG, CXR, ABGs, Hct, polysomnogram
GI	Hepatic dysfunction Full stomach NIDDM	Angina Jaundice, bleeding disorders, ascites Heartburn; hiatus hernia Polydipsia, polyuria	Hepatomegaly, ascites, spider angiomas, jaundice	LFTs, PT, PTT Fasting glucose
ENDO	Obesity Hypothyroidism Acromegaly		Mental function Reflexes BMI	Free T_4 estimate TSH level; GH level
HEME	Polycythemia		Plethoric clubbing; cyanosis	Hypoxemia Hct
CNS	Disturbed sleep Memory problems Irritability	Daytime sleepiness Complaints of disrupted sleep		Polysomnogram

Key Reference: Fletcher EC, Proctor M, Yu J, Zhang J, Guardiola JJ, Hornung C, Bao G: Pulmonary edema develops after recurrent obstructive apneas. Am J Respir Crit Care Med 1999; 160:1688–1696.

PERIOPERATIVE IMPLICATIONS

Preoperative Preparation
- Avoid sedatives
- Assess CV status
- Histamine H_2 blockers, metoclopramide, and antacids for morbidly obese patients

Monitoring
- Routine
- Volume status if RV dysfunction present
- Consider arterial catheter if BP cuff doesn't fit or takes too long to inflate

Airway
- Airway obstruction with induction—see HEENT
- Awake intubation in those with potentially difficult airway
- Consider elevating shoulders on bolsters

Induction
- Airway obstruction
- Exacerbation of pulm Htn by hypoxemia and hypercarbia

Maintenance
- Volume status may change precipitously with position change
- Oxygenation may deteriorate with upper abdominal surgery or increased abdominal pressure

Extubation
- Only when patient fully awake
- Airway obstruction from residual anesthetics
- Avoid opioids and sedatives
- Monitor for airway obstruction and apnea

Adjuvants
- Very sensitive to CNS-depressant drugs

ANTICIPATED PROBLEMS/CONCERNS

- Airway obstruction at induction and after extubation
- 13% risk of perioperative complications especially of pneumonia; avoided by minimal sedation, appropriate pain control, early ambulation
- Worsening pulm Htn and right-sided heart failure
- Aspiration risk in morbidly obese
- Postop thromboembolism
- Poor motivation resulting in poor ambulation. Avoided by intensive preop teaching and postop coaching.

SPASMODIC TORTICOLLIS

Peter S. Staats, M.D.

RISK

- Incidence within USA: 1/100,000
- Race with highest prevalence: Caucasian
- Affects young women more frequently than men: 1.6:1
- Average age of onset 40–50 y

PERIOPERATIVE RISKS

- Morbidity related to airway difficulty

WORRY ABOUT

- Airway difficulties due to hypertrophy of sternocleidomastoid and splenius capitis muscles
- Associated with jaw dystonia leading to involuntary jaw closure (trismus), jaw opening, lateral deviation of vocal cords (adductor spasmodic torticollis)
- Associated with cervical spine injuries or toxicities from various drugs
- Theoretical risk of increased K^+ release with depolarizing muscle relaxants if Rx with extensive botulism toxin injections due to denervation injury

OVERVIEW

- Second most common dystonia, characterized by sustained muscle contractions causing twisting and repetitive movements or abnormal posture resulting in sustained abnormal head postures
- May result from basal ganglia dysfunction

ICD-9-CM Code: 333.83

ETIOLOGY

- Idiopathic
- Status post cervical trauma
- Drug-induced, e.g., neuroleptics, antiemetics (metoclopramide)
- Brain lesions, metabolic and neurodegenerative disorders

USUAL TREATMENT

- Medical: anticholinergic drugs, benzodiazepines, muscle relaxants, anticonvulsants
- Intervention: botulinum toxins (provides 3–4 mo relief), and neurosurgical stabilization and/or ablative procedures
- Avoid inciting agents

ASSESSMENT POINTS

SYSTEM	EFFECT	PE
HEENT	Hypertrophy of neck muscle	ROM of neck Abnormal phonation
RESP	Associated adductor spasmodic torticollis Restrictive lung disease	Have patient phonate
GI	Liver dysfunction, associated Wilson's disease	
ENDO	Can be associated with thyroid dysfunction (both hypo- and hyperthyroid reported) or Wilson's disease	
CNS	Wilson's disease	Kayser-Fleischer rings Serum ceruloplasmin
MS	Impaired joint mobility due to development of contractures Associated hemidystonia in ipsilateral arm	

Key Reference: Jankovic J, Brin MF: Therapeutic uses of botulinum toxin. N Engl J Med 1991; 324:1186–1194.

PERIOPERATIVE IMPLICATIONS

Preoperative Preparation

- Consider perioperative botulinum toxin injection

Monitoring

- Placement of invasive lines can be difficult because of associated hemidystonia

Airway

- Assess ability to ventilate and intubate
- Rule out cervical spine pathology

Preinduction/Induction

- Routine

Maintenance

- Nondepolarizing muscle relaxants can lead to improved ability to ventilate and secure an airway

Extubation

- Consider inability to clear secretions from associated cranial nerve pathology

Adjuvants

- Avoid use of neuroleptics in patients who have demonstrated a hypersensitivity

Postoperative Period

- Routine

ANTICIPATED PROBLEMS/CONCERNS

- Development of contractures from longstanding dystonia. After patient is maximally relaxed, ability to ventilate and visualize cords during intubation can be compromised.
- Associated cervical spine instability
- Inability of patient to communicate concomitant disorders
- Can be confused with akinetic disorders (parkinsonian syndromes) or other hyperkinetic movement disorders (tremor, choreoathetosis, myoclonus, asterixis)
- Placement of monitors can be compromised owing to dystonia

SUBCLAVIAN STEAL SYNDROME

Jackie Martin, M.D.
Dolores B. Njoku, M.D., F.A.A.P.

RISK

• Uncommon entity with a variably reported clinical significance
• Male:female preponderance 3:1

PERIOPERATIVE RISKS

• Stroke from a plaque originating from vertebral artery system

WORRY ABOUT

• Worsening neurologic symptoms

OVERVIEW

• Variant of cerebrovascular insufficiency
• Occlusion of subclavian or innominate artery proximal to vertebral artery results in reversal of flow from ipsilateral vertebral artery into distal subclavian
• Left subclavian involved more than right
• Frequently asymptomatic
• CNS ischemia precipitated by exercise of ipsilateral arm or plaques from vertebral artery system
• Arm claudication precipitated by exercise of ipsilateral arm
• Symptoms may be obscured by concomitant carotid insufficiency

ICD-9-CM Code: 435.2

ETIOLOGY

• Atherosclerosis, primarily
• Rare causes include congenital atresia of first portion of left subclavian, hypoplastic arch with severe coarctation, or stenosis of left subclavian at old suture site of a coarctation repair

USUAL TREATMENT

• Surgical
  – Common carotid to subclavian artery bypass graft
  – Subclavian to subclavian artery bypass graft
  – Axillary to axillary artery bypass graft
• Nonsurgical
  – Percutaneous transluminal angioplasty and stent placement

ASSESSMENT POINTS

SYSTEM	ASSESSMENT BY HX	PE	TEST
CV	Claudication	Bruit	Difference in brachial systolic BP of at least 30 mmHg Bruit at base of neck or supraclavicular area on affected side Vascular structures well demonstrated by contrast-enhanced MRA Flow reversal well demonstrated by flow-encoded MRI
CNS	Vertigo Rarely cortical visual disturbances, ataxia, syncope, dysarthria		Retrograde catheter Angio
MS	Paresis/paresthesias		See CV

Key Reference: Mannick J: Subclavian steal syndrome. *In* Sabiston D (ed): Textbook of Surgery, 14th ed. Philadelphia, WB Saunders, 1991, p 1584.

PERIOPERATIVE IMPLICATIONS

Preoperative Preparation

• Bilateral upper extremity BP in patients undergoing surgery characterized by large variations in hemodynamic status or in patients with previous internal mammary-coronary bypass grafts

Monitoring

• Consider arterial catheterization since BP maintenance may be essential for cerebral perfusion
• Consider CVP monitoring and/or PA catheterization if contributing factors in patient

Maintenance

• Consider maintaining arterial BP and heart rate near preop levels to facilitate cerebral perfusion

Extubation

• None

Postoperative Period

• Neurologic evaluation at end of surgery

ANTICIPATED PROBLEMS/CONCERNS

• Patients with internal mammary grafts may experience a similar syndrome of coronary-subclavian steal: there is a gradient in systolic brachial blood pressure of 60 mmHg. In such situations myocardial ischemia that is refractory to medical management occurs. Assessment points and perioperative implications are as stated above but also include myocardial protection concerns.

SUBPHRENIC ABSCESS

James R. Hebl, M.D.

RISK

- Prior abdominal surgery
- Blunt or penetrating trauma
- Gastrointestinal perforation (malignancy, appendicitis, diverticulitis)
- Inflammatory bowel disease
- Immunocompromised patient
- Race/gender predilection: none

PERIOPERATIVE RISKS

- Developing or impending sepsis
- Multiorgan dysfunction syndrome (MODS)

WORRY ABOUT

- Respiratory compromise (pleural effusion, atelectasis, V/Q mismatching, ARDS)
- High-output cardiac failure/LV dysfunction
- Septic shock
- Renal failure and/or coagulopathy associated with sepsis
- Increased capillary permeability (hypovolemia)
- Electrolyte and acid-base disturbances
- Preop ileus/bowel obstruction; aspiration risk

OVERVIEW

- Classic findings include fever, leukocytosis, and abdominal pain
- Associated findings include atelectasis, pleural effusions, elevated diaphragm, ipsilateral shoulder pain, and/or hiccoughs secondary to diaphragmatic irritation
- May be right- or left-sided, or both; above or below the liver or spleen
- Fistulas may form to any abdominal or thoracic organ including pericardium or bronchi
- Disease severity ranges from mild to moribund

ICD-9-CM Code: 567.2

ETIOLOGY

- Primary: associated with perforated viscus such as duodenal ulcer, diverticulitis, appendicitis, primary liver abscess, immunocompromised state. (Pathogens include *Escherichia coli, Enterococcus* spp, *Bacteroides fragilis, Clostridium* spp.)
- Secondary: following surgical intervention, critical illness, or blunt abdominal trauma. (Pathogens include *Candida* spp, *Enterococcus* spp, *Enterobacter* spp, *Staphylococcus epidermidis, E. coli.*)

USUAL TREATMENT

- Broad-spectrum antibiotics based on culture and sensitivity
- Percutaneous or surgical abscess drainage (80–90% successful resolution)
- Supportive therapy: appropriate monitoring, nutrition, oxygenation, hydration, vasopressors as indicated

ASSESSMENT POINTS

SYSTEM	EFFECT	ASSESSMENT BY HX	PE	TEST
CV	*Early:* Hyperdynamic state, high cardiac output associated with low SVR *Late:* Septic shock, low output associated with high SVR, LV dysfunction		Tachycardia Bounding pulses Warm, ruberous skin Tachycardia Diminished pulses Cool integument Peripheral cyanosis	ECG CVP *or* PA catheter ECHO
RESP	Atelectasis, elevated diaphragm, pleural effusion, abdominal distention, pain, or ARDS ↓ Diaphragm excursion	Dyspnea Ipsilateral shoulder pain	Tachypnea Cyanosis ↓ or abnormal breath sounds, dullness to percussion	CXR; fluoroscopy ABGs CT scan
HEME	Anemia due to suppressed marrow Coagulopathy associated with sepsis	Fatigue	Pallor Oozing around old incisions or IV sites Petechiae Ecchymoses	Hgb, Hct Plt count PT/APTT Fibrinogen, FSPs, D-dimer Thromboelastogram
GU	↓ Perfusion due to hypovolemia or sepsis		↓ UO	BUN, Cr Lytes Acid-base balance
CNS	Mental status changes associated with sepsis		Range from mild confusion to coma	Must exclude other possible causes (e.g., CVA, CNS infection)

Key Reference: Feldman H (ed): Sleisenger & Fordtran's Gastrointestinal and Liver Disease, 6th ed. Philadelphia, WB Saunders, 1998, pp 357–363.

PERIOPERATIVE IMPLICATIONS

Preoperative Preparation

- Appropriate antibiotics
- Restore intravascular volume
- Optimize respiratory function: PEEP, thoracentesis, bronchodilators
- NG tube for ileus and/or obstruction
- Tenuous CV status may require vasopressors and/or inotropes
- Assess coagulation status

Monitoring

- Tailor to severity of illness

Airway

- Rapid-sequence induction or awake fiberoptic intubation (aspiration risk)

Preinduction/Induction

- Titrate agents to severity of disease

Extubation

- Tenuous pulmonary status may require prolonged mechanical ventilation

Postoperative Period

- NPO until intestinal function returns
- Analgesia important for adequate respiratory function
- Monitor for postinterventional complications (transient sepsis, organ injury, hemorrhage, pneumothorax, peritonitis, wound dehiscence)

ANTICIPATED PROBLEMS/CONCERNS

- Recurrent abscess formation or sepsis (57% in high-risk patients)
- At risk for MODS (resp/ARDS, renal, hepatic, GI bleed)
- High mortality rate (23–50%) in the presence of multiple organ dysfunction
- Periop pneumonia/empyema/pleural effusion
- Fistula formation
- Ototoxicity and nephrotoxicity of aminoglycosides

SUPRATENTORIAL BRAIN TUMORS
Robert F. Bedford, M.D.

RISK
- 35,000 USA adults diagnosed with primary brain tumors annually (increasing in rate considerably since 1950)

PERIOPERATIVE RISKS
- Presenting symptoms: seizures, neurologic deficit/dementia
- Endocrinopathy/visual deficits if pituitary tumor

WORRY ABOUT
- Seizure medications: Dilantin, Tegretol
  – Need adequate levels to avoid postop seizures

- Brain edema: may lead to herniation
  – Dexamethasone Rx may lead to hyperglycemia
  – Hyperglycemia may cause more retractor-induced ischemic injury to adjacent brain tissues
- Endocrinopathy, particularly diabetes insipidus if near pituitary

OVERVIEW
- Portion of brain superior to tentorium cerebelli
- Majority of intracranial surgeries
- Frequently metastatic lesions; pulmonary and GI most common

ICD-9-CM Code: 239.6 (Tumor, brain)

ETIOLOGY
- Many supratentorial tumors are lung or GI tumor metastases
- Brain edema surrounding malignant tumors causes initial Sx; often improve initially after corticosteroids
- Seizures due to local neuronal irritation
- Obstructive hydrocephalus if tumor near 3rd ventricle or foramen of Monro

USUAL TREATMENT
- Dexamethasone for initial Sx
- Diagnostic extirpation/biopsy
- Radiation/gamma knife
- Chemotherapy
- Surgery

ASSESSMENT POINTS

SYSTEM	EFFECT	ASSESSMENT BY HX	PE	TEST
HEENT	Cartilaginous overgrowth in acromegaly		Acromegalic features	Lat neck x-ray
CV	CHF, ASCVD Age effect	DOE, edema, angina	Gallop, rales, jugular distention	CXR, ECG, ECHO, scan
RESP	COPD, primary tumor with cerebral metastases	Dyspnea, cough, sputum	Signs of COPD	FEV$_1$, FVC (if indicated) ABGs CXR
ENDO	Iatrogenic Cushing's syndrome due to Decadron	Improved level of consciousness	Cushingoid appearance	Glucose levels
HEME	Anemia	Occult GI bleeding caused by tumor	Pale conjunctiva, positive occult fecal blood	Hct, Hgb
CNS	Seizures Somnolence	Headache, confusion	Papilledema Hemiparesis	MRI, CT
PNS	Hemiparesis	Clumsiness	Weakness	Nerve transmission

Key Reference: Drummond JC, Patel PM: Neurosurgical anesthesia. *In* Miller RO (ed): Anesthesia, 5th ed. Philadelphia, Churchill Livingstone, 2000, pp 1895–1933.

PERIOPERATIVE IMPLICATIONS

Preoperative Preparation
- Level of consciousness evaluation: is patient candidate for awake stereotaxic surgery?
- Is there elevated ICP to start with?
- Dexamethasone: may lower ICP initially, but ICP on knee of curve at time of operation
- Head scan report:
  – Temporal lobe lesion with impending herniation?
  – Massive peritumor edema with shift of midline?
  – May want to treat more as a head-trauma case than an elective case
- Antiseizure drugs adequate? Beware postop seizure.

Monitoring
- Consider arterial line: BP control, frequent ABGs, glucose
- End-tidal CO$_2$ as rough guide only, rely on Paco$_2$
- ICP:
  – If lumbar CSF drains are used, connect to transducer
  – Fiberoptic ICP monitors for postop measurement
  – Optimize hyperventilation, mannitol Rx
  – Diagnostic if patient slow to awaken from anesthetic
- NMB: ↑ receptor density in paretic extremities gives false twitch data: use nonparetic arm/leg

Airway
- Cushingoid facies may result in difficult mask ventilation
- Acromegaly causes laryngeal compromise by cartilaginous overgrowth. Anticipate difficult intubation. Consider lateral neck x-ray for airway abnormalities such as enlarged epiglottis, narrowed cricoid ring.

Preinduction/Induction
- Induction with agents that act to ↓ cerebral blood flow
- Opioids prn to avoid hemodynamic responses early on
- Avoid ↑ BP with intubation/head pins
- Avoid brain swelling due to venous outflow occlusion: do not permit overflexion or rotation of neck
- Goggles: eye protection while face covered by drapes, instruments

Maintenance
- Recheck Paco$_2$, especially with COPD
- Mannitol: 0.5–1 mg/kg: empirical or prn?
- No painful structures below dura: minimal anesthetic requirement with brain manipulation; low-dose inhalation agent and/or propofol infusion
- N$_2$O:
  – Suspected antiprotective effect
  – ↑ CBF can usually be overridden by hyperventilation
- Allow temp to ↓ spontaneously to ~34°C.

Extubation
- Awake: normocarbia, early neuro assessment
  – Risk of coughing, straining, possible hematoma formation
  – Perhaps ↑ postop Htn
- Deep: avoids coughing, maybe Htn
  – Transient Paco$_2$ about 50 mmHg until patient awakens
  – Use only if no brain edema during craniotomy and no anticipated airway problems

Adjuvants
- Muscle relaxants
  – Profound paralysis: may minimize need for inhalation agents
  – Monitor NMB on nonparetic extremity to avoid confusion due to increased cholinergic receptor density
- Regional drugs
  – Expect hemodynamic effects from epinephrine in local infiltrated into scalp incision site
- Drug interactions
  – Expect to use more nondepolarizing NMB if patient taking Dilantin, most other antiseizure medications
- Vasoactive compounds
  – Postop Htn common
  – Consider treatment with labetalol, enalaprilat
  – Consider avoiding cerebral vasodilators: hydralazine, sodium nitroprusside

ANTICIPATED PROBLEMS/CONCERNS
- Postexcision brain swelling; seizures
- Postop arterial Htn

SUPRAVENTRICULAR TACHYCARDIA (TACHYARRHYTHMIAS)

John L. Atlee, M.D.

RISK

- SVT has a paroxysmal (PSVT) or gradual onset/termination (sinus tachycardia, automatic and multiform atrial tachycardia—AAT, MAT). Distinction important for treatment.
- Aside from congenital heart disease or mitral valve prolapse, WPW, no special predilection for PSVT
- AAT ($\pm$ AV block) rare in adults, except with digitalis toxicity, hypokalemia, alkalosis
- AAT causes up to 20% of SVT in children but has no special associations
- MAT is common in critically ill patients with chronic pulmonary disease

PERIOPERATIVE RISKS

- Circulatory compromise or myocardial ischemia with tachycardia
- Chronic sustained PSVT/AAT/MAT can cause irreversible cardiomyopathy

WORRY ABOUT

- Status of CV, pulm, other major systemic disease with MAT
- Status of digitalization, K^+ and Mg^{2+} balance, and alkalosis in patients with AAT
- AFIB/AFLT and very rapid ventricular rates (>250 bpm) with WPW or Lown-Ganong-Levine (LGL) syndrome

OVERVIEW

- Aside from adverse effects of tachycardia, PSVT confers no special perioperative risks
- With AAT/MAT, concern is with associated cardiomyopathy and other systemic disease

ICD-9-CM Code: 427.89

ETIOLOGY

- PSVT, esp with WPW or LGL, may have a congenital predilection
- Most (80–90%) PSVT is due to AV node $\pm$ accessory pathway re-entry; SA node and atrial re-entry account for 10–15% and $\sim 5\%$, respectively; structural heart disease is required

- AAT and MAT are acquired automatic or triggered arrhythmias, except for AAT in children, which may be automatic, triggered, or re-entrant

USUAL TREATMENT

- PSVT: drugs that increase conduction/refractoriness in the atria (class 1A or 1C and class 3), AV node (class 2 or 4 and amiodarone), or accessory pathways (class 1A or 1C and class 3) may terminate tachycardia
- AAT: amiodarone, sotalol, flecainide, moricizine, and propafenone and β-blockers are most effective for suppressing AAT. β-Blockers and vagal maneuvers may slow AAT or ↑AV block.
- MAT: β-blockers and Ca^{2+}-channel blockers usually slow the heart rate and improve function, but treating the underlying CV or pulm disease is the mainstay of Rx. With hypomagnesemia, magnesium may suppress MAT.
- Cardioversion or pacing will terminate PSVT but not AAT or MAT

ASSESSMENT POINTS

SYSTEM	EFFECT	ASSESSMENT BY HX	PE	TEST
CV	Arrhythmia	Palpitations, dizziness, fatigue, failure to thrive (infants/young children), dyspnea, angina, syncope	Regular pulse (PSVT, AAT), irregular pulse (MAT), signs of CHF, diaphoresis	ECG, Holter monitoring Exercise ECG, cardiac electrophysiologic study
	LV function Ischemia	Exercise intolerance, CHF Sx of angina	S_3, rales, wheezes	CXR, ECHO, scintigraphy, coronary angio
RESP	CHF, COPD	Dyspnea, orthopnea, cough	S_3, rales, wheezes	CXR, PFTs
GI	↓Perfusion	GI distress, diarrhea		
RENAL	↓Perfusion	Polyuria	UO	BUN/Cr

Key References: Atlee JL: Management of perioperative dysrhythmias. Anesthesiology 1997; 86:1397–1424; Kastor JA: Arrhythmias, 2nd ed. Philadelphia: WB Saunders, 2000, pp 164–268.

PERIOPERATIVE IMPLICATIONS

Preoperative Preparation

- PSVT: adenosine, esmolol, or edrophonium on hand; also procainamide or amiodarone if WPW or LGL patient
- AAT: check for digitalis toxicity; is there K^+, Mg^{2+}, or acid-base imbalance?
- MAT: optimize cardiopulmonary and metabolic status, treat infections or other pathophysiology

Monitoring

- ECG/ST trending; strip-chart recorder
- Consider direct arterial and PA catheter monitoring

Induction

- With cardiomyopathy or LV dysfunction, there is ↑risk of circulatory deterioration during anesthetic induction

- AAT and MAT: caution with drugs that increase heart rate (antimuscarinics, β-agonists, ketamine, pancuronium, desflurane)

Maintenance

- With possible exception of desflurane, volatile agents are not conducive to PSVT and are expected to have little effect on AAT/MAT
- Prophylactic β-blockers may be useful in patients with AAT/MAT during surgical stimulation

Extubation

- At ↑risk for tachyarrhythmias during emergence as a result of sympathetic hyperactivity
- Use drugs/means to reduce/avoid effects of airway stimulation and hyperdynamic circulation
- Consider prophylactic use of β-blockers (if tolerated) for patients with AAT and MAT

Adjuvants

- With AAT or MAT, avoid or use caution with sympathomimetic or histamine-releasing drugs

Postoperative Period

- Attention to adequate sedation and pain control will reduce likelihood of PSVT
- AAT and MAT are suppressed with β-blockers and by optimizing treatment of underlying cardiopulmonary disease

ANTICIPATED PROBLEMS/CONCERNS

- In patients with WPW or LGL and Hx of tachyarrhythmias, be prepared to treat AFIB/AFLT with rapid ventricular rate or ventricular fibrillation (DC cardioversion/defibrillation)
- DC cardioversion is not effective for treatment of AAT/MAT and may cause worse arrhythmias

SWALLOWING DISORDERS

Shiroh Isono, M.D.

- 10+% of elderly individuals have an absent gag reflex
- Patients with bulbar paralysis of any etiology

PERIOPERATIVE RISKS

- Malnutrition and dehydration due to inadequate oral intake
- Presence of pneumonia due to chronic aspiration
- ↑ Risk of aspiration pneumonia postop
- ↑ Retained bronchial secretions

WORRY ABOUT

- Aspiration pneumonia

OVERVIEW

- Condition usually associated with impairment of any part of swallowing reflex arc, such as sensory receptors in pharynx and larynx, afferent nerves, CNS, efferent nerves, muscles
- High risk for aspiration pneumonia pre- and postop can be evaluated by video fluoroscopy
- Associated with abnormal hygiene of upper and bronchial airways

ICD-9-CM Code: 787.2 (Dysphagia)

ETIOLOGY

- Depressed CNS by sedation, sleep, coma, or light anesthesia
- Neuromuscular disorders such as polymyositis, progressive muscular dystrophy, multiple sclerosis, myasthenia gravis, Eaton-Lambert syndrome

- Regional anesthesia to upper airway
- Tracheotomy or prolonged ET intubation; surgery on the head and neck
- Precurarization
- Peripheral nerve disorders such as Guillain-Barré syndrome, acute porphyria, laryngeal nerve injury; parkinsonism; advanced age

USUAL TREATMENT

- Control for underlying disorders if possible
- Cricopharyngeal myotomy sometimes indicated
- Nasogastric balloon tube reported useful

ASSESSMENT POINTS

SYSTEM	EFFECT	ASSESSMENT BY HX	PE	TEST
HEENT	Aspiration	Cough	Check gag reflex Chest exam	Videofluoroscopy
CV	Dehydration		Skin, orthostatic vital signs	UO
RESP	Pneumonia	Dyspnea, sputum production	Fever	CXR, ABGs
GI	Dysphagia GE reflux	Salivation Repeated pneumonia Heartburn	UA inspection Laryngeal movement	Fluoroscopy, manometry CT, MRI, endoscopy
CNS	Cranial nerve IX or X or others dysfunctional	Eating/swallowing pattern	Cranial nerve examination	

Key Reference: Nishino T: Swallowing as a protective reflex for the upper respiratory tract. Anesthesiology 1993; 79:588–601.

PERIOPERATIVE IMPLICATIONS

Preoperative Preparation

- Control underlying disorders and complications (pneumonia, dehydration)
- Correct malnutrition and dehydration by tube feeding, gastrostomy, or parenteral alimentation
- Consider metoclopramide or domperidone as a part of preop medication to treat prolonged retention of stomach contents
- H_2 blocker to decrease effects of silent regurgitation due to use of anticholinergic drug
- Avoid deep sedation

Monitoring

- Routine

Airway

- Tracheal intubation with cuffed ET tube
- Suction of secretions above the tracheostomy tube
- Do not apply local anesthetics to upper airway

Preinduction/Induction

- Rapid induction/intubation of trachea after cricoid pressure
- Avoid precurarization, possibly leading to severe dysphagia or pharyngeal obstruction

Maintenance

- Minimize NMB

Extubation

- Aspirate stomach contents and clear the oronasal cavity before extubation
- Eliminate or reverse residual anesthetics and muscle relaxants before extubation
- Check recovery of swallowing reflex

Possible Drug Interactions

- Light sedation may impair swallowing reflex
- Precurarization and residual muscle relaxants can severely impair swallowing
- Possible synergistic effect of low concentration of enflurane and vecuronium on impairment of upper airway muscles
- Regional anesthesia impairs other upper airway protective reflex (closure of the larynx, cough reflex)

Postoperative Period

- Fowler position if possible
- Prophylaxis of and/or treat N/V
- Evaluate for presence of aspiration pneumonia

ANTICIPATED PROBLEMS/CONCERNS

- Aspiration pneumonia (chemical or infectious)

SYNDROME OF INAPPROPRIATE ANTIDIURETIC HORMONE SECRETION (SIADH)

Philippa Newfield, M.D.
Rukaiya K.A. Hamid, M.D.

RISK

- Increased in patients who have cancer, pneumonia, intracranial disorders

PERIOPERATIVE RISKS

- Increased risk of neurologic dysfunction: altered level of consciousness, seizures, coma from hyponatremia and cerebral swelling
- Risk of volume overload and CHF

WORRY ABOUT

- Volume overload
- Hyponatremia
- Changing level of consciousness, seizures, coma
- Neurologic complications of overly rapid correction of hyponatremia (central pontine myelinolysis or osmotic demyelination syndrome, cerebral hemorrhage) with behavioral disturbances, seizures, pseudobulbar palsy, quadriparesis
- Rate of decrease of [Na$^+$], which influences clinical manifestations

OVERVIEW

- ADH normally released in response to 1–2% ↑ in serum osmolality or 7% ↓ in intravascular volume
- SIADH is characterized by sustained endogenous release of ADH or ADH-like substances in the absence of physiologic stimuli
- Serum sodium is ↓, urinary sodium is ↑, and urine is hyperosmolar relative to plasma
- Results primarily in water retention with excretion of non–maximally dilute urine in the face of hyponatremia
- Patients reach a volume-expanded steady state in which output equals input
- ADH is released in cranial disorders because of direct hypothalamic stimulation

ICD-9-CM Codes: 259.3 (Ectopic); 259.6 (Neurohypophysial)

ETIOLOGY

- Disease states: pulmonary disease; cancer; cranial disorders (head trauma, skull fractures, subdural hematomas, brain tumors, infections of CNS, cerebral thrombosis, removal of pituitary macroadenomas); myxedema; acute intermittent porphyria; stress situations (emotional upheaval)
- Drug-induced ADH release (chemotherapy, tricyclics, barbiturates)
- Drug-induced enhancement of ADH effect on collecting ducts
- Drugs that mimic action of ADH in renal tubules
- Exogenously administered ADH
  – DDAVP for perioperative hemostasis
- Postop with impaired water secretion and hypervolemia

USUAL TREATMENT

- Fluid restriction to 800–1000 ml/d for plasma [Na$^+$] > 120–125 mEq/L
- Urea, 40 g/150 ml NS IV over 2 hr. Repeat q8h over 48 h until [Na$^+$] > 130 mEq/L.
- Diuretics (furosemide up to 1 mg/kg)
- Replace urinary sodium losses with 0.9% saline
- 3.0% hypertonic saline if [Na$^+$] < 115–120 mEq/L at a rate of 1–2 ml/kg/h to increase [Na$^+$] by 1–2 mEq/L/h and to bring [Na$^+$] to 125 mEq/L (or ≤ 12 mEq/L in 24 h or 25 mEq/L in 48 h)
- Hemodialysis
- Demeclocycline (dimethylchlortetracycline), lithium, diphenylhydantoin
- Thyroid hormone replacement

ASSESSMENT POINTS

SYSTEM	EFFECT	ASSESSMENT BY HX	PE	TEST
CV	CHF	DOE, PND	Peripheral edema, gallop JVD, weight gain	Oral water load if plasma [Na$^+$] > 124 mEq/L and no symptoms
RESP	CHF	DOE, PND	Bibasilar rales	CXR
GI	Hyponatremia	Nausea, anorexia, vomiting		[Na$^+$] < 130 mEq/L
RENAL	Dilutional hyponatremia ↓ Serum osmolality ↑ Urine osmolality ↓ Urine output ↑ Urine sodium Normal hydration	↓ Urine output	No edema	Urine osmolality > 300–400 mOsm/L Urine [Na$^+$] > 25–30 mEq/L Plasma [Na$^+$] < 130 mEq/L Serum Osm < 280 mOsm/L Low Cr, albumin Low BUN, uric acid
CNS	Brain swelling from ↑ extracellular and intracellular brain water Depletion of brain electrolytes	Lethargy, weakness, somnolence Mental confusion, seizures Personality changes Coma	Areflexia, weakness, altered level of consciousness, pseudobulbar palsy, asterixis, Babinski	[Na$^+$] < 130 mEq/L
MS	Hyponatremia → changes in action potential	Cramps Muscle weakness	Skeletal muscle weakness	↑ Plasma arginine, vasopressin by RAI

Key Reference: Tommasino C: Fluid management. *In* Newfield P, Cottrell JE (eds): Handbook of Neuroanesthesia, 3rd ed. Philadelphia, Lippincott Williams & Wilkins, 1999, pp 381–383.

PERIOPERATIVE IMPLICATIONS

Preoperative Preparation
- Correction of hyponatremia
- Discontinuation of drugs enhancing or mimicking action of ADH or ↑ secretion of ADH
- Treatment of underlying disorder (e.g., hypothyroidism, pneumonia)

Monitoring
- PA or CVP catheter for large fluid shift operations or patients with LV dysfunction
- Intraoperative serum [Na$^+$] and Osm
- Urinary output

Airway
- None

Preinduction/Induction
- May develop volume overload with fluid administration
- Avoid drugs known to lower seizure threshold

Maintenance
- Avoid hypotonic fluids
- Limit stress response, which may increase ADH secretion
- Limit drugs that induce ADH release (morphine, barbiturates, β-adrenergics)
- Limit total fluids if patient has received DDAVP or other ADH analogues

Extubation
- Period of risk for patients who have CHF

Adjuvants
- 0.9% saline, 3.0% saline, furosemide, urea

Postoperative Period
- Monitor serum [Na$^+$] and Osm closely, especially in patients who have received DDAVP
- Monitor urine [Na$^+$] and Osm
- Monitor volume status and urinary output
- Treat hypervolemia and hyponatremia

ANTICIPATED PROBLEMS/CONCERNS

- Symptoms of acute hyponatremia are more severe than those of chronic hyponatremia for same plasma [Na$^+$]
- Free water losses (renal, skin, GI) must exceed free water intake to ↑ serum [Na$^+$]
- Acute water intoxication is a medical emergency

SYNDROME X

Jonathan Moss, M.D., Ph.D.

RISK

- True incidence unknown, but occurs commonly in Europe
- Postmenopausal or posthysterectomy women most often at risk
- Most common cause of chest pain in women with angiographically normal coronary arteries

PERIOPERATIVE RISKS

- Acute withdrawal of sex hormone replacement for reasons of ↑ coagulation (thrombophlebitis risk) can potentially lead to coronary vasospasm

WORRY ABOUT

- Women on hormone replacement may be subject to acute vasospasm upon withdrawal
- Estrogen patches or therapy may be useful in alleviating chest pain

OVERVIEW

- Clinical example relating chronic sex hormone status to acute vascular responsiveness to estrogen
- First described by Kemp (1973) but includes exertional angina, positive exercise test, and angiographically normal coronary arteries

ICD-9-CM Code: 413.9

ETIOLOGY

- Impairment of vasodilator reserve in peripheral and coronary vessels due to estrogen deficiency
- Estrogen appears to act as Ca^{2+}-channel antagonist at high doses and facilitates nitric oxide effects on coronary endothelial cells at low doses
- Acute withdrawal of estrogen appears to be more significant factor than chronic withdrawal

USUAL TREATMENT

- Estrogen patch has been found to significantly improve exercise tolerance

ASSESSMENT POINTS

SYSTEM	EFFECT	ASSESSMENT BY HX	PE	TEST
CV	Myocardial ischemia	Exertional angina, prior hysterectomy, acute withdrawal of estrogen, physical examination, and flushing		Normal coronary angiogram in presence of chest pain without Prinzmetal's angina or valvular heart disease
DERM	Vasodilation seen during menopause also seen in this syndrome; migraine headache may occur coincidentally		Flushing	17β-Estradiol levels are lowest and angina most frequent and severe during luteal phase of menstrual cycle

Key References: Egashira K, Inou T, Hirouka Y, Yamuda A, Urabe Y, Takeshita A: Evidence of impaired endothelium-dependent coronary vasodilation in patients with angina pectoris and normal coronary angiograms. N Engl J Med 1993; 328:1659–1664; Kao CH, Hsieh JF, Tsai CS, Ho YJ, Lee JK: Evidence of abnormal esophageal motility in syndrome X by radionuclide esophageal transit test. Digestion 2000; 62:26–30.

PERIOPERATIVE IMPLICATIONS

Preoperative Preparation

- Estrogens are withdrawn because of possible thrombophlebitis. Patients with this syndrome may experience significant angina upon such withdrawal.
- Distinguish chest pain due to this syndrome from chest pain due to coronary insufficiency from other causes

Monitoring

- ST-segment analysis

Preinduction/Induction

- Contingent upon type of surgery; may consider maintaining estrogen therapy. No data as to effects on preinduction and induction and maintenance of anesthesia.

ANTICIPATED PROBLEMS/CONCERNS

- Occurs most commonly in postmenopausal or posthysterectomy women (4× greater incidence than that of age-matched population); successfully treated with exogenous estrogen. A major concern may be that acute discontinuation of estrogen may lead to coronary vasoconstriction. Vessels may still dilate in presence of IV nitroglycerin, but with a Hx of menopausal flushing and coincident chest pain clinicians should weigh risks and benefits of continued estrogen therapy versus withdrawal.

SYSTEMIC LUPUS ERYTHEMATOSUS
David M. Robinson, M.D.

RISK

- Average incidence 1/1000; 1/250 high-risk populations
- Females >> males
- African-American >> Caucasian
- Majority diagnosed at age 30–40: 20% diagnosed as children

PERIOPERATIVE RISKS

- N/V, abdominal pain
- Vasculitis, pancreatitis, lupoid hepatitis
- Endocarditis (nonbacterial), myocarditis, thrombophlebitis
- Precipitation of relapse related to surgery not uncommon

WORRY ABOUT

- Pituitary-adrenal chronic steroid suppression
- Antibiotic prophylaxis if valvular disease present
- Restrictive PFTs with A-a gradient and effusions
- Lupus nephritis and renal insufficiency
- Splenomegaly, thrombocytopenia
- Lupus anticoagulant may be present
- Thrombosis and hemorrhage
- Neuropathy, confusion, psychosis

OVERVIEW

- Multisystem disease requiring evaluation of each organ system
- 10 y survival is 90%
- Fibrinoid substances are deposited in multiple tissues, causing inflammation. Development of thrombocytopenia, anemia, leukopenia, and decreased complement heralds relapses.

- Drugs that can precipitate relapse include procainamide, hydralazine, phenytoin, penicillin, isoniazid

ICD-9-CM Code: 710.0

ETIOLOGY

- Unknown
- Autoimmune process possibly following trauma to mast cells and association with an X chromosome factor

USUAL TREATMENT

- Aggressive treatment limited to therapy during relapses and prevention of exacerbations. Treatments include rest, steroids, salicylates, azathioprine, cyclosporine, plasmapheresis.

ASSESSMENT POINTS

SYSTEM	EFFECT	ASSESSMENT BY HX	PE	TEST
CV	Pericarditis Endocarditis Myocarditis CHF, conduction blocks	Chest pain Palpitations	Pericardial friction rub Murmur Effusion Diastolic noncompliance	ECG CXR ECHO
RESP	Infiltrates Restrictive PFTs ↑ A-a gradient Atelectasis	Pleuritic chest pain Dyspnea Cough Hemoptysis	Friction rub Effusion Cyanosis Normal peak flow	CXR PFTs ABGs
GI	Perforated viscus Pseudo-obstruction Liver congestion Lupoid hepatitis	N/V Peritonitis and pancreatitis Abdominal pain Ileus	Dilated loops of bowel Peritoneal free air Hepatomegaly Jaundice	GI series LFTs Bilirubin A/G ratio
HEME	Hemorrhage infrequent Thromboembolism Anemia	Bruising Thrombosis	Lymphadenopathy Splenomegaly Anemia	CBC Plt count PT/PTT
RENAL	Glomerulitis Nephrotic syndrome Renal insufficiency Renal failure	Polyuria Oliguria Hematuria Fever	Costophrenic tenderness Edema	Urinalysis Renal US Renal scan BUN, Cr, TP, albumin
CNS	Confusion Hallucinations Psychoses Seizures	Paranoid states Hyperirritability Numbness Hemiparesis	Psychosis Nystagmus, ptosis, diplopia Aphasia Peripheral neuropathy	EEG CT scan Neuro and psychiatry evaluations
MS/ DERM	Vasculitis and ulceration Symmetric arthritis Joint immobility Aseptic necrosis	Photosensitivity Atrophic or scarred area Ecchymosis or purpura Joint pain or immobility	Malar or butterfly rash Perioral ulcerations Reduced ROM Hip pain	Hip x-rays ANA

Key Reference: Cuenco J, Tzeng G, Wittels B: Anesthetic management of the parturient with systemic lupus erythematosus, pulmonary hypertension, and pulmonary edema. Anesthesiology 1999; 91:568–570.

PERIOPERATIVE IMPLICATIONS

Preoperative Preparation

- Stress steroid dose if on chronic steroid therapy. Hydrocortisone 100 mg IV q 6–8 h prior to induction and tapered as stress reduces over several days.

Monitoring

- Consider arterial line for blood gases; consider PA catheter for pulmonary Htn
- Consider arterial line and PA line if evidence of CHF
- Foley catheter and careful titration of fluid replacement (consider CVP/PA catheter) if renal involvement

Airway

- Occasionally reduced TMJ ROM and narrowed larynx with immovable arytenoids
- Consider fiberoptic intubation

Maintenance

- No specific agents indicated or contraindicated. Regional acceptable if no coagulopathy.
- If renal insufficiency present, avoid renally excreted drugs and renal toxins

Adjuvants

- Corticosteroids, supplemental O_2, careful titration of fluids with renal involvement

Extubation/Postoperative Period

- Reassess respiratory, renal, CV status prior to extubation

ANTICIPATED PROBLEMS/CONCERNS

- Pituitary-adrenocortical axis suppression
- CHF and arrhythmias
- Resp insufficiency and nephritis
- Renal function and volume management
- CNS dysfunction, seizure, neuropathy
- Thrombosis and abnormal coagulation tests
- Vasculitis injury, especially GI tract
- Fulminant hepatitis

TETANUS

Roy D. Cane, M.B., B.Ch.

RISK

- Incidence in USA: 60–80 cases/y
- Female of any age; males >50 y and African-Americans from rural South

PERIOPERATIVE RISKS

- Focal/generalized muscle spasms occurring spontaneously or in response to external stimuli
- Autonomic nervous system instability
- Case mortality rate in USA is 30%

WORRY ABOUT

- Autonomic nervous system instability
- Toxic myocarditis
- Respiratory failure due to muscle spasms or treatment
- Inadequate bronchial hygiene

OVERVIEW

- An exotoxin, tetanospasmin, produced by *Clostridium tetani,* enters CNS by intraneuronal transport via peripheral nerves and inhibits release of γ-aminobutyric acid and glycine, resulting in disinhibition of motor and autonomic nervous system
- Characterized by muscle rigidity with intermittent, usually generalized, spasms; localized spasms of muscle groups close to site of skin penetration

ICD-9-CM Code: 037

ETIOLOGY

- Infection of deep penetrating wounds with anaerobic spore-producing organism, *C. tetani*

USUAL TREATMENT

- Primary infection treated by debridement of wound and high-dose penicillin therapy (tetracycline or erythromycin if penicillin-allergic)
- Neutralization of circulating toxin by single dose of human tetanus immune globulin
- Spasms controlled by heavy sedation and/or neuromuscular relaxation or blockade
- Ventilatory and nutritional support as needed

ASSESSMENT POINTS

SYSTEM	EFFECT	ASSESSMENT BY HX	PE	TEST
HEENT	Rigidity of masseter and cervical muscles	Dysphagia, excessive salivation, drooling	Limitation of mouth opening and ROM of neck	
CV	Toxic myocarditis		Hypotension	ECG
RESP	Hypoventilation, diminished bronchial hygiene	Poor cough, SOB	Limited chest excursion, ↓ breath sounds, rhonchi	ABGs, CXR
CNS	Autonomic nervous system overactivity	Flushing, palpitations	Fluctuating BP with episodic Htn, arrhythmias, sudden cardiac death	ECG
MS	Generalized or localized rigidity and spasms	Stiffness, painful muscle spasms	Rigidity, spasm leading to opisthotonos and risus sardonicus	

Key Reference: Tobias JD: Anesthetic implications of tetanus. South Med J 1998; 91:384–387.

PERIOPERATIVE IMPLICATIONS

Preoperative Preparation

- Adequate sedation with benzodiazepines or control of generalized spasms by NMB with vecuronium or atracurium
- Consider avoiding pancuronium (potential for ANS stimulation) and (reported to be less effective) rocuronium

Airway

- Masseter and cervical muscle rigidity and spasms can make intubation difficult. If patient not already intubated, consider fiberoptic intubation.
- Elective tracheotomy recommended for long-term support of ventilation and bronchial hygiene

Induction

- None. Most patients will already be heavily sedated or intubated with NMB.

Maintenance

- Usually GA with inhalational anesthetic agents and NMB has been described
- Monitor for ANS overactivity. Consider adding continuous spinal/epidural anesthesia for controlling ANS overactivity.

Postoperative Period

- Usually managed in ICU. Maintain intubation, NMB, sedation, mechanical ventilatory support.
- Provide nutritional support via nasoenteric feeding
- Continue surveillance and therapy of ANS overactivity

- Observe for toxic myocarditis manifesting as ST-segment and T-wave changes on ECG and hypotension due to drug therapy
- Hypotension with bradycardia, indicative of brainstem involvement, associated with very poor prognosis

ANTICIPATED PROBLEMS/CONCERNS

- Extremes in BP, arrhythmias, cardiac arrest may occur
- Morphine, magnesium sulfate, β-blockers are used to control ANS overactivity
- Propranolol, labetalol, and phentolamine associated with ↑ risk of sudden cardiac arrest

TETRALOGY OF FALLOT

Winnie Y. Ruo, M.D.

RISK

- 2/10,000 live births
- 15% of infants with congenital heart disease
- Race with highest prevalence: none

PERIOPERATIVE RISKS

- Risk of "tet spell" if unrepaired
- Mortality in tetralogy of Fallot (TOF) repair: 6–8%
- ↑Mortality if co-existing PA hypoplasia

WORRY ABOUT

- Avoid increases in PVR resulting in ↑ R → L shunt
- Avoid ↓ in SVR resulting in ↑ R → L shunt
- Crying and agitation leading to "tet spell," resulting in more hypoxemia, hypercarbia, acidosis
- Air bubbles in IV tubing
- Polycythemia and associated thrombocytopenia

- RV failure after inadequate repair
- Residual VSD causing difficulty in separation from CPB
- May need temporary pacemaker after repair because of AV conduction system injury

OVERVIEW

- Anatomy
  - RV outflow tract obstruction
  - Infundibular narrowing
  - Pulm valve stenosis
  - PA hypoplasia
  - VSD: may be single or multiple
  - Overriding aorta
  - RV hypertrophy
  - 5% have anomalous origin of LAD from right coronary artery
- Degree of R → L shunting determined by fixed factors (degree of infundibular obstruction, size of pulmonary valve annulus, size of PA) and reactive factors (PVR and SVR)
- Avoid hypoxia, acidosis, high airway pressures, excitement, agitation
- 96% 10-y survival after complete repair
- Dx by ECHO and cardiac catheterization

ICD-9-CM Code: 745.2

USUAL TREATMENT

- Palliative shunts to increase pulmonary blood flow (Blalock-Taussig shunt, aortopulmonary shunts)
- Surgical repair consists of RV outflow tract enlargement, closure of VSD, PA conduits
- β-blockers to decrease infundibular spasm
- Treatment of "tet spell"
  - 100% O_2
  - Propranolol
  - Bicarbonate to correct metabolic acidosis
  - Phenylephrine to ↑ SVR
  - Sedation
  - Squatting to ↑ SVR
  - Aortic compression by abdominal pressure to ↑ SVR

ASSESSMENT POINTS

SYSTEM	EFFECT	ASSESSMENT BY HX	TEST
CHEST			CXR with dominant RV, concave PA segment
CV	See Overview: Anatomy	Frequency and severity of "tet spells"	ECHO/cath ECG-RVH, RA
HEME	Polycythemia from chronic hypoxemia Plt count may be low from polycythemia		Hct, plt count

Key Reference: Lake CL: Pediatric Cardiac Anesthesia, 2nd ed. Norwalk, CT, Appleton & Lange, 1993, pp 243–252.

PERIOPERATIVE IMPLICATIONS

Preoperative Preparation

- Heavy premedication to avoid agitation, crying

Monitoring

- Arterial line to monitor blood gases
- Central line for drugs and right-sided pressures
- TEE to assess adequacy of repair

Airway

- None

Induction

- Avoid ↑ in PVR and ↓ in SVR
- Consider IM ketamine if no IV present

Maintenance

- Avoid high-dose inhalational agents to maintain stable SVR
- Narcotics may be used

Separation from CPB after Tetralogy Repair

- Measure ratio of RV to LV pressures to judge adequacy of repair. If ratio < 0.8, repair adequate. If RVP > LVP, need RV patch.
- Ventilation
  - Avoid high airway pressures
  - Keep $Paco_2$ 30–35 mmHg
  - Keep pH 7.5
- May need to ↓ PVR pharmacologically (nitroglycerin, dobutamine, amrinone, phentolamine, PGE_1)
- May need temporary pacemaker if AV conduction system injury

ANTICIPATED PROBLEMS/CONCERNS AFTER COMPLETE REPAIR

- Intraoperative "tet spell"
- RV failure
- Residual VSD
- Arrhythmias

THALASSEMIA

Eric Weissend, M.D.
Ronald S. Litman, D.O.

RISK

- People in USA with severe disease: 1000
- 3–5% incidence among people of Mediterranean, African, or Asian descent

PERIOPERATIVE RISKS

- High-output CHF common with severe anemia
- Iron loading from chronic therapy can result in diabetes, adrenal insufficiency, liver dysfunction, coag abn, hypothyroidism, hypoparathyroidism, arrhythmias, intractable cardiac failure
- Hypersplenism can result in thrombocytopenia and ↑ risk of infection
- Alloimmunization 2° to multiple blood transfusions. Obtaining appropriately cross-matched blood may require prolonged testing.

WORRY ABOUT

- Difficult airway 2° to maxillary deformation
- Cardiac arrhythmias or CHF
- Coagulopathy

OVERVIEW

- Diverse group of microcytic anemias characterized by absence or ↓ synthesis of normal globin chains of Hgb (α, β, δ, and γ). Decrease or absence of α or β chains most common.
- Beta thalassemia major, Cooley's anemia (homozygous)
  - Absent β-chain synthesis. Results in severe anemia requiring aggressive intervention. Median survival 31 y.
- Beta thalassemia minor (heterozygous)
  - Clinical manifestations range from asymptomatic to mild anemia, depending on severity of β-chain deficiency. Usually does not require intervention.
- Thalassemia intermedia (heterozygous)
  - Results in milder form of anemia than homozygous type. May require transfusion therapy for aplastic crisis or folate deficiency or when hypersplenism occurs.
- Alpha thalassemia
  - Four α genes: two on each chromosome 16
  - One-gene deletion = silent carrier
  - Two-gene deletion = α thalassemia minor—mild microcytic anemia
  - Three-gene deletion = α thalassemia major—severe hemolytic anemia due to formation of unstable β globin tetramer (Hgb H). Most complications 2° to iron overload, which results from compensatory GI absorption and chronic transfusion therapy.
  - Four-gene deletion = hydrops fetalis—incompatible with life. Absent Hgb F replaced with Hgb Barts (γ tetramer). Intrauterine death from high-output CHF and tissue anoxia.

ICD-9-CM Code: 282.4

ETIOLOGY

- Deletions of point mutations of one or all of the α and/or β globin genes

USUAL TREATMENT

- Supportive transfusions and folate replacement for mild forms
- Chronic transfusions and iron chelation therapy for major forms
- Splenectomy when indicated
- Bone marrow transplantation in selected patients

ASSESSMENT POINTS

SYSTEM	EFFECT	ASSESSMENT BY HX	PE	TEST
HEENT	Prominent maxilla and malar eminences, frontal bossing		Airway examination	
CV	CHF, arrhythmias, pericarditis, effusion	DOE Orthopnea PND Palpitations	Rales Rub S_3 gallop	ECG ECHO
RESP	Restrictive defects, small airway obstruction, chronic PE/pulm Htn	Poor exercise tolerance Dyspnea, fatigue, syncope, angina	Wheezing, peripheral edema, elevated JVP, hepatosplenomegaly	CXR, ECHO
GI	Liver dysfunction Cholelithiasis	RUQ pain	Hepatomegaly	LFTs
ENDO	Diabetes, hypothyroidism, hypoparathyroidism	Polyuria, polydipsia, cold intolerance, growth retardation		Glucose Ca^{2+} TSH
HEME	Coagulopathy, mild to severe anemia	Bleeding or bruising	Splenomegaly	Plt count Hgb, PT/PTT
RENAL	Enlarged kidneys	Dark brown urine (heme products)		UA
MS	Cortical thinning, Fx of long bones	Acute pain	X-ray	

Key Reference: Weatherall DJ: The thalassaemias. BMJ 1997; 314:1675–1678.

PERIOPERATIVE IMPLICATIONS

Preoperative Preparation

- Search for co-existing conditions
- Careful airway evaluation
- Early type and cross-match if large blood loss anticipated

Monitoring

- Routine
- Consider invasive hemodynamic monitors if CHF

Airway

- May have distorted anatomy 2° to extramedullary hematopoiesis; may need awake and/or fiberoptic intubation

Preinduction/Induction

- Hemodynamic compromise with induction agents if low cardiac reserves

Maintenance

- Routine care; depends on organ system involvement
- Care with moving and positioning; bones easily fractured

Extubation

- Awake if difficult intubation

Adjuvants

- Will depend on organ system involvement (e.g., hepatic insufficiency)

ANTICIPATED PROBLEMS/CONCERNS

- Difficult intubation
- Regional anesthesia contraindicated if coagulopathy exists
- Potential cardiac disease including pericardial effusion
- Type and cross-match may be difficult 2° to alloimmunization

THROMBOCYTOPENIA

Nauder Faraday, M.D.

RISK
- Common in both adults and children, especially in critical illness
- Often associated with systemic illness and pathologic conditions of pregnancy

PERIOPERATIVE RISKS
- May lead to massive bleeding

WORRY ABOUT
- Excessive perioperative bleeding
- Concurrent anemia or hypovolemia
- Concurrent hemodynamic instability from hypovolemia or infection
- Implications of specific drug therapies and potential for anesthetic interaction
- Implications of pregnancy
- Concurrent liver disease

OVERVIEW
- Definition: $< 150,000$ plt/mm^3
- Spontaneous bleeding does not generally occur unless the plt count $< 20,000$/mm^3
- Adequate surgical hemostasis achieved with plt counts between 50,000 and 100,000/mm^3, depending upon site and extent of procedure

- Generalized petechiae, purpura, and bleeding from mucous membranes denotes high risk of bleeding from other sites
- Dx of cause of thrombocytopenia is key to successful treatment; begins with CBC, PT/PTT, fibrinogen, and D-dimer
- Bleeding time has not been shown to correlate with risk of surgical bleeding

ICD-9-CM Code: 287.5

ETIOLOGY
- ↑ Plt destruction, immune: drug-induced, idiopathic thrombocytopenic purpura (ITP), rheumatologic disorders, post-transfusion purpura, neonatal immune thrombocytopenia
- ↑ Plt destruction, nonimmune: infection with or without overt DIC, preeclampsia/HELLP syndrome, thrombotic thrombocytopenic purpura (TTP), hemolytic uremic syndrome (HUS)
- ↓ Plt production
- Marrow failure: cancer infiltration, chemo- or radiation therapy, ethanol

- Hypersplenism: cirrhosis, portal or splenic vein thrombosis
- Dilution: generally plt counts maintained until intravascular replacement $> 1.5-2$ blood volumes

USUAL TREATMENT
- Treat underlying cause:
  – Discontinue offending drug, antibiotics for infection, splenectomy
  – Immunologically mediated syndromes generally respond to corticosteroids and IgG therapy
  – TTP and HUS may respond to plasmapheresis or to corticosteroids and IgG
- Decision to transfuse plts depends on etiology of thrombocytopenia and relative risks of bleeding vs. risks of transfusion
- Each unit of transfused plts should raise count $\sim 10,000$/mm^3 if there has not been immediate plt destruction, sequestration, or dilution, but increases risk of future thrombocytopenia (alloimmunization occurs in 50% of patients transfused with plts)

ASSESSMENT POINTS

SYSTEM	EFFECT	ASSESSMENT BY HX	PE	TEST
HEENT	Mucosal hemorrhage		Petechiae, purpura, and ecchymoses of skin, oral mucosae, and conjunctivae	
CV	Hypovolemia, anemia, hemorrhagic pericardial effusion	Lightheadedness, syncope, palpitations	Vital signs, orthostasis, pericardial friction rub, pulsus paradoxus	ECG, CXR
RESP	Pulm hemorrhage	Cough, hemoptysis		CXR
GI	GI bleeding	Hematemesis, hematochezia, melena		Stool guaiac
RENAL	Potential prerenal or renal azotemia, glomerulonephritis with specific disease entities	UO		BUN, Cr, urinalysis
CNS	Intracranial hemorrhage	Change in mental status	Neuro exam: mental status, focal findings	Head CT

Key Reference: Slaughter TF, Greenberg CS: Heparin-associated thrombocytopenia and thrombosis: implications for perioperative management. Anesthesiology 1997; 87:667–675.

PERIOPERATIVE IMPLICATIONS

Preoperative Preparation
- Assess volume status and Hct
- Qualitative assessment of bleeding risk from physical exam, extent of thrombocytopenia, type of surgical procedure
- Ensure that blood bank has adequate cross-matched PRBCs and plts available
- Plt transfusion immediately prior to surgical procedure for plt count $< 50,000$/mm^3
- DDAVP 0.3 μg/kg IV beneficial only in patients with concurrent renal failure or von Willebrand's disease

Monitoring
- Routine
- Plt count

Airway
- ↑ Risk of mucosal bleeding demands gentle laryngoscopy—lubrication of ET and laryngoscope blade may be helpful
- Nasal intubation relatively contraindicated

Induction
- None

Maintenance
- ↑ Risk of blood loss makes vigilance to volume status and replacement essential

Extubation
- Airway trauma/bleeding can occur with extubation

Adjuvants
- Regional: epidural and spinal anesthetics can be safely administered with plt counts $\geq 100,000$/mm^3. Risk of bleeding increases as the plt count falls below this level, although relationship is not linear. A few dozen cases of epidural anesthesia in patients with plt counts $< 100,000$/mm^3 have been reported by retrospective review without neurologic sequelae.

ANTICIPATED PROBLEMS/CONCERNS
- Excessive perioperative bleeding
- Physical exam, plt count, type of surgical procedure are best predictors of bleeding risk

THYROID NEOPLASMS
Alisa C. Thorne, M.D.

RISK

- In the USA: 11,300 new thyroid cancer cases/y; 8300 female, 3000 male
- Ranks among the 5 most frequent cancers in the 15–40 y age group
- Hispanics, African-Americans—lower rate; Caucasians—moderate rate; Japanese, Chinese, Hawaiian, Filipinos—higher rate
- Overall incidence 2–3 times higher in women than in men, but varies with age group

PERIOPERATIVE RISKS

- Large thyroid mass may produce airway compression, deviation, or vocal cord paralysis
- ↓BP, ↓HR, asystole with manipulation of carotid sinus
- Postop complications: phrenic n. injury, pneumomediastinum, pneumothorax, tracheomalacia and tracheal collapse post extubation, hematoma or laryngeal edema → airway compromise; bilat laryngeal n. injury → tracheotomy; superior laryngeal n. injury → aspiration
- Accidental removal/injury of parathyroid glands causes ↓Ca^{2+}

WORRY ABOUT

- Occult pheochromocytoma: bilateral lobe medullary thyroid cancer is associated with MEN IIA and IIB

OVERVIEW

- 4 types—papillary, follicular, medullary, undifferentiated
- Prognosis of well-differentiated papillary cancer excellent, especially for age <40 y with small tumors
- Prognosis worsens for large tumors with poorly differentiated, anaplastic histology
- Age at Dx, tumor burden, gender, extrathyroidal invasion, and distant metastases: important prognostic factors
- Latest research: define subcellular and molecular prognostic factors

ICD-9-CM Code: 193

ETIOLOGY

- Factors include previous radiation, dietary iodine deficiency, goitrogens (chemical or dietary), pre-existing benign thyroid disease, and genetic factors (Gardner's syndrome, Cowden's disease)
- Association between primary thyroid cancer and an ↑ incidence of subsequent breast cancer

USUAL TREATMENT

- Surgery initial therapy of choice
- Lobectomy with or without isthmectomy, near-total or total thyroidectomy as indicated
- Radical debulking procedure (palliative) for large tumors invading airway and causing esophageal obstruction and bleeding
- Combined chemo- and radiation therapy for poor prognosis cases
- Doxorubicin: most active single agent; medullary thyroid cancer responds poorly
- Doxorubicin combined with cisplatin possibly better for anaplastic malignancies

ASSESSMENT POINTS

SYSTEM	EFFECT	ASSESSMENT BY HX	PE	TEST
HEENT	Vocal cord dysfunction Tracheal obstruction	Dysphonia SOB, DOE Wheeze/stridor	Neck mass	Indirect laryngoscopy CXR CT of neck
CV	Mediastinal mass	SOB, DOE Wheeze, may be asymptomatic	Facial swelling	CXR CT/MRI
RESP	Lung metastases Lower airway obstruction	SOB, DOE Wheeze, hemoptysis		CXR CT/MRI
GI	Esophageal obstruction Liver metastases	Dysphagia		LFTs
ENDO	MEN IIA/IIB Pheochromocytoma	Htn, especially episodic Flushing Palpitations, episodic Sweating		CT/MRI 24 h urine epinephrine ↑ Epinephrine/norepinephrine
	Hyperparathyroidism			↑Ca^{2+} Hypercalciuria
	Ganglioneuromatosis	Colic Cramping Diarrhea Obstruction	Mucosal neuromas in tongue, subconjunctival areas, or GI tract Thickened lips Marfanoid features	Provocative test for calcitonin release
MS	Bone metastases PTH-induced bone disease	Bone pain		Bone scan

Key Reference: Lo Gerfo P: Local/regional anesthesia for thyroidectomy: evaluation as an outpatient procedure. Surgery 1998; 124:975–978.

PERIOPERATIVE IMPLICATIONS

Preoperative Preparation
- Assess thyroid gland/tumor size
- Assess larynx/trachea compression
- May need smaller or armored ETT to prevent kinking (check CT scan)
- Record description of voice preop
- Correct abnormal Ca^{2+}, TFTs prior to surgery
- Check serum calcitonin level if medullary cancer suspected; rule out pheochromocytoma

Monitoring
- Routine

Airway
- Anticipate difficult airway

Induction
- Consider awake fiberoptic intubation for large thyroid masses

Maintenance
- No one agent or technique shown superior
- CV instability may occur with manipulation of carotid sinus

Extubation
- May develop tracheomalacia
- May require reintubation owing to hematoma

Postoperative Period
- Metabolic: ↓Ca^{2+}, hypoparathyroidism
- Nonmetabolic: unilateral or bilateral n. injury, hemorrhage, airway obstruction

Adjuvants
- May be performed under local anesthesia with IV sedation in selected cases
- Antiemetics, including dexamethasone, effective in reducing postop N/V

ANTICIPATED PROBLEMS/CONCERNS
- Patients with medullary thyroid cancer: rule out occult pheochromocytoma
- Thyroid tumor can invade larynx, trachea, pharynx, or esophagus
- If esophageal wall invaded, reconstruction often by free microvascular jejunal transfer or gastric pull-up

TRANSFUSION-RELATED ACUTE LUNG INJURY

Christine S. Rinder, M.D.

• All patients receiving packed RBC, plt, FFP, cryo, or whole blood
• Incidence probably <1%, but being recognized with increasing frequency, probably because of greater awareness by clinicians

PERIOPERATIVE RISKS

• Noncardiogenic pulm edema within 2–6 h after transfusion
• Mortality reported, but rare

WORRY ABOUT

• Oxygen toxicity
• Barotrauma
• Should be suspected from signs of pulm edema after transfusion when little clinical suspicion of volume overload

OVERVIEW

• Classic presentation is acute development of respiratory compromise indistinguishable from ARDS 2–6 h after transfusion. Sx include acute hypoxemia, bilateral pulm edema (noncardiogenic), fever, possible hypotension.
• Dx one of exclusion (rule out fluid overload, CHF, sepsis)

ICD-9-CM Code: 999.8 (Transfusion, complication)

USUAL TREATMENT

• Supportive care: oxygen, pressure support. No clear indications for steroids. Generally resolves within 1–4 days with appropriate care and no supervening complications.

ASSESSMENT POINTS

SYSTEM	EFFECT	ASSESSMENT BY HX	PE	TEST
CV	Pulm edema			PA catheter, ECHO
RESP	Pulm edema	Recent transfusion	Rales, S_3, S_4	CXR—bilateral infiltrates, SpO_2
HEME	Leukoagglutination			Agglutination of recipient leukocytes by donor plasma: contact blood collection agency

Key Reference: Popovsky MA, Chaplin HC, Moore SB: Transfusion-related acute lung injury: a neglected, serious complication of hemotherapy. Transfusion 1992; 32:589–592.

PERIOPERATIVE IMPLICATIONS

Perioperative Concerns

• Acute respiratory compromise that may occur shortly after transfusion in healthy patient, but more typically 2–4 h after transfusion

Monitoring

• PA catheter may aid in the exclusion of cardiac etiology

Postoperative Considerations

• Most require ventilatory support for several days
• Ventilator management appropriate for ARDS

ANTICIPATED PROBLEMS/CONCERNS

• Oxygen toxicity and barotrauma

TRANSVERSE MYELITIS

John A. Ulatowski, M.D., Ph.D

RISK

- Incidence 1–1.7/1 million population

PERIOPERATIVE RISKS

- Few data available (usually grouped with multiple sclerosis)
- Anesthetic effect (worsening) unknown
- Sequelae of hypotension or Htn (dysautonomia)
- Urinary retention and UTI

WORRY ABOUT

- Autonomic dysfunction (midthoracic and above)
  - Acute: hypotension from spinal shock
  - Chronic: Htn, bradycardia from mass reflex
- Hyperkalemia from succinylcholine

OVERVIEW

- Inflammatory disease of spinal cord causing demyelination/necrosis
- Ascending paralysis and sensory level usually T8–12 associated with pain and urinary retention
- Spinal cord swelling; ↑ CSF protein, WBC 10–200 (higher if culture positive)
- Onset over hours to days
- Antecedent febrile illness (33%)
- Variable recovery
- Multiple sclerosis (other demyelinating lesions) occurs in 5–10% of cases

ICD-9-CM Code: 323.9 (Encephalitis, unspecified cause)

ETIOLOGY

- Viral (polio, HSV, HIV)
- Bacterial, fungal, parasitic
- Noninfectious (postinfectious, postvaccine, lupus)

USUAL TREATMENT

- High-dose steroids
- Long-term antibiotics if frequent UTI

ASSESSMENT POINTS

SYSTEM	EFFECT	ASSESSMENT BY HX	PE	TEST
HEENT	Eyes (MS, Devic's syndrome)	↓ Visual acuity	Optic neuritis, ophthalmoscope	Visual EPs
CV	↑ BP, ↓ BP	Syncope, headache	BP changes	Orthostasis
RESP	Pulm embolism	Dyspnea, tachycardia	DVT, cord sign	Doppler, V/Q scan
GI	Gastric atony	N/V, dyspepsia, early satiety	Tympany, CXR	Stomach bubble
CNS	Brain Spine	Encephalitis presenting symptoms	Mental status changes Paraplegia	MRI MRI, LP
RENAL	Bladder paralysis	Retention, oliguria	Palpation, catheterization	UA, residual

Key Reference: Jones RM, Healy TEJ: Anaesthesia and demyelinating disease. Anaesthesia 1980; 35:879–884.

PERIOPERATIVE IMPLICATIONS

Preoperative Preparation
- Relieve gastric ileus

Monitoring
- Routine

Airway
- Avoid succinylcholine

Induction
- Adequate hydration because of dysautonomia

Maintenance
- GA or epidural; spinal with caution, possible toxicity with usual doses

Extubation
- Return of airway reflexes if demyelinating lesions in brain/brainstem

Adjuvants
- Resistance to nondepolarizing muscle relaxants

ANTICIPATED PROBLEMS/CONCERNS

- Unstable hemodynamics
- Possible hyperkalemia following succinylcholine

TREACHER COLLINS SYNDROME

Daniel Siker, M.D.
James Armstrong, M.D.

RISK

• People within USA: 1/8000–10,000 live births

PERIOPERATIVE RISKS

• Difficult airway management from mandibular dysostosis

WORRY ABOUT

• Difficult intubation
• Risk of obstructive sleep apnea or death postop
• Difficult mask induction of anesthesia

OVERVIEW

• Form of mandibulofacial dysostosis characterized by hypoplasia of mandible, maxilla, and malar bones as well as bilateral deformities of pinnae and lateral downward sloping of palpebral fissures
• Pharyngeal hypoplasia, esp in lateral diameter and to lesser extent in AP dimension
• Dimensions of pharynx are reduced by hypoplastic facial bones. Base of tongue may have narrowest opening.
• Hyoid bone displaced anteriorly and inferiorly

ICD-9-CM Code: 756.0

ETIOLOGY

• Autosomal dominant with variable expressivity
• First branchial arch defect (Franceschetti's syndrome) caused by loss of blood supply to area during 3rd and 5th wk of development

USUAL TREATMENT

• Operations include tympanoplasty, cleft lip and palate repair, palatoplasty

ASSESSMENT POINTS

SYSTEM	EFFECT	ASSESSMENT BY HX	PE	TEST
HEENT	Limited airway	Inspiratory stridor Coughing during feeding Diaphoresis during feeding Snoring	Narrow pharynx	
CV	Cor pulmonale ↑ Association with congenital heart defects	Easy fatigability Chest discomfort	S_3, hepatomegaly ↑ Jugular venous pulsations Heart murmur	ECG: RAE P waves in II, IIIa, VF RAO CXR: RVH ECHO
RESP	Obstructive sleep apnea	Loud nasal snoring Frequent arousal during sleep Daytime hypersomnolence		Polysomnography
CNS	Usually intellectually normal May have learning disability			

Key Reference: Marsh KL, Dixon MJ: Treacher Collins syndrome. Adv Otorhinolaryngol 2000; 56:53–59.

PERIOPERATIVE IMPLICATIONS

Preoperative Preparation

• Preoperative sedation may cause upper airway obstruction
• Antisialagogue may be of benefit

Monitoring

• Communication between surgeon and anesthesiologist

Airway

• Mask ventilation may be difficult. Consider large, clear, pliable facial mask.
• Consider fiberoptic bronchoscope or Bullard laryngoscope or laryngeal mask airway, tactile guides, or retrograde techniques
• Airway may become more difficult to secure following pharyngeal surgery
• Tracheotomy may be considered for patient requiring multiple procedures

Preinduction/Induction

• Avoid sedatives if obstructive symptoms
• Consider direct laryngoscopy if obstructive symptoms
• Consider deep inhalation induction or ketamine induction with maintenance of spontaneous ventilation during laryngoscopy

Maintenance

• Avoid heavy use of opioids because of postop resp depression

Extubation

• Extubate when fully awake
• Risk of upper airway obstruction and negative pressure pulm edema

Adjuvants

• IV steroids for treatment of edema

Postoperative Period

• Possibility of hypersomnolent state
• Monitor for airway obstruction
• Obstructive sleep apnea
• Post palatoplasty, airway obstruction may be ameliorated by suture through tongue to relieve airway obstruction

ANTICIPATED PROBLEMS/CONCERNS

• Failure to thrive
• Significant hearing loss may be present
• Obstructive sleep apnea
• Cor pulmonale
• Removal of all oral packing

TRICUSPID ATRESIA

Susan C. Nicolson, M.D.

RISK

- Occurs in ~1/10,000 live births
- Third most common cause of cyanotic congenital heart disease
- Slight male predominance

PERIOPERATIVE RISKS

- Sequelae of chronic hypoxemia or CHF
- Surgical shunt complications
- Issues unique to patients with univentricular heart undergoing staged reconstructive surgery

WORRY ABOUT

- Associated CV anomalies
- Extracardiac anomalies (GI, musculoskeletal systems)

OVERVIEW

- Congenital cardiac malformation with agenesis of the tricuspid valve resulting in no communication between right atrium and hypoplastic RV
- Survival depends on interatrial communication and L → R shunt at ventricular (VSD) or great vessel (PDA) level
- Types of tricuspid atresia (frequency)
  - Type I—normally related great vessels (70%)
  - Type II—D-TGA (transposition of the great arteries) (30%)
  - Type III—L-TGA (rare)

Each type further subdivided depending on presence of pulmonic stenosis/atresia and the absence or size of VSD
- Clinical presentation and treatment depend on associated cardiac anomalies that are responsible for pulm blood flow being increased, decreased, or normal

ICD-9-CM Code: 746.1

ETIOLOGY

- Postulated to result from malalignment of the ventricular septum in relation to the atria and AV canal

USUAL TREATMENT

- Palliative surgery usually within 1st year of life intended to
  - Increase pulm blood flow when it is diminished (small VSD, pulmonary stenosis [PS]) via systemic to PA shunt or systemic venous to pulm anastomosis or
  - Decrease pulm blood flow when it is excessive (large VSD) via PA band and/or
  - Eliminate major interatrial obstruction
- Ultimate physiologic correction via modification of Fontan's operation (see Transposition of the Great Vessels [TGV], Repair of, in Procedures section)

ASSESSMENT POINTS

SYSTEM	EFFECT	ASSESSMENT BY HX	PE	TEST
CV	↓ Pulm blood flow – Hypoxemia – Acidosis ↑ Pulm blood flow		Cyanosis	ABGs/ SpO$_2$
	Heart failure	Poor weight gain, frequent URIs	Tachycardia, tachypnea Hepatosplenomegaly	
	Endocarditis			ECHO
	Dysrhythmias			ECG
RESP	Pulm vascular obstructive disease			ECHO ECG SpO$_2$
HEME	Polycythemia			Hgb; coag tests
CNS	Stroke Brain abscess	Hemiplegia		CT/ MRI

Key Reference: Okanlami O, Nichols DG, Nicolson SC, et al: Tricuspid atresia and the Fontan operation. *In* Nichols DG, Cameron DE, Greely WJ, et al (eds): Critical Heart Disease in Infants and Children. St. Louis, Mosby-Year Book, 1995, pp 737–769.

PERIOPERATIVE IMPLICATIONS

Preoperative Preparation

- PGE$_1$ infusion in neonate with ductal dependent pulm circulation
- Anticongestive measures for rare infant presenting with CHF
- Preanesthetic medication appropriate for age and physical status

Monitoring

- Routine
- Consider intra-arterial and/or central venous catheter when patient condition or procedure indicates

Airway

- Meticulous attention to maintain patency

Preinduction/Induction

- Carefully titrated anesthetic appropriate for age and procedure, taking into consideration physiology of individual patient

Maintenance

- Keep warm
- Maintain euvolemia

Adjuvants

- Consider heparin (100 U/kg) prior to systemic to pulm artery shunt placement

ANTICIPATED PROBLEMS/CONCERNS

- Manipulating physiology through appropriately timed and precisely executed palliative procedures to maximize the potential for the child to ultimately be good candidate for Fontan's procedure

RISK

• Trigeminal neuralgia (TN) is a symptom and not a disease
• 15/100,000 of population are affected. 1–3% of multiple sclerosis (MS) patients have TN.
• 45% of patients are male

PERIOPERATIVE RISKS

• Carbamazepine and phenytoin used in treatment of TN may cause enzyme induction
• Patients on baclofen requiring GA may have severe bradycardia and hypotension due to unknown mechanism
• Potential for drug abuse with anxiolytic and opioid preparations

WORRY ABOUT

• Side effects of drug therapy
• Worsening MS after surgery
• Airway problems due to associated cranial nerve involvement
• Associated sensory or motor deficits of eyes, face

OVERVIEW

• TN is a common painful condition of the face; peak occurrence in 6th decade. The most common division of cranial nerve V involved, in order of frequency, is mandibular, or 3rd division; combination of mandibular and maxillary, or 2nd division; maxillary and rarely ophthalmic, or 1st division. Pathognomonic features of TN are

– *Pain:* Abrupt onset of paroxysmal, sharp, electric shock–like, brief, lancinating pains lasting a few seconds to 1 min. In between flashes, patient is pain-free, 50% have remission lasting 6 mo. TN with MS rarely has spontaneous remission. Pain is unilateral, confined to anatomic pathways of cranial nerve V, brought about by non-noxious stimuli (light touch, cold breeze, talking, vibrations). Pain bilateral in 5% of cases, right > left, and seldom at night. Pain is of burning type, when chronic, and supersedes tic.
– *Neurologic findings (NF):* No NF in idiopathic TN. Abnormal NF in symptomatic TN. CT scans or MRI yields <5% positive results. 45% of patients show structural abnormalities on posterior cranial fossa surgery (PCFS). Patients with previous ganglion neurolysis may show areas of sensory deficits or other cranial nerve involvement.
– *No pathologic findings post mortem*
– *Trigger zones:* Trigger zones are present on same side as facial pain in 91%. Trigger zones are present in more than one division of the trigeminal nerve, predominantly in central part of face.
• *Recurrence:* In similar areas of face with intervals decreasing over time

ICD-9-CM Code: 350.1

ETIOLOGY

Idiopathic

• Degeneration of myelin sheath of Vth nerve root over petrous temporal bone
• Compression by aberrant vessel

Symptomatic

• Cancer of maxillary antrum or nasopharynx, tumors of cranial nerves, vascular anomalies, and mass lesions
• Painful paroxysm of TN caused by combination of ↑ afferent activity and ↓ segmental inhibition in delta and C fibers, resulting in excessive response of wide dynamic range neurons to tactile stimulation

USUAL TREATMENT

• *Pharmacologic:* Carbamazepine (Tegretol), phenytoin (Dilantin), baclofen (Lioresal) are used for TN. Chlorphenesin and mephenesin less commonly used.
• *Anesthesiologic:* Mandibular and/or maxillary nerve blocks under fluoroscopy. Glycerol chemical or percutaneous radiofrequency lesioning of trigeminal ganglion under CT scan.
• *Surgical*
– Microvascular decompression (MVD) involving posterior cranial fossa surgery with 92% success rate
– Gamma knife radiation first developed in Sweden is being used by some centers in USA as first-line therapy for TN. A maximal radiosurgical dose of 70 Gy is delivered to ipsilateral side of brain where trigeminal nerve root exits the brainstem. Success rate is 88% with minimal incidence of numbness (10%).
– Radio-frequency lesioning reported to provide pain relief in 85% of TN cases

ASSESSMENT POINTS

SYSTEM	EFFECT
CNS	Assess other cranial nerve involvement and sensory deficit in face, cornea, and areas of dysesthesia; sensory Sx

Key References: Barry J, Sessle S: Trigeminal pain: nociceptive pathways and mechanisms. Pain Digest 1991; 1:78–91; Maciewicz R, Scrivani S: Trigeminal neuralgia: gamma radiosurgery may provide new options for treatment. Neurology 1997; 48:565–566.

PERIOPERATIVE IMPLICATIONS

Preoperative Preparation

• Patients on baclofen requiring GA may have severe bradycardia and hypotension due to unknown mechanism. Potential for drug abuse with anxiolytic and opioid preparations.

Monitoring

• Monitored anesthesia care for anesthesiologic procedures. For posterior cranial fossa surgery, A-line, CVP, Doppler US, esophageal stethoscope, and end-tidal CO_2 monitor may aid detection and treatment of air embolism and hypotension.

Airway

• Caution if patient has other cranial nerve involvement or MS (assess for intraoperative airway obstruction due to brainstem stimulation)

Induction

• Avoid succinylcholine in patients with MS

Maintenance

• Sitting posture associated with hypotension, air embolism, and hemodynamic instability intraoperatively with posterior cranial fossa surgery. Prevention, early detection, and treatment of hypotension, airway obstruction, and air embolism.

Extubation

• Consider for loss of protective reflexes

Adjuvants

• Be prepared to treat bradycardia, hypotension, or air embolism efficiently
• Carbamazepine and phenytoin used in treatment of TN may cause enzyme induction. These agents may increase dosage requirements of drugs metabolized by cytochrome P-450 such as NM blockers (see also Carbamazepine [Tegretol] and Phenytoin in Drugs section)

Postoperative Period

• Consider ventilator support if difficult posterior cranial fossa craniotomy

TRUNCUS ARTERIOSUS

Chandra Ramamoorthy, F.F.A.R.C.S.
Jeffrey P. Morray, M.D.

RISK

- Rare anomaly, 2.8% of all congenital heart defects
- No gender predilection

PERIOPERATIVE RISKS

- Thrombosis if prolonged NPO
- CHF
- Myocardial contractile depression by volatile agents
- Inadvertent hyperventilation resulting in reduced PVR with excess PBF and worsening CHF
- Infective endocarditis
- Risks of CPB

WORRY ABOUT

- Difficult intubation
- Heart failure
- Hypocalcemia
- Air embolus

OVERVIEW

- Common trunk is the only great artery arising from heart
- VSD always present
- Dominant physiology is a L → R shunt at the level of great vessels leading to excessive PBF; CHF
- Obligatory mixing of systemic and pulm venous blood at level of VSD and truncal valve. High SaO_2 suggests excess PBF.
- Abnormal truncal valve, with regurgitation in half, stenosis in a third. Anomalies of coronary artery and aortic arch may be present.
- Early development of pulm vascular obstructive disease due to excessive pulm blood flow
- 33% have DiGeorge's anomaly (congenital absence of thymus, parathyroid hypoplasia, great vessel anomaly, micrognathia, low-set ears, short philtrum)
- 20% with 22q11 deletion; part of CATCH 22 syndrome (cardiac defect, abnormal facies, thymic hypoplasia, cleft palate, hypocalcemia)

- Uniformly fatal without surgical correction (50% die by 1 mo and 80% within 1 y)

ICD-9-CM Code: 745.0

ETIOLOGY

- Congenital heart defect arising from partial or complete absence of truncoconal septum. Embryonic truncus fails to separate into a pulm and aortic trunk.
- Maternal diabetes predisposes to truncoconal abnormalities

USUAL TREATMENT

- Medical therapy is temporizing (digoxin, loop diuretics, inotropes) to treat CHF
- Surgical repair in the neonatal period is the definitive treatment. On hypothermic CPB, the pulmonary trunk is separated from the truncal artery. VSD is closed, and an RV-to-PA (Rastelli) conduit is placed.

ASSESSMENT POINTS

SYSTEM	EFFECT	ASSESSMENT BY HX	PE	TEST
HEENT	Difficult laryngoscopy and intubation		Small mandible, small mouth	
CV	CHF—truncal valve regurgitation Pulm Htn	Difficulty feeding Sweating during feeds Failure to thrive	Cyanosis ± single S_2 Murmur—systolic or diastolic	Pulse oximeter, ECG, ECHO Cardiac cath ±
RESP	CHF—excessive pulm blood flow	Difficulty breathing	Tachypnea Retraction	CXR (↑ pulm markings, cardiomegaly)
ENDO	Parathyroid hypoplasia	Seizures, tetany		Serum ionized Ca^{2+}, parathyroid hormone level
IMMUNO	Cellular immunodeficiency	Recurrent infections Chronic diarrhea		CBC, T-cell function
MS	Dysmorphic facies		Hypertelorism, low-set ears	

Key References: Garson A Jr, Bricker JT, Fisher DJ, Neish SR: The Science and Practice of Pediatric Cardiology. Baltimore, Williams & Wilkins, 1998, pp 1421–1430; Lake CL: Pediatric Cardiac Anesthesia. Norwalk, CT, Appleton & Lange, 1998, pp 360–363.

PERIOPERATIVE IMPLICATIONS

Perioperative Preparation

- Avoid long NPO as thrombosis risk
- Treat CHF
- If intubated, adjust to normocapnia and normoxemia
- Avoid hyperventilation—↑ PBF
- Check electrolytes and Ca^{2+}

Monitoring

- Arterial catheter and CVP
- TEE valuable to assess truncal valve function, VSD patch leak, assess ventricular function, pulm blood flow
- Consider LA line

Airway

- Difficult airway precautions

Preinduction/Induction

- Meticulous air bubble exclusion
- Antibiotic SBE prophylaxis
- SVR decrease with induction may result in hypotension with stenotic truncal valve
- Monitor for myocardial ischemia due to PA runoff; temporary PA band after sternotomy may help

Maintenance

- More sensitive to the effects of volatile agents
- Deep hypothermia and circulatory arrest or low-flow CPB

Extubation

- Postop ventilation usually required (resp acidosis will reduce PBF and impair myocardial function)

Postoperative Period

- CHF: poor RV function (right ventriculotomy and Rastelli conduit placement); LV dysfunction (circulatory arrest, long bypass, myocardial ischemia, truncal valve abnormalities)
- Increased PVR and pulm Htn (low CO and low SaO_2) responds to hyperventilation, metabolic alkalosis, vasodilators (milrinone, PGE_1, NO), sedation (analgesia, paralysis)
- AV block requiring pacemaker
- Bleeding, tamponade

ANTICIPATED PROBLEMS/CONCERNS

- CHF
- Truncal valve regurgitation and/or stenosis
- Pulm Htn
- Infective endocarditis

TUBERCULOSIS (TB)

Karen B. Traber, M.D.

- 8 million cases/y
- Increased risk of exposure to infected adult in homeless, the elderly (especially in nursing homes), minorities, immigrants (especially from Asia and Latin America), and prisoners
- Increased likelihood once infection occurs in HIV co-infection, immunosuppressive therapies, malnutrition, body wt ≥ 10% below ideal, infants, and with certain medical conditions (silicosis, diabetes mellitus, carcinoma)

PERIOPERATIVE RISKS

- Depends on pulmonary and systemic dysfunction and type of surgery
- CDC recommends delay of elective surgery until infected individual has had adequate course of chemotherapy

WORRY ABOUT

- Co-morbidities of patient, extent of organ system impairment, toxicity of TB therapy

OVERVIEW

- *Mycobacterium tuberculosis* is one of most significant worldwide pathogens, causing estimated 8 million new cases and 3 million deaths each year
- Number of cases in USA declined prior to 1985 but is now on the rise (poverty, drug and alcohol abuse, HIV infection, immigration of infected persons)

ICD-9-CM Codes: 013-017

ETIOLOGY

- Transmitted by droplet nuclei produced by coughing, sneezing, talking
- Primary and exogenous reinfection now more common than reactivation, especially with HIV

USUAL TREATMENT

- 6 mo of isoniazid plus rifampin, supplemented by pyrazinamide for first 2 mo
- Same therapy used for HIV-positive patients with TB, but for longer duration (at least 9 mo, or 6 mo after negative cultures)
- Streptomycin and ethambutol can be used in resistant infections

ASSESSMENT POINTS

SYSTEM	EFFECT	ASSESSMENT BY HX	PE	TEST
GENERAL		Night sweats, wt loss	Fever	PPD (purified protein derivative [tuberculin])
CV	Pericardial effusion, myocarditis, heart block		Muffled heart sounds, friction rub	ECHO, ECG, biopsy
RESP	Apical infiltrates, caseation necrosis, hilar adenopathy	Cough, possible hemoptysis	Often normal	CXR, sputum culture
GI	Peritonitis, enteritis, colitis	Diarrhea, hematochezia	Ascites	Endoscopy, biopsy
GU	Chronic cystitis and epididymitis, pyelonephritis	↑ Urine frequency and urgency when advanced Painless hematuria		Urinalysis and culture
CNS	TB meningitis	Headache, dizziness, confusion		Lumbar puncture for CSF and culture
MS	Long bone and vertebral involvement	Pain		X-ray, bone scan

Key Reference: Tait AR: Occupational transmission of tuberculosis: implications for anesthesiologists. Anesth Analg 1997; 85:444–451.

PERIOPERATIVE IMPLICATIONS

Preoperative Preparation

- Evaluate for possible toxic response to anti-TB therapy (hepatitis, thrombocytopenia, ototoxicity, optic neuritis, nephrotoxicity, peripheral neuropathy) and extent of organ system involvement
- Restrict spread of organism by removing unnecessary OR equipment, limiting traffic to OR, using disposable equipment, and wearing protective clothing including special surgical mask with tight face seal that prevents penetration of aerosolized particles in 1–5 μm range
- Use ultraviolet lights (often in old orthopedic OR) as *M. tuberculosis* sensitive to UV radiation

Monitoring

- Depends on extent of systemic involvement and surgical procedure

Extubation

- Restrict exposure of perioperative personnel to aerosolized TB

Adjuvants

- Isoniazid may increase defluorination of volatile anesthetics. Increased plasma fluoride levels in patients on isoniazid after exposure to enflurane anesthesia has been reported.

ANTICIPATED PROBLEMS/CONCERNS

- TB a contagious disease with significant consequence to general public. Drug resistance and patient noncompliance with therapy are major public health problems. Universal infection precautions should be taken when managing patients in high-risk groups.

ULCERATIVE COLITIS, CHRONIC

Jeffrey Dodd-o, M.D.

RISK

- Prevalence in USA: 45–80/100,000, with static incidence of 5–10/100,000/y
- Incidence in two peaks: first at age 20–30 y and again at age 60 y
- More common in Caucasians than African-Americans
- Jews > non-Jews
- Nonsmokers > smokers
- About 5–10% have family Hx

PERIOPERATIVE RISKS

- Adrenal insufficiency if preop corticosteroid use
- Infection and delayed wound healing, especially with stress steroids
- Resp compromise from abdominal incision, malnutrition, or associated seronegative spondyloarthropathy (ankylosing spondylitis)

WORRY ABOUT

- If surgery for Sx unresponsive to medical management, patient is more likely to be anemic, dehydrated, malnourished, and with lyte imbalance

OVERVIEW

- Inflammatory reaction limited to mucosal layers of all or part of colon. Results in impaired intestinal absorption, bleeding, and colonic dilation.
- Can lead to diarrhea and its complications (dehydration, hypokalemia, metabolic acidosis, malnutrition, hypoalbuminemia), anemia, and impaired colonic motility resulting in distention and perforation
- Pharmacologic adjuncts include sulfasalazine and steroids. Sulfasalazine can lead to hemolytic anemia (which worsens anemia from GI bleeding) and hepatitis. Corticosteroids can lead to uremia and adrenal insufficiency.

ICD-9-CM Code: 556.9

ETIOLOGY

- Unknown, though genetics may be contributory

USUAL TREATMENT

- Mild disease—sulfasalazine. Begun at 500 mg bid and increased over 1–2 wk to 2–4 g/d. Can be continued indefinitely. Steroid retention enemas for 4–6 wk may help proctosigmoiditis.
- Severe disease—corticosteroids, lyte repletion, parenteral nutrition. Corticosteroids may make abdominal exam unreliable.
- Uncontrolled symptoms or threat of malignancy—surgery to remove colon and rectum. Panulcerative colitis has ↑ risk of dysplasia, with malignancy risk as high as 10% per decade.

ASSESSMENT POINTS

SYSTEM	EFFECT	ASSESSMENT BY HX	PE	TEST
HEENT	Difficult positioning if associated ankylosing spondylitis	Ankylosing spondylitis		
CV	Hypovolemia Sepsis Aortic regurgitation		Orthostatic vital signs	BUN/ Cr
RESP	Apical fibrosis Associated ankylosing spondylitis	Exertional dyspnea		CXR
GI	Bowel obstruction/perforation	Constipation, vomiting		Abd x-ray
HEME	Anemia	Bloody stools	Pale conjunctiva	Hgb
RENAL	Diarrhea	Diarrhea Muscle cramps		Lytes BUN/Cr

Key Reference: McGill DB, Hoffman HN II: Gastroenterology. *In* Kochar M (ed): Concise Textbook of Medicine, 2nd ed. Norwalk, CT, Appleton & Lange, 1990, pp 320–323.

PERIOPERATIVE IMPLICATIONS

Preoperative Preparation

- Fluid resuscitation; consider stress steroids
- Anticholinergics may ↑ risk of toxic megacolon

Monitoring

- Routine; consider UO
- Consider CVP catheter for fluid management

Airway

- Consider full stomach

Maintenance

- If surgery for uncontrolled symptoms, expect large intraoperative fluid requirements
- Technically difficult surgery if abdominal adhesions from prior surgeries
- Potential for progression of underlying sepsis
- Avoid nitrous oxide if intestinal obstruction

Extubation

- Keep warm

Postoperative Period

- Early parenteral nutrition and postop neuraxial analgesia may be beneficial

ANTICIPATED PROBLEMS/CONCERNS

- If prior steroid use, may be addisonian and require supplemental steroids

UPPER RESPIRATORY TRACT INFECTION Susan C. Nicolson, M.D.

RISK

- Children suffer 5–8 URIs/y (higher incidence in children in day care and whose parents smoke)
- 6% of pediatric surgical candidates present for anesthesia with an active URI

PERIOPERATIVE RISKS

- Phase of URI (onset, active, resolution) may influence risk
- Potential respiratory complications 2° to secretions and/or irritable airway
  - Laryngospasm (other risk factors: young age, airway surgery, inexperienced anesthesiologist)
  - Bronchospasm (intubated patients)
  - Postextubation stridor
  - Perioperative arterial desaturation
- No data to show respiratory complications are associated with morbidity

WORRY ABOUT

- Cost of complication: prolonged day surgery stay, unexpected admission of outpatient, unexpected ICU admission
- Cost of cancellation: repeat preoperative evaluation and testing (if needed), inconvenience and lost income to patient and family, lost revenue from inefficient use of OR

OVERVIEW

- At least 2 of the following Sx must exist for a child to have a URI: (1) sore or scratchy throat, (2) sneezing, (3) rhinorrhea, (4) congestion, (5) malaise, (6) nonproductive cough, (7) temp < 38.5°C, and (8) laryngitis
- Combination of items 1 and 5, 2 and 3, 3 and 6, and 4 and 6 require the presence of at least 1 additional symptom
- Higher temp, constitutional symptoms, and/or signs of lower respiratory tract involvement are not consistent with diagnosis of URI

ICD-9-CM Code: 465.9

ETIOLOGY

- Viral

USUAL TREATMENT

- Time, self-limited
- Treatment of symptoms

ASSESSMENT POINTS

SYSTEM	EFFECT	ASSESSMENT BY HX	PE	TEST
RESP	URI	Sore or scratchy throat Sneezing Rhinorrhea Congestion Nonproductive cough	Wheezing	CXR (if indicated)

Key Reference: Nicolson SC, Steven JM: Child with upper respiratory tract infection. *In* Atlee JL (ed): Complications in Anesthesia. Philadelphia, WB Saunders, 1999, pp 707–709.

PERIOPERATIVE IMPLICATIONS

- Age of child
- Frequency of URIs—Is there likely to be an interval when the child does not have an active process or is not within a few weeks of having one?
- Type and urgency of surgery—Is the operation directed at ameliorating chronic upper respiratory tract symptoms? Is the procedure urgent or emergent?
- Child's other medical problems—Patients with reactive airway disease have a higher likelihood of respiratory complications
- Anesthesiologist's skill and experience
- Attitude of parents—ability to make informed decision
- Miscellaneous issues (designated or autologous blood availability, surgeon availability)

Preoperative Preparation

- Obtain CXR if evidence of lower respiratory pathology
- Consider administration of an anticholinergic (nebulized ipratropium, atropine) to block muscarinic receptors and as antisialagogue

Monitoring

- Continuous perioperative SpO_2

Airway

- Use of a smaller ET tube, if intubation is indicated
- Consider regional technique or sedation with natural airway

Induction

- Consider IV rather than inhalational to minimize airway reactivity
- Consider avoiding ketamine because of the copious secretions that may result

Maintenance

- Use heated humidified inspired gases

Extubation

- Fully awake or deep

Adjuvants

- Consider use of lidocaine and/or opioids to ↓ airway reflexes

Postoperative Period

- Administration of supplemental O_2 when appropriate

ANTICIPATED PROBLEMS/CONCERNS

- Pulmonary changes may last 4–7 wk after resolution of symptoms

URINARY LITHIASIS
Terri G. Monk, M.D.

RISK

- Annual incidence of stone disease: 16.4/10,000
- 12% of all individuals will experience calculous disease
- Male:female ratio is 3:1
- Race with highest prevalence: Caucasians; rare in North American Indians and African-Americans
- Peak incidence: 3rd to 5th decade of life

PERIOPERATIVE RISKS

- Morbidity/mortality very low

WORRY ABOUT

- ↓ Renal function from partial or complete renal obstruction
- Sepsis, possibly septic shock, if surgical procedure performed in presence of UTI
- Perinephric hematoma if bleeding diathesis

- Pregnancy testing of women of child-bearing age because urologic procedures often utilize radiation, and lithotripsy is contraindicated during pregnancy

OVERVIEW

- Urolithiasis refers to abnormal concretions occurring anywhere along collecting system of urinary tract
- Most stones seen in industrialized countries contain calcium oxalate (75%); remainder are composed of uric acid, struvite, or cystine
- If properly treated, urolithiasis does not adversely affect life expectancy
- Calculi < 4 mm in diameter usually pass without intervention
- ~20% of stones cause enough symptoms to require surgical removal

ICD-9-CM Codes: 592.0 (Calculus of kidney); 592.1 (Calculus of ureter)

ETIOLOGY

- Intrinsic factors: renal tubular acidosis, cystinuria, primary hyperparathyroidism
- Lesch-Nyhan syndrome
- Extrinsic factors: ↑ environmental temperatures resulting in ↑ perspiration and hyperconcentration of urine (southeast and southwest regions of USA); low-intake drinking habits resulting in low UO; diet rich in calcium, animal fat (uric acid), or leafy vegetables (oxalate); immobility, including sedentary occupations

USUAL TREATMENT

- Observation and symptomatic pain Rx until spontaneous passage
- If surgical intervention necessary (20%), choice based on stone size and location
  - Lithotripsy
  - Percutaneous nephrolithiasis
  - Ureteroscopy

ASSESSMENT POINTS

SYSTEM	EFFECT	ASSESSMENT BY HX	PE	TEST
CV	↑ Heart rate or BP 2° to pain		Tachycardia Htn	
RESP	Grunting respiration during renal colic		Normal chest exam	
GI	Abdominal pain	N/V "Moving irritation" in abdomen	Tenderness to deep palpation of abdomen	
RENAL	Renal colic characterized by unusually severe pain localizing to affected flank; pain may radiate to groin or abdomen	Sudden onset of flank pain	Flank tenderness to palpation over affected kidney	UA (hematuria) Abdominal film (KUB)

Key Reference: Drach GW: Urinary lithiasis: etiology, diagnosis and medical management. *In* Walsh PC, Retik AB, Stamey TA, Vaughan ED Jr (eds): Campbell's Urology, 6th ed. Philadelphia, WB Saunders, 1992, pp 2085–2156.

PERIOPERATIVE IMPLICATIONS

Perioperative Preparation

- If obese, require acid aspiration prophylaxis and airway evaluation

Monitoring

- Routine
- Temp monitoring during immersion lithotripsy essential because water temp may produce hyperthermia or hypothermia
- Shock waves synchronized to ECG to avoid dysrhythmias

Preinduction

- Adequate padding to avoid nerve damage

Induction

- Many anesthetic techniques employed, but sedation adequate for lithotripsy and minor ureteroscopy procedures

Maintenance

- Central blood volume increases
- May become hypotensive 2° to warm water ↓ SVR
- Vital capacity ↓ and work of breathing ↑
- Pleural effusion or hydropneumothorax may occur during percutaneous renal procedures

Adjuvants

- Visualization of stone may require iodine-containing contrast material
- Anticholinergic agents (atropine) occasionally given to shorten lithotripsy treatments; however, tachycardia can occur, resulting in myocardial ischemia in high-risk patients
- Most patients receive prophylactic antibiotics prior to urinary tract procedures

ANTICIPATED PROBLEMS/CONCERNS

- Allergic reactions in 5% receiving IV contrast media
- Steinstrasse, ureteral obstruction by fragmented calculi, may cause ureteral colic following lithotripsy
- Htn may occur following lithotripsy
- Septic complications occur in 1% after lithotripsy
- Ureteral injury occurs in 9% of ureteroscopy procedures, with 1.6% requiring further surgical intervention

URTICARIA, COLD

Richard R. Bartkowski, M.D., Ph.D.

RISK

- Prevalence is very low (< 1/100,000)
- Appears in all races and genders, reported between ages 3 mo and 74 y but seen typically at 18–25 y

PERIOPERATIVE RISKS

- Can develop urticaria or angioedema with skin cooling and rewarming
- Shocklike reactions can occur with whole-body cold exposure
- Cooling with cardiopulmonary bypass can induce symptoms

WORRY ABOUT

- Cold exposure of patient (e.g., cold room, cold fluids, cold instruments or devices to cool skin)

OVERVIEW

- Characterized by appearance of urticaria or angioedema after cold exposure
- Usually acquired condition—seen typically by 18–25 y
- Can be primary or 2° to underlying disease such as malignancy or infection
- Symptoms often last 5–9 y and undergo remission or recede with primary disease
- Diagnosis by cold stimulation test
- Not related to cold serum factors

ICD-9-CM Code: 708.2

ETIOLOGY

- Primary cold urticaria appears related to skin mast cells sensitized to cold by a serum factor, very likely antibodies
- Sensitized skin mast cells (not blood basophils) release histamines on interaction with cold
- Similar activation by cryoglobulins appears in secondary cold urticaria

USUAL TREATMENT

- Antihistamines, both H_1 and H_2, successful at reducing occurrences even for hypothermic cardiopulmonary bypass

---

ASSESSMENT POINTS

SYSTEM	EFFECT	ASSESSMENT BY HX
SKIN	Urticaria or angioedema	Hx of cold reactions
RESP	Angioedema	Hx of swelling on cold exposure

Key Reference: Shephard RJ, Shek PN: Cold exposure and immune function. Can J Physiol Pharmacol 1998; 76:828–836.

PERIOPERATIVE IMPLICATIONS

Preoperative Preparation

- Antihistamines H_1 and H_2 only if a cold challenge anticipated during surgery

Monitoring

- Temperature, skin condition

Maintenance

- IV fluids; keep room and patient warm

ANTICIPATED PROBLEMS/CONCERNS

- Localized areas of urticaria/angioedema not of great concern, but serious widespread edema can compromise the airway or lead to fluid extravasation or shock
- Maintain temperature
- Pretreatment with antihistamines if cold is unavoidable

UTERINE RUPTURE

Judith Ruiz-Lachica, M.D.

- Reported incidence varies: 1/1280–1/3000 vaginal deliveries
- Incidence of uterine rupture in women with prior C-section 0.2–0.8%, in two recent series
- Incidence may increase as more women with previous C-section are undergoing trial of labor for subsequent pregnancies
- May develop as result of pre-existing injury or anomaly; may complicate labor in a previously unscarred uterus

PERIOPERATIVE RISKS

- Uncommon but potentially catastrophic for mother and fetus: in USA, maternal morbidity ~0.1% when rupture occurs vs. 1:12,000 in all deliveries. Uterine rupture usually found at site of previous operation or injury.
- In traumatic or spontaneous rupture with no uterine scar, maternal mortality significantly higher (22 and 66% in two recent studies), likely because of low index of suspicion, inadequate resuscitation, delayed laparotomy

WORRY ABOUT

- Massive bleeding in mother
- Lack of blood/oxygen supply to fetus

OVERVIEW

- Split in walls of uterus, often due to separation of a C-section scar in trial of labor with uterine scar along most of its length, with rupture of fetal membranes so that uterine and peritoneal cavity communicate; bleeding often massive
- If dehiscence of previous scar, fetal membranes not ruptured, peritoneum overlying defect intact, bleeding is usually minimal. Dehiscence may take place gradually, whereas rupture takes place suddenly and is symptomatic.
- Advantages of vaginal delivery over repeat C-section include ↓ maternal blood loss, ↓ incidence of febrile morbidity, earlier ambulation after delivery
- ACOG publishes specific guidelines on trial of labor after C-section; currently recommended that patients with low transverse uterine scar be considered candidates for trial of labor; ACOG guidelines specifically exclude patients who have prior classic C-section
- Normally, lower uterine segment at term consists mostly of connective tissue and does not contain placental tissue. Dehiscence does not usually produce maternal or fetal compromise.

- Sx include vaginal bleeding, severe lower abdominal pain, ± shoulder pain from diaphragmatic irritation with blood, severe maternal hypotension/shock, disappearance of fetal heart tones

ICD-9-CM Code: v22.2 (Pregnancy)

ETIOLOGY

- Separation of scar from previous C-section, often during trial of labor
- Rupture of myomectomy scar due to precipitous or tumultuous labor
- Prolonged labor with excessive oxytocin stimulation or CPD
- Weak or stretched uterine muscles such as in grand multipara, multiple gestation, polyhydramnios
- Traumatic rupture (iatrogenic) from intrauterine manipulations, difficult forceps application, excessive suprafundal pressure, intra-amniotic fluid instillation

USUAL TREATMENT

- Emergent delivery with repair or hysterectomy is only treatment
- Most common finding is fetal distress: occasionally, loss of intrauterine pressure or cessation of labor

ASSESSMENT POINTS

SYSTEM	EFFECT	ASSESSMENT BY HX	PE	TEST
CV	Shock with massive blood loss		BP, HR Orthostatic VS if slow	
RESP	Difficulty breathing due to diaphragmatic irritation			
GU	Vaginal bleeding Fetal distress Rupture	Lower abdominal pain followed by severe abdominal pain, absence of contractions, and shoulder pain	Rigid abdomen if not receiving epidural anesthesia	Hct

Key Reference: Amata AO: Anaesthetic and intensive care management of rupture of the gravid uterus: a review of 50 cases. Trop Doct 1998; 28:214–217.

PERIOPERATIVE IMPLICATIONS

Preoperative Preparation

- If trial of labor for patient with previous C-section, monitor FHR, uterine tone and pattern prior to initiation of epidural analgesia using lowest effective concentration of local anesthetic
- Epidural for labor advantageous and may be used for surgical anesthesia if trial of labor fails and repeat C-section required
- If no epidural, GA indicated for emergent repeat C-section in case of suspected uterine scar, rupture, fetal distress, or other
- Anesthetic management similar to management of actively bleeding, acutely hypovolemic parturient:
  - Preparation includes nonparticulate oral antacid, oxygen, 2 large-bore peripheral IV catheters, blood warmer
  - Preinduction: crystalloid, colloid, and packed red blood cells infused as rapidly as

indicated to treat hypovolemia (uterine blood flow at term—~700 ml/min). Do not delay to obtain vital sign stability as it will not occur in a living patient in most emergent cases of rupture.

Monitoring

- Consider arterial and central venous catheters if time permits or as soon as aortic/bleeding control obtained

Induction/Airway

- ET intubation with cricoid pressure
- If severely hypovolemic, peripheral vasoconstriction already maximal, direct cardiac depressant effect of ketamine may contribute to hypotension. In severe situations consider intubation with succinylcholine only.

Maintenance

- 100% predelivery; consider low-dose halogenated agents if hemodynamically stable until delivery to ↓ incidence of maternal recall

- Restore blood volume based on BP, UO (CVP?)
- After delivery, when blood volume restored, consider narcotics, muscle relaxants as indicated
- Neonate may require intensive resuscitation at birth

Extubation

- Awake

Postoperative Period

- EBL: 3000–6000 ml
- Pain score: 6–8; consider postop epidural or epidural PCA

ANTICIPATED PROBLEMS/CONCERNS

- Other more common causes of antepartum hemorrhage: placenta previa and placental abruption
- Symptoms may be misleading; high index of suspicion critical to preventing morbidity and mortality
- Rupture of classic scar much more likely to result in severe hemorrhage

VARICELLA-ZOSTER VIRUS

Lee A. Fleisher, M.D.

RISK

- Prevalence: <10% of adults seronegative
- Usually contracted during childhood

PERIOPERATIVE RISKS

- Minimal additional risk to patient unless immunocompromised
- Risk of infection to caregivers

WORRY ABOUT

- Encephalitis in immunocompromised patient
- Potential nosocomial transmission
- Acyclovir-induced nephrotoxicity
- Transmission to pregnant woman

OVERVIEW

- Viral cause of varicella (chickenpox) and herpes zoster (shingles)
- Both nosocomial transmission and direct contact
- Development of herpes zoster common in immunocompromised patient and may be forerunner of AIDS
- Zoster is reactivated form of varicella from neural ganglion cells
- May lead to congenital abnormalities if contracted during 1st trimester of pregnancy

ICD-9-CM Code: 053.9

ETIOLOGY

- Herpes group of viruses

USUAL TREATMENT

- Varicella immune globulin
- Vaccine currently available but controversial
- Acyclovir decreases severity if initiated within 24 h of herpes zoster infection
- Corticosteroid controversial for postherpetic neuralgia

ASSESSMENT POINTS

SYSTEM	EFFECT	ASSESSMENT BY HX	PE	TEST
RESP	Pneumonia	Dyspnea	Rhonchi	CXR
HEME	Thrombocytopenic purpura	Bleeding		Plts
DERM	Rash		Erythematous macules, papules, vesicles	
RENAL	Acyclovir nephrotoxicity			Cr
CNS	Encephalitis Optic neuritis; transverse myelitis	MS changes Vision changes		CT scan
PNS	Zoster shingles		Shingles in single dermatome Multiple dermatomes in immunocompromised	
IMMUNO	Associated with AIDS			HIV tests; CD4 titer

Key Reference: Dunkle LM, Arvin AM, Whitley RJ, et al: A controlled trial of acyclovir for chickenpox in normal children. N Engl J Med 1991; 325:1539–1544.

PERIOPERATIVE IMPLICATIONS

Preoperative Preparation
- Consider isolation precautions

Monitoring
- Routine

Airway
- Routine

Induction/Maintenance
- Routine

Extubation
- Routine

ANTICIPATED PROBLEMS/CONCERNS

- Multiple dermatomes may indicate immunocompromised individual
- Avoid exposing pregnant individuals to virus

VENTRICULAR FIBRILLATION

Randy H. Steadman, M.D.

RISK

- VFIB/VTach: most frequent rhythm in sudden cardiac arrest
- At risk are the 1.5 million/y in USA who have acute MIs: about 540,000 will die, 350,000 before they reach hospital (this includes death from dysrhythmia and myocardial failure)
- 1-y mortality in near–sudden death survivors: 20–30% if nonresponsive to antiarrhythmics (20–50% of near–sudden death survivors)

PERIOPERATIVE RISKS

- Primary VFIB, if associated with acute infarction, when treated promptly with defibrillation, may not affect prognosis
- Secondary VFIB (preceded by pump failure or hypotension) associated with 75–80% mortality during hospitalization

WORRY ABOUT

- Hypoxemia, hypercarbia, hyper- or hypokalemia, hypomagnesemia, digitalis toxicity, acid-base abnormality
- Antiarrhythmic drug levels
- Availability of defibrillator, myocardial ischemia

OVERVIEW

- Asynchronous, chaotic contraction of ventricles characterized by no organized ventricular depolarization and therefore no QRS; no cardiac output

- Coarse VFIB indicates recent onset, readily correctable with prompt defibrillation
- Fine VFIB ("coarse asystole") indicates delay since collapse; successful resuscitation more difficult

ICD-9-CM Code: 427.41

ETIOLOGY

- Usually ischemic, often associated with LV aneurysm
- Idiopathic cardiomyopathy
- Coronary spasm
- Hypothermia
- Long QT syndrome is associated with VTach, esp torsades de pointes (one type of polymorphic VTach; other types not associated with long QT)

USUAL TREATMENT

- Definitive emergency Rx is always electrical defibrillation: external—either manual or automatic (AEDs)—or internal: internal may be implanted (ICDs)
- Time to defibrillation major determinant of survival, with chances of success reduced by 10% each minute
- Early bystander CPR and early defibrillation are the only factors that have been proven to increase the rate of return of spontaneous circulation (ROSC) and decrease mortality
- Vasopressors such as epinephrine and vasopressin are indicated after 3 successive countershocks fail to terminate VFIB. Vasopressors improve coronary and cerebral perfusion pressures; ↑ coronary perfusion pressure is associated with ↑ likelihood of ROSC.

- Vasopressin may have fewer side effects than epinephrine, while being equally or more effective, particularly in acidotic patients. Vasopressin's longer duration of action (10–20 min) has led to the recommendation of a single, 1-time dose for VFIB.
- Amiodarone is the only antiarrhythmic associated with improved resuscitation rates from VFIB; it is recommended after 3 successive shocks, an IV vasopressor (epinephrine or vasopressin), and a subsequent 4th shock are unsuccessful in restoring a perfusing rhythm
- Prospective trials of lidocaine and bretylium in VFIB patients have shown no benefit on outcome. However, based on historical use and the lack of side effects, lidocaine is considered an alternative to amiodarone in VFIB.
- Due to inconsistent availability, side effects, and lack of confirmed benefit, bretylium is no longer recommended for VFIB
- Evidence supporting procainamide use in VFIB is limited, while the need for slow infusion makes it less than ideal
- Magnesium may be beneficial in torsades de pointes (polymorphic VTach associated with prolonged QT), but routine use does not improve outcome

ASSESSMENT POINTS

SYSTEM	EFFECT
HEENT	Right radical neck dissection assoc with increasing QT interval
CV	No effective cardiac output
RESP	Apnea should be anticipated
CNS	Glucose administration may worsen CNS outcome

Key Reference: Guidelines 2000 for cardiopulmonary resuscitation and emergency cardiovascular care. Circulation 2000; 102(Suppl):I86–I157.

PERIOPERATIVE IMPLICATIONS

Preoperative Preparation

- Antiarrhythmic drug levels in optimal therapeutic range
- If for EPS, ablation, or ICD, antiarrhythmic drugs withdrawn on ECG monitoring
- Avoid anticholinergic premedication or sympathetic stimulation
- For patients with prolonged QT syndrome consider β-blockers or prophylactic left stellate ganglion block

Monitoring

- Consider ECG and pulse oximetry en route to OR
- Consider arterial catheter for transport and in OR

Airway

- Apnea expected with acute VFIB; ventilation should be supported with 100% O$_2$
- Airway secured with ET tube if 3 successive countershocks fail to restore perfusing rhythm

Induction

- Avoid ketamine; intubate after adequate depth of anesthesia

Maintenance

- Suppress sympathetic responses to stimulation

Extubation

- Suppress sympathetic stimulation; extubate when spontaneous ventilation with oropharyngeal reflexes has been restored
- Reversal of NMBs acceptable
- Regional: Serum levels of local anesthetics given epidurally may affect intraoperative defibrillation threshold testing during ICD placement
- Defibrillator should be available with sterile defibrillator paddles on surgical field; pharmacologic therapy for dysrhythmia conversion/maintenance, for treating Htn and tachycardia, which frequently follow defibrillation; bradycardia may require pacing

Postoperative Period

- Cardiac monitoring; resumption of preop antiarrhythmics, maintaining oxygenation
- Avoid lyte abnormalities
- Post defibrillation pain score: 1–3 from chest wall and psychic disturbances
- Psychiatric counseling if disturbed by shock or "out of body" experience

ANTICIPATED PROBLEMS/CONCERNS

- PA catheter insertion may induce VTach or VFIB in dysrhythmia-prone patients; if PA catheter necessary consider central venous placement with advancement after ventricular dysrhythmia procedure completed
- For patients with prolonged QT syndrome avoid drugs that prolong the QT interval (class Ia antiarrhythmic drugs such as quinidine and procainamide)
- Psychic disturbances from defibrillation in "aware state"

VENTRICULAR PREEXCITATION SYNDROME   John L. Atlee, M.D.

RISK

• Incidence of Wolff-Parkinson-White (WPW) syndrome, short P-R interval with ventricular preexcitation and tachyarrhythmias: 1–3/1000 persons
• While WPW patients have accessory AV pathways, other types of anomalous pathways may cause pre-excitation or participate in re-entry tachycardia, but these are rarely diagnosed. In addition, patients may have accessory pathways that do not conduct to the ventricles during normal sinus rhythm to produce ventricular preexcitation. However, these pathways may participate in re-entry supraventricular tachycardia (SVT).
• Short P-R interval in patients with the Lown-Ganong-Levine (LGL) syndrome usually reflects conduction through an intranodal fast pathway that either is anatomically short or, more frequently, has a shorter refractory period and conducts faster in the antegrade and retrograde directions. Re-entrant SVT is favored in patients with LGL syndrome who also have slow AV nodal pathways (e.g., evidence of normal AV conduction times), because of large differences in conduction and refractoriness between the fast and slow pathways.
• Rate of paroxysmal SVT is usually faster in patients with LGL syndrome than in patients with normal P-R intervals. In addition, there is capacity for more rapid conduction during AFIB/AFLT.

PERIOPERATIVE RISKS

• WPW per se carries no added risk, but danger of misdiagnosis-mistreatment of tachyarrhythmias with potentially devastating consequences
• Antidromic (preexcitation) AV reciprocating tachycardia or AFIB easily mistaken for VTach
• Drugs used to slow the ventricular rate with AFIB/AFLT may dangerously accelerate rate in WPW (>300 bpm)

WORRY ABOUT

• Hyperadrenergic states and other imbalance that might provoke or aggravate tachyarrhythmias
• Ca^{2+}-channel blockers (diltiazem, verapamil), digitalis, or adenosine, which slow AV nodal conduction and terminate PSVT, either do not affect or may enhance conduction over accessory pathways. Because PSVT may deteriorate into AFIB/AFLT, there is danger of extremely rapid ventricular rates during AFIB/FLT with ensuing VTach/VFIB.
• AFLT/AFIB in a patient with ventricular preexcitation and potential for extremely rapid ventricular rates and sudden deterioration into VFIB

OVERVIEW

• During PSVT sustained in accessory pathways, the QRS complexes usually look like non-preexcited supraventricular beats (narrow QRS; absence of δ wave) because, in most cases (>90%), the ventricles are activated via the normal pathway (atria → AV node → His bundle) to cause orthodromic PSVT
• In patients with accessory pathways and WPW or LGL syndromes, AFLT with antegrade conduction down accessory pathways is the most frequent cause of regular tachycardias with wide (>0.12 sec) QRS complexes. Ventricular rate exceeds 240 bpm in many patients. Next in frequency comes antidromic PSVT, in which case the ventricles are activated via accessory pathways. Usually, the ventricular rate is faster in patients with ventricular preexcitation and AFLT compared with those with antidromic PSVT.
• Orthodromic and antidromic PSVT account for 70–80% of all paroxysmal tachycardia with WPW syndrome. AFIB and AFLT account for 15–25% and 5–10%, respectively. Primary VTach/VFIB is rare, but VTach/VFIB may arise as a consequence of rapid SVT.
• The first episode of PSVT appears in > half of patients with accessory pathway re-entry

(regardless of whether they have manifest pre-excitation during sinus rhythm) before the age of 20 y, seldom after middle age, and occasionally after the age of 50 y. Frequency of paroxysms of PSVT increases with age in patients with WPW.

ICD-9-CM Codes: 426.7 (WPW); 426.81 (LGL)

ETIOLOGY

• Preexcitation may be familial. Characteristic ECG of patient with WPW syndrome (short P-R interval; δ wave) appears in greater number of first-degree relatives of those with preexcitation than would be expected in the general population.

USUAL TREATMENT

• PSVT in patient with WPW: caution with adenosine, Ca^{2+}-channel blocker (diltiazem, verapamil), or digitalis since they may enhance conduction over accessory pathways to increase rate of tachycardia and precipitate AFIB/AFLT
• Most patients with WPW or LGL syndrome and recurrent tachyarrhythmias will have undergone definitive catheter ablation of their accessory pathway(s). However, if a drug is required to terminate PSVT, consider a β-blocker or amiodarone, since neither facilitates accessory pathway conduction. With destabilizing PSVT, immediate cardioversion is advised, and a β-blocker or amiodarone to prevent recurrences.
• Disopyramide, procainamide, and quinidine prolong refractoriness in accessory pathways, thereby encouraging conduction through the AV node and slower ventricular rates with AFLT/AFIB. These drugs may convert some AFLT/AFIB to sinus rhythm in patients with WPW. However, amiodarone may be a better choice, since not only does it ↑ accessory pathway refractoriness, but also it prevents recurrences of AFLT/AFIB and subsequent deterioration to VTach/VFIB.

ASSESSMENT POINTS

SYSTEM	EFFECT	ASSESSMENT BY HX	PE	TEST
CV	Arrhythmia	Palpitations, dizziness, syncope or near-syncope, angina, chest pain, cardiac arrest; sometimes asymptomatic	Monitor BP; variable S_1-pulse amplitude; fast regular, irregular, and/or weak pulse; S_3; rales	12-lead ECG, Holter ECG, cardiac EP study ECHO and possible further study
	LV function	Weakness, lassitude, exercise intolerance, CHF		

Key Reference: Kastor JA: Arrhythmias, 2nd ed. Philadelphia, WB Saunders, 2000, pp 39–163, 198–268.

PERIOPERATIVE IMPLICATIONS

Preoperative Preparation

• Consult to cardiology re patient's status, type/risk of arrhythmias, management goals
• Assemble drugs for tachycardia; cardioverter-defibrillator on hand

Monitoring

• ECG monitoring (strip-chart recorder) and arterial line if patient at high risk for tachycardia

Induction

• Patients with ventricular dysfunction 2° to tachycardiomyopathy may not tolerate usual doses of IV anesthetic induction or potent

volatile agents. Consider etomidate (not ketamine) and regional or balanced anesthetic techniques.
• Drugs to reduce pain and stress, and β-blockers (especially, prior to laryngoscopy and tracheal intubation) may reduce risk of tachyarrhythmias

Maintenance

• Volatile anesthetics ↑ accessory pathway/AV node refractoriness; droperidol and fentanyl ↑ accessory pathway refractoriness

Extubation

• β-blockers may be useful prior to emergence/extubation; try to avoid adrenergic hyperactivity

Adjuvants

• Drugs that directly or indirectly ↑ adrenergic tone/heart rate should be used with caution

Postoperative Period

• Adequate pain control may help reduce likelihood of paroxysmal tachycardia

ANTICIPATED PROBLEMS/CONCERNS

• Possibility of dangerous ventricular rates with AFIB/AFLT, with early deterioration into VFIB
• Antidromic PSVT or AFLT/AFIB with preexcited (wide) QRS complexes masquerading as VTach/VFIB

VENTRICULAR SEPTAL DEFECT (CONGENITAL)

David L. Reich, M.D.

RISK

- Incidence is ~2/1000 live births
- Prevalence is 1/1000 school-age children
- 10% of congenital heart disease in adults

PERIOPERATIVE RISKS

- Mortality higher in patients >5 y, PVR >7 Wood's units, and surgery complicated by CHB
- RV or LV failure postoperatively related to preop status

WORRY ABOUT

- Worsening of L → R shunt with hyperventilation and increased FIO_2
- Paradoxical embolization
- Hypothermia
- Post-CPB pulmonary Htn and RV failure

OVERVIEW

- Small defects asymptomatic, present with murmur, usually close spontaneously
- Larger defects result in CHF symptoms, poor weight gain, URIs beginning at 3–12 wk of age as decreases in PVR cause massive L → R shunting
- Untreated massive L → R shunting results in fixed pulmonary Htn (Eisenmenger's syndrome) by 2–6 y

ICD-9-CM Code: 745.4 (Ventricular septal defect)

INDICATIONS/USUAL TREATMENT

- 75% of small defects close spontaneously and require only antibiotic prophylaxis
- Large defects usually result in hospitalization for CHF by 2–4 mo of age
- Medical therapy includes digoxin and furosemide
- Cardiac catheterization only for measurement of pulmonary vascular resistance
- Surgery when CHF not amenable to medical treatment, or if failure to thrive
- Surgical repair contraindicated if PVR >10 Wood's units

ASSESSMENT POINTS

SYSTEM	EFFECT	ASSESSMENT BY HX	PE	TEST
CV	Low forward cardiac output due to L → R shunt Pulmonary Htn due to excessive flow	CHF symptoms, failure to thrive Age of patient	Loud holosystolic murmur and thrill Cyanosis	Auscultation, ECHO ECHO, cardiac cath
RESP	Congestion/edema due to L → R shunt	Frequent URI	Rhonchi	CXR
HEME	Anemia in massive L → R shunt; polycythemia in R → L shunt	Pallor or cyanosis	Paleness or plethora	Hct
MS	Chronic hypoxemia due to late reversal of shunt flow (Eisenmenger's syndrome)	Cyanosis	Clubbing of digits	Pulse oximetry

Key Reference: Kidd L, Driscoll DJ, Gersony WM, et al: Second natural history study of congenital heart defects. Results of treatment of patients with ventricular septal defects. Circulation 1993; 87 (2 Suppl):I38–51.

PERIOPERATIVE IMPLICATIONS

Preoperative Preparation

- May withhold digoxin and furosemide on day of surgery
- May not be possible to delay operation until free of upper respiratory symptoms

Anesthetic Techniques

- Limit FIO_2 to minimum necessary prior to CPB to restrict excessive pulmonary blood flow
- Maintain normal to slightly high $PaCO_2$ to restrict excessive pulmonary blood flow
- Patients may receive inhalational, IV, or combined techniques
- Avoid nitrous oxide to prevent sequelae of paradoxical air embolization
- Antifibrinolytic therapy

Monitoring

- Intra-arterial line (cut-downs often required when patient is <5 kg)
- Secure peripheral IV or central venous line (ultrasonic vessel finder desirable)
- Pulse oximetry, capnometry, multiple-site temp monitoring
- Transesophageal ECHO

Induction/Maintenance

- IV, mask, IM, rectal inductions all possible

Surgical Stages

- Pre-CPB
  - Low FIO_2, normal to high $PaCO_2$
  - Maintain intravascular volume using crystalloid/colloid
- CPB
  - Whole blood usually necessary for pump prime under 10 kg
  - Prevent movement and intraoperative awareness during rewarming by supplementing anesthetic and NMB
- Post-CPB
  - Rule out residual shunting by transesophageal ECHO or direct measurement of arterial saturation "step-up" between SVC (or right atrium) and PA
  - Maintain Hct >25–30% using residual CPB reservoir blood or fresh whole blood <48 h old (platelets in fresh whole blood improve hemostasis) and modified ultrahemofiltration

Postoperative Considerations

- Most patients can be extubated at end of surgery
- Mechanically ventilate, sedate, and maintain intense analgesia using opioids in neonates and older children prone to pulmonary hypertensive crises (e.g., Down syndrome)
- Indefinite infective endocarditis prophylaxis
- EBL: 200–800 ml

ANTICIPATED PROBLEMS/CONCERNS

- Imbalance in pulmonary to systemic blood flow ratio:
  - Excessive pulmonary blood flow results in high arterial saturation but with diminished tissue perfusion and metabolic acidosis
  - Diminished pulmonary blood flow results in good tissue perfusion but with cyanosis and potential injury due to hypoxia
- Postop ventricular dysfunction, coagulopathy, renal/hepatic dysfunction, CNS dysfunction

VENTRICULAR SEPTAL RUPTURE (DEFECT), POST MYOCARDIAL INFARCTION

David L. Reich, M.D.

RISK

- Occurs in 1–3% of acute MIs
- Majority occur within 1 wk; 20–30% in first 24 h post MI
- Rarely occurs >2 wk post MI

PERIOPERATIVE RISKS

- Accounts for 5% of MI-related deaths
- Nearly 100% die without surgery
- Surgical short-term survival 42–75%
- Results worse with inferior MI or RV/septal dysfunction

WORRY ABOUT

- Associated papillary muscle rupture
- Poor systemic perfusion and end-organ dysfunction
- Pulm congestion with massive L → R shunt

OVERVIEW

- Sudden onset of holosystolic murmur with thrill and hemodynamic deterioration (hypotension and pulmonary congestion)
- Associated with high morbidity and mortality because emergency surgery after extensive recent MI
- Prolonged postop ventilation and ICU stay

ICD-9-CM Codes: 429.71 (Acquired cardiac septal defect); 410.00–410.92 (Associated MI)

USUAL TREATMENT

- Repair of new VSD with hemodynamic deterioration using pericardial or prosthetic patch material
- Support preop with inotropic agents/nitroprusside/intra-aortic balloon counterpulsation

ASSESSMENT POINTS

SYSTEM	EFFECT	ASSESSMENT BY HX	PE	TEST
CV	Low forward cardiac output due to massive L → R shunt	Sudden onset of hypotension and shock	Loud holosytolic murmur and thrill Auscultation	ECHO, cardiac catheterization
RESP	Congestion/edema	Resp distress	Rales	CXR
RENAL/ HEPATIC	Dysfunction due to hypoperfusion	Anuria		ABGs Foley catheter

Key Reference: Held AC, Cole PL, Lipton B, et al: Rupture of the interventricular septum complicating acute myocardial infarction: A multicenter analysis of clinical findings and outcome. Am Heart J 1988; 116:1330–1336.

PERIOPERATIVE IMPLICATIONS

Preoperative Preparation

- Consider elective tracheal intubation and PEEP
- Support cardiac output using inotropic agents
- Lower resistance to forward cardiac output using nitroprusside (if not already hypotensive) and/or intra-aortic balloon counterpulsation

Anesthetic Technique

- High-dose opioid muscle relaxant technique common
- Prior to CPB, use minimal FIO_2 (maximizes pulm vascular resistance) to decrease L → R shunt across VSD

Monitoring

- Intra-arterial line and PA catheter
- Thermodilution cardiac outputs falsely elevated
- Step-up in saturation between right atrium and PA indicates shunting
- Transesophageal ECHO (TEE) to define anatomy, diagnose associated papillary muscle rupture, monitor ventricular function, assess adequacy of surgical repair

Airway

- Frequent suctioning if pulm edema

Induction

- Avoid vasodilation associated with benzodiazepine/opioid combinations

Maintenance

- Titrate low doses of benzodiazepines if Htn

Surgical Stages

- Pre-CPB
  - Median sternotomy with aortic and biatrial cannulation
  - May require vein or internal mammary artery harvest for concomitant myocardial revascularization
  - Lowest FIO_2 consistent with adequate oxygenation
- CPB
  - Maintain Hct using hemofiltration and transfusion
- Post-CPB
  - Inotropic support almost universally required for LV failure
  - RV failure common
  - Assess ventricular repair using TEE or right atrial-to-pulm O_2 saturation ratio
  - FIO_2: 1.00 to minimize pulm vascular resistance
  - May require ventricular assist devices

Blood Loss/Volume Concerns

- Plt and FFP may be necessary owing to DIC-like syndrome
- Aprotinin and antifibrinolytic therapy (beginning pre-CPB) controversial
- Pain score: 7–9

Postoperative Considerations

- Postop renal/hepatic/neurologic dysfunction
- Postop LV, RV, or biventricular failure

ANTICIPATED PROBLEMS/CONCERNS

- Cardiogenic shock
- Prolonged ventilatory dependency and ICU stay

VENTRICULAR TACHYARRHYTHMIAS

John L. Atlee, M.D.

RISK

• Ventricular tachycardia (VTach) is an uncommon arrhythmia that occurs more frequently in men than women, with CAD being the most common cause
• VTach also occurs in patients with cardiomyopathy, RHD, or no structural heart disease (e.g., exercise/catecholamine-induced VTach)
• Many drugs, including antiarrhythmics, can cause VTach, a proarrhythmic effect (2–8% incidence with classes 1 and 3 antiarrhythmics)
• Polymorphic VTach may occur in association with IHD or drugs that prolong the QT interval. If the latter, it is termed torsades de pointes (TDP). Incessant monomorphic VTach may also result from drug-caused proarrhythmia.
• Polymorphic VTach in association with congenital or acquired QT interval prolongation is termed TDP
• Most Vtach is transient/nonsustained (lasts ≤ 30 sec) and does not produce symptoms or hemodynamic deterioration
• New-onset, sustained VTach after coronary surgery is rare. When it occurs, it carries a poor prognosis, because it is usually associated with periop MI.

PERIOPERATIVE RISKS

• Catecholamine-induced ventricular arrhythmias with halothane, enflurane, and isoflurane. This is not known to occur with desflurane or sevoflurane.
• Volatile inhalation anesthetics tend to oppose ventricular arrhythmias with acute and chronic MI. Effect on VTach in other circumstances is unknown.

WORRY ABOUT

• Is cardiopulmonary function optimal? What about acid-base, lyte, and metabolic balance?
• Sympathomimetics and drugs that ↑ the QT interval (e.g., classes 1A and 3 antiarrhythmics; nonsedating antihistamines; some tranquilizers, tricyclic antidepressants, and antipsychotic drugs; erythromycin; organophosphate insecticides)

OVERVIEW

• VTach hemodynamic impact minimal or profound: rate is most important determinant; others are LV function, AV dissociation, degree of mitral regurgitation, ventricular activation pattern
• VTach and VFIB often due to proarrhythmic effects of type 1A and C drugs, amiodarone, sotalol
• R-on-T or complex ventricular extrasystoles do not cause VTach in absence of acute MI

ICD-9-CM Codes: 427.1 (Ventricular tachycardia); 427.41 (Ventricular fibrillation)

ETIOLOGY

• Except for adrenergic TDP, most VTach is result of acquired, structural heart disease
• Structural heart disease provides substrate for re-entry or initiates triggered or automatic VTach
• Since VTach is due to multiple mechanisms, there can be no uniform treatment

USUAL TREATMENT

• Monomorphic VTach: immediate cardioversion for destabilizing VTach. IV amiodarone and procainamide now recommended ahead of lidocaine or bretylium for initial drug treatment. Chronic treatment includes drugs (guided by results of EP testing), ablation, and ICD.
• Polymorphic VTach (without long QT): same as treatment for monomorphic VTach. Also, indicated treatment for underlying CAD. Drugs used to treat polymorphic VTach, may convert disturbance to monomorphic VTach or VFIB. Pacing does not suppress disturbance.
• TDP (with long QT): MgSO$_4$ suppresses TDP in many cases. Although bolus MgSO$_4$ is acutely effective, slow IV infusion reduces incidence of untoward side effects. MgSO$_4$ does not shorten prolonged QT. Temporary atrial or ventricular pacing is very reliable for suppressing TDP, whether with acquired or congenital long QT. D/C offending drugs.
• Nonsustained VTach (< 30 sec): at least initially, do not treat with antiarrhythmic drugs (proarrhythmia risk), unless disturbance recurs so frequently as to be destabilizing. Treat the underlying cause.

ASSESSMENT POINTS

SYSTEM	EFFECT	ASSESSMENT BY HX	PE	TEST
CV	Arrhythmia	No symptoms, palpitations, dizziness, syncope or near-syncope, cardiac arrest	Monitor BP, cannon A waves, variable S$_1$ and pulse amplitude, regular or weak irregular pulse S$_3$, rales, findings of specific heart disease	12-lead ECG (if possible), Holter ECG, cardiac electrophysiologic studies ECHO, exercise ECG, MRI
	LV function	Weakness, lassitude, exercise intolerance, CHF		
	Ischemia	Symptoms of angina, CHF		Scintigraphy, cardiac catheter, angio
RESP	CHF, COPD	Dyspnea, orthopnea, cough	S$_3$, rales, wheezes	CXR, PFTs
CNS	Ischemia	Syncope, near-syncope	Altered mental status	See CV assessment

Key Reference: Kastor JA: Arrhythmias, 2nd ed. Philadelphia, WB Saunders, 2000, pp 342–508.

PERIOPERATIVE IMPLICATIONS

Preoperative Preparation

• Monomorphic/polymorphic VTach (by history): optimal treatment for underlying heart disease and to improve hemodynamic function
• TDP: with acquired long QT, remove offending drug(s) and correct imbalance (especially, low K$^+$ and/or Mg^{2+}). Consider temporary pacing and/or MgSO$_4$ to suppress TDP. β-blockers, left cardiac sympathetic denervation, and ICDs are mainstays of chronic treatment for congenital long QT with TDP.

Monitoring

• ECG, ST-T trending, strip-chart recorder and that indicated for underlying heart condition

Induction/Maintenance

• Use drugs compatible with patient's CV status; control exaggerated sympathetic responses with airway or surgical manipulation; avoid sympathomimetic, sensitizing, or QT-prolonging drugs

Extubation

• Consider using β-blockers and/or vasodilators to control circulatory lability

Adjuvants

• Bupivacaine may cause further ↑ in QT with long QT syndromes (avoid)
• Caution with chronotropes and sympathomimetic drugs

Postoperative Period

• Adequate sedation and pain control, maintain as near normal physiology as possible; be mindful of VTach etiology and conditions, factors, or interventions that might trigger or worsen it

ANTICIPATED PROBLEMS/CONCERNS

• Do not treat ventricular extrasystoles or nonsustained VTach based solely on appearance or assumption they will precipitate sustained VTach or VFIB due to proarrhythmia risk with drugs

VENTRICULAR TACHYCARDIA

Edelberto Perez, M.D.
Kenneth J. Tuman, M.D.

RISK

• Structural heart disease (most commonly chronic phase of MI)
• Most common cause of mortality with CHF

PERIOPERATIVE RISKS

• Endogenous or exogenous catecholamines trigger VTach in susceptible patients
• Central venous and pulmonary artery catheters and intubation can trigger VTach
• Hyperventilation may ↓ serum K^+
• Precipitation of polymorphic VTach with agents that alter QT interval

WORRY ABOUT

• Possible effect of antiarrhythmics on cardiac and pulm function
• Perioperative ventricular dysfunction and/or ischemia
• Progression of VTach to VFIB
• Reduction of LV function due to IV antiarrhythmic

OVERVIEW

• Defined as 3 or more consecutive ventricular beats (usually at a rate > 100 bpm)
• Sustained VTach persists for > 30 sec or requires an intervention for termination
• Nonsustained VTach is ≤ 6 consecutive beats terminating spontaneously within 30 sec
• Possible signs of VTach include a wide QRS (> 140 msec), presence of fusion beat, AV dissociation, LBBB morphology
• Must rule out SVT with aberrant conduction or pre-existing bundle branch block
• Torsades de pointes refers to VTach characterized by polymorphic QRS complexes that undulate in a regular fashion about baseline. Often associated with prolonged QT interval.

ICD-9-CM Code: 427.42

ETIOLOGY

• CAD—acute myocardial ischemia or MI or old MI with LV scar or aneurysm
• Cardiomyopathies, esp with ventricular dilation/enlargement
• Myocarditis
• Mechanical irritation (catheters)
• Metabolic (hypokalemia, hypomagnesemia)
• Hypertrophic cardiomyopathy or mitral valve prolapse may present with VTach
• Acquired polymorphic VTach (torsades) may result from lyte imbalances (K^+, Mg^{2+}) or drugs that prolong repolarization (phenothiazines, tricyclic antidepressants, class Ia antiarrhythmics, erythromycin, pentamidine, terfenadine, astemizole)
• Congenital QT prolongation may be associated with left-sided cardiac sympathetic dominance
• Rare association with right radical neck dissection

USUAL TREATMENT

• Removal or manipulation of catheter if patient hemodynamically stable
• Chronic PO therapy includes Ia—quinidine, procainamide, disopyramide; Ib—mexilitene, tocainide; Ic—propafenone; II—β-blockers; III—amiodarone, sotalol
• Intravenous therapy includes procainamide, phenytoin, lidocaine, amiodarone, bretylium (less commonly quinidine) as well as Mg^{2+} and/or K^+ when necessary
• Digoxin antibodies if digitalis-induced VTach
• Class I antiarrhythmics generally contraindicated in presence of polymorphic VTach (torsades de pointes)
• Electrical cardioversion for VTach with hemodynamic instability
• Nonpharmacologic management includes ablative techniques, myocardial revascularization, implantable cardioverter-defibrillators
• Treatment of torsades includes withdrawal of offending agent, correction of lyte abnormality (K^+, Mg^{2+}), and/or electrical defibrillation to terminate episode. Accelerating HR with isoproterenol or cardiac pacing may terminate rhythm. Empirical Mg^{2+} treatment may be lifesaving.
• Treatment of congenital QT prolongation includes β-blockers to blunt sympathetic activity, Mg^{2+}, and/or left cervicothoracic sympathectomy

ASSESSMENT POINTS

SYSTEM	EFFECT	ASSESSMENT BY HX	PE	TEST
CV	Myocardial ischemia Hypotension	Angina/anginal equivalent (syncope, SOB, palpitations, and exercise intolerance)	Cardiomegaly, JVD Cannon A waves; S_3, S_4	ECG, CXR Electrophysiologic studies
	Cardiac arrest	CHF		Ambulatory ECG
RESP	Pulm edema Amiodarone effects (fibrosis)	Shortness of breath	Rales (wet or dry)	CXR, PFTs (A-a)O_2 gradient
CNS	Syncope	Dizziness or loss of consciousness		

Key Reference: Shenasa M, Borggrefe M, Haverkamp W, Hindricks G, Berithardt G: Ventricular tachycardia. Lancet 1993; 341:1512.

PERIOPERATIVE IMPLICATIONS

Preoperative Preparation

• Ascertain etiology of VTach and associated problems
• Evaluate for Hx of palpitations, SOB, VTach, dizziness, syncope, chest pain
• Evaluate ECG for morphology of PVCs, QT interval, underlying BBB (important for Dx and therapy of wide complex tachycardia)
• Review electrophysiologic studies to determine optimal treatment of VTach
• Assess K^+ and Mg^{2+} levels, digoxin level if indicated
• Pulmonary and thyroid function tests may be indicated for chronic amiodarone therapy
• Continue PO antiarrhythmic therapy
• Have defibrillator immediately available (nearby) whenever inserting central venous catheters

Monitor

• ECG for ischemia or QT prolongation
• Consider invasive hemodynamic monitor if suspect serious concomitant cardiac disease and major anesthetic/surgical intervention

Induction/Maintenance

• Avoid myocardial ischemia (maintain O_2 supply and minimize O_2 demand)
• Minimize surgical stimulus response and subsequent catecholamine release
• Avoid sympathomimetics, which may aggravate ventricular dysrhythmias
• Avoid hypokalemia, excessive hyperventilation

Postoperative Period

• Consider continuous arrhythmia monitoring
• Continue parenteral antiarrhythmics until able to resume PO
• Treat Mg^{2+} and K^+ deficits (common postop, esp after major surgical procedures)

VITAMIN B$_{12}$/FOLATE DEFICIENCY   Donald D. Koblin, M.D., Ph.D.

RISK

- 5–20% of elderly
- Predisposed by prolonged exposure to N$_2$O, ICU patients, ileal resections, chemotherapy with antifolates, ethanol abuse, AIDS, pregnancy

PERIOPERATIVE RISKS

- Worsening of pre-existing megaloblastic anemia and neuropathies after exposure to N$_2$O (infrequent)
- Anemia and limited oxygen-carrying capacity
- Limb (positioning) injuries associated with pre-existing neuropathy

WORRY ABOUT

- Delayed onset of hematologic and neurologic abn after N$_2$O exposure—several weeks may pass before Sx develop
- Untoward outcomes (e.g., death, infection) in critically ill patients with megaloblastic anemia undergoing anesthesia and surgery

OVERVIEW

- Folate metabolism requires vitamin B$_{12}$-dependent enzyme methionine synthase, which converts methyltetrahydrofolate and homocysteine to free tetrahydrofolate and methionine and is rapidly inactivated (T$_{1/2}$ ~ 1 h) by N$_2$O
- Vitamin B$_{12}$ required for two enzymes in humans: methionine synthase and methylmalonyl-CoA mutase (which converts L-methylmalonyl-CoA to succinyl-CoA)
- Tetrahydrofolate (in its free form and derivatives) needed for many metabolic processes, including pyrimidine, purine, DNA synthesis; amino acid metabolism; formate elimination
- Vitamin B$_{12}$/folate required for synthesis and maturation of blood cells, integrity of CNS, GI function, growth of fetus and child
- Associated with ↑ serum homocysteine levels and atherosclerosis

ICD-9-CM Codes: 281.0–281.2

ETIOLOGY

- Pernicious anemia (antibodies to gastric cells and lack of intrinsic factor) is most common cause
- Impaired nutritional intake, malabsorption (e.g., ileal resection), ↑ folate demand (e.g., pregnancy), treatment with antifolate drugs (e.g., methotrexate, prolonged N$_2$O exposure)

USUAL TREATMENT

- Daily oral supplements of folate/weekly IM injections of vitamin B$_{12}$
- Folate treatment alone may produce partial hematologic remission due to vitamin B$_{12}$ deficiency but mask vitamin B$_{12}$ deficiency and result in irreversible neurologic abnormality
- Deficiencies associated with N$_2$O exposure have been successfully treated with IM injections of vitamin B$_{12}$, IV administration of folinic acid, oral methionine

ASSESSMENT POINTS

SYSTEM	EFFECT	TEST
HEENT	Glossitis and painful tongue (infrequent)	
CV	Angina and palpitations 2° to anemia DOE 2° to anemia	
GI	Anorexia, diarrhea	Schilling test for malabsorption of vitamin B$_{12}$.
HEME	Megaloblastic anemia	Serum levels of vitamin B$_{12}$ and folate. RBC folate considered better indicator of tissue folate levels than serum folate. ↑ Urinary levels of methylmalonic acid in vitamin B$_{12}$ deficiency. Hematologic variables may be normal or abnormal; anemia, ↑ mean corpuscular volume. Hypersegmented neutrophils may be present
GU	Impotence	
CNS	Subacute combined degeneration of spinal cord Gait ataxia Romberg's sign, memory deficits, psychosis	
PNS	Diminished vibratory sense, proprioception, and sensation; paresthesias, loss of deep tendon reflexes	

Key Reference: Koblin DD: Toxicity of nitrous oxide (N$_2$O). *In* Rice SA, Fish KJ (eds): Anesthetic Toxicity. New York, Raven Press, 1994, pp 135–155.

PERIOPERATIVE IMPLICATIONS

Preoperative Preparation

- If elective procedure, postpone to correct vitamin deficiencies and hematologic/neurologic abnormalities

Monitoring

- Myocardial ischemia may occur with anemia and is associated with ↑ homocysteine levels

Airway

- Large and painful tongue may be present

Induction/Maintenance

- Avoid nitrous oxide if patient known to be vitamin B$_{12}$/folate–deficient and has hematologic/neurologic abnormalities

Adjuvants

- Regional: documentation of pre-existing neurologic deficits is required before proceeding with regional anesthesia

Postoperative Period

- Worsening of hematologic and neurologic abn may not occur until several weeks after N$_2$O exposure

ANTICIPATED PROBLEMS/CONCERNS

- Anemia may result in impaired oxygenation of tissues and be associated with myocardial ischemia
- CNS and PNS abnormalities may exist
- Nitrous oxide may exacerbate pre-existing hematologic/neurologic abnormality associated with vitamin B$_{12}$/folate deficiency

VITAMIN D DEFICIENCY

Alexandre N. Chapochnikov, M.D., Ph.D.

RISK

- Large prevalence of deficiency: prevalent in elderly and nursing home residents (25–54%), premature infants of VLBW, in rigid vegetarian macrobiotic diet consumers
- Prescribed for rickets, osteomalacia
- Two types of vitamin D–dependent rickets: Type I—inherited autosomal recessive trait (defect in the $25OH-D_3$ conversion into calciferol [true vitamin D]). Type II—autosomal dominant disorder, where single amino acid change in vitamin D receptor results in nonfunctional state.
- Osteomalacia—metabolic disease with inadequate/delayed mineralization of osteoids in mature bone. Remodeling of bone normal, but mineral calcification/deposition of calcium is diminished. Bone volume is the same, density is decreased.

WORRY ABOUT

- Vitamin D–deficient patients are *probably* hypocalcemic; low total body magnesium and phosphorus levels also likely
- Chronic vitamin D deficiency may lead to impaired mineralization of cervical spine (↑ incidence of abnormal neck mobility; pediatric patients with deformed chest wall may experience lowered FRC; ↑ incidence of respiratory infections)

OVERVIEW/PHARMACOLOGY

- Involved in functioning of hemopoietic cells, skin cells, cancer cells of various origins, islet cells of the pancreas, immune response, as well as CV function (via serum Ca^{2+})
- Synthesis of active vitamin D requires Mg^{2+}, molecular oxygen, NADPH, renal ferredoxin reductase, renal ferredoxin, cytochrome P450, hydroxylase (key enzyme)

- 7-Dehydrocholestrol (skin supply) is photolysed under UV into vitamin D_3, which is transported to the liver by vitamin D–binding protein (globulin). Then, $25OH-D_3$ formed in the liver is transported by the same protein to the kidneys, where it is hydroxylated into 1,25-dihydroxycalciferol (active vitamin D_3).

ICD-9-CM Code: 268.9

DRUG CLASS/MECHANISM OF ACTION/USUAL DOSE

- Produced by a complex series of enzymatic reactions (its precursors are transported to different tissues), then the ultimate product—1,25-dihydroxycalciferol—goes to different organs (prominent effect on proofreader genes, gut, bone, kidney) and activates processes via its receptor, where binding is saturable, specific, reversible
- Fat-soluble

ASSESSMENT POINTS

SYSTEM	EFFECT	ASSESSMENT BY HX	PE	TEST
MS	Impaired mineralization Increased arthritis due to bone spur formation	Bone pain, fracture Joint pain	Dry, scaly skin Brittle nails Coarse hair Neck immobility Osteoarthritis	Bone density
CV	Irregular heart beat Orthostatic hypotension			ECG
CNS/PNS	NM irritability	Depression Muscle stiffness, rigidity	Seizure	Calcium levels

Key Reference: Thomas M, Demay M: Vitamin D deficiency and disorders of vitamin D metabolism. Endocrinol Metab Clin North Am 2000; 29:611–627.

PERIOPERATIVE IMPLICATIONS/POSSIBLE DRUG INTERACTIONS

- Both PTH and vit D_3 (calcitriol) work to keep the level of ionized Ca^{2+} within tight range (±0.1 mg/dl).
- Perioperative considerations are related to
  - Level of ionized Ca^{2+} (regulation of muscle contraction)
    - Neurotransmitter release
    - Hormone secretion/enzyme action
    - Energy metabolism
    - Blood coagulation
- ECG changes: compare to previous tracing! Prolonged QT interval (adjusted to R-R interval; 2:1 intraventricular heart block)
- CHF symptoms and signs
- Monitors: easy availability of blood sample for immediate serum calcium assessment (art cath vs. vein stick). ECG continuous monitoring is essential. $ETCO_2$: Avoid hyperventilation (alkalosis shifts ionized Ca^{2+} into the cells). Acute hypocalcemia ↑ chance of tetany. Laryngeal spasm on extubation in fully awake patient is also likely. Predictor may be distal extremity paresthesia.
- Replete Mg^{2+} as well
- Older people with fracture of the proximal femur should be treated with vit D

- Chronic anticonvulsant Tx (phenobarbital/phenytoin) may lead to hypocalcemia (↓ Ca^{2+} absorbtion from the intestine) and diminished vit D biosynthesis in the liver
- Vit D serum concentration is ↓ when PTH is ↓ (may occur with thiazide medications)
- Cimetidine—this hepatic P450-mediated-metabolism inhibitor leads to decreased vit D plasma concentration
- Antibiotics: rifampin, isoniazid

ANTICIPATED PROBLEMS/CONCERNS

- Disorders of small bowel, hepatobiliary system, pancreas (bile salt deficiency, pancreas insufficiency, poor intestinal absorption of fat-soluble vitamins [A, D, K, E]) may cause maldigestion/malabsorption states
- Liver diseases, isoniazid therapy
- CRI/ESRD (GFR < 25% of nml); moderate to severe impairment of renal phase synthesis of vit D with reduction of serum albumin
- Uremia suppresses vit D action on gut
- Chronic renal failure acidosis leads to negative calcium balance; typical patients have ↑ phosphorus/↓ calcium serum levels

- Nephrotic syndrome causes vit D deficiency related to chronic proteinuria (loss of circulating 25 vit D_3–binding globulin). Symptoms present are secondary hyperparathyroidism, low serum Ca^{2+}, osteomalacia.
- Vit D_3 (1,25 dihydroxycalciferol) directly facilitates Ca^{2+}, Mg^{2+}, and $(PO_4)^{3-}$ uptake by intestinal mucosa, their transport through intestinal cells and efflux
- Primary regulators of vit D synthesis are hypocalcemia (↑); hypophosphatemia (↑); PTH (↑); its own plasma concentration(↓)
- Active vit D_3 enhances the bone resorptive effects of PTH
- Vit D_3 requires transportation in the blood via its vit D–binding globulin
- Dose: current adult (19–50 y) RDA for vit D—5 mg (or 200 IU); 51–70 y—400 IU; >71 y—600 IU. By age 70 y, skin makes 50% of vit D of 20-year-old patient. Broiled salmon: 3 oz (90 g)—11 mg; broiled herring: 3 oz—15 mg; fortified milk: 150 ml—2.5 mg.
- Toxicity: safety margin is large. Prolonged intake of doses >40,000 IU/d promotes bone demineralization, leads to hypercalcemia, enhances CV calcification.

VITAMIN K DEFICIENCY

Ronald P. Chavez, M.D.

PERIOPERATIVE RISKS

- ↑ Risk of bleeding

WORRY ABOUT

- Prolongation of prothrombin time
- Inadequate surgical hemostasis
- May need to give FFP
- Vitamin K administered to correct problem may take several hours to days to take effect

OVERVIEW

- Major Sx: ↑ bleeding tendency; GI bleeding, epistaxis, hematuria, ecchymoses, intracranial hemorrhage, operative bleeding

ICD-9-CM Code: 269.0

ETIOLOGY

- Inadequate intake of vitamin K
- Prolonged use of drugs that inhibit intestinal bacterial growth
- Inadequate absorption due to intra- or extrahepatic biliary obstruction
- Inadequate utilization due to hepatocellular disease
- Drug-induced owing to anticoagulants such as warfarin
- Malabsorption syndromes such as sprue or ulcerative colitis, or induced by Olestra
- Newborn infants: due to inadequate dietary intake and unestablished normal intestinal flora

USUAL TREATMENT

- Administration of vitamin K; poor liver function may have inadequate response
- Phytonadione (vitamin K_1, AquaMEPHYTON) is the only natural form available for therapeutic use. (Oral and IM routes are less likely than IV routes to cause side effects such as allergic reactions or bronchospasm.)
- Menadione (vitamin K_3) (water-soluble) is an artificial provitamin converted to menaquinone (vitamin K_2) by liver. Does not require presence of bile salts for systemic absorption, useful when malabsorption of vitamin K is due to biliary obstruction.
- Dosage
  – Vitamin K deficiency induced by warfarin: 2.5–10 mg PO or slow IV (1 mg/min)
  – Hyperalimentation: 10 mg IM or IV q wk
  – Vitamin K deficiency in newborn: 0.5–1 mg phytonadione to infant immediately after delivery
  – Preoperative: if immediate treatment needed, give 10 mg SQ/d for 3 days; response should be seen within 24 h

ASSESSMENT POINTS

SYSTEM	EFFECT	ASSESSMENT BY HX	PE	TEST
HEENT	Bleeding	Epistaxis		PT/PTT
GI	GI bleeding	Hematemesis Melena Hematochezia	Tenderness Masses Ascites/hepatomegaly	UGI endoscopy
HEME	↑ Bleeding 2° to ↓ factor VII, IX, X, prothrombin	Easy bruising Bleeding gums Drug use such as warfarin		
RENAL	Hematuria			Urinalysis
CNS	Intracranial hemorrhage	Injury	CNS exam	CT scan

Key Reference: Vermeer C, Hamulyak K: Pathophysiology of vitamin K deficiency and oral anticoagulants. Thromb Haemost 1991; 66:153–159.

PERIOPERATIVE IMPLICATIONS

Perioperative Preparation

- If immediate surgery is obligatory, consider transfusing 2–4 U FFP and follow PT/PTT
- Factor VII has $T_{1/2}$ of 6–12 h and is metabolized quickly; repeat treatment may be needed 6–12 h later. Begin treatment with vitamin K 10 mg SQ/d for 3 days; response should be seen after 24 h. (Liver disease may have poor response to vitamin K.)

Monitoring

- Routine

Airway

- ↑ Risk of bleeding trauma with direct laryngoscopy
- Potential difficult airway 2° to bleeding

Maintenance

- Observe for clot in surgical field

Extubation

- Watch for blood in oropharynx

ANTICIPATED PROBLEMS/CONCERNS

- ↑ Bleeding and problems associated with decreased RBC mass
- Trauma to oropharynx with direct laryngoscopy may obscure vision during laryngoscopy and result in difficult intubation

VON WILLEBRAND'S DISEASE
Thomas M. McLoughlin, Jr., M.D.

RISK

- People within USA: 1 million (severe disease 1/10,000–1 million)
- Race/gender with highest prevalence: none

PERIOPERATIVE RISKS

- ↑ Risk if hepatic dysfunction from prior plasma product transfusions
- Significant risk of bleeding if untreated

WORRY ABOUT

- Excessive perioperative hemorrhage
- Adverse reactions to desmopressin therapy (seizures due to hyponatremia, hypotension, anaphylaxis)

OVERVIEW

- Coagulopathy characterized by quantitative/qualitative alterations in von Willebrand factor (vWF), which molecularly bridges plts and vascular subendothelium and prolongs $T_{1/2}$ of circulating factor VIII
- Presents as defect in primary hemostasis—mucocutaneous hemorrhage
- Highly variable severity
- Classified by band pattern of radiolabeled vWF after gel electrophoresis (multimeric analysis)
- Type I: quantitative decrease in vWF of all sizes; type II: quantitative/qualitative alterations primarily in largest molecular weight vWF multimers (many type II subtypes exist depending on abnormality); type III: severe quantitative reductions or absence of vWF

ICD-9-CM Code: 286.4

ETIOLOGY

- Autosomal dominant trait; variable penetrance and expression leads to unpredictable clinical severity; most severe disease in homozygotes
- Rarely, acquired disorder due to autoimmune disease or induced alterations in vWF function

USUAL TREATMENT

- *Must* know disease subtype prior to therapy
- Desmopressin acetate (DDAVP), 0.3 µg/kg IV, stimulates release of endothelial vWF, variably effective in types I and II disease
- Desmopressin absolutely contraindicated in type IIB
- Recombinant vWFs
- Pasteurized pooled factor VIII concentrates that preserve vWF (Humate-P) are mainstay of therapy, if recombinant vWFs not available
- Cryoprecipitate best alternative if Humate-P unavailable
- Antifibrinolytics often useful adjuncts

ASSESSMENT POINTS

SYSTEM	EFFECT	ASSESSMENT BY HX	TEST
HEENT		Epistaxis	
GI	GI bleeding	Melena, hematochezia	Stool guaiac
HEPATIC	Requirement for transfusion therapy	Random donor exposures	LFTs, hepatitis panel
HEME	Coagulopathy, principal defect in primary hemostasis	Easy bruising, menorrhagia, epistaxis Patient's experience during prior surgery or hemostatic challenge (e.g., dental extraction) vital to assessing periop risk, given variable severity of disease among individuals	Prolonged bleeding time; PT, PTT, plt count often normal; quantitative vWF antigen; ristocetin cofactor activity; multimeric analysis

Key Reference: Cameron CB, Kobrinsky N: Perioperative management of patients with von Willebrand's disease. Can J Anaesth 1990; 37:341–347.

PERIOPERATIVE IMPLICATIONS

Preoperative Preparation

- Collaboration with consultant hematologist and blood bank
- Desmopressin 1 h preop in all but IIB subtype
- Antifibrinolytics for dental procedures

Monitoring

- Bleeding time/vWF activity periodically in prolonged procedures; $T_{1/2}$ of administered vWF about 8–12 h

Airway

- Laryngoscopy can lead to tissue trauma
- Nasotracheal route best avoided

Induction

- No specific recommendations

Maintenance

- Meticulous surgical hemostasis

Extubation

- Avoid coughing if possible; gentle orotracheal suction best performed under direct vision

Adjuvants

- Consider regional anesthetics with caution
- Repeat desmopressin doses likely to be less effective than initial; reaccumulation of endothelial stores takes time

ANTICIPATED PROBLEMS/CONCERNS

- Excessive intra- and postoperative blood loss
- Increased likelihood of infectious bloodborne disease

WALDENSTRÖM'S MACROGLOBULINEMIA Kamla K. Prasad, M.D.

RISKS

- Incidence in USA: 1/100,000
- Racial preponderance: Caucasians >> African-Americans
- Males > females 3:2
- 100% fatality rate; median survival 5 y
- Median age at diagnosis: 63 y

PERIOPERATIVE RISKS

- Hyperviscosity syndrome
- Hemorrhage

WORRY ABOUT

- Hyperviscosity syndrome
- Multifactorial coagulopathy
- Pre-existing peripheral neurologic deficits
- Difficulties in evaluation and treatment of anemia

OVERVIEW

- Plasma cell dyscrasia characterized by neoplastic proliferation of clone of IgM-producing B cells
- Pathology from excessive monoclonal IgM production
- Potentially severe adverse neurologic, hemostatic, CV problems perioperatively
- Anesthetic concerns similar to those in multiple myeloma except that hypercalcemia and bone lesions are rare; renal failure and Bence Jones proteinuria less common

ICD-9-CM Code: 273.3

See also Multiple Myeloma in Diseases section

ETIOLOGY

- Cause unknown; possible genetic predisposition; possible occupational exposure (leather, rubber dyes, paints)

USUAL TREATMENT

- Alkylating agents (chlorambucil), nucleoside analogues (fludarabine, cladribine), rituximab, and prednisone
- Plasmapheresis prior to transfusion and to treat hyperviscosity syndrome

ASSESSMENT POINTS

SYSTEM	EFFECT	ASSESSMENT BY HX	PE	TEST
CV	Hyperviscosity syndrome (microvascular sludging)	Angina Fatigue CHF	Venous thrombosis	Serum viscosity >5 cp (nml: ≤1.8)
RESP	Pulm involvement	Dyspnea	Pleural effusion	CXR (pleural effusion, diffuse pulm infiltrates)
HEME	Impaired plt aggregation Inhibition of factors V, VII, VIII Impaired clot formation	Episodic epistaxis Episodic mucosal and gum bleeding		Bleeding time PT, PTT, TT
	Normocytic/normochromic anemia	Fatigue	Pallor	CBC
	Cryoglobulinemia	Cold intolerance Raynaud's syndrome Arthralgia	Purpura	Cryoglobulin assay
RENAL	Glomerulonephritis			BUN/Cr
CNS	Leukoencephalopathy Abnormal cerebrovascular permeability		Mental status changes	
PNS	Demyelinating peripheral neuropathy		Symmetric peripheral neuropathy, legs > arms	

Key Reference: Dimopoulos MA, Panayrotidis P, Moulopoulos LA, Sfikakis P, Dalakas M: Waldenström's macroglobulinemia: clinical features, complications, and management. J Clin Oncol 2000; 18:214–226.

PERIOPERATIVE IMPLICATIONS

Preoperative Preparation

- Consider plasmapheresis and transfusion

Monitoring

- Normothermia to prevent cryoglobulin precipitation

Airway

- Macroglossia if amyloidosis (5%)

Adjuvants

- All drugs: theoretical unpredictable pharmacokinetics due to alterations of relative proportions of globulins and albumin in blood; unpredictable pharmacodynamics due to increased cerebrovascular permeability

Postoperative Period

- Transient postop paresis due to disease rather than anesthetic management

ANTICIPATED PROBLEMS/CONCERNS

- Hyperviscosity syndrome (20% incidence perioperatively)
  – Develops from markedly increased concentration of large, asymmetric IgM molecule
  – Capillary blood flow impaired, reducing O_2 delivery through microcirculation
  – Expanded plasma volume, ↑ ICP, and ↑ cerebrovascular permeability
  – Findings include fatigue, dizziness, headache, visual blurring, mucosal bleeding, impaired mentation, CHF, dilated, segmented retinal and conjunctival vessels
  – Plasmapheresis mainstay of therapy
- Anemia
  – Hgb value may be artificially reduced by as much as 2 g/dl because of increased plasma volume
  – Transfusion may precipitate CHF or hyperviscosity syndrome (by increasing serum viscosity) and actually decrease O_2 delivery
  – Consider plasmapheresis before transfusion
- 5% at risk for cryoglobulinemia. At cold blood temp, cryoglobulins precipitate, triggering complement activation, causing immune complex vasculitis, and resulting in ischemia of skin, nerve, and renal tissues. Raynaud's syndrome, arthralgia, purpura, peripheral neuropathy, hepatic dysfunction, and renal failure may ensue.

WILMS' TUMOR

Peter J. Davis, M.D.

RISK

- Most common malignant renal tumor in childhood
- 6% of all childhood malignancies
- 5–7.8 / million children < 15 y
- M = F
- Peak age 1–3 y
- 5% bilateral
- Relapse-free survival rate at 2 y, 90%

PERIOPERATIVE RISKS

- ↑ Intra-abdominal pressure
- Immunocompromised
- Tumor extension into renal vein, IVC, and heart
- Some treated with chemotherapy prior to surgery
- Associated Htn

WORRY ABOUT

- Anomalies
  - Aniridia 1%, hemihypertrophy 2%
  - Neurofibromatosis
  - Beckwith-Wiedemann syndrome
  - GU abnormalities, horseshoe-shaped kidney, cryptorchidism, gonadal dysgenesis, hypospadias, duplication of collecting systems
- Metastatic disease
  - Lymph nodes, lung, liver, brain

OVERVIEW

- Most common abdominal tumor of childhood; prognosis related to staging
- Because of location of tumor, blood loss can be significant
- Tumor is also associated with other congenital abnormalities, which may affect anesthetic/surgical management
- Tumor extension into IVC and heart carries ↑ morbidity and mortality

ICD-9-CM Code: 189.0

ETIOLOGY

- Embryonal neoplasm
- No consistent chromosome abnormality, although abnormalities in chromosomes 1 and 11 are common
- 3 Genes associated with Wilms'
  - 11p13 interstitial deletion associated with Wilms'-aniridia-growth retardation
  - 11p15.5 deletion associated with Beckwith-Wiedemann syndrome
  - 3rd locus not determined associated with familial Wilms'

USUAL TREATMENT

- Chemotherapy (with vincristine, actinomycin D, and Adriamycin)
- Radiotherapy
- Surgical removal of tumor. If tumor bilateral, surgery has focused on nephron-sparing procedures. (Procedure includes biopsy followed by chemo and delayed definitive resection.)

ASSESSMENT POINTS

SYSTEM	EFFECT	ASSESSMENT BY HX	PE	TEST
HEENT	Beckwith-Wiedemann syndrome	Obstructive airway 2° to large tongue	Direct examination	Blood glucose levels
CV	Htn Tumor extension into heart	Asymptomatic	Htn	ECG CT abdomen US renal vein/IVC Cardiac ECHO
RESP	Respiratory compromise	Abdominal distention Metastatic disease Tumor embolization	↑ RR Hypoxemia	Pulse oximetry CT abdomen US renal vein/IVC Possible cardiac ECHO
GI	Gastric reflux	↑ Intraoperative pressure History of reflux	Abdominal distention	Review CT scan

Key Reference: Przybylo HJ, Stevenson GW, Backer C, et al: Anesthetic management of children with intracardiac extension of abdominal tumors. Anesth Analg 1994; 78:172–175.

PERIOPERATIVE INDICATIONS

Preoperative Preparation

- Htn—controlled
- R/O renal vein/IVC tumor involvement

Monitoring

- Arterial catheter may be indicated
- CVP catheter may be needed esp if IVC and tumor extend mid-heart
- Pre-existing hematuria—Foley catheter to aid in fluid balance
- IV catheters above diaphragm, large-bore catheters preferable
- ETCO$_2$ to rule out air and/or tumor embolus

Airway

- May be a problem if Beckwith-Wiedemann syndrome present

Preinduction/Induction

- Age-appropriate use of sedation
- Rapid-sequence if ↑ intra-abdominal pressure
- Regional anesthesia, for postop pain—epidural
- Pre-existing chemotherapy may have cardiac depressant effect
- IV access above diaphragm

Maintenance

- Prolonged procedure
- Avoid N$_2$O
- Maintain temperature
- Increased third space fluid requirements
- Procedure may be associated with large blood loss
- Pulm function may be compromised, 2° to metastasis/tumor embolization, abdominal distention, and/or surgical traction

Extubation

- Expected if temp maintained and patient hemodynamically stable

Postoperative Period

- Pain control
- Third space fluid requirements
- Htn may still be present

ANTICIPATED PROBLEMS/CONCERNS

- Risk of tumor and/or air embolus. If tumor extends into renal vein, IVC may have to be crossclamped, the IVC opened, and the tumor removed.
- Intraop blood loss can be extensive
- Periop implications

WOLFF-PARKINSON-WHITE (WPW) SYNDROME

Jeffrey R. Balser, M.D., Ph.D.

RISK

- Prevalence: 3/1000 in general population

PERIOPERATIVE RISKS

- Paroxysmal supraventricular tachycardia (PSVT): rapid heart rate impairs LV filling. May cause hypoperfusion if LV failure, LV hypertrophy, aortic stenosis, or mitral stenosis.
- AFIB occurs in 10–35% of patients with WPW, with ↑ incidence with age. Major concern is rapid ventricular response due to antegrade conduction over accessory pathway (AP) and induction of VFIB.

WORRY ABOUT

- Perioperative hypotension in patients with LV failure (systolic or diastolic dysfunction)
- Ischemia in patients with CAD if PSVT or AFIB occurs
- Induction of VFIB

OVERVIEW

- AP is congenital auxiliary electrical connection between atria and ventricles. WPW present when this AP is manifested on surface ECG and when it participates in PSVT. Other patients may have concealed APs (not apparent on surface ECG) that also underlie PSVT and ↑ tendency to develop AFIB.
- APs may conduct antegrade or retrograde. During sinus rhythm, antegrade conduction through AP may produce ventricular preexcitation on ECG with a short P-R interval (<0.12 sec), a slurred QRS upstroke (δ wave), and wide QRS complex. These abnormalities in QRS complex may vary in magnitude and depend on relative contribution of normal AV nodal system and AP to ventricular depolarization.
- PSVT results from re-entrant circuit involving AV node AP. QRS complex during PSVT matches the usual QRS morphology when conduction is antegrade through AV system and retrograde over AP (orthodromic). 5–10% of time, conduction over AP is antegrade (antidromic), producing wide QRS complex. This rhythm may be confused with VTach.

- AFIB/AFLT more common in patients with WPW. Usually, but not always, AFIB precipitated by episode of PSVT. Rapid (≥300 bpm) ventricular rates may occur in patients with APs with short refractory periods. These patients at risk for developing VFIB and hemodynamic collapse.

ICD-9-CM Code: 426.7

See also Supraventricular Tachycardia and Ventricular Tachycardia in Diseases section

USUAL TREATMENT

- With severe hemodynamic compromise: DC cardioversion (50–100 J)
- PSVT: usually terminated by vagal maneuvers or adenosine. Small incidence of induction of AFIB with adenosine therapy for PSVT in WPW has been described.
- Agents that reduce the accessory bundle refractory period (digoxin, Ca^{2+}-channel blockers, β-blockers, and adenosine) ↑ the risk of causing VFIB and hemodynamic collapse in patients with WPW and AFIB. WPW patients who experience AFIB should not be treated with these AV nodal blockers; rather, IV procainamide and amiodarone are preferred agents for slowing the rate and to achieve conversion.

ASSESSMENT POINTS

SYSTEM	EFFECT	ASSESSMENT BY HX	PE	TEST
CV	Tachycardia, hypotension	Palpitations, diaphoresis, angina, vague chest discomfort, neck pounding	Prominent jugular venous pulsations due to atrial contraction against closed tricuspid valve	12-lead ECG; Electrophysiologic study and catheter ablation
RESP	CHF exacerbation if PSVT + poor LV function	Dyspnea, orthopnea	Rales, wheezing, S_3	CXR
CNS	Lightheadedness			

Key Reference: Wellens HJJ, Smeets JLRM, Rodriguez LM, Gorgels APM: Atrial fibrillation in Wolff-Parkinson-White syndrome. *In* Falk RH, Podrid PJ (eds): Atrial Fibrillation: Mechanisms and Management. New York, Raven Press, 1992, pp 333–344.

PERIOPERATIVE IMPLICATIONS

Preoperative Preparation

- If preexcitation on ECG or Hx of WPW, consider cardiology evaluation
- If symptomatic, consider electrophysiologic study and catheter ablation

Monitoring

- ECG for detection of perioperative PSVT or AFIB
- Consider arterial line and CVP catheter if LV dysfunction or valve disease because of high dependence on preload and atrial kick

Induction/Maintenance/Extubation

- Avoid tachycardia, light anesthesia, hypoxia, and lyte abnormalities

Adjuvants

- Limit use of vagolytic agents such as pancuronium and atropine

Postoperative Period

- Pain management to avoid catecholamine excess

ANTICIPATED PROBLEMS/CONCERNS

- AV nodal blockers (digoxin, Ca^{2+}-channel blockers, adenosine, and β-blockers) may shorten refractoriness in the AP and thereby provoke VFIB in WPW patients with AFIB
- Hemodynamic collapse may occur when verapamil or β-blockers used in VTach mistaken for antidromic (wide-complex) PSVT in patient with WPW

SECTION II

PROCEDURES

ABDOMINAL AORTIC ANEURYSM REPAIR

Garry V. Walker, M.D.
Charles Beattie, M.D., Ph.D.

RISK

- Incidence: 3% of males aged >55 y, autopsy incidence of 1.8–6.6%
- Most Dx in 6th, 7th decades
- Male:female, 4:1
- Predominantly caused by atherosclerosis, Htn, tobacco abuse

PERIOPERATIVE RISKS

- Depends on patient condition, level of aortic occlusion
- Mortality: 1.5–8%, elective; 25–60% emergent/ruptured
- Morbidity: strongly depends on level of aortic crossclamp: infrarenal, suprarenal, supraceliac
- Nonlethal MI 4–15%
- Resp 5–10%
- Renal insufficiency 2–5% (infrarenal), 17% (suprarenal)
- Bowel complications 3–4%
- Paraplegia <1% (infrarenal), 1–5% (supraceliac)

WORRY ABOUT

- Myocardial ischemia/MI with aortic clamping; postop MI
- Renal failure/insufficiency
- Blood loss, hypothermia, acid-base abnormal with supraceliac clamp release

OVERVIEW

- High incidence of co-existing Htn (40–60%), CAD (30–40%), carotid bruits (10–30%)
- Emergent repair has much higher associated mortality
- Significant cardiac stress can occur with aortic crossclamp
- Anesthesia goals are to keep normal intrachamber cardiac size; optimize coronary, renal, cerebral O_2, esp during aortic crossclamp

ICD-9-CM Code: 441.4

INDICATIONS AND USUAL TREATMENT

- Asymptomatic aneurysms of <5 cm may be followed by quarterly exams
- Elective repair for aneurysms >5 cm
- Evidence of leak or rupture; documented recent ↑ in size
- Prompt repair of all aneurysms that become symptomatic (sudden severe abd pain that may radiate to back associated with faintness or syncope)

ASSESSMENT POINTS

SYSTEM	EFFECT	ASSESSMENT BY HX	PE	TEST
CV	Previous MI, CAD with poss ventricular dysfunction	<70 y, angina, ventricular arrhythmia, Q-wave, PND	Pedal edema, S_3	Stress ECG, ECHO, dipyridamole thallium or dobutamine ECHO
RESP	COPD, pulm edema	Dyspnea	Barrel chest, bronchospasm	CXR, ABGs, ?PFTs
RENAL	Renal insufficiency	Renal vascular Htn		Cr
CNS	Carotid/vertebral disease	TIA, stroke	Neuro deficits, carotid bruits	Neuro assessment, carotid Doppler

Key Reference: Ellis JE, Roizen MF, Youngberg JA: Anesthesia for abdominal aortic revascularization. *In* Youngberg JA, Lake CL, Roizen MF, Wilson RS (eds): Cardiac Vascular and Thoracic Anesthesia. New York, Churchill Livingstone, 2000, pp 538–566.

PERIOPERATIVE MANAGEMENT

Preoperative Preparation

- Assess co-existing morbidities, prepare to maintain homeostasis
- Consider epidural placement for pre-emptive, perioperative analgesia

Monitoring

- Invasive arterial pressure monitoring, large-bore vascular access essential
- A-line, CVP for all, PA cath for suprarenal and supraceliac aortic crossclamps and those with infrarenal who have cardiac disease (LVEF <35%, and/or significant CAD-ischemia on preop Holter, coronary stenosis >70%)
- Consider intraoperative TEE for patients with significant LV dysfunction

Anesthetic Technique/Induction

- Stable induction technique essential
- All variations of carefully conducted general or regional-supplemented general anesthesia
- Influence of anesthesia technique on perioperative morbidity is equivocal

SURGICAL STAGES

Dissection

- Ability to transfuse blood products must be immediate and blood scavenging is indicated
- For suprarenal and supraceliac consider establishing brisk UO; mannitol (25 g) well before aortic crossclamping, or dopamine 3 μg/kg/min for suprarenal and supraceliac, and infrarenal with pre-existing renal dysfunction
- Consider heparin 100 U/kg 5 min prior to aortic crossclamping

Aortic Clamping

- Control BP with nitroprusside, nitroglycerine, and/or inhalation agent
- Consider fluid loading at end of aortic crossclamping to prep for clamp release
- Cerebral, renal, myocardial protection depend on adequate perfusion pressure, maintaining normal cardiac chamber size during operation

Aortic Unclamping

- Normalize preload, discontinue vasodilators before unclamping to effect stable hemodynamics

- Acidosis with supraceliac aortic crossclamping release can be profound; consider treating with bicarbonate during clamp period, esp if long surgical technique (>1 h); may need Ca^{2+} Rx for blood transfusion, if liver is "out of circ" during aortic crossclamping. With good surgical technique, these problems do not occur.
- EBL: 600–4000 ml

Postoperative Considerations

- BP and HR control
- Many routinely extubate at end of case, but postop fluid shifts/requirement may be significant
- Pain score: 6–9; depends on incision type
- Postop analgesia: epidural or IV PCA

ANTICIPATED PROBLEMS/CONCERNS

- Combined regional/general can be associated with hypotension
- Desirable to maintain body temperature, but not with lower extremity warming during aortic crossclamping
- Controversies include need for renal protection; use of nitroprusside for supraceliac aortic crossclamping; prompt extubation; need for routine ICU care

ABDOMINOPERINEAL RESECTION
Randolph B. Gorman, M.D.

RISK

- Rectal cancer: 40,000 cases/y; abdominoperineal resection used in ~10% of operations for condition; remainder, low anterior resection, sparing anus, sphincter
- Males:females, 1.4:1
- Racial predominance: none

PERIOPERATIVE RISKS

- Perioperative mortality 2–3%
- Mortality mostly related to cardiopulm issues, older patients
- Morbidity mainly urol, pulm, wound dehiscence

WORRY ABOUT

- Perioperative fluid deficit (bowel prep, leaky capillaries)
- Poss blood loss during pelvic dissection
- Poss ureteral, bladder injury
- Patient position in lithotomy or jackknife position
- Co-existing disease in elderly

OVERVIEW

- Surg involves removal of distal colon, rectum; closure of anus, creation of permanent colostomy

ICD-9-CM Code: 154.1

INDICATIONS AND USUAL TREATMENT

- In curative, palliative resections of tumors of middle and lower 3rd of rectum, some tumors of anus
- Occasionally used for severe inflammatory bowel disease
- Use of operation ↓ in favor of low anterior resection or local excision in absence of invasive lesion
- Chemo/radiotherapy may be employed pre- or postop

ASSESSMENT POINTS

SYSTEM	EFFECT	ASSESSMENT BY HX	PE	TEST
CV	Impairment due to advanced age	Chest pain, SOB, exercise tolerance	CV exam	ECG
RESP	Metastasis	Cough, SOB	Auscultation	CXR, CT
GI	Hepatic metastases Bowel obstruction	Pain N/V	Palpation Distention, pain	CT Abd x-ray
ENDO	Malnutrition	Wt loss	Cachexia	Lytes, albumin
HEME	Bleeding	Weakness	Pallor, tachycardia	CBC
GU	Obstruction	Pain, oliguria		BUN, Cr IVP

Key Reference: Rothenberger DA, Wong WD: Abdominoperineal resection for adenocarcinoma of the low rectum. World J Surg 1992; 16:478–485.

PERIOPERATIVE IMPLICATIONS

Preoperative Preparation
- Worry about occult dehydration, consider H_2 blockers if bowel obstruction

Anesthesia Technique
- Performed with general anesthesia or combined regional/general

Monitoring
- Routine monitors
- Consider arterial line in patients with CV or pulm disease
- Monitor UO for volume status, indicator of bladder, ureter injury
- Consider CVP or PA cath

Airway
- If bowel obstruction, consider rapid-sequence induction

Induction
- Replace volume deficit from bowel prep, NPO, esp in patients admitted on the day of surgery

SURGICAL STAGES

- Dissection: 2 stages: abdominal and perineal; patients usually in lithotomy position

Definitive Surgery
- Abdominal phase: mobilization of rectum, sigmoid colon, creation of descending colostomy
- Perineal phase: dissection beginning with elliptical incision from perineum to coccyx; dissection in posterior, lateral planes for 270°; specimen then pulled through perineal wound, final dissection done
- Abdominal perineal wounds closed; colostomy is matured
- EBL: 1000 ml

Postoperative Considerations
- Pain score: 7–8
- Pain management: PCA IV; epidural
- Morbidity: urol (bladder/ureter injury, sexual dysfunction), wound dehiscence/infection, blood loss, adhesions (late)

ANTICIPATED PROBLEMS/CONCERNS

- Hypovolemia from bowel prep, capillary leak
- Ureter/bladder injury
- Surg technically more difficult in males (narrow pelvis) with ↑ morbidity

PATHOLOGY

- Dukes' classification:
  - A—limited to bowel wall
  - B—invading through bowel wall
  - C—B plus node involvement
  - D—distant metastasis (liver, lung)
- 5-y survival:
  - A—>90%
  - B—60–80%
  - C—20–50%
  - D—<5%

ADRENALECTOMY FOR PHEOCHROMOCYTOMA

Michael F. Roizen, M.D.

RISK

- People within USA: 0.03%–0.04% (~ 80,000) by autopsy of nonselected individuals; 0.1%–1.0% of individuals with sustained Htn
- Race with highest prevalence: Caucasian

PERIOPERATIVE RISKS

- Major goal to avoid pheo crisis; pre-, intraop goals of management of extra-adrenal surgery no different from those of adrenal surgery; if α blockade not present before surg, try to delay operation until degree of α blockade judged appropriate by:
  - No BP > 165/90 mmHg for 48 h
  - Presence of orthostatic hypotension, but BP on standing should not be < 80/45 mmHg
  - An ECG free of ST-T changes due to cardiomyopathy
  - Absence of Sx of catecholamine excess; and signs of α blockade (e.g., nasal stuffiness)
- If emergency use α-blockers, β-blockers, nitroprusside; keep in ICU till most painful time has passed or adrenergic control attained

- ↑ Risk of Htn crisis with bleeding into myocardium, brain, kidney or ischemia
- Mortality rate to 3% even with appropriate preparation for tumor resection, in "good" hands
- 25–50% of those who die in hospitals of pheo crisis do so during induction of anesthesia/stressful periop periods, or in labor, delivery
- Associated with cholelithiasis, renal stones

WORRY ABOUT

- Catecholamine crisis with hemorrhage/infarcts in vital organs, hypotension due to ↓ levels of catecholamines postop (uncommon more than 3 days postop if all pheo tissue removed)

OVERVIEW

- Tumor of catecholamine-producing tissue (90% in adrenals): painful (stressful) events often cause exaggerated stress response
- For patients with pheo, even small stresses can lead to blood catecholamine levels of 2000–20,000 pg/ml; infarction of tumor, with release of products on retroperitoneal surfaces, surgical, or other pressure causing release of products, can result in blood levels of 200,000–1 million pg/ml

- Need α-blockers before β blockade lest vasoconstrictive effects of latter go unopposed, causing ↑ risk of dangerous Htn. β blockade suggested if persistent arrhythmias or tachycardia not resolving α-adrenergic effects or when aggravated by α-adrenergic effects.
- If appropriate, α blockade preop can lower risk of crisis by >90%

ICD-9-CM Code: 194.0

INDICATIONS AND USUAL TREATMENT

- 90% spont arise; 10% familial (autosomal dominant genetics involving chromosome 7 implicated)
- Assoc with MEA IIA (medullary thyroid cancer, primary hyperparathyroidism), IIB (medullary thyroid cancer, mucosal neuromas; assoc with neurofibromatosis, von Hippel–Lindau syndrome, and retinal and cerebellar hemangioblastoma, ataxia-telangiectasia, Sturge-Weber syndrome)
- "Prehydrate" liberally over 6–60 days if CV status tolerates; expand with high salt/fluid diet while ↑ α blockade over 7–60 day period

ASSESSMENT POINTS

SYSTEM	EFFECT	ASSESSMENT BY HX	PE	TEST
HEENT		Nasal stuffiness (from α-adrenergic blockade)		
CV	Htn, dysrhythmias, AFIB, sinus tachycardia, mitral valve prolapse, CHF, myocardial fibril necrosis or myocarditis	SOB, exercise tolerance, palpitations, Htn (50% sustained, 40% paroxsymal)	Standard exam plus measurement of BP q1min in stressful environment plus orthostatic maneuvers with BP/HR measurement q1min	ECG, ECHO (if cardiomyopathy suspected)
GI	90% tumors adrenal or abdominal Wt loss, diarrhea, dehydration		Be careful when palpating abdomen not to trigger pheo crisis	No different from normal
HEME		Mild polycythemia, thrombocytopenia		Hgb (way to judge volume expansion)
CNS	↑ Catecholamine effects	Headache, tremor, anxiety, ↓ pain threshold, fatigue		
METAB	Assoc with hyperparathyroidism	Glucose intolerance due to α-adrenergic gluconeogenesis, ↓ insulin secretion		Glucose often ↑ (insulin Rx prescribed before correct Dx of cancer made)

Key Reference: Roizen MF: Pheochromocytoma in anesthetic implications of concurrent disease. *In* Miller's Anesthesia. New York, Churchill Livingstone, 2000, pp 924–927.

PERIOPERATIVE MANAGEMENT

Monitoring
- Temperature
- Art line placement before induction difficult
- Consider PA cath and/or TEE if CV system severely affected; CVP rarely used

Anesthetic Care/Technique
- No technique assoc with better or worse outcome; use of droperidol controversial. Agents that block catecholamine reuptake (ketamine) or cause release might be avoided.

Induction/Maintenance
- Prehydrate liberally if tolerated
- Gentle induction with nitroprusside available
- Dopamine infusion in reserve
- Painful or stressful events often cause exaggerated stress response caused by release of catecholamines from nerve endings "loaded" by reuptake

SURGICAL STAGES

Initial Dissection
- Transabd incision preferred if localization does not exclude bilat tumors; flank/post approach with nephrectomy/jackknife position if unilateral adrenalectomy without paraganglionoma exploration planned
  - Laparoscopic approach assoc with same intra- and postop CV events. Faster bowel recovery.

Adrenal Removal
- Dissection to secure venous drainage, double ligature with transection between; then arterial supply; then complete mobilization, liberation
- After predominant tumor removed, palpation of paraganglionic chain with observation to monitor for sudden ↑ in BP or HR
- Goal in resection is securing venous supply from tumor(s). Pressure on tumor causing release can result in blood levels of 200,000–1 million pg/ml (ask for temporary stay of surgery while nitroprusside infusion ↑).
- Good communication essential

- Relative hypotension often develops after venous drainage of tumor or its removal. If perfusion adequate can let BP stay at 80/40. Massive infusions of catecholamines occasionally required.
- EBL: 100–400 ml; cell saver use not advised
- Often hypovolemic if < 2–3 wk has been allowed for ↑ titration of α-blocking drugs; guide volume replacement with PCWP or TEE vol estimates

POSTOPERATIVE CONSIDERATIONS

- Postop, do not force high UO with crystalloid infusions, as pts have tendency to CHF
- Postop, ~50% remain hypertensive for 1–3 days, when all but 25% become normotensive
- Usually use epidural, PCA, IV narcotics for 2–4 days postop (1 day if laparoscopic)

ANTICIPATED PROBLEMS/CONCERNS

- Pheo crisis a life-threatening illness, manifest by ↑ temp, ↑ HR, alterations in consciousness

ADVANCED CARDIAC LIFE SUPPORT (ACLS)

Alan Jay Schwartz, M.D., M.S.Ed.

RISK

- People within USA: 1000 cardiac arrests/d
- Risk factors: male sex, Htn, cigarette smoking, older age, elevated blood cholesterol, diabetes mellitus, Hx of premature artherosclerosis
- No racial predominance

PERIOPERATIVE RISKS

- 1.7 cardiac arrests/10,000 anesthetics
- Associated pathology: ischemic, valvular, or hypertensive heart disease; congestive cardiomyopathy
- Uncommon associated conditions: preexcitation syndromes, hereditary or acquired prolonged QT disorders, metabolic abnormalities, adverse drug reactions

WORRY ABOUT

- Cardiac pathology
- Perioperative ischemic changes, metabolic abnormalities
- Subsequent episodes postresuscitation
- Postresuscitation end-organ ischemic damage

OVERVIEW

- Morbidity and mortality decreased when ACLS initiated promptly
- Outcome dismal if initiation of ACLS is delayed >8 min or lasts >30 min
- Other factors associated with decreased survival: age >70 y, unwitnessed, sepsis, cancer, renal failure, prearrest hypotension
- Survival rate for in-hospital cardiac arrest is 14%

ICD-9-CM Code: 997.1 (Resulting from procedure)

INDICATIONS AND USUAL TREATMENT

- ACLS indicated for treatment of potentially life-threatening arrhythmias and fatal arrhythmias or cardiac arrest, e.g., supraventricular bradycardias and tachycardias, ventricular fibrillation, bradyasystole and electrical mechanical dissociation
- Treatment depends on the arrhythmia or cause of cardiac arrest and the hemodynamic stability of the patient. (Spinal anesthetics associated with hypotension and bradycardia.)
- The quicker the restoration of normal rhythm, the more likely survival. The watchword is defibrillate early and often.

ASSESSMENT POINTS

SYSTEM	EFFECT	ASSESSMENT BY HX	PE	TEST
CNS	Arrhythmia may cause hypotension	Syncope	CNS exam	ECG, MRI
CV	Arrhythmia, Htn, valvular disease	CV status, Hx angina, SOB, palpitations	CV exam	ECG, ECHO
RESP	Pulmonary edema	SOB, orthopnea	Chest exam	SaO_2, CXR

Key Reference: Guidelines 2000 for Cardiopulmonary Resuscitation and Emergency Cardiovascular Care. Circulation 2000; 102 (Suppl 8) I140–I141.

INTRAOPERATIVE MANAGEMENT

Monitoring

- Routine, with SpO_2; confirmation of ETT position using qualitative end-tidal CO_2 indicator, capnographic and capnometric and esophageal detector devices
- Invasive monitoring as indicated by the patient's condition

Management

- Dependent upon type of rhythm and hemodynamic status
- Emergency drugs, including epinephrine, lidocaine, and atropine, must be immediately available
- Cardiac defibrillator and means of cardiac pacing must be available
- Initiate BLS with attention to maintenance of airway, ventilation, and circulation via chest compressions until definitive treatment established
- Supraventricular bradyarrhythmias
  - Treat if significant decrease in BP or cardiac output or in the presence of PVCs; atropine 1 mg IV, repeat 3–5 min, if needed, to total of 0.04 mg/kg; transcutaneous or transvenous pacing; dopamine or epinephrine infusion; isoproterenol infusions used with extreme caution as last resort
- Supraventricular tachyarrhythmias
  - Paroxysmal supraventricular tachycardia (PSVT) with severe hypotension and atrial fibrillation or flutter with hemodynamic compromise

  - If stable in PSVT, vagal maneuvers followed by adenosine 6 mg IV, then adenosine 12 mg IV after 1–2 min if PSVT persists; try procainamide and amiodarone. If PSVT recurs and BP remains stable, verapamil 2.5–5.0 mg IV.
  - If stable in AFIB or atrial flutter, consider diltiazem, β-blockers, or verapamil
  - If unstable, cardioversion with 100, 200, 300, and 360 J may be used in succession until converted
  - Atrial flutter responds to lower energy (25 J)
- Ventricular bradyarrhythmias
  - CHB with slow idioventricular escape rhythm treated with transvenous or external pacing
  - Atropine or isoproterenol tried until pacing instituted. Beware of precipitating VTach or VFIB.
- Premature ventricular beats
  - Look for treatable cause
  - Suppress with lidocaine 1.0–1.5 mg/kg IV; may repeat 0.5–0.75 mg/kg every 5–10 min to total 3 mg/kg, then procainamide
- Ventricular tachycardia
  - If stable, lidocaine 1.0–1.5 mg/kg IV; may repeat 0.5–0.75 mg/kg every 5–10 min to total of 3 mg/kg; then procainamide and amiodarone 150 mg IV over 10 min
  - If unsuccessful or hemodynamically unstable, cardioversion with 100, 200, 300, and 360 J in progressive increments
- Ventricular fibrillation (VFIB)

  - Rapid defibrillation with 200, 200–300, and 360 J shocks in rapid sequence if VFIB persists
  - If persistent, intersperse defibrillation with epinephrine 1.0 mg IV, vasopressin 40 U IV, then lidocaine 1.0–1.5 mg/kg IV followed by amiodarone, magnesium, and procainamide
- Bradyasystole
  - High mortality, suspect hypoxia
  - Consider immediate transcutaneous pacing
  - Epinephrine is drug of choice along with atropine
  - Defibrillation may be tried with asystole as unrecognized VFIB is alternative diagnosis
- Pulseless electrical activity
  - Caused by acute derangements in preload (hypovolemia, cardiac tamponade, tension pneumothorax), afterload (pulmonary embolism), myocardial performance (acidosis, hypoxemia)
  - Treatment dependent on cause
  - Epinephrine and atropine may be given

ANTICIPATED PROBLEMS/CONCERNS

- Following resuscitation, continued support of vital organ function often required: CNS insult may cause increase in ICP or seizures; myocardial damage may result in persistent dysrhythmias or decreased contractility; renal damage may result in acute renal failure

AMPUTATION, ABOVE-KNEE (AKA) Caridad Bravo-Fernandez, M.D.

RISK

- 22/100,000 people undergo amputations, 49% above knee
- Mean age 70 y
- Male:female, 3–9:1
- Cause: vascular insufficiency, DM, malignant neoplasm, trauma
- Htn dominant underlying medical condition

PERIOPERATIVE RISKS

- Operative mortality 5–30% (within 30 days)
- Morbidity includes myocardial ischemia, infarction, CHF, arrhythmias
- Pulmonary emboli: 6–10%
- Nonhealing, infection common surgical problems

WORRY ABOUT

- Underlying disease → AKA
- Associated infection, gangrene
- CVD
- Perioperative pulmonary emboli
- Flexion contractures of involved limb
- Decubiti
- Phantom limb pain/stump pain

OVERVIEW

- Associated with high operative mortality
- Vascular insufficiency to limb limits viability, ↑ risk of sepsis and complications of immobility; viability evaluated by Doppler, blood flow studies to determine level of amputation
- Preop epidural narcotics to eliminate rest pain
- Regional anesthesia, postop analgesia frequently used; contraindicated in patients receiving anticoagulants

- Rehabilitation less optimal than with below-knee amputation; AKA avoided if possible

ICD-9-CM Codes: 747.64 (PVD); 897.2 (Trauma)

INDICATIONS AND USUAL TREATMENT

- Amputations for trauma done early to ↓ contamination
- Control infection, sepsis with antibiotics
- Control blood sugar with regular insulin in diabetic patients
- Smoking should be discontinued 1 wk before operation
- Consider limited revascularization to improve changes for good results
- Below-knee amputation preferred for better rehabilitation

ASSESSMENT POINTS

SYSTEM	EFFECT	ASSESSMENT BY HX	PE	TEST
CV	CAD, Htn	CV status, chest pain, previous MI, SOB	CV exam	ECG, stress test ECHO
RESP	Emphysema	SOB, smoking, exercise tolerance	Chest exam	O_2 sat, CXR, ABGs
ENDO	DM	Polyuria, polydipsia Cardiomyopathy, neuropathy Autonomic neuropathy Delayed gastric emptying	Sensory exam	Glucose, orthostatic BP
HEME	Thrombophlebitis, bleeding	Pain, bruising, bleeding	Ulcerations, ecchymoses	PT, PTT, Hct
RENAL	Renal insufficiency/failure			BUN/Cr
CNS	CVA, TIA	CNS deficits	CNS exam	Carotid studies
PNS	Poor circulation Posterior cerebral circ	Claudication	Peripheral pulses Neck extension	Doppler, flow studies, angio
INFECTION	Malaise, swelling, gangrene	Fever, chills	Extremity ulcers, swelling, calor, rubor	Temp, cultures for organism

Key Reference: Mayfield, JA, Reiber GE, Maynard C, et al: Trends in lower limb amputation in the Veterans Health Administration, 1989–1998. J Rehab Res Dev 2000; 37:23–30.

INTRAOPERATIVE MANAGEMENT

- Volume status monitoring—blood loss without tourniquet

Preoperative Preparation

- Antibiotics for trauma
- Ensure availability of blood products

Anesthetic Technique

- Either regional or GA appropriate

Monitoring

- Routine monitors including ST-segment analysis
- Consider arterial, CVP, or PA line if long surgery, depending on CV status

Airway

- In trauma, diabetes, dialysis, consider "full stomach"

SURGICAL STAGES

Induction

- Spinal or epidural acceptable in patients with normal coagulation profile
- If GA, worry about myocardial ischemia and ventricular dysfunction

Skin Incision

- Circular incision at the level of amputation
- Observe blood loss; need for ligation of large vessels

Dissection

- Identify femoral artery, vein for clamping, division, ligation; sciatic nerve for ligation
- Assessment of viability of tissue by observing blood loss

Definitive Surgery/Closure

- Femur is divided with a saw, filed
- Wound closed in 2 layers

- Sterile dressing applied
- Immediate postop prosthesis can be applied
- Approximate duration: 1–2 h
- EBL w/o tourniquet: 250–500 ml

POSTOPERATIVE CONSIDERATIONS

- Blood loss may continue; replace as indicated by Hct
- Venous thrombosis associated with prolonged hosp, immobilization, venous stasis
- Aggressive pulmonary toilet to prevent atelectasis, pneumonia
- Phantom limb sensation in 100% of patients; usually resolves in 1 y
- Pain score: 5–10
- Pain relief by PCA if epidural is contraindicated

ANTICIPATED PROBLEMS/CONCERNS

- CV morbidity, mortality common 5–30%

AMPUTATION, LOWER EXTREMITY (LEA) Robert H. Bode, Jr., M.D.

RISK

- 100,000 patients undergo LEA annually
- Racial/gender predominance: none
- 40–70% of patients diabetic

PERIOPERATIVE RISKS

- Mortality 3–15%; usually CV-related
- ↑ Risk of MI, CHF, cardiac ischemia
- Survival in diabetic amputees <50% at 3 y
- Postop phantom limb pain common

WORRY ABOUT

- Perioperative cardiac morbidity/mortality
- Phantom limb pain
- Blood glucose control in diabetic patient

OVERVIEW

- Vast majority of LEAs performed for vasc insufficiency complicated by secondary infections and/or chronic pain
- Below-knee/above-knee amputations in USA 20:1
- >70% of patients undergoing below-knee amputations can be rehabilitated vs. only 30% of patients receiving above-knee amputations
- Postop phantom limb pain may ↓ with use of continuous regional anesthesia/analgesia techniques
- High incidence of assoc cardiac morbidity, mortality
- Co-existing diseases common, e.g., CAD, CHF, ↓ LV function, sepsis, diabetes

ICD-9-CM Code: 433.9 (PVD)

INDICATIONS AND USUAL TREATMENT

- Most common condition requiring LEA: vasc insufficiency with lower extremity infections and/or chronic pain (other indications include severe trauma, malignancy, congenital deformities)
- Preservation of knee joint important for rehab; creation of adequate stump flap essential
- Circumferential guillotine amputations are used in cases of severe infection/gangrene and battlefield injuries; guillotine amputations require extensive revision

ASSESSMENT POINTS

SYSTEM	EFFECT	ASSESSMENT OF HX	PE	TEST
CV	Co-existing CAD, CHF Autonomic neuropathy	SOB, angina	Rales S_3 JVD	ECG, stress test, or Holter, ECHO
RESP	Diabetes/difficult intubation	Chart review	Airway exam Prayer test (see Diabetes, Type I in Diseases section)	
	Co-existing COPD	SOB/bronchospasm	Auscultation	CXR
GI	Diabetes/gastroparesis	Vomiting, early satiety		
ENDO	Diabetes			Blood sugar, urinalysis
HEME	Patients on antithrombotic agents or aspirin	Bleeding		?Bleeding time
GU	Diabetes/nephropathy			BUN/serum Cr
MS	Infections/sepsis	Chart review	VS	WBC with differential, blood/wound cultures

Key Reference: Humphrey LL, Palumbo PJ, Butters MA, et al: The contribution of non-insulin-dependent diabetes to lower-extremity amputation in the community. Arch Intern Med 1994; 154:885–892.

PERIOPERATIVE MANAGEMENT

Preoperative Preparation

- CV assessment for all
- If patients diabetic consider need to control blood glucose, preserve renal function, provide prophylaxis against aspiration
- Regional anesthesia may be contraindicated if patients septic and/or on antithrombotic Rx

Anesthetic Technique

- Can be performed with regional, general, or combined anesthetic techniques

Monitoring

- Rare need for arterial line, CVP, and/or PA line, except in patients with active and significant heart disease

Airway

- Consider possibility of difficult airway in diabetics

Induction/Maintenance

- Vigilant control of hemodynamic variables and limiting fluids indicated in patients with heart disease

SURGICAL STAGES

Definitive Surgery

- Min blood loss during dissection (100–200 ml)
- Procedure <2 h

Postoperative Considerations

- Both early and late postop pain problems common
- Pain scores: 6–10
- Continuous regional anesthesia/analgesia techniques assoc with less phantom limb pain. Other modalities include PCA, TENS, TCA.
- If significant CAD, consider need for postop monitored care for 24–48 h

- Blood glucose control in diabetic patients may be difficult to achieve; keep <200 ml/dl to preserve renal, CNS autoregulation, <250 mg/dl for WBC phagocytic function

ANTICIPATED PROBLEMS/CONCERNS

- ↑ Incidence of CV morbidity/mortality
- Phantom limb pain common after LEA; may be ↓ with continuous regional anesthesia/analgesia, dilantin premedication

ANTERIOR CERVICAL FUSION
Laurel E. Moore, M.D.

RISK

- 70,000–80,000 procedures/y (underestimated in literature); 12,000 deaths/y from cervical spine disease in USA
- Racial predominance: none
- Male > female, 3:2

PERIOPERATIVE RISKS

- <1% 30-day mortality
- Recurrent nerve injury: 5%

WORRY ABOUT

- Airway management
- Risk of injury to esophagus, carotid artery, jugular vein
- Postop tracheal edema, recurrent laryngeal nerve injury, ↑ radicular pain or myelopathy, dysphagia

OVERVIEW

- Repair of degenerative, congenital, or traumatic injury to cervical spine or disks
- Anterior approach permits supine position with neutral head position
- Anterior approach provides good access to vertebral bodies, transverse processes of C2–C7
- Generally low blood loss procedure
- Good fusion rate at 12 wk postop

ICD-9-CM Code: 722.0 (Cervical herniated disc)

INDICATIONS AND USUAL TREATMENT

- Cervical herniated disk or spur
- Degenerative hypermobility or subluxation
- Radiculopathy with foraminal stenosis
- ↓ AP diameter of spinal canal
- Compressive myelopathy
- Degenerative kyphoscoliosis
- Alternative Rx includes posterior cervical approach and conservative care with NSAID, rest

ASSESSMENT POINTS

SYSTEM	EFFECT	ASSESSMENT BY HX	PE	TEST
HEENT	Access limited 2° to pain, anatomy, prior fusion, neurologic Sx	↑ Neurologic Sx or pain with movement	Oral opening, cervical ROM, neuro exam	Review of cervical x-ray studies
PNS	Radicular Sx, myelopathy	Onset of pain, numbness, weakness, bowel or bladder Sx	Motor, sensory assessment, ? single root vs. cord compression	Review of cervical x-ray studies (MRI, CT, myelogram)

Key Reference: Miller JI, Parsa AT: Neurosurgical disease of the spine and spinal cord: surgical considerations. *In* Cottrell JE (ed): Anesthesia and Neurosurgery, 3rd ed. St. Louis, Mosby, 1994, pp 543–567.

PERIOPERATIVE IMPLICATIONS

Anesthetic Technique

- General endotracheal due to surgical traction on trachea, esophagus

Monitoring

- Generally routine
- If multiple levels with instrumentation, consider invasive monitoring
- Arms, neck inaccessible during procedure, so invasive monitoring placed prospectively
- Consider neurologic monitoring (somatosensory or MEP)

Airway

- Consider awake intubation based on presence, absence of neurologic Sx with cervical motion
- Light wand alternative to awake intubation
- Radiologic evidence of cord compression
- Frequently position requires greater neck extension than for direct laryngoscopy

Maintenance

- Consider narcotic-based anesthesia, particularly if neurologic monitoring
- Muscle relaxation assists in distraction of cervical spine
- Generally not stimulating procedure except with placement of vertebral spreading retractor; removal of iliac bone for interbody fusion graft

Emergence

- Rapid awakening for neurologic assessment optimal

SURGICAL STAGES

- 10–15 lb traction applied by Gardner-Wells tongs or head brace for cervical distraction
- Combination of weighted traction, muscle paralysis, vertebral spreading retractor gives access to disk space

Exposure

- Trachea and esophagus retracted medially
- Carotid artery retracted laterally
- Recurrent laryngeal nerve retracted inferiorly
- Sup laryngeal, hypoglossal nerves retracted superiorly
- Vertebral artery ascends via foramina of transverse processes
- Disk space cleaned; interbody fusion performed with autologous (iliac crest) or cadaveric bone graft
- EBL, third space losses generally small

POSTOPERATIVE CONSIDERATIONS

- Pain at iliac graft site (pain score: 6–8), can be attenuated with local anesthetic injection pre-emergence
- Dysphagia common postop 2° to traction on esophagus

- Complications include
  - Recurrent laryngeal nerve injury
  - ↓ HR, BP with carotid sinus manipulation
  - ↑ Radicular pain or myelopathy
  - Postop hematoma formation
  - Transient tracheal or esophageal edema, dysmotility from prolonged retraction
  - Nonunion of fusion

ANTICIPATED PROBLEMS/CONCERNS

- Airway management
- Vital structures close to operative site causing hemodynamic changes intraoperatively or nerve injury postoperatively
- Fusions involving >1 or 2 levels have ↑ risk of nonunion or pseudarthrosis

AORTIC VALVE REPLACEMENT

Patricia Satitpunwaycha, M.D.
James G. Ramsay, M.D., F.R.C.P.C.

RISK

- Number of operations in USA/y: 26,000 (1997)
- Gender predominance: M > F, 3:2

PERIOPERATIVE RISKS

- For isolated AS, 3–8% perioperative mortality for pts <70 y, 3–16% for pts >70 y
- Mortality for elective AVR in pts with chronic AR is 4–10%
- ↑ Mortality with ↑ age, ↓ LV function, co-existing CAD, AFIB, renal failure
- Morbidity includes heart block, CVA

WORRY ABOUT

- Maintaining optimal hemodynamic variables for valvular lesion

- ↓ LV function preop, especially with AR
- Arrhythmias
- Myocardial preservation in hypertrophied ventricle during bypass
- De-airing before discontinuation of CPB

OVERVIEW

- Operative mortality for isolated AVR <5%, ↑ mortality with ↑ age, ↓ LV function, co-existing CAD, and ↓ exercise tolerance
- Patients with AS generally have better prognosis than those with AR, especially when ↓ LV function present
- Choice of porcine bioprosthesis or mech valve based on pt's expected longevity, risks of chronic anticoagulation
- Homograft valve is alternative if active infection, young woman desiring pregnancy, or anticoagulation is contraindicated

- Arrhythmias/heart block—atrial contribution to CO very important after AVR, especially in hypertrophied heart. Bundle of His prone to injury; atrial, ventricular pacing wires often used.

ICD-9-CM Codes: 424.1 (AS); 424.1 (AR); 35.22 (AVR—other)

INDICATIONS AND USUAL TREATMENT

- Symptomatic AS (angina, syncope, CHF) or AR (fatigue, DOE, CHF)
- Asymptomatic AS with aortic valve area <0.7 cm² or pressure gradient >50 mmHg at rest (with normal LV function)
- Acute severe AR
- Optimal timing in chronic AR controversial; benefit greatest before onset of LV dysfunction

ASSESSMENT POINTS

SYSTEM	EFFECT	ASSESSMENT BY HX	PE	TEST
HEENT	Co-existing dental infection—↑ risk for postop endocarditis	Oral hygiene	Oral exam	
CV	Aortic valve dysfunction Arrhythmia Ischemia LV dysfunction	Angina, syncope, CHF Palpitation, syncope Angina DOE, fatigue	CV exam – Rhythm – Murmur – Gallop	ECG ECHO Cardiac cath
RESP	Pulmonary vascular congestion from ↑ LVEDP	Dyspnea Orthopnea PND	Rales S₃	CXR SaO₂
RENAL	Renal insufficiency			BUN, Cr
CNS	TIA, RIND, CVA Syncope	Chronic AFIB Endocarditis Carotid disease	Carotid bruit Neuro deficit	Carotid Doppler TEE (atrial thrombus, valvular vegetations)

Key Reference: Torsher LC, Shub C, Rettke SR, Brown DL: Risk of patients with severe aortic stenosis undergoing noncardiac surgery. Am J Cardiol 1998; 81:448–452.

INTRAOPERATIVE MANAGEMENT

Preoperative Preparation

- Cautious premed; prevent anxiety but avoid acute changes in HR, preload, and afterload
- Adequate vascular access, blood products available

Anesthetic Technique—AS

- Perioperative hemodynamic goals: (1) maintain preload, afterload, (2) avoid ↓ BP (coronary perfusion pressure essential for LVH), (3) maintain sinus rhythm, normal rate, (4) aggressive Rx for dysrhythmias (loss of atrial click/rapid rate poorly tolerated) may require synchronized cardioversion

Anesthetic Technique—AR

- Perioperative hemodynamic goals: (1) maintain preload, (2) maintain arterial dilation (nitroprusside, nicardipine), (3) avoid significant myocardial depression, (4) maintain high-normal HR (90–100/min); bradycardia results in ↑ regurgitation LVEDP, (5) inotropic support frequently required post bypass if ↓ LVEF
- IABP contraindicated in presence of AR
- For uncomplicated AVR with good LV function, may combine smaller narcotic dose with sedative and inhalational agents to permit early extubation

Monitoring

- A-line, ECG with ST-segment analysis

- CVP vs. PAC (CVP may grossly underestimate LVEDP, but placement of PAC has potential for dysrhythmias)
- Consider TEE to monitor LV filling, contractility, regional wall motion, adequacy of de-airing, and postop valve function
- Consider external defibrillation pads with capability of transthoracic pacing
- Consider esophageal stethoscope with atrial pacing capacity

SURGICAL STAGES

Induction/Prebypass

- AS
  – Maintain preload, afterload (phenylephrine)
  – Avoid ↓ BP: coronary perfusion pressure essential with LVH (CPP = diastolic BP – LVEDP)
  – Maintain sinus rhythm, normal rate
  – Aggressive Rx for dysrhythmias
  – Surgeon and perfusionist available
- AR
  – Maintain preload
  – Afterload reduction to improve forward flow (nitroprusside, nicardipine)
  – Avoid significant contractile depression
  – Maintain high-normal HR (90–100/min); bradycardia results in ↑ regurgitation
  – IABP contraindicated in presence of AR
- Antifibrinolytic drug

Cardiopulmonary Bypass

- Cardioplegia: antegrade ± retrograde to allow infusion without interruption
- In AR, prevent LV distention at initiation of CPB by maintaining sinus rhythm:
  – IV esmolol 1–2 mg/kg
  – IV lidocaine 1–1.5 mg/kg
  – Defibrillation or urgent aortic crossclamping/LV venting poss necessary
- Evacuate air and assess valve function with TEE before discontinuing CPB
- Inotropic support frequently required post bypass if ↓ LVEF (AR)

Postoperative Considerations

- Compliance of hypertrophic ventricles after AVR unchanged, need adequate preload NSR
- Control hypertension to avoid bleeding and dissection
- Anticoagulation for mechanical valves; coumadin usually begun 2–3 days postop

ANTICIPATED PROBLEMS/CONCERNS

- ↓ Preop LV function may require support
- AFIB/AFLT poorly tolerated with LVH; consider low-dose β-blocker to prevent arrhythmias
- Heart block can develop on postop day 1. Atrial, ventricular pacing wires recommended. Bundle of His prone to injury, permanent pacemaker possibly required.

AORTOPULMONARY WINDOW

Howard Alan Zucker, M.D.

RISK

- 0.2–0.6% of congenital HD
- Associated with secundum ASD, PDA, VSD, aortic origin of right PA, type A interrupted aortic arch, tetralogy of Fallot, anomalous origin of coronary arteries
- No gender predilection

PERIOPERATIVE RISKS

- Perioperative mortality rate < 3%

WORRY ABOUT

- ↑ Pulmonary flow 2° to L → R shunt preop
- Development of preop CHF
- Pulmonary Htn with associated reactive pulmonary vascular bed; of concern if repaired later in life

OVERVIEW

- Manifests similarly to VSD or PDA with overcirculation of pulmonary vascular bed
- Sx of CHF include failure to thrive, diaphoresis, dyspnea

ICD-9-CM Code: 745.0

INDICATIONS AND USUAL TREATMENT

- Surg correction indicated in all cases using CPB with patch closure (Dacron or glutaraldehyde-treated pericardium)
- Associated congenital heart lesions may result in postop problems unrelated to the aortopulmonary window repair
- Eisenmenger's syndrome with physiologic changes from long-standing L → R shunting only contraindication to surg closure

ASSESSMENT POINTS

SYSTEM	EFFECT	ASSESSMENT BY HX	PE	TEST
CV	CHF, pulmonary Htn, Eisenmenger's syndrome	Exercise tolerance, dyspnea, cyanosis	CV exam	ECG ECHO CXR
RESP	Reactive pulmonary vascular bed	Tachypnea	Auscultation	O$_2$ sat

Key Reference: van Son JA, Hambsch J, Mohr FW: Anatomical reconstruction of aorta and pulmonary trunk in patients with an aortopulmonary window. Ann Thorac Surg 2000; 70:674–675.

PERIOPERATIVE IMPLICATIONS

Anesthetic Technique

- General anesthesia with narcotic-based technique usual
- Avoid extubation in neonatal patient or those with reactive pulmonary vascular bed

Monitoring

- Arterial line
- Two peripheral IVs
- Right and left atrial lines placed by surgeon at conclusion of CPB

Airway

- No associated airway anomalies

Induction

- If IV access available can use opioids, ketamine, or etomidate
- If patient without IV access, halothane or sevoflurane mask induction acceptable
- Use principles applied to VSDs, PDAs, other L → R shunting lesions

SURGICAL STAGES

Dissection

- Under CPB through midline sternotomy

Definitive Surgery

- Involves placement of pericardial or Dacron patch
- Performed under moderately hypothermic conditions

- Deep hypothermic circulatory arrest used in certain situations
- Modifications of reconstruction may occur in patients with associated coronary anomalies
- Consider use of aprotinin

Postoperative Considerations

- Significant postop pain
- Use of duramorph in caudal space to control pain with associated postop monitoring for respiratory compromise may be helpful
- Pain score: 6–8
- Reactive pulmonary vascular bed with associated pulmonary Htn; often seen with tube suctioning
- Postop blood loss 2° to CPB
- Packed RBC, platelets, cryoprecipitate, and/or FFP replacement as indicated

APPENDECTOMY

Joseph Rosa III, M.D.

RISK

- Consider in any patient with abd pain
- Rare in infants, more common in childhood; max incidence in teens, 20s; thereafter declines; 1 in 7 sometime in their lifetime (15% of USA population)
- M:F 3:2
- Etiology: 60%, hyperplasia of submucosal lymphoid follicles; 35%, fecal stasis (fecalith); 4%, other foreign bodies; 1%, tumors

PERIOPERATIVE RISKS

- Mortality: overall, < 1/100,000; in acute but not gangrenous, < 0.1%; gangrenous, 0.6%; perforated, 5%
- Morbidity: pelvic, intra-abd, subphrenic abscess with perforation, ~20%; wound abscess, < 5%; fecal fistula, < 1%; wound hematoma, < 0.5%; ileus, variable
- Greater morbidity and mortality in children, 2° to absence of fully developed omentum, subsequent spread of infection, with development of peritonitis after perforation

WORRY ABOUT

- Intravascular vol status 2° to poor oral intake, ± vomiting, 3rd spacing with peritonitis
- Aspiration: ileus, full stomach
- Electrolyte abnormalities
- Perioperative sepsis
- If laparoscopic, usual concerns with pneumoperitoneum, CO_2 insufflation
- Differential Dx: consider more catastrophic etiologies of abd pain, incl rupturing aneurysm, intestinal ischemia, acute pancreatitis
- Postop infection, sepsis

OVERVIEW

- Obstruction of appendiceal opening
- Perioperative infection a concern with perforated appendix, peritonitis
- ↑ Morbidity, mortality with perforation
- Fewer normal appendixes removed since US, laparoscopy used for Dx

ICD-9-CM Code: 540

INDICATIONS AND USUAL TREATMENT

- Suspected appendicitis
- Differential Dx in young children: acute gastroenteritis, mesenteric lymphadenitis, pyelitis, Meckel's diverticulitis, intussusception, pneumonia
- Differential Dx in teenagers and adults depends on gender: in F, ruptured ectopic pregnancy, mittelschmerz, endometriosis, salpingitis, regional enteritis; in M, regional enteritis, renal calculi, testicular torsion, acute epididymitis
- Differential Dx in older adults: diverticulitis, perforated ulcer, acute cholecystitis, pancreatitis, intestinal obstruction, perforating cecal cancer, torsion of ovarian cyst, mesenteric vascular occlusion, rupturing abd aortic aneurysm
- Differential Dx made easier with ultrasound or spinal CT

ASSESSMENT POINTS

SYSTEM	EFFECT	ASSESSMENT BY HX	PE	TEST
CV	Age-related considerations; dehydration 2° to fever, emesis; ↓ PO intake	CV status, Hx of angina, SOB, exercise tolerance	CV exam	ECG if indicated, orthostatics to assess vol
RESP	Resp impaired 2° to abd pain/splinting in elderly; tachypnea, hyperpnea may suggest perforation/sepsis; full-stomach considerations		Chest exam	CXR if indicated
HEME	Leukocytosis, with left shift hemoconcentration; 4% of patients have normal WBC, differential			CBC with differential
RENAL/CNS	Mental status changes associated with dehydration; electrolyte abnormalities, early sepsis; ↓ UO 2° to ↓ IV vol	UO, mental status	CNS exam	UA

Key Reference: Sabiston DC, Jr: Textbook of Surgery: The Biological Basis of Modern Surgical Practice, 15th ed. Philadelphia, WB Saunders, 1997, pp 964–970.

PERIOPERATIVE MANAGEMENT

Preoperative Preparation

- Restore IV vol/temperature management

Anesthetic Technique

- General ET with rapid-sequence intubation with Sellick's maneuver or awake if difficult airway
- Regional: spinal vs. epidural if no absolute contraindications; patient adequately hydrated, cooperative; high abdominal exploration unlikely

Monitoring

- Routine

Airway

- Usual considerations apply

Induction

- Consider IV volume status when choosing induction agents
- Consider possibility of myopathy in children if choosing succinylcholine

Maintenance

- Usually volatile agent ± N_2O, narcotic, relaxant

SURGICAL STAGES

- Skin incision: McBurney's incision (RLQ)
- Dissection: extent depends on appendix location, degree of inflammation; 3rd space volume a consideration
  - Retrocecal position, 65%
  - 30% tip in pelvis

- Closure: perforated ± skin closure if abscess present, surgeon may place drain; minimal if laparoscopic
- EBL: < 75 ml
- Vol requirements: replace deficit and 5–8 ml/kg/h with normal saline or lactated Ringer's solution
- Some done laparoscopically

Postoperative Considerations

- Pain score: 5–7; PCA for postop pain

ANTICIPATED PROBLEMS/CONCERNS

Complications

- Sepsis, paralytic ileus, atelectasis
- Aspiration risk
- Prolongation of NMB drugs 2° to interaction with antibiotics, esp aminoglycosides

ATRIAL SEPTAL DEFECT, REPAIR OF

Susan B. McDonald, M.D.
Charles W. Hogue, Jr., M.D.

RISK

- Ostium secundum occurs in 7% and 40% of all congenital heart disease in children and adults, respectively
- Female:male ratio 2:1, except for ostium primum ASD, for which ratio is 1:1
- ASD is most common congenital heart defect

PERIOPERATIVE RISKS

- Risk dependent on age, degree of reversibility of ↑ PVR; mortality usually < 1%
- Supraventricular arrhythmias including atrial flutter, AFIB
- AV conduction block possible if ASD close to AV node

WORRY ABOUT

- Paradoxical venous embolism
- Right heart volume overload with RV dysfunction
- MVP, regurgitation with ostium secundum

- Partial anomalous pulmonary venous drainage with sinus venosus
- Cleft anterior mitral valve leaflet with ostium primum defect
- Endocarditis prophylaxis
- L → R shunt leading to pulmonary hypertension and Eisenmenger's syndrome; concern greater with large defects (> 1 cm diameter)

OVERVIEW

- Classified by location: *ostium secundum* (70% of ASDs) involves midseptal fossa ovalis; *sinus venosus,* high in RA, close to RA/SVC junction; *ostium primum,* in inferior septum, is an endocardial cushion defect
- Unless heart murmur heard, usually not diagnosed until symptomatic in 3rd–4th decade of life
- Degree of L → R shunting dependent on size of ASD, relative compliance of ventricles, relative SVR, PVR

- MVP in 10–30% of patients; may be 2° to shift of interventricular septum from RV volume overload; usually reversed with closure of ASD
- RV diastolic dimensions ↑, interventricular septum shifted; normal resting but ↓ LVEF with exercise possible

ICD-9-CM Code: 745.5

INDICATIONS AND USUAL TREATMENT

- Surgical closure for uncomplicated ASD with pulmonary-to-systemic flow ratio > 1.5
- Optimal age of repair may be < 5 y
- PVR at rest > 8 U/m^2 that fails to ↓ to < 7 U/m^2 with pulmonary vasodilators usually contraindication to surgery
- Lung Tx considered with correction of ASD or heart and lung Tx for irreversibly ↑ PVR
- Transcatheter closure possible in some centers

ASSESSMENT POINTS

SYSTEM	EFFECT	ASSESSMENT BY HX	PE	TEST
CV	Pulmonary Htn, RHF	SOB, DOE, fatigue	↑ RV impulse, JVD	ECG (R axis deviation in ostium secundum vs. L axis deviation in ostium primum)
			Fixed split S$_2$, hepatomegaly, ascites, edema	ECHO (RAE, RVE; paradoxical septal motion; Qp:Qs calculation from R- and L-sided stroke volumes; color-flow Doppler; check for anomalous pulmonary veins and MVP/mitral valve regurgitation) Cardiac catheterization
RESP	Infection	Cough, sputum	Rhonchi, wheezing, consolidation	CXR, CBC, cultures
HEPATIC	Passive edema		Hepatomegaly, jaundice, ascites	Liver enzymes, albumin, PT, PTT

Key Reference: Skorton DJ, Garson A: Congenital heart diseases in adolescents and adults. Cardiol Clin 1993; 11:717–720.

PERIOPERATIVE IMPLICATIONS

Anesthetic Technique
- General

Monitoring
- CVP
- Arterial line
- Consider TEE with color-flow Doppler, LAP

Induction/Maintenance
- Anesthetic technique guided by preferences, age, condition; extubation early after surgery in most patients
- Maintain HR, preload, contractility
- Avoid large increases in PVR or large decreases in SVR to minimize R → L shunt

SURGICAL STAGES

- Median sternotomy, but anterior lateral thoracotomy, cosmetic submammary incision appropriate at times
- Cardioplegic arrest
- Direct suture closure if ASD small, pericardial patch closure otherwise. Dacron graft, Gore-Tex CV patch suitable substitutes for pericardial patch in some cases.
- Anomalous pulmonary venous drainage repaired with pericardial patch "baffle," redirecting pulmonary venous flow into LA
- Mitral valve repair for some patients with ostium primum

Postoperative Considerations

- LAP/PCWP may be high, 2° to MR, LV diastolic dysfunction from co-existing disease or shift of I-V septum
- RV dimension, hemodynamics improve shortly after surgery
- Supraventricular arrhythmias including AFIB/flutter
- Reoperation uncommon, but occasional dehiscence of atrial baffle
- Pulmonary and peripheral thromboembolism with AFIB (warfarin commonly started 2nd day after surg for 8–12 wk)
- Risk of heart block, especially in ostium primum repairs

AV GRAFT FOR HEMODIALYSIS

Irene E. Leonard, M.B., F.F.A.R.C.S.I.
Anthony J. Cunningham, M.D., F.R.C.P.C.

RISK

- End-stage renal disease with Cr clearance < 10 ml/min likely to require hemodialysis within 3 mo
- > 300,000 treated for ESRD in USA
- > 192,000 on hemodialysis in USA

PERIOPERATIVE RISKS

- Perioperative mortality low related to complications of ESRD (electrolyte-induced arrhythmias, cardiac decompensation)
- ESRD increases risk of CAD
- Fistula failure 10–15%
- Other surgical complications: thrombosis, infection, poor venous outflow, venous aneurysm, venous Htn, reduced arterial inflow, or steal

WORRY ABOUT

- Adequate preoperative Rx of Htn, CAD, DM

- Hypovolemia and hypokalemia (esp if recently dialyzed)
- Hypervolemia, hyperkalemia, acidosis (esp if not recently dialyzed)
- Possible marked Htn to surgical stimuli
- Adequate intravascular volume and BP to preserve patency of graft

OVERVIEW

- 66% with ESRD are dialysis-dependent
- Causes of ESRD: glomerulonephritis, diabetes, Htn, pyelonephritis, polycystic disease, collagen vascular diseases
- Associated conditions: CAD, PVD, diabetes, platelet dysfunction, neuropathy, electrolyte abnormalities
- Autonomic neuropathy, e.g., Stokes-Adams attacks grade III–IV

ICD-9-CM Code: 586 (Renal failure)

INDICATIONS AND USUAL TREATMENT

- ESRD: Cr clearance ≤ 5 ml/min or serum Cr > 1200 μmol/L
- Methods of dialysis: peritoneal dialysis (PD) vs. hemodialysis depends on patient's general condition and preference
- PD preferred in young children, elderly, difficult vascular access, patient's preference for independent self-care
- Contraindications to hemodialysis: psychosis/severe mental retardation, carcinomatosis, difficulty with CHF or hemodynamic instability, multiple nonrenal complications, e.g., blindness, diabetic neuropathy
- AV fistula fashioned 1–2 mo prior to expected start of hemodialysis to allow adequate maturation period

ASSESSMENT POINTS

SYSTEM	EFFECT	ASSESSMENT BY HX	PE	TEST
CV	CAD, CHF, LVH, arrhythmias	Exercise tolerance, Htn, palpitations	CV	ECG, CXR
RESP	Pulm edema, uremic pleuritis	SOB, orthopnea, PND	Resp	CXR
GU/ ENDO	↓ Concentrating ability, uremia, electrolyte/ acid-base abn Oliguria/anuria	Anorexia, N/V, diarrhea, diabetes, hiccoughs	Wt, hypotension, resp BP	Cr, BUN HCO$_3^-$ Glucose
HEME	Anemia Plt dysfunction	Fatigue, SOB, bruising	Pallor Bruising	Hgb Plts
CNS/ PNS	Encephalopathy Autonomic/peripheral neuropathy	↓ Mental acuity Postural hypotension Paresthesias	MS	
GI	↓ Gastric emptying GI bleeding	Regurgitation, N/V		

Key Reference: Marx AB, Landmann F, Harder FH: Surgery for vascular access (Review). Curr Probl Surg 1990; 27:1–48.

PERIOPERATIVE MANAGEMENT

Anesthetic Technique

- Monitored anesthesia care (MAC)/regional, or GA
- Regional—advantage: vasodilation (esp sparse venous network); contraindication: patient objection, anticipated technical difficulty
- GA—prolonged drug effects, electrolyte/ acid-base abn + potential drug interactions, exaggerated hypertensive responses

Monitoring

- Place IV, BP cuff, pulse oximeter on nonoperated arm
- Fluids: non-K^+-containing, careful fluid balance monitoring
- End-tidal CO_2, esp for MAC if sedative drugs given

Induction/Maintenance

- ↓ Protein binding: prolonged and ↑ effect of highly protein bound drugs
- Uremia: ↑ permeability of BBB
- Acidemia: ↑ nonionized, unbound drug, so active portion of drug also mostly nonionized
- Muscle relaxants
  - Avoid succinylcholine if K^+ ≥ 5.5
  - Delayed excretion + ↑ duration of action of pancuronium (atracurium/vecuronium—duration not significantly prolonged)
- Opioids
  - ↑ Magnitude and prolonged duration
  - Accumulation of morphine glucuronide → respiratory depression

- Accumulation of normeperidine (meperidine metabolite) may → seizure
  - Fentanyl useful
- Local anesthetics
  - ↑ Duration of action due to ↓ elimination
  - ↑ Susceptibility to myocardial toxicity with bupivacaine

Surgical Stages

- Location
  - Should be easily accessible
  - First fistula: as far peripheral as possible
  - Nondominant arm if possible (self-cannulation for home dialysis)
  - Forearm (most common first site): radial/ulnar/brachial art to brachial vein
  - Wrist: "snuff-box"—radial art to antebrachial cephalic vein
  - Upper arm: brachial art to basilic/axillary vein
- Blood flow
  - 200–300 ml/min immediately after anastomosis formed (up to 600–1200 ml/min after maturation); > 200 ml/min required to complete dialysis in 3–4 h
- Types of access
  - Fistulas, e.g., Brescia-Cimino (side-to-side), or art-side-to-vein-end
  - Prosthetic graft, e.g., polytetrafluoroethylene (Teflon)
- Procedure duration—variable, ~ 1–2 h
- Blood loss—depends on access and ease

Postoperative Considerations

- Operated arm
  - Elevated for several hours and avoid constrictive clothing to minimize surgical swelling
  - Avoid venipuncture/BP measurements
  - Important: monitoring of fistula for blood flow (palpate thrill, auscultate, Doppler)
  - Early surgical revision for fistula dysfunction
- Pain management
  - PO analgesia usually adequate

ANTICIPATED PROBLEMS/CONCERNS

- Maturation process: blood flow ↑ with time, with resultant venous wall thickening—prevents venous tears, infiltration during dialysis. Maturation period variable—longer for smaller vessels.
- Avoid fistula use for initial 3 wk to prevent aneurysm formation
- Thrombosis most common complication with Brescia-Cimino fistula
- Graft fistulas: infection rate depends on site and material used

PROGNOSIS

- Fistulas have a finite life span—revisions and repeat procedures are common
- Renal transplantation is the optimal treatment for ESRD in suitable patients

BLALOCK-TAUSSIG (BT) SHUNT

Richard D. Alessi, Jr., M.D.

- For patients (usually neonates or infants) with severely ↓ pulmonary blood flow due to congenital heart disease, including infants with tetralogy of Fallot, pulm atresia, pulmonary stenosis, tricuspid atresia, some cases of TGV

PERIOPERATIVE RISKS

- 30-day mortality: 5.5% for all cases, probably closer to 2% for tetralogy of Fallot
- Other complications include Horner's syndrome, chylothorax, phrenic nerve damage, acute arm ischemia when subclavian arterial flow is diverted

WORRY ABOUT

- Maintain saturation prerepair by continued prostaglandin E_1 or physiologic ↑ pulmonary blood flow, avoiding hypoxemia, hypercarbia, hypotension, acidosis
- Possible severe hypoxemia while PA clamped
  - See Postoperative Period

OVERVIEW

- One of multiple types of systemic pulm shunts to ↑ pulmonary blood flow
- Familiarity with underlying anatomy and physiology is essential to management, including ductal patency, VSD, ASD
- Subclavian (opposite side of arch to limit kinking) to PA anastomosis performed directly (classic), or using Gore-Tex tube graft (modified)

- Goal: adequate but not excessive pulmonary blood flow
- Followed by mechanical or pharmacologic closure of ductus, if still open
- Nonconfluence of pulmonary arteries or distal pulmonary artery stenosis may require bypass, more extensive surgery

ICD-9-CM Code: 745.2 (Tetralogy of Fallot)

INDICATIONS AND USUAL TREATMENT

- Palliatively for cyanotic congenital heart defects not surgically correctable or in infants as part of a staged procedure to allow development of pulmonary vasculature or heart: including tetralogy of Fallot, pulm atresia, pulm stenosis, tricuspid atresia, some cases of TGV

ASSESSMENT POINTS

SYSTEM	EFFECT	PE	TEST
HEENT	↑ Incidence of craniofacial defects	Airway	
CV	Congestive heart disease		ECHO or angio
RESP	↓ Pulmonary blood flow	Cyanosis	O_2 sat ABGs

Key Reference: Smith VC, Caggiano AV, Knauf DG, Alexander JA: The Blalock-Taussig shunt in the newborn infant. J Thorac Cardiovasc Surg 1991; 102:602−605.

PERIOPERATIVE MANAGEMENT

Preoperative Preparation

- Patients often already intubated due to cyanosis, acute or chronic
- Maintain ↓ PVR to max pulmonary blood flow (hyperventilate, high FIO_2)
- Arterial line usually should be placed to monitor contralateral upper extremity, femoral, umbilical pressures

Intraoperative Period

- May use inhalation induction but effect may be delayed with ↓ pulmonary blood flow (despite faster rise in Fa/Fi)
- Lateral thoracotomy classic, but CPB possible, median sternotomy may be used

- Heparin sometimes used (1 mg/kg)
- Anticipate worsened hypoxia with PA clamping
- Transfusion not usually required

Postoperative Period

- Goal is adequate but not excessive pulmonary blood flow; shunt should be slightly restrictive to avoid CHF; check, compare pressure in subclavian or aortic artery with PA (should be almost equal), or flows compared with ECHO Doppler (usually aim for 3:1 Qp:Qs ratios)
- Cyanosis or clotting possible if shunt too small or systemic vessel kinks
- CHF or pulmonary edema possible (may be unilateral) if pulmonary blood flow is too great

- Shunt flow usually restricted by shunt orifice, therefore adequate pulmonary blood flow, oxygenation require normal pressure (i.e., avoid hypotension)
- EBL: 50−100 ml
- Pain score: 8−10

PROGNOSIS

- Ultimate prognosis depends on underlying congenital defects
- Recent advances, techniques in surgery allow many patients to undergo primary (complete) repair, avoiding BT shunts

BLOOD COMPONENTS

Linda Stehling, M.D.

RISK

- Estimated utilization in USA: 22 million
- RBC: 12; plt: 7; FFP: 2; Cryo: 1 (million)

PERIOPERATIVE RISKS

- Overtransfusion
- Undertransfusion

WORRY ABOUT

- Transfusion-transmitted disease (e.g., HIV, hepatitis)
- Hemolytic reaction due to RBC incompatibility
- Nonhemolytic reactions (fever, urticaria)
- Immunosuppression (infection, cancer recurrence)

OVERVIEW

- RBC: To increase oxygen-carrying capacity in chronic anemia and acute blood loss
- Plt: To prevent or treat bleeding due to thrombocytopenia or impaired platelet function
- FFP: To prevent or treat bleeding due to coagulation factor depletion; urgent reversal of warfarin if insufficient time for vit K therapy
- Cryo: For bleeding due to hypofibrinogenemia or dysfibrinogenemia; also used in treating some patients with von Willebrand's disease and hemophilia if virus-inactivated or recombinant Factor VIII, IX not available; used in preparing fibrin glue

DOSE

- RBC: 3 ml/kg ↑hematocrit 3% (Hgb 1 g/d)
- Plt: 1 concentrate/10 kg [1 apheresis unit = ±6 concentrates]
- FFP: 10–15 ml/kg
- Cryo: 1 unit/7–10 kg

ASSESSMENT POINTS

COMPONENT	EFFECT	ASSESSMENT BY HX	PE	TEST
RBC	Oxygen delivery	Anemia; blood loss; cardiopulmonary reserve, oxygen consumption	Pallor; blood loss	Hgb, Hct, O_2 extraction ratio
PLT	Coagulation	Petechiae, mucosal bleeding; disease, drugs affecting plt function; blood loss ≥ 1 blood volume	Microvascular bleeding	Plt count
FFP	Coagulation	Ecchymoses, bleeding; liver disease; warfarin therapy; blood loss ≥ 1 blood volume	Microvascular bleeding	PT, PTT
CRYO	Coagulation	von Willebrand's disease, hemophilia, congenital fibrinogen disorders; blood loss ≥ 1 blood volume	Microvascular bleeding	Fibrinogen

Key Reference: American Society of Anesthesiologists Task Force on Blood Component Therapy: Practice guidelines for blood component therapy. Anesthesiology 1996; 84:732–747.

PERIOPERATIVE IMPLICATIONS

Preoperative Preparation

- RBC: Hct/Hgb may be indicated
- Plt, FFP, Cryo: Labs not required in absence of Hx, PE suggestive of hemostatic abnormality

Induction/Maintenance

- RBC: Inability to ↑ cardiac output in response to lower O_2 delivery can cause myocardial ischemia
- Plt: Clinically significant thrombocytopenia (plt count < 50 × 10⁹/L) may occur with ≥ 1 blood volume replacement

- Use autologous (rather than allogeneic) blood whenever possible
- FFP: Bleeding may occur if PT, PTT > 1.5 × mean normal value and/or ≥ 1 blood volume replacement. 1 unit of plts on average increases plt count by 7 × 10⁹/L.
- Cryo: Bleeding may occur with fibrinogen < 100 mg/dl and with von Willebrand's disease unresponsive to DDAVP

Regional Anesthesia

- RBC: Hypotension may further impair O_2 delivery
- Plt, FFP, cryo: Epidural hematoma can occur in patients with coagulopathy

Postoperative Period

- Continued bleeding may necessitate additional component therapy

ANTICIPATED PROBLEMS/CONCERNS

- Indications for transfusion should be documented
- Fear of tranfusion-transmitted disease should not lead to withholding of necessary transfusion
- Use autologous (rather than allogeneic) blood whenever possible

BLOWOUT ORBITAL FRACTURE

Kathryn E. McGoldrick, M.D.

RISK

- Rare
- Patients subjected to blunt trauma with a nonpenetrating object (e.g., fist)
- Racial predominance: none

PERIOPERATIVE RISKS

- In absence of serious associated injuries, rare perioperative mortality (<0.1%)
- Postop risk of visual disturbances, including blindness, infection, and cosmetic deformity

WORRY ABOUT

- Intraocular damage (ruptured globe rare in isolated orbital blowout fracture owing to release of compressive forces into the maxillary sinus)

- Associated nonophthalmic injuries (intracranial injury, cervical spine fracture or subluxation, Le Fort fractures with basilar skull fracture)
- Prolapse and incarceration of orbital soft tissues
- Preop systemic steroids (to distinguish neuromuscular edema or related motility disturbance from true entrapment, unmask enophthalmos, and reduce discomfort) predispose to sinus-orbital infections
- Hemostasis for delicate surgery

OVERVIEW

- Fractures of orbital floor are repaired by various surgical approaches
- Intraoperative infiltration with lidocaine with 1:100,000 epinephrine for hemostatic effect

- Entrapped tissues freed with care taken to avoid infraorbital neurovascular tissue trauma
- Autologous or alloplastic implant material placed over fracture site

ICD-9-CM Code: 802.6

SURGICAL INDICATIONS/USUAL TREATMENT

- The three standard indications for surgical intervention are enophthalmos, motility disturbance secondary to entrapment, hypoophthalmos
- Timing of surgical intervention depends on associated injuries and patient's age, general health, and preference; preferable to delay in order to permit some resolution of edema and bleeding; technical ease and functional result typically enhanced by surgery in 5–14 days

ASSESSMENT POINTS (in addition to evaluation of co-existing disease)

SYSTEM	EFFECT	ASSESSMENT BY HX	PE	TEST
HEENT	Trauma may produce orbital subcutaneous emphysema, restriction of globe motility, globe ptosis, enophthalmos, retinal or choroidal injury		Inspection Palpation Funduscopic exam	CT scan
CNS	Trauma may produce head injuries	CNS Hx	CNS exam	CT scan
MS	Trauma may produce assorted MS and organ injuries	Pain	Palpation	Plain films as indicated

Key Reference: Mead MD: Evaluation and initial management of patients with ocular and adnexal trauma. *In* Albert DM, Jakobiec FA (eds): Principles and Practice of Ophthalmology. Philadelphia, WB Saunders, 1994, pp 3362–3382.

PERIOPERATIVE IMPLICATIONS

Preoperative Preparation
- None

Anesthetic Technique
- GA usual; also local

Monitoring
- Routine

Airway
- Other facial injuries may complicate airway management

Induction/Maintenance
- Without associated injuries, few hemodynamic perturbations
- Avoid Htn (to minimize bleeding)
- Adequate depth of anesthesia to prevent patient movement during delicate surgery
- Consider antiemetic prophylaxis

SURGICAL STAGES

Dissection
- Minimal blood loss

Definitive Surgery
- Minimal blood loss (<100 ml) and fluid shifts
- Approximate duration: 2 h

Postoperative Considerations
- Mild postop pain
- IV PCA usually not necessary
- Without other injuries, discharge on day of surgery

ANTICIPATED PROBLEMS/CONCERNS

- Blindness
- Infraorbital paresthesia
- Implant extrusion
- Diplopia and delayed extraocular muscle restriction
- Obstructive sinus disease
- Infection
- Return to potentially violent environment

BONE MARROW TRANSPLANTATION (HARVEST PROCEDURE)

Charles D. Boucek, M.D.

RISK

- Autologous: patients with malignancies that respond to chemotherapy (9740 cases 1989–1993, North American Autologous Bone Marrow Transplant Registry)
- Allogeneic: HLA-matched healthy donors for (usually related) recipient with malignancy or marrow failure (16,905 cases worldwide 1964–1993, International Bone Marrow Transplant Registry)

PERIOPERATIVE RISKS

- Postop morbidity high 2° to underlying malignant disease (autologous donor)
- Life-threatening complications extremely rare (0.27%) for allogeneic (healthy) donor

WORRY ABOUT

- Volume status/blood loss
- Position-related injuries (prone)
- Anesthetic drug interactions with prior chemotherapy ↓ adrenal reserve
- Puncture of intrathoracic structures if sternal harvest necessary

OVERVIEW

- Multiple needle aspirations of marrow from post iliac crest (occasionally other sites) made to obtain stem cells for reinfusion following marrow ablative chemotherapy for malignancy
- Operating physician usually hematologist (not surgeon)

ICD-9-CM Code: V59.3 (Bone marrow donor)

See also Chemotherapeutic Agents and individual chemotherapeutic agents (e.g., Bleomycin Sulfate, Alkylating Agents) in Drugs section

INDICATIONS AND USUAL TREATMENT

- Marrow failure, hematologic malignancy, selected chemotherapy-responsive solid tumors
- Recipient anticipates prolonged hospitalization in major medical center, aggressive support for anemia, thrombocytopenia, neutropenia, GVHD
- Autologous transplantation may follow first or subsequent remission for hematologic malignancy or be performed prior to chemotherapy for solid tumor of sites remote from bone marrow stores
- Usually performed as outpatient procedure without general anesthesia for healthy allogeneic donors

ASSESSMENT POINTS

(applies primarily to autologous donors)

SYSTEM	EFFECT	ASSESSMENT BY HX	PE	TEST
CV	CHF, dysrhythmias	Doxorubicin, pericardial effusions	CV exam	ECG, consider ECHO/MUGA
GI	Electrolyte imbalance	Vomiting, melena	Edema, orthostasis	Na^+, K^+, Ca^{2+}
HEME	Blood loss, infection	Recent chemotherapy	Petechiae, ecchymosis	CBC, platelets

Key Reference: Armitage JO: Bone marrow transplantation. N Engl J Med 1994; 330:827–838.

INTRAOPERATIVE MANAGEMENT

Monitoring

- Large-bore IV (×2)
- Consider CVP, if access difficult
- Check availability of irradiated blood
- Urinary cath may be necessary (large fluid shifts)
- Arterial access may result in hematoma (thrombocytopenia); useful if BP is labile
- Pulse oximetry may guide O_2 requirements: acutely reduced end-tidal CO_2 may indicate embolism from marrow space

Induction

- ↓ Dose of induction agent if there is Hx of cardiotoxic chemotherapy

SURGICAL STAGES

- Establishment of adequate venous access
- Induction of general anesthesia (spinal/epidural possible for homologous donors)
- Establish prone position
- Supine to prone position change requires minimum of 4 persons
- Wt supported on chest/pelvis with arms extended on armboards
- Avoid pressure on eyes, throat, genitals
- Abd position for free excursion
- Aspiration of marrow
- Cell count of marrow determines volume needed ($1–4 \times 10^8$ cells/kg recipient body wt frequently > 1000 ml)
- Return to supine position
- Approximate duration 2–4 h
- Postop pain score 1–4; usually PO drugs (acetaminophen with codeine) adequate

ANTICIPATED PROBLEMS/CONCERNS

- Familiarity with patient's specific chemotherapy protocols
- Volume replacement with irradiated RBCs, crystalloid, albumin
- Avoid starch (interferes with processing of marrow)
- Avoid nonirradiated RBCs (potential engraftment of random donor nucleated cells)
- Prior steroid Rx may result in ↓ adrenal reserve
- Avoid unnecessary O_2 enrichment if prior chemotherapy included bleomycin
- Air/O_2 may be used (N_2O inhibits methionine synthetase resulting in marrow toxicity)

BOWEL RESECTION

Kevin Stierer, M.D.

RISK

• Incidence: colon cancer: 30/100,000; Crohn's: 1–6/100,000
• Gender predominance: male:female 1.3:1 for colon cancer

PERIOPERATIVE RISKS

• Perioperative mortality of 0.5–5% due mainly to underlying disorder
• Perioperative morbidity: prolonged ileus: 5–10% with small-bowel resection; small-bowel obstruction: 5–10% with large-bowel resection; anastomotic leak: 2–4%; wound dehiscence: 1–2%; bleeding: 1%; splenic injury: 1%

WORRY ABOUT

• Preop bowel preparation leading to hypovolemia, hypokalemia
• ↑ Risk for pulmonary aspiration
• Bowel obstruction, especially small bowel, at risk for bowel necrosis, perforation, septic shock

OVERVIEW

• Removal of bowel: performed for a variety of malignant, nonmalignant processes
• Small-bowel resection involves varying amounts of mesentery; may include regional lymph nodes if malignancy suspected with primary anastomosis
• Large-bowel resection involves mobilization prior to resection
  – Ureter possibly transected during mobilization of pelvic colon

– Primary anastomosis via creation of colostomy depends on number of factors (local ischemia, inflammation, unprepped bowel)

ICD-9-CM Codes: 153.9 (Neoplasm, large intestine); 555.9 (Crohn's disease)

INDICATIONS AND USUAL TREATMENT

• Small-bowel resection: intestinal obstruction, volvulus, intussusception, Crohn's disease, small-bowel tumors, trauma
• Large-bowel resection: colon cancer, diverticulosis, Crohn's disease, ulcerative colitis, lower GI bleed, trauma
• Usual medical Rx varies. Depends on underlying cause (see Diseases section).

ASSESSMENT POINTS

SYSTEM	EFFECT	ASSESSMENT BY HX	PE	TEST
CV	Hypovolemia	Lightheadedness	Orthostatic VS, capillary refill	BUN/Cr, ABGs (acidosis)
RESP	Aspiration risk Hypoventilation or hypoxemia 2° to intra-abdominal process	N/V Splinting (due to pain)	Abdominal exam Observation, auscultation	SpO$_2$, ABGs
RENAL	Electrolyte abnormality			ECG, serum electrolytes

Key Reference: Grief R, Akca O, Horn EP, Kurz A, Sessler DI.: Supplemental perioperative oxygen to reduce the incidence of surgical-wound infection. Outcomes Research Group. N Engl J Med 2000; 342:161–167.

PERIOPERATIVE MANAGEMENT

Preoperative Preparation

• Volume replacement before induction due to bowel preparation and/or third space fluid loss with intra-abdominal process
• Consider H$_2$ antagonist for aspiration prophylaxis
• Metoclopramide contraindicated if bowel obstruction/perforation suspected

Anesthetic Technique

• General anesthesia may combine technique with epidural for postop analgesia

Monitoring

• Routine
• Consider Foley catheter if of long duration

Airway

• High incidence of gastric aspiration
• Consider secure airway with rapid-sequence or awake technique

Induction

• Hemodynamic instability 2° to hypovolemia

SURGICAL STAGES

Dissection

• Hypotension after peritoneum opened, especially if intra-abd bleeding tamponaded
• Hypotension, ↑airway pressure may be encountered during surgical manipulation of secretory small-bowel tumors
• Hypotension during manipulation of strangulated or perforated small bowel

Definitive Surgery

• Anticipate large third space fluid loss, depending on degree of bowel exposure, amount resected (10–15 ml/kg/h of crystalloid)
• Additional fluid requirements if suction enterostomy of obstructed bowel performed
• Monitor for ureteral injury during pelvic dissection

• EBL usually <500 ml but may ↑ significantly for reoperation or inflammatory bowel disease
• Maintain normothermia

Postoperative Considerations

• Significant postop pain: pain score 5–8
• Epidural analgesia or IV PCA
• Pulmonary dysfunction 2° to splinting with inadequate analgesia
• Paralytic ileus usually related to amount of bowel manipulation, not narcotic analgesia

ANTICIPATED PROBLEMS/CONCERNS

• Preop hypovolemia with hemodynamic instability unless proper volume resuscitation instituted before induction

BRAIN CORTEX RESECTION (FOR EPILEPSY)   Patricia H. Petrozza, M.D.

RISK

- 39,000 patients in USA with drug-resistant epilepsy
- 3000 ablative operations/y
- Racial predilection: none

PERIOPERATIVE RISKS

- Depends on procedure—potential unintentional interruption of neural pathways
- Combined morbidity, mortality rates <5% for epileptogenic focus resection, <11% for corpus callosotomy, <17% for functional hemispherectomy
- Blood loss diathesis (functional hemispherectomy)
- Risk of craniotomy includes hypercoagulable state (PE, thromboembolism), intracerebral hemorrhage, air emboli

WORRY ABOUT

- Intraop seizures
- Aspiration

- Tailoring anesthetic technique for appropriate intraoperative testing, responsiveness
- Favorable cranial conditions
- N/V
- Blood loss diathesis
- Awareness

OVERVIEW

- Used for intractable seizures
- Requires discussion with surgeons and neurologists; concerns about intraop electrocorticography (ECoG), patient responsiveness
- Concerns about seizures, possible status epilepticus
- Concerns about craniotomy, including blood loss, adequate operating conditions, postop responsiveness
- Patient may have co-morbid conditions—e.g., psychiatric disorders, tuberous sclerosis, neurofibromatosis

- Patients on anticonvulsants often require larger doses of narcotics, muscle relaxants than expected
- Hepatic enzyme induction and drug interactions are common

ICD-9-CM Code: 345.91

INDICATIONS AND USUAL TREATMENT

- Patients recommended for cortical resection for epilepsy have met these criteria:
  - Have focal seizure not responding to adequate trial of antiepileptic agents
  - Seizures significantly interfere with patient's overall function
  - Surgery appears to offer reasonable opportunity for improvement of overall function
- Medical Rx is first-line Rx with max Rx with 1 drug before multiple-drug Rx, then surgery

ASSESSMENT POINTS

SYSTEM	EFFECT	ASSESSMENT BY HX	PE	TEST
HEENT	Gum hypertrophy related to phenytoin		Airway exam	
GI/HEPATIC	Hepatitis	Rx with mephenytoin, valproic acid, trimethadione	Hepatomegaly, jaundice	LFTs, bilirubin, SGOT, SGPT
HEME	Blood dyscrasias related to antiepileptic drugs	Weakness, fatigue, Rx with carbamazepine, ethosuximide, mephenytoin, phenytoin, trimethadione, lamotrigine	Petechiae, rash	CBC
RENAL	Nephritis	Trimethadione therapy		BUN, Cr
NEURO	Lethargy, depression, etc., related to anticonvulsants		MS exam	

Key Reference: Kofke WA, Tempelhoff R, Dasheiff RM: Anesthetic implications of epilepsy, status epilepticus, and epilepsy surgery. J Neurosurg Anesthesiol 1997; 9:349–372.

PERIOPERATIVE MANAGEMENT

Intraoperative Electrocorticography/Conscious Analgesia

- Discussion by surgeon, anesthesiologist about specific patient's suitability
- Patients position themselves as comfortably as possible; O_2 delivered by nasal prongs
- Avoid benzodiazepines if intraop ECoG is planned

Monitoring

- Capnography by nasal prongs
- Urinary cath
- 1 large-bore IV line

Airway

- Careful inspection mandatory: difficult intubation anticipated in lateral position with preexisting airway abn
- Rigid head pin fixation may be used

Induction

- If intraop ECoG, general anesthesia chosen, induction can be with ultra–short-acting barbiturate—e.g., thiopental, maintenance with N_2O, narcotic technique supplemented with low-dose isoflurane 0.25%. Avoid N_2O if craniotomy for electrode placement within previous 2 wk.

  - NMB used
  - Anesthesia maintenance with fentanyl infusion often satisfactory for intraop ECoG recording
  - Discontinue propofol/inhalation agents 20 min prior to ECoG
- Fentanyl, NMB agent requirements may be ↑
- During closure of craniotomy, care must be taken to avoid Htn, movement by patient
- For craniotomy, conscious analgesia under local anesthesia, 2 generally accepted techniques: (1) fentanyl 0.5–1.0 μg/kg/min, droperidol 0.15 mg/kg with additional fentanyl boluses 25–100 μg IV or (2) propofol, initial bolus 1 mg/kg IV followed by infusion at 25–100 μg/kg/min
- Infusions discontinued 20 min before patient needs to be responsive to ECoG recordings
- Local infiltration of scalp by surgeons (careful attention to local anesthesia overdose)

SURGICAL STAGES

- Scalp incision: should be comfortable with adequate local anesthesia
- Removal of bone flap: patient may be bothered by drilling (should be warned)
- Stripping of dura: may cause N/V
- Meningeal vessel manipulation: may cause pain
- Blood loss: while usually not large, replaced to avoid hypovolemia
- N/V: can be controlled with metoclopramide 5–10 mg or droperidol 1.5–2.5 mg
- Patient at risk for seizures
  - May require therapy with IV methohexital 0.5–1.0 mg/kg if ECoG anticipated; following ECoG, benzodiazepines acceptable

Postoperative Considerations

- Fluctuating blood levels of anticonvulsants
- Monitoring for seizure activity
- Control of hemodynamics, possibility of recurrent seizures
- Pain score ~5–10; careful narcotic titration

ANTICIPATED PROBLEMS/CONCERNS

- Difficulties with seizure control
- Possible brain swelling or intracranial hematoma related to resection
- Patient anxiety related to lengthy operation time
- Intraoperative N/V

BRONCHOSCOPY, FIBEROPTIC

Andranik Ovassapian, M.D.

RISK

- Technique for evaluation of tracheobronchial tree
- Has virtually replaced rigid bronchoscopy
- First performed 1966 by Ikeda
- Available in a range of sizes applicable to pediatric and adult populations
- Better tolerated than rigid bronchoscopy

PERIOPERATIVE RISKS

- Depends on nature of disease for which bronchoscopy performed
- ↑ Risk in patients with cardiac disease, severe hypoxemia, and bleeding diathesis

WORRY ABOUT

- Coughing, breath holding, hypoxemia
- ↑ Airway resistance when performed through endotracheal or tracheostomy tube
- Postbronchoscopy airway irritation, coughing, airway obstruction, hypoxemia if not treated with O_2

OVERVIEW

- Fiberoptic bronchoscopy enables endoscopist to go deeper into bronchial tree for evaluation of lesions not commonly accessible to rigid bronchoscopy
- Fiberoptic bronchoscopy associated with repeated coughing, Htn, tachycardia often due to inadequate topical or general anesthesia
- Hypoxemia common when performed without supplemental O_2 Rx
- Blood loss from biopsy site of lower airway lesions can be troublesome
- Tracheal and sometimes bronchial intubation, separation of lungs possibly necessary for major hemoptysis

ICD-9-CM Code: 162.9 (Lung cancer)

INDICATIONS AND USUAL TREATMENT

- Evaluation of upper, lower airway problems, Dx of pulm disease
- Most useful for diagnosis and staging of lung cancer
- Has diagnostic, therapeutic, and problem-solving indications
- Rx of acute atelectasis performed by saline lavage, aspiration of thick secretions
- Transbronchoscopic bronchial biopsy, brushing cytology, transbronchial needle aspiration biopsy, bronchoalveolar lavage performed
- Absolute contraindications include acutely unstable CV system, current life-threatening cardiac arrhythmias, severe hypoxemia

ASSESSMENT POINTS

SYSTEM	EFFECT	ASSESSMENT BY HX	PE	TEST
HEENT	Upper airway obstruction due to tumor, edema Limitation of movement	Degree of compromise Airflow pattern Snoring Stridor	Mandibular subluxation Size of tongue Head and neck anatomy Mouth opening Neck ROM	Lateral x-ray CT scan Barium swallow Flow-volume loop
CV	Ischemic CAD potential	CAD Hx: chest pain CHF Sx	Heart rate and rhythm, S_3, rales	ECG with stress
GI	Aspiration potential	GE junction integrity by Hx of regurgitation Nighttime cough Sour nighttime taste	Evaluate nutritional status	Esophagoscopy Examination of larynx
CNS	Sleep dysfunction due to obstruction	Sleep history	CNS exam	MRI
RESP	Upper airway obstruction due to tumor	Tumor Hx	Wheezing Cyanosis Clubbing	Flow-volume loop, ABGs

Key Reference: Ovassapian A: Fiberoptic assisted airway management. Acta Anaesthesiol Scand Suppl 1997; 110:46–47.

PERIOPERATIVE MANAGEMENT

Preoperative Preparation

- Dependent on indication:
  – If laryngeal tumors, evaluate for degree of airway compromise
  – If stridor present, closely observe, preferably in ICU. Humidified O_2 and steroids may be given to avoid severe/complete airway obstruction.
- Patient lies supine with head and neck in sniffing position when laryngoscopy performed for tracheal intubation. When performed by otolaryngologist for Dx and therapy, head and neck hyperextended.

Monitoring

- Routine

Anesthetic Technique

- Done with great caution and with spontaneous ventilation if Sx of compromised upper airway
- Secure airway with patient awake under topical anesthesia if resp failure due to airway obstruction
- Short-acting IV drugs (e.g., alfentanil, midazolam, esmolol) may provide analgesia and attenuate CV response to rigid laryngoscopy
- Surgical blood loss negligible

Postoperative Concerns

- CV hyperactivity
- Status of upper airway

ANTICIPATED PROBLEMS/CONCERNS

- Difficult mask ventilation and difficult intubation in immediate postop period common

BRONCHOSCOPY, RIGID
Andranik Ovassapian, M.D.

RISK

- First performed by Killian in 1895. Its use has declined continuously after introduction of fiberoptic bronchoscope.
- Performed for removal of foreign body, massive hemoptysis, to dilate tracheobronchial strictures, laser bronchoscopy, and stent placement

PERIOPERATIVE RISKS

- Depends on nature of disease
- Cardiac arrhythmias, hypoxemia, increased blood pressure and heart rate, myocardial infarction
- Incidence of reintubation reported at 0.39% when panendoscopy performed for upper airway path

WORRY ABOUT

- Ventilation, oxygenation in patients with chronic pulm disease, airway pathology
- Endoscopist, anesthesiologist share airway, complicating ventilatory management
- Massive hemorrhage

OVERVIEW

- Associated with severe CV response manifested with tachycardia, Htn
- Bleeding from biopsy site could be troublesome
- Level of the lesion critical
- Ventilation performed through side arm
- Requires communication with surgeon throughout procedure

ICD-9-CM Code: 146.9 (Oropharyngeal cancer)

INDICATIONS AND USUAL TREATMENT

- Removal of foreign bodies
- Management of major hemoptysis
- Dilation of tracheobronchial stricture
- Laser surg
- Bronchoscopy in infants, small children
- Bronchoscopy, esophagoscopy, laryngoscopy for staging of oropharyngolaryngeal malignant lesions
- Biopsy of endobronchial lesion
- Establishing emergency airway
- Placement of stent

ASSESSMENT POINTS

SYSTEM	EFFECT	ASSESSMENT BY HX	PE	TEST
HEENT	Airway compromise	Wheezing, stridor	Lung, airway exam	CXR
CV		Exercise intolerance, angina, Hx of CV disease	S_3, rales	ECG Stress test
RESP		Wheezing, exercise tolerance impairment, Hx of smoking	Clubbing, cyanosis, wheezing	PFTs ABGs CXR
AIRWAY	Tumors Infections Compressions	Shortness of breath Hemoptysis	Wheezing Use of accessory muscles	X-ray studies PFTs ABGs

Key Reference: Prakash UBS: Bronchoscopy. New York, Raven Press, 1994, pp 53−89.

PERIOPERATIVE MANAGEMENT

- Usually done as outpatient with patient in sitting or supine position
- Antisialagogue (glycopyrrolate 0.2 mg IV or 0.4 mg IM) to minimize secretions, enhance topical anesthesia of airway
- Appropriate size bronchoscope, ancillary equipment should be available

Monitoring

- Routine

Anesthetic Technique

- Usually done under sedation, topical anesthesia
- Lidocaine 4% spray of oropharynx followed by translaryngeal injection of 3 ml 4% lidocaine provides excellent topical anesthesia

- Spray-as-you-go technique used to anesthetize rest of bronchial tree
- Laryngeal mask airway can provide passageway for fiberoptic bronchoscopy
- Short-acting IV drugs used during fiberoptic bronchoscopy
- Jet ventilation can be applied through fiberscope but not commonly practiced

Postoperative Concerns

- Hypoxemia treated with supplemental O_2 Rx
- Irritable airway, coughing, tachycardia, Htn common during early recovery
- Bleeding from biopsy site

ANTICIPATED PROBLEMS/CONCERNS

- Inadequate ventilation, hypoxemia when sedation heavy
- Airway obstruction, hypoxemia, barotrauma of lungs possible
- Consider precautions to minimize fire hazards during laser surgery

BURR HOLE

Jonathan D. Halevy, M.D.

RISK

- 470,000 people/y sustain traumatic brain injury in USA
- 15% die before reaching a medical facility
- 10% have severe brain injury
- Average age: 30 y
- M:F ratio 2:1

PERIOPERATIVE RISKS

- Mortality 25–30%
- Clinical good outcome in only 60%

WORRY ABOUT

- Complex injury presentation
- Establishment of airway may be complicated by associated cervical spine injury (~10%)
- Hemorrhagic shock related to other injury

- Air embolism, esp if burr hole over/near major sinus
- Intracranial pressure

OVERVIEW

- Types of head injuries include:
  - Skull fractures
  - Intracranial lesions (56% diffuse vs. 42% focal injury)—e.g., *subdural hematoma* (in 24% of closed head injuries, CT shows high-density crescent-shaped lesion); *epidural hematoma* (in 6% of closed head injuries, often temporal [91% with skull fractures], CT shows biconvex hyperdense lesion); *intracranial hematoma* (in 3% of closed head injuries, often frontal or temporal lobes, poss delayed Dx on CT scan); *diffuse brain injury* (no focal mass lesion, 60% with diffuse axonal injury if duration of unconsciousness >6 h)

- Anesthetic techniques: local with monitored anesthesia care with or without IV sedation according to patient's LOC
- On Glasgow Coma Scale, >12 is rough guide for tolerating some sedation; otherwise GA

ICD-9-CM Codes: 851–854

INDICATIONS AND USUAL TREATMENT

- For evacuation and/or drainage of subdural/epidural/intracranial hematoma
- May be Dx as well as Rx: brain biopsy
  - ICP monitoring: implantation of ventricular catheter/reservoir or EEG electrodes
  - Stereotactic surgery
  - Brain cyst/abscess

ASSESSMENT POINTS

SYSTEM	EFFECT	ASSESSMENT BY HX	PE	TEST
HEENT	Cervical spine injury in 10%; full stomach in most cases; ↑ blood alcohol levels in 50%	Based on cause of injury; usually patient not good source of info	Airway exam; assume unstable, not cooperative	C-spine series
CV	Autonomic dysfunction, blunt chest trauma concerns		Auscultation VS	CXR
RESP	Resp distress issues, neurogenic pulm edema, blunt chest trauma concerns	Neuro dysfunction	Auscultation	ABGs, pulse oximetry, CXR
ENDO	Hyperkalemia, hyperglycemia, hyponatremia, diabetes insipidus			Na$^+$, K$^+$, glucose Serum, urine osmolality
HEME	May have large blood loss from many causes; watch for DIC			CBC, PT, FSP, plts
GU	ARF due to hypotension			BUN, Cr
CNS	Impaired LOC	Glasgow Coma Scale assessment	Neuro exam	CT, MRI
MS	Special positioning concerns in OR, look for long bone fractures			Radiologic evaluation

Key Reference: Gopinath SP, Robertson CS: Management of severe head injury. *In* Cottrel JE, Smith DS (eds): Anesthesia and Neurosurgery, 3rd ed. St. Louis, Mosby–Year Book, 1994, pp 661–684.

PERIOPERATIVE MANAGEMENT

Preoperative Preparation

- Look at CT/MRI scans (if available) to confirm side of lesion
- Consider need for preop steroids, anticonvulsants, antiemetics, H$_2$ antagonists, and/or antibiotics

Anesthetic Technique

- Local anesthesia with monitored anesthesia care or GA

Monitoring

- Consider large-bore IV access, art line, central line
- Consider ICP monitoring, Foley catheter (esp if osmotic diuretics to be used)
- Nasal end-tidal CO_2 monitoring with anesthesia care technique
- Blood glucose levels (keep <250 mg/dl; >50 mg/dl)

Airway

- Patient often already intubated
- Assume C-spine injury if post trauma (motor vehicle accident)
- Secure ET tube well

Induction/Maintenance

- Consider ↑ ICP issues
- Neuro prep/drape time possibly lengthy; watch for low BP during minimal stimulation period

SURGICAL STAGES

Dissection

- Definite risk for complications during drilling—e.g., plunging into, through dura
- If hit major sinus, watch for air embolism

Definitive Surgery

- Hemodynamic changes if brainstem herniation
- May need intraop ICP monitoring early instead of late (CPP >90 mmHg; higher Glasgow Coma Scale score → better neuro outcome)
- Observe surgical site for excessive brain swelling (impending disaster)

Closure/Postoperative Considerations

- Goal to have patient as awake as possible
- May require intubation postop to assess CNS status (esp if starting from poor LOC)
- Postop pain difficult to assess due to MS problems
- Neuro exam of paramount importance to assist in management in neuro ICU
- Use vasoactive medications to control BP/HR at end of procedure
- Pain Rx: codeine and/or narcotic; PCA not appropriate due to CNS derangement
- EBL: 50–100 ml (may be more)

ANTICIPATED PROBLEMS/CONCERNS

- Outcome depends on severity of injury, presence of focal lesion, duration of unconsciousness, ICP course
- Goal to avoid secondary neuronal insults (48% of comatose patients postop)
- Expect impaired autoregulation of cerebral vasculature
- Assess realistic postop LOC in view of preop condition
- Intensive management of hemodynamic/metabolic/neuro/other issues required in neuro ICU

BYPASS, FEMORAL-FEMORAL

Alexandru Gottlieb, M.D.

RISK

• ~ 8000/y performed in USA. ↓ With ↑ number of aortic and iliac stents.

PERIOPERATIVE RISKS

• Related to diffuse arteriosclerosis, CV disease
• Perioperative MI as high as 10%
• Mostly geriatric patients with age-related risk factors and accompanying diseases: DM, COPD, Htn, renovascular
• Potential for improvement and/or more distal occlusion with risk of need for amputation

WORRY ABOUT

• Thrombosis and embolism of leg or graft
• Blood loss
• The groin is considered a "dirty" location, rendering prosthetic graft infection relatively common

OVERVIEW

• Femoral-femoral bypass is suggested for patients too risky to undergo abdominal procedure (ABI, ABF)
• Done with prosthetic graft. This is a nonanatomic graft that might be "fed" by a nonoptimal vessel.
• Regional anesthesia can be beneficial in its effect on coagulation and graft patency
• Procedure sometimes can be performed also under monitored anesthesia care

ICD-9-CM Code: 440.2x (Atherosclerosis, peripheral)

INDICATIONS AND USUAL TREATMENT

• An extra-anatomic procedure
• Performed in patients with lower extremity ischemia, gangrene, or severe short-distance claudication; in one limb more than the other
• Replace the standard anatomic bypass of ABI or ABF in patients with the following conditions:
  – S/P abdominal procedure
  – S/P extensive abdominal radiation
  – Intestinal stoma
  – Abdominal infection
  – Poor medical condition
  – S/P iliac–aortic stent graft
  – Ischemic limb from thoracic dissection

ASSESSMENT POINTS

SYSTEM	EFFECT	ASSESSMENT BY HX	PE	TEST
RESP	High incidence of lung disease that could have caused this procedure to be selected	Smoking, chronic cough, dyspnea	Chest exam, wheezing, clubbing cyanosis	CXR, ABGs, spirometry
CV	High incidence of CAD, myocardial ischemia, and/or infarction	Angina, MI, CHF, dysrhythmia, PTCA, CABG, exercise tolerance, activity level	Chest auscultation, VS	ECG, stress test— dipyridamole, thallium dobutamine Cardiac cath
	Chronic Htn	BP Rx, drug interaction, LVH	BP	ECG, CXR, retinal funduscopy
RENAL	Renal insufficiency 2° to age, arteriosclerosis, and multiple dye studies	Hx edema and intolerance to salt load	Edema, anuria	Urea, Cr lytes
CNS	Possible carotid disease	Syncope, stroke, or TIAs	Neuro exam Carotid bruit	Carotid angiogram, CT, MRI
ENDO	DM	Infections, stress/gestational DM, polydipsia, polyuria, coma/ stupor, abnormal glucose	Skin infections	CNS exam, urine output; glucose
HEME	Perioperative heparin, t-PA, or aspirin	Petechiae, nasal bleed	Petechiae or bruising	PT, PTT, ACT

Key Reference: Ellis JE, Roizen MF, Mantha S, Tzeng G, Desai T: Anesthesia for vascular surgery. *In* Barash PG, Cullen BF, Stoelting RK (eds): Clinical Anesthesia. Philadelphia, Lippincott Williams & Wilkins, 2000, pp 929–968.

PERIOPERATIVE MANAGEMENT

Perioperative Evaluation

• A detailed H & P, drug Hx, evaluation of cardiovascular status
• Dysrhythmias, CAD, CHF
• Hypertensive and valvular heart disease
• Noninvasive and invasive cardiac evaluation tests such as cardiac cath

Anesthetic Techniques

• General anesthesia, regional anesthesia, or MAC. Regional anesthesia preferred by some clinicians because of lack of systemic effect on the respiratory, CV, and GI systems. There is some positive effect of regional anesthesia on coagulation, preserving fibrinolysis and graft patency.

Monitoring

• ECG, arterial BP, urine output
• Consider CVP or PA line in patients with severe CAD or severely ↓ EF
• Monitoring for myocardial ischemia; ECG with continuous 3-lead ST-segment analysis, PA catheter, or TEE
• Monitoring of vol replacement: CO, CVP, PAOP or with TEE

SURGICAL STAGES

• Groin area should be thoroughly prepped and draped; procedure can be lengthy, 2–4 h. Minimal third space or blood loss.
• Avoid ↓ in BP—femoral-femoral bypass can thrombose easily with lack of flow

Postoperative Period

• Mild postop pain: 5–7
• Ischemic leg pain should improve
• Epidural extended for postop pain control

ANTICIPATED PROBLEMS/CONCERNS

• High incidence of periop cardiac and respiratory complications
• Inappropriate blood flow from donor side tends to make the bypass not functional
• Infection of prosthetic graft at the groin is relatively frequent, compared to other prosthetic graft locations
• If the femoral-femoral bypass is not functional, a bypass such as axillary femoral-femoral or amputation may be needed

BYPASS GRAFT PROCEDURE, INFRAINGUINAL

Rose Christopherson, M.D., Ph.D.

RISK

- Operations/y: 300,000
- Risk factors for atherosclerotic vascular disease include smoking, Htn, diabetes
- Demography: no known racial predominance; slightly more prevalent among males than females

PERIOPERATIVE RISKS

- Death: 0–5%
- Major cardiac morbidity, including MI, unstable angina, ischemic pulm edema, significant dysrhythmias: 6–33%

WORRY ABOUT

- Perioperative cardiac morbidity
- Concomitant diseases, including COPD, diabetes, Htn, vascular disease

OVERVIEW

- ↓ Graft failure associated with regional and/or regional-supplemented GA, or with optimization of cardiac performance using PA cath
- Work-up, monitoring, Rx appropriate for patients at high risk for CAD

ICD-9-CM Code: 440.2 (Atherosclerosis)

INDICATIONS AND USUAL TREATMENT

- Severe claudication, ischemic pain at rest, nonhealing foot or leg ulcers if due to poor circulation
- At some institutions, laser endarterectomy performed as alternative to infrainguinal bypass grafting
- Graft materials including native vein, Gore-Tex, other artificial grafts; vein considered superior except for femoral-femoral bypass grafting; vein may be used either in situ or reversed

ASSESSMENT POINTS

SYSTEM	EFFECT	ASSESSMENT BY HX	PE	TEST
CV	Associated CAD	MI, CHF, angina, palpitations	CV	ECG ECHO Holter, dipyridamole thallium imaging, or dobutamine ECHO, if indicated
RESP	COPD 2° to smoking	Dyspnea, wheezing	Chest auscultation	PFT if indicated CXR
ENDO	Diabetes	Hx of diabetes		Glucose
RENAL	Renal insufficiency	Renal failure		Cr, BUN
CNS	Cerebrovascular disease	TIA, CVA	CNS	Carotid Doppler (if indicated)

Key Reference: Bode RH Jr, Lewis KP, Zarich SW, Pierce ET, Roberts M, Kowalchuk GJ, Satwicz PR, Gibbons GW, Hunter JA, Espanola CC: Cardiac outcome after peripheral vascular surgery: comparison of general and regional anesthesia. Anesthesiology 1996; 84:3–13.

PERIOPERATIVE MANAGEMENT

Anesthetic Technique
- Performed under spinal, epidural, general, or combined techniques; evidence supports neuraxis blockade for improved surgical outcome, but not for ↓ cardiac morbidity

Monitoring
- Routine
- ST-segment analysis (computerized if possible)
- Intra-arterial cath in most cases
- CVP or PA cath, depends on CV work-up

Induction/Maintenance
- GA: depends on cardiac, other medical status
- Regional: block at T8–T10 adequate, but good sacral blockade necessary. If pure regional, motor blockade necessary.
- Maintain normothermia

SURGICAL STAGES

- Vein harvest: if previous CABG, vein sometimes from dorsum of leg; patient may be turned prone, then supine for arterial surgery
- Heparin usually given (~ 70 U/kg) before clamping femoral artery
- Crossclamp
- Blood loss usually controlled by pressure on or clamping of femoral artery
- Patency of graft tested intraoperatively with Doppler and/or angio
- EBL: ~ 500 ml, but highly variable
- Third spacing minimal
- Hypovolemia may be conducive to clotting of graft

Postoperative Considerations

- Not extremely painful: pain score 3–6
- Routinely admitted to PACU, step-down ICU, or intermediate care unit for 18–24 h for pulse, cardiac monitoring, especially if diabetic with autonomic neuropathy (see Diabetes, Type I [Insulin Dependent] in Diseases section)
- Body temp <35°C immediately after surgery associated with ↑ cardiac morbidity

ANTICIPATED PROBLEMS/CONCERNS

- Continuing epidural may ↓ early graft occlusion
- Perioperative MI, ischemia, CHF common

CARCINOID, EXCISION OF

Randy H. Steadman, M.D.

RISK

- Incidence: 1.5 cases/100,000/y; 1/300 appendectomies; 1/2500 proctoscopic exams
- Race/gender predominance: none
- Age with highest incidence: 5th or 6th decade; range: 10 y–ninth decade
- Indications for operation: ability to identify; primary should be treated with resection regardless of metastases; local complications—e.g., obstruction, intussusception—frequent

PERIOPERATIVE RISKS

- CV collapse due to release of vasoactive peptides
- Severe bronchospasm
- 1.5–10% perioperative mortality reported before use of somatostatin analogue

WORRY ABOUT

- Crisis consisting of flushing and hemodynamic changes, usually hypotension, but rarely Htn
- Severe bronchospasm
- Stimulation or sympathomimetics precipitating crisis

- Midgut (ileal, jejunal) carcinoids associated with fibrosis of mesentery (can result in shortgut syndrome if too extensive resection)
- Tricuspid, pulmonic valve regurgitation, stenosis, right heart failure

OVERVIEW

- Slow-growing malignancies capable of metastases, derived from APUD cells of embryonic neuroectoderm originating in GI tract 85% (most commonly, appendix; next, rectum, ileum); 10% from lung
- Release vasoactive peptides; in 10% these peptides access systemic circulation due to hepatic metastases (or primary tumor when drainage not portal); carcinoid syndrome can develop
- The peptides include serotonin, bradykinin, histamine, others; common Sx include facial flushing (94%), watery diarrhea (78%), asthma (19%); right heart involvement can also result in tricuspid insufficiency, pulmonic valve stenosis or insufficiency requiring valve replacement. Dx made as incidental finding during appendectomy, upper GI endoscopy, proctoscopic exam.
- Even without carcinoid syndrome, serotonin metab 5-HIAA may be elevated in 50% of patients with GI carcinoid tumors

- Prognosis related more to location, size of primary than to pathologic findings
- Patients with noninvasive appendiceal, rectal tumors < 2 cm have 5-y survival rates near 100%; if tumor is > 2 cm, survival declines to 40%; with liver metastases, 5-y survival 21–42%

ICD-9-CM Codes: 199.1 (Tumor); 259.2 (Syndrome)

INDICATIONS AND USUAL TREATMENT

- Surgery only potentially curative Rx
- With distant metastases, cure by resection of all tumor
- When resection not possible, palliative procedures may be needed for obstruction or to debulk tumor, ↓ quantity of vasoactive peptides released, or replace heart valves
- Medical Rx for symptomatic relief from flushing, diarrhea with advanced disease
- Octreotide (Sandostatin), a somatostatin analogue, inhibits synthesis, release, binding of vasoactive peptides; can control Sx, retard tumor growth, and prolong survival by as much as 3 years

ASSESSMENT POINTS

SYSTEM	EFFECT	ASSESSMENT BY HX	PE	TEST
CV	Carcinoid crisis, right heart valve involvement	Hx carcinoid syndrome, fatigue, ascites, edema	Hemodynamic collapse; JVD, murmur	ABGs ECHO
RESP	Bronchospasm	SOB	Wheezing	O$_2$ sat
GI	Diarrhea	Abd pain, wt loss	Flushing	Electrolytes, 5-HIAA
ENDO	10% MEN (hyperplasia of parathyroid, pancreas, pituitary) associated with carcinoid	Ulcers, renal calculi	Lipomas	Glucose Ca^{2+}, PO$_4$$^{2-}$, prolactin, gastrin
CNS	Postop sedation			
NUTRITION	Pellagra due to niacin deficiency if large amt serotonin produced	Diarrhea	Dermatitis, dementia	None Rx niacin

Key Reference: Vaughan DJA, Brunner MD: Anesthesia for patients with carcinoid syndrome. Int Anesthesiol Clin 1997; 35:129–142.

OPERATIVE MANAGEMENT

Preoperative Preparation

- Adequate sedation to avoid sympathetic stimulation resulting in carcinoid crisis
- Pretreatment for minimum of 24 h with subcutaneous octreotide

Monitoring

- Arterial catheter
- Consider CVP cath for vol monitoring (substitute PA cath or TEE if valvular lesions)

Airway

- Gastric emptying may be delayed
- Occasional laryngeal tumors

Anesthesia Technique

- Attempt to avoid histamine-releasing drugs (thiopental, succinylcholine, atracurium, cisatracurium, morphine) although they have been used without incident
- Adrenergic agonists—e.g., epinephrine, norepinephrine—stimulate release of vasoactive substances

- Etomidate or propofol appropriate for induction, maintenance with volatile agent (isoflurane), narcotic (fentanyl)
- Succinylcholine may, by causing fasciculations of abd wall, cause mechanical compression of tumor with release of vasoactive peptides
- Epidural techniques controversial since hypotension may lead to sympathetic stimulation, precipitating a carcinoid crisis, which may be difficult to treat without use of sympathomimetics

SURGICAL STAGES

Skin Incision

- Site varies according to location
- Sympathetic and/or mechanical stimulation with skin preparation has caused crisis

Dissection

- May be extensive if small-bowel fibrosis has occurred
- Manipulation of tumor may release vasoactive substances

Definitive Surgery

- En bloc resection of ileal carcinoids justified due to freq presence of multiple tumors

Closure and Postoperative Considerations

- About 1/3 of patients with advanced (hepatic) disease require blood transfusions intraoperatively
- Postop PCA usual
- Subcutaneous octreotide resumed with IV supplement for hypotensive episodes
- Pain score depends on location: abd 4–7

ANTICIPATED PROBLEMS/CONCERNS

- Carcinoid crisis can result in abrupt CV collapse or severe bronchospasm
- Sympathomimetics should not be used; IV octreotide (somatostatin analogue), miracle drug for aborting or prophylaxis of CV, bronchospastic effects
- Htn may be treated by IV ketanserin (a 5-HT antagonist)

CARDIOPULMONARY BYPASS

Marvin L. Appel, M.D., Ph.D.
Lori Heller, M.D.

RISK

- 800,000 open heart operations/y in North America

PERIOPERATIVE RISKS

- Heavily dependent on patient's underlying condition requiring bypass
- Stroke occurred in 0–13% in different studies
- Neuropsychiatric deficits common perioperatively, but 0–5% of patients have persistent deficits 6 mo postop (bubble membrane oxygenator)

WORRY ABOUT

- Underlying HD may make it difficult to maintain patient until CPB can start; may predispose to difficulty separating from bypass
- Condition of arterial cannulation site; aneurysmal, calcified, severely atheromatous areas may be unsuitable (evaluate with CXR, ECHO, catheterization)
- Dilutional anemia from 2 L fluid to prime pump; may obligate RBC transfusions in small patients

- Air embolism
- Clot formation in pump, with arterial embolization
- Awareness during bypass, especially during rewarming
- Protamine reaction (H_2-mediated hypotension, anaphylaxis, pulmonary Htn)
- Coagulopathy post bypass
- Spontaneous recooling of patient post bypass
- Repeat surgery concerns—chest wall adhesions make sternal incision more risky with potential for lacerating RV or previous graft. Check blood and have in room. Check retrosternal airspace on lateral CXR.

OVERVIEW

- CPB involves passively draining blood from venous system into pump, forcing it through oxygenator, back into patient's arterial circulation. Bypass machine assumes functions of heart and lung.
- Safety features include air detectors to prevent pumping air into arterial circ, continuous measurement of patient's mixed venous O_2 sat to detect inadequate tissue O_2 delivery, continuous monitoring of hydrostatic pressure within pump circuit to detect obstruction, prevent rupture of circuit
- Bypass associated with post bypass myocardial dysfunction, lung injury, hematologic derangements; usually reversible in perioperative period
- Significant 3rd space fluid shifts during bypass and for several days post bypass

ICD-9-CM Code: 414.0 (Atherosclerotic heart disease)

INDICATIONS AND USUAL TREATMENT

- CAB, valve surg, heart Tx, some lung Tx, removal of intracardiac tumors or those involving great vessels, rewarming from severe hypothermia, resection of some intracranial aneurysms
- Treatment of local anesthetic toxicity (bupivacaine)

ASSESSMENT POINTS

SYSTEM	EFFECT	ASSESSMENT BY HX	PE	TEST
CV	Underlying cardiac disease dictates anesthetic management pre and post bypass, affects ability to separate from bypass	Angina, CHF, arrhythmias, etc.	Cardiac	ECG, ECHO, cath, CXR
ENDO	CPB elicits hormonal stress response; glucose control may worsen in diabetics	Diabetes		May choose to check glucose during CPB
HEME	Preop plt dysfunction (including ASA, other plt inhibitor use) or coagulopathy may obligate transfusion post-CPB	Bleeding problems, anticoagulation, aspirin use, recent cardiac cath	Skin: bruises, petechiae esp at cath site	PT, PTT, plt count, bleeding time
RENAL	Preop renal dysfunction predisposes to postop problems Preop diuretic use may require diuresis during CPB to maintain UO	Renal dysfunction, diuretic use		BUN, Cr, UA
CNS	Prior CVA ↑ risk of intraop CVA	CVA, TIA	Neuro exam	Carotid US

Key Reference: Kaplan JA (ed): Cardiac Anesthesia, 4th ed. Philadelphia, WB Saunders, 1999, pp 1061–1110.

INTRAOPERATIVE MANAGEMENT

- Arterial line mandatory: CPB flow is insufficiently pulsatile for BP cuff; maintain mean arterial BP from 40–80 mmHg using anesthesia, pressors, vasodilators as needed
- Periodically sample ABGs to treat acidosis, abnormal K^+, Ca^{2+} values
- Foley cath: keep UO at least 1 ml/kg/h using mannitol, diuretics, dopamine as needed
- If PA line present, pull back during CPB to prevent its drifting into wedge position
- Ventilation and/or pulse oximetry mandatory during partial bypass (i.e., when some of venous return is allowed to pass through lungs instead of all going to pump)
- Consider priming pump with FFP to correct pre-existing coagulopathy or RBCs for severe anemia
- Consider giving antifibrinolytics (e.g., ε-aminocaproic acid, aprotinin) for patient at high risk for bleeding complications (long pump runs, redo operations)

SURGICAL STAGES

- Sternal incision/spread
- Dissection
- Heparinization
- ECHO of proposed aortic cannulation site
- Arterial cannulation—site chosen should be free of atherosclerosis
- Venous cannulation
- Bypass
- Crossclamp, cardioplegia (if used)
- Circulatory arrest (if used)
- Rewarming
- ECHO of LV to ensure no bubbles
- Separation from bypass
- Reversal of anticoagulation (usually with protamine)

Anesthesia During Bypass

- Opiates, benzodiazepines, nondepolarizing muscle relaxant, potent inhalational agent (delivered into pump oxygenator with a standard vaporizer)
- Anticoagulation: heparin or LMW heparins common

Checklist Before Separation from Bypass

- Venous reservoir volume sufficient to fill heart (usually > 1 L)
- Acceptable lab values (Hgb > 7, K^+ > 4.0, Ca^{2+} > 1.0)
- SVR: 800–1600
- ECG with rate of 60–120, with sinus rhythm, pacing, or AFIB, and free of ischemia
- Myocardial contractility acceptable (inotropes and/or mechanical assistance as needed)
- Patient warm (rectal or bladder temp > 34°C, nasal temp > 36°C)

CARDIOVERSION

Ross H. Zoll, M.D., Ph.D.

RISK

- Usually performed electively for AFIB
- Incidence: 2% over 20 y
- Occasionally urgent or emergent; also routine with other diseases or surgery—e.g., acute MI or CV surgery

PERIOPERATIVE RISKS

- Greatest risk is embolization from stagnant blood in atria (2%)
- ↑ In presence of mitral valve disease
- Long duration of arrhythmia or left atrial size >4.5 cm indicates poor response to conversion—either failure to convert or rapid recurrence

WORRY ABOUT

- Coag status, poss presence of clot with duration of arrhythmia >24 h
- NPO status, presence of CHF or ischemia
- Poss arrhythmias—e.g., VFIB, asystole, or presence of permanent pacemaker wires (poss damaged by defibrillation)
- Poss of recall
- Digitalis toxicity may predispose to refractory VFIB; synchronized shock ↓ risk of shock during vulnerable phase of recovery of ventricles; ↓ risk of VFIB. In WPW, digoxin, Ca^{2+}-channel blocker contraindicated.

OVERVIEW

- Term *cardioversion* applied to synchronized shock for AFLT, AFIB, SVT, VTach
- Cardioversion of AFLT, VTach usually easy; requires small energy
- Cardioversion of AFIB, like VFIB, requires depolarizing significant no. of muscle fibers at once and large dose of electrical current. Reasonable therapeutic ratio exists, but actual delivered current (dose) unpredictable. Defibrillators store a set amount of energy, and most delivered to patient, but current delivered to the heart is relevant variable, depending on geometric factors, impedance that varies widely, etc.
- Underdosing ineffective
- Overdose may cause myocardial damage, dysfunction, persistent arrhythmia. Rx should begin at low energy (50 J) but may proceed to 400 J unless complications evident or current is known to be adequate by measurement.
- New rectilinear biphasic waveform cardioverts much more reliably with less energy and no variation in dose for different impedances
- To obtain a reasonably uniform current density in atria, AP paddle placement preferred

ICD-9-CM Code: 427.31 (AFIB)

INDICATIONS AND USUAL TREATMENT

- AFIB
- Many patients tolerate AFIB well and may need rate control with digoxin, β-blocker, or Ca^{2+}-channel blocker
- 5% yearly incidence of stroke; therefore anticoag indicated if tolerated; if atrium small, so that cardioversion likely successful, it is preferable
- Cardioversion with drugs such as quinidine or procainamide often attempted while anticoag being established
- Cardioversion indicated if rate control difficult (often exercise rate response not well controlled); hyperthyroidism, Htn, CHF, lyte disturbances, COPD all predispose to AFIB; Rx before cardioversion likely successful, NSR sustained
- Atrial contribution to contractility may be needed to prevent CHF

ASSESSMENT POINTS

SYSTEM	EFFECT	ASSESSMENT BY HX	PE	TEST
CV	Valve disease	SOB	Auscultation	ECG
	CHF	Palpitations	Edema	
		Chest pain		ECHO
HEME	Anticoag			PT, PTT
CNS	CVA	Duration of abn rhythm	Neuro	Cardiac ECHO
	TIA	Coag status		

Key Reference: Mittal S, Ayati S, Stein KM, et al: Transthoracic cardioversion of atrial fibrillation: comparison of rectilinear biphasic versus damped sine wave monophasic shocks. Circulation 2000; 101:1282–1287.

PERIOPERATIVE MANAGEMENT

Anesthetic Technique

- Usually brief; requires only IV induction agent titrated to LOC; propofol, benzodiazepines, thiopental, methohexital, etomidate, ketamine, etc., may be used
- If ET intubation indicated for preventing aspiration or because of difficult mask fit, succinylcholine may be added

- In CHF or ischemia, short-acting narcotic may be added; inhalation agents not useful (may predispose to arrhythmias; are longer acting)

Postoperative Considerations

- Pain: minimal

ANTICIPATED PROBLEMS/CONCERNS

- Recall can be a problem, esp in severely compromised patient or in emergency cardioversion when adequate anesthesia not well tolerated
- CNS function should be assessed on waking
- Ischemia or Htn may be induced by electrical stimulation
- Arrhythmias can be induced by shock or absence of atrial electrical activity
- Hypotension, ↓ CO poss from anesthetic drugs or effect of electrical shock on myocardium; atrial mechanical systole may not be effective immediately after a period of fibrillation

CAROTID ENDARTERECTOMY

John A. Youngberg, M.D.

RISK

- TIAs in ~ 0.5/1000 population
- 150,000 procedures in 1998; 91,000 in 1992; ↑ due to establishment as most beneficial Rx for TIAs, nonsymptomatic > 70% carotid atherosclerosis
- Asymptomatic bruit in ~ 4–5% of patients > 40 y
- Smoking, DM, Htn, male, high cholesterol, high triglycerides, obesity, family Hx, stress, plt function, alcohol use may be associated with ↑ risk

PERIOPERATIVE RISKS

- Periop mortality 0–2.6%
- Periop permanent neuro deficit 0–6.3%
- Risk of periop MI
- Risk of associated nerve injury

WORRY ABOUT

- Co-existing CAD
- CBF/oxygenation during carotid clamping/shunting
- Htn/hypotension postop
- Associated nerve injury
- Postop hematoma
- Postop CNS assessment
- Hyperperfusion syndrome

OVERVIEW

- Plaque removed from carotid artery
- Significant risk of embolization of plaque debris
- Significant risk of cerebral ischemia/hypoxia during surgery from both surgical and anesthetic techniques
- Significant percentage of patients have known, unknown CAD
- Periop mortality highest from cardiac event, followed by cerebrovascular event
- Regional anesthesia does not appear to lower cardiac or CNS event rate
- Regional anesthesia may be associated with shorter period of Htn postop, shorter ICU/hosp stay

ICD-9-CM Code: 443.1 (Arteriosclerosis of carotid artery)

INDICATIONS AND USUAL TREATMENT

- Patients who have experienced RIND, TIA, or stroke are candidates
- According to ACAS data, asymptomatic patients with stenosis > 60–70% are candidates if surgeon has low periop risk of morbidity/mortality (< 3%)
- Surgical removal of plaque in carotid artery by endarterectomy with or without vein patch graft
- Intravascular removal of plaque by mechanical device—e.g., Simpson's atherectomy cath
- Minimally invasive techniques such as balloon dilation or stent placement
- Stroke risk 1–2%/y in asymptomatic patient vs. 6–10% if patient has TIAs; stroke risk ↑ significantly in asymptomatic patient if stenosis > 75%
- Significant ↓ in stroke rate in "at risk" patients following surgery

ASSESSMENT POINTS

SYSTEM	EFFECT	ASSESSMENT BY HX	PE	TEST
CV	Patients often have known or unknown CAD Htn	Chest pain, MI, CHF, SOB, dyspnea, exercise tolerance	HR and BP, both arms; lying, standing murmur; S_3 or S_4 dysrhythmia	ECG, ECHO, stress test, Holter
RESP	Often smoker with COPD	SOB, cough, exercise tolerance	Auscultation	CXR
ENDO	Often co-existing DM	Ketoacidosis, diet/insulin control		Glucose
CNS	Reversible ischemic neurologic deficit, TIAs, stroke, asymptomatic bruit	RIND, TIA, stroke, ringing in ears, dizziness, changes in vision, weakness, slurred speech, paralysis	Bruit, evidence of weakness	CT EEG Angio

Key Reference: Larson CP, Youngberg JA: Cerebral vascular surgery. *In* Youngberg JA (ed): Cardiac Vascular and Thoracic Anesthesia. New York, Churchill Livingstone, 2000, pp 567–589.

INTRAOPERATIVE MANAGEMENT

Monitoring

- Art line in nondominant arm for ABGs, glucose, BP measurement
- ECG leads II, V_5
- Monitor CNS well-being:
  - Awake patient: mentation, speech quality, motor function
  - Asleep patient: raw or processed EEG, SSEP, near-infrared monitoring, transcranial Doppler, JV O_2; stump pressure usually not helpful
- Monitoring as indicated for patients with co-existing CAD
- TCD differentiates hemodynamic from embolic neurologic events, uninterpretable in 15–20% of cases

CNS Protection

- Avoid exogenous glucose unless indicated by serum hypoglycemia
- Maintain normocarbia
- Maintain patient's usual BP; in Htn patients, cerebral autoregulation curve has shifted to right
- Consider use of barbiturates, hypothermia, etc., to ↓ $CMRO_2$
- Shunts may increase flow or produce emboli or dissection. Flow in different types of shunts not the same.

Anesthetic Technique

- Regional: local, superficial with or without deep cervical plexus block, epidural, etc.
- Avoid oversedation of patient due to loss of cooperation and inability to assess CNS status
- General: few to no outcome data to recommend one technique over another; isoflurane can ↓ critical CBF from 20 ml/100 g/min to 8–10 ml/100 g/min, but may not be achievable in clinical setting
- Use of pure α-1 agents may result in wall motion abnormalities during moderately deep levels of inhaled anesthetics

SURGICAL STAGES

Induction

- CV instability due to possible co-existing CAD
- Blood loss usually not of major concern
- Crossclamping of carotid
  - Assess adequacy of cerebral perfusion in awake patient or by changes in monitors in asleep patient
    - Consider use of shunt
    - Consider use of barbiturates, etc., for CNS protection
    - Maintain patient's normal BP, CO_2 levels
- EBL: < 200 ml; keep vol replacement < 1 L to avoid postop Htn

Postoperative Considerations

- Htn
- Hypotension (from hyperactive carotid sinus)
- Hematoma formation (possible airway compromise)
- Associated cranial nerve injury (hypoglossal, recurrent, etc.)
- Phrenic nerve block in regional anesthesia in patient with COPD
- Hyperperfusion syndrome, esp in patients with high-grade stenosis
- CNS deficit (ischemia, emboli, intimal flap, thrombosis, etc.)
- Residual effects of regional anesthetic on carotid sinus or carotid sinus denervation may result in Htn

ANTICIPATED PROBLEMS/CONCERNS

- Htn/hypotension postop
- Ability to assess neuro deficit vs. residual anesthetic effects
- Myocardial ischemia in patients with co-existing CAD
- Associated nerve injury or residual from regional anesthesia
- Airway edema 2° to venous and lymphatic congestion

CARPAL TUNNEL RELEASE

Scott Mittman, M.D., Ph.D.

RISK

- 1.5% of adults in USA
- Racial predominance: white > African-Americans
- Gender predominance: female > male

PERIOPERATIVE RISKS

- Morbidity very rare
- Perioperative exacerbation of median neuropathy

WORRY ABOUT

- Flexion of the wrist during long procedures
- ↑ Risk of exacerbation with cannulation of neighboring radial artery

OVERVIEW

- A compression neuropathy of the median nerve at the wrist

ICD-9-CM Code: 354.0

ETIOLOGY

- Numerous factors → compression of median nerve in the carpal tunnel or ↑ susceptibility of nerve to compression:
  - ↓ In size of the carpal tunnel (e.g., bony abnormalities of the carpal bones, thickening of transverse carpal ligament)
  - ↑ Volume of contents of carpal tunnel (e.g., neuroma, lipoma, pregnancy, hemodialysis, myxedema)
  - ↑ Susceptibility (e.g., diabetes, alcohol abuse)
  - Position and use of the wrist (e.g., flexion of wrist during sleep, repetitive use injuries)

USUAL TREATMENT

- Treatment of any underlying medical condition
- Avoidance of exacerbating wrist positions or repetitive movements; splinting
- Steroid injections
- Release of the transverse carpal ligament

ASSESSMENT POINTS

SYSTEM	EFFECT	ASSESSMENT BY HX	PE	TEST
PNS	Median neuropathy	Sensory or motor symptoms in median nerve distribution	Sensory and motor function of median nerve distribution	Phalen's and Tinel's tests Nerve conduction velocities

Key Reference: Szabo RM, Madison M: Carpal tunnel syndrome. Orthop Clin North Am 1992; 23:103–109.

PERIOPERATIVE IMPLICATIONS

Anesthetic Technique

- Can be performed under axillary block, Bier block, MAC, or GA techniques

Monitoring

- Routine
- For non–carpal tunnel decompression surgery, consider sites other than the radial artery of an affected hand for arterial catheters

Positioning

- Avoid flexion of either wrist (bilateral disease is common)

Airway

- No special considerations

Induction

- No special considerations

SURGICAL STAGES

Postoperative Considerations

- EBL: minimal
- Minimal fluid shifts
- Pain score: 2–4
- Oral medications usually adequate

ANTICIPATED PROBLEMS/CONCERNS

- Exacerbation of median neuropathy

CATARACT ± IOL

Kathryn E. McGoldrick, M.D.

RISK

- > 1.5 million cataract operations/y in USA
- Gender predominance: none
- Advanced age
- Direct trauma
- Response to other intraocular conditions, including chronic uveitis, glaucoma, retinal detachment
- Systemic diseases (diabetes mellitus, myotonic dystrophy, galactosemia)
- Chronic use of topical or systemic corticosteroids
- Congenital (idiopathic, familial, associated with prenatal infection)

PERIOPERATIVE RISKS

- Perioperative mortality exceedingly rare
- Surgical morbidity: bleeding into anterior chamber; capsule rupture; posterior dislocation of lens into degenerative vitreous; loss of vitreous, producing retinal detachment and macular edema; expulsive hemorrhage

WORRY ABOUT

- Anesthetic morbidity following retrobulbar block
  - Retrobulbar hemorrhage (1–3%)
  - Perforation of globe (0.1% or less)
  - Central spread of local anesthesia that may affect brainstem (0.1%)
  - Intra-arterial injection with immediate seizures (< 0.1%)
  - Optic nerve injury (< 0.1%)

OVERVIEW

- Removal of cloudy lens with small incision(s), with aspiration or ultrasonic fragmentation
- Associated with extremely low mortality, although complications of retrobulbar block (e.g., brainstem anesthesia) can be life threatening
- Morbidity can include blindness in operated eye

- Topical anesthesia for selected patients (cooperative and able to control eye movements, not photophobic, appropriate-size pupil) avoids potentially serious complications of regional anesthesia. Topical anesthesia has become increasingly popular in recent years.

ICD-9-CM Code: 366.9

INDICATIONS AND USUAL TREATMENT

- Based on degree of visual impairment in relation to visual needs of the individual, as well as anticipated visual improvement and risk of serious complications
- With congenital cataracts, risk of amblyopia dictates that surgery be performed within the first few months of life

ASSESSMENT POINTS

SYSTEM	EFFECT	ASSESSMENT BY HX	PE	TEST
OCULAR	Determination of lens power of intraocular implant			Ultrasonic measurement of axial length of eye; optical measurement of corneal curvature
CARDIOPULM	Impaired ability to lie flat; chronic coughing	SOB, orthopnea	Inspection Auscultation	
CNS	Impaired ability to follow instructions and remain motionless because of age, anxiety, claustrophobia, deafness, tremors	CNS Hx	CNS exam	

Key Reference: Friedman DS, Bass EB, Lubomski LH, et al: Synthesis of the literature on the effectiveness of regional anesthesia for cataract surgery. Ophthalmology 2001; 108:519–529.

PERIOPERATIVE IMPLICATIONS

Preoperative Preparation

- None

Anesthetic Technique

- Can be performed under regional (peribulbar or retrobulbar), general, sub-Tenon's, or topical anesthesia

Monitoring

- Routine
- Invasive monitoring seldom indicated

Regional Techniques

- Eye in neutral gaze to minimize risk of optic nerve injury
- Small-gauge needle, no longer than 31 mm (1¼ inch) to ↓ risk of globe perforation
- Consider general or topical anesthesia if high risk (e.g., extreme myopia; severe enophthalmos; staphyloma; previous ocular complications of regional anesthesia; severe vascular disease; bleeding diathesis; one-eyed patient) for complications associated with retro- or peribulbar block
- Avoid deep orbital penetration
- Avoid heavy sedation

General Anesthesia

- Meticulously secure endotracheal tube to prevent intraoperative extubation
- Neuromuscular paralysis with appropriate monitoring to avoid coughing or bucking that can cause loss of intraocular contents
- Consider prophylactic antiemetic

SURGICAL STAGES

- Two basic techniques of cataract extraction—intracapsular and extracapsular
- Majority extracapsular because an intact posterior capsule may reduce posterior segment complications: retinal tear, retinal detachment, macular edema

Incision for Extracapsular Procedure

- With the pupil fully dilated, an anterior capsulotomy is performed

Definitive Surgery

- Central anterior capsule removed, with expression or irrigation of lens nucleus through wound. Alternatively, nucleus may be fragmented ultrasonically (phacoemulsification) behind iris plane to avoid corneal epithelial damage. Phacoemulsification is generally considered the preferred technique.

- Incision partially closed and every precaution taken to maintain normal anterior chamber depth (by air infusion, fluid infusion, or injection of viscoelastic solution) to prevent corneal endothelial damage during intraocular lens insertion
- Supporting loops of posterior chamber lens inserted into capsular bag or ciliary sulcus
- Minimal hemodynamic disturbance
- Approximate duration: 1 h or less

Postoperative Considerations

- EBL: negligible
- Minimal postop pain
- Patients instructed to avoid bending, lifting, straining

ANTICIPATED PROBLEMS/CONCERNS

- Ptosis
- Postop wound dehiscence
- Iris prolapse
- Infectious endophthalmitis
- Retinal tear or detachment
- Cystoid macular edema
- Delayed posterior capsule opacification

CEREBRAL ANEURYSM CLIPPING
Frederick E. Sieber, M.D.

RISK

- Prevalence: 2–5% of general population
- ~28,000 cases/y of subarachnoid hemorrhage, only 18,000 surviving to receive medical attention
- Gender predominance: M:F ratio, 3:2

PERIOPERATIVE RISKS

- Perioperative morbidity and mortality for unruptured intracranial aneurysms 12–17%; for bleeding intracranial aneurysms, mortality is ~20%
- Leading causes of death and disability are vasospasm and/or CNS effects of initial subarachnoid hemorrhage

WORRY ABOUT

- Intraoperative aneurysmal rupture
- CNS ischemic episodes

OVERVIEW

- Congenital aneurysmal dilation, usually at branch points of circle of Willis
- Surgical position and technique may vary according to location, configuration of aneurysm
- Most aneurysms are managed by placement of metal clip on aneurysm base
- Use of temporary clip may eliminate the need for intraoperative controlled hypotension during aneurysmal dissection

ICD-9-CM Codes: 437.3; 430 (A-V, ruptured)

INDICATIONS AND USUAL TREATMENT

- Unruptured aneurysms >5 mm in diameter in patients with life expectancies justifying expected surgical risks
- Ruptured cerebral aneurysms with Hunt-Hess grade 1, 2, or 3 subarachnoid hemorrhage
- Controversial whether clipping of aneurysms with grade 4 or higher subarachnoid hemorrhage should be performed because of poor CNS outcome
- Nimodipine may be used to reduce risk of vasospasm

ASSESSMENT POINTS

SYSTEM	EFFECT	ASSESSMENT BY HX	PE	TEST
CV	ECG changes	Rule out angina		Lytes ECG, ECHO, CK-MB (rarely required)
RESP	Pulm edema	Dyspnea SOB	Rales, rhonchi on auscultation	CXR Consider ABGs
CNS	Hydrocephalus ↑ ICP	↓ Consciousness	Neuro	CT scan

Key References: Dangor AA, Lam AM: Anesthesia for cerebral aneurysm surgery. Neurosurg Clin N Am 1998; 9:647–659.

PERIOPERATIVE IMPLICATIONS

Anesthetic Technique

- Performed under GA; deliberate hypotension may be required
- Mild hypothermia may be cerebroprotective

Monitoring

- Arterial line
- CVP to direct fluid management
- Consider EEG, SSEP

Airway

- Routine

Induction

- Aneurysm rupture rare, but can follow sudden BP ↑ during laryngoscopy

SURGICAL STAGES

Dissection

- BP control to prevent aneurysm rupture
- Brain relaxation to assist visualizing aneurysm may be accomplished by using diuretics, elevation of head, barbiturates, or hyperventilation
- Spinal fluid drainage possibly required to assist visualizing aneurysm

Definitive Surgery

- Temporary clip placement may require CNS monitoring, administration of cerebral metabolism depressants—i.e., barbiturates, etomidate, or propofol
- Aneurysmal rupture may require induced hypotension
- Confirmation of correct placement of aneurysm clip may require intraoperative angiography

Postoperative Considerations

- Significant risk of vasospasm requires Rx with Ca^{2+}-channel blockers and hypervolemic, hypertensive, hemodilutional Rx
- If aneurysm unclipped, significant risk of rebleed exists
- Rapid emergence from anesthesia desired to assess immediately CNS status
- EBL: 200–500 ml

ANTICIPATED PROBLEMS/CONCERNS

- Cerebral ischemia possible during temporary clip placement, with inadequate maintenance of CPP, or with incorrect clip placement

CEREBRAL AVM REPAIR

Armin Schubert, M.D.

RISK

- ~2000–3000/y
- More common in young and middle-aged adults
- Risk of bleeding 2–4%/y; higher after 1st bleed
- Mortality 1%/y; 10% after 1st bleed
- Racial predominance: none

PERIOPERATIVE RISKS

- Preop embolization ↓ bleeding, facilitates resection, and ↓ hyperemic complications
- 30-Day operative morbidity 20–40%; worse with higher clinical grade
- 30-Day mortality <5%
- Unique complication: normal perfusion pressure breakthrough (NPPB) syndrome; overall risk = 1–18%; at highest risk are high-flow lesions, border-zone AVM location, large AVMs (19–37% risk); lesions with severe hypoperfusion or steal around AVM; severe CNS deficit (may significantly improve over time)
- Postop CNS deficits may predispose to airway obstruction, aspiration

WORRY ABOUT

- Blood availability
- Effect of preop embolization: new neuro deficit; bleeding; pulmonary embolus
- Emergence: to allow early CNS assessment
- Massive brain swelling; cerebral hemorrhage
- High-dose barbiturate Rx to prevent edema, intracranial Htn
- Tight BP control on emergence, early postop

OVERVIEW

- Congenitally abnormal connections between arterial and venous cerebral circulation, without intervening capillaries; 80% are supratentorial
- Mass of thin-walled vessels with abnormal vasomotor response and chronically ischemic surrounding brain tissue
- Associated with cerebral aneurysms in 5-10%; in neonates and infants, shunt usually causes high-output heart failure. Excision can be associated with substantial blood loss.
- After extirpation of nidus, may get hyperemic brain swelling

ICD-9-CM Code: 747.81 (Cerebral AVM)

INDICATIONS AND USUAL TREATMENT

- Surg excision: small surface AVMs; large AVM if resectable with low risk of deficit; progressive Sx; refractory seizures; <40 y
- Alternate Rx: stereotactic radiosurgery or embolization for older population, location in eloquent area, symptom control. Embolization is palliative, not curative.

ASSESSMENT POINTS

SYSTEM	EFFECT	ASSESSMENT BY HX	PE	TEST
CV	Hyperdynamic CHF in small children, failure to thrive	Recurrent respiratory failure, prolonged ventilatory support Diaphoresis with feeding	Auscultation, hepatomegaly JVD, diaphoresis	CXR, ECHO
RESP	May aspirate during seizure, hemorrhage	Review with family; records from ER, ICU	Auscultation	CXR, pulmonary compliance, ABGs, oximetry
GU	Dehydration and/or mild renal insufficiency from multiple CNS imaging	Chart review		BUN, Cr
CNS	Seizures, chronic ischemia of brain surrounding AVM; hydrocephalus, intracranial Htn	LOC, headache, diplopia, nausea; family to describe Sx	MS CNS exam (esp hemiplegia, cranial nerves)	MRI, angio, clinical AVM grade: size, location, drainage (deep vs. superficial)

Key Reference: Black S, Sulek CA, Day A: Cerebral aneurysm and arteriovenous malformation. *In* Cucchiara RF, Black S, Michenfelder JD (eds): Clinical Neuroanesthesia, 2nd ed. New York, Churchill Livingstone, 1998, pp 265–318.

INTRAOPERATIVE MANAGEMENT

Preoperative Preparation

- Avoid premedication if mental status impaired or ICP high
- Determine risk of NPPB

Anesthetic Technique

- Requirements include brain relaxation, BP control, early emergence (or in patients at high risk for NPPB, high-dose barbiturates)
- Hyperventilation to $PaCO_2$ of 25–30 mmHg
- Avoid glucose-containing fluid

Monitoring

- Routine
- Direct arterial pressure routine; CVP for larger, deeper AVMs; PA catheter, ECHO for CV compromise
- Consider EPs
- Consider EEG for barbiturate effect
- ICP for emergence and postop

SURGICAL STAGES

Induction

- Avoid succinylcholine with hemiplegia, ↑ICP
- Maintain BP control; avoid coughing

Skeletal Fixation

- Avoid BP spike during fixation

Skin Incision

- Avoid Htn; may see effects of local anesthesia, epinephrine
- Consider beginning mannitol 0.5–2.0 g/kg

Dissection

- Arterial supply resected 1st; severe episodic bleeding, especially if dural sinuses involved
- After resection, test for bleeding by normalizing BP
- Consider barbiturate infusion to prevent NPPB

Definitive Surgery

- May develop brain swelling (NPPB) with occlusion of AVM
- Rx for NPPB: hyperventilation, diuretics, propofol, mild hypothermia, BP control

Closure/Postoperative Period

- EBL: 300–2000 ml; depends on AVM size, location; no need for 3rd space allowance
- Control BP, often to <130 systolic
- Assure normal coag status
- Pain score: 3–5
- Rx small doses of IV opioid, if CNS status OK

ANTICIPATED PROBLEMS/CONCERNS

- Intraoperative concerns: bleeding, brain volume control; CNS assessment at end of procedure
- Postoperative concerns: brain swelling (NPPB); bleeding into surgical site; hydrocephalus, seizure

CESAREAN SECTION, EMERGENT

Gertie F. Marx, M.D.

RISK

- Total USA C-sections: 1,000,000/y
- Emergent C-sections: 5–10%
- Racial predominance: none

PERIOPERATIVE RISKS

- Anesthesia-related mortality: 0.6/100,000 live births
- Most maternal deaths from anesthesia occur during emergent C-sections
- Most freq causes: failed intubation, pulm inhalation of gastric contents, drug misuse
- Nonanesthetic perioperative risks: amniotic fluid embolism, PE, preeclampsia-eclampsia

WORRY ABOUT

- Limited time for preanesthetic evaluation
- Airway and recent solid food intake
- Hypovolemia
- Coagulopathy

OVERVIEW

- Truly emergent C-sections—threatening life or essential functions of mother, fetus—are performed immediately, within minutes after recognition of complications
- Regional block safer for mother, less depressant for fetus than GA
- Incision-delivery interval:
  – Skin incision to delivery interval: with appropriate uterine displacement, admin of suppl O_2—no bearing on fetal outcome
  – Uterine incision to delivery interval: deterioration of 1-min Apgar score after 189 sec with regional anesthesia vs. 90 sec with GA

ICD-9-CM Code: 656.31 (Fetal distress resulting in delivery)

INDICATIONS AND USUAL TREATMENT

- Maternal: massive hemorrhage (placenta previa, abruptio placentae, trauma) associated with deteriorating maternal and/or fetal VS, uterine rupture, nonabating uterine tetany (cocaine overdose)
- Fetal: severe distress, prolapsed umbilical cord, associated (usually) with late decelerations (often prolonged), sometimes preceded by loss of beat-to-beat variability

ASSESSMENT POINTS

SYSTEM	EFFECT	ASSESSMENT BY HX	PE	TEST
HEENT	Engorged oropharynx		Airway exam	
CV	↓ MAP ↑ HR, ↑ CO		CV	ECG monitor
RESP	Compensated respiratory alkalosis ↑ Minute ventilation, ↑ FRC		Tachypnea	SaO_2
GI	Gastroesophageal reflux	Heartburn		
HEME	Dilutional anemia			Hgb, Hct

Key References: Marx GF, Luykx WM, Cohen S: Fetal-neonatal status following caesarean section for fetal distress. Br J Anaesth 1984; 56:1009–1013; van Zundert A: Emergency cesarean deliveries: how urgent are they? Acta Anaesthesiol Belg 1999; 50:227–228.

PREOPERATIVE PREPARATION

- Administer oral antacid (e.g., 10–30 ml cooled, pH-adjusted sodium citrate)
- Position mother with uterine displacement
- Maintain fetal HR monitoring until onset of surgery

Anesthetic Technique

- Hemorrhage: GA
- Uterine rupture: GA or extension of epidural block
- Uterine tetany: GA
- Fetal distress: spinal block, extension of epidural block, GA
- Prolapsed umbilical cord: GA or extension of epidural block

Monitoring

- Routine unless significant blood loss

Airway

- Consider full stomach, edematous oropharynx

Induction/Maintenance

- Spinal anesthesia: give IV preload of crystalloid solution rapidly but do not delay block because of as-yet insufficient amount of solution; continue IV infusion; use moderate-size needle—i.e., 22-gauge—to obtain CSF readily
  – Inject hyperbaric bupivacaine for average duration of surgery or hyperbaric lidocaine for duration of less than 1 h
  – Treat falling BP immediately with ↑ IV fluid, ↑ uterine displacement, ephedrine 5–10 mg doses: if no improvement, use phenylephrine 0.1–0.5 μg IV
- Epidural anesthesia: extend pre-existing block with 3% 2-chloroprocaine or 2% pH-adjusted lidocaine for fast action; can supplement with 10-mg doses of ketamine IV; for incomplete analgesia, have obstetrician perform local infiltration with 1% 2-chloroprocaine or 0.5% lidocaine
- GA: rapid-sequence IV induction with ketamine, 1–4.5 mg/kg, or ketamine, 0.5 mg/kg, followed by thiobarbiturate, 2.0 mg/kg, except in uterine tetany when barbiturate preferable (ketamine thought less cardiodepressant than barbiturates, especially in hypovolemia)
  – Maintenance until birth with at least 60% but preferably 100% O_2 + low concentration ($\frac{1}{2}$ MAC) of halogenated agent

SURGICAL STAGES

- Uterine incision (2 techniques):
  – Horizontal (lower segment)—stronger scar, less blood loss, less infection, T4 blockade required
  – Vertical (classic)—faster delivery of fetus, T6 blockade sufficient
- EBL: 800–1200 ml
- Volume concerns: patients freq hypovolemic

Postoperative Pain Management

- Pain severity: varies; Rx 24–48 h: IM, IV, or epidural opioid bolus injections or IV or epidural opioid infusion, PCA
- Postpartum depression more likely to develop if emergent C-section vs. vaginal delivery

ANTICIPATED PROBLEMS/CONCERNS

- After GA: pulmonary inhalation of gastric contents, Htn, arrhythmia, awareness
- After regional anesthesia: hypotension, failed block, high block, systemic toxicity

CESAREAN SECTION, PLANNED

Andrew P. Harris, M.D., M.H.S.

RISK

- Increasing again in USA: 1995, 785,000/y; 1998, 900,000/y
- Racial predominance: none

PERIOPERATIVE RISKS

- Perioperative pulmonary morbidity varies by type of anesthesia—GA is associated with ↑ pulmonary morbidity
- Low mortality, but anesthesia (5–24/100,000) significant contributor to mortality

WORRY ABOUT

- Inability to intubate
- Unintentional high regional block
- Unanticipated blood loss
- Spinal headache
- Embolism—thromboembolism, air embolism, amniotic fluid embolism
- Postoperative endometritis

OVERVIEW

- "Significant other" frequently accompanies patient to the OR
- Hysterotomy usually through the lower uterine segment
- Occasional uterine atony after delivery Rx with oxytocic agents, occasionally progressing to cesarean hysterectomy
- Exteriorization of the uterus during closure associated with greater intraop discomfort if regional anesthesia
- Regional anesthesia preferred to avoid risk of airway mishaps and postop pulm morbidity

ICD-9-CM Code: V22.2 (Pregnancy)

See also Pregnancy, Maternal Physiology, in Diseases section and Pregnant Surgical Patient in Procedures section

INDICATIONS AND USUAL TREATMENT

- Conditions that would result in ↑ perinatal morbidity for mother or fetus if vaginal delivery attempted; most common examples include Hx of classic (or maybe any) C-section, macrosomia, Hx of CPD, twin gestation
- May also be emergent (see Cesarean Section, Emergent, in Procedures section)
- Vaginal birth after C-section may be attempted in lieu of elective repeat C-section, but now risks seem to be greater than benefits

ASSESSMENT POINTS

SYSTEM	EFFECT	HX ASSESSMENT	PE	TEST
AIRWAY	Engorgement of vessels and breast		Airway exam Mallampati class	
PULM	↑ Minute ventilation ↑ O$_2$ consumption	Shortness of breath		
CV	↑ Cardiac output ↑ Dilutional anemia Vena caval obstruction	Cardiac failure Supine hypotensive syndrome		Hgb Antibody screen
GI	Delayed gastric emptying	Regurgitation		
MS	↑ Back pain	Back pain, sciatica		

Key Reference: Reisner LS, Lin D: Anesthesia for cesarean section. *In* Chestnut DH (ed): Obstetric Anesthesia Principles and Practice, 2nd ed. St. Louis, Mosby–Year Book, 1999, pp 465–492.

PERIOPERATIVE MANAGEMENT

Preoperative Preparation

- Antacids or H$_2$ blocker/metoclopramide
- Left uterine displacement

Anesthetic Technique

- Any: general, local, spinal, epidural; regional preferred due to potential airway problems

Monitoring

- Fetal HR monitoring during induction
- Consider air embolism monitoring

Airway

- Engorgement leads to easy bleeding, difficult intubation
- ~ 1/300 unanticipated difficult intubation
- Airway cart/equipment available

Induction/Maintenance

- 33% Less local anesthetic required for regional anesthesia
- T4 level during regional anesthesia desirable
- If GA, discontinue halogenated agents (if possible) after delivery to ↓ blood loss
- Prophylactic antibiotic after cord clamp
- Oxytocin, methylergonovine, carboprost available for uterine atony after delivery

SURGICAL STAGES

- Skin incision to delivery: venous air embolism or amniotic fluid embolism possible
- Closure: uterine atony or hemorrhage possible
- EBL: 750–1000 ml normal; can be much greater with uterine atony

Postoperative Considerations

- Uterine atony possible
- Pain score: typically 4–8
- IV PCA or epidural PCA for 1–2 days

ANTICIPATED PROBLEMS/CONCERNS

- Inability to intubate
- High block with hypotension, sudden bradycardia
- Hemorrhage
- Postoperative headache

CHOLECYSTECTOMY, LAPAROSCOPIC Sorin J. Brull, M.D.

RISK

- 20 million in USA with gallstones
- 600,000 cholecystectomies/y
- Prevalence ↑ with age; higher incidence in women, 17%; men, 8%
- Among Pima Indian women, 75% affected
- Incidence in African-Americans higher than in Caucasians

PERIOPERATIVE RISKS

- Perioperative mortality ~0.1%, morbidity 4–6× lower than in open procedure (2–9%)
- Most benefits derived from avoidance of large abdominal incision

WORRY ABOUT

- Intraoperative hemorrhage
- Visceral damage
- Bacterbilia, sepsis
- PE, arrhythmias (CO_2 absorption)
- SQ emphysema from improperly placed CO_2 insufflating needle
- Hemodynamic consequences of pneumoperitoneum
- CO_2 absorption, position changes; CO_2 embolism

OVERVIEW

- Laparoscopic procedure ↑ in freq
- Lower incidence of complications than with open
- Freq short stay; outpatient procedure in appropriate patients

ICD-9-CM Code: 574.0 (Cholelithiasis)

INDICATIONS AND USUAL TREATMENT

- Indications: chronic cholecystitis, symptomatic cholelithiasis
- Early contraindications: large stones in common bile duct, acute inflammation, pregnancy, obesity, but now used in acute cholecystitis and pregnancy
- Considered technique of choice in octogenarians
- Alternative Rx: open procedure, stone/contact dissolution, biliary lithotripsy, cholecystolithotomy

ASSESSMENT POINTS

SYSTEM	EFFECT	ASSESSMENT BY HX	PE	TEST
CV	Likely co-morbidities: PVD, CAD		CV	ECG
RESP	Co-morbidity likely: COPD (elderly)		Chest	CXR O_2 sat
HEME	Intraoperative blood loss (cystic artery liver laceration)	Preop dehydration (N/V, elderly)	Orthostasis	Hct, electrolytes
GU	Impairment 2° to age, co-morbidity	CNS Hx	CNS	BUN/Cr

Key Reference: Cunningham AJ, Brull SJ: Laparoscopic cholecystectomy: anesthetic implications. Anesth Analg 1993; 76:1120–1133.

INTRAOPERATIVE MANAGEMENT

Monitoring

- Routine, UO (Foley catheter)
- End-tidal CO_2 not good substitute for arterial P_{CO_2}

Airway

- Change in position from head-up to head-down may displace ET tube into endobronchial position

Anesthetic Technique

- GA, controlled ventilation with cuffed ET tube (prevent aspiration during pneumoperitoneum); regional (axial) anesthesia not advocated

SURGICAL STAGES

Induction

- CV instability if co-existing disease, elderly
- Trocar insertion: injury to viscera
- Trendelenburg position:
  – CV effects: improves venous return, CO, BP; pulmonary effects: reduced VC, atelectasis, shunting

- Pneumoperitoneum creation:
  – Subcutaneous emphysema from poorly placed insufflating needle
  – CV effects: intra-abd pressure <15 mmHg associated with minimal CV changes (slight increase in MAP, no change in CO)
  – Pulmonary effects: hypoventilation, respiratory acidosis, hypoxemia, tension pneumothorax (via patent pleuroperitoneal canal), atelectasis, shunting; exogenous CO_2 insufflation—rapid absorption, necessitating controlled ventilation; arrhythmias, catecholamine release; poss CO_2 pulmonary embolism, especially at release of pneumoperitoneum

Definitive Surgery

- Postop N/V high (42%); prophylaxis recommended: metoclopramide, droperidol, ondansetron
- Avoiding neostigmine, ↓ narcotic requirements by using NSAIDs (ketorolac) also effective
- Narcotic-induced sphincter of Oddi spasm reversed with narcotic antagonists, local anesthetic infiltration, glucagon

- Use of N_2O controversial due to ? bowel distention, ? postop N/V
- Pre-emptive/adjuvant anesthesia with local anesthetic infiltration of skin, gallbladder bed may reduce postop pain
- Blood loss: minimal
- Surg duration: ~1–3 h
- Fluid shifts: minimal
- Pain score: 2–5; same day or next day hospital discharge

ANTICIPATED PROBLEMS/CONCERNS

- Intraoperative: tension pneumothorax, CO_2 absorption, arrhythmias, hemodynamic compromise from pneumoperitoneum, visceral damage from surgical trocar, CO_2 embolism
- Conversion to open procedure (1–7% incidence) due to technical factors
- Gasless (traction) laparoscopic techniques under trial

CHOLECYSTECTOMY, OPEN

Sorin J. Brull, M.D.

RISK

- 20 million in USA have gallstones
- 600,000 cholecystectomies/y
- Prevalence ↑ with age; in women incidence is 17%, in men 8%
- Pima Indian women, incidence is 75%
- African-Americans affected more often than Caucasians

PERIOPERATIVE RISKS

- Perioperative mortality: 0–0.5% (0.1% in patients <50 y)
- In elderly: up to 10%
- Morbidity: 5–25%, especially 2° to impairment of pulmonary mechanics (abdominal incision)

WORRY ABOUT

- Intraoperative hemorrhage
- Hepatic failure
- Bacterbilia, sepsis

OVERVIEW

- Becoming rare mode of cholecystectomy
- Antibiotic prophylaxis; midline, paramedian, or subcostal surg incision
- Identification of cystic duct, common hepatic duct, common bile duct, cystic artery
- Operative cholangiogram performed for choledocholithiasis
- US ~98% sensitivity, specificity

ICD-9-CM Code: 574.0 (Cholelithiasis)

INDICATIONS AND USUAL TREATMENT

- Chronic cholecystitis and symptomatic cholelithiasis
- Biliary colic treated with parenteral narcotics; antibiotic therapy for patients over age 60 with chronic cholecystitis, and for patients with acute cholecystitis or with concomitant common duct stones
- Nasogastric suction and low-fat diet not proven beneficial
- Other Rx: gallstone dissolution; percutaneous shock wave lithotripsy; contact dissolution; percutaneous cholecystolithotomy; laparoscopic cholecystectomy

ASSESSMENT POINTS

SYSTEM	EFFECT	ASSESSMENT BY HX	PE	TEST
CV	Rule out angina vs. cholecystitis ECG changes and arrhythmias	Rule out CAD Relief by nitroglycerin (relieves both angina and biliary colic)		ECG, coronary angio; exercise tolerance test if unable to differentiate
RESP	Co-morbidity likely: COPD (elderly)	Pulmonary reserve Exercise tolerance	Auscultation	CXR
GI	N/V	N/V		

Key Reference: Nahrwold DL: The biliary system. *In* Sabiston DC Jr (ed): Textbook of Surgery, 15th ed. Philadelphia, WB Saunders, 1997, pp 1126–1131.

PERIOPERATIVE MANAGEMENT

Perioperative Evaluations
- Assess CV system, CAD

Anesthetic Technique
- GA
- Regional (axial) anesthesia may not be appropriate due to high level of sensory denervation required (at least T4)
- Local anesthesia for cholecystostomy
- Adjunct techniques: interpleural cath, intercostal nerve block
- Prophylaxis for postop N/V

Monitoring
- Routine

Airway
- Consider rapid-sequence induction if preop N/V

Induction
- Narcotic-induced sphincter of Oddi spasm reversed with narcotic antagonists, injection of local anesthesia, or glucagon
- Use of N_2O controversial because of nausea, bowel distention

SURGICAL STAGES
- Skin incision: large, usually subcostal

Dissection
- Possible bleeding from cystic artery, liver laceration/damage
- Possible pneumothorax if diaphragmatic or pleural damage

Definitive Surgery
- Exposure, bowel manipulation/traction may lead to hypotension (release of vasoactive substances from gut and/or ↓venous return)

- Approximate duration: 0.5–3.0 h
- Fluid shift: can be marked if bowel exposed for long periods
- Hypothermia a concern if prolonged procedure, esp in elderly
- EBL: 50–150 ml

Postoperative Considerations
- N/V: consider prophylaxis
- Pain score: 6–10; narcotic requirements ↓ by "pre-emptive analgesia," adjunct techniques (interpleural cath, intercostal nerve block), local anesthetic infiltration of gallbladder bed

ANTICIPATED PROBLEMS/CONCERNS
- Severe postop pain (incisional) may lead to ↓ ambulation; splinting; ↓ cough, mobilization; atelectasis, pulmonary infection

CIRCUMCISION

Stanley W. Stead, M.D.

RISK

- ~2 million/y
- Generally performed in neonatal period

PERIOPERATIVE RISKS

- Considered minimal 0.2% (aspiration, bleeding, hematoma, malignant hyperthermia reported 1 series [2/476], postop fever); complications from local anesthesia rare
- Local skin necrosis after dorsal penile nerve block (<0.5%)

WORRY ABOUT

- Complicated preop neonatal course: sepsis, hypospadias, immaturity

OVERVIEW

- Most common surgical procedure in USA. Uncommon in most other parts of the world. Religious followers of Jewish and Islamic faiths practice circumcision for religious and cultural reasons. Circumcision rates also vary among racial and ethnic groups, with whites being much more likely to be circumcised.
- ↑ From 1985–1992; largest increment following 1989 American Academy of Pediatrics statement of "potential benefits and advantages" of procedure
- According to unpublished data, 64.1% of male infants were circumcised in 1995; however, some estimate the percentage even higher
- Risk from UTI in uncircumcised males is 4–10 times greater than in circumcised males, with the greatest risk in infants <1 y. Absolute risk of developing UTI in an uncircumcised male infant is low (~1%).

ICD-9-CM Codes: V50.2 (Circumcision [no medical indication, ritual, routine]); 605 (Phimosis); 607.1 (Balanitis)

INDICATIONS AND USUAL TREATMENT

- Parental choice
- Coincidence with other surg
- Recurrent balanoposthitis
- Difficulty retracting foreskin: "tight prepuce"
- UTIs
- True phimosis (obstruction of urine flow)
- Three methods used in the newborn male all use an associated device: Gomco clamp, the Plastibell device, or the Mogen clamp. After the newborn period, a more formal surgical procedure is used, necessitating hemostasis and suturing of the skin edges; frequently performed with GA

ASSESSMENT POINTS

SYSTEM	EFFECT	PE	TEST
GU	Hypospadias	Urethra ventral surface of penis	
	Balanoposthitis, phimosis	Nonretractile prepuce or tight ring	
	Urinary tract infections		UA, microscopic
OVERALL	Immaturity, sepsis		

Key Reference: American Academy of Pediatrics Task Force on Circumcision: Circumcision policy statement. Pediatrics 1999; 103:686–693.

INTRAOPERATIVE MANAGEMENT

- Considerable evidence that newborns circumcised without analgesia experience pain and physiologic stress, manifested by changes in heart rate, blood pressure, oxygen saturation, and cortisol levels
- In the past, the procedure was performed without analgesia or anesthesia. Current recommendations now emphasize procedural analgesia.
- Subcutaneous ring block: A subcutaneous circumferential ring of 0.8 ml of 1% lidocaine without epinephrine injected at the midshaft of the penis was found to be more effective than either EMLA cream or dorsal penile nerve block (DPNB)
- 1–2 g of EMLA cream is applied to the distal half of the penis and wrapped in an occlusive dressing, 60–90 min before the procedure. There is a risk of methemoglobinemia from a metabolite of prilocaine, which can oxidize hemoglobin to methemoglobin (see Prilocaine in Drugs section).

- DPNB: a 27-gauge needle is used to inject 0.4 ml of 1% lidocaine, administered at the 10- and 2-o'clock positions at the base of the penis. The needle is directed posteromedially 3–5 mm on each side until Buck's fascia is entered. After aspiration, the local anesthetic is injected. Bruising may be seen from the injection.
- GA may be preferred in children

Monitoring

- Routine

Airway

- Routine: mask, laryngeal mask airway, intubation

SURGICAL STAGES

Skin Incision/Definitive Surgery

- Two methods, "sleeve" or "freehand," in which ring incision made around prepuce, or using a clamp (Plastibell, Gomco, or Mogen). In either, maximum surgical stimuli at this point; no dissection. Bleeding controlled with compression or electrocautery; suture placement rare.

- Commonly, petrolatum-based gauze used to dress wound edges, which are brought together

Postoperative Considerations

- Pain score: 2–4
- Pain relief by rectal acetaminophen in neonates
- Older individuals may require opiates

ANTICIPATED PROBLEMS/CONCERNS

- Newborn infants experience pain manifested by physiologic changes (↑in BP, HR, sweating, ↓oxygenation), behavioral changes, which persist for at least 22 h; physiologic, behavioral effects attenuated by local or regional anesthesia
- Pain often undertreated
- Infection remains a possibility in neonates, since hygiene may be compromised

RISK

- ~ 1/1000 live births
- Racial predominance: Caucasian:black infants 2:1:
- More frequently male than female
- Very frequently associated with cleft palate
- Associated with maternal phenytoin or alcohol ingestion

PERIOPERATIVE RISKS

- Extremely low morbidity/mortality; no deaths reported in recent literature with cleft lip repair alone
- When associated with cleft palate repair, the most significant risk is postop airway obstruction

WORRY ABOUT

- Difficult airway when associated with syndromes—e.g., EEC, Mohr's, Shprintzen's, Wolf-Hirschhorn, or Pierre Robin
- Undiagnosed associated congenital heart, renal disease
- Intraoperative dysrhythmias caused by surgical infiltration of epinephrine
- Timing of surgery coinciding with physiologic anemia of infancy
- Postop airway obstruction by forgotten pharyngeal pack
- Associated with cleft palate, risks of preop anemia due to poor feeding; intrainduction laryngospasm due to chronic otitis media, URI; intrainduction airway obstruction due to tongue wedged in cleft palate; postop airway obstruction due to lingual edema

OVERVIEW

- Congenital condition by 7th wk intrauterine life
- Strong genetic influence; $\frac{1}{4}$ cases bilateral cleft lip
- Traditionally done at ~ 3 mo, but recently done neonatally

ICD-9-CM Code: 749.10

INDICATIONS AND USUAL TREATMENT

- If in good health, cheiloplasty electively performed
- Primary indications are aesthetic: early repair encourages maternal bonding
- Should be done by 18 mo to assure normal speech, social integration

ASSESSMENT POINTS

(inclusive for associated cleft palate)

SYSTEM	EFFECT	ASSESSMENT BY HX	PE	TEST
HEENT	Otitis media Clear rhinorrhea, difficult airway	Ear pain Snore, grunt	TM distance Airway exam	
CV	Associated CHD	SOB, cyanosis, poor growth	CV exam Club feet	ECG, ECHO
RESP	URI aspiration	Cough/fever SOB, cyanosis	Auscultation Chest exam	CXR, ABGs
GI	Impaired deglutition Malnutrition	Nasal regurgitation Poor growth		Observe feeding Albumin
HEME	Anemia	Malnutrition	Pallor	Hgb/Hct
GU	Associated congenital defects	UTI	Club feet	UA, BUN/Cr

Key Reference: Prabhu KP, Wig J, Grewal S: Bilateral infraorbital nerve block is superior to peri-incisional infiltration for analgesia after repair of cleft lip. Scand J Plast Reconstr Surg Hand Surg 1999; 33:83–87.

PERIOPERATIVE IMPLICATIONS

Preoperative Preparation

- During neonatal period ascertain associated birth defects
- Establish postconceptional age to exclude premature neonates

Anesthetic Technique

- GA, anticholinergic agent usual
- Oral intubation using appropriate-sized RAE tube well secured to mandible
- Maintenance with inhalational agent; NMB not usual

Monitoring

- Well-placed precordial stethoscope especially important since intraoperative access to airway severely limited
- If neonate, aggressively prevent heat loss

SURGICAL STAGES

- Placement of pharyngeal pack
- Local anesthetic and epinephrine infiltration
- Minimal tissue mobilization, direct closure of defect
- Procedure time usually brief
- EBL: usually minimal

Postoperative Considerations

- Check that pharyngeal pack removed before extubation
- If patient premature continue apnea monitoring for at least 24 h postop
- Pain score: 2–5
- Oral or rectal acetaminophen usually sufficient
- Oral feeding can start after ~ 2 h with clear liquids

ANTICIPATED PROBLEMS/CONCERNS

- Undiagnosed cardiac anomalies in neonate
- Postop airway obstruction due to forgotten pack or airway edema

CLEFT PALATE REPAIR

C. Dean Kurth, M.D.

- Incidence of cleft palate is about 1/1000 live births
- Repaired before speech develops, usually at age 8–12 mo

PERIOPERATIVE RISKS

- Perioperative mortality rare in pediatric centers

WORRY ABOUT

- Associated deformities, their risks: congenital heart disease (SBE prophylaxis, cyanosis, CHF), micrognathia (difficult intubation), retroglossia (difficult mask airway), upper airway congestion (laryngospasm)
- Tracheal tube: difficult intubation; tube occlusion, extubation, endobronchial during surgery
- Intraoperative arrhythmias and Htn
- Postoperative airway obstruction

OVERVIEW

- Usually isolated deformity; it can also be part of syndrome (e.g., Pierre Robin)
- Repaired to separate oral, nasal cavities; improve feeding, speech; prevent middle ear disease, hearing loss; aspiration
- Surgical position: supine, head extended, mouth open (Dingman gag), pharyngeal packs in
- Before incision, palate is infiltrated with epinephrine for hemostasis
- Surgery involves undermining tissues around defect to create flap to cover it; soft palate edema; opioid administration may contribute to postop obstructive apnea

ICD-9-CM Codes: 749.0; 749.2

INDICATIONS AND USUAL TREATMENT

- Defects are surgically repaired if life expectancy reasonable
- Bottle-fed with special nipple before defect closed; caloric intake, growth monitored
- Otitis media often occurs; antibiotic prophylaxis common preop
- Myringotomy tubes frequently placed concomitantly with repairs

ASSESSMENT POINTS

SYSTEM	EFFECT	ASSESSMENT BY HX	PE	TEST
HEENT	Palate defect, other deformities, rhinorrhea	Apnea, known syndrome	Defect size, airway exam, nasal secretions	
CV	Cardiac defect	Slow feeding, diaphoresis	Murmur, liver size, cyanosis, HR, RR	ECG/CXR ECHO
RESP	Bronchitis, chronic aspiration	Cough, fever, feeding problem	Rhonchi, wheeze	O_2 saturation CXR
HEME	Anemia	Age 3–9 mo	Pallor	Hct

Key Reference: Kharkov LV: Evolution of methods of uranostaphyloplasty exemplified by the analysis of 1118 primary operations for congenital palatal defects. Br J Oral Maxillofac Surg 2000; 38:104–106.

PERIOPERATIVE MANAGEMENT

Preoperative Preparation

- Premedication: if no obstructive apnea, then midazolam PO
- Consider cross-match, depending on surgeon, patient's Hct

Anesthetic Technique

- No special techniques

Monitoring

- Routine

Airway

- Secure tracheal tube at midline, flat against chin, bend of tube at lip; use water-resistant tape, oral RAE tube
- Flex, extend head to check for bronchial intubation or inadvertent extubation

SURGICAL STAGES

- Palate infiltrated with epinephrine before incision; keep dose < 10 μg/kg
- Tissue on both sides of defect mobilized to create flap
- During dissection, observe wound for bleeding, but transfusion rarely required
- After defect, check palate for edema, gauge airway caliber
- At end, heavy ligature may be placed through tongue, or NP airway may be inserted
- Wound may be injected with bupivacaine for postop analgesia; keep dose < 2 mg/kg
- Surgical duration: 2–4 h
- Blood loss variable

Emergence

- Before extubation, ensure that the pharyngeal pack is gone and that the oral cavity is dry
- Extubation best done when patient is awake
- Restrain arms to prevent child from pulling at oral suture line

POSTOPERATIVE CONSIDERATIONS

- Analgesia with acetaminophen, COX-2 inhibitors, or opioid; careful with opioid dose (obstructive apnea)
- Pulse oximetry, cardiorespiratory monitoring recommended for 24–48 h

COLOSTOMY

Kevin P. Limp, M.D.*

RISK

- Approximately 70,000/y in USA
- Racial predominance: colostomy for colon cancer: none; Crohn's/ulcerative colitis: white > African-American
- Gender predominance: colostomy for colon cancer: M:F, 3:1; Crohn's: M ≤ F; ulcerative colitis: M ≤ F; trauma: M:F, 3:1; diverticulitis: M:F, 1:1

PERIOPERATIVE RISKS

- Perioperative morbidity related to concurrent medical diseases, associated surgical procedure(s)
- Colostomy performed to ↓ perioperative complications
- Specific periop mortality rare (<0.5%)
- Specific periop morbidity: infection (<5%), stomal ischemia/necrosis (<2%), stomal retraction, parastomal fistula, stomal stenosis, parastomal hernia, stomal prolapse, bleeding

WORRY ABOUT

- Malnutrition, hypoproteinemia, lyte disturbances
- Intravascular volume depletion (bleeding, NPO status, vomiting, bowel prep, 3rd spacing, poor PO intake)
- Anemia (bleeding, chronic disease)
- Aspiration risk (obstruction, NPO status, urgent surgery, pain, debilitation)
- Complications, metabolic derangements of hyperalimentation
- Perioperative corticosteroid supplementation (inflammatory bowel disease)
- Associated trauma lesions
- Extracolonic manifestations of inflammatory bowel disease (e.g., arthritis, anemia)

OVERVIEW

- A type of enterostomy that creates an opening in the colon, the proximal end of which is exteriorized and fashioned as a stoma to form an abdominal anus
- Patients present electively (e.g., inflammatory bowel disease), urgently (e.g., colon cancer with obstruction), or emergently (penetrating abdominal trauma)

- Performed in association with surgical procedure(s) for patient's underlying condition (e.g., large bowel resection for ulcerative colitis, abdominoperineal resection for colon cancer)

ICD-9-CM Codes: 555–569

INDICATIONS AND USUAL TREATMENT

- General indications: to replace anus as distal opening of GI tract, to divert fecal stream from more distal pathologic process, to decompress obstructed colon
- Specific indications: colon cancer, Crohn's disease, ulcerative colitis, abdominal trauma, diverticulitis, Hirschsprung's disease
- Usual Rx: colon CA: primary resection (chemotherapy, radiation therapy 2°)
  – Inflammatory bowel disease: sulfasalazine, corticosteroids, bowel rest, resection
  – Penetrating abdominal trauma with bowel injury: laparotomy, resection

ASSESSMENT POINTS

SYSTEM	EFFECT	ASSESSMENT BY HX	PE	TEST
HEENT	Ankylosing arthritis of inflammatory bowel disease can affect ability to intubate	Spine immobility	Airway exam	Spine imaging
CV	Intravascular volume depletion	Bleeding, vomiting, diarrhea, NPO, bowel prep, poor PO intake	VS Cardiac exam	ECG
RESP	Pulm metastases (colon CA)	Cough, hemoptysis, dyspnea	Chest exam	Chest imaging
GI	Potential for aspiration	Obstruction, NPO status	Abd exam	Abd imaging
HEME	Anemia (hemorrhage, chronic disease)	Orthostasis, ↓ exercise tolerance	Cardiac exam	Hct

Key Reference: McGinnis LS: Surgical treatment options for colorectal cancer. Cancer 1994; 74:2147–2150.

PERIOPERATIVE MANAGEMENT

Preoperative Preparation

- Restoration of intravascular volume; correction of electrolyte, metabolic disturbances
- Corticosteroid supplementation if appropriate
- Consider H_2 blocking agents, antacids

Anesthetic Technique

- Balanced GA with ET intubation provides protection from aspiration of gastric contents; allows use of muscle relaxants for optimal surgical conditions
- Combined general, epidural anesthesia may facilitate rapid extubation, excellent postop analgesia, early return of bowel function, ↓ intraoperative blood loss, ↓ incidence of postop DVT, pulmonary emboli

Monitoring

- Consider Foley catheter
- Consider CVP based on volume status, anticipated bleeding, 3rd spacing, need for postop access
- Consider arterial line for co-existing disease or hemodynamic instability

Airway

- ET intubation preferred

Induction

- If at risk for aspiration, rapid-sequence induction with cricoid pressure or awake intubation
- In combined epidural/GA, administer epidural drug slowly if intravascular volume repletion not assured

Maintenance

- Prudent to avoid N_2O until wound closure
- Anticipate large 3rd space losses, potential bleeding if other procedures planned

Emergence

- For patients at risk for aspiration, extubate after full recovery of airway reflexes

Postoperative Considerations

- ICU for co-existing disease, extensive surgery, hemodynamic instability
- Corticosteroid supplements for inflammatory bowel disease
- Ongoing fluid shifts, hemodynamic instability
- Pain score: 5–8 (for laparotomy)
- EBL: <100 ml for stoma creation; often 200–300 ml for primary surgical procedure
- Anticipate significant 3rd space fluid shifts, possible blood loss

ANTICIPATED PROBLEMS/CONCERNS

- None

* Deceased

CORONARY ARTERY BYPASS GRAFT

Daniel M. Thys, M.D.

RISK

- 360,000 CABG operations/y
- Risk factors for CAD: cigarette smoking, Htn, diabetes, ↑cholesterol, high LDL, low HDL, age, male sex, family Hx

PERIOPERATIVE RISKS

- 30-Day mortality: 1.5–5%
- Risk factors for poor outcome: age, reoperation, disaster/emergent surg, EF <30%
- Cardiac outcomes: cardiac failure, MI, arrhythmias, cardiac death
- Severe perioperative morbidity: stroke (1–25%) dependent upon condition of aorta, degree of neuropsychiatric testing

WORRY ABOUT

- Perioperative ventricular function
- Myocardial protection, perioperative ischemia
- Completeness of surg revascularization
- Bleeding with reoperations

OVERVIEW

- Occluded or severely diseased coronary arteries bypassed with venous or arterial grafts
- Anesthesia technique, monitoring, postop ventilatory care affected by patient's physical condition
- Early extubation and discharge are goals if good preop condition, but safety of "fast-tracking" and effects of rapid temperature normalization upon stroke rate is under investigation

ICD-9-CM Code: 414.0

INDICATIONS AND USUAL TREATMENT

- High-grade (>75%) stenosis of left main coronary artery
- Severe angina with multivessel disease, poor LV function
- Angina after failed medical therapy, PTCA, or previous CABG

ASSESSMENT POINTS

SYSTEM	EFFECT	ASSESSMENT BY HX	PE	TEST
CV	Cardiac failure	Exercise tolerance	Auscultation	Radionuclide stress test, ECHO
	Atheromata bruits	Asymptomatic, TIA, etc.	Auscultation	ECHO, Doppler, angio
	Htn	None to SOB	BP measurement	ECG for LVH, ECHO, radionuclides for diastolic function
ENDO	Diabetes	Medical Rx, autonomic dysfunction: gastroparesis, etc.	BP lying, standing	Glucose, BUN, Cr
HEME	Bleeding diathesis	Bleeding, bruising	Ecchymosis	PT, PTT, plt

Key Reference: Kaplan JA, Wynands JE: Anesthesia for myocardial revascularization. *In* Kaplan JA (ed): Cardiac Anesthesia, 3rd ed. Philadelphia, WB Saunders, 1999, pp 689–726.

INTRAOPERATIVE MANAGEMENT

Preoperative Preparation

- Maintain all preop meds, including IV heparin

Anesthetic Technique

- Narcotics, relaxants, amnesics in patients in poor physical condition
- Hypnotics, volatile agents, ↓narcotic doses in patients in good physical condition

Monitoring

- Multilead ECG for detection of ischemia
- Invasive arterial pressure in all patients because of nonpulsatile CPB flow
- Central venous access for assessment of CVP, drug administration
- Activated clotting or heparin levels to assess adequate coag paralysis, reversal with protamine
- PA cath and/or TEE if ↓LV function, high risk of intraop ischemia, or associated cardiac disease (e.g., ischemic mitral regurgitation)

Induction

- Minimize imbalance between myocardial O_2 supply, demand
- Avoid intraoperative awareness

SURGICAL STAGES

Conventional CABG

Skin Incision

- Large, midline chest incision

Graft Dissection

- During dissection of internal mammary art, potential for occlusion of an ipsilateral radial artery line

Heart Cannulation

- Cannulation of aorta associated with Htn, ischemia, emboli
- Cannulation of right atrium with arrhythmias

Cardiopulmonary Bypass (CPB)

- Concerns are
  - Potential for awareness
  - Management of acid-base status to optimize cerebral perfusion
  - Management of anticoagulation
  - Management of perfusion press flow
  - Temperature control

Termination of CPB

- Inotropes, vasoactive agents, IABP may be needed to optimize ventricular function
- Post-CPB ventricular function determined by preop ventricular function, myocardial protection during CPB, completeness of revascularization; mech assist devices (e.g., IABP) will often be used

Postoperative Considerations

- Less severe than after other chest incisions
- Use of regional analgesic techniques (spinal or epidural) not widespread due to potential for complications with heparinization

New Surgical Approaches

- MIDCAB: Mediastinum is reached through smaller incisions
- OPCAB: CABG is performed without CPB
- Port access: small incisions to reach mediastinum; CPB is achieved by using endovascular devices

ANESTHETIC IMPLICATIONS

- As above, except that lung separation using a double-lumen tube may be necessary

ANTICIPATED PROBLEMS/CONCERNS

- Presence of myocardial ischemia, MI suggests incomplete revascularization or inadequate protection during CPB
- In reoperations, antifibrinolytics, aprotinin, other drugs that influence coagulation under intense evaluation

CRANIOTOMY

Scott M. Eleff, M.D.
Robert McPherson, M.D.*

RISK

- Head trauma
- Intracranial tumors
- Vascular lesions

PERIOPERATIVE RISKS

- Periop risk of poor CNS outcome highly depends on disease process
- Concurrent C-spine trauma
- Increased risk of stroke, coma, paralysis

WORRY ABOUT

- Perfusion pressure = inflow pressure (usually MAP) less outflow resistance (can be ICP, cerebral venous pressure, or tissue pressure caused by tumor or brain retractor)
- Brain herniation when dura opened
- Blood gases: avoid hypoxia, hypercapnia (even mild)

OVERVIEW

- Craniotomies performed for variety of lesions, both space-occupying and vascular
- Nervous system accommodates well to chronic processes; even mild CNS Sx indicate exhaustion of compensatory mechanisms in patients with chronic diseases
- Decompensation can occur from ↑ ICP, hypoxia, hypercapnia, ↓ venous return, or ↓ MAP

ICD-9-CM Codes: 239.6 (Brain tumor); 437.3 (Nonruptured cerebral aneurysm); 854.x (Head injury)

ETIOLOGY

- Brain tumor: benign, malignant
- Vascular lesion, aneurysm, AVM, Htn, hemorrhage
- Head trauma, epidural hematoma, subdural hematoma

INDICATIONS AND USUAL TREATMENT

- Evacuation of hematoma
- Debulking of malignant tumors
- Complete removal of benign lesions
- Ablation of aneurysm
- Ablation, removal of AVM

ASSESSMENT POINTS

SYSTEM	EFFECT	ASSESSMENT BY HX	PE	TEST
HEENT	Trauma may cause concurrent airway and C-spine injuries	Hx of acute trauma	Fractured mandible/maxilla; blood in oropharynx; pain on palpation of C-spine	CT scan of head and neck
CV	Usually none, unless intracranial Htn (bradycardia, dysrhythmias)	Hx of CV disease, systemic hypertension diabetes	Blood pressure Heart rate	ECG
RESP	Brainstem pressure causes apnea	Cushing's response	Pupils dilate	Brain CT demonstrating midline shift
GI	Arterial bleed 2° to steroids	Hx of steroid use	Blood in stool, gastric ulcer	
CNS	Change in consciousness	Acute vs. chronic	Focal motor/sensory dysfunction; awake/lethargic/comatose Papilledema	MRI or CT of brain

Key Reference: Schubert A, Mascha EJ, Bloomfield EJ, DeBoer GE, Gupta MK, Ebrahim ZY: Effect of cranial surgery and brain tumor size on emergence from anesthesia. Anesthesiology 1996; 85:513–521.

PERIOPERATIVE IMPLICATIONS

Preoperative Preparation

- Emergency/trauma: maintain MAP
  - Control airway to prevent hypoxia/hypercapnia
  - If Cushing's response present, maintain MAP until hyperventilation established

Elective

- Avoid preop sedatives/narcotics if ICH present
  - Preop steroids and diuretics (mannitol, Lasix)
- Evaluation for midline shifts
  - Indicates ↑ sensitivity to ↓ MABP

Monitoring

- Invasive art pressure
- Consider CVP/(rarely PA) catheter, depending on surg procedure
- Urine output
- EEG/EPs

Airway

- Trauma victims may have associated neck injury
- Avoid even brief periods of relative hypoxia

Preinduction/Induction

- IV induction with barbiturate, narcotics
- NM blocker to avoid bucking; use succinylcholine if any airway concerns
- Support MAP with phenylephrine

Maintenance

- Support MAP until any compression relieved
- Low-dose (< 1 MAC) volatile agent
- ± N_2O (may interfere with EP monitoring if waves small)
- Preincision mannitol (0.5–1.0 g/kg)
- Hyperventilation to $PaCO_2$ of ~30 mmHg until beginning of dural closure

Extubation

- Prompt awaking and extubation important
- May need to remain intubated if comatose preop
- If level of arousal less than anticipated, immediate study (CT scan, MRI) frequently indicated
- Patient with posterior fossa surg may have loss of airway reflexes despite ability to respond to commands

Adjuvants

- β-blockers and phenylephrine ideal for BP control and do not effect cerebral vessels
- Barbiturates ↓ ICP; narcotics are ICP neutral

ANTICIPATED PROBLEMS/CONCERNS

- Postop brain swelling
- Hypovolemia from preop fluid restriction and intraop diuretics

* Deceased

PROCEDURES   391

CRANIOTOMY, SITTING POSITION

Thomas J. Toung, M.D.

RISK

- Patients with infratentorial tumors (pineal, floor of 4th ventricle, pontomedullary junction, vermis, cerebellopontine angle)
- Trend ↓, but still used in 50% of USA institutions

PERIOPERATIVE RISKS

- Venous air embolism (as high as 80%)
- Paradoxical air embolism (probe patent foramen ovale in 25% of adult population)
- Hypotension
- Brainstem/cervical spinal cord ischemia
- Airway obstruction
- Tension pneumocephalus
- Macroglossia

WORRY ABOUT

- Subdural hematoma due to major brain shift (excessive CSF drainage)
- Venous and/or paradoxical air embolism
- Brainstem, lower cranial nerve injury
- Poor cerebral venous drainage with acute flexion of head on neck

OVERVIEW

- Acoustic neuroma most common infratentorial tumor in adults
- 2 mmHg reduction in cerebral BP with every inch of elevation above heart
- Head, neck markedly flexed for better exposure
- Operation is performed around brainstem centers vital to respiration and circulation
- N_2O avoided during closure of dura
- Muscle relaxant avoided by some because of facial nerve monitoring; when used, 2–3 twitches of train-of-four usually maintained

ICD-9-CM Code: 239.6 (Brain tumor)

INDICATIONS AND USUAL TREATMENT

- Surgical indications
  - Supracerebellar infratentorial approaches to pineal region, midline, 4th ventricular lesions, CP angle tumor
- Contraindications
  - Ventriculoatrial shunt in place and open
  - Cardiac diseases
  - Hydrocephalus
  - Autonomic dysfunction
  - Extremes of age
  - Cerebral ischemic disease (stroke)

ASSESSMENT POINTS

SYSTEM	EFFECT	ASSESSMENT BY HX	PE	TEST
HEENT	Dysphagia, facial paralysis	Choking, hoarseness	ENT exam	Cine x-ray
CV	Patent foramen ovale predisposes to paradoxical air embolism	Easy fatigability	Auscultation	CXR Cardiac cath
RESP	Aspiration	Coughing	Auscultation	CXR
CNS	Ventriculoatrial shunt predisposes to venous air embolism Hydrocephalus predisposes to tension pneumocephalus	Shunt surgery	CNS exam	Head CT scan

Key Reference: Matjasko J, Petrozza P, Cohen M, Steinberg P: Anesthesia and surgery in the seated position: analysis of 554 cases. Neurosurgery 1985; 17:695–702.

PERIOPERATIVE IMPLICATIONS

Preoperative Preparation

- Antishock trouser (MAST suit)
- Precordial Doppler
- Multiorificed RA catheter
- Adequate hydration

Anesthetic Technique

- General with controlled ventilation

Monitoring

- PA catheter or CVP
- End-tidal CO_2 arterial catheter
- Precordial Doppler or TEE

Airway

- ETT may be kinked by acute flexion of neck
- Allow at least 2 fingerbreadths between chin, sternum

Induction/Maintenance

- Isoflurane, N_2O, low-dose fentanyl most common technique
- Use of short-acting NMB (for quick reversal for facial nerve monitoring)

SURGICAL STAGES

Dissection

- Sudden onset of tachycardia/bradycardia, PVCs, hypotension

Definitive Surgery

- Except for extra-axial lesions in cerebellopontine angle, surgery for pathologic Dx, and/or to reduce mass effect
- Blood loss usually not significant
- Chemo/radiation Rx

Postoperative Considerations

- Pain score: 0–5
- Minimize coughing, straining on ETT
- Cranial nerve dysfunction
- Extubation determined by extent of surgery
- Postop Htn possibly caused by brainstem compression

ANTICIPATED PROBLEMS/CONCERNS

- CV complications resulting from venous air embolism
- Tension pneumocephalus
- Cranial nerve paresis
- Macroglossia
- Failure to awaken from anesthesia: ? brainstem or subdural hematoma

ELECTROCONVULSIVE THERAPY (ECT) Laurel E. Moore, M.D.

RISK

- Prevalence of major depression: 3.2% of males, 4.5–9.3% of females
- 4% of all psychiatric admissions are for ECT

PERIOPERATIVE RISKS

- Perioperative mortality rare
- Dysrhythmias, Htn common

WORRY ABOUT

- Sympathetic stimulation producing myocardial ischemia
- Risk of dysrhythmia as a result of parasympathetic, sympathetic stimulation
- Confusion, short-term memory loss from Rx
- Adequate medical Hx frequently difficult to obtain

OVERVIEW

- Induced seizures produce multiple neuroendocrine changes ($\uparrow$ ACTH, cortisol, epinephrine, norepinephrine) effective in Rx of depression; but exact mechanism unclear

- Seizure time may be related to clinical response: $>25-<120$ sec/Rx; patients undergo $\sim 6–10$ ECT Rx (200–1000 sec of cumulative seizure time)
- Seizure induces sympathetic response, $\uparrow$ myocardial O_2 requirements in elderly
- Use of antidepressants complicates anesthesia management:
  – TCAs block reuptake of serotonin, norepinephrine, causing acute release, depleting central adrenergic stores, causing unpredictable response to indirect-acting sympathomimetics. Direct-acting sympathomimetics may cause exaggerated response; most TCAs have anticholinergic effects.
- MAOIs form irreversible complex with MAO, preventing breakdown of intraneuronal norepinephrine, serotonin, dopamine; use of an indirect-acting sympathomimetic can produce Htn crisis; direct-acting agents may also produce exaggerated response
- Lithium may prolong effects of depolarizing, certain nondepolarizing relaxants, sedatives (barbiturates). It may also $\uparrow$ incidence of confusion, memory loss from ECT; is generally discontinued before ECT.

ICD-9–CM Codes: 296.2 (Major depression, single episode); 296.3 (Major depression, recurrent episode); 311 (Depressive disorder, not elsewhere classified)

INDICATIONS AND USUAL TREATMENT

- Clinical indications:
  – Failure to respond to conventional pharmacologic Rx
  – Medical contraindication to pharmacologic Rx (e.g., cardiac conduction defect)
  – Profound depression if delay in Rx places patient at unacceptable risk for suicide
  – Controversial indications include forms of schizophrenia, mania, eating disorders, catatonia
- Relative contraindications include intracranial space–occupying lesion, recent MI, recent CVA, pheochromocytoma, longbone fractures, pregnancy
- Alternative therapies include use of antidepressants, psychotherapy

ASSESSMENT POINTS

SYSTEM	EFFECT	ASSESSMENT BY HX	PE	TEST
CV	CAD	Angina, prior MI		ECG as indicated
	$\downarrow$ LV function	$\downarrow$ Exercise tolerance	Enlarged heart	ECG/ECHO
		PND, orthopnea	JVD	as indicated
	Conduction defect	Syncope or near-syncope	Rales	Holter as indicated
			? Rhythm	
GI	GE reflux	Reflux Sx		
MS	Fracture or vertebral collapse	Pain or trauma	Palpation	X-ray of back
NS	Confusion/delirium	?Clear prior to ECT	CNS exam	Routine work-up for change in MS
PSYCHIATRIC	Competent for consent			Determined by psychiatric exam

Key Reference: Avramov MN, Husain MM: The comparative effects of methohexital, propofol, and etomidate for electroconvulsive therapy. Anesth Analg 1995; 81:596–602.

ANESTHETIC MANAGEMENT

Monitoring

- Routine
- EEG to determine adequacy, duration of seizure
- In high-risk patients consider invasive monitoring, esp for 1st few Rx

Induction/Maintenance

- GA, usually by mask
- IV induction with methohexital ($\downarrow$ seizure threshold, rapid awakening), thiopental ($\uparrow$ seizure threshold, delayed awakening), or propofol ($\downarrow$ seizure duration, rapid awakening)
- Muscle relaxation achieved with small dose of succinylcholine (0.5 mg/kg) to $\downarrow$ potential for injury from seizure

- Hyperventilation with 100% O_2 by mask before stimulus $\downarrow$ seizure threshold, possibly prolongs seizure
- Stimulus produces initial parasympathetic stimulation assoc with bradycardia, hypotension; asystole possible
- Subsequent sympathetic stimulation assoc with $\uparrow$ HR, $\uparrow$ BP, $\uparrow$ CO, $\uparrow$ myocardial O_2 consumption
- Other physiol effects include $\uparrow$ CMRO$_2$, $\uparrow$ CBF, $\uparrow$ ICP, $\uparrow$ intragastric pressure, $\uparrow$ IOP
- Vasodilators (sodium nitroprusside, nitroglycerin) and β-blockers, esmolol effective
- Bradycardias rarely require Rx

ECT Management

- Waveform, frequency, duration of stimulus adjusted to produce desired seizure
- Bilat Rx, prolonged seizure associated with $\uparrow$ memory loss

- Place, inflate BP cuff on extremity before succinylcholine admin to monitor seizure
- Seizures ideally 25–120 sec but controversial whether clinical efficacy related to seizure duration
- Patients may complain of headache or myalgias post ECT

ANTICIPATED PROBLEMS/CONCERNS

- Elderly patient in whom thorough preop interview difficult if not impossible
- Repetitive short anesthetics require efficient system to record medical Hx, allergies, drug dosages, complications, etc.
- Rx produces sympathetic activation in patient population deemed medically unfit to tolerate conventional pharmacologic Rx

ENDOSCOPIC SINUS SURGERY (ESS)

C. Daniel Chou, M.D.
Michael J. Peck, M.D.

RISK

- Common procedure
- M:F ratio, 1:1

PERIOPERATIVE RISKS

- 1.1% incidence of major complications including orbital hematoma, blindness, diplopia, CSF leak, CNS infection, stroke, carotid arterial injury, death
- 5.4% incidence of minor complications including periorbital emphysema, ecchymosis, lip pain or numbness, bronchospasm, epistaxis

WORRY ABOUT

- Asthma control preop
- Bronchospasm
- Aspiration of blood, secretion
- Blood vessel injury/bleeding
- Postop N/V

OVERVIEW

- Procedure aims to eliminate chronic infection of sinuses, allowing aeration, restoring mucociliary flow, clearance
- Major complications may result from
  - Perforation of ethmoid sinus roof
  - Dehiscence or breaking of lamina papyracea
  - Injury to optic nerve or carotid artery during sphenoidectomy
- Advantage of MAC
  - Possibility of early discharge
  - Maintain sensation of orbit, base of skull as warning signals
  - ↓ Blood loss

ICD-9-CM Code: 473.9 (Chronic sinusitis)

INDICATIONS AND USUAL TREATMENT

- Recurrent sinusitis refractory to medical Rx
- Chronic hyperplastic sinusitis with obstructive nasal polyposis
- Chronic sinusitis with mucocele formation
- Fungal sinusitis esp in immunocompromised patients including diabetics; Dx of neoplasm, orbital cellulitis (abscess unresponsive to medical Rx)
- Usual medical treatments
  - Identify and control the suspected allergen
  - Steroid
  - Antihistamine
  - Antibiotics
  - Decongestant

ASSESSMENT POINTS

SYSTEM	EFFECT	ASSESSMENT BY HX	PE	TEST
HEENT	Postnasal drip	Cough/aspiration in AM	Airway	Direct laryngoscopy
CV	Impairment due to age Toxicity from medication (e.g., theophylline)	SOB; exercise tolerance Hx of chest pain, palpitation	CV	Theophylline level ECG
RESP	40–50% of patients with Hx of asthma, 30% with multiple allergy Laryngotracheal bronchitis from chronic drip	Wheezing, allergen, systemic steroid Hx of intubation Hx of hospitalization, ER visit Voice strength and hormone Hx	Chest; listen to voice	Spirometry
GI	Theophylline toxicity	NVD, epigastric pain		Theophylline level
CNS	Rule out meningitis from sinusitis Theophylline effect	Headache, fever, N/V, double/blurred vision, mental status change Headache, irritability, reflex hyperexcitability, muscle twitching, convulsion	Neuro	Spinal tap Theophylline level

Key Reference: Levin HL, May M: Endoscopic Sinus Surgery. New York, Thieme Medical Publishers, 1993.

PERIOPERATIVE MANAGEMENT

Preoperative Preparation

- Continue bronchodilator, antihypertensive medication
- Consider stress steroid
- Topical decongestion with oxymetazoline

Anesthetic Technique

- MAC or general ET anesthesia
- Supine position with shoulder roll, head extended, flexed, or neutral (dependent on surgeon preference)

Monitoring

- Routine

Airway

- Oropharyngeal packing before surgery; removal before extubation

Induction/Maintenance

- Ketamine may potentiate effects of cocaine, epinephrine
- Avoid histamine-releasing medications
- Achieve deep anesthesia before intubation to prevent bronchospasm and optimize airway protection
- Controlled hypotension to avoid excessive blood loss

SURGICAL STAGES

- Lidocaine, epinephrine injection may cause arrhythmia, tachycardia, Htn
- Nasal septoplasty may be needed to gain access to osteomeatal complex
- Orbit palpated to prevent injury to orbit from maxillary sinus ostium seeker

- Roof of ethmoid sinus may be perforated when mucosa removed from posterior ethmoid cell
- Lamina papyracea may be breached during exposure
- Sphenoidotomy associated with injury to brain, optic nerve, carotid artery

Closure and Postoperative Considerations

- Nasal packing placed after surgery
- Remove oropharynx packing; suction oropharynx, stomach before extubation
- EBL: 100 ml
- Pain score: 4–5
- Oral opiates, NSAIDs

ENDOVASCULAR AORTIC STENT REPAIRS

Alexandru Gottlieb, M.D.

RISK

• About 10,000 aortic stents in USA/y. The number is increasing dramatically (originally was reserved only for high-risk patient, is now indicated for all patients)

PERIOPERATIVE RISKS

• Mostly related to the diffuse arteriosclerotic CV disease, unknown long-term mortality/morbidity
• Perioperative MI 5–10%
• Geriatric patients with age and other related risk factor: Htn, DM, and COPD
• Potential for thrombosis, embolization, occlusion, or bleeding

WORRY ABOUT

• Failure of deployment and need to convert to open procedure
• Leak to aortic sack—repeat endovascular intervention
• Device cost may be limiting
• Dissection of the aortic wall

OVERVIEW

• Open repair is still the "gold standard." Aortic stent repair was initially suggested for high-risk patients, but successful enough that it is currently recommended for all reconstructive aortic patients, provided that they do not have contraindication for the operation (see Indications)
• MAC, regional or general anesthesia
• Applicability will be determined by safety, efficiency, durability, cost, and patient demand

ICD-9-CM Code: 44.4 (AAA [Unruptured])

INDICATIONS AND USUAL TREATMENT

• Indication: AAA, occlusive disease, or aortic dissection
• Contraindications: 1) young patient (long-term prognosis—unknown); 2) aneurysm neck: 4 cm long, >3.5 cm wide irregular, calcified, mural circumferential thrombus; 3) renal or visceral involvement; 4) iliac artery disease: occlusive, calcified; 5) dominant inferior mesenteric artery

ASSESSMENT POINTS

SYSTEM	EFFECT	ASSESSMENT BY HX	PE	TEST
RESP	High incidence of lung disease that could have caused this procedure to be selected	Smoking, chronic cough, dyspnea	Chest exam, wheezing, clubbing, cyanosis, dyspnea	CXR, ABGs, spirometry
CV	High incidence of CAD, myocardial ischemia, and/or infarction	Angina, MI, CHF, dysrhythmia PTCA, CABG, exercise tolerance, activity level	Chest auscultation Vital signs	ECG stress test: dipyridamole, thallium, dobutamine Cardiac cath
	Chronic Htn	BP Rx, drug interaction LVH	Blood pressure	ECG, CXR Retinal funduscopy
RENAL	High incidence of renal insufficiency 2° to age, arteriosclerosis, and multiple dye studies	History of edema and intolerance to salt load	Presence of edema Anurea	Urea, Cr, electrolytes
CNS	Possible carotid disease	Syncope, stroke, or TIAs	Neuro exam Carotid bruit?	Carotid angiogram CT, MRI
ENDO	High incidence of DM	Hx of infections Stress-related/gestational DM Polydipsia, polyuria, coma/ stupor Hx of abnormal glucose	Skin infections	CNS exam Urine output Serum glucose
HEME	Some patients on perioperative heparin, t-PA, or aspirin	Hx of petechiae, nasal bleed	Presence of petechiae or clinical bleeding	PT, PTT, ACT

Key Reference: Baker B: Anesthesia for endovascular surgery. Probl Anesth 1999;11:179–192.

PERIOPERATIVE MANAGEMENT

Perioperative Evaluation

• A detailed H & P of the CVS, and medication history
• Dysrhythmias, CAD, CHF
• Hypertensive and valvular heart disease
• Noninvasive and invasive cardiac evaluation tests such as stress test and cardiac catheterization

Anesthetic Techniques

• GA, regional anesthesia, or MAC can be performed. Regional anesthesia preferred by some clinicians because of lack of systemic effect on the respiratory, cardiovascular, and gastrointestinal systems. There is some positive effect of regional anesthesia on coagulation, preserving fibrinolysis and graft patency.

• Set for possible immediate conversion to open procedure: IVs, arterial line, and CVP

Monitoring

• ECG, arterial BP, urine output
• Consider CVP or PA line in patients with severe CAD or LV impairment
• Monitoring for myocardial ischemia: ECG with continuous 3-lead ST-segment analysis, PA catheter, or TEE
• Monitoring vol replacement, CVP, PAOP, cardiac output

SURGICAL STAGES

• Percutanous or open access to both groins (femoral artery) and/or L brachial artery in case of diseased iliac artery
• Thoroughly prep, drape area (procedure can be 2–4 h, but with minimal 3rd space or blood loss)

• Involves multiple fluoroscopy and contrast injection

Postoperative Considerations

• Mild postop pain (3–4)
• Groin hematoma, seroma, or bleeding

ANTICIPATED PROBLEMS/CONCERNS

• Periop cardiac, pulmonary complications
• Thrombosis/embolization of lower limb
• Leak around aortic stent
• ↓ UO

PATHOLOGY FINDINGS

• Continuous persistent leak
• Potential for ↓ renal function
• Long-term prognosis after stent repair unavailable

ESOPHAGECTOMY

Ronald W. Pauldine, M.D.

RISK

Esophageal Carcinoma

• Squamous cell more common among African-Americans, M (3:1), tobacco abusers (4:1), alcohol abusers (6:1), Hx of achalasia, caustic burns to esophagus, Paterson-Kelly syndrome (iron-deficiency anemia, esophageal webs, glossitis)
• Adenocarcinoma more common among M; associated with Barrett's esophagus

PERIOPERATIVE RISKS

• Operative mortality less than 5%
• Periop complication rate of 10–27% including anastomotic disruption (leading to sepsis), pulmonary insufficiency, delayed emptying of intrathoracic stomach, diaphragmatic herniation of abdominal viscera, chylothorax, massive aspiration, pancreatitis, delayed splenic rupture

WORRY ABOUT

• Aspiration risk
• Hemodynamic effects of blunt dissection
• Consequences of N_2O technique if colonic interposition performed
• Recurrent laryngeal nerve injury if cervical anastomosis performed
• Consequences of perioperative TPN (hypoglycemia, $\uparrow CO_2$ production)

OVERVIEW

• Midline laparotomy to explore for metastases
• Mobilization of stomach (Kocher's maneuver), pyloromyotomy
• Mobilization of esophagus: depends on site of lesion, surgeon's preference; may occur via transhiatal approach, right (Ivor-Lewis) or left thoracotomy
• Reconstruction: stomach is preferred conduit, but colon or jejunum may be used

• Endoscopic resection more common but not completely accepted

ICD-9-CM Code: 150.9 (Esophageal carcinoma)

INDICATIONS AND USUAL TREATMENT

• Surgery only curative treatment (5-y survival as high as 70% if limited to stage I disease)
• At presentation disease is usually advanced with overall 5-y survival of only 10–15%
• Palliative Rx includes chemotherapy, combined chemo/radiation, or radiation alone
• Postop chemotherapy has not resulted in improved survival
• Preop (neoadjuvant) chemotherapy with irradiation may downstage tumors before resection; role in possible improved survival not clearly established
• If albumin low, consider preop enteral nutrition

ASSESSMENT POINTS

SYSTEM	EFFECT	ASSESSMENT BY HX	PE	TEST
HEENT	Aspiration risk, esophagorespiratory fistula, Tracheal compression	Dysphagia, heartburn, N/V		Barium swallow, CT, flow loops
CV	Chemotherapy-induced cardiomyopathy	DOE, PND, orthopnea, exercise tolerance	Auscultation, JVD, edema, hepatojugular reflex	CXR, ECHO, MUGA
RESP	Chronic aspiration	Wheezing, dyspnea	Auscultation	CXR, spirometry
GI	Malnutrition	Wt loss, fatigue	Cachexia	Serum protein, Albumin, pre-albumin
RENAL	Dehydration, Electrolyte wasting, Renal failure (nephrotoxic chemotherapy)		Orthostatic VS	BUN, Cr, Serum electrolytes
HEME	Anemia, Impaired immune function			CBC

Key Reference: Weissman C: Pulmonary function after cardiac and thoracic surgery. Anesth Analg 1999; 88:1272–1279.

PERIOPERATIVE MANAGEMENT

Anesthetic Technique

• General or combined technique
• If transhiatal or left thoracotomy approach, single-lumen ETT is adequate. Right thoracotomy approach requires placement of a double-lumen tube or bronchial blocker.

Monitoring

• Large-bore intravenous access
• Consider arterial catheter
• Consider central venous catheter

Airway

• Full-stomach precautions
• Possibility of tracheal compression if significant mediastinal lymphadenopathy
• Possible esophagorespiratory fistula (may need to maintain spontaneous ventilation)

Induction

• Potential for significant hypotension if dehydrated
• If esophagorespiratory fistula: avoid PPV, vent stomach if necessary, isolate fistula with appropriate double-lumen ETT

SURGICAL STAGES

Dissection

• Initial laparotomy
• Depending on approach may have right or left thoracotomy
• Cervical incision if cervical anastomosis to be performed (necessary with transhiatal approach)

Definitive Surgery

• Blunt dissection during transhiatal approach may result in compression of vena cava or heart with resultant hypotension or dysrhythmias

• Impaired gas exchange may occur during 1-lung ventilation if required
• EBL: 500–1500 ml

Postoperative Considerations

• High perioperative mortality due to cardiorespiratory complications, sepsis
• Significant postop pain, esp with approaches employing thoracotomy
• Pain management may include IV PCA, epidural PCA, epidural and subarachnoid narcotics, intrapleural techniques
• High likelihood of disruption of cervical anastomosis if reintubation required immediately postop; consider delayed extubation and maintenance of muscle relaxation of selected high-risk patients

ANTICIPATED PROBLEMS/CONCERNS

• Possibility for unrecognized pneumothorax with transhiatal approach

EXTRACORPOREAL MEMBRANE OXYGENATION (ECMO)

Suanne M. Daves, M.D.

RISK

- Proven utility in newborn respiratory failure
- Common causes of newborn respiratory failure are meconium aspiration, persistent fetal circulation, persistent pulmonary hypertension (PPH), congenital diaphragmatic hernia, sepsis
- May be indicated in children and adults with potentially reversible respiratory failure unresponsive to conventional therapy
- Currently used for cardiac and pulmonary support after cardiac surgery in infants and children

PERIOPERATIVE RISKS

- Survival depends on the underlying condition
- Neonatal respiratory failure has an 80% survival for those thought to have a 20% survival without ECMO

- Survival after repair of CHD in infants is largely dependent on the severity of the underlying lesion (43–54% in TOF, 14% in HLHS)

WORRY ABOUT

- Mechanical complications (cannula dislodgment, clot in circuit, air in circuit)
- Bleeding complications (particularly intracranial hemorrhage)
- Multisystem organ failure

OVERVIEW

- Provides total respiratory support with venovenous or venoarterial bypass
- Venoarterial bypass also provides total hemodynamic support
- Patient is anticoagulated to maintain an activated clotting time (ACT) of ~200 sec

ICD-9-CM Code: 756.6 (Congenital diaphragmatic hernia; 769 [RDS])

INDICATIONS AND USUAL TREATMENT

- Criteria vary among institutions
- Contraindications: congenital abnormalities not compatible with meaningful life, profound neurologic impairment, irreversible lung disease, prolonged ventilatory support (>7–10 days), estimated gestational age <35 wk, evidence of intracranial hemorrhage

ASSESSMENT POINTS

SYSTEM	EFFECT	ASSESSMENT BY HX	PE	TEST
CV	Myocardial dysfunction	Hypoxemia, acidosis	CV exam	ECHO Hemodynamic variables ABGs
	PPH	Hypoxemia R → L shunt through PDA or PFO	CV exam	ECHO Hemodynamic variables ABGs
NEURO	Hemorrhage	Intracranial hemorrhage	Neuro exam	Cranial US

Key Reference: Rais-Bahrami K, Short BL: The current status of neonatal extracorporeal membrane oxygenation. Semin Perinatol 2000; 24:406–417.

INTRAOPERATIVE MANAGEMENT

Monitoring

- ECG, temp, UO
- Arterial and central venous pressures
- Arterial and mixed venous blood gases
- Pulse oximetry if cardiac ejections present

SURGICAL STAGES

Anesthetic Choice

- Cannulation often performed at the bedside in ICU with local anesthetic infiltration. Narcotics and muscle relaxants may be used and continued while cannulas in place.
- ECMO may be initiated in OR after failure to wean from CPB

Initiating ECMO

- Venoarterial ECMO can be done with extrathoracic cannulation (carotid artery and internal jugular vein or femoral artery and vein) or by transthoracic cannulation through a median sternotomy (aorta and right atrium)
- Original cannulation sites are used after failure to wean from CPB in OR
- Right internal jugular vein is commonly used for venovenous bypass
- Heparin (100–150 units/kg) is given and the vessels are cannulated
- Bypass is initiated slowly by increasing extracorporeal flow rate
- After reaching full flow rates, ventilate at nontraumatic settings

ECMO MANAGEMENT

- Heparin to maintain ACTs at approximately 200 sec. If bleeding occurs, the ACT can be maintained at lower levels (140–180 sec).
- Platelets transfused to maintain 100,000/mm³
- As cardiopulmonary function improves, the pump flow is decreased. Prior to decannulation, the patient is given a trial without ECMO support.
- After decannulation, the vessels are usually ligated

ANTICIPATED PROBLEMS/CONCERNS

- Hypoxia and hemodynamic instability prior to bypass
- Bleeding complications
- Multiorgan failure
- Mechanical problems with ECMO circuitry

EXTRACORPOREAL SHOCK WAVE LITHOTRIPSY (ESWL)

Christopher D. Beatie, M.D.

RISK

- Incidence of urolithiasis: 1.5/1000

PERIOPERATIVE RISKS

- Shock waves can trigger cardiac dysrhythmias if not delivered during ventricular refractory period
- Shock waves can damage kidney resulting in renal hematoma, parenchymal injury with loss of renal function, hematuria, new-onset Htn
- Shock waves can cause pancreatic, hepatic injury resulting in elevations in amylase, lipase, bilirubin, lactic dehydrogenase, transaminases, CK; changes are usually mild, transient
- Hemodynamic changes associated with immersion in water bath may precipitate myocardial ischemia, MI in high-risk patients

WORRY ABOUT

- Cardiac dysrhythmias
- Cardiopulmonary derangements resulting from immersion
- Electrical safety
- Renal insufficiency
- Platelet dysfunction

OVERVIEW

- Shock waves propagated through body to pulverize urinary stones. Older lithotriptors require immersion in water bath, which complicates monitoring, airway management; regional (usually epidural) anesthesia preferred for procedures in these machines. Immersion also induces changes in cardiac/pulmonary physiology, which may be detrimental to patients with concurrent cardiac and/or pulmonary disease.
- Newer, 2nd-generation (dry) lithotriptors eliminate these problems, generate less powerful shock waves, so lighter planes of anesthesia or sedation combined with topical anesthesia may be effective

- Newest (3rd-generation) lithotriptors use piezoelectric crystals, are essentially painless; may also be used to pulverize gallstones

ICD-9-CM Codes: 592.0 (Kidney stones); 592.1 (Ureteral stones); 592.9 (Urinary stones)

INDICATIONS AND USUAL TREATMENT

- Rx of choice for upper urinary tract stones. Contraindicated in presence of morbid obesity, pacemakers, pregnancy, coagulopathy; in patients with orthopedic implants in lumbar/pelvic areas, those with intra-abd calcific processes—e.g., AAAs.
- Urolithiasis may also be Rx by adjustments in urinary pH using weak bases such as sodium bicarbonate or weak acids such as ammonium chloride
- Urinary stones can be extremely painful; patients may be taking variety of analgesic drugs including NSAIDs, opioids

ASSESSMENT POINTS

SYSTEM	EFFECT	ASSESSMENT BY HX	PE	TEST
GI	Delayed gastric emptying, gastritis, PUD	Reflux Sx, dyspepsia, abdominal pain		Hgb, endoscopy, upper GI x-ray Stool heme
HEME	Anemia (due to renal failure, GI losses) Platelet dysfunction (due to analgesia or uremia)	Fatigue Bruising, bleeding	Pallor Ecchymoses, petechiae	Hct Bleeding time
GU	Obstructive uropathy, analgesic nephritis	Oliguria, anuria, CHF Sx	Rales, edema	BUN/Cr UA, CXR

Key Reference: Tritrakarn T, Lertakyamanee J, Koompong P, et al: Both EMLA and placebo cream reduced pain during extracorporeal piezoelectric shock wave lithotripsy with the Piezolith 2300. Anesthesiology 2000; 92:1049–1054.

INTRAOPERATIVE MANAGEMENT

Preoperative Preparation

- Evaluate renal function
- Evaluate platelet function
- R/O anemia

Anesthetic Technique

- Regional anesthesia usually preferred for immersion-type lithotriptors
- Platelet dysfunction may influence decision to use regional anesthesia
- If GA used, small TV should be used to keep stone at focal point of shock wave
- Patient position in gantry requires care to avoid peripheral nerve damage
- Local anesthesia, topical anesthesia (e.g., EMLA) and/or IV sedation may be used with newer (dry) lithotriptors

Monitoring

- Easier if patient's arms not immersed
- Cover ECG leads with waterproof tape; usually lead placed on each shoulder with 3rd on left arm or high on chest wall

- If BP cuff to be immersed, use clip-type cuff (Velcro will not work)
- Pulse oximetry probes may be placed on ear or nose if fingers immersed

Airway

- Intubation or LMA indicated for GA if immersion required

Induction/Maintenance

- T4–T6 level required for regional block
- Cover epidural cath with waterproof dressing; avoid air bubbles under dressing and foam tapes (attenuate shock wave energy)
- Euthermic water bath to prevent hyperthermia or hypothermia/shivering
- 1000–4000 shocks/Rx
- Since shock waves synchronized to ECG, bradycardia can prolong Rx
- HR higher than lithotriptor's max firing rate also prolongs Rx by forcing shock waves to be triggered by every other QRS complex

EBL/Volume Concerns

- Effects of immersion in water bath
  - ↑ Venous return due to hydrostatic pressure, resulting in ↑ CO
  - Afterload, FRC, TV ↓
  - ↓ Renin, ADH secretion result in diuresis, kaliuresis, natriuresis
- Hypotension possible on emergence from water bath
- Diuretics, hydration may be used to encourage passage of stone fragments

Postoperative Considerations

- Pain scale: 1–3; NSAIDs usually sufficient
- Hematuria frequent postop—usually resolves spontaneously over several days

ANTICIPATED PROBLEMS/CONCERNS

- Lithotripsy suite often noisy, dimly lit: use caution to maintain adequate monitoring, patient safety

EYE ENUCLEATION

RISK

- 7000–10,000 operations/y in USA
- Racial predominance: none
- More common in older age group, males

PERIOPERATIVE RISKS

- Morbidity, mortality 0.1%; mortality rate related to patient's other diseases
- Oculocardiac reflex may result in bradycardia, asystole

WORRY ABOUT

- Other associated diseases of patient (DM, Htn)
- Postop N/V, pain

OVERVIEW

- Age, co-morbidity of patient
- Age of patient varies with disease of eye, but enucleation more common in older group

ICD-9-CM Code: 190.5 (Retinoblastoma)

INDICATIONS

- Tumor (melanoma, retinoblastoma)
- Blind painful eye
- Trauma

ASSESSMENT POINTS

SYSTEM	EFFECT	ASSESSMENT BY HX	PE	TEST
HEENT		Snoring	Airway exam	
CV	Associated diseases			
RESP	Co-existing diseases	SOB, exercise tolerance		O_2 sat

Key Reference: Blanc VF, Hardy JF, Milot J, Jacob JL: The oculocardiac reflex: a graphic and statistical analysis in infants and children. Can Anaesth Soc J 1983; 30:360–369.

INTRAOPERATIVE MANAGEMENT

Anesthetic Technique
- General anesthesia

Monitoring
- Routine

SURGICAL STAGES

Induction/Dissection
- ECG monitoring for oculocardiac reflex during dissection of eye muscles
- Deep level of anesthesia needed during dissecting, cutting optic nerve
- Recovery/extubation: avoid bucking, coughing that leads to venous congestion, bleeding (fentanyl, lidocaine, deep extubation an option)

Postoperative Considerations
- Postop N/V, pain
- Psychological issues
- Pain score: 3–5

ANTICIPATED PROBLEMS/CONCERNS

- Bradycardia, asystole: treat by stopping surgical stimulation with atropine, lidocaine to nerve beforehand
- Postop N/V

GAS EMBOLISM

Richard E. Moon, M.D.
Bryant W. Stolp, M.D., Ph.D.

RISK

- Injection of gas into a blood vessel during diagnostic or therapeutic procedures: cardiopulmonary bypass, cardiac catheterization, angiography, hemodialysis, pressurization of an IV bottle using air, CO_2 angiography
- Entrainment of air into a vein during surgical procedures in which venous pressure at the wound site is subatmospheric (wound higher than heart): sitting craniotomy, spine surgery, total hip replacement, dental implant surgery, C-section
- Surgery in which gas is injected into tissues: intrauterine laser surgery, laparoscopy, arthroscopy
- Other forceful instillation of gas into tissues: injury due to industrial compressed air, blowing air intravaginally during oral sex in pregnancy
- Pulmonary overexpansion, in which gas enters the pulmonary capillaries: breath-holding or regional gas-trapping during ascent from a scuba dive, positive pressure ventilation
- Hydrogen peroxide irrigation or ingestion

PERIOPERATIVE RISKS

- Gas in blood vessels or tissues can expand, if N_2O used, to 2–4 times its original volume, compounding the original injury. After initial equilibration, the ↑ in gas volume can be approximated by the following:

$$\frac{V_{new}}{V_{old}} \approx \frac{1}{1 - F_{N_2O}}$$

WORRY ABOUT

- Stroke
- Myocardial infarction
- Pulmonary edema

OVERVIEW/ETIOLOGY

- Immediate effect: obstruction of blood flow and tissue ischemia; pulm Htn if venous gas
- Secondary effect: increased permeability of vascular endothelium, tissue edema (pulm edema from venous gas)
- Tertiary effect: leukocyte accumulation on vascular endothelium, resulting in release of mediators and late reduction in blood flow
- While small venous gas emboli are prevented by the pulm capillary network from entering the arterial circulation, large volumes of gas can exceed its filtration capacity. Air can also enter the left heart via intracardiac R → L shunts.
- Venous gas embolism can cause sudden hypotension, hypoxemia, pulm Htn, or cardiac arrest. Awake individuals may experience dyspnea or tachypnea or cough.
- Arterial gas embolism is manifested by altered consciousness, acute onset of focal neurologic deficit, arrhythmias, and ST-segment elevation or depression
- Venous gas embolism is suggested by a sudden change in cardiac sounds on precordial Doppler monitor or abrupt reduction in end-tidal CO_2. If inspired gas contains no nitrogen, venous gas emboli may manifest as nitrogen in expired gas, detectable by mass spectrometer or Raman gas analyzer. Intracardiac bubbles can be detected using transthoracic or transesophageal ECHO, and cerebral bubbles by transcranial Doppler.
- Rarely, a mill-wheel murmur (a "whoosh" in both systole and diastole) can be heard by precordial stethoscope

ICD-9-CM Codes: 434.1; 958.0; 999.1

USUAL TREATMENT

- If possible, prevent further ingress of gas
- If surgical gas embolism
  - Flood surgical field with fluid
  - Lower surgical site with respect to heart
  - Elevate venous pressure (application of PEEP hazardous, as PEEP may augment R → L shunt if patient has an intracardiac defect, e.g., patent foramen ovale)
- 100% inspired O_2 to enhance oxygenation of ischemic tissues and increase nitrogen diffusion gradient from bubble into blood
- IV fluid administration to maintain intravascular volume
- Hyperbaric O_2 to effect reduction in size and rapid resolution of bubbles. Hyperbaric O_2 may inhibit endothelial leukocyte adherence. Immediate recompression treatment is most efficacious; delayed treatment can also be effective.
- Indications for hyperbaric O_2 include neurologic deficit, myocardial ischemia, or evidence of residual intravascular gas
- Experimental studies suggest that IV lidocaine infusion may be helpful
- Radiographic imaging (e.g., brain CT, MRI) to confirm the diagnosis plays no useful role

ASSESSMENT POINTS

SYSTEM	EFFECT	ASSESSMENT BY HX	PE	TEST
CV	Filling of cardiac chambers with air ↑ Permeability of vascular endothelium Tissue edema		Hypotension Mill-wheel murmur ↑ Third space fluid requirement, cerebral edema	ECG, ECHO, precordial Doppler, $ETCO_2$, ETN_2
RESP	Pulm Htn Pulm edema	Dyspnea Tachypnea Cough	↑ P_2 heart sound Crepitations on auscultation of chest	PA pressure CXR
CNS	Arterial gas embolism or transpulmonary/transcardiac passage of venous gas emboli	Mental status Acute onset of focal neurologic deficits	Neuro exam	

Key Reference: Moon RE, Camporesi EM: Clinical care at altered environmental pressure. *In* Miller RD (ed): Anesthesia, 5th ed. New York, Churchill Livingstone, 1999, pp 2271–2301.

PERIOPERATIVE IMPLICATIONS

- Consider in patients at high risk for venous gas embolism: direct arterial pressure monitoring, precordial Doppler or continuous mass spectrometry (ETN_2 and $ETCO_2$), TEE
- If gas embolization occurs, immediately discontinue N_2O
- Individuals requiring surgery who have recently suffered gas embolism or decompression sickness (in situ gas formation due to nitrogen supersaturation) from diving or compressed air exposure should not be administered N_2O anesthesia

GASTRECTOMY

Michael Webb, M.D.

RISK

• Incidence of gastric cancer in USA: 8/100,000
• Male predominance (3:1)
• ↓ Incidence 2° to ↓ incidence of gastric cancer and to medical Rx of Zollinger-Ellison syndrome

PERIOPERATIVE RISKS

• Mortality in hospital from 0−11.7% for early cancer to 25% for advanced cancer at esophagogastric junction
• Pulmonary complication: 15%
• High mortality, complication rate result from poor nutritional status of patient

WORRY ABOUT

• Malnutrition (see Diseases section)
• Anemia
• Perioperative hypovolemia
• Large third space losses

OVERVIEW

• Resection of all or part of stomach for malignant or benign conditions is common
• Periop hypovolemia from N/V, diarrhea, or GI bleeding
• Anemia may be masked by dehydration
• Regional anesthesia as an adjuvant to GA, postop epidural analgesia offers potential benefits in pulmonary mechanics, ↓ periop catabolism, effects of stress on immune system

ICD-9-CM Codes: 151.9 (Gastric cancer); 531 (Gastric ulcer)

INDICATIONS AND USUAL TREATMENT

• Total gastrectomy
  – Gastric cancer
  – Hemorrhagic gastritis
  – Zollinger-Ellison syndrome; medical management more common using H_2 blocker, misoprostol
• Partial gastrectomy
  – Gastric cancer
  – Gastric ulcers

ASSESSMENT POINTS

SYSTEM	EFFECT	ASSESSMENT BY HX	PE	TEST
CV	Hypovolemia	N/V, diarrhea Poor oral intake	Low BP, UO, orthostatic hypotension	
GI	Pulmonary aspiration	N/V	Abdominal exam	Radiologic studies
HEME	Anemia	GI bleeding	Pallor	Hct
GU	Prerenal vs. renal	↓ UO	Hydration status	BUN, Cr
MS	Malnutrition	Weight loss	Muscle wasting	Albumin

Key Reference: Komatsu H, Matsumoto S, Mitsuhata H, Abe K, Tonyabe S: Comparison of patient-controlled epidural analgesia with and without background infusion after gastrectomy. Anesth Analg 1998; 87:907−910.

PERIOPERATIVE MANAGEMENT

Preoperative Preparation

• Aspiration prophylaxis with H_2 blocker, nonparticulate antacids, metoclopramide
• Preop rehydration
• Consider preop transfusion to maintain Hct at 30 if CV disease
• Consider preop hyperalimentation if albumin < 2.1

Anesthetic Technique

• General anesthesia
• Consider adjuvant Rx intra-/postoperatively; may include epidural local anesthesia/opioids or intrathecal opioids

Monitoring

• Volume status monitoring important concern 2° to periop hypovolemia, large intraoperative third spacing, potential blood loss
• Consider CVP or PA catheter depending on co-existing disease, but frequently not needed
• Foley catheter for urine output
• Consider arterial line

Airway

• Intubation awake or using rapid-sequence induction with cricoid pressure if there is aspiration concern

Induction/Maintenance

• Prevention of hypothermia by forced warm air, warming IV fluids, using warmed humidified gas
• Epidural anesthesia/analgesia is placed preferably in low thoracic region, tested prior to induction to ensure correct placement

SURGICAL STAGES

• Exploration of abdomen before removal of malignant tumor to search for hepatic, serosal, pelvic implants; dictates procedure of choice: palliative vs. curative
• Palliative surgery indicated for pyloric stenosis, bleeding, impending perforation
• Incision upper midline, unilateral or bilateral subcostal
• Left lobe of liver retracted for exposure; ↑ peak airway pressures may occur during retraction, packing

• Omentum resected
• Splenectomy performed in total gastrectomy
• Vessels supplying stomach ligated first; stomach then resected
• Intestinal continuity restored
• Drains inserted before closure
• EBL: >500 ml for total gastrectomy
• Third space losses: ~10 ml/kg/h

Postoperative Considerations

• Pain score: 8−9
• Consider postop mechanical ventilation 2° to diaphragmatic impairment following abdominal procedure, severe abdominal discomfort, hypothermia, CV instability
• Consider ICU postoperatively
• IV PCA or epidural analgesia

ANTICIPATED PROBLEMS/CONCERNS

• Pulmonary complications from ↓ functional residual capacity (general anesthesia, abdominal surgery), poor nutrition: 15%
• Reoperation: 0−5%

GASTRIC BYPASS STAPLING FOR MORBID OBESITY

John C. Alverdy, M.D., F.A.C.S.

RISK

- 30,000/y undergo procedure
- Gender predominance: F > M (2:1)

PERIOPERATIVE RISKS

- In mild to moderate obesity (250–350 lbs), risks depend on medical co-morbidities; procedure itself does not impose any greater risk
- In the severely obese (>400 lbs), significant cardiopulmonary problems arise intraop and postop, including fluid shifts, abd closure under tension, high peak airway pressure, prolonged ventilator dependence due to need for complete muscle relaxation
- Severe sleep apnea
- Pulmonary Htn
- Cardiomyopathy of obesity
- Morbidity (~10% with 1 of following): anastomotic leak; dilation of bypassed stomach; bleeding; wound dehiscence; obstruction; postop apnea from combination of underlying sleep apnea, narcotic use
- Mortality: ~0.5%

WORRY ABOUT

- Positioning patient
- Proper OR table
- Airway
- Adequate relaxation
- Adequate anesthesia

OVERVIEW

- Gastric bypass is surgical Rx of morbid obesity designed to limit food intake, also limits desire for food
- Medical Rx of obesity in USA has recidivism rate of 98%
- Americans spend ~30 billion dollars/y trying to lose weight
- Accumulated data with 10-y follow-up demonstrate that gastric bypass achieves sustained weight loss (>50% excess wt lost) in ~75% of patients

ICD-9-CM Code: 278.0

INDICATIONS AND USUAL TREATMENT

- Patients 100 lbs over ideal body wt who have one or more of following medical co-morbidities:
  – Weight-bearing osteoarthritis, stress urinary incontinence, pseudotumor cerebri, sleep apnea syndrome, pulmonary insufficiency, cardiomyopathy, gastroesophageal reflux, Htn, diabetes mellitus, thromboembolism

ASSESSMENT POINTS

SYSTEM	EFFECT	ASSESSMENT BY HX	PE	TEST
HEENT	Tight airway	Snoring, hoarseness	Airway exam	
CV	CAD, Htn	Angina	BP	ECG, stress test
RESP	Restrictive lung disease	SOB	CV	PFTs
PERIPHERAL VASC	DVT	PE	None	

Key Reference: NIH Consensus Development Conference Proceedings: Gastrointestinal surgery for severe obesity. Am J Clin Nutr 1992; 55:478s–619s.

PERIOPERATIVE MANAGEMENT

- Patient position: check position of all extremities; do not hyperabduct arms; elevate arms on cushions so AP position physiologic
- If shoulders fall back during muscle paralysis, brachial plexopathy likely; problem in superobese when shoulders, arms very anterior to trunk
- Venodynes must be fitted preop and work before induction

Monitoring

- Consider central line after induction in superobese
- Consider PA cath if cardiopulmonary problems such as sleep apnea
- CO in superobese ranges from 10–18 L/min
- Arterial cath due to unreliable automatic devices

Airway

- Intubate; most intubations straightforward as airway is usually widely patent
- Fiberoptic intubation sometimes difficult due to large tongue, bulky hypopharynx

SURGICAL STAGES

- Induction: watch for inadequate anesthesia/muscle relaxants shortly after induction (tendency to underestimate dose requirements)
- Skin incision: midline incision from xyphoid to umbilicus
- Dissection: stomach mobilized along greater curvature to GE junction; large self-retaining retractors used; can press on RV at diaphragm; watch for ectopic ventricular beats. Spleen injury can cause sudden blood loss. Following evisceration, tendency to volume load; but upon closure CVP may be elevated.
- Definitive surgery: stomach stapled; small (30-ml) pouch created; ~100–200 cm of small intestines bypassed. Jejunojejunostomy performed to re-establish continuity; total operation usually 3 h.

- Watch for mesenteric traction syndrome as cause of sudden hypotension
- Closure/postop considerations: because of fluid shifts, extensive volume expansion may be necessary. On closure of abdomen significant ↑ in intra-abdominal pressure may impose restrictive elements to pulmonary circulation. Under these circumstances it is recommended that patient be transported to recovery facility, intubated, anesthetized.
- EBL: <500 ml
- Pain score: 6–8

ANTICIPATED PROBLEMS/CONCERNS

- Thromboembolism, infection/prophylaxis routine
- Epidural analgesia, narcotic use, sleep apnea syndrome can result in unanticipated postop apnea/respiratory arrest
- Prolonged postop ventilation needed in select cases; minimally invasive surgery may be associated with less need for prolonged postop ventilation

GASTROSCHISIS SURGERY

Peter J. Davis, M.D.

RISK

- Rare abdominal wall abnormality
- Occurs in 1/20,000 births

PERIOPERATIVE RISKS

- Increased risk of infection
- 90–100% survival reported

WORRY ABOUT

- Large fluid requirements
- Temperature instability
- Cardiopulmonary compromise 2° to ↑ intra-abdominal pressure
- Postop ventilation
- Postop nutrition
- Postop infection
- Other congenital abnormalities

OVERVIEW

- Extrusion of abdominal contents through a defect *TO THE RIGHT* of the umbilical cord. Must be differentiated from omphalocele.
- True surgical emergency
- Abdominal contents not covered by sac
- Abdominal viscera matted together and thickened 2° to amniotic fluid exposure and chemical peritonitis
- 60% of patients are premature
- Associated abnormalities (other than GI) rare, but their presence may affect patient morbidity and mortality
- GI abnormalities include intestinal atresia and stenosis

ICD-9-CM Code: 756.7 (Congenital)

USUAL TREATMENT

- Medical management
  – Wrap exposed viscera in saline-soaked gauze
  – NG tube to decompress abdominal contents
  – Antibiotics
  – Treat CV and resp instability
- Increased fluid requirements, large 3rd space fluid losses
- Temperature instability
- Surgery definitive treatment
  – Spring-loaded silo may obviate surgery

ASSESSMENT POINTS

SYSTEM	EFFECT	ASSESSMENT BY HX	PE	TEST
CV	Impaired transitional circulation	Cyanosis and acidosis	Poor capillary refill	CXR, ECHO
	Hypotension 2° to hypovolemia	Poor UO	Poor perfusion	SaO$_2$
		Poor tissue perfusion		BP
			Poor UO	ABGs
	Hypotension 2° to ↑ intra-abdominal pressure	Poor UO		
		Poor tissue perfusion; cold lower extremities; vascular congestion; Cyanosis		
RESP	Surfactant deficiency 2° to prematurity	Tachypnea	Auscultation	ABGs
	Restrictive lung disease 2° to ↑ intra-abdominal pressure	Hypoxemia		↓ Pulm compliance
METAB	Large 3rd space fluid requirements	Review of volume replacement	Skin perfusion	BP
	Hyper-/hyponatremia		UO	Electrolytes
TEMP	Hypothermia 2° to large heat loss from large 3rd space fluid requirements			

Key Reference: Snyder CL: Outcome analysis for gastroschisis. J Pediatr Surg 1999; 34:1253–1256.

PERIOPERATIVE IMPLICATIONS

Anesthetic Technique

- GA
- Endotracheal intubation
- Avoid N$_2$O

Monitoring

- Pulse oximeters on both the right upper extremity and a lower extremity
- Adequate venous access preferably above the diaphragm
- Consider arterial catheter
- Consider central venous catheter
- Foley catheter

Airway

- Expect usual neonatal variants
- Endotracheal intubation
- Avoid distention of bowel by bag/mask ventilation
- Muscle relaxation required

Induction

- CV instability 2° to hypovolemia
- Avoid N$_2$O

SURGICAL STAGES

Dissection

- Care in bowel manipulation
- Blood loss 2° to adhesions
- Hypotension from bowel manipulation, blood loss, and large 3rd space fluid requirements

Definitive Surgery

- Four surgical options:
  – Primary fascial closure,
  – Skin closure,
  – Prosthetic silo with delayed closure, *or*
  – Insertion of Silastic spring-loaded silo
- All options associated with ↑ intra-abdominal pressure. With abdominal closure: if intragastric pressure > 20 mmHg and CVP changes by > 4 mmHg, consider silo. If intragastric pressure < 20 mmHg and CVP changes < 4 mmHg, consider primary repair.
- All surgical closure options associated with ↑ risk of sepsis
- Spring-loaded silo may obviate surgery

POSTOPERATIVE CONSIDERATIONS

- Need for mechanical ventilation
- Need for hyperalimentation
- In patients with silo, gradual reduction of abdominal contents, ↑ risk of sepsis, and prolonged ventilatory requirements

ANTICIPATED PROBLEMS/CONCERNS

- Hypovolemia 2° to large 3rd space fluid requirements
- Instability 2° to ↑ intra-abdominal pressure following abdominal wall closure
- Decrease in lung compliance 2° to impaired diaphragmatic movement from reduced abdominal contents and ↑ intra-abdominal pressure
- Prolonged postop pain relief may be required
- ↑ Risk of necrotizing enterocolitis

GERIATRIC SURGERY

Timothy M. Bittenbinder, M.D.
Charles H. McLeskey, M.D.

RISK

- 13% of USA population > 65 y, 17–20% by 2030

PERIOPERATIVE RISKS

- Multiple concomitant diseases are the rule, not the exception
- Atherosclerosis, Htn, renal disease, mental dysfunction most common concomitant diseases

WORRY ABOUT

- ↑ Risk for perioperative morbidity/mortality, more dramatic in emergent surgery

- Physiologic changes with aging result in ↑ pharmacologic sensitivity of elderly to many anesthetic drug classes

OVERVIEW

- Most commonly refers to patients > 65 y
- Aging changes important in perioperative period including cardiac, pulmonary, CNS, renal, hepatic decrement in function, loss of physiologic reserve
- Age-related disease combines with age-related ↓ in basic organ function to contribute to ↑ risk for perioperative complications, death

ETIOLOGY

- Birth a long time ago
- Degree of management of environmental exposure, resulting in ↑ or ↓ physiologic age (RealAge) in relation to chronologic age

USUAL TREATMENT

- None specific other than specific disease-related Rx and age-reduction strategies such as keeping BP at 115/75, physical fitness, strength, dietary fat restriction; antioxidant or vitamin E, C, folate, and D use still somewhat experimental

ASSESSMENT POINTS

SYSTEM	EFFECT	ASSESSMENT BY HX	PE	TEST
HEENT	Inadequate mask fit, difficult laryngoscopy	Presence of dentures	State of dentition ROM of cervical spine and TMJ, facial contour changes	
CV	↑ Systolic BP, concentric hypertrophy of LV, mild aortic dilation, ↑ SVR, ↑ PAP, ↓ max HR, ↓ responsiveness to atropine and sympathomimetics Incidence of concomitant CAD very high in elderly; many subclinical Age-dependent ↓ in CO, cardiac reserve found in all but active, healthy geriatric patients; CO maintained in "healthy" elderly patients but at cost of ↑ filling pressure	Exercise tolerance, CAD Hx, Sx of CAD		ECG Stress test as indicated ↑ HR may be less reliable test of an intravascular epidural catheter with epinephrine-containing test doses
RESP	Reduction in vital capacity, total lung capacity, max breathing capacity, ↓ FVC Age-induced parenchymal changes mimic emphysema, creating V/Q mismatch, age-related ↓ in resting PaO_2 Ventilatory response to hypoxia or hypercapnia ~ ½ that seen in young patients Above physiologic changes of aging greatly affected by concomitant pulm disease	Exercise tolerance		Consider CXR, PFT Anticipated: PaO_2 = 100 − [0.4 × age (y)] mmHg
GI	↓ Hepatic size, blood flow			
RENAL	Age-related ↓ in glomerular filtration, tubular function			Small elevations in serum Cr may represent large ↓ in renal function in elderly due to age-related reduction in muscle mass, Cr production
CNS	↓ Requirement for anesthetic agents, both inhalation, IV Greater sensitivity to inhalation agents, benzodiazepines, opioids due to pharmacodynamic changes Risk of postop delirium ↑ with ↑ age	Preop mentation		"Test dose" of pentothal before induction

Key Reference: McLeskey CH (ed): Geriatric Anesthesiology. Philadelphia, Lippincott Williams & Wilkins, 1996.

PERIOPERATIVE IMPLICATIONS

Preoperative Preparation

- Light or no sedative premed

Monitoring

- Generally should be more intense
- Individual patient assessment critical

Airway

- Laryngeal, pharyngeal, airway reflexes less effective in older patients
- Optimal head position important because laryngoscopy is more difficult, and vertebrobasilar insufficiency more common

Induction

- Consider regional anesthesia (reduce dose 4–5%/decade)
- All common induction agents require smaller dose (4–5%/decade of RealAge) for induction of GA; injecting IV induction agents slowly permits titration of dose for required effect

Maintenance

- MAC of inhalational agent ↓ in elderly (4–5%/decade after 20 y)
- Keep warm: periop hypothermia more common due to ↓ BMR, ↓ shivering threshold, ↓ compensatory peripheral vasoconstriction

Extubation

- ↑ Risk for hypothermic complications
- At ↑ risk for passive aspiration
- Consider supplemental O_2

Adjuvants

- Muscle relaxants: initial dosing is same as with younger patients; duration of action longer with all agents other than atracurium, cisatracurium

ANTICIPATED PROBLEMS/CONCERNS

- Starting low, going slow with all drugs critical to safe perioperative care

GI ENDOSCOPY/EGD, NON–OPERATING ROOM ANESTHESIA

Aisling Conran, M.D.

RISK

- Children may have this procedure due to Hx of N/V, abdominal pain, GE reflux
- Gender predominance: none

PERIOPERATIVE RISK

- Aspiration risk
- Risk of perforation: rare

WORRY ABOUT

- Sharing the airway with endoscopist
- Maintaining the same standards as in the OR

OVERVIEW

- Endoscopy and biopsies of esophagus, stomach, and duodenum for evidence of ulcers, bleeding

INDICATIONS AND USUAL TREATMENT

- Diagnostic exam to evaluate Hx of N/V, abdominal pain, or reflux; or a follow-up exam to evaluate the effects of drug Tx

ASSESSMENT POINTS

SYSTEM	EFFECT	ASSESSMENT BY HX	PE	TEST
HEENT				
CV				
RESP		Asthma	Wheezing	Peak expiratory flow rate
GI	Aspiration risk	GE reflux, N/V		
HEME	Anemia	Hematemesis or blood in stools		
CNS				

Key Reference: Mackenzie RA, Southorn PA, Stensrud PE: Anesthesia at remote locations. *In* Miller RD (ed): Anesthesia, 5th ed. New York, Churchill Livingstone, 1999, pp 2241–2269.

PERIOPERATIVE MANAGEMENT

Preoperative Preparation

- Both patients and parents may be very anxious
- Consider premedication with metoclopramide and famotidine
- Consent for sedation/GA

Anesthetic Technique

- Consider IV sedation in ≥10 y olds, mask induction/GA in younger children

Monitoring

- Same standards as in OR. O_2 sat, NIBP, ECG standard. $ETCO_2$ used if GA.

Airway

- Decision to intubate based on patient Hx, risk of aspiration, and age of child. With infants and smaller children, maintaining the airway during EGD without an ETT is fraught with difficulty.

Induction/Maintenance

- Mask vs. IV. Consider EMLA cream for IV and parental presence at induction.

SURGICAL STAGES

- Short procedures; in children biopsy almost always done due to difficulty of repeating the exam

Blood Loss and Volume Concerns

- Minimal, even if biopsy done

Postop Considerations

- N/V. Recovery area nearby. Monitoring and O_2 if transporting to PACU. Discharge criteria.

ANTICIPATED PROBLEMS/CONCERNS

- Parental and patient anxiety

GIFT PROCEDURE
Bernard Wittels, M.D., Ph.D.

RISK

- Infertility affects 3 million couples in USA

Age (y)	Male Factor	Live Deliveries (%)
<35	Absent	36
35–39	Absent	28
>39	Absent	15
<35	Present	34
35–39	Present	34
>39	Present	17

PERIOPERATIVE RISKS

- Perioperative mortality nil
- Anesthetic morbidity:
  - Local: none
  - Spinal: headache   2–37%
  - Epidural: headache   0.5–5%
  - General: nausea   18–78%
             emesis   16–92%
- Failed fertilization   65%
- Successful fertilization   35%
  - Ectopic pregnancy   0.4%
  - Multiple delivery   33%
  - Birth defects   2%
  - Neonatal death   1%

WORRY ABOUT

- Drug effects on oocyte fertilization, implantation, growth, development
- CO_2 insufflation requires hyperventilation
- Residual peritoneal CO_2 causes diaphragmatic, subscapular pain
- CO_2 can be insufflated/injected into unintended areas: air embolism possible

OVERVIEW

- Young, female outpatients have ↑ risk of postop N/V
- ↑ Ventilatory demands with regional, GA

ICD-9-CM Code: 628.9 (Infertility, female)

INDICATIONS

- Primary or secondary infertility:
  - Endometriosis
  - Ovulatory disorders
  - Male-factor infertility
  - Unexplained infertility
- Criteria:
  - Ovulation (serum LH, US)
  - Adequate luteal phase (serum progesterone)
  - Normal endometrium (biopsy)
  - Normal TSH, T_4, prolactin
  - Tubal patency (laparoscopy or hysterosalpingogram)
  - Normal semen analysis

USUAL TREATMENT

- Clomiphene, hCG, Gn-RH analogues
- Chromotubation, tuboplasty
- In vitro fertilization

ASSESSMENT POINTS

SYSTEM	EFFECT	ASSESSMENT BY HX	PE	TEST
RESP	↑ Workload	Asthma, smoking, obesity	Auscultation	Pulse oximetry
GI	Adhesions	Previous abdominal surgery	Scar survey	
GU	Tubal patency	Previous infection, surgery		Hysterosalpingogram

Key Reference: Beilin Y, Bodian CA, Mukherjee T, et al: The use of propofol, nitrous oxide, or isoflurane does not affect the reproductive success rate following gamete intrafallopian transfer (GIFT). Anesthesiology 1999; 90:36–41.

PERIOPERATIVE MANAGEMENT

Anesthetic Technique

- Local anesthetic with US
- Spinal, epidural, or GA for laparoscopy or laparotomy

Monitoring

- Routine

Induction/Maintenance

- Propofol, N_2O, midazolam, and isoflurane do not alter success rates for pregnancy or delivery

SURGICAL STAGES

Trocar Introduction

- Adhesions of intestines to anterior abdominal wall ↑ risk of bowel perforation
- Traumatic trocar placement may perforate bowel, bladder, blood vessel

CO_2 Insufflation

- ↑ Intragastric pressure, ↑ CO_2 absorption requires ↑ ventilation (↑ rate to avoid barotrauma with ↑ PIP)

Postoperative Considerations

- Mild abdominal pain after laparoscopy
- EBL: minimal
- Pain score: 2–4
- Residual peritoneal CO_2 may cause subdiaphragmatic or subscapular discomfort
- Ibuprofen may suffice

ANTICIPATED PROBLEMS/CONCERNS

- Excessive postop pain warrants evaluation for peritoneal trauma

HEART TRANSPLANT (ADULT)
Leonard Firestone, M.D.

- ~ 14,000 candidates/y with end-stage heart disease (HD) in USA; most common Dx ischemic cardiomyopathy
- ~ 1800 orthotopic procedures/y in USA, limited by suitable donor organ availability
- Overwhelmingly male; no unambiguous racial predominance for end-stage HD

PERIOPERATIVE RISKS

- Early (30-day) mortality: ~ 8% due to surgical technique complications; fulminant rejection or infection; reperfusion injury
- Early morbidity from nosocomial bacterial infection (*Pneumococcus* pneumonia, *Pseudomonas* sepsis); later opportunistic infection with *Pneumocystis carinii*, *Candida* spp, CMV

WORRY ABOUT

- *Recipient heart* usually compromised by low cardiac index; ventricular irritability; mediastinal adhesions from prior cardiac surgery; chronic pulmonary Htn (but transpulmonary

gradient [= MPAP−MLAP] must be < 15 mmHg)
- *Donor heart* (allograft) function may be compromised after CPB by transient pulmonary vasospasm, reperfusion injury, prolonged ischemia, atypical drug responses (see Anticipated Problems/Concerns)
- Mural thromboembolism before CPB or systemic air embolism after CPB from completely "open" heart
- Allograft dysfunction from prolonged ischemia (function ↓ after 4–6 h); may be due to technical problems or poor coordination of donor-recipient teams
- Hyperacute rejection (rare with ABO matches)
- Pulmonary gastric aspiration (all procedures emergencies)

OVERVIEW

- Transplantation markedly improves survival of end-stage heart disease patients
- In standard midatrial orthotopic procedure, native heart (except for post atrial walls) re-

placed by donor heart in normal anatomic location
- Rejection, infection, reperfusion injury, hemorrhage are major causes of perioperative morbidity/mortality
- Stroke from air or thromboembolism may also occur

ICD-9-CM Code: 425.40 (Cardiomyopathy)

INDICATIONS AND USUAL TREATMENT

- *Specific indication:* End-stage heart disease (NYHA Class IV = severely compromised status with guarded prognosis) unimproved by maximal medical Rx
- *Maximal medical Rx* usually includes oral inotropes, ACE, PDE III inhibitors, diuretics, antiarrhythmics
- Only *absolute contraindication:* irreversible pulmonary Htn (transpulmonary gradient > 15 mmHg)

ASSESSMENT POINTS

SYSTEM	EFFECT	ASSESSMENT BY HX	PE	TEST
CV	Biventricular failure	Exercise intolerance Orthopnea PND	JVD Liver edge ↓	R & L heart cath
RESP	Pulmonary edema	Orthopnea	Rales	CXR
RENAL	Prerenal azotemia	PND, nocturia		BUN/Cr
CNS	Poor perfusion	Confusion?	Mental status	
HEPATIC	Chronic congestion	RUQ fullness/pain	Liver edge	LFTs

Key Reference: Firestone L: Heart transplantation. *In* Firestone L, Firestone S (eds): Transplantation, Anesthesia and Critical Care Medicine Procedures at the University of Pittsburgh. Boston, Butterworth, 1996.

INTRAOPERATIVE MANAGEMENT

Monitoring

- PA cath with long sheath (to facilitate withdrawal during cardiac anastomoses, use of caval snares); placement may be complicated by AFIB, TR, RV dilation, low CO; RIJ vein appropriate location
- TEE useful to optimize vol; rule out mural thrombus pre-CPB; assist in de-airing during CPB; rule out mediastinal tamponade postop

Airway

- To minimize nosocomial pneumonia risk, bacterial filter placed in anesthesia circuit

Blood Products

- Only CMV-neg blood products used for seroneg recipients, to avoid CMV sepsis
- Leukocyte-filtered or γ-irradiated blood unnecessary to avoid alloimmunization during transplant
- FFP and/or vit K may be required if on chronic warfarin
- Bleeding may be profuse, lead to coagulopathy, if transplant follows a prior cardiac procedure

Anesthetic Technique

- IV premed judiciously
- Azathioprine often infused ASAP after arrival in OR

- GA regimen should be least perturbing to precarious CV status; also, full-stomach precautions essential during induction
- Phenylephrine, inotrope, judicious vol infusion may then be required to optimize CO

SURGICAL STAGES

Dissection

- Cardiomegaly and/or prior cardiac surgery ↑ risk of RV or innominate vein laceration
- Epicardial irritability can lead to VFIB
- Redo surgery is associated with protracted pre-CPB interval
- With LV mural thrombus, cardiac manipulation can lead to systemic embolism

Definitive Surgery

- Bicaval cannulation for CPB mandatory due to atrial anastomoses; SVC pressure must be scrupulously monitored to avoid intracranial Htn
- Cardiectomy not performed until just before donor organ arrival
- After atrial, great vessel anastomoses, aortic crossclamp removed ASAP to end ischemia; methylprednisolone 500 mg IV used to prevent hyperacute rejection

Weaning/Post-CPB Considerations

- Inotrope usually required to support HR (due to denervation, contractility (due to mild reperfusion injury)

- Pulmonary vasospasm possibility transiently seen; treated with PGE_1 infusion (0.025−0.1 μg/kg/min)
- Typical transfusion requirement 2–4 units of packed RBCs
- Pain management same as that following CABG

ANTICIPATED PROBLEMS/CONCERNS

- Atypical responses to cardioactive drugs by denervated donor heart—e.g., indirect-acting agents (e.g., atropine) fail to produce expected cardiac effects (tachycardia); thus only direct-acting agents should be used (e.g., isoproterenol); but, denervation supersensitivity to catecholamines, a theoretical concern, is NOT clinically relevant
- Persistently slow junctional rhythms lead to need for permanent pacemakers in ~ 5% of recipients
- Rejection marked by low CO and arrhythmias

Pathology Findings

- Myocardial fibrosis, edema, necrosis, or (in appropriate cases) infiltration with amyloid deposits; coronary atherosclerosis
- May also see patent foramen ovale; congenital cardiac lesions leading to Eisenmenger's physiology

HEART TRANSPLANT (PEDIATRIC)

Susan Firestone, M.D.
Leonard Firestone, M.D.

See also Heart Transplant (Adult) in Procedures section

RISK

• ~3000 neonatal candidates/y with hypoplastic heart syndrome or equivalent; that number does not include older children with complex congenital end-stage heart disease, or idiopathic or viral cardiomyopathy
• ~250 orthotopic pediatric procedures/y in USA, limited by organ availability
• No unambiguous gender or racial predominance; bimodal age distribution, with peaks in those < 1 y, adolescents

PERIOPERATIVE RISKS

• Early (30-day) mortality: ~25% in patients < 1 y due to technical complications; ~10% in adolescents due to same factors as in adults
• Early morbidity in patients < 1 y from acute rejection; viral infection (CMV, adenovirus)

WORRY ABOUT

• Pulm Htn common in neonatal recipients
• Mediastinal adhesions from prior cardiac surgery and chronic pulm Htn

• Donor heart (allograft) intrinsic rate often too slow in neonatal recipients, necessitating mech or pharmacologic chronotropic support
• Deep hypothermic circulatory arrest always needed for neonatal procedures
• Cardiac index may be compromised after CPB
• Systemic air embolism after CPB

OVERVIEW

• Treatment alternative to complete repair of complex lesions with superior early real survival (70%, vs. < 60% at 1 y for complex repairs)
• Standard midatrial orthotopic procedure as for adults, except aortic arch reconstruction necessary in neonates with hypoplastic left heart syndrome
• Surgical technical difficulties, hemorrhage, reperfusion injury, rejection, infection cause perioperative morbidity/mortality
• Seizures common in infant recipients, especially after circulatory arrest

ICD-9-CM Codes: 746.9 (Congenital HD); 425.40 (Cardiomyopathy)

INDICATIONS AND USUAL TREATMENT

• Specific indications: univentricular anatomy, esp hypoplastic left heart syndrome; pulm atresia with intact ventricular septum in neonates; end-stage heart disease for adolescents with cardiomyopathy (NYHA class IV = severely compromised status with guarded prognosis) unimproved by max medical Rx
• No long-term alternative medical Rx for hypoplastic left heart syndrome; alternative surgical Rx is Norwood's procedure (neoaortic reconstruction, creation of central aortic-to-pulm artery shunt), but high mortality
• Max medical Rx for cardiomyopathy in adolescents is similar to that for adults
• Same general conditions for other organ transplant candidates apply, as in adults
• Only absolute medical contraindication is irreversible pulm Htn (transpulmonary gradient > 15 mmHg); unfavorable social milieu may also contraindicate pediatric transplantation

ASSESSMENT POINTS

SYSTEM	EFFECT	ASSESSMENT BY HX	PE	TEST
Neonates with Hypoplastic Left Heart Syndrome:				
CV	Systemic hypoperfusion	Poor systemic perfusion Cyanosis rarely	Low BP, tachypnea	ECHO Cath (rare) ABGs: low pH
RESP	Pulm overperfusion	Tachypnea	Rales Resp distress	CXR
GU	Prerenal axotemia	Oliguria		BUN/Cr
HEPATIC	Systemic hypoperfusion	Liver		LFTs abn

Key Reference: Firestone S, Firestone L: Pediatric organ transplantation. *In* Churchill-Davidson HC (ed): Wylie and Churchill-Davidson's A Practice of Anesthesia, 6th ed. Chicago, Mosby, 1995, pp 1190–1204.

INTRAOPERATIVE MANAGEMENT

Monitoring

• Neonates with hypoplastic left heart syndrome require a short, high internal jugular cath (bicaval cannulation obligatory)
• Frequent ABGs to detect inadequate systemic perfusion
• Management of older children with cardiomyopathy analogous to that of adults

Blood Products

• Only CMV-neg blood products, organs used for neonates, to avoid CMV sepsis
• Plt dysfunction, clotting factor consumption may lead to profuse bleeding after hypothermic circulatory arrest

Anesthetic Technique

• Management of children with cardiomyopathy analogous to that for adults
• In neonates with hypoplastic left heart syndrome, overriding goal is to maintain proper balance between systemic and pulm perfusion. Hyperventilation, high FIO_2 must be avoided, otherwise pulm overperfusion results; admin of hypoxic gas mixtures ($FIO_2 = 0.15–0.18$) with exogenous CO_2 may be necessary; targets are $SaO_2 = 75\%$, pH = 7.3–7.4.

• Azathioprine is usually infused ASAP after arrival in OR
• Induction, maintenance of GA is frequently accomplished with narcotics (e.g., fentanyl 25–50 μg/kg), supplemented with vagolytic muscle relaxants to avoid bradycardia

SURGICAL STAGES (with hypoplastic left heart syndrome)

Dissection

• Branch PA isolated early, to allow tight control of pulmonary blood flow
• For CPB, arterial cannula placed in main PA; venous cannulation is bicaval

Definitive Surgery

• Long segment of donor aorta used to reconstruct aortic arch to level of ductal insertion
• Arterial cannula removed during circulatory arrest; after arch reconstruction, replaced in neoaorta, CPB resumed
• SVC pressure must be scrupulously monitored to avoid intracranial Htn

• After atrial and great vessel anastomoses, aortic crossclamp removed ASAP to end ischemia; methylprednisolone 10 mg/kg IV used to prevent hyperacute rejection

Weaning/Post-CPB Considerations

• Inotrope (e.g., dobutamine 5 μg/kg/min) usually infused to support HR (due to denervation), contractility due to mild reperfusion injury
• Pulm vasospasm may be seen transiently; Rx with PGE_1 infusion (0.025–0.1 μg/kg/min) or N_2O
• Typical transfusion requirement: 1–2 U pRBCs; 2 U platelets; 2 U cryoprecipitate

ANTICIPATED PROBLEMS/CONCERNS

• Donor HR commonly requires support after neonatal transplantation to preserve CO
• Atypical responses to cardioactive drugs similar to those in adults. Denervation supersensitivity to catecholamines *not* clinically relevant.
• Rejection episodes (low CO, low ECG voltage) common, Rx with glucocorticoid boluses, poss OKT3
• Late morbidity from accelerated coronary atherosclerosis; lymphoproliferative disorders; nephrotoxicity from immunosuppressants

HERNIORRHAPHY

Douglas S. Snyder, M.D.

RISK

- Groin hernias: 680,000/y
- Gender predominance:
  - Inguinal: M:F 9:1
  - Femoral: M:F 1:3
  - Abdominal: M:F 7:13

PERIOPERATIVE RISKS

- Perioperative mortality rare ($< 0.3\%$)
- Higher mortality/morbidity if strangulated bowel
- Risk related to co-morbidities
- Morbidity: wound abscess, hematoma

WORRY ABOUT

- Appropriateness of surgery as outpatient
- Possible strangulated bowel, sepsis
- Vagal stimulation with retraction, resultant bradycardia
- Postop urinary retention
- Spinal headache: incidence $\leq 3\%$ with 25-gauge needle

OVERVIEW

- Procedure performed for repair of abd wall (epigastric, femoral, incisional, umbilical)
- May be uncomplicated or may be complicated with bowel contents
- Strangulated hernia with necrotic bowel can be associated with sepsis syndrome
- May require bowel resection if necrotic
- Laparoscopic hernia repair currently performed; exact role poorly defined

ICD-9-CM Codes: 550–553.9

INDICATIONS AND USUAL TREATMENT

- Uncomplicated hernia: elective surgery, binder, truss
- Incarcerated hernia: urgent surgery
- Strangulated hernia: emergent surgery

ASSESSMENT POINTS

SYSTEM	EFFECT	ASSESSMENT BY HX	PE	TEST
CV	Potential of sepsis		HR, BP	Invasive monitor
GI	Reflux, obstruction	Reflux Sx, emesis		
HEME	Coagulation DIC if necrotic bowel	ASA use		PT, PTT, fibrinogen, FSP

Key Reference: Rutkow IM: A selective history of groin herniorrhaphy in the 20th century. Surg Clin North Am 1993; 73:395–411.

PERIOPERATIVE IMPLICATIONS

Preoperative Preparation

- Determine appropriateness of outpatient procedure

Anesthetic Technique

- Local, regional, GA, or combined anesthetic technique
- Local anesthesia ± sedation preferred for appropriate cases
- Local anesthesia permits patient to strain, cough during procedure if desired by surgeon
- Consider local wound or nerve infiltration for postop pain control
- Laparoscopic surgery, strangulated hernia require GA

Monitoring

- Routine
- Consider arterial line, CVP, PA cath if signs of sepsis

Airway

- Routine

Induction

- Require level of at least T8 for regional
- Local infiltration of ilioinguinal, iliohypogastric nerves

SURGICAL STAGES

Dissection

- Depends on hernia site

Definitive Surgery

- Inguinal hernia most common: transversalis aponeurosis, internal oblique fascia sutured to shelving edge of inguinal ligament
- Prosthetic mesh can be used for all sites to relieve tension
- Incisional hernia may require intraperitoneal approach
- EBL: 50–100 ml

Postoperative Considerations

- Postop pain depends on site, use of local infiltration
- Pain score: 3 (local)–6

- Important to void before discharge if outpatient
- Consider stool softener for inguinal hernias to avoid strain

ANTICIPATED PROBLEMS/CONCERNS

- Bradycardia during peritoneal retraction
- Potential for necrotic bowel

HIP FRACTURE REPAIR

Meg A. Rosenblatt, M.D.

RISK

- Elderly patients (femoral neck, intertrochanteric, subtrochanteric, intracapsular Fx through osteoporotic bone)
- Young patients (traumatic Fx)
- Pathologic Fx
- 5–100 Fx/100,000
- M:F ratio 1:4–5

PERIOPERATIVE RISKS

- Cardiac, CNS, accident/fall–seek cause of Fx
- Perioperative fluid deficiency—large volumes of blood in leg or thigh after Fx
- Fat embolism syndrome
- Geriatric patients with multiple co-morbidities

OVERVIEW

- Commonly performed procedures
- Goal is reduction and stabilization of Fx to allow mobilization
- 7-Day mortality 1.3–1.6%
- 30-Day mortality 4.4–5.4%

ICD-9-CM Code: 820.x

INDICATIONS AND USUAL TREATMENT

- Nondisplaced neck Fx treated with closed reduction and percutaneous pinning
- ORIF with dynamic hip screws or other sliding nail fixations for inter- or subtrochanteric Fx
- Cemented or uncemented hemiarthroplasty prostheses for intracapsular Fx

ASSESSMENT POINTS

SYSTEM	EFFECT	PE	TEST
CV	Hypotension 2° to hypovolemia vs. fat embolism	Tachycardia Right-sided heart failure	ECG ST-segment abnormalities PA pressures, ECHO
RESP	Fat embolism syndrome	Tachypnea Pulmonary Htn	Pulmonary infiltrates on x-ray ABGs O_2 sat
HEME	Blood loss 2° to Fx	Orthostatic hypotension	Hct
CNS	Senile dementia vs. fat embolism syndrome	Confusion, agitation, stupor, coma, cerebral edema	Neuro assessment CT scan
GU	Fat embolism syndrome		Fat globules in urine
DERM	Fat embolism syndrome	Petechiae on chest, extremities, conjunctivae	

Key Reference: O'Hara DA, Duff A, Berlin JA, Poses RM, Lawrence VA, Huber EC, Noveck H, Strom BL, Carson JL: The effect of anesthetic technique on postoperative outcomes in hip fracture repair. Anesthesiology 2000; 92:947–957.

PERIOPERATIVE MANAGEMENT

Preoperative Preparation

- Early surgery indicated in premorbidly fit patients
- Surgery delayed if correctable co-morbidities
- Considerable preoperative pain—consider femoral nerve block, analgesics

Anesthetic Technique

- No association between type of anesthesia and postop mortality
- ↑ Use of vasopressors and arrhythmia associated with neuraxial anesthesia
- Isobaric spinal anesthesia may limit level of sympathectomy, thus hypotension
- Regional anesthesia reduces incidence of DVT, intraop blood loss, and need for airway manipulations
- Paramedian approach to neuraxial blocks 2° to inability to reduce lumbar lordosis
- Prophylactic antibiotics strongly suggested

Monitoring

- Consider arterial monitoring if underlying severe Htn, pulmonary Dx, or hypovolemia
- PA cath if significant cardiac disease
- Urinary drainage catheters—retention vs. UTI

SURGICAL STAGES

- Performed on Fx table, which allows manipulation of Fx and radiographic evaluation
  - Arms frequently across chest or in overhead slings—avoid antecubital IVs
  - Avoid compression injuries from perineal post
- Lateral position for hemiarthroplasty
  - Dependent shoulder compresses brachial plexus—place axillary roll
  - Meticulous padding of pressure points
  - Embolism of air, fat, or bone fragments during insertion of femoral prosthesis with associated systemic hypotension and pulmonary Htn
- Aggressive warming to decrease blood loss
- EBL < 100 to > 500 ml

Postoperative Considerations

- Thromboembolic prophylaxis
- Mortality rate varies in association with poorly controlled systemic disease, cognitive disorders, and absence of DVT prophylaxis
- Multidisciplinary approach using skilled medical, nursing, and paramedical care to maximize rehabilitation potential

ANTICIPATED PROBLEMS/CONCERNS

- Be wary of elderly patients with normal-range hematocrits
- Fat embolism syndrome may be 2° to direct release of fatty acids, which cause capillary endothelial breakdown. Pericapillary hemorrhagic exudates are found in the lungs and brain. Require supportive care, often including mechanical ventilation, and vigilant fluid management.

HYPOSPADIAS REPAIR

M. Emily White, M.D.

RISK

- 8/1000 male births
- May require multiple operative procedures to correct

PERIOPERATIVE RISKS

- Patients usually otherwise healthy

WORRY ABOUT

- Associated congenital anomalies: inguinal hernia and cryptorchidism are the most common
- Alteration of prognosis when associated with a syndrome such as Smith-Lemli-Opitz syndrome, Opitz-Frias syndrome, trisomy 13 or 18, or intersex state
- Association with intersex state and adrenal dysfunction

OVERVIEW

- Urethral meatus is located on the ventral penile surface proximal to its normal position at the tip of the glans penis. Classification is based on the location of the meatus (perineal, penoscrotal, penile, coronal, or glandular).
- In addition remnants of the corpus spongiosum distal to the urethral meatus form fibrous bands called chordee, producing ventral penile curvature of varying degrees
- Penoscrotal and perineal forms (those more proximal) are more commonly associated with other organ system abnormalities

ICD-9-CM Code: 752.6

ETIOLOGY

- Unclear for routine hypospadias
- Defective androgen stimulation of the developing penis when associated with an intersex condition
- Environmental and genetic factors have also been implicated

USUAL TREATMENT

- Surgical repair ideally performed between ages 6 and 12 mo to minimize the psychologic effects of genital surgery

ASSESSMENT POINTS

SYSTEM	EFFECT	ASSESSMENT BY HX	PE	TEST
RENAL	Associated anomaly such as solitary kidney may not require further work-up, or it may be a surgically significant upper tract anomaly	History of UTI, upper or lower tract obstructive symptoms, hematuria, strong family Hx of urinary tract abnormalities	Locate the hypospadias	As directed by H & P ± voiding cystourethrogram, renal US, IVP
ENDO	Rarely associated with intersex state, which may be accompanied by adrenal dysfunction		↑ Risk of association when failure of testicular descent, micropenis, penoscrotal transposition present	Lytes, blood glucose ± karyotype screening

Key Reference: Chhibber AK, Perkins FM, Rabinowitz R, Vogt AW, Hulbert WC: Penile block timing for postoperative analgesia of hypospadias repair in children. J Urol 1997; 158:1156–1159.

PERIOPERATIVE MANAGEMENT

Preoperative Preparation

- Use of midazolam effective especially for patients undergoing multistep repairs

Monitoring

- Routine
- If the reconstruction is very involved (more proximal meatus) and the case long with a potentially high EBL, consider an art cath

Airway

- LMA for shorter, more straightforward repairs
- GETA for procedures of longer duration and complexity

Induction

- Standard mask induction with sevoflurane or halothane/N_2O/O_2

Maintenance

- Either inhalation only or balanced
- Caudal epidural block is optimal because of complete intraop and postop analgesia
  – In children having outpatient surgery, use one shot caudal after induction (0.25% bupivacaine with 5 μg/ml epinephrine at 0.5–1 ml/kg). Repeat the caudal after surgery if duration > 2 h using $\frac{1}{2}$–$\frac{2}{3}$ original volume or use 0.125% bupivacaine and inject original volume.
  – In children being admitted to the hospital, use continuous caudal epidural
- Penile block less effective for postop analgesia especially when hypospadias is proximally located

SURGICAL GOALS

- Straightening of the penis by release of fibrous chordee—artificial erection by injecting saline in the corpora during the operation allows for determination of the exact degree of curvature
- Placing meatus at the tip of the glans by glans channeling or glans splitting techniques
- Forming a symmetric conical glans
- Constructing a neourethra uniform in caliber and of appropriate size for age using free or vascularized pedicle flaps
- Completing a satisfactory cosmetic skin coverage while maintaining good vascularization

ANTICIPATED PROBLEMS/CONCERNS

- Bleeding
- Infection
- Urethrocutaneous fistulas
- Stricture
- Devitalized skin flaps
- Recurrent complications resulting in multiple repairs

HYSTERECTOMY, VAGINAL

Robert K. Parker, D.O.

RISK

- Hysterectomy within USA/y: 600,000, 1988; 580,000, 1992
- Vaginal hysterectomy: 133,000 (22%), 1988; 177,000 (31%), 1992
- Laparoscopy-assisted ↑ 3-fold from 1991–1993
- Cost estimated at $1.7 billion/y

PERIOPERATIVE RISKS

- Mortality very rare
- Risks: 20–30% associated morbidity with abdominal hysterectomy, 6–10% with vaginal hysterectomy
- More common risks (laparoscopy-assisted) include unintended laparotomy (1.4%), hemorrhage (1.3%), bowel or UT injury (0.9%)

WORRY ABOUT

- Indication for procedure (abnormal bleeding?)
- Effects of positioning
- Effects of CO_2 insufflation (laparoscopic-assisted)
- Unrecognized, underestimate of blood loss

OVERVIEW

- Laparoscopy-assisted not necessarily a replacement for vaginal hysterectomy
- Laparoscopy-assisted considered when vaginal hysterectomy contraindicated, e.g., pelvic endometriosis, PID, previous uterine suspension, nulliparity with insufficient prolapse, significant pelvic pain requiring abd-pelvic exploration

ICD-9-CM Codes: 618.1 (Prolapse); 625.3 (Dysmenorrhea)

INDICATIONS AND USUAL TREATMENT

- Uterine prolapse with other organ compromised, dysmenorrhea, dysfunctional uterine bleeding, premalignant endometrial lesion, CIN, uterine myomas, failed medical Rx of endometriosis, uterine cancer
- Usual medical Rx includes oral contraceptives, prostaglandin inhibitors, Danocrine or Gn-RH analogues

CONTRAINDICATIONS

- Multiple previous abdominal laparotomies (relative contraindication)
- Uterine fibroids exceeding size comparable to 16-wk gestation (relative contraindication)
- Significant medical problems that would be exacerbated by a lengthy procedure in dorsal lithotomy or Trendelenburg position and/or abdominal CO_2 insufflation

ASSESSMENT POINTS

SYSTEM	EFFECT	ASSESSMENT BY HX	PE	TEST
HEENT	Obesity hinders airway management	Prior difficult intubation	Airway	
CV	Obesity/CO_2 insufflation/ Trendelenburg position inhibit venous return/CO	CV status Hx CHF/cardiopulmonary disease/ SOB, exercise tolerance	CV	ECG Stress test if indicated
RESP	Obesity/CO_2 insufflation/ Trendelenburg position inhibit respiratory excursion	Orthopnea	Chest	O_2 sat
HEME	Chronic/acute blood loss due to uterine bleeding	Orthostatic changes		Hct Tilt table test

Key Reference: Nezhat F, Nezhat CH, Admon D, et al: Complications and results of 361 hysterectomies performed at laparoscopy. J Am Coll Surg 1995; 180:307–316.

INTRAOPERATIVE MANAGEMENT

Monitoring

- Routine
- End-tidal CO_2 should be followed during CO_2 insufflation under GA as end-tidal CO_2 may rise, requiring alteration in ventilation
- Peak airway pressure may rise considerably during Trendelenburg positioning, CO_2 insufflation; obesity may markedly exaggerate these changes
- Subcutaneous emphysema due to tissue extravasation of insufflated CO_2 may occur

Anesthetic Technique

- GA may be used for vaginal hysterectomy; often preferred for laparoscopy
- Regional anesthesia may be used for vaginal hysterectomy; for laparoscopy, regional anesthesia may be considered for highly motivated patients

Airway

- Risk of aspiration of gastric contents increased 2° to Trendelenburg position, CO_2 insufflation
- Laryngeal mask airway anesthesia may be contraindicated
- Orogastric tube to ↓ abdominal content may be indicated

SURGICAL STAGES

Induction

- CV instability 2° to preop blood loss
- Rapid onset of regional anesthesia (esp if large intra-abdominal mass) may exacerbate instability
- Sensory level of T6 may need to be achieved with regional anesthesia

CO_2 Insufflation

- Observe for CO_2 extravasation—e.g., subcutaneous emphysema, sudden increase in airway pressure (laparoscopy-assisted)
- Trauma to major vessels may occur with introduction of trochar with laparoscope; unrecognized hemorrhage can occur

Positioning

- Observe, protect pressure points
- Trendelenburg position may lead to cephalad spread of local anesthetic during regional anesthesia
- Sacral anesthesia may be difficult to reestablish with epidural redosing in Trendelenburg position

Intraoperative

- Hemorrhage may occur during ovarian, uterine artery dissection
- Ureters need to be identified and isolated to avoid inadvertent ligation
- During laparoscopy, surgical stimulation variable; stimulus high during laparoscopy, low during vaginal approach; high again during repeat laparoscopy just prior to completion of procedure. Consider IV infusion to titrate to surg stimulus.
- Approximate duration: 1–5 h

Closure/Postoperative Considerations

- Evacuation of CO_2 may be aided by Valsalva maneuver
- Postop nausea, shoulder pain from CO_2 irritation of diaphragm ↓ by adequate CO_2 evacuation, avoidance of early semi-Fowler position
- Blood loss generally 250–1000 ml; ~1% require transfusion. In isolated cases, traumatic injury to major vessels may cause massive, rapid blood loss.
- Pain score: 3–6 (generally lower than for abdominal hysterectomy)
- Postop pain relief plans may include PCA or epidural (if used during surgery), although most patients tolerate oral pain med in early postop period; use of NSAIDs may depend upon degree of bleeding, exposed surfaces

HYSTEROSCOPY

David Wlody, M.D.

RISK

- Performed diagnostically, therapeutically in women of all ages

PERIOPERATIVE RISKS

- Overall risk 0.28%
- 0.13% for diagnostic procedures
- 0.95% for operative procedures

WORRY ABOUT

- Fluid overload
- Hyponatremia
- Hypo-osmolality
- Anaphylaxis to dextran 70 (rarely used)
- CO_2 embolization
- Uterine perforation
- Bowel/urinary tract injury
- Hemorrhage

OVERVIEW

- Direct examination of uterine cavity for evaluation of uterine bleeding or treatment of uterine pathology
- Distending medium necessary to adequately visualize endometrium
- CO_2 used for diagnostic procedures; excess pressure can lead to embolization
- Electrolyte solutions (LR, NS) preferred for procedures avoiding electrosurgery
- Nonelectrolyte solutions (dextran, glycine, sorbitol, mannitol) used when electrosurgery performed
- Dextran 70 has been associated with anaphylaxis; pretreatment with dextran 1 may prevent allergic reactions
- Glycine and sorbitol associated with hyponatremic encephalopathy with hypo-osmolality

- Risk of permanent brain damage after hyponatremic encephalopathy is 25 times greater in premenopausal women than in men or postmenopausal women—hormonal effect?
- Mannitol can produce hyponatremia without hypo-osmolality, which is associated with fewer neurologic symptoms

ICD-9-CM Code: 626.2 (Menometrorrhagia)

INDICATIONS

- Evaluation of infertility
- Evaluation of abnormal uterine bleeding
- Resection of submucosal myomas, polypectomy, adhesiolysis, endometrial ablation

ASSESSMENT POINTS

SYSTEM	EFFECT	ASSESSMENT BY HX	PE	TEST
HEME	Blood loss	Abn bleeding, syncope	Orthostasis	Hgb/Hct

Key Reference: Cooper JM, Brady RM: Intraoperative and early postoperative complications of operative hysteroscopy. Obstet Gynecol Clin North Am 2000; 27:347–366.

PERIOPERATIVE MANAGEMENT

Preoperative Preparation

- If Hx of reaction to dextran, consider alternative distending medium; alternatively, pretreatment with monovalent dextran ↓ frequency of anaphylaxis

Anesthetic Technique

- Diagnostic procedures commonly performed under paracervical block with sedation as needed
- Operative procedures performed under regional or general anesthesia

Monitoring

- Routine
- Significant cardiopulmonary disease, consider invasive monitoring because absorption of large vol of distending fluid

Airway

- Since no pneumoperitoneum, mask anesthesia or LMA acceptable

Induction/Maintenance

- Usually performed on ambulatory basis: any technique allowing rapid emergence, recovery

Postoperative Concerns

- Monitor for excess bleeding
- EBL: minimal
- Pain score: 3–5
- Postop pain can be managed with NSAID

ANTICIPATED PROBLEMS/CONCERNS

- Monitor for anaphylaxis if dextran 70 used
- Monitor input/output of distending fluid to avoid hypervolemia, hyponatremia, hypo-osmolality
- If CO_2 used as distending medium, use insufflator designed for hysteroscopy (laparoscopic insufflators produce flow rates high enough to lead to gas embolization via endometrial vessels)
- Carefully evaluate level of consciousness after surgery, especially if large volumes of distending fluid were used
- Electrolyte determination mandatory if level of consciousness is abnormal

ILEOSTOMY

Michael S. Higgins, M.D.

RISK

- Relatively common procedure for adults 20–65 y
- Male/female predominance: none. For cancer, men ≥ women; for inflammatory bowel disease, women > men
- Racial predominance: none
- Usually performed for intestinal obstruction (60–70%) or diseases requiring a total proctocolectomy (10–15%); often associated with intestinal adhesions, inflammatory bowel disease, abdominal cancer, trauma

PERIOPERATIVE RISKS

- Mortality: varies widely with co-existent disease, generally < 1%
- Procedural morbidity: ileus 5%, wound infection < 5%, intestinal obstruction 2–3%, fistula formation 1–3%, ostomy necrosis < 0.5%

WORRY ABOUT

- Pulm aspiration
- Perioperative intravascular volume deficiency
- Hemorrhage
- Postop pulm atelectasis
- Sepsis

OVERVIEW

- Co-morbid diseases include malnutrition, hypovolemia, lyte abn, effects of chronic steroid therapy, effects of primary oncologic process, associated traumatic injuries
- Often ↑ risk of gastric regurgitation and pulm aspiration
- Associated with preop hypovolemia and continuing intravascular volume shift to extravascular tissues (third spacing) perioperatively
- Intraoperative monitoring modalities determined by patient age and co-existing disease

ICD-9-CM Code: 560.9 (Bowel obstruction)

INDICATIONS AND USUAL TREATMENT

- Ileal disease: inflammatory bowel disease, small bowel obstruction, volvulus, intussusception, mesenteric vascular occlusion, radiation enteritis, intestinal fistulae, small bowel tumors, Crohn's disease, trauma (if reanastomosis contraindicated by infection)
- Large bowel disease: proctocolectomy for inflammatory bowel disease, ulcerative colitis, familial polyposis, neoplasm, trauma
- Surgical intervention for inflammatory bowel disease and Crohn's disease may follow prolonged steroid therapy
- Surgical alternatives include both incontinent and continent ileostomy (Kock pouch)

ASSESSMENT POINTS

SYSTEM	EFFECT	ASSESSMENT BY HX	PE	TEST
CV	Hypovolemia from ↓ fluid intake, bowel prep, third spacing	PO status, vomiting, bowel prep, UO	Hypotension with tachycardia, orthostatic BP, skin turgor	BUN/Cr, urine output, electrolytes, consider ECG
RESP	Resp insufficiency from abdominal distention/splinting and reduced FRC	Dyspnea, Abdominal pain	Rales, Abdominal distention and rigidity	CXR, Pulse oximetry, Consider ABGs
GI	Possible ↑ intragastric pressure, volume, acidity, Possible perforation with peritonitis	Abdominal pain	Peritoneal signs	X-ray—dilated bowel
HEME/ IMMUNO	Hemoconcentration from dehydration, DIC possibly associated with sepsis, Immune suppression from chronic steroid therapy, Potential malnutrition from malabsorption, Bacteremia and sepsis	GI losses, Abnormal bleeding, Hemodynamic instability	See under CV, Febrile, hypotensive	PCV, plt, PT/PTT, WBC count with differential
RENAL	Possible hypokalemic, hypochloremic metabolic alkalosis with vomiting, lyte abn from lower GI losses/bowel prep, hemoconcentration, Associated renal insufficiency in elderly	Vomiting, bowel prep	See under CV	Serum lytes

Key Reference: Binderow SR, Wexner SD: Current surgical therapy for mucosal ulcerative colitis. Dis Colon Rectum 1994; 37:610–624.

PERIOPERATIVE MANAGEMENT

Premedication

- Consider H_2 antagonists and oral nonparticulate antacid
- Consider metoclopramide—contraindicated if intestinal obstruction
- Consider steroid coverage if on chronic steroid therapy (hydrocortisone 100 mg IV over 24 h)
- Consider NSAIDs to reduce incidence of mesenteric traction syndrome

Monitoring

- Consider arterial catheter if hemodynamically unstable or severe cardiopulmonary disease
- Foley catheter
- Volume status monitoring a major concern—consider CVP, PA cath, or transesophageal ECHO monitoring if renal insufficiency or significant cardiac dysfunction with intravascular volume or prolonged surgical procedure

Airway

- Routine; consider awake intubation, rapid-sequence or modified rapid-sequence intubation (aspiration risk)

Induction

- Consider peri-induction intravascular volume expansion (10–20 ml/kg) if hypovolemic

Maintenance

- May be performed under regional, general, or combined anesthetic techniques; NG tube placed to suction reduces gastric distention
- Usual blood loss: < 300 ml
- Consider convective air warming

Emergence

- Extubation depends on usual criteria with emphasis on volume status, body temp
- Pain score: 5–8
- Consider epidural or IV PCA
- Postop volume requirements moderate

IMPERFORATE ANUS REPAIR
Ronald S. Litman, D.O.

RISK

- Minor abnormalities in 1/500 live births
- Major abnormalities in 1/5000 live births
- Slight male predominance

PERIOPERATIVE RISKS

- Relate to other significant congenital anomalies (mainly cardiac disease), if present

WORRY ABOUT

- Accompanying congenital malformations of the heart or lungs: VACTERL syndrome (sometimes called VATER syndrome):
  - Vertebral anomalies (including sacrum)
  - Anal malformations
  - Cardiac malformations
  - Tracheal anomalies (tracheoesophageal fistula)
  - Esophageal atresia
  - Renal and urinary tract anomalies
  - Limb malformations

OVERVIEW

- Congenital anal malformations are typically divided into high (above the levator ani muscle) and low (below the levator ani muscle) lesions
- Low lesions are usually associated with fistulas that drain to the skin of the perineum or vaginal vestibule
- Presenting symptoms include abdominal distention and failure to pass 1st stool within 24–48 h

ICD-9-CM Code: 751.2

INDICATIONS AND USUAL TREATMENT

- Transverse colostomy is performed, usually on the 1st day of life
- Surgically corrected some time within the 1st year of life. Most common corrective procedure is posterior sagittal anorectoplasty (Pena procedure).
- Surgery for the low type involves closure of the fistula, creation of an anal opening, and repositioning the rectal pouch into the anal opening
- Major challenge: finding, using, or creating adequate nerve and muscle structures around the rectum and anus to provide the child with the capacity for bowel control

ASSESSMENT POINTS

SYSTEM	EFFECT	ASSESSMENT BY HX	PE	TEST
CV	Wide variety of possible cardiac malformations, VSD most common		Murmur, cyanosis, CHF, absent femoral pulses	ECHO if murmur heard
RESP	May also have tracheoesophageal fistula, usually corrected at the same time		Wheezing, ↓ breath sounds	CXR
GU	Renal and ureteral anomalies possible			US
GI	May also have esophageal atresia	Gagging and vomiting of 1st feeding		Unable to pass orogastric tube
MS	Possibility of limb anomalies		Visual inspection	

Key Reference: Pena A, Hong A: Advances in the management of anorectal malformations. Am J Surg 2000; 180:370–376.

INTRAOPERATIVE MANAGEMENT

Monitoring

- Routine
- Attempt to place IV catheters and pulse oximeter on the upper extremities because patient is often situated at the far end of the operating room table
- Esophageal temp probe is required. Hypothermia is likely unless precautions are taken. Use forced warm air blanket underneath or around patient during surgical procedure. Also advisable to use IV fluid warmer if available.
- Anticipate insensible fluid loss of 7–10 ml/kg/h during major portions of the procedure
- Foley urinary catheter should be placed before surgery

SURGICAL STAGES

- Posterior sagittal dissection is most often done with patient in the prone position, toward the end of the operating room table—must plan to move the patient after induction
- Some surgeons may operate with patient in lithotomy or supine position
- Usually very little blood loss

Anesthetic Technique

- GETA, without special considerations
- Rapid-sequence intubation is indicated for newborn colostomy, unless stomach is emptied first with an oro- or nasogastric tube.
- Consider postop "one-shot" epidural analgesia via the caudal approach after colostomy

- For Pena procedure, consider preop (but after induction of GA) insertion of a caudal epidural cath for intraop and postop pain management
- Surgeons often prefer NMB throughout procedure
- Usually awaken patient and extubate trachea at end of procedure unless influenced by other medical problems. No special postop concerns.

ANTICIPATED PROBLEMS/CONCERNS

- Management of associated CHD or other existing medical problems

IMPLANTABLE CARDIOVERTER-DEFIBRILLATORS (ICDs), IMPLANTATION

Paul D. Eckenbrecht, M.D.

RISK

- 400,000/y in USA suffer sudden cardiac death
- Pharmacologic Rx for *near* sudden death is ineffective in 20–50%; 1-y sudden death rate is 30%
- 50,000 undergo ICD implantation annually, after which the 1-y sudden death rate is 2%
- Gender predominance: 76% male
- Associated diseases: CAD—65%; cardiomyopathy—19%; valvular disease—8%; LV dysfunction with mean LVEF—35 ± 10%; tetralogy, transposition, long QT syndrome—1%

PERIOPERATIVE RISKS

- Surgical (thoracotomy) mortality is 3.3%; varies inversely with LVEF (2.3% when performed separately from cardiac surgery)
- Factors increasing surgical mortality: LVEF <30%; concomitant cardiac surgery; postop device deactivation; preop amiodarone
- 72% of surgical deaths are cardiac (24%—sudden; 17%—tachydysrhythmic/nonsudden; 31%—cardiac nondysrhythmic), and 28% are noncardiac
- Surgical cardiac morbidity: sustained VTach/VFIB—5–15%; AFIB—10–19%; CHF—2%; MI—1%
- Surgical pulmonary morbidity (with thoracotomy approach): pleural effusion/atelectasis/pneumonia—3–27%; ARDS—2–21%
- Surgical noncardiopulmonary morbidity: CVA—1–2%; renal failure—1%
- Percutaneous, transvenous implantation (nonsurg) has a lower mortality: 0.05–0.12%

- Nonsurgical mortality includes CHF—33%; cardiorespiratory arrest—33%; cardiogenic shock—13%; EMD—6%; ischemic—6%; pneumonia—6%
- Nonsurgical morbidity includes lead dislodgment—5.3%; AFIB—2%; pneumothorax—1.7%; hematoma—0.7%; respiratory failure—0.7%; infection—0.7%

WORRY ABOUT

- Myocardial ischemia, low CO, ↓ BP during defibrillation threshold (DFT) testing
- Increase DFT: antiarrhythmics (class IA, B, C—including lidocaine, propranolol, amiodarone, verapamil); halogenated hydrocarbons; hypothermia; myocardial ischemia; acidosis
- Increased incidence of intraoperative conduction defects, atropine-resistant bradycardia, CHB, pacemaker and inotropic dependency, α-blockade with low SVR and hepatic, thyroid, and pulm dysfunction if taking chronic amiodarone

OVERVIEW

- ICDs have two interrelated functions: dysrhythmia detection and dysrhythmia therapy
- Dysrhythmia detection may be based on morphology (ECG shape) or rate
- For dysrhythmia therapy, all devices implanted since 1993 have programmable, tiered therapy options: programmable single, dual-chamber, or rate-responsive pacing for bradycardia; antitachycardia pacing (ATP) and low-energy cardioversion for VTach; and high-energy defibrillation for VFIB

- Before 1993, surgical implantation of epicardial patch electrodes was most common (~90%)
- Since 1993, multiple percutaneous transvenous or subpectoral sense/pace and defibrillating leads are usually implanted (95%)
- Surgical approaches: left anterolateral thoracotomy—67%; median sternotomy—27%; subcostal—6%
- Nonsurgical approaches: submuscular or subcutaneous generator implantation in the pectoral region and a subcutaneous patch and/or multiple transvenous sense/pace and defibrillating leads
- DFT testing is performed after both initial lead placement and generator implantation

ICD-9-CM Codes: 427.1 (for VTach); 427.41 (for VFIB)

INDICATIONS AND USUAL TREATMENT

- Survivors of cardiac arrest presumably due to VT/VFIB not associated with acute MI
- Patients with sustained VTach at EPS are noninducible; nonsuppressed by drug or surgical therapy; intolerant of drugs
- Patients with nonsustained VTach with CAD, prior MI, LV dysfunction, and inducible VFIB or sustained VTach at EPS that is not suppressed by a class I antiarrhythmic
- ICDs considered first-line therapy for poorly tolerated VTach with impaired LV function, or VTach in pts not inducible at EPS
- 80% of ICD patients receive concomitant antiarrhythmic therapy

ASSESSMENT POINTS

SYSTEM	EFFECT	ASSESSMENT BY HX	PE	TEST
CV	Myocardial ischemia LV dysfunction Rate, mechanism of VTach	Angina symptoms Exercise tolerance, DOE	S₃, rales	ECG, Ex thallium ECHO, MUGA, cath EPS, ambulatory ECG
RESP	Amiodarone toxicity	Exercise tolerance, DOE		CXR, PFTs, ABGs
RENAL	Renal insufficiency		Edema	BUN, Cr
NEURO	CV disease	Stroke, TIAs	Bruits	Carotid duplex
LYTES	Reversible VTach/VFIB	Diuretic Rx		Serum K^+ and Mg^{2+}

Key Reference: Singer I, Barold SS, Camm AJ (eds): Nonpharmacological Therapy of Arrhythmias for the 21st Century: The State of the Art. Armonk, NY, Futura Publishing Co., 1998.

PERIOPERATIVE MANAGEMENT

Anesthetic Technique
- GA required for surgical approaches
- Local with sedation is used for nonsurgical, transvenous implantation
- Opioid-hypnotic-relaxant techniques least effect on hemodynamics and EPS or DFT testing
- Halogenated hydrocarbons may increase DFT, so keep concentrations <1.0 MAC

Monitoring
- PA cath if LVEF <35% but may dislodge hardware positioned in SVC

Airway
- A left double-lumen tube for thoracotomy

SURGICAL STAGES

- Implantation of sense/pace and defibrillation lead systems (usually transvenous)

- Determine R-wave amplitude from sensing and defibrillating leads (5 mV and 1 mV, respectively)
- Determine pacing threshold for ATP capable devices (<1.5 V endocardial, <2.0 V epicardial)
- DFT testing of implanted ICD leads using external cardioverter-defibrillator (≤15–25 joules)
- Creation of the ICD generator pocket
- Tunnel and connect leads to ICD, implant generator, and repeat DFT testing using ICD
- Inactive ICD during closure of pocket, then reactivate at end of procedure
- EBL and volume shifts are minimal

Postoperative Considerations
- Significant postop pain with thoracotomy approach (pain score 6–10)
- Consider epidural/spinal narcotics
- Inappropriate device discharge due to postsurgical atrial tachydysrhythmias can be prevented by device deactivation; however, a number of studies suggest an association between postsurgical tachydysrhythmic death and intentional, postsurgical device deactivation
- Studies suggest association between chronic, presurgical amiodarone administration and postsurgical ARDS

ANTICIPATED PROBLEMS/CONCERNS

- 1–2% of transvenous implants require conversion to thoracotomy due to high DFTs (>25 joules)
- 3–18% of all implants result in high DFTs. This results in a 1-y sudden death rate 15× greater than in implants with acceptable DFTs.
- Sustained VFIB during DFT testing should be promptly treated with rescue shocks and CPR/ACLS as needed. Because lidocaine raises DFT, IV bretylium, which has no effect on DFT, is drug of choice.

INGUINAL HERNIORRHAPHY

Lucinda L. Everett, M.D.
Surinder K. Kallar, M.D.

RISK

- 700,000 groin hernias repaired in USA/y
- Congenital: 1–2% of live births
- Age predominance: congenital, especially premature infants; elderly
- Sex: 80–90% of adult repairs in males; incidence in congenital hernias quoted as 4–10× higher in males

PERIOPERATIVE RISKS

- Mortality: <0.01% elective repairs; up to 5% in emergency cases and very elderly
- Morbidity: hematoma, 2–3%; infection, 1–2%; entrapment of ilioinguinal or genitofemoral nerve with neuralgia; ischemic orchitis, 0.03–0.5% in primary hernias; recurrence, 10–15%

WORRY ABOUT

- Straining or bucking with emergence may damage repair
- Bowel obstruction with incarcerated hernia
- Apnea risk in ex–premature infants

OVERVIEW

- Groin hernias represent defect of transversalis fascia
- Classification includes location (medial [direct], lateral [indirect], femoral) and size; also sliding, recurrent, or incarcerated
- Chronically increased abdominal pressure thought to be predisposing factor, as in obesity, COPD, prostatic hyperplasia, ascites, pregnancy, constipation, colonic stenosis
- Most inguinal hernias can be diagnosed by palpation, though clinical exam distinguishes direct from indirect with only 70% accuracy
- US exam useful in patients with symptoms but no signs

ICD-9-CM Code: 550.9

INDICATIONS AND USUAL TREATMENT

- Early elective surgery recommended to prevent incarceration/strangulation; "broad direct bulges" have lower incidence of incarceration (some manage this type conservatively, but others endorse repair in all, as preop differentiation of direct vs. indirect is not absolute by clinical exam); recurrence depends on size and location
- Mesh repair indicated for multiple recurrences and bilateral hernias, particularly in elderly
- Laparoscopic repair may ↓ postop pain but may require longer surgical time

ASSESSMENT POINTS

SYSTEM	EFFECT	ASSESSMENT BY HX	PE	TEST
CV	Ischemic heart disease prevalent in elderly	Exercise tolerance Chest pain/discomfort		ECG >50 y or with Hx Testing for myocardium at risk if Hx suggests
RESP	Obstructive pulm disease may predispose	Dyspnea, wheezing	Auscultation Forced exhalation Chest diameter Clubbing, cyanosis Periodic breathing	O₂ saturation CXR if infection suspected PFTs if etiology unclear or to evaluate Rx
	Postop apnea risk in ex–premature infants	Postconceptual <56 wk Hx apnea; caffeine Rx		
GI	Bowel obstruction if hernia incarcerated	N/V	Abdominal distention	KUB Electrolytes
CNS	Ability to tolerate procedure under local anesthesia	Orientation/cooperation	Mental status exam	
SOCIAL	Most procedures done on outpatient basis	Adequate home support for elderly		

Key Reference: Song D, Greilich NB, White PF, Watcha MF, Tongier WK: Recovery profiles and costs of anesthesia for outpatient unilateral inguinal herniorrhaphy. Anesth Analg 2000; 91:876–881.

PERIOPERATIVE MANAGEMENT

Preoperative Preparation

- Consider caffeine citrate, 20 mg/kg in ex–premature infants at risk for apnea
- Avoid sedatives in premature infants having procedure under spinal anesthesia
- Fluid resuscitation and aspiration prophylaxis if bowel obstruction present

Anesthetic Technique

- Local infiltration effective for repair; potentially fewer side effects than field block/nerve block
- Spinal or epidural (T8)
- Paravertebral block (T10–L2)
- GA by mask or LMA
- General endotracheal (especially if obstructed or if large/recurrent hernia)

Monitoring

- Routine
- Consider postop apnea monitoring for ex–premature infants

SURGICAL STAGES

Skin Incision

- Above inguinal ligament

Dissection

- To identify type of hernia and vital structures

Definitive Surgery

- Management of peritoneal sac; repair of fascial defect

Postoperative Considerations

- Minimal blood loss; minimal fluid shifts unless incarcerated hernia with bowel obstruction
- Pain management: local infiltration; nerve block; caudal (pediatric); NSAIDs
- Pain score: 4–5

ANTICIPATED PROBLEMS/CONCERNS

- Potential complications of laparoscopy with laparoscopic repair
- Occasional vagal response to traction
- Femoral nerve palsy with leg weakness possible after "blind" ilioinguinal block

INTESTINAL OBSTRUCTION

David A. Rosen, M.D.
Kathleen R. Rosen, M.D.

RISK

- Operations counted in millions if all etiologies included
- Small bowel obstructions predominate by 60–80%
- Etiology of most cases is adhesions from factors such as previous surgery, inflammatory processes, and endometriosis. Other etiologies include neoplasms, hernias ± strangulation, volvulus, foreign body, and treatment with NSAIDs.
- Race and gender predilection: none

PERIOPERATIVE RISKS

- Apache II scores >8 correlate with ↑ risk
- Mortality: SBO associated with adhesions 5–10%. SBO associated with cancer or bowel gangrene and LBO 15–28%.
- ↑ Risk (bowel factors): strangulation, malignancy, high obstruction, delay in treatment >24 h, nonviable strangulation, bowel resection
- ↑ Risk (general): sepsis, CV instability (especially hypovolemia and hypotension prior to surgery), extremes of age, co-existing disease, suboptimal nutritional state

- Complication rate ~25%. ↑ Rate associated with advanced age, co-morbid illness, treatment delay, and previous abdominal surgery. ↓ Occurrence of death and complications when lesion is amenable to laparoscopic treatment.

WORRY ABOUT

- Co-existing medical conditions: especially cardiopulmonary disease if >75 y. Bowel pathology requiring resection: gangrene, perforation, malignancy.
- Volume status: acid-base, lytes
- Perfusion: systemic, pulmonary, regional
- Sepsis
- Physiologic problems can persist or worsen after surgery

OVERVIEW

- Indications for surgery: strangulation of vascular supply or complete obstruction of lumen. Functional or partial obstructions may be amenable to conservative management.
- Patients may need aggressive management prior to surgery (see Worry About)

ICD-9-CM Code: 560.9

INDICATIONS AND USUAL TREATMENT

- Any intrinsic or extrinsic lesions that obstruct the intestinal lumen or strangulate the vascular supply require urgent surgery
- Prophylactic surgery may be indicated if an abnormality that predisposes to obstruction is detected
- If diagnosis is uncertain, water-soluble contrast material may be used to distinguish partial from complete obstruction
- Hemodynamic resuscitation can occur prior to surgery in virtually all cases
- Many advocate an initial laparoscopic approach in a select patient population: probable etiology, adhesion. Successful treatment is reported in 60–80% of patients. Laparoscopy is not recommended for patients with malignancy, gangrene, or perforation.

ASSESSMENT POINTS

SYSTEM	EFFECT	ASSESSMENT BY HX	PE	TEST
CV	Hypotension Tachycardia Poor peripheral perfusion Venous return impeded	Orthostasis, edema	BP (positional) Skin color Capillary refill Pulse quality, HR	As indicated by pre-existing disease and age as well as present condition
RESP	Restrictive defect	SOB (positional)	Resp rate/pattern, skin color Resp work/effort	ABGs, pulse oximetry
GI	Loss of fluids, lytes, or blood	I/O, vomiting (amount, description) BM (timing, character) Abdominal pain ± distention Prior operations	Abdominal scars Mass Rectal tenderness Abdominal girth Bowel sounds Hernias	Abdominal CT ± enhancement NG drainage
RENAL/HYDRATION	↓ UO ↑ Other fluid, ↓ Electrolytes	I/O	Skin turgor Dry mouth	BUN, Cr, Na^+, K^+, Cl^-, HCO_3^-, UA
IMMUNO	Contamination of GI flora, sepsis or peritonitis	Fever, chills	Temperature (see above, CV and GI)	CBC with differential

Key Reference: Fevang BT, Fevang J, Stangeland L, Sorerde O, Svanes K, Viste A: Complications and death after treatment of small bowel obstruction. Ann Surg 2000; 231:529–537.

PERIOPERATIVE IMPLICATIONS

Preoperative Preparation
- Restoration of intravascular volume
- Correction of acid-base and lyte abnormalities
- Decompression of stomach
- Antibiotic coverage

Anesthetic Technique
- Usually GA
- Hemodynamic concerns mandate careful selection of anesthetic, relaxant, and analgesic medication

Monitoring
- Required: routine + Foley catheter
- Consider: arterial line, CVP, PAC, TEE

Induction/Maintenance
- Rapid-sequence
- CV instability 2° to volume status
- Avoidance of nitrous oxide
- Muscle relaxation
- Large-bore intravenous access

SURGICAL STAGES

- Laparoscopy in a selected population
- Laparotomy accompanied by more profound physiologic changes
- Large fluid shifts on opening of abdomen
- Tumors or mass manipulation may cause hemodynamic alterations
- Restriction of pulmonary function or cardiac performance 2° to placement of surgical retractors
- Release of hemodynamically active substances when the bowel is manipulated
- Relaxation until abdomen closed
- Body heat and fluid loss due to exposed bowel
- Blood loss ranges from minimal to significant depending on etiology
- Abdominal closure may be difficult or contraindicated

POSTOPERATIVE PERIOD

- Delay extubation if pulm and CV status in question
- Continued fluid and lyte abnormalities
- ARDS a potential if large fluid volumes were required
- Pulmonary atelectasis, pneumonia, or aspiration
- DVT ± pulm emboli
- Infection: general or local
- Pain management may be vital to ensure deep breathing and coughing
- PCA for 3–5 days (pain score: 2–9)
- Coagulopathies
- Renal failure
- Malnutrition
- Antiemetics

ANTICIPATED PROBLEMS/CONCERNS

- Hemodynamic, fluid, lyte, pulm alterations
- Sepsis

INTRA-AORTIC BALLOON COUNTERPULSATION (IABCP)

Carole Vannier, M.D.

RISK

- Used in > 75,000 patients/y worldwide (1992)

PERIOPERATIVE RISKS

- Frequency of complications: 14–45% (4–9% major; 22–41% minor); vascular (9–22%); infectious (1–22%); failure to place balloon pump (5–11.7%; no difference between percutaneous and surgical); bleeding (4–10%). Rare complications include excessive bleeding, balloon catheter leak, perforation or entrapment, gas embolism, small bowel infarction, aortic dissection leading to paraplegia.

WORRY ABOUT

- Timing of balloon inflation
- Dysrhythmias including sinus tachycardia
- Bleeding at insertion site
- Distal extremity ischemia

OVERVIEW

- Cardiac assist device placed surgically or percutaneously for management of acute LV dysfunction or unstable angina
- Removes volume from central aorta prior to and during LV ejection (reduces aortic pressure and therefore LV work by decreased afterload)
- Returns volume to central aorta during diastole (increases aortic pressure and therefore improves coronary blood flow and myocardial oxygen delivery)
- IABP system consists of drive unit; balloon catheter (30–40 ml displacement volume) placed surgically or percutaneously. Helium most effective inflating gas.
- Beneficial effects: ↓ time-tension index 20–40% (reflects ↓ myocardial O_2 ventilation rate); ↑ diastolic pressure–time index (reflects ↑ myocardial blood flow); ↓ LVEDP 25–40% while maintaining CO; ↓ LV work 18–50% while maintaining perfusion; improves CO (10–100%); improves EF; improves subendocardial perfusion as assessed by endocardial viability ratio; ↑ coronary blood flow (5–100%); ↑ cerebral blood flow (56%); ↑ myocardial O_2 supply (56%); ↓ myocardial O_2 consumption; ↓ lactate production

INDICATIONS/CONTRAINDICATIONS

Indications

- LV failure or ischemia refractory to pharmacologic intervention: status post MI, precardiac transplant (bridge), post cardiac transplant, acute mitral regurgitation, unstable angina
- May also be useful in high-risk patients undergoing PTCA, refractory ventricular dysrhythmia, high-risk cardiac patients undergoing noncardiac surgery

Contraindications

- Aortic insufficiency, aortic dissection
- Relatively contraindicated in patients with prosthetic thoracic aorta graft (may be considered if graft is > 12 mo old)

ASSESSMENT POINTS

SYSTEM	EFFECT	PE	TEST
CV	Dysrhythmias	Pulse	ECG
	Volume status	BP	CVP, PCWP
	Bleeding	Inspect site	CT, Hgb (retroperitoneal bleed)
	Vascular insufficiency	Inspect distal extremities	Doppler

Key Reference: Sanborn TA, Sleeper LA, Bates ER, et al: Impact of thrombolysis, intra-aortic balloon pump counterpulsation, and their combination in cardiogenic shock complicating acute myocardial infarction: a reprint from the SHOCK trial registry. Should we emergently revascularize occluded coronaries for cardiogenic shock? J Am Coll Cardiol 2000; 36:1123–1129.

PERIOPERATIVE MANAGEMENT

- Femoral insertion
  - Select site with greater pulse
  - Monitoring to include radial arterial pressure catheter and PA catheter
  - Heparinize if not contraindicated (LMW dextran or alternative can be used otherwise)
  - Cannulate femoral artery
  - Sheath and wire left in place, balloon advanced either under fluoroscopic guidance or to estimated angle of Louis. Final position should be 1 cm below origin of left subclavian artery. Central lumen can be connected to pressure transducer and used for balloon pump timing. Confirm with CXR and ECHO.
- Usual balloon volume approximates that of failing LV, ~ 20–40 ml
- Usual balloon diameter occludes 75–90% of cross-sectional area of descending aorta during inflation (overinflation can damage intima and lead to hemodynamic compromise)
- Inflation timing is critical to ensure benefit. Improper timing can worsen hemodynamics.
- Central aortic pressure tracing is related to ECG to determine interval between R wave of ECG and aortic valve opening (pressure wave upstroke) and aortic valve closure (dicrotic notch). This is used to program drive unit.

- Usual inflation initiated at the dicrotic notch on the central aortic BP waveform
- Deflation occurs at the end of diastole
- Incorrect timing can be recognized by examination of assisted pressure tracings and includes
  - Early inflation: augmented wave superimposed over systolic component of pressure trace
  - Late inflation: augmented wave initiated after valve closure
  - Early deflation: deflation occurs before isovolumetric contraction
  - Late deflation: inflation extends into systolic component
- At HR > 120, balloon may not be able to fill and empty completely. Consider augmentation at alternate beats (1:2 timing).
- Dysrhythmias may cause difficult or impossible adequate timing. Treatment of underlying dysrhythmia is a must. Avoid hypovolemia.
- Assess balloon timing frequently, esp with changes in HR. Wean vasopressors ASAP.
- Maintain APTT 1.5–2.0 × control if possible
- Check extremities frequently for evidence of ischemia
- Monitoring to include HR, BP, CVP, PAP, PCWP, CO, UO, electrolytes, ABGs, pH, CBC, temp. ECHO may also be useful.

- Consider weaning if CI > 2.2 L/min/m², PCWP < 18 mmHg, BP normal, and no ongoing ischemia
- Frequency weaning involves decreasing ratio of assisted beats to total number of beats (1:1, 1:2, 1:3, 1:4)
- Volume weaning involves decreasing balloon volume gradually (opponents of volume weaning cite risk of clot formation on balloon; proponents cite minimal risk if balloon volume maintained 10–15% stroke, and this method is more physiologic)
- Prior to removing IABP, heparin should be stopped for at least 4 h. Balloon is deflated and Doppler monitoring of distal leg vessels is performed. Catheter and sheath are removed as one unit while pressure is applied distal to puncture site to prevent distal embolization. Proximal pressure applied to encourage distal back-bleeding and to flush thrombi.

ANTICIPATED PROBLEMS/CONCERNS

- Timing may be difficult in patients with changing HR. Assess frequently.

INTUSSUSCEPTED BOWEL REPAIR

David A. Rosen, M.D.
Kathleen R. Rosen, M.D.

RISK

Pediatric Population

- 80–90% of infantile bowel obstruction
- 0.3% of live births
- 50% first year of life
- Greatest incidence at 3–10 mo
- Male predominance 3:2
- Typically ileocolic location
- Possible association with rotavirus vaccine

Adult Population

- 2–5% of bowel obstruction
- Associated with bowel abnormalities
- Malignant lead point common in patients >60 y
- Common in underdeveloped nations (idiopathic)

PERIOPERATIVE RISKS

- Prolapse of bowel and passage of necrotic tissue are grave signs

Pediatric Population

- Mortality <1%
- Increased morbidity and mortality if delayed diagnosis
- Preoperative perforation risk if <6 mo or symptoms >3–4 days
- Difficult to differentiate from necrotizing enterocolitis in preterm infants
- Bowel perforation risk during hydrostatic or pneumatic reduction

Adult Population

- Site and extent of intussusception influences risk
- Ileocolic intussusception greatest risk of bowel strangulation

WORRY ABOUT

- Hydration and electrolyte status
- Sepsis
- Viral illness (URI or GI)
- Co-existing disease at extremes of age: neonates and elderly

OVERVIEW

- Definition: invagination of one portion of intestinal tract into adjacent portion
- Lead point: anatomic abnormality that is drawn into distal bowel
- Bowel lymphadenopathy (Peyer's patches) in idiopathic cases

Pediatric Population

- 90% idiopathic (no lead point)
- Lead point present in neonates <3 mo
- Seasonal peaks parallel seasonal occurrence of viral illness
- Classic triad: pain, abdominal mass, intestinal bleeding
- Currant jelly stool in 65% of those <2 y
- Associations: Henoch's purpura, cystic fibrosis, Meckel's diverticulum, polyps

Adult Population

- Lead point in 75–90%
- Peutz-Jeghers syndrome (pigmentation of face/oral mucosa) + acute abdominal pain = intussusception
- Colic-colic intussusception associated with primary bowel neoplasm
- Ileocolic or appendiceal intussusception: metastatic (melanoma, lymphoma, lung) neoplasm, cystic fibrosis, endometriosis
- Ileoileo intussusception: benign tumors, Meckel's diverticulum, inflammatory process, prior gastric bypass surgery

- Other associations: Meckel's, Crohn's disease, eosinophilic granuloma, foreign body, AIDS, intra-abdominal adhesions
- Presentation variable: 70% crampy, recurrent, or steady abdominal pain
- Intraoperative diagnosis in majority

ICD-9-CM Code: 560.0 (Intussusception)

INDICATIONS AND USUAL TREATMENT

Pediatric Population

- Nonsurgical reduction with air, barium, iodine contrast, or saline—75% success rate
- Sedation/GA may facilitate reduction
- Recurrence rate 4–10%
- Contraindications: bowel perforation, strangulation, sepsis, or hemodynamic instability
- Surgery: failed closed reduction
  - Bowel resection uncommon
  - Many advocate laparoscopy ± saline enema
  - Competent ileocecal valve may prohibit preop documentation of reduction
  - Laparotomy if <3 mo; pathologic lead point, bowel compromise, or perforation

Adult Population

- Rarely amenable (idiopathic) to hydrostatic Rx
- Surgery first line of treatment
- Bowel resection likely
- Enterostomy unusual
- Laparoscopy or hydrostatic reduction in only a few select patients

ASSESSMENT POINTS

SYSTEM	EFFECT	ASSESSMENT BY HX	PE	TEST
GI	Bowel obstruction Bowel compromise	Nausea and vomiting Diarrhea (bloody), currant jelly stools Abdominal pain	Increased peristalsis RUQ abdominal mass Legs drawn up	US, x-ray ± contrast, spiral CT, endoscopy, UGI in adults
RENAL/ HYDRATION	Dehydration	I/O, vomiting	Decreased UO Decreased skin turgor	Electrolytes BUN, Cr, UA
HEME	Anemia Sepsis	Listlessness/pallor Fever	Tachycardia, hypotension (orthostasis)	Hgb, Hct CBC

Key Reference: Begos DG, Sandor A, Modlin IM: The diagnosis and management of adult intussusception. Am J Surg 1997; 173:88–94

PERIOPERATIVE MANAGEMENT

Preoperative Preparation

- Restore intravascular volume
- Decompression of stomach
- Antibiotics if sepsis is suspected

Anesthetic Technique

- General anesthesia is preferred
- Hemodynamics mandate careful selection of anesthetic, relaxant, and analgesics

Monitoring

- Routine plus Foley catheter
- Consider invasive monitors if septic

Induction/Maintenance

- Rapid sequence
- CV instability 2° to volume status
- Nitrous oxide can aid in reduction if bowel is not ischemic
- Relaxation usually needed

SURGICAL STAGES

Pediatric Population

- Initial laparoscopy in selected patients
- Laparotomy via right transverse incision
- Gentle proximal milking on nonischemic bowel
- Bowel manipulation may produce hemodynamic changes
- 25% require resection

Adult Population

- Etiology and location determine surgical approach
- Resection of lead point with primary anastomosis

Postoperative Period

- Recurrence or adynamic ileus
- Fluid shifts
- Opiates required for 2–3 days
- Pain score: 6–8
- Fever

ANTICIPATED PROBLEMS/CONCERN

- Maintenance of intravascular volume
- Sepsis
- Decrease in body temperature
- Pediatric anesthesia

JOINT REPLACEMENT CEMENTING
(METHYLMETHACRYLATE CEMENTING)

Jonathan L. Parmet, M.D.

RISK

- Cemented knee arthroplasty >141,000/y
- Cemented hip arthroplasty >250,000/y
- Racial predominance: none
- Gender predominance: none

PERIOPERATIVE RISKS

- 30-Day mortality (1–5%)
- DVT (no prophylaxis 72% and 50%, respectively, for TKR and THR; 45% and 20% with prophylaxis)
- Myocardial ischemia (31%)
- Fat embolism syndrome (10–20%)
- Pulm embolism (5%)

WORRY ABOUT

- ↑ PA pressures after cementing
- Intraoperative arterial desaturation (30%) with FIO_2 <50%
- Hypotension in 34% of hypovolemic patients. Euvolemia seems to reduce incidence of hypotension.
- Fatal pulm embolism (1–5%)
- Transient third degree heart block (?)

OVERVIEW

- An acrylic bone cement is freshly prepared and inserted into reamed bony cavities.
- Cementing associated with echogenic emboli regardless of joint (100%)
- ↓ Amount of echogenic emboli released for uncemented joints

- Intraoperative CV collapse
- Hypotension due to monomer and release of emboli
- Regional anesthesia ↓ postop DVT but does not ↓ echocardiographic emboli

ICD-9-CM Code: 820.x (Hip fracture)

INDICATIONS AND USUAL TREATMENT

- Cemented joint replacement (DJD, obesity, connective tissue diseases), distal and proximal femoral fracture, revision joint replacement; rare in craniotomy
- Treatment: NSAIDs (D/C >24 h prior to central neural axis blockade; for aspirin D/C >2 days), steroids (stress dose for surgery), subcutaneous heparin, LMW heparin (D/C >24 h prior to spinal or epidural)

ASSESSMENT POINTS

SYSTEM	EFFECT	TEST
HEENT	Taste of monomer after cementing	
CV	Cardiac output (no Dx, ↓ hypovolemia), preload (↓), afterload (↓), PVR (↑), third degree heart block, pericardial effusion Heart failure from pulm Htn If PFO, risk for paradoxical emboli	MAP, ECG, TEE CVP, PA catheterization
HEME	↑ Plt aggregation, ↑ thrombosis	Venography, duplex US, impedance plethysmography
CNS	↓ Cognitive function, stroke, confusion	Quick baseline neuro exam
RESP	V/Q mismatch, ↑ pulm pressure, pulm emboli Atelectasis	V/Q scan, PA catheterization Pulm angio, SaO_2, ABGs End-tidal CO_2, TEE, electrolytes

Key Reference: Parmet JL, Horrow JC, Singer R, Berman AT, Rosenberg H: Echogenic emboli upon tourniquet release during total knee arthroplasty. Anesth Analg 1994; 79:940–945.

INTRAOPERATIVE MANAGEMENT

Monitoring

- Volume status: Foley catheter, CVP (revision procedures, THR lateral approach)
- Consider PA catheter or transesophageal ECHO (↓ ventricular function, pulm Htn, age >70 y, severe connective tissue disease)
- If bilateral joint replacement, consider PA catheter to assess ↑ in PA pressure after cementing first joint
- Cardiac status: continuous monitoring of BP at time of cementing (A-line or NIBP 1-min cycle), end-tidal CO_2. Consider PA catheter (as above), TEE (intravascular volume, RV function, severity of emboli released after cementing, paradoxical emboli), ECG with ST-segment trending.
- Exhaled gas analysis: ↓ end-tidal CO_2 if significant pulm embolism; ↑ end-tidal N_2 if air embolus
- Pulm: blood gas analysis, pulse oximetry

SURGICAL STAGES

Pre-Cement

- THR: insidious blood loss due to irrigation
- TKR: tourniquet-induced Htn (tourniquet time >45 min)
- Maintain intravascular volume
- Upon mixing of cement and cementing, volume load with colloid, crystalloid, or autologous blood
- Discontinue N_2O during mixing of polymer
- Have inotrope available

Cementing

- Hypotension can result from monomer-induced vasodilation, open IV fluids
- FIO_2 100% to combat ↑ PVR from emboli
- If GA, lighten anesthetic and discontinue N_2O, maintain NMB
- Give inotrope (epinephrine or dobutamine) if 20% ↓ MAP

ANTICIPATED PROBLEMS/CONCERNS

- Intraoperative hypovolemia
- Impaired cardiopulmonary function leads to ↓ tolerance to cementing
- Fat embolism syndrome (hypoxemia, petechiae, neuro change)
- Neurocognitive changes due to paradoxical emboli

KASAI PROCEDURE
Nishan G. Goudsouzian, M.D.

RISK

- Incidence of biliary atresia: 1/15,000 live births
- Very rare association with other anomalies

PERIOPERATIVE RISKS

- Impaired liver function and coagulation disorders (late manifestation)
- Malnutrition, vitamin deficiencies (vit K and E)

WORRY ABOUT

- Other causes of jaundice such as viral hepatitis or cholangitis
- Alagille's syndrome (arteriohepatic dysplasia) in which jaundice is associated with hypercholesterolemia, pulmonary stenosis, pointed chin, and frontal bossing

OVERVIEW

- Performed to correct biliary atresia
- Entire extrahepatic biliary system consists of fibrous tissue
  – Perinatal type: most common, manifests at 4–8 wk of life with persistent and progressive cholestasis and jaundice
  – Embryonic or fetal type: infrequent, early onset, no jaundice-free interval after birth, may be associated with CV or GI anomalies
- Diagnosis with US, radionuclear scanning, MRI, and/or liver biopsy

ICD-9-CM Code: 751.61 (Congenital biliary atresia)

ETIOLOGY

- Unknown
- Leading cause for liver transplantation in children

INDICATIONS AND USUAL TREATMENT

- Biliary atresia
- Phenobarbital 5 mg/kg to enhance bilirubin conjugation and excretion (choleretic effect)
- Correction of nutritional and vitamin deficiencies
- Portoenterostomy (Kasai procedure)
- Liver transplantation

ASSESSMENT POINTS

SYSTEM	EFFECT	ASSESSMENT BY HX	PE	TEST
DERM	Jaundice	Progressive increase	Deep greenish-bronze color	Conjugated hyperbilirubinemia
GI	Cirrhosis	Abdominal discomfort	Abdominal distention Firm, enlarged liver Splenic enlargement	Hypoalbuminemia
	Stools	White or clay-colored		Acholic stools
RENAL	Urine	Greenish color		Bile stained
NUTRITIONAL	Weight loss	Poor appetite	Failure to thrive	Vitamin deficiency
CNS	Vit E deficiency	Ataxia	Hyporeflexia Ophthalmoplegia	
HEME	Blood loss	Weakness	Bloody stool	Endoscopy for esophageal varices

Key Reference: Howard ER: Biliary atresia: *In* Stringer MS (ed): Pediatric Surgery and Urology. Philadelphia, WB Saunders, 1998, pp 402–416.

PERIOPERATIVE IMPLICATIONS

Preoperative

- Correct coagulation defects with vit K and transfusion of FFP. If coagulation is normal, epidural block is helpful.
- Broad-spectrum antibiotics
- Nasogastric tube
- If vascular access is difficult, consider a central line

Monitoring

- Expect prolonged surgery
- A good IV in an upper limb is useful
- Arterial line is helpful. Not necessary if a central line is present for sampling.

Maintainance

- Avoid N$_2$O
- Maintain temperature, humidity, and urine output

SURGICAL STAGES

Surgery: Kasai Portoenterostomy

- Right subcostal incision extended to the left
- Cholangiogram and wedge biopsy of the liver to confirm diagnosis
- Meticulous dissection of the porta hepatis
- Roux-en-Y loop, the antimesenteric side of jejunum is sutured to the porta hepatis for biliary drainage
- If the gallbladder is present (5%), it can be used for the enterostomy

Postoperative Period

- Stomach decompression by nasogastric tube
- Prednisone 2 mg/kg/d for its choleretic effect, tapered after 1 mo
- If there is poor bile flow, absorption of fat and fat soluble vitamins will be impaired; must be supplemented

ANTICIPATED PROBLEMS/CONCERNS

- Cholangitis is frequent; recurrence of jaundice, elevation of liver enzymes, leukocytosis, and acholic stools
- Long-term survivors delayed development (nutritional deficiencies)
- Eventually will require liver transplantation
- Better to delay liver transplantation until the infant grows up
- Portoenterostomy prolongs transplantation surgery but does not affect outcome

KIDNEY TRANSPLANTATION
Dennis W. Coalson, M.D.

RISK

- 46,000 patients with ESRD on waiting list in USA in 2000
- 8100 cadaveric, 4400 living donor kidney transplantations performed in USA in 1999
- Recipients 60% male, 87% between 18–64 y
- Recipients 61% Caucasian, 23% African-American, 11% Hispanic, 4% Asian

PERIOPERATIVE RISKS

- 1–2% 30-day patient mortality
- Patient survival 1 y/4 y: cadaveric 93%/85%, living donor 97%/92%
- Allograft survival 1 y/4 y: cadaveric 83%/67%, living donor 92%/81%
- Hyperacute rejection, cardiac events, infection

WORRY ABOUT

- Hypovolemia or hypervolemia depending on dialysis-surgery interval
- Hyperkalemia with long interval since dialysis
- Prolonged duration of drugs excreted by kidneys
- Protection of hemodialysis access site, AV shunt or fistulas
- Noncardiogenic pulm edema with perioperative administration of OKT3
- Complications of IDDM (gastroparesis, CAD, autonomic neuropathy)
- Positioning: diabetics at increased risk for perioperative nerve injuries

OVERVIEW

- Extraperitoneal graft placement results in less fluid loss
- Potential for rapid blood loss
- Blood volume expansion desired to promote diuresis and early graft function
- Diuretics (furosemide), osmotic agents (mannitol), and dopamine agonists (dopamine, fenoldopam) given to promote diuresis

ICD-9-CM Code: 585

INDICATIONS AND USUAL TREATMENT

- Treatment of choice for patients with ESRD. Improves quality of life and increases life expectancy.
- Cause of ESRD: IDDM (31%), chronic glomerulonephritis (28%), polycystic kidney disease (12%), nephrosclerosis (9%), systemic lupus erythematosus (3%), interstitial nephritis (3%), IgA nephropathy (2%), Alport's syndrome (1%)
- Most common cause by race: type I diabetes in Caucasians, hypertensive nephrosclerosis in African-Americans, and chronic glomerulonephritis in Hispanics and Asians
- Alternative therapies: hemodialysis, peritoneal dialysis

ASSESSMENT POINTS

SYSTEM	EFFECT	ASSESSMENT BY HX	PE	TEST
CV/RESP	Hypervolemia Hyperkalemia	SOB	Rales, tachypnea Irregular HR	CXR, ABGs, ECG, electrolytes
HEME	Anemia		Systolic murmur, pale mucous membranes	Hct
PNS	Peripheral neuropathy, gastroparesis, autonomic neuropathy	Early satiety, nausea, postural syncope	↓ Peripheral sensation	Tilt table test, gastric emptying studies
MS	Osteopenia	Fractures		Bone density

Key Reference: Lazowski T: The influence of type of anaesthesia on postoperative pain after kidney transplantation. Ann Transplant 2000; 5:28–29.

PERIOPERATIVE MANAGEMENT

- Administration of antibiotics and attention to sterile technique in catheter placement
- Volume status monitoring and potential blood loss a concern
- Consider invasive arterial and CVP measurement
- UO absent or unreliable marker of volume status
- Administration of immunosuppressives prior to graft reperfusion
- Maximize renal blood flow at time of graft reperfusion with blood volume expansion and pharmacologic promotion of diuresis with mannitol, furosemide, and dopamine (2–4 μg/kg/min)

Anesthetic Technique

- General or regional (epidural) acceptable
- Rapid-sequence induction if full stomach or gastroparesis present

SURGICAL STAGES

- Skin incision
  – Adults: oblique lower abdominal incision for placement of graft in extraperitoneal iliac fossa
  – Small children: midline abdominal incision for retroperitoneal placement of graft
- Renal artery anastomosed end-to-end to recipient's artery or end-to-side to internal or common iliac artery
- Renal vein anastomosed to external iliac vein in adults and to IVC in children
- Donor ureter inserted by creating submucosal tunnel in recipient's bladder

POSTOPERATIVE CONSIDERATIONS

- Maintain normal to elevated art pressure and CVP to maximize renal blood flow
- Pain relief with PCA or epidural analgesia. If graft does not have early function, avoid prolonged use of meperidine/morphine.
- Watch for fluid overload and pulm edema

ANTICIPATED PROBLEMS/CONCERNS

- Noncardiogenic pulm edema if OKT3 given intraoperatively
- Sudden BP drops with administration of vasodilators in renal arteries by surgeon
- Sudden increase in stimulation with closure of fascia

KNEE ARTHROSCOPY

Nigel E. Sharrock, M.B., Ch.B.

RISK

- Arthroscopy of knee: in USA, >700,000/y
- Arthroscopic anterior cruciate (ligament) repair: in USA, 100,000/y
- Patients primarily <60 y—related to athletic injury
- No racial or gender predominance

PERIOPERATIVE RISKS

- Mortality rate <1:10,000
- Morbidity
  - Rare
  - Infection (esp with allografts)
  - Deep vein thrombosis/pulm embolism in patients >40 y if tourniquet used
  - Nerve injury to superficial branches of femoral nerve resulting in neural trauma—associated, sympathetically maintained pain
  - Popliteal artery injury

WORRY ABOUT

- Risk of bradycardia/asystole following tourniquet deflation or with regional anesthesia
- Risk of dural puncture in young patients
- Ability to discharge ambulatory patients
- Whether patient has an empty stomach
- Technical problems with obese or very muscular patients

OVERVIEW

- Arthroscopy is rapid ambulatory procedure in which arthroscope and repairing instruments/medications are inserted into joint; anatomic defects are viewed and recorded; and repair is initiated
- Very low perioperative mortality and morbidity
- Regional anesthesia preferred: early discharge, reduced pain, patients able to participate by viewing surgery on monitor

- Postop pain control an issue, esp following ACL repair
- MRI diagnosis

ICD-9-CM Codes: 717.83 (Anterior cruciate ligament tear); 836.0 (Medial meniscus tear)

INDICATIONS AND USUAL TREATMENT

- Meniscectomy or meniscal repair for torn medial or lateral meniscus
- Removal of loose bodies
- Reconstruction of torn ACL
- Debridement of osteochondral defects or osteoarthritis
- Synovectomy for inflammatory arthritis
- Nonsurgical treatment includes NSAIDs, physical therapy to increase strength of quadriceps, intra-articular steroids

ASSESSMENT POINTS

SYSTEM	EFFECT	ASSESSMENT BY HX	PE	TEST
CV	Risk of bradycardia/asystole due to tourniquet deflation, conduction anesthesia, emotional reaction	Hx of athletic state	Slow resting HR	ECG
HEME	Bleeding diathesis contraindication to regional anesthesia	Bleeding or bruising with injury or tooth extraction	Bruises	PT, APTT, plt count, bleeding time as indicated by Hx
GU	Postop urinary retention	Nocturia Hx of prior catheterization	Size of prostate	
CNS	Risk of bradycardia/ hypotension and nausea with sight of blood/surgery	Fainting or stress with prior surgery Rx with anxiolytic medication	Visibly anxious	

Key Reference: Mulroy MF, Larkin KL, Hodgson PS, Helman JD, Pollock JE, Liu SS: A comparison of spinal, epidural, and general anesthesia for outpatient knee arthroscopy. Anesth Analg 2000; 91:860–864.

PERIOPERATIVE IMPLICATIONS

Preoperative Issues

- Does patient want to watch procedure?
- Focus on early discharge
- Potential length of procedure

Monitoring

- Routine

Anesthetic Technique

- Local infiltration of portals + intra-articular injection of 20–30 ml 0.25% bupivacaine (often requires additional sedation). Cannot tolerate thigh tourniquet.
- Femoral nerve block: limited by tourniquet and surgery in back of knee
- Epidural, spinal, or combined spinal epidural. Issues are dural puncture headache, duration of surgery, and rate of onset and resolution of blockade.
- Choice of local anesthetic for spinal
  - Lidocaine (risk of transient radicular irritation)
  - Lidocaine plus fentanyl (problem of nausea and itching)
  - Other long-acting agents
- Conscious to deep sedation to GA: issues are short-acting agents (e.g., propofol/desflurane), airway problems, N/V, orthostatic dizziness postop

- Choice depends on duration of surgery, use of thigh tourniquet, the surgeon, patient preference, ease of discharge
- Induction: infiltration, blocks, intra-articular local anesthetic usually performed 15 to 20 min before surgery
- Spinal/epidural: control hemodynamic state
- GA: airway/full stomach

SURGICAL STAGES

Incisions

- Multiple portals around knee
- Tourniquet: pain may limit use if surgery is long—advantage of epidural or combined spinal epidural
- Irrigation can distend soft tissues around knee
- Rotation of leg can stress hip joint or lumbar spine (figure 4 position)

POSTOPERATIVE CONSIDERATIONS

- Control of pain and side effects can lead to early discharge
- N/V and orthostatic dizziness limit discharge, esp after deep sedation or GA, excessive sedation, or use of narcotics (less of a problem after regional anesthesia)
- Options—intra-articular drugs, e.g., bupivacaine ± morphine

- Local infiltration of portals with bupivacaine
- Femoral nerve blocks helpful after ACL repair, synovectomy, debridement, or lateral release. Requires knee brace for discharge
- IV or IM NSAIDs reduce narcotic requirement
- Narcotics: IV morphine (2-mg boluses) or oral medications every 3–4 h
- Urinary retention usually not limiting factor in young patients
- Follow-up phone call helps define and treat problems

ANTICIPATED PROBLEMS/CONCERNS

- Postop back pain (with or without regional anesthesia)
- Dural puncture headaches: should be followed and treated
- Postop pain usually controlled with oral medication and hypothermia
- Late urinary retention
- Transient radicular irritation with spinal lidocaine

LABOR, EPIDURAL BLOCK

Raymond S. Sinatra, M.D., Ph.D.

- In USA, ~20–22% of laboring women receive epidural analgesia
- Higher rates of use occur in hospitals with >1500 deliveries/y; placement dependent upon availability of skilled anesthesia caregivers

PERIOPERATIVE RISKS

- Hypotension 2° to sympathetic blockade; incidence as high as 17% in parturients not given adequate prehydration
- Inadequate analgesia 2° to unilateral block, dermatomal "window," rapid progression of labor
- Intravascular injection (risk of seizure and cardiotoxicity) 2° to needle insertion or catheter migration into epidural vein
- Other risks include excessive sensorimotor block, backache, dural puncture, intrathecal injection, headache, transient and persistent paresthesias

WORRY ABOUT

- Reduction in uteroplacental perfusion, fetal hypoxia/acidosis

- CV collapse/convulsions 2° to intravascular injection of local anesthetic
- Early placement of labor epidural block (e.g., primiparas <3–4 cm cervical dilation) or use of concentrated local anesthetic may slow progress of labor and increase incidence of dystocia and C-section
- High level of anesthesia "total spinal" with loss of airway (incidence 1/4500) related to excessive dose or to subarachnoid or subdural injections; hypoxemia and acidosis develop rapidly in parturients, and cardiopulmonary resuscitation is difficult
- Epidural hematoma/epidural abscess may occur with abnormal hemostasis (pre-eclampsia, abruption, ITP), underlying sepsis
- Post–dural puncture headache, incidence ~70% with 17-gauge epidural needle. Frequently requires epidural autologous blood patch.

OVERVIEW

- During 1st stage of labor, combinations of dilute local anesthetics and opioids effectively block pain impulses from uterus and cervix that travel via visceral afferent fibers (T10–T12, L1)

- During 2nd stage, epidural analgesia extended caudally to block input from S2–S4, controlling pain associated with vaginal and perineal distention

ICD-9-CM Code: V22 (Pregnancy)

INDICATIONS/CONTRAINDICATIONS

- Nearly complete pain relief with greater uniformity, duration, and patient satisfaction than other forms of labor analgesia; reduces maternal stress response and may improve uteroplacental perfusion
- Facilitation of vaginal delivery of twins and preterm infants; control of catecholamine release and maternal BP in preeclampsia and cardiac disease
- Contraindications include patient refusal, infection at site of placement, uncooperative patient, ↑ICP, coagulopathy, uncorrected hypovolemia, certain cardiac conditions. Alternatives include parenteral opioids, intrathecal opioids, distraction, TENS, hypnotherapy

ASSESSMENT POINTS

SYSTEM	EFFECT	ASSESSMENT BY HX	PE	TEST
CV	Aortocaval compression	Dizziness, syncope ↓FHR	Hypotension in supine position	Assess UO, provide left uterine displacement
RESP	↓FRC ↑Minute ventilation and O$_2$ consumption	Rapid development of hypoxemia	Tachypnea	Avoid high spinal blockade; provide supplemental O$_2$
CNS	↓MAC Epidural vein distention	Exaggerated effect of local anesthetics	Sedation; ↑sensory and motor block	Assess dermatomal blockade frequently
COAG	↓Plt count, abnormal function	Abnormal hemostasis	Oozing at IV site Bruising	Assess plt count Fibrinogen, FSPs, check bleeding time
FHR	Sensitive to maternal hypotension	Bradycardia, ↓HR variability	↓Movement HR variability; meconium	FHR monitoring, tocodynograph, fetal scalp blood sampling

Key Reference: Halpern SH, Leighton BL, Ohlsson A, Barrett JF, Rice A: Effect of epidural vs. parenteral opioid analgesia on the progress of labor: a meta-analysis. JAMA 1998; 280:2105–2110.

PERIOPERATIVE MANAGEMENT

Monitoring

- Establish BP and continuous maternal/fetal HR monitoring
- Assess airway; have resuscitation drugs and equipment immediately available
- Prehydrate with 750–1000 ml Ringer's lactate

Induction

- Epidural needle and subsequent catheter insertion at the L2–3 or L3–4 interspace. Test dose 3 ml local anesthetic solution containing 5 μg/ml epinephrine (epinephrine test dose controversial in labor).
- Maintain left uterine displacement; treat maternal hypotension with small doses of ephedrine (5–10 mg IV)

SURGICAL STAGES

- Very dilute LA/opioid solutions indicated for primiparas <5-cm cervical dilatation

- "Single shot" epidural and more concentrated solutions may be provided to multiparas
- Epidural induction: (1) bupivacaine 0.125–0.25% (8–12 ml) + fentanyl 50–75 μg, sufentanil (10–20 μg), or hydromorphone (100 μg). (2) Ropivacaine 0.2% (8–12 ml) or ropivacaine 0.1–0.2% + fentanyl 50–75 μg. (3) Levo-bupivacaine 0.125–0.25% + fentanyl (50–75 μg). Options 2 and 3 may lower the risk of maternal cardiotoxicity
- Epidural infusion: (1) Bupivacaine 0.0625–0.125% with fentanyl 1.0–3 μg/ml at 10–14 ml/h (higher concentrations of fentanyl are required with the most dilute bupivacaine infusions and may increase the incidence of pruritus). (2) Ropivacaine 0.2% alone or ropivacaine 0.1% + fentanyl 1.6–2 μg/ml at 10–14 ml/h. (3) Levo-bupivacaine 0.0625–0.125% with fentanyl (as described for bupivacaine).
- Epidural PCA: Reduce epidural infusion rate by ⅓. Add patient-controlled bolus dose of 2–3 ml of infusate solution q 10 min (prn). Useful for covering increased pain intensity during transition and 2nd stage labor.

- Anesthesia personnel should be immediately available 20–30 min after epidural induction/initiation of epidural infusion. Vital signs should be charted regularly.
- Epidural analgesia/anesthesia may be maintained for episiotomy repair or to facilitate removal of retained placenta
- Dermatomal blockade may be extended with lidocaine 2% with epinephrine (15–25 ml) or ropivacaine 0.5%–0.75% (15–25 ml) for C-section

ANTICIPATED PROBLEMS/CONCERNS

- Technical difficulty 2° to obesity, edema, patient movement; multiple attempts ↑risk of dural puncture, backache, paresthesia
- Fetal hypoxia 2° to ↓uteroplacental blood flow. Neonatal CNS depression related to opioid/local anesthetic exposure.
- Motor blockade, excessive relaxation of pelvic floor, ↓ability to push, need for oxytocin augmentation, possible ↑length of 1st and 2nd stages of labor

LABOR, PERIPHERAL BLOCKS

Manuel C. Vallejo, M.D.
Sivam Ramanathan, M.D.

RISK

• Pregnant women in labor who request analgesia where epidural or spinal analgesia is contraindicated

PERIOPERATIVE RISKS

• Periop mortality from anesthetic technique: rare
• Morbidity—accidental maternal IV local anesthetic (LA) injection: risk of seizures, cardiotoxicity, and fetal bradycardia

WORRY ABOUT

• Accidental IV injection
• Hypotension
• Fetal bradycardia (paracervical block)
• Neuropathy (nerve damage)
• Infection
• Hematoma formation

OVERVIEW

• Lumbar sympathetic block (LSB)—analgesia for the 1st stage of labor
• Paracervical block—analgesia for the 1st stage of labor
• Pudendal block—analgesia for the 2nd stage of labor
• Perineal infiltration—supplemental analgesia for the 2nd stage of labor

ICD-9-CM Code: V22.2 (Pregnancy)

INDICATIONS AND USUAL TREATMENT

• Indications—parturient in whom regional, parental, or other means of analgesia are not possible (i.e., coagulopathy, previous back surgery, spine pathology, failed or inadequate neuraxial analgesia)
• LBS may accelerate both 1st and 2nd stages of labor. Avoid in parturients with a history of uterine hyperstimulation.
• Paracervical block may produce fetal bradycardia

ASSESSMENT POINTS (Potential Complications)

SYSTEM	EFFECT	ASSESSMENT BY HX	PE	TEST
CV	Cardiac arrest Hypotension (LSB) Hematoma	IV injection Vessel puncture	Unresponsive Peripheral vasodilatation Swelling	ECG BP
CNS	Total spinal anesthesia Nerve damage	Subarachnoid injection	Loss of consciousness Neuropathy	 EMG
FETAL	Bradycardia	Fetal absorption		FHR
INFECTIOUS	Retropsoas abscess Subgluteal abscess	Poor aseptic technique	Fever, pain	MRI

Key Reference: Richardson MG: Regional anesthesia for obstetrics. Anesthesiol Clin North Am 2000; 18:383–406.

PERIOPERATIVE MANAGEMENT

Monitoring

• BP, pulse, O$_2$ saturation, FHR

Anesthetic Technique

• Lumbar sympathetic block
 – Prone position
 – Bilateral L1 or L2 transverse process
 – Needle advanced approximately 9 cm to anterolateral surface of L1 or L2 vertebral body
 – Inject bilaterally 10 ml of LA (bupivacaine 0.5% + fentanyl 25 μg + epinephrine 50 μg)
 – Will block entire lumbar sympathetic chain
 – Analgesia for 2–3 h

• Paracervical block
 – Blocks the paracervical ganglion (Frankenhauser's plexus)
 – Modified lithotomy position
 – 3–5 ml of LA each side
 – 1st injection—lateral fornix of vagina at 4-o'clock position, 0.5 cm deep
 – 2nd injection at 8-o'clock position
 – Epinephrine with LA may increase incidence of fetal bradycardia
 – Analgesia for 2–3 h
• Pudendal block
 – Perineal anesthesia for 2nd stage of labor, episiotomy, forceps or vacuum delivery
 – Transvaginal approach
 – Bilateral (10 ml) injections 1 cm posteromedial to ischial spines
• Perineal infiltration
 – Supplemental analgesia for vaginal delivery, episiotomy, forceps or vacuum delivery
 – Infiltration of several milliliters of LA into the posterior fourchette

ANTICIPATED PROBLEMS/CONCERNS

• Aspirate before injection to avoid IV bolus
• Lumbar sympathetic block
 – Hypotension
 – Retroperitoneal hematoma
 – Horner's syndrome
• Paracervical block
 – Fetal bradycardia
 – Fetal scalp injection
• Perineal infiltration
 – Fetal scalp injection

LAPAROSCOPY, GYNECOLOGIC

Susan Chan, M.D.

RISK

- >400,000 patients undergo gynecologic laparoscopy in USA yearly; female > male (50:1)
- Most common gyn surgical procedure

PERIOPERATIVE RISKS

- Mortality: 1.6–11/100,000
- CV complications (e.g., air embolus): 1–10/100,000
- Intra-abdominal complications—1%
- Postop pain necessitating hospitalization—0.5–2%

WORRY ABOUT

- Hypercarbia, resp acidosis, hypoxemia, pulm Htn, systemic vasodilation
- Pressure of pneumoperitoneum
- Hypothermia
- Pulm—atelectasis, ↓ FRC, high peak airway pressure, CO_2 embolus
- CV— ↓ venous return, ↓ cardiac output, cardiac dysrhythmia
- Gastric reflux—esp in patients with gastroparesis, hiatal hernia, obesity, or gastric outlet obstruction

OVERVIEW

- Endoscopic technique to visualize pelvic structure
- Adhesions and endometriosis can be treated endoscopically
- A small incision below umbilicus is made to insufflate CO_2 and 2 or more slightly larger incisions for insertion of visualization devices and instruments
- Duration of hospital stay significantly reduced. Most performed on outpatient basis, but duration of procedure may exceed that for open technique.
- Surgical complications include misplacement of Veres needle or trocar resulting in acute hemorrhage; bowel, bladder, uterus perforation; subcutaneous emphysema

ICD-9-CM Code: 54.21

INDICATIONS

- Tubal ligation, ectopic pregnancy, vaginal hysterectomy, PID, infertility
- Question of PID vs. appendicitis

ASSESSMENT POINTS

SYSTEM	EFFECT	ASSESSMENT BY HX	PE	TEST
CV	CV arrhythmia; ↓ venous return; ↑ level of stress hormones	Chest pain, SOB, Hx of CAD, DM, arrhythmia	CV exam	ECG
RESP	If pre-existing lung disease, hypercarbia, acidosis, hypoxia not tolerated well	SOB, ↓ exercise tolerance	Chest exam	O_2 sat ?ABGs
GI	↑ Intra-abdominal pressure; Trendelenburg position may ↑ chance of aspiration	DM, gastroparesis, hiatus hernia, obesity, gastric outlet obstruction	Airway exam	
HEME	Minimal blood loss normally	Hx of anemia, exercise tolerance	Vital signs	?Hct

Key References: Chi IC, Potts M, Wilkens L: Rare events associated with tubal sterilizations: an international experience. Obstet Gynecol Surv 1986; 41:7–19; Leonard F, Lecuru F, Rizk E, Chasset S, Robin F, Taurelle R: Perioperative morbidity of gynecological laparoscopy: a prospective monocenter observational study. Acta Obstet Gynecol Scand 2000; 79:129–134.

INTRAOPERATIVE MANAGEMENT

Monitoring

- Postop course more benign than in open procedure, yet intraoperative period may have much physiologic derangement
- Routine with end-tidal CO_2 waveform

Airway

- ↑ Risk of passive regurgitation and aspiration due to Trendelenburg position and ↑ intra-abdominal pressure. GA with ET intubation most common.
- Laryngeal mask airway satisfactory alternative in nonobese patients undergoing relatively short procedures

Anesthetic Technique

- No advantage of less physiologic stress has been shown by using regional anesthesia
- With ↑ intra-abdominal pressure, ↑ ventilatory pressures required to ventilate
- Nasogastric tube recommended to minimize gastric reflux
- Complete relaxation of abdominal muscle

Postoperative Considerations

- Pain score: 2–8 depending on procedure
- Potent opioid analgesics (fentanyl) most commonly used. NSAID ketorolac, 60 mg IM or IV, shown to decrease postop analgesic requirement.

ANTICIPATED PROBLEMS/CONCERNS

- Hypercarbia and acidosis most common physiologic complications when CO_2 used
- Subcutaneous emphysema, pneumothorax, pneumopericardium, pneumomediastinum, gas embolism less common
- Hypothermia and cardiac arrhythmia may be due to ↑ ventricular irritability, ↓ venous return, ↓ cardiac output, hypoventilation, gas embolism, or profound vagal response
- Blind insertion of the Veres needle or trocar associated with injuries to hollow viscera, major vessels, abdominal wall vessels

LARYNGOSCOPY

Andranik Ovassapian, M.D.

- Procedure used in millions of patients, to visualize pharynx and larynx for diagnostic/therapeutic purposes
- All age groups

PERIOPERATIVE RISKS

- Depends on nature of complaint and underlying disease
- Htn and tachycardia common because of pain and stimulation of airway reflexes
- Higher incidence of postextubation airway obstruction and reintubation than without tracheal intubation
- Incidence of reintubation when laryngoscopy performed for upper airway pathology: 0.39%

WORRY ABOUT

- CV response to laryngoscopy
- Postextubation laryngeal spasm and airway obstruction
- Establishing airway in postextubation period

OVERVIEW

- Rigid laryngoscopy associated with severe CV responses and increase in plasma catecholamine concentrations
- If difficult laryngoscopy associated with difficult mask ventilation, can cause cerebral damage and death in paralyzed patient

INDICATIONS AND USUAL TREATMENT

- Routinely applied for tracheal intubation during GA
- In combination of esophagoscopy and bronchoscopy, is applied for diagnosis and staging of oropharyngolaryngeal malignant lesions

ASSESSMENT POINTS

SYSTEM	EFFECT	ASSESSMENT BY HX	PE	TEST
HEENT	Limited neck flexion/extension Rule out unstable C-spine	Pain upon neck movement	ROM of neck, opening of mouth, pain on motion	C-spine x-ray
CV	Underlying cardiac disease common in elderly	Angina, arrhythmias Exercise tolerance	Cardiac evaluation Heart sounds Pulse rate and rhythm	ECG Stress test Thallium imaging angiogram
RESP	Hx of smoking	Wheezing; coughing; SOB; exercise tolerance	Wheezing, cyanosis	CXR PFTs with flow-volume loop
Airway	Tumors, infections Compression	SOB Difficulty in breathing Hemoptysis	Wheezing Use of accessory muscles	PFTs (flow-volume loop) X-rays ABGs

Key Reference: Atlee JL, Dhamee MS, Olund TL, George V: The use of esmolol, nicardipine, or their combination to blunt hemodynamic changes after laryngoscopy and tracheal intubation. Anesth Analg 2000; 90:280–285.

PERIOPERATIVE MANAGEMENT

Preoperative Preparation

- Observe patients with lower airway obstruction, preferably in ICU
- Communicate with endoscopist, as airway shared with anesthesiologist
- Check size of bronchoscope, ventilating side port attachment

Monitoring

- Routine

Anesthetic Technique

- Consider maintaining spontaneous ventilation if signs and symptoms of compromised airway are present
- Short-acting IV analgesics attenuate CV response to rigid bronchoscopy
- For jet ventilation, patient often totally paralyzed
- Surgical blood loss negligible, unless patient with hemoptysis, bleeding endobronchial lesions
- For laser operation, low concentration O_2 (<30%) in combination with N or He, special laser ET tube cuff inflated with saline used to minimize danger of fire; patient paralyzed to avoid movement

SURGICAL STAGES

- Patient supine with head and neck extended
- Bronchoscope is entered through right side of the mouth going midline to visualize the larynx
- Biopsy may be taken through bronchoscope
- Steroid considered if airway is compromised or if manipulation was extensive

Postoperative Concerns

- Continue observation of airway

ANTICIPATED PROBLEMS/CONCERNS

- Postbronchoscopy hypoxemia common; supplemental O_2 Rx recommended
- Coughing, secretions, SOB common
- Severe limitation of cervical spine precludes extension
- Contraindicated if unstable CV system
- Manipulation of the foreign body carries the risk of total airway obstruction
- Removing the bronchoscope and foreign body together endangers control of the airway

LASER SURGERY OF AIRWAY

Ira J. Rampil, M.D.

RISK

- People within USA: 3000–5000/y
- Race/gender predominance: none

PERIOPERATIVE RISKS

- Postop airway compromise
- Airway fires (5–70 reported/y)

WORRY ABOUT

- Loss of patent airway
- Displacement or ignition of ET tube
- Postop laryngospasm
- Residual NMB
- Misdirected laser beam igniting drapes
- Infection of OR personnel by vaporized but competent papillomavirus

OVERVIEW

- Focused, coherent far-infrared (CO_2) laser light can precisely vaporize superficial tissue lesions at a distance through free air
- Shorter wavelength (i.e., Nd:YAG) laser light can coagulate and necrose deeper lesions

ICD-9-CM Code: 478.4 (Laryngeal polyp)

INDICATIONS

- Many heterogeneous conditions, including laryngeal papilloma, tracheal scarring, webs or synechiae, vascular malformations, neoplasms, idiopathic subglottic stenosis

ASSESSMENT POINTS

SYSTEM	EFFECT	ASSESSMENT BY HX	PE	TEST
HEENT	Glottic or tracheal stenosis	DOE Stridor	Mallampati exam	Indirect laryngoscopy PFTs (flow-volume loop)
RESP	Neoplasia (V/Q mismatch)	Hemoptysis	Auscultation	CT or MRI of chest ABGs

Key Reference: Rampil IJ: Anesthetic considerations for laser surgery. Anesth Analg 1992; 74:424–435.

PERIOPERATIVE IMPLICATIONS

Preoperative Preparation

- Consider antisialagogue
- Eye protection for OR personnel appropriate to laser wavelength

Anesthetic Technique

- GA
- FIO_2 ≤40% to retard combustion, consider FIO_2 of 21%
- Avoid N_2O as it supports combustion
- Complete neuromuscular blockade

Monitoring

- Routine

Airway

- Use protected ET tubes, either commercial or smoothly wrapped with metal foil
- To allow surgical access, use smallest diameter tube consistent with adequate ventilation, i.e., 5.5 to 6.5 mm outside diameter for adults

Maintenance

- Maintain close communication with surgeon as procedure may conclude without significant lead time
- Be ready to emergently extubate trachea and provide mask ventilation in event of airway fire

Extubation

- Despite suctioning, pharynx may contain blood that may promote laryngospasm
- Some surgeons have strong preference for "deep" extubation following vocal cord surgery in order to avoid cough-induced injury

Postoperative Period

- Stridor, excess coughing, or bronchospasm warrants immediate investigation

Adjuvants

- Topical lidocaine ointment on ET tube and/or saline in cuff may retard ignition
- Surgeons may place moist pledgets in airway—be sure to retrieve them

ANTICIPATED PROBLEMS/CONCERNS

- Airway fire: clamp ET tube and remove; then reintubate with new ET tube

LIVER RESECTION

Steven M. Frank, M.D.

RISK

- Primary neoplasms: 5% of hepatic tumors
- Incidence: 4/100,000
- Males > females: 2:1
- Racial predominance: Asian
- Metastatic neoplasms: 95% of hepatic tumors, mostly from GI tract

PERIOPERATIVE RISKS

- 1–10% perioperative mortality, dependent on institution and co-morbidities of patient
- CV collapse from hypovolemia or vena cava crossclamp
- Morbidity: hepatic failure (5%), intra-abdominal infection (10–15%)

WORRY ABOUT

- Blood loss and proximity of blood bank
- IV access
- Need for vena cava crossclamp, and inability of liver to clear fibrin degradation products

OVERVIEW

- Surgical removal of tumors if no end-stage liver disease and potential to increase longevity or quality of life
- Potential for blood loss is increased with inexperienced surgical staff, large tumors, tumors located near porta hepatis or vena cava
- Consider intraoperative hemodilution to ↓ need for banked blood
- Consider venovenous bypass when IVC crossclamp may be required

ICD-9-CM Code: 235.3 (Neoplasm)

INDICATIONS AND USUAL TREATMENT

- Benign tumors: liver cell adenoma, hemangioma
- Malignant
  - Metastatic—GI tract, lung, breast, esophagus
  - Primary—hepatocellular carcinoma, cholangiocarcinoma, hepatoblastoma, angiosarcoma, lymphoma

ASSESSMENT POINTS

SYSTEM	EFFECT	ASSESSMENT BY HX	PE	TEST
RESP	Restrictive lung disease due to ascites	Dyspnea		Pericentesis
GI	Ascites	Ability to lie flat	Fluid wave Abd girth	Pericentesis
HEME	Splenomegaly can ↓ plt count	Bleeding Hx	Petechiae	Plt count, Hct
RENAL	Hepatorenal syndrome	UO	Uremia signs	BUN/Cr

Key Reference: Beebe DS, Carr R, Komanduri V, Humar A, Gruessner R, Belani KG: Living liver donor surgery: report of initial anesthesia experience. J Clin Anesth 2000; 12:157–161.

INTRAOPERATIVE MANAGEMENT

Preoperative Preparation

- Check availability of blood in bank or blood collection bags for hemodilution
- Check availability of FFP, plts, RBCs

Monitoring

- If large blood loss expected, consider arterial, CVP, and large-bore venous lines
- Clinical suspicion for venous air embolus
- Air embolism is more likely if the surgical field is situated at a level higher than the heart or in the presence of hypovolemia and resultant ↓ venous pressures

SURGICAL STAGES

Induction

- Consider rapid-sequence technique if ascites
- Limit doses of opioids and NM blockers in case of "open and close" situation—if the lesion is unresectable

Skin Incision

- Large RUQ incision

Dissection

- Cavitron (US), scalpel, finger dissection, cautery (electro- or argon beam)
- Wedge resection: least invasive; segmentectomy: moderately invasive; lobectomy: very invasive; trisegmentectomy: most invasive

Intraoperative Problems

- Vena cava crossclamp needed for tumor invasion into cava— ↓ venous return
- Need for venovenous bypass—from iliac vein to internal jugular
  - Best accomplished through extra large-bore percutaneously placed introducer (8.5–9 Fr)
- Venovenous bypass can be accomplished with a centrifugal (Biomedicus) pump

Closure and Postoperative Considerations

- Patients often remain intubated postop if large amount of IV fluid given or if hemodynamically unstable
- Can observe for postop bleeding through drains
- Analgesia can be by IV or epidural PCA
- EBL: 500–2000 ml
- Pain score: 8–10

ANTICIPATED PROBLEMS/CONCERNS

- Blood loss/hypovolemia—ensure IV access, blood availability; titrate anesthesia
- Need for plt after ~1 blood volume transfusion (~10 U)
- Need for FFP after ~1–2 blood volumes (>10 U)

PROCEDURES

LIVER TRANSPLANTATION

Phillip Mushlin, M.D.
Simon Gelman, M.D., Ph.D.

RISK

- Within USA: 16,000 people on waiting list
- Age range: neonate to >75 y; M:F, 1:1
- Only 4700 transplants/y (85% adults; 15% children), owing to shortage of donors (1999–2000 data)

PERIOPERATIVE RISKS

- Infection, renal failure, Htn, nerve injury
- Graft failure (primary nonfunction or rejection): allograft survival: 1-y = 80%
- Patient survival: 1-mo = 94%; 3-y = 76%

WORRY ABOUT

- Cardiomyopathy (alcoholism, hemochromatosis)
- Multisystem organ disease; infection, hepatorenal syndrome
- Severe coagulopathy; massive hemorrhage
- CV instability; metabolic derangements
- Embolism; VAE and thromboembolism
- Pulm Htn; RV failure on liver reperfusion
- Nerve injuries from positioning

OVERVIEW

- Native liver is removed and replaced with a whole liver, split liver, or liver segment
- Usually occurs in 24 h of removal from donor

INDICATIONS AND USUAL TREATMENT

- Noncholestatic cirrhosis (HCV, alcoholic, HBV, cryptogenic, postnecrotic)
- Cholestatic cirrhosis (1° biliary cirrhosis, 1° sclerosing cholangitis)
- Biliary atresia
- Fulminant hepatic failure (viral, drug)
- Inborn errors of metabolism, malignant neoplasms

ASSESSMENT POINTS

SYSTEM	EFFECT	ASSESSMENT BY HX	PE	TEST
CV	Hyperdynamic circulation Splanchnic hypervolemia Cardiomyopathy, pericardial effusion	SOB, palpitations, fatigue, poor exercise tolerance Symptoms of CHF	CV exam, ankle edema	ECG, ECHO, cardiac stress test, MUGA, coronary angiography
RESP	Restrictive lung disease, ARDS; pleural effusion, atelectasis Hepatopulmonary syndrome Portopulm Htn	Shortness of breath, dyspnea on exertion	$\downarrow$ SpO$_2$ Tachypnea, $\downarrow$ breath sounds Platypnea, orthodeoxia Clubbing of digits	CXR, ABGs, PFTs, pulmonary angiography
GI	Portal Htn, esophageal varices, GI bleeding Ascites; gastric emptying often delayed Cholestasis	Hematemesis Refractory ascites N/V, pruritus	Firm liver, hepatomegaly Palpable spleen Jaundice	Liver profile (SGOT, SGPT, albumin, INR), UGI endoscopy, mesenteric angiography
HEME	Anemia, coagulopathy, hypercoagulability (Budd-Chiari syndrome)	Bleeding diathesis, DVT, pulmonary embolism		CBC, PT, PTT, fibrinogen, DIC evaluation, TEG
RENAL	Oliguria; acute tubular necrosis (rare) Hepatorenal syndrome	Overly aggressive diuresis, fluid restriction, hypotension		BUN, Cr; CrCl, urinary osmolality and sodium
CNS	Encephalopathy, ICP increase (FHF)	Mental status changes	Pupillary signs, posturing Lethargy to coma	ICP monitor, EEG, MCA Doppler
INFECTION	Sepsis Spontaneous bacterial peritonitis		Fever	WBC, HTV test, hepatitis B vaccine Fungal, parasite, viral serologies
NUTRITION	Malnutrition, cachexia			Albumin, INR
FLUID/ LYTES	Hypervolemia, hyponatremia, $\uparrow$ K$^+$, $\uparrow$ or $\downarrow$ glu			Glucose, Na$^+$, K$^+$, Ca^{2+}

Key Reference: Alfrey EJ, Dafoe DC, Esquivel CO, et al: Liver transplantation. *In* Jaffe RA, Samuels SI (eds): Anesthesiologist's Manual of Surgical Procedures, 2nd ed. Philadelphia, Lippincott Williams & Wilkins, 1999, pp 494–504.

PERIOPERATIVE MANAGEMENT

Preoperative Preparation

- Correct coagulopathy and lyte imbalances
- Dialysis in patients with renal failure
- Drain pleural effusions if hypoxemia

Monitoring

- Use meticulous sterile technique when placing vascular catheters
- Large-bore IV lines, usually right-sided; left side often reserved for venovenous bypass
- Two arterial lines
- Central access—two 8.5-Fr percutaneous sheaths: distal for PA cath; proximal for vol
- TEE; be cautious if esophageal varices
- UO (Foley cath), lytes and glucose, coagulation status, Hgb, ABGs, ETCO$_2$

Induction

- Aspiration pneumonia prophylaxis (sodium citrate: IV metoclopramide and ranitidine)
- Rapid-sequence induction preferred

Maintenance

- Consider low-dose dopamine ± mannitol
- PEEP may improve oxygenation
- Monitor K$^+$ and Ca^{2+}

SURGICAL STAGES

Preanhepatic (Hepatectomy, Dissection)

- Major hemorrhage can occur; hemodynamic instability, metabolic acidosis, oliguria often occur

Anhepatic Stage (Implantation of Liver Allograft)

- Portal vein and hepatic artery are clamped
- Clamping IVC markedly $\downarrow$ VR, CO, and BP
- VVB stabilizes hemodynamics; it reroutes blood from portal vein and femoral vein to an axillary vein, which maintains VR and CO
- Complications of VVB: thromboembolism, VAE, fibrinolysis, brachial plexus injury, and infection
- Without a liver, likelihood of transfusion-induced citrate toxicity is $\uparrow$: treat with calcium

- Flushing donor liver with cold solution (5% albumin) removes most of preserving solution (145 mEq/L K$^+$)

Neohepatic Stage (Postrevascularization)

- Profound, usually transient, CV instability ($\downarrow$ BP, $\downarrow$ HR, $\downarrow\downarrow$ SVR, ± high CVP) can occur
- Severe coagulopathy can result
- To $\downarrow$ risk of hepatic art thrombosis, keep Hct <35

Postoperative Considerations

- Observe for postop bleeding
- Severe postop pain: treat with IV opioids
- Observe for graft dysfunction: e.g., $\downarrow$ production of bile, persistence of coagulopathy, CV instability, hypocalcemia, hyperglycemia, lactate

ANTICIPATED PROBLEMS/CONCERNS

- Potential for massive hemorrhage
- Avoid salvaged blood if infection
- Careful attention to positioning, hypothermia

LIVER TRANSPLANTATION (PEDIATRIC) Ashwani K. Chhibber, M.D.

RISK

- 567 liver transplants in patients < 18 y
- Approximately 1100 awaiting

PERIOPERATIVE RISKS

- 30-Day mortality < 10%

WORRY ABOUT

- Anemia
- Coagulation disorder
- Moderate to massive ascites
- Possibility of renal dysfunction or failure
- Pulmonary disorders 2° to ascites (restrictive lung disease) or decrease in A-a gradient
- ↑ Risk of systemic air embolization in patients with R → L shunts
- Encephalopathy
- Renal insufficiency
- Immunosuppression
- Peripheral nerve injuries due to positioning
- Hemodynamic instability
- Metabolic derangement

OVERVIEW

- 15% of all liver transplant recipients in USA are children
- About 70% of these patients are under 5 y
- Majority of pediatric liver transplants have been performed in pts with primary liver failure; most common cause, biliary atresia (~ 60%)
- Other patients requiring liver transplant include patients with α antitrypsin deficiency, inborn errors of metabolism, or acute liver failure due to acute viral illness and toxic or drug induced failure
- Due to shortage of organs, recent increase in living-related and split-liver transplantation

INDICATIONS AND USUAL TREATMENT

- Different indications than adults
  - Biliary atresia, biliary hypoplasia, and Alagille syndrome most common
  - Inborn error of metabolism (tyrosinemia, glycogen storage disease, urea cycle defects)
  - Metabolic disorders (e.g., Wilson's disease, cystic fibrosis, α_1 antitrypsin)
- Liver failure 2° to viral illness or toxic or drug-induced failure

ASSESSMENT POINTS

SYSTEM	EFFECT	ASSESSMENT BY HX	PE	TEST
CV	High CO, low SVR, high EF, dysrhythmias, pericardial effusion, ↑ AV shunting	Palpitations		ECG, ECHO
RESP	Hypoxia 2° to pleural effusion, atelectasis and ascites, V/Q mismatch, intrapulmonary shunting Pulmonary Htn, hepatopulmonary syndrome	Dyspnea, SOB		Chest x-ray, ABGs, PFTs (in older children, if indicated)
RENAL	Renal dysfunction due to prerenal azotemia Hepatorenal syndrome		UO	BUN, Cr, electrolytes, CrCl if indicated
HEME	Anemia, coagulopathy: thrombocytopenia, DIC, hypofibrinogenemia, dysfibrinogenemia, fibrinolysis			Bleeding time, PT, APTT, thrombin time, FDPs
CNS	Encephalopathy Cerebral edema in fulminant hepatic failure	Sx of ↑ ICP		Ammonia level ↑ ICP in fulminant failure
GI	Hepatic dysfunction; portal hypertension Delayed gastric emptying		Edema	Bilirubin, serum albumin, SGOT, SGPT
FLUID, LYTE, ACID-BASE STATUS	Intravascular volume depletion Hypokalemia, hyponatremia (hyperkalemia in hepatorenal syndrome), metabolic alkalosis			ABG analysis, electrolytes, glucose

Key Reference: Kelley SD, Cauldwell CB: Anesthesia for transplantation. *In* Gregory GA (ed): Pediatric Anesthesia, 3rd ed. New York, Churchill Livingstone, 1994.

PERIOPERATIVE IMPLICATIONS

Preoperative Preparation
- Judicious use of low-dose premedications
- Avoid intramuscular injections

Anesthetic Technique
- GA with volatile agents and narcotics
- Rapid-sequence or modified rapid-sequence
- Benzodiazepines for amnesia

Monitoring and Positioning
- Right and left arterial cannulation for BP monitoring and blood specimen collection
- CVP via internal jugular or subclavian
- In older children, PA cath to manage hemodynamics
- Consider TEE to monitor cardiac functions and air embolism
- ICP is measured if hepatic failure
- Two large-bore IV cannulas above diaphragm and fluid warmers
- Rapid infusing system is used
- Coagulation assessed with TEG, PT, PTT, INR, plt count, fibrinogen, and FDPs
- Urine output and electrolytes
- Pts wrapped in plastic to minimize heat loss; warmers are used along with humidification

Fluid and Blood Requirements for the Procedure
- Normal saline and/or plasmalyte
- Blood and FFP available in the room
- Maintain Hct 25–30%
- Excessive use of crystalloids should be avoided to avoid pulmonary edema

- Generally, blood-saving and rapid-infusion devices and VVB are not practical alternatives for reducing blood loss and maintaining CV stability in young infants

SURGICAL STAGES

Dissection Phase
- Skin incision to remove recipient's liver
- ↓ In CI and CVP in this phase 2° to blood loss, 3rd spacing, and vascular compression
- If patient has severe portal Htn and adhesions, can have massive blood loss
- Blood loss is replaced by PRBCs and FFP
- Frequent coagulation testing
- Massive blood transfusion associated with ↑ citrate load, ↓ calcium, ↑ potassium
- Hyperkalemia treated with hyperventilation, correcting acid-base status using glucose, insulin, and washed cells
- UO maintained
- Calcium replaced and inotrope started
- Consider aprotonin infusion

Anhepatic Stage
- Clamping of hepatic vessels and IVC
- Portal and IVC crossclamping just before removal of recipient's liver leads to ↓ venous return, low CO, low CVP, acidosis, ↓ renal function, and intestinal swelling
- Maintain normal to low-normal intravascular volume

Reperfusion/Neohepatic Phase
- Reperfusion of donor liver after unclamping portal vein and IVC
- Initial decrease in heart rate and BP, dysrhythmias, lactic acidosis
- Rapid ↑ in K^+ level may cause cardiac arrest
- Post-reperfusion hypotension syndrome is composed of sudden ↓ in BP, HR accompanied by coagulopathy, acid-base and lyte disturbance; correct quickly
  - Epinephrine infusion administered to maintain adequate BP and HR. CO is usually maintained
- With return of liver functions, improvement in coagulation, ↓ in lactic acid, and normalization of acid-base status and lytes

Postoperative Period
- Transferred to PICU intubated
- Hepatic functions monitored and PT maintained 1.5–2.0 times normal to avoid hepatic artery thrombosis

ANTICIPATED PROBLEMS/CONCERNS

- Bleeding and neurologic deficits
- Hepatic artery and/or portal vein thrombosis
- Bile leaks
- Rejection; primary or delayed
- Renal failure
- Electrolyte abnormalities
- Pulmonary complications

LUMBAR LAMINECTOMY

Sally C. Palmon, M.D.

- Up to 80% of USA population have at least temporary disability from low back pain. Majority without neurologic deficit recover with conservative therapy; <5% undergo surgery.
- Laminectomy for ruptured disk is most common major neurosurgical procedure
- Most common site of herniated nucleus pulposus is L4–L5 or L5–S1. Spinal cord ends at L2; therefore problems related to cord dysfunction are extremely rare.

PERIOPERATIVE RISKS

- Mortality rate ≤0.02%
- Continuing or recurrent pain is most common postop complication
- Life-threatening complications: hemorrhage from major vascular injury (0–1.6%); pulm embolism, thrombophlebitis, visceral injuries (0–0.5%)

WORRY ABOUT

- Hemorrhage due to perforation of major blood vessel (rare)
- Positioning complications: blindness, brachial plexus injury (esp when horseshoe headset used), meralgia paresthetica or other peripheral nerve injuries, quadriplegia, and Horner's syndrome from hyperextension of neck
- Chest wall and abdominal compression: at risk for resp embarrassment or hypotension due to ↓ preload
- Spinal cord compromise by extruded intervertebral disk
- Period of "monitoring blackout" during which ECG leads and BP monitor disconnected; prone position causes ↓ right heart filling, resulting in ↓ BP

OVERVIEW

- Operative procedures: can be done in prone, lateral, or kneeling position (prone-sitting frame). Last is associated with venous pooling and may cause hypotension. In posterior approaches, midline incised to detach and mobilize paraspinous muscles through subperiosteal technique. Removal of posterior neural arch in piecemeal fashion is termed laminectomy.

ICD-9-CM Codes: 722 (Herniated disk); 724 (Spinal stenosis)

INDICATIONS AND USUAL TREATMENT

- Rest, antispasmodics, NSAIDs
- For lumbar stenosis: a brief course of epidural steroid injections, physical therapy, or lumbar corset
- When medical therapy fails, surgery is indicated
- Laminectomy for decompression of lumbar stenosis indicated for recurrent intolerable pain associated with leg weakness or radiculopathy that restricts or prevents activities of daily living
- LOS shorter if microdiskectomy, some as outpatients

ASSESSMENT POINTS

SYSTEM	EFFECT	ASSESSMENT BY HX	PE	TEST
CV	Deconditioning	↓ Exercise tolerance— difficult to assess Smoking Hx, pulm disease	Heart murmur, gallop	ECG, ?ECHO
RESP	Restrictive diaphragm or other rib cage movement		Lung exam—signs of failure?	PFTs if severe lung disease
CNS/PNS	Peripheral neuropathy, paraplegia, myelopathy or sensory deficit, compromised by prone position	Pain, inability to ambulate, bowel or bladder dysfunction	Sensory deficit, ?motor deficit	Preop evoked potentials, EMG, or MRI/CT
MS	Skeletal metastasis from primary cancer	Primary tumor from breast, lung, kidney, thyroid, prostate Chemotherapy Hx		?CXR, electrolytes (Ca^{2+}), bone scan
PSYCH	Chronic pain, possible substance abuse (opioids)	Multiple medications (narcotics, NSAIDs, antidepressants)		

Key Reference: Olympio MA, Youngblood BL, James RL: Emergence from anesthesia in the prone versus supine position in patients undergoing lumbar surgery. Anesthesiology 2000; 93:959–963.

PERIOPERATIVE IMPLICATIONS

Preoperative Preparation

- Preload patient before turning to prone position to avoid CV effects of ↓ preload

Anesthetic Technique

- Need to know if single- or multilevel decompressive laminectomy to estimate blood loss, monitoring, and time to awakening to obtain neurologic exam
- General ET intubation with inhalational or N_2O/narcotic anesthesia and muscle relaxants is preferred but spinal, epidural, or local anesthesia has been used
- If regional chosen, preop evaluation for pre-existing neurologic deficit is important
- To evaluate nerve root stimulation, no muscle relaxant used. Avoid succinylcholine if severe neurologic deficit present (paraplegia).

- If cord compromised with neurologic deficit, attempt to maintain spinal cord perfusion pressure by maintaining BP at preop level

Monitoring

- Consider intra-arterial catheter if severe spinal stenosis or neurologic deficit present

Airway

- Patient in prone position after hours of surgery for multilevel laminectomy with more than usual fluid requirements and blood loss may have airway edema and facial swelling. Be aware of co-existing cervical spine disease. Consider postop ventilation if breathing cannot occur around ET tube when cuff is down.

SURGICAL STAGES

Dissection

- Cauda equina injury (0.01–0.02%) and root injury rare during dissection
- Major vascular injury during dissection also rare (0–1.6%)

Definitive Surgery

- Hypotension may develop from unrecognized blood loss or ↓ preload in prone position
- Air embolism can occur in spinal surgery in prone position (rare)

Postoperative Considerations

- Early neurologic assessment required; consider anesthetic tailored to prompt awakening
- PCA or epidural or spinal analgesia

ANTICIPATED PROBLEMS/CONCERNS

- Problems with prone positioning
- Need for reoperation

LUNG VOLUME REDUCTION SURGERY (PNEUMOPLASTY)

Brett A. Simon, M.D., Ph.D.

RISK

- Severe, activity-limiting pulm emphysema; given prevalence of emphysema (13.5 million Americans affected), the number of potential candidates for this operation is enormous
- Average preop FEV_1 25–30% predicted
- Controversy over patient selection, long-term outcomes, optimal surgical procedure, and cost-benefit tradeoffs have prompted a joint HCFA/NIH clinical study (National Emphysema Treatment Trial [NETT]), randomizing patients to medical or surgical treatment with 5 years of follow-up. Medicare will pay for this procedure only within the NETT.

PERIOPERATIVE RISKS

- In-hospital mortality: 3–6%
- 25% morbidity includes prolonged air leaks, resp failure, pulm embolism, pneumonia
- Greatly increased risk of complications in patients with reactive airway disease, CAD, pulm Htn

WORRY ABOUT

- Hypotension due to air trapping with controlled ventilation
- Difficulty with ventilation and oxygenation (less so) during one-lung ventilation
- Exaggerated resp depressive effects of narcotics (IV and neuraxial)
- Minimizing airway pressures and smoothly extubating spontaneously ventilating patient in OR to avoid creating or worsening air leaks

OVERVIEW

- Palliative procedure for severe, activity-limiting emphysema with 20–30% of lungs resected to reduce lung volume and reshape diaphragm and chest wall
- Bovine pericardial or Gore-Tex strips used to reinforce staple lines and reduce air leaks
- Variety of unilateral, bilateral, open, and thoracoscopic techniques being explored. Open, bilateral lung volume reduction via median sternotomy is original approach and has best documented results to date.
- Benefit thought to result from improving mechanical function of chest wall and diaphragm by reducing total lung volume, combined with reduction and reshaping of lung tissue; results in increase in lung recoil at this lower volume and increased expiratory flows
- Patients typically require a great deal of attention to keep them extubated during first several hours postop

- Successful outcome requires team approach including experienced pulmonologists, pulm rehab, thoracic surgeons, anesthesiologists, pain service, chest PT, ICU physicians. Sophisticated pulm function testing and lung imaging facilities should be available.

ICD-9-CM Code: 492.8 (Emphysema)

INDICATIONS AND USUAL TREATMENT

- Alternative to lung transplantation for patients with primarily pure emphysema that significantly limits their activity
- Exclusion criteria include pulm Htn (mean PAP >35 at rest), bronchospasm, LV dysfunction, bronchitis or excessive sputum production, persistent smoking, previous thoracotomy or pleurodesis, obesity, or cachexia
- All patients required to undergo at least 6 wk of preop pulm rehab, with supplemental O_2 if necessary. Poor results expected if cannot perform at least 800 ft in standard 6-min walk test.
- Successful procedures typically result in 60–70% increase in FEV_1 by 3 mo sustained at least 1 y, ↓ TLC and residual volume, improved exercise tolerance, and significant reductions in O_2 requirements at rest and during exercise. Data suggest improvements are sustained for at least 2–3 y.

ASSESSMENT POINTS

SYSTEM	EFFECT	ASSESSMENT BY HX	PE	TEST
CV	LV/RV dysfunction Pulmonary Htn	CHF, PND, palpitations	Peripheral edema, JVD, S_3	MUGA, ECHO may be unreliable with COPD
RESP	Emphysema	SOB, exercise tolerance and performance with rehab, bronchospasm, sputum production	Wheezing	PFTs, CT, plethysmography, quantitative V/Q scan

Key Reference: Cooper JD, Lefrak SS: Lung reduction surgery: 5 years on. Lancet 1999; 353:S1, 26–27.

PERIOPERATIVE MANAGEMENT

Preoperative Preparation
- Successful completion of pulm rehab program
- Maximize bronchodilator therapy

Anesthetic Technique
- Thoracic epidural placement at ~T4 interspace for intraop and postop use; test and verify onset of segmental block prior to induction
- Minimize narcotics because of risk of resp depression
- Goal of anesthetic is to maximize possibility of extubation in OR
- Chest tubes placed to water seal only, unless suction required

Monitoring
- Arterial line required
- Consider central line for intraoperative infusions and postop fluid management

Airway
- Left-sided double-lumen tube placed for bilateral procedures

Induction/Maintenance
- Anticipate hypotension due to air trapping with chest closed
- Ventilate with low pressures and low rates; tolerate hypercapnia if necessary
- Maintain on low-dose inhaled agent
- Use of epidural depends on hemodynamic stability; consider waiting until chest open before dosing; use of straight local may require phenylephrine infusion for BP maintenance; if narcotics used, limit dose
- Continue bronchodilator therapy in OR if necessary

SURGICAL STAGES
- Bronchoscopy: flexible bronchoscopy
- Resection: "better" side, usually right, resected first to improve tolerance of one-lung ventilation when second side resected
- Emergence: switch to single-lumen tube, LMA, or mask while patient is deep to facilitate emergence
- Elevate head; optimize pain control; suctioning; bronchodilators for emergence
- Patients require 30–90 min observation, encouragement, and "fine-tuning" in OR prior to transport to ICU; first ABG in ICU has P_{CO_2} >70 mmHg in >50% of patients

Fluid Considerations
- Typically run "dry"
- Significant blood loss requiring transfusion unusual

Postoperative Considerations
- Make every effort to extubate in OR and avoid reintubation and ventilation; if required, use minimum pressure support without mandatory breaths if possible
- Use epidural infusion ($1/8$–$1/4$% [0.0625–0.125%] bupivacaine ± 1–3 μg/ml fentanyl) supplemented with non-narcotic pain relievers
- Pain score: 6–8

ANTICIPATED PROBLEMS/CONCERNS
- Extremely marginal patients susceptible to even mild postop insults (pneumonia, pulm embolism, oversedation, pneumothorax, bronchospasm)
- Reintubation and mechanical ventilation associated with high morbidity

MENINGOMYELOCELE REPAIR
Madelyn Kahana, M.D.

RISK

- 2/1000 live births
- Most common in lumbar and lumbosacral segments

PERIOPERATIVE RISKS

- Failure to surgically close in a timely fashion results in ↑ risk of infection
- Co-existing congenital defects largely determine operative risk

WORRY ABOUT

- Co-existing congenital abnormality
- Intraoperative temp instability
- Proper prone positioning

OVERVIEW

- Defect in closure of bony spine at any level associated with defects of meninges and spinal cord
- Associated with high frequency of other abnormalities
- Prenatal diagnosis possible with amniocentesis and US
- Gestational age important as predictor of co-existing pulm insufficiency
- Postop apnea not uncommon following GA in newborn, esp if premature

ICD-9-CM Codes: 741.9 (Without hydrocephalus); 741.0 (With hydrocephalus)

INDICATIONS AND USUAL TREATMENT

- Prompt closure of meningomyelocele with preservation of viable neural tissue after careful evaluation of infant for associated abn, esp significant cardiac defects
- Initial resuscitation generally unnecessary; wound covered with sterile saline-soaked dressings until operative closure possible

ASSESSMENT POINTS

SYSTEM	EFFECT	ASSESSMENT BY HX	PE	TEST
CV	Associated cardiac defect		Murmur Cyanosis	ECG ECHO O$_2$ saturation
RESP	Possible IRDS Resp failure	Prematurity High thoracic or cervical lesion		CXR
RENAL	Associated renal anomalies	Abdominal mass		US
CNS	Varying degrees of paralysis Associated Chiari deformity Associated hydrocephalus Associated hydromyelia/ diastematomyelia		Careful neurologic exam	CT US

Key Reference: Viscomi CM, Abajian JC, Wald SL, Rathmell JP, Wilson JT: Spinal anesthesia for repair of meningomyelocele in neonates. Anesth Analg 1995; 81:492−495.

INTRAOPERATIVE MANAGEMENT

Preoperative Management

- Meticulous debubbling of lines in patients with septal defects
- Infection control—postop sepsis a major concern

Anesthetic Technique

- Performed under general anesthesia in prone position

Monitoring

- Temp maintenance can be problematic
- Consider a warming mattress and lamps
- Resp status determines need for arterial catheter
- Foley catheter indicated if preop bladder distention

Airway

- Associated proximal bowel atresias may dictate precautions for full-stomach intubation

SURGICAL STAGES

Induction

- Consider co-existing cardiac and intestinal malformations in the choice of agents
- Infants prone to hypotension with deep inhalation anesthesia
- Atropine as premedication recommended by some

Dissection and Definitive Surgery

- Minimal blood loss

Postoperative Considerations

- Recovered in prone position
- Apnea a frequent problem, associated with prematurity, GA, Chiari malformation
- Pain postop influenced by sensory level associated with defect
- CSF leaks not uncommon

ANTICIPATED PROBLEMS/CONCERNS

- Associated congenital malformations, especially of heart, brain, intestinal tract
- Co-morbidity of prematurity
- Eventual development of latex allergy common

MITRAL VALVE REPLACEMENT

David L. Berger, M.D.

RISK

- Majority of cases are post-rheumatic
- Associated with advancing age and myxomatous degeneration
- Ischemia increasingly a cause
- Gender predominance: none
- Age: 40–75 y

PERIOPERATIVE RISKS

- Perioperative 30-day mortality: 5–8%
- Morbidity
  - CNS complications: transient neurologic dysfunction 5–10%; CVA 1–2%
    - Pneumonia: 10–15%
    - Infection: < 1%

WORRY ABOUT

- Cardiac failure
- Dysrhythmias
- Hemorrhage
- Tamponade
- Conduction defects
- AV disruption

OVERVIEW

- Mitral valve repair or replacement typically done for correction of post-rheumatic degenerative mitral insufficiency, or repair after endocarditis
- Normal valve area is 4–6 cm^2
- Symptoms occur at 50% decrease in area, with severe symptoms at 1 cm^2
- Severe symptoms if regurgitant fraction > 0.6

ICD-9-CM Codes: 394.0 (Stenosis); 424.0 (Insufficiency)

INDICATIONS AND USUAL TREATMENT

- For mitral regurgitation (MR) from posterior leaflet abnormality (myxomatous degeneration, torn chordae) or pure annular dilatation, most valves can be repaired
- For severe rheumatic calcific mitral stenosis (MS), replacement with preservation of subannular structures may be necessary
- Transesophageal echocardiography now routine to assess repair/replacement prior to leaving OR

ASSESSMENT POINTS

SYSTEM	EFFECT	ASSESSMENT BY HX	PE	TEST
CV	MS: DOE, pulm edema MR: acute: CHF; chronic: DOE, paroxysmal nocturnal dyspnea	Exertional dyspnea, fatigue	Rales S$_3$	ECG ECHO
RESP	Pulm congestion, SOB	SOB	Chest exam	CXR
GI	Hepatic congestion Coagulation problems		Hepatomegaly	LFTs
HEME	May be on anticoagulants			PT, PTT
RENAL	↓ CO may lead to renal failure			BUN, Cr, electrolytes
CNS	CVA due to thrombus in AFIB		Neuro exam	CT scan, ECHO

Key References: Kaplan JA (ed): Cardiac Anesthesia, 4th ed. Philadelphia, WB Saunders, 1999, pp 755–768; Youngberg JA (ed): Cardiac, Vascular and Thoracic Anesthesia. Philadelphia, Churchill Livingstone, 2000, pp 394–398.

PERIOPERATIVE MANAGEMENT

Preoperative Preparation

- Assess status of ventricular function

Monitoring

- Arterial line
- CVP, PA catheter
- Urinary catheter
- ST-segment analysis
- TEE (for volume management, regional wall motion, assessment of valve repair)

Anesthetic Technique

- GA with low- to moderate-dose narcotic

SURGICAL STAGES

Induction

- MS: hypotension treated with fluid; maintain SVR with phenylephrine if necessary. Avoid tachycardia and treat with increased anesthesia (esmolol if cardiac function adequate). Sinus rhythm should be maintained.
- Treat new-onset AFIB/AFLT with defibrillation. Avoid increases in PVR.
- MR: maintain or augment preload based on response to fluid load. Inotropic agents may be necessary for contractility. Fenoldopam is a favorite drug. Afterload reduction to improve forward flow. IABP may be useful if acute MR due to MI.

Maintenance

- MS: avoid tachycardia, exacerbation of pulm Htn; maintain preload
- MR: maintain mild tachycardia, low SVR, adequate preload

Post-Bypass

- Patients with MR usually do well after valve replacement. Minimal inotropes necessary for separation from CPB.
- Patients with MS, especially late in disease, may require significant inotropes on separation from CPB

Emergence

- Transport to ICU intubated and ventilated
- Consider continuation of hypnotic infusions into ICU
- Pain scores: 5–10
- Manage pain with small doses of opioids; hypnotic/anxiolytic infusions or small doses for sedation while intubated
- EBL: 300–400 ml

ANTICIPATED PROBLEMS/CONCERNS

- Postop ventilation usually necessary; may be a candidate for "fast-tracking" if cardiac function adequate and uncomplicated operative course
- Inotropic support or vasodilator therapy may be needed
- IABP for mitral incompetence, especially with infarction-associated MR
- Postop neurologic deficit

MYRINGOTOMY AND TYMPANOSTOMY   Kenneth B. Fickling, M.D.

RISK

- Most common pediatric surgical procedure in USA requiring anesthesia
- No racial or gender predominance

PERIOPERATIVE RISKS

- Perioperative mortality extremely low ($\ll 1\%$)
- Concurrent URI symptoms not associated with increased perioperative morbidity

WORRY ABOUT

- Upper airway obstruction 2° to or worsened by hypertrophied adenotonsillar tissue, lateral head positioning, nonpatent nasal airways
- Laryngospasm
- Immediate IV access usually not available
- Cardiac dysrhythmias and suppression 2° to inhalational anesthesia (usually halothane or sevoflurane)

OVERVIEW

- Procedure to remove infection potential of fluid and to allow pressure equalization
- Vast majority of procedures performed in children aged 12 mo–5 y
- May be performed on anyone 6 mo to adult
- Associated with chronic or recurrent middle ear infections (otitis media [OM]) 2° to eustachian tube dysfunction
- Eustachian tube dysfunction etiologies include viral URI infections, congenital obstruction, adenotonsillar hypertrophy
- 30–40% present with URI symptoms at time of surgery (URI not contraindication to surgery without airway intubation in absence of productive cough; may increase risk of postop airway problems)

ICD-9-CM Code: 382.9

INDICATIONS AND USUAL TREATMENT

- Pressure equalization (PE) tubes are generally placed only if
  - Episodes of acute OM are frequent, recurrent, and poorly responsive to conventional antibiotic therapy
  - A chronic OM ensues that is refractory to antibiotic prophylaxis
  - A chronic middle ear effusion associated with hearing loss develops

ASSESSMENT POINTS

SYSTEM	EFFECT	ASSESSMENT BY HX	PE	TEST
HEENT	Ear pain, effusions, concurrent URI symptoms	Tugging at ears, hearing loss, nasal congestion or discharge, sneezing, snoring	Ear exam, adenotonsillar enlargement	Audiogram
CV		Hx of heart murmur or congenital heart disease	Murmur	
RESP	URI symptoms	Cough, wheezing	Auscultation for wheezing	CXR, O₂ sat

Key Reference: Paradise JL, Feldman HM, Campbell TF, et al: Effect of early or delayed insertion of tympanostomy tubes for persistent otitis media on development outcomes at the age of three years. N Engl J Med 2001; 344:1179–1187.

PERIOPERATIVE MANAGEMENT

Preoperative Preparation

- Age-appropriate NPO modifications to avoid mask induction in dehydrated child
- Potential need for preop sedation with midazolam (rectal or nasal) in extremely anxious child; best if avoided because procedure extremely brief

Monitoring

- Routine including precordial stethoscope
- IV unnecessary unless significant co-existing disease mandates use

Airway

- Mask induction with O₂, N₂O, inhalational agent
- Maintenance with mask anesthesia often easier with oral airway in place, as nasal passages are frequently obstructed. Consider LMA placement.
- Lateral head positioning can compromise airway

SURGICAL STAGES

Induction

- Potential for CV instability 2° to volume status
- Deep anesthesia generally maintained until after final myringotomy

Postoperative Considerations

- Emergence generally rapid if procedure is brief
- Minimal to moderate postop pain
- Acetaminophen 30–40 mg/kg rectally prior to emergence may be helpful
- EBL: minimal

ANTICIPATED PROBLEMS/CONCERNS

- Speed and experience of surgeons inversely and duration of anesthetic directly proportional to airway complication rate
- SpO₂ desaturation with even brief periods of airway obstruction or in presence of co-existing lung disease (e.g., former premature infants with bronchopulmonary dysplasia)
- Laryngospasm if adequate depth of anesthesia not achieved prior to myringotomy

NEPHRECTOMY/RADICAL NEPHRECTOMY Vinod Malhotra, M.D.

RISK

- Radical nephrectomy (>half of all nephrectomies) performed for renal carcinoma. Incidence: 24,000 cases/y.
  – Male:female ratio: 2:1
  – Urban dwellers > rural dwellers
  – 3–7% of lesions extend into IVC
- Simple nephrectomy: indicated for nonfunctioning obstructed kidney, polycystic kidney, donor transplants, uncontrollable renal Htn

PERIOPERATIVE RISKS

- Perioperative mortality rare (<1%)
- Considerable risk (22%) of DVT, pulm embolism, pulm atelectasis, renal dysfunction

WORRY ABOUT

- Massive blood loss (injury to renal vein, vena cava, renal artery, liver, spleen)
- Pneumothorax in thoracoabdominal approach
- Hypotension in flank position with kidney rest (bar) up

- Preservation of remaining kidney function
- Thrombus in IVC/hepatic vein
- Renal artery/vein avulsion during laparoscopic surgery

OVERVIEW

- Kidney with its pedicle removed in simple nephrectomy
- Kidney, adrenal, perinephric fat, and Gerota's fascia removed en bloc in radical nephrectomy
- Monitoring requirements depend upon IVC involvement and patient's medical status
- Excessive bleeding may occur if IVC involved
- CPB indicated if large atrial thrombus (right heart catheterization to be avoided)
- Venous return impeded by tumor thrombus in IVC leads to hypotension and falsely ↑ CVP
- Pulm embolization may occur during mobilization of tumor thrombus

- Pneumothorax likely
- Epidural analgesia for postop pain relief preferred by many. *Note*: With vena caval obstruction, epidural veins are dilated and space is narrowed.
- Laparoscopic-assisted nephrectomy becoming more common, associated with shorter length of stay

ICD-9-CM Codes: 593.89 (Obstructed kidney); 189.0 (Renal neoplasm); V59.4 (Donor kidney)

INDICATIONS AND USUAL TREATMENT

- Radical nephrectomy only effective treatment for renal carcinoma
- Pre- and postop radiation therapy as adjunct of questionable value
- Nonfunctioning, obstructed kidney must be removed to prevent sepsis, renovascular Htn, dysfunction of contralateral kidney
- Donor nephrectomies are elective and in healthy subjects

ASSESSMENT POINTS

SYSTEM	EFFECT	ASSESSMENT BY HX	PE	TEST
CV	Thrombus extending into IVC and right atrium	SOB	Lower limb edema Collateral prominent abdominal wall veins Varicocele	MRI MRA MRV
RESP	Pulm metastases Pleural effusion Pulm embolus	SOB	Auscultation	CXR CT
HEPATIC	Portal vein occlusion (Budd-Chiari syndrome)			CT Venogram
CNS	Brain metastasis	Altered neural function		CT
MS	Metastasis	Bone pain	Bone deformity in advanced cases	X-ray, bone scan, CT

Key Reference: Shah N: Radical cystectomy, nephrectomy, RBLD. *In* Malhotra V (ed): Anesthesia for Renal and Genitourinary Surgery. New York, McGraw-Hill, 1996, pp 209–211.

PERIOPERATIVE MANAGEMENT

Preoperative Preparation

- US, CT, MRI, metastatic work-up
- Cardiorespiratory, renal evaluation

Anesthetic Technique

- GA with controlled ventilation
- Combined epidural/general or epidural for postop analgesia
- CPB may be required
- Blood salvage and transfusion may be used

Monitoring

- Consider arterial line and ECHO if renal vein–IVC involvement
- Consider CVP/right heart catheter (right heart catheter contraindicated if intra-atrial thrombus)
- Foley catheter

SURGICAL STAGES

- Bleeding during renal dissection, renal vein/IVC injury, or injury to spleen/liver
- Hypotension during positioning in kidney position
- Decreased venous return during removal of IVC/intra-arterial thrombus
- Pulmonary embolus during thrombectomy
- Pleura may be entered through diaphragm
- EBL: 500–2000 ml

Postoperative Considerations

- Pain score: 5–10 for open cases
- Epidural analgesia may improve resp function, or IV PCA for 3 days
- May develop DVT or pulmonary embolism
- Atelectasis due to splinting
- Head and neck edema from head-down positioning
- Shorter length of stay if laparoscopic

ANTICIPATED PROBLEMS/CONCERNS

- Blood loss, pulmonary embolism, pneumothorax

OFFICE-BASED ANESTHESIA

Angela Gailey, M.D.

RISK

- \>3.5 million office-based procedures performed/y
- ~20% of all elective surgeries are performed in an office-based setting
- No race/gender predominance

PERIOPERATIVE RISKS

- Procedure-specific—risks are in accordance with planned procedure and condition of the patient
- Absence of adequate number of well-trained personnel to support procedure
- Sufficient support and equipment available to handle an emergency
- Inability to rapidly get to another health care facility, e.g., a hospital

WORRY ABOUT

- Loss of airway
- Unforeseen operative and/or anesthetic complications
- Lack of proper emergency equipment and help
- Systems to transfer patient to acute care facility in emergency situation

OVERVIEW

- Procedures that occur at a site physically removed from both the hospital and surgical center that use IV or inhalational agents of psychotropic drugs to provide varying degrees of sedation/anesthesia, amnesia, and analgesia
- Delivery of high-quality patient care in the office makes for lower overhead, thereby decreasing the cost of providing surgical services

- Improvements in anesthesia techniques and new surgical technologies continually push the limits of what can be safely performed in office surgery suites

INDICATIONS

- Many elective and low-risk or minimally invasive procedures in otherwise healthy individuals, i.e., ASA classes I and II, usually between the ages of 7 and 70
- Office-based surgery is useful when convenience, comfort, and privacy are desired

ASSESSMENT POINTS

SYSTEM	EFFECT	ASSESSMENT BY HX	PE	TEST
HEENT	Difficult intubation	Difficult airway Sleep apnea/snoring	Mallampati exam	
RESP	Desaturation Hypoxia	Smoker, SOB Asthma/emphysema Significant obesity	Chest exam	CXR
CV	CAD	MI/Htn/arrhythmia Angina/CHF/orthopnea Past cardiac surgery Exercise tolerance	Chest exam	ECG
GI	N/V	Postop N/V		
HEME	Tachycardia Hypotension	Anemia, bleeding disorder Sickle cell disease		Hct/Hgb
RENAL	Hyperkalemia Fluid overload	Renal insufficiency		BUN, Cr
HEPATIC	Bleeding Hepatic dysfunction	Jaundice	Abdominal exam	LFTs PT, PTT

Key Reference: Guidelines for Office-Based Anesthesia. American Society of Anesthesiologists, 1999.

PERIOPERATIVE IMPLICATIONS

Preoperative Preparation

- Adequate emergency plans and equipment
- Instruct patient about preprocedure fasting

Anesthetic Technique

- Most common technique involves use of local anesthesia in combination with rapid- and short-acting intravenous (propofol) and inhaled anesthetics (N_2O, sevoflurane, and/or desflurane)
- Short-acting potent opioid analgesics are normally used, e.g., fentanyl, remifentanil, sufentanil, alfentanil

Monitoring

- Routine

Airway

- Supplemental oxygen via face mask or nasal cannula

- Have available oral airways, nasopharyngeal airways, COPA, and/or LMAs
- Appropriate-size ET tubes readily available

Induction/Maintenance

- Administration of incremental doses of intravenous sedative-analgesic drugs until the desired level of sedation and/or analgesia is achieved
- Mask inhalational anesthetic may be necessary
- Local anesthetic (short- and long-acting)

Emergence/Extubation

- Most office procedures performed under local with minimal sedation; patients able to transfer themselves from the OR table to recovery
- Watch for airway obstruction, respiratory depression, and excessive sedation

Postoperative Period

- Monitor until patient is alert and oriented
- Vital signs should be stable
- Sufficient time should have elapsed after last administration of reversal agents or last drug administration to ensure that patient does not become resedated
- Discharge in the care of a responsible adult who will accompany patient home
- Patients provided with written instructions regarding postprocedure diet, medications, and activities along with a phone number in case of an emergency

ANTICIPATED PROBLEMS/CONCERNS

- Postoperative N/V may necessitate longer recovery period and even hospitalization
- If regional anesthetic technique is used, a proactive approach should be taken to address pain after discharge home as the anesthetic wears off

OMPHALOCELE SURGERY

Wendy B. Binstock, M.D.

RISK

- Incidence varies from 1/6000 to 1/10,000 live births
- Racial predominance: none

PERIOPERATIVE RISKS

- Significant heat losses
- Major fluid shifts
- Infection
- Complications related to associated congenital abnormalities

WORRY ABOUT

- Blood glucose, especially with possibility of Beckwith-Wiedemann syndrome
- Possibility of cardiac defects and CV compromise
- Possibility of respiratory compromise, postop ventilation difficulties
- Metabolic problems

OVERVIEW

- Congenital abdominal wall defects that result in herniation of the intestine into base of umbilical cord
- Translucent avascular sac consisting of peritoneum and amniotic membrane at base of umbilical cord
- Vary in size: may contain only small bowel or may contain liver, spleen, stomach, and other abdominal organs
- Associated congenital anomalies occur in approximately 67% of infants (GI, CV, GU, CNS)
- Often associated with other known syndromes, particularly trisomies 13 and 18, and Beckwith-Wiedemann syndrome
- 25–30% of infants with an omphalocele are premature or of low birth weight

ICD-9-CM Code: 756.7

ETIOLOGY

- Congenital failure of embryonic lateral folds, or persistent body stock in the region normally occupied by somatopleure
- Amniotic sac present, although it may have been ruptured during birth or shortly thereafter

INDICATIONS

- Prompt surgical repair, either primary or staged, depending on size

ASSESSMENT POINTS

SYSTEM	EFFECT	ASSESSMENT BY HX	PE	TEST
HEENT	Beckwith-Wiedemann syndrome: macroglossia, microcephaly		Head exam	
CV	Congenital heart disease: tetralogy of Fallot, ASD		CV exam	Transthoracic ECHO
RESP	If associated with prematurity, may have immature lungs	Gestational age	Chest exam and signs of respiratory distress	O_2 saturation If available, predelivery lecithin/sphingomyelin ratio
GI	Gastric and intestinal distention, small abdominal cavity		Size of omphalocele	
ENDO	Possibility of Beckwith-Wiedemann syndrome			Blood glucose
RENAL/ HEPATIC	Immaturity of hepatic and renal systems Possibility for ↓ hepatic blood flow and impaired renal perfusion post closure			

Key Reference: Bikhazi GB, Davis PJ: Anesthesia for neonates and premature infants. *In* Motoyama EK, Davis PI: Smith's Anesthesia for Infants and Children, 6th ed. St. Louis, Mosby, 1996, pp 455–457.

PERIOPERATIVE MANAGEMENT

Preoperative Preparation

- IV access and restoration of intravascular volume
- Fluid losses tend to be isotonic; therefore, balanced salt solutions often used (lactated Ringer's or 5% albumin)
- Up to 10–15 ml/kg/h of fluid often necessary initially
- Maintain normothermia by wrapping abdomen in moist, warm, sterile dressing; lower body can be placed in plastic bag
- Decompression of the stomach to prevent regurgitation/aspiration
- Antibiotics to prevent sepsis

Monitoring

- Consider arterial line depending on extent of defect and ventilatory status
- Consider CVP if defect is large
- Adequate temp and glucose monitoring

Airway

- After decompression of the stomach, anesthesia may be induced with inhalation or IV agents. Paralysis should be used to facilitate intubation. Awake intubation may also be performed after premedication with atropine but is not necessary.

- ET tube should be secured in a manner suitable for prolonged postop ventilation

Maintenance

- Nitrous oxide usually avoided
- A suitable mixture of O_2 and air to produce adequate oxygenation (PaO_2 50–70 mmHg, SaO_2 97–98% for term infants, 87–92% for preterm infants); will vary as surgeons attempt to replace bowel in abdomen
- Maximal muscle relaxation
- Increases in CVP more than 4 mmHg during surgical closure associated with reduction in venous return, cardiac index, anuria
- Ability to tolerate primary closure assessed by measuring BP in lower extremities, or by following lower extremity circulation with pulse oximeter
- Primary closure may cause ventilatory, circulatory, and renal dysfunction and bowel necrosis if abdomen is too tense
- Placing bowel in a silo associated with higher infection rate
- If vital signs are abnormal after the expected respiratory changes associated with hernia reduction, it is usually impossible to achieve adequate ventilation and oxygenation until intra-abdominal pressure and distention diminish

Extubation

- Postop care varies with magnitude of defect, type of repair, and associated pathology
- Healthy patients treated with a silo or a small primary closure often tolerate extubation in OR
- In patients with large defects (especially those with compromised circulation), postop intubation, ventilation, and maximal muscle relaxation continued until abdominal pressure results in little resp or circ compromise

ANTICIPATED PROBLEMS/CONCERNS

- Ventilatory care: similar to that for other neonates with respiratory distress
- Fluid requirements: may remain high until abdominal venous pressure decreases, at which time fluid restriction and diuresis probably indicated
- FIO_2: adjust to maintain a normal PaO_2
- PEEP: appropriate levels used to ↑ FRC
- Nutritional status: because bowel function is usually compromised and slow to resume, TPN requirements are often extended
- Circulatory and renal dysfunction common
- Infection: common, especially if silo used instead of primary closure

ORCHIOPEXY

W. Casey Lenox, M.D.

RISK

- Premature infants: risk is 30% for one or both testicles to be undescended
- Full-term infants: risk is 3%
- 60% of undescended testicles found in inguinal position; 8% intra-abdominal; only 24% in the easily operable low inguinal/high scrotal position
- Progressive injury occurs when testicle is left undescended: decreased sperm production after age 6 y, impaired hormonal production, ↑ risk of malignant degeneration
- Risk of malignant degeneration may not be improved following orchiopexy, but self-examination becomes more reliable

PERIOPERATIVE RISKS

- Perioperative mortality rare in term infants ($<0.01\%$)
- Risks in ex–premature children dependent upon co-existing morbidity (e.g., bronchopulmonary dysplasia, reactive airway disease, subglottic stenosis, hydrocephalus and seizure due to intraventricular hemorrhage, GI dysfunction due to necrotizing enterocolitis, malnutrition, anemia, RV hypertrophy/failure, poor IV access)
- Operative risks of testicular atrophy or hypotrophy: 8% for those beyond external ring, 13% when canalicular, 26% for intra-abdominal locations

WORRY ABOUT

- Co-morbidity associated with prematurity
- Venous air embolism, aspiration, diaphragmatic embarrassment if laparoscope utilized for repair

OVERVIEW

- Testicle(s) located and spermatic cord and accompanying vasculature freed and mobilized so that testicle can be relocated within hemiscrotum. Spermatic vessels may be sacrificed, with vasculature of vas deferens supplying collaterals.
- Operative laparoscope increasingly utilized for relocating intra-abdominal or high inguinal testicles
- Operative time: 1 h (open, low testicular location) to 3 h (laparoscopic)

ICD-9-CM Code: 752.5 (Cryptorchidism)

INDICATIONS AND USUAL TREATMENT

- Testicle will not descend beyond 1 y of age and ultrastructural changes have been demonstrated by 2 y, so that most repairs should occur at 12–24 mo of age
- Some evidence that hCG may promote testicular descent, so this may be attempted prior to operation

ASSESSMENT POINTS (IN EX–PREMATURE INFANTS)

SYSTEM	EFFECT	ASSESSMENT BY HX	PE	TEST
HEENT	Subglottic stenosis		Stridor, wheezing, croup	CXR, bronchoscopy
CV	Pulm Htn, PDA, RV hypertrophy	Failure to thrive	↑ S_2, murmurs	ECG Cardiac ECHO/catheter
RESP	Bronchopulmonary dysplasia, blebs	Asthma, oxygen? Apnea monitor alarms Diuretics		CXR
RENAL	Nephrocalcinosis	Htn		BP, electrolytes, BUN, Cr
CNS	Intraventricular hemorrhage Seizures, hydrocephalus	Mental status Development Seizure type, frequency Ventriculoperitoneal shunt		Shunt evaluation Anti-epilepsy drug levels

Key Reference: Hannallah RS, Broadman LM, Belman AB, et al: Comparison of caudal and ilioinguinal/iliohypogastric nerve blocks for control of post-orchiopexy pain in pediatric ambulatory surgery. Anesthesiology 1987; 66:832–834.

PERIOPERATIVE MANAGEMENT

Preoperative Preparation

- May have clear liquids up to 2 h before induction
- No lab work necessary if otherwise normal
- If uncomplicated, may be done as outpatient procedure

Anesthetic Technique

- Combined general and regional anesthetic in open case
- Usually regular mask or laryngeal mask airway (LMA) and caudal injection of local anesthetic or ilioinguinal/iliohypogastric nerve block for analgesia intra- and postoperatively
- Combined technique in laparoscopic procedures but with trachea intubated (usually; LMA now being used by some)

Monitoring

- Routine

Induction

- Inhalational mask induction, then maintenance with halothane or sevoflurane and nitrous oxide
- IV, then single-injection caudal placed following induction of anesthesia

SURGICAL STAGES

Dissection

- Caudal usually not effective in blocking visceral pain that occurs with pulling on spermatic cord; may require increasing volatile anesthetic concentrations temporarily
- Possible respiratory compromise if laparoscopic procedure
- Minimal blood loss

Postoperative Considerations

- If 0.025% bupivacaine used for caudal, 4–6 h of analgesia usual
- Most children need enteral opioids for 2–3 days
- Incidence of emesis postop 45%; usually self-limited

ANTICIPATED PROBLEMS/CONCERNS

- Ex–premature children have an ↑ incidence of wheezing and desaturation intra- and postoperatively. May need to be observed overnight.

ORIF OF HIP

Kevin V. Sanborn, M.D.

RISK

- 200,000/y in USA
- Predominantly elderly women
- Racial predominance: none

PERIOPERATIVE RISKS

- 30-Day mortality: 7%
- Anemia and hypovolemia
- Multiple trauma victims—other injuries?
- Perioperative confusion—etiology of fall in elderly: TIA, stroke, MI
- Decubitus ulcers

WORRY ABOUT

- Etiology of fracture: reason for falling—syncope
- Drug abuse, including ethanol
- Anemia, hypovolemia, hypothermia
- Pulmonary emboli

OVERVIEW

- Break in bone supporting weight with pain and fluid/blood collection in leg
- Early treatment to stabilize associated with better functional recovery and fewer perioperative complications
- Usually occurs in elderly with co-morbidities: dehydration, anemia, at least mild CNS disturbances
- Both regional and general anesthesia are supported in literature. Meta-analysis failed to show any significant benefit of one vs. the other.
- With good preop assessment of medical problems, preinduction resuscitation of fluid and blood losses, and appropriate monitoring, choice of light GA or cautiously induced regional anesthesia can be based on anesthesiologist's preference and patient's condition
- Pin fixation of hip fracture does not violate major body cavities and is not associated with massive bleeding or fluid shifts; usually reasonably well tolerated

ICD-9-CM Code: 820.8 (Closed fracture of hip)

INDICATIONS AND USUAL TREATMENT

- Fracture of femoral neck results in pain and disability corrected by pin fixation under x-ray guidance
- Severe fracture involving femoral head may require replacement with cemented femoral prosthesis
- In elderly patients, treatment of fracture with traction results in high morbidity and mortality due to pulmonary and septic complications
- Co-existing chronic medical problems and acute disturbances of physiology of vital organs should be rapidly assessed and treated. Delay in surgical treatment associated with poorer outcome.

ASSESSMENT POINTS

SYSTEM	EFFECT	ASSESSMENT BY HX	PE	TEST
CV	Htn, CAD, MI, heart block or AS → syncope?	Htn, CAD, TIA	Chest exam, VS	ECG, ECHO
RESP	Atelectasis, pneumonia, fat embolism, pulm edema	CHF, ?SOB, chest pain	Chest exam	SpO_2, ABGs, CXR
ENDO	Diabetes	Adult-onset DM	Peripheral pulses	FBS, UA
HEME	Anemia, thrombocytopenia (2° to fat embolism)	Dyspnea, GI bleeding	Pallor, petechiae	CBC
RENAL	Dehydration, electrolyte imbalance, UTI	?Nursing home, NPO × ?h	Jugular veins	BUN, Cr, electrolytes
CNS	Stroke, TIA, confusion, delirium, syncope	Previous stroke, TIA, medications	Auscultation of carotid	Neuro exam

Key Reference: Urwin SC, Parker MJ, Griffiths R: General versus regional anaesthesia for hip fracture surgery: a meta-analysis of randomized trials. Br J Anaesth 2000; 84:450–455.

INTRAOPERATIVE MANAGEMENT

- Early surgical treatment associated with fewer postop complications. Assessment and treatment of medical problems and fluid resuscitation can be completed within 24 h.
- Spinal, epidural, or light general anesthesia
- Analgesia ± sedation needed for positioning and transfers
- Lateral decubitus position preferred for induction of spinal or epidural anesthesia

Monitoring

- Routine
- Consider arterial line, CVP, PA catheter depending on co-existing disease

Induction

- Consider fluid resuscitation, vasopressors before induction of spinal or epidural anesthesia
- Consider warming blanket, warmed fluids to offset heat losses due to advanced age and exposure
- Minimize sedation during regional anesthesia to avoid postop delirium

SURGICAL STAGES

Positioning

- Use of fracture table and x-ray image intensifier adds 30–60 min to setup
- Fracture table makes it difficult to avoid exposure to drafts → hypothermia
- Consider positioning ipsilateral arm carefully out of field

X-ray

- Consider wearing lead apron and thyroid collar

Pin or Screw Fixation

- Add 1 U of hematoma to EBL
- Minimally invasive procedure, well-tolerated even by sick patients

Replacement of Femoral Head

- Cemented femoral prosthesis—problems similar to total hip replacement

Postoperative Period

- Pain score: 3–5
- IV PCA well tolerated

ANTICIPATED PROBLEMS/CONCERNS

- Anemia, hypovolemia, hypotension, hypothermia
- Pulm edema due to too-aggressive fluid replacement; may not be evident until recovery from sympathetic blockade after regional anesthesia
- Confusion, delirium
- Sensitivity to narcotics and sedatives
- Postop pulmonary complications (pulmonary embolism, pneumonia, bone marrow fat embolism, ARDS)
- Postop urinary sepsis
- Postop GI disturbances (intestinal obstruction, GI bleeding)

PACEMAKER IMPLANTATION FOR SICK SINUS SYNDROME

Carl Lynch III, M.D., Ph.D.

RISK

- Accounts for ~50% of pacemaker implantations, or about 200/1 million population/y
- Typically seen in older patients, although rarely may be familial or follow surgery for congenital heart defects

PERIOPERATIVE RISKS

- Perioperative bradycardia (unpaced) or tachycardia, with potential for CV compromise, including pulm edema

WORRY ABOUT

- Previously undiagnosed or early disease (see Etiology), with modest early symptoms
- In the absence of pacemaker or with pacemaker dysfunction, severe bradycardia or asystole may occur, especially with ↑ vagal tone
- Rhythm will always recover in time, and sudden cardiac death is not an important risk in pure sinus node dysfunction
- In the presence of pacemaker, sustained paroxysmal tachycardia may require control

OVERVIEW

- Sick sinus syndrome divided into three types: (1) simple sinus bradycardia; (2) sinus arrest or SA block with or without sinus bradycardia; (3) bradycardia with paroxysmal tachycardia ("tachy-brady syndrome")
- Tachycardia may be caused by AFIB/AFLT
- Syncope or severe lightheadedness results from prolonged sinus or atrial pause following termination of tachycardia; atrial pause frequently caused by SA exit block
- Sinus or atrial pauses may rarely be 15-sec duration
- May be associated with high-degree AV block (pan-conduction defect)
- Increased likelihood of stroke in patients who are paced ventricularly (VVI) and more prone to develop AFIB

ICD-9-CM Code: 427.81

ETIOLOGY

- Usually due to degenerative (possibly familial), sclerotic, or fibrotic changes of sinus node
- May be manifestation of cardiac disease: ischemia, pericarditis, cardiomyopathy
- May be 2° to cardiac involvement by other diseases (typically infiltrative):
  – Muscular dystrophy, collagen disease, hemochromatosis, amyloidosis, metastatic disease

INDICATIONS AND USUAL TREATMENT

- Permanent cardiac pacemaker placement in symptomatic patients, or in asymptomatic patients who need β-blockers or antiarrhythmic drugs
- For previously undiagnosed disease, temporary transvenous pacing may be appropriate
- Sinus rate and atrial conduction may be enhanced by stimulation with β-adrenergic agonists (isoproterenol, epinephrine, ephedrine) and parasympathetic blocking agents (atropine, glycopyrrolate)

ASSESSMENT POINTS

SYSTEM	EFFECT	ASSESSMENT BY HX	PE	TEST
CV	Bradycardia, tachycardia	Pacemaker implantation	Low (or high) HR	ECG, electrophysiologic testing
CNS		Unexplained episodic lightheadedness, confusion, syncope		Holter CT scan

Key Reference: Pavia S, Wikoff B: The management of surgical complications of pacemaker and implantable cardioverter-defibrillators. Curr Opin Cardiol 2001; 16:66–71.

PERIOPERATIVE IMPLICATIONS

Monitoring
- ECG
- Monitor of perfusion if pacemaker (Doppler, SpO_2, ECHO, arterial line)

Airway
- None

Maintenance
- Volatile agents, especially enflurane, may suppress SA function
- If pacemaker is not implanted, high doses of fentanyl or sufentanil or maneuvers that ↑ vagal tone may worsen bradycardia, requiring treatment with atropine

Extubation/Emergence
- Emergence excitation may contribute to development of paroxysmal tachycardia

Adjuvants
- Calcium-channel blockers, especially verapamil, contraindicated in the absence of pacemaking capability
- With pacemaker present, paroxysmal tachycardia may be treated acutely with IV verapamil; digoxin may be added for longer duration control

ANTICIPATED PROBLEMS/CONCERNS

- Severe bradycardia (or tachycardia) 2° to anesthetic agents or autonomic imbalance associated with perioperative period. Since problems may arise from parasympathetic dominance, atropine or glycopyrrolate is indicated.

PANCREAS TRANSPLANTATION Dennis W. Coalson, M.D.

RISK

- 12,000–19,000 new cases of type I diabetes/y
- 1500 pancreas transplants in USA in 1999
  – 76% simultaneous pancreas-kidney transplant (SPK)
  – 24% isolated pancreas transplant
- Recipients 59% male, 73% Caucasian, 8% African-American, 4% Hispanic, 89% age 18–49 y

PERIOPERATIVE RISKS

- 30-Day mortality: 1–2%
- Morbidity of SPK is 15% > kidney transplant alone
- Recipient 1–4-y survival: 92–84%
- Pancreatic graft 1–4-y survival: 77–64%
- Cardiac events, acute rejection, infections

WORRY ABOUT

- Positioning for long surgical time (4–8 h)
- Diabetics at ↑ risk for perioperative nerve injuries
- Potential rapid blood loss
- Complications of IDDM (gastroparesis, CAD, autonomic neuropathy)
- Noncardiogenic pulm edema with perioperative OKT3
- For SPK, hypovolemia if recently dialyzed; hyperkalemia and hypervolemia if long since last dialysis. Protection of hemodialysis access site, AV shunt, or fistulas. Prolong duration of drugs renally excreted.

OVERVIEW

- Only treatment of type I diabetes mellitus that establishes insulin-independent euglycemic state

- Improvement in quality of life primary reason for transplant. Potential for favorable effect on secondary complications of diabetes is additional goal.
- Usually performed along with kidney transplant

ICD-9-CM Code: 250.01

See also Diabetes, Type I (Insulin Dependent), in Diseases section

INDICATIONS AND USUAL TREATMENT

- Usually uremic diabetic patients who need kidney transplant or have received prior kidney transplant
- For nonuremics, problems of diabetes considered more serious than potential side effects of immunosuppression therapy (diabetics with extreme lability in metabolic control and hypoglycemic unawareness)

ASSESSMENT POINTS

SYSTEM	EFFECT	ASSESSMENT BY HX	PE	TEST
HEENT	Difficult laryngoscopy Joint immobility	Hx of difficult airway Joint contractures	Airway exam Palm or prayer sign	Test palms together to estimate joint mobility
CV/RESP	CAD Hypervolemia Hyperkalemia	SOB	Rales, tachypnea	CXR, ABGs, ECG, lytes
HEME	Anemia		Systolic flow murmur, pale mucous membranes	Hct
PNS	Peripheral neuropathy, gastroparesis, autonomic neuropathy	Early satiety, nausea, postural syncope	↓ Peripheral sensation	Tilt table test, R-R interval with breathing or Valsalva's maneuver
MS	Osteopenia	Fractures		Bone density

Key Reference: Stratta RJ, Larsen JL, Cushing K: Pancreas transplantation for diabetes mellitus. Annu Rev Med 1995; 46:281–298.

PERIOPERATIVE MANAGEMENT

Preoperative Preparation

- Absence of infection, dental evaluation
- Administration of preop antibiotics

Anesthetic Technique

- Usually general or combined technique because of length of case
- Rapid-sequence induction for full stomach or gastroparesis

Monitoring

- Consider arterial and central venous catheters
- Frequent blood glucose measurements

Airway

- High incidence (30%) of difficult laryngoscopy in type I diabetics
- ↑ Risk for aspiration

Induction/Maintenance

- Blood glucose assessment as pancreatic graft function occurs rapidly; in most patients, blood glucose levels decrease to normal within several hours
- Administration of immunosuppressant agents prior to graft reperfusion

SURGICAL STAGES

- Preservation times up to 30 h safe for cadaveric pancreas

Dissection

- Midline incision. Mobilization of iliac artery and vein bilaterally. Intraperitoneal placement in side opposite renal graft.

Definitive Surgery

- Graft superior mesenteric and splenic arteries anastomosed to recipient iliac artery via donor iliac artery Y graft. Graft portal vein anastomosed to recipient iliac vein.
- Most commonly exocrine drainage provided by anastomosing a graft duodenal segment to bladder. Can also have enteric exocrine drainage.

Postoperative Considerations

- Pain relief with PCA or epidural analgesia
- Occasional postoperative anticoagulation to decrease graft thrombosis
- Rejection after SPK transplantation determined by serum Cr and kidney biopsy

- 90% of rejection episodes: kidney dysfunction manifests earlier than pancreatic dysfunction
- Rejection in isolated pancreas transplants diagnosed by ↓ urine amylase activity in urinary bladder, drained pancreas grafts, and graft biopsy
- Delayed complication with urinary drainage related to pancreatic juice in the bladder, such as hematuria, UTI, chemical cystitis, metabolic acidosis, and reflux pancreatitis

ANTICIPATED PROBLEMS/CONCERNS

- Positioning problems associated with long surgical time
- Noncardiogenic pulm edema with intraoperative administration of OKT3
- Early return to euglycemic state after surgery requiring ↓ in exogenously administered insulin

PARATHYROIDECTOMY

Eli M. Brown, M.D.

RISK

- Incidence: 0.1–0.2%
- Peak incidence 5th–6th decades
- Females > males
- Racial predominance: none

PERIOPERATIVE RISKS

- Hypercalcemia produces symptoms related mainly to renal, skeletal, neuromuscular, GI systems
- Perioperative mortality rare
- Most common postop complications are injury of recurrent laryngeal nerve(s), hematoma, eye injury, hypocalcemia

WORRY ABOUT

- Parathyroid crisis (Ca^{2+} > 14 mg/dl) accompanied by marked dehydration and coma
- Positioning—presence of osteoporosis or simple diffuse osteopenia may result in pathologic fracture
- Skeletal muscle weakness
- Renal insufficiency
- Nerve injury, hematoma, hypocalcemia postop

OVERVIEW

- Low incidence of morbidity (<1%)
- 85% of primary hyperparathyroidism caused by benign adenoma in a single gland. Localization techniques include sestamibi scanning, US, MRI, CT scan.
- Most asymptomatic when diagnosed by routine screening. Major Sx result from severe hypercalcemia when Dx is delayed.

ICD-9-CM Code: 252.0 (Hyperplasia)

ETIOLOGY

- Hyperparathyroidism present when secretion of parathormone is increased
- Classified as primary, secondary, or ectopic

INDICATIONS AND USUAL TREATMENT

- Complete removal of gland containing adenoma with biopsy of 1 or 2 normal-appearing glands
- For known hyperplasia, 3 glands are removed and 4th gland partially excised
- Guidelines for surgery include serum calcium > 12 mg/dl, hypercalciuria, presence of classic symptoms, ↓ bone density, ↓ creatinine clearance, age < 50 y

ASSESSMENT POINTS

SYSTEM	EFFECT	ASSESSMENT BY HX	PE	TEST
CV	Conduction disturbances (short QT_c; prolonged P-R intervals associated with hypercalcemia) Htn			ECG BP
GI	Disorders of stomach and pancreas Zollinger-Ellison syndrome	Vague abdominal pain	Abdominal exam	Endoscopy (if indicated)
RENAL	Calculi Insufficiency	Flank pain Polyuria Polydipsia	Flank tenderness	X-ray (if indicated) GFR (if indicated) Cr
NM	Peripheral muscle weakness Atrophy of muscles	Easy fatigability	Extremity exam	Ca^{2+} level
MS	Osteitis fibrosa cystica Osteopenia	Frequent fractures Bone pain	Skeletal exam	X-ray; CT (if indicated) Quantitative digital radiography (if indicated)

Key Reference: Kaplan EL, Yashiro T, Salti G: Primary hyperparathyroidism in the 1990s: choice of surgical procedures for this disease. Ann Surg 1992; 215:300–317.

PERIOPERATIVE MANAGEMENT

Preoperative Preparation

- Treat hypercalcemia—primarily hydration and diuresis accompanied by phosphate repletion
- Glucocorticoids, mithramycin, calcitonin may be used if necessary
- Correct hypovolemia and electrolyte imbalance
- Check ECG for P-R, QT changes

Monitoring

- Routine

Airway

- None

Preinduction/Induction

- Careful positioning to avoid bone fracture
- Patient may exhibit unpredictable response to muscle relaxants

- No specific anesthetic agent or technique is advantageous or contraindicated
- Local or regional anesthesia may be appropriate for poor-risk patients or limited surgery
- Protect eyes

Maintenance

- Check ECG for prolonged P-R and short QT_c intervals
- Tracheal manipulation may cause bucking if patient inadequately anesthetized or partially paralyzed

Extubation

- Be aware of possibility of damage to recurrent laryngeal nerves or presence of bullous glottic edema producing airway obstruction

ANTICIPATED PROBLEMS/CONCERNS

- Airway obstruction 2° to damage to recurrent laryngeal nerves, hematoma, bullous glottic edema
- Hypocalcemia or hypomagnesemia may occur. Severe hypocalcemia may result in laryngeal spasm and seizure.
- Perform serial determinations of serum Ca^{2+}, inorganic phosphate, magnesium, parathyroid hormone
- Chvostek's sign and Trousseau's sign are classic indications of latent tetany
- Primary hyperparathyroidism may be due to adenoma or hyperplasia, or rarely may be due to carcinoma. Symptoms are similar, so type must be confirmed by frozen section.

PATENT DUCTUS ARTERIOSUS, LIGATION OF

Eugenie Heitmiller, M.D.

RISK

- Full-term infants: 1/2500 live births
- Premature infants: 45% <1750 g; 80% <1200 g
- Overall incidence: 8/1000 live births
- Female preponderance, 2–3:1 male
- High incidence in congenital rubella syndrome

PERIOPERATIVE RISKS

- Perioperative mortality rare (0.4%)
- Residual ductal patency 0.4–3.1%
- Rare complications: chest wall deformity, recurrent nerve injury, ligation of left pulmonary artery or aorta

WORRY ABOUT

- Hypothermia
- Adequate venous access and blood products readily available for uncontrolled hemorrhage

- Vagal reflex with lung and vessel retraction
- Fluid status of premature infant on diuretics and fluid restriction
- Hypoxia and hypercarbia with lung retraction during surgery

OVERVIEW

- L → R shunt between aorta and PA that causes increased pulmonary blood flow with pulm edema and cardiac failure in premature infants. Uncorrected PDA in older patients can result in cyanosis in lower half of body with R → L shunt.
- Antibiotics required to prevent bacterial endocarditis in all patients
- Air embolism can occur with bidirectional shunting
- Massive hemorrhage may occur during ductal ligation

ICD-9-CM Code: 747.0 (Patent ductus arteriosus)

See also Patent Ductus Arteriosus in Diseases section

INDICATIONS AND USUAL TREATMENT

- Premature infants: initial treatment with fluid restriction and diuretics; administration of indomethacin (a prostaglandin inhibitor) usually causes ductal closure in 24 h; surgery indicated if trial of indomethacin fails; procedure performed in NICU at some hospitals
- Full-term infants and older children: ligated electively after age 6 mo if asymptomatic
- Standard surgical treatment is via open thoracotomy. Other procedures for closure of PDA include transcatheter device closure and a video-assisted thoracoscopic approach.

ASSESSMENT POINTS

SYSTEM	EFFECT	ASSESSMENT BY HX	PE	TEST
CV	L → R shunt Diastolic runoff Heart failure	CHF Failure to grow	Rales Murmur Low diastolic BP Bounding pulses	ECHO
RESP	↑ Pulm blood	Failure to wean from ventilator		CXR

Key Reference: Rosen DA, Rosen KR: Anomalies of the aortic arch and valve. *In* Lake C (ed): Pediatric Cardiac Anesthesia, 2nd ed. Norwalk, CT, Appleton & Lange, 1993, p 347.

PERIOPERATIVE MANAGEMENT

Preoperative Preparation

- Monitor premature infants during transport to OR
- Adequate vascular access. Blood products available prior to incision.
- Warm OR prior to patient arrival
- IV lines cleared of air bubbles

Anesthetic Technique

- Combined GA with regional block for thoracotomy pain

Monitoring

- Pulse oximetry on right hand (preductal) and on one lower extremity (postductal) to confirm that correct vessel is ligated
- Use invasive monitors if in ICU
- Temp closely monitored

Airway

- May have associated congenital anomalies of airway
- Mechanical ventilation

Induction/Maintenance

- May require fluid resuscitation at induction because of fluid restriction and diuretics

SURGICAL STAGES

- Incision
  – Usually left thoracotomy incision; can have right-sided PDA
- Dissection
  – Lung retraction can produce hypoxemia and hypercarbia
  – Vagal reflex produced by surgical traction on lung; may require atropine, since bradycardia poorly tolerated in infants
- Definitive surgery
  – Major blood loss can occur if ductal vessel injured or if clip/suture on vessel is inadequate or slips off vessel
  – Chest tube placed prior to chest closure
- Fluid shift: can have ↑ systemic volume after ductus arteriosus is ligated

Postoperative Considerations

- CXR immediately postop to check for pneumothorax
- EBL: usually minimal
- Pain score: 6–9
- Continuous regional technique or intercostal blocks with parenteral narcotics for thoracotomy pain management

ANTICIPATED PROBLEMS/CONCERNS

- Shunt predominantly L → R
- Large shunts can result in heart failure and pulm Htn
- Cyanosis of lower half of body indicative of a R → L shunt
- Development of necrotizing enterocolitis due to ↓ intestinal blood flow
- Intracranial hemorrhage in preterm babies with ↑ blood pressure after ligation

PITUITARY RESECTION, TRANSSPHENOIDAL APPROACH

Stephen M. Rupp, M.D.

RISK

- Pituitary adenoma: 14–20/100,000
- Males > females, 1:2

PERIOPERATIVE RISK

- <1% immediate perioperative mortality
- 8–15% morbidity (transient [1–3 days] diabetes insipidus is most frequent); hypopituitarism in large resections
- Microadenomas of all types can have up to 90% cure rates in some surgical series
- 50% of untreated acromegalics die before age 50 y
- Untreated Cushing's disease has a 50% 5-y mortality

WORRY ABOUT

- Airway in acromegalics and Cushing's syndrome

- Intraoperative injection of epinephrine-containing local anesthetics to vasoconstrict nasal mucosa (precipitate dysrhythmias or myocardial ischemia); severe Htn if β-blocker present
- Hemorrhage intraoperatively (cavernous sinus intrusion)
- Air embolism reported
- Saddle deformity of nose postop
- Blood in airway at end of procedure
- Diabetes insipidus postop

OVERVIEW

- Pituitary microadenoma usual indication for surgery; in descending order of frequency, tissue types/most common presenting symptoms are
  – Nonsecreting adenoma/visual field defect, headache, CN III–VI may be affected by pressure

  – Prolactin-secreting adenoma/amenorrhea; galactorrhea, lost libido
  – ACTH-secreting tumor/Cushing's disease; obesity, Htn, diabetes, sleep apnea
  – Growth hormone–secreting tumor/acromegaly, Htn, cardiomyopathy, diabetes, sleep apnea

ICD-9-CM Codes: 253.0 (Acromegaly); 255.0 (Cushing's syndrome)

INDICATIONS AND USUAL TREATMENT

- Bromocriptine is first line of Rx for prolactin-secreting tumors and can suppress GH tumors
- Irradiation used as single treatment and surgical adjuvant in selected cases
- Surgical treatment is choice for macroadenomas (>10 mm in diameter) ± radiation later

ASSESSMENT POINTS

SYSTEM	EFFECT	ASSESSMENT BY HX	PE	TEST
HEENT	Airway in acromegalics; glottic fixation or narrowing in GH excess Airway in Cushing's CN III–VI impingement	Hoarseness, sleep apnea? Tongue size, stridor/DOE? Visual disturbance, field cut	Airway Visual field	
CV	Htn in acromegaly and Cushing's	CV status, LVH? Exercise tolerance Chest pain, sleep apnea?		ECG
RESP	↓ FRC in obese	SOB, DOE		ABGs
ENDO	Diabetes mellitus Hypercortisolism	Glucose intolerance		Glucose
RENAL	Hypertensive or diabetic kidney disease			Cr
CNS	↑ ICP in severe suprasellar extension	Headache, N/V	Visual field	Funduscopic exam

Key Reference: Smith M, Hirsch NP: Pituitary disease and anaesthesia. Br J Anaesth 2000; 85:3–14.

PERIOPERATIVE MANAGEMENT

Preoperative Preparation

- Evaluate for significant CAD (Hx, ECG, exercise tolerance); may suffer myocardial stress from exogenous epinephrine, sleep apnea?
- Airway assessment requires oral ET tube; plan fiberoptic intubation if indicated
- Surgeon may request lumbar subarachnoid drain to inject saline or air or N_2O intraoperatively to outline and monitor progress of suprasellar extension of adenoma. Postop, CSF catheter may be placed to drain if CSF leak anticipated.

Anesthetic Technique

- GA required

Monitoring

- Routine + air embolism
- If plan to have patient in >30° upright sitting position, consider multiorificed single-lumen CVP for air aspiration and plan Doppler monitoring/end-tidal N_2

Airway

- In acromegalics, hypertrophy of facial bones, jaw, nose, turbinates, soft palate, tonsils, epiglottis, and larynx may occur: mask fit/intubation may be difficult. Fiberoptic intubation may be indicated.

Induction/Maintenance

- Rapid-acting induction agent acceptable
- Maintain anesthetic with narcotic, volatile anesthetic (isoflurane good choice because of favorable profile of ↓ sensitivity of myocardium to exogenous epinephrine), ± N_2O and relaxant
- Target $PaCO_2$ = 34–38 mmHg
- Aim to have patient comfortable and cooperative (awake) prior to extubation
- Mouth and pharynx packed with gauze to prevent blood in stomach or airway
- ± Subarachnoid drain prior to positioning

SURGICAL STAGES

- Surgical positioning: semi-sitting 5–35° head-up
- Placement of tongs: watch for adrenergic/hypertensive response
- Injection of epinephrine containing local anesthetic to vasoconstrict: watch for dysrhythmias, Htn, myocardial ischemia
- Nasal septal and sublabial incision (blood loss)
- Placement of transsphenoidal speculum: bone work, needs fluoroscopic control to ensure midline approach (high anesthetic requirement for this stage)
- Adenoma removal under direct visualization with microscope
- If suprasellar extension, surgeon may want saline or air injected: if air, discontinue N_2O

- If lateral extension of tumor occurs, excessive bleeding may ensue from invasion of cavernous sinus. Induced hypotension via high-concentration isoflurane may reduce venous pressure to allow adequate hemorrhage control.
- Rebuilding sella turcica (part of nasal septum used)
- Pack with fat pad (abdominal wall donor site)
- Close
- EBL: 150–400 ml

Postoperative Considerations

- Pain score: 2–3

ANTICIPATED PROBLEMS/CONCERNS

- Extubate awake
- Diabetes insipidus in 8–15%, usually transient. Dx via analysis of high volume (3–6 ml/kg/h) of dilute urine (<200 mOsm/L, specific gravity = 1.001–1.005). May require aqueous vasopressin 0.5 ml (10 U) q4–6h SQ. Replace urinary losses. If serum >320 Osm/L, replace H_2O loss.
- CSF rhinorrhea: lumbar CSF drain to reduce CSF pressure
- If excessive packing needed to control cavernous sinus bleeding, CN II, IV, or VI compression can occur. Impingement of cavernous internal carotid can result in carotid spasm.
- If air has been injected subarachnoid, tension pneumocephalus can occur

PNEUMONECTOMY

Paula Craigo, M.D.

RISK

- Vast majority of malignancy: lung or metastatic tumor; male:female 2:1
- 10–30% of curative resections for lung CA are pneumonectomies
- Benign: mycobacteria, fungus, infection/necrosis

PERIOPERATIVE RISKS

- Mortality 5–10% within 30 days
- Cardiac morbidity significant
- Morbidity/mortality higher after right pneumonectomy, more complex procedure (sleeve 12%/completion 20%), some benign diseases
- Mortality for trauma 60–100%

WORRY ABOUT

- Pulm reserve/pulm Htn, edema, after resection
- Concomitant CV disease
- Cardiac arrhythmias common postop
- Perioperative thromboembolic events in 26%
- Benign diseases: neovascularization, high-pressure bronchial system bleed; soiling of contralateral lung

OVERVIEW

- Mortality of untreated non–small cell lung CA is 100%; effective treatment is surgery
- Paraneoplastic syndromes not a contraindication

- Effective treatment for drug-resistant TB
- Last resort for traumatic injury: resection in hypovolemic shock → persistent high PVR in R heart failure: pulmonary vasodilators, nitric oxide may be tried

ICD-9-CM Codes: 162.2–9 (Primary lung cancer)

INDICATIONS AND USUAL TREATMENT

- Non–small cell lung CA (T2) with hilar involvement, no distant mets; main stem bronchus involvement or crossing major fissure
- T3 lesions: plus resection of involved chest wall/diaphragm/mediastinal pleura/pericardium
- Sleeve pneumonectomy: resection of carina, ipsilateral lung, and bronchial tree; anastomosis of contralateral main stem bronchus to distal trachea

ASSESSMENT POINTS

SYSTEM	EFFECT	ASSESSMENT BY HX	PE	TEST
HEENT	Recurrent laryngeal nerve involvement	Hoarseness	HEENT exam	
CV	RV dysfunction due to PA Htn LV function, valvular disease Arrhythmias	Chest pain/SOB Exercise tolerance, palpitations	CV exam	ECG; possible ECHO, Doppler studies, PA catheterization
RESP	Sputum, bronchospasm; ability to tolerate loss of lung	SOB, exercise tolerance, sputum, smoking Hx	Resp exam Clubbing	Chest CT; ABGs; PFTs: FEV_1, DL_{CO} Quantitative VQ scan; VO_2 max; *See note*
ENDO	Hypercalcemia; SIADH → hyponatremia; Cushing's syndrome	Somnolence, anorexia, N/V Wt loss, signs of water intoxication		Check Ca^{2+}, Na^+; SIADH → hypotonic plasma, relatively hypertonic urine; Cushing's: hypokalemic alkalosis
HEME	Anemia, polycythemia Migratory thrombophlebitis	Hx of thrombophlebitis		Hct
NM	Eaton-Lambert syndrome (E-L) Polymyositis		Muscle wasting	E-L: sensitivity to nondep muscle relaxants

Note: Acceptable risk: $DL_{CO}\% > 60$; PFTs: $FVC > 2.5$ L, $FEV_1 > 1.8$ L if no pulm Htn; quantitative V/Q scans predict postop $FVC > 1.3$ L, $FEV_1 > 900$ ml; $VO_2max > 10$ ml/kg/min. Test values are used to define risk to the patient to aid in informed decision-making, not as rigid limits prohibiting attempted surgical cure.

Key Reference: Ferguson MK: Assessment of operative risk for pneumonectomy. Chest Surg Clin N Am 1999; 9:339–351.

PERIOPERATIVE IMPLICATIONS

Preoperative Preparation
- Bronchodilators
- If sputum: antibiotics, hydration, mobilization
- Prophylactic digoxin prob not warranted

Monitoring
- Arterial line; CVP not routine intraop, but may be useful postop
- PA: requires placement on nonoperative side; fluoroscopy helpful; consider TEE

Airway
- If difficult airway or unable to intubate orally: bronchial blocker, nasal intubation
- Aspiration devastating

Induction/Maintenance
- Lateral decubitus positioning: check ear and eye on down side, axillary roll, arm positioning
- Potent inhalational agents bronchodilate but ↓ LV function, attenuate hypoxic vasoconstriction; ↑ in Qs/Qt not clinically significant at 1.0 MAC
- Problems with one-lung ventilation techniques: trauma, malposition, hypoxemia

SURGICAL STAGES

Dissection
- Posterolateral thoracotomy incision in 5th or 6th intercostal space for best exposure
- Venous drainage may be temporarily occluded to ↓ theoretical dissemination of tumor cells, while avoiding engorgement
- PA may be divided first to ↓ blood loss in specimen
- Closure tested with positive pressure breath
- Video-assisted thoracoscopy indicated only in rare cases due to current limits of technique

Definitive Surgery
- Limit volume administration
  – EBL: <500 ml
  – Capillary leak and ↑ PVR due to loss of pulm tissue → pulm edema
- Routine chest tube drainage not recommended; if used, keep tube clamped to avoid excess mediastinal shift, except briefly to evacuate air/fluid to underwater seal system

Postoperative Considerations
- Cardiac arrhythmias >20%, usually supraventricular
- Postpneumonectomy pulm edema
  – High mortality
- Risk of pulm insufficiency
- Significant postop pain: epidural analgesia probably most effective

ANTICIPATED PROBLEMS/CONCERNS
- Hypotension from unrecognized blood loss; cardiac tamponade; MI/ischemia with low CO
- Postop pulm edema: R/O myocardial dysfunction; volume overload; correct dysrhythmias, hypoalbuminemia; atelectasis, pneumonitis
- Wound dehiscence and infection rare
- DVT and pulm embolism common (20%)
- Persistent air leak
- Early excess mediastinal shift life-threatening
- Contralateral shift: ↓ remaining lung function and venous return
- Ipsilateral shift: arrhythmia, ↓ BP, cardiac herniation, pulm edema
- Empyema in 5%
- Bronchopleural fistula in 4%

PREGNANT SURGICAL PATIENT

Rhonda Zuckerman, M.D.

RISK

- 50,000 pregnant patients/y undergo non-delivery procedures in USA
- Most common: trauma-related procedures, cervical suture, appendectomy, biliary tract disease−related procedures, breast biopsy, ovarian cystectomy

PERIOPERATIVE RISKS

- ↑ Maternal anesthetic risk for hypoxemia/pulmonary aspiration due to failed ET intubation
- Potential risk to fetus
  − Preterm delivery (preterm labor incidence 8−11%, higher for pelvic procedures)
  − Teratogenicity

WORRY ABOUT

- Maternal airway precautions
- Gastric chemoprophylaxis
- Prevention and treatment of maternal hypoxemia
- Avoidance of aortocaval compression (after 20 wk of gestation) and hypotension
- Detection and treatment of preterm labor

OVERVIEW

- If surgery must be performed during pregnancy, 2nd trimester is preferred period, since organogenesis is complete and risk of preterm delivery relatively low
- Acute exposure to anesthetic agents has not been associated with fetal malformations at birth
- Depressant effects of anesthetic agents are mainly of concern if fetus is delivered perioperatively

ICD-9-CM Code: V22.2 (Pregnancy)

INDICATIONS AND USUAL TREATMENT

- Cervical suture placement for prevention of preterm delivery due to cervical incompetence (performed at 12−16 wk of gestation)
- Other procedures performed only when risks of postponement outweigh benefits of avoiding increased maternal anesthetic risk and potential fetal harm

ASSESSMENT POINTS

SYSTEM	EFFECT	ASSESSMENT BY HX	PE	TEST
HEENT	Engorged, fragile mucosa, difficult intubation		Airway exam	Mallampati class
CV	Supine hypotensive syndrome	Nausea, diaphoresis while supine	Assess for hypotension, bradycardia while supine	
RESP	↑ O_2 consumption; ↓ FRC ↑ Pao_2, ↓ $Paco_2$			ABGs (if indicated)
GI	Full stomach, decreased LES tone	Reflux symptoms		
CNS	↓ MAC, ↓ intraspinal local anesthetic requirements			

Key Reference: Cohen SE: Nonobstetric surgery during pregnancy. *In* Chestnut DH (ed): Obstetric Anesthesia: Principles and Practice, 2nd ed. St. Louis, Mosby−Year Book, 1999, pp 279−299.

PERIOPERATIVE IMPLICATIONS

Anesthetic Technique

- Regional anesthesia: ↓ risk of maternal airway problems, ↑ risk of hypotension (compared with GA)
- General anesthesia: inhalation agents are tocolytic—may prevent contractions in OR; however, preterm labor may occur in recovery period

Monitoring

- Viable-gestational-age fetus: consider pre-, intra-, postoperative fetal heart tone and uterine activity monitoring
- Nonviable-gestational-age fetus: pre- and postoperative fetal heart tone documentation; consider pre-, intra-, and postoperative uterine activity monitoring
- Obstetric consultation recommended; pediatric notification indicated if delivery of a viable fetus is possible

Airway

- Edema and engorgement: ↑ risk of failed intubation, ↑ risk of bleeding, especially during nasal intubation
- ↑ Risk of pulm aspiration

Induction

- Regional anesthesia: spinal, epidural, or other block may be appropriate depending on location of surgical site
- General anesthesia: full stomach—awake intubation vs. denitrogenation followed by rapid-sequence induction

Maintenance

- Maintain left uterine displacement
- General anesthesia: inhalation agent—consider nitrous oxide, opioid, benzodiazepine (last often avoided in 1st trimester, although acute exposure not thought to be teratogenic). Muscle relaxants—minimal placental transfer.

Extubation

- After patient awake, able to protect airway

Postoperative Considerations

- Pain: consider IV or epidural PCA (opioids should not be withheld)
- Left uterine displacement in PACU
- Document fetal viability
- Consider monitoring for preterm labor

ANTICIPATED PROBLEMS/CONCERNS

- Pulm aspiration, failed intubation
- Preterm labor
- Fetal distress

PYLORIC STENOSIS REPAIR

J. Lance Lichtor, M.D.

RISK

- 1.5–3/1000 Caucasian births
- Lower incidence in African-Americans, Puerto Ricans, Asians
- Male > female, 4:1
- Tends to run in families (children of affected parents have higher incidence [3–5%])
- 2.5–5.5 times higher incidence for first-born

PERIOPERATIVE RISKS

- Hypotension due to preop hypovolemia and volume shifts common
- Hypoglycemia common with postop apnea or convulsions due to cessation of IV glucose and inadequate glycogen stores
- Mortality <1%
- Wound infection 5–20%

WORRY ABOUT

- Fluid and electrolyte deficiency (hypochloremic metabolic alkalosis, hypokalemia)
- Not a surgical emergency

OVERVIEW

- Gross thickening at circular smooth muscle of pylorus resulting in gradual obstruction of gastric outlet
- Projectile vomiting usually 2–4 wk; can have severe dehydration and acid-base abnormality

ICD-9-CM Code: 750.5

INDICATIONS AND USUAL TREATMENT

- Persistent vomiting usually after or toward the end of a feed with inability to feed
- Pyloromyotomy is treatment of choice
- No successful medical therapy

ASSESSMENT POINTS

SYSTEM	EFFECT	ASSESSMENT BY HX	PE	TEST
GI	Pyloric thickening	Vomiting	Olive-size mass, upper abdomen	GI series with barium or US
HEME	Hemoconcentration		Volume status measures; orthostatic vital signs Vasoconstriction	Hct
LYTES	Dehydration Acid-base abnormalities		Volume status measures; orthostatic vital signs; area with cold skin	Electrolytes
RENAL	Alkaline urine Acid urine	Persistent vomiting, volume depletion		

Key Reference: Bissonnette B, Sullivan PJ: Pyloric stenosis. Can J Anaesth 1991; 38:668–676.

PERIOPERATIVE IMPLICATIONS

- Correct electrolyte and acid-base abnormalities. Gastric sections are lost; therefore, hypochloremic alkalosis results.
- Stop oral feeds, replace ECF volume, replace K^+

Monitoring
- Routine

Airway
- Risk of aspiration: evacuate stomach contents. Consider rapid-sequence induction.
- Nasogastric tube after induction

Maintenance
- Avoid narcotics: rarely needed, prolong awakening. Local anesthetics (in addition to GA) useful.

SURGICAL STAGES

Induction
- Consider emptying stomach before induction

Skin Incision
- Abdomen opened through right transverse skin incision above liver edge or a right paramedian incision

Dissection
- Pylorus delivered into wound; incision through serosa and extended through circular muscle the length of tumor; circular muscle spread bluntly

ANTICIPATED PROBLEMS/CONCERNS

- Hypotension due to altered volume status
- Hypoglycemia, apnea, and convulsions, possibly due to cessation of IV glucose and depletion of liver glycogen
- Postop vomiting if early feeds
- Wound infection not uncommon
- Duodenal perforation may occur during myotomy; not a problem if recognized intraoperatively

RADICAL NECK DISSECTION

Noel Lee Chun, M.D.

RISK

- Performed for a variety of cancers, both local and metastatic from head and thorax
- Frequency ↑ with age, peaking in 7th decade
- Male > female, 3:1

PERIOPERATIVE RISKS

- Mortality rare, related to preop medical condition
- Morbidity includes MI, CVA, cranial nerve injury (20+%), pneumothorax, chylothorax, vascular injury, venous air embolism

WORRY ABOUT

- Tumor may distort airway and cause obstruction

- Associated cigarette use affecting CV and pulmonary systems
- Associated alcohol use affecting hepatic, hematologic, neurologic systems
- Malnutrition

OVERVIEW

- A complete cervical lymphadenectomy and sacrifice of sternocleidomastoid muscle, internal jugular vein, and spinal accessory nerve (cranial nerve XI). A functional neck dissection preserves these three structures; many modifications in between attempt to preserve some of these structures (termed modified).

ICD-9-CM Code: 144 (Malignant neoplasm of floor of mouth)

INDICATIONS AND USUAL TREATMENT

- To remove neoplastic tissue. In 80%, cancer is metastatic from another site. In 85%, primary tumor is supraclavicular.
- Often performed in conjunction with an operation to remove primary tumor (glossectomy, laryngectomy)
- Often performed in conjunction with flap reconstruction or skin graft to cover surgical defect
- Patient management often includes a course of preop or postop radiation therapy

ASSESSMENT POINTS

SYSTEM	EFFECT	ASSESSMENT BY HX	PE	TEST
HEENT	Tumor may affect airway	Dyspnea, dysphagia, dysarthria	Airway exam Headlight exam Fiberoptic exam	CXR CT/MRI Flow-volume loops
CV	Smoking and alcohol related	Angina/PND/orthopnea Htn/CHF/MI Exercise tolerance	Chest exam	CXR ECG Stress test ECHO/angio
RESP	Smoking related	SOB Cough/sputum Exercise tolerance	Chest exam	ABGs, ?PFTs CXR
HEME	Anemia, coagulopathies, cirrhosis	Fatigue Bleeding, bruisability Abdominal distention	Inspection for evidence of same	CBC PT, PTT, BT LFTs
NEURO	Alcohol withdrawal, nutritional deficiencies (see Malnutrition in Diseases section)	Anxiety, tachycardia, diaphoresis, seizures, peripheral neuropathy	Neuro exam	Treatment based on Hx and PE

Key Reference: Dougherty TB, Nguyen DT: Anesthetic management of the patient scheduled for head and neck cancer surgery. J Clin Anesth 1994; 6:74–82.

INTRAOPERATIVE MANAGEMENT

Monitoring

- Consider 2 major IVs at a minimum, as blood loss can be significant (esp with flap reconstruction), and usually both arms are tucked with head 180° away
- Blood loss usually < 800 ml; volume shifts usually not hemodynamically significant
- Consider precordial Doppler, end-tidal CO_2/N_2, TEE to monitor for venous air embolism (head usually elevated 30–45°)
- Consider arterial catheter and CVP/PA catheters for monitoring pressures and checking laboratory tests and monitoring volume status if CV unstable

Airway

- Head and neck tumors can compromise airway. Consider awake intubation or elective tracheotomy.
- Nasal and oral airways may be impossible to use because of airway distortion or tumor
- Patient usually 180° away from anesthesiologist
- Often a tracheotomy placed at beginning or end of procedure; airway control crucial at this stage

SURGICAL STAGES

Induction

- Once airway secured, routine

Skin Incision

- Many variations of neck incisions with an apron of dermis and epidermis stripped of subcutaneous fat and reflected upward

Dissection

- During dissection, all lymphatic tissue and fat removed en bloc and major anatomy defined
- Large neck vessels and important structures can be damaged with significant blood loss, cranial nerve paralysis, chyle leak

Definitive Surgery

- If performed in conjunction with excision of primary, extensive flap reconstruction, microvascular reanastomosis, laryngectomy, and tracheotomy may be necessary
- If flap reconstruction, avoid peripheral vasoconstrictors
- LMW dextran or other anticoagulation with postop monitoring for ischemia/thrombosis may be desirable
- Approximate duration: 4–10 h
- Occasionally carotid artery must be sacrificed because of tumor invasion; it may be ligated, anastomosed to external carotid, or reconstructed with graft material

Closure and Postoperative Considerations

- Airway considerations are first concern: have tracheotomy obturator available at all times
- Disfiguring procedure; if laryngectomy, patients often unable to communicate. Need sensitivity.
- Pain score: 2–6

ANTICIPATED PROBLEMS/CONCERNS

- Extent of surgery and preop medical condition determine complications
- If bilateral neck dissection performed, and both internal jugular veins are sacrificed, ↑ ICP with blindness has been reported
- Majority, even patients in poor medical condition, tolerate procedure well
- Postop pulm toilet and nutritional support crucial to short-term recovery, but patients must remember that recovery can be prolonged

RADICAL PROSTATECTOMY (RETROPUBIC) Lee A. Fleisher, M.D.

RISK

- 50,000 patients/y
- Racial predominance: none

PERIOPERATIVE RISKS

- Perioperative mortality rare ($<1\%$)
- Increased risk of DVT, pulmonary embolism
- 25% risk of impotence with nerve-sparing procedure; 75% risk without nerve-sparing procedure

WORRY ABOUT

- Venous air embolism
- Massive blood loss
- Nerve injury from position and surgical manipulation
- Often in flexed position with head down, increasing risk of aspiration

OVERVIEW

- Prostate, bladder, and seminal vesicles are removed
- Significant blood loss associated with transection of dorsal vein
- Regional anesthesia may be associated with lower blood loss and lower incidence of DVT
- Laparoscopic procedure rarely being performed
- Although autologous predonation common, becoming less widely used
- Consider hemodilution techniques to ↓ blood loss
- Myocardial ischemia ↑ if Hct $<28\%$

ICD-9-CM Code: 185.0 (Cancer of prostate)

INDICATIONS AND USUAL TREATMENT

- The following conditions should be met:
  - Isolated and localized prostatic malignancy
    - Anticipated life expectancy of ≥10 y
    - Good general health
    - Absence of indication of metastatic disease by work-up
- If co-existing disease, orchiectomy and hormonal therapy primary treatment
- Radiation therapy has similar 5-y survival rates
- "Smart bomb" radiation therapies also have similar 5-y survival rates with less surrounding tissue toxicity than classic radiation therapy
- Herbal therapies are alternative—8 hydroxy compounds in green teas have effectiveness in experimental animal models

ASSESSMENT POINTS (in addition to evaluation of co-existing disease)

SYSTEM	EFFECT	ASSESSMENT BY HX	PE	TEST
RESP	Pulmonary metastases	SOB	Auscultation	CXR, CT scan
MS	Skeletal metastases	Bone pain	Palpation	X-ray, bone scan, prostate-specific antigen (PSA)
RENAL	Chronic obstruction			Cr and/or BUN

Key Reference: Shir Y, Raja SN, Frank SM: The effect of epidural versus regional anesthesia on postoperative pain and analgesic requirements in patients undergoing radical prostatectomy. Anesthesiology 1994; 80:49–56.

PERIOPERATIVE IMPLICATIONS

Anesthetic Technique

- Can be performed under regional, general, or combined anesthetic techniques

Monitoring

- Large-bore IV lines for blood loss
- Consider arterial line depending on extent of surgery
- Consider CVP, PCWP, or TEE if co-existing disease
- Consider monitoring for air embolism

Airway

- None

Induction

- Requires level of at least T8 for regional
- Continuous regional techniques offer excellent pain management
- Consider blood conservation strategies

SURGICAL STAGES

Dissection

- Steady blood loss during dissection

Definitive Surgery

- May have significant blood loss during control of dorsal vein complex
- Hypotension may develop from blood loss or air embolism
- Indigo carmine frequently given to facilitate repair—incidence of anaphylaxis after indigo carmine and disturbance of pulse oximetry
- EBL: 1000–2000 ml
- Moderate volume shifts

Postoperative Considerations

- Significant postoperative pain
- Epidural may lead to fewer complications
- Pain score: 4–8
- IV PCA or epidural PCA for 2–3 days; newer modalities with education are associated with discharge on postop day 2 or 3
- May develop pulmonary embolism or DVT
- May develop peroneal nerve injury from lithotomy position

ANTICIPATED PROBLEMS/CONCERNS

- Air embolism may occur because of large open veins and patient position

RADIOTHERAPY/CT SCAN

Vivian H. Porche, M.D.

RISK
- CT
  - Intracranial imaging
  - Studies of the thorax and abdomen
  - IV contrast media can cause adverse reaction in 5–8% of cases
- Radiotherapy
  - External beam and intraop radiation
  - Impossible to directly observe the patient; watch on closed-circuit television

WORRY ABOUT
- Location of suction, oxygen, and electricity
- Compromise of thoracic structures with an anterior mediastinal mass
- Severe contrast reactions
- Aspiration with oral contrast
- Hypothermia, especially in children

OVERVIEW
- Goal: to provide a surgical level of safety in the radiologic suite
- Complicated by technique required
  - Radiotherapy patients scheduled for a series of daily treatments over several weeks

INDICATIONS
- Young children
- Disorders causing uncontrolled movements
- Patients with whom communication is impossible (e.g., language barrier, obtundation, mental retardation)
- Patients who are very ill or in severe pain

ASSESSMENT POINTS

PROCEDURE	PATIENT TYPE	ANESTHESIA TYPE	CONCERNS	MONITORING	COMMENTS
CT	Pediatric—less than 3 mo—with contrast	Deep sedation or MAC or GA	Keep patient warm to prevent hypothermia (neurologic dysfunction ↑ thermoregulation problems)	BP, pulse oximeter, $ETCO_2$ (if no $ETCO_2$, verify ventilation rate) ECG, consider temp monitoring	Position sedated child to avoid airway obstruction; mobile cart equipped for emergencies
	Pediatric—less than 3 mo—no contrast	No sedation—have infant suck on bottle of formula or allow to sleep	As above	No monitoring required Consider temp monitoring	As above
	Pediatric—under age 8, and/or mental handicap and/or contrast	Deep sedation—MAC or GA	If oral contrast given, treat patient as with full stomach	As above	As above
	Pediatric—over age 8, and/or no contrast	No sedation required; usually conscious sedation if unable to hold still	Maintain thermal stability	For conscious sedation: BP, pulse oximeter, ECG; consider temp monitoring	As above
	Adult—healthy	No sedation	If oral contrast is given, treat patient as with full stomach	None	If suspected ↑ in ICP, use caution to avoid ↑ arterial CO_2 or ↓ arterial O_2, which can further ↑ ICP
	Adult—difficulty holding still	Conscious sedation or MAC/GA	If oral contrast given, treat patient as with full stomach	BP, ECG, pulse oximeter, $ETCO_2$, FIO_2	Positioning of gantry or table during procedure may result in kinking or disconnection of anesthesia circuit
RADIO-THERAPY	Pediatric—esp under age 8	Sedation or MAC: use short-acting, easily titratable drugs; for repeated treatments, patient needs central indwelling catheter	Temp maintenance Airway management and ventilation Positioning of the gantry during procedure may result in kinking or disconnection of the anesthesia circuit Observe patient prior to each treatment for sepsis or ↑ ICP	ECG, $ETCO_2$, pulse oximeter, BP Make sure closed-circuit TV shows patient and monitors	Immobility is the primary goal of anesthesia IV anesthesia technique may avoid transporting agent vaporizers and other bulky equipment
	Adult	None Conscious sedation or easily titratable drugs		Same as above	

Key Reference: Porche VH: Anesthetic considerations in radiologic procedures performed outside the operating room. Int Anesthesiol Clin 1998; 36:9–19.

PERIOPERATIVE IMPLICATIONS

Preoperative Preparation
- Same careful preanesthesia evaluation as for any other surgical patient
- Know layout of area in advance
- Have warm blankets available

Anesthetic Technique
- Conscious sedation, MAC, or GA

Monitoring
- Routine; may need to add temperature

Positioning
- Airway and ventilation must be maintained
- May need long circuits or long IV tubing (watch for ↑ fluid volumes in pediatric patients)

POST-PROCEDURE CONSIDERATIONS
- Make sure of standard discharge criteria

RETAINED PLACENTA, REMOVAL OF

Mark C. Norris, M.D.

RISK

- Manual extraction needed in 5% of vaginal deliveries
- 3rd stage of labor is complete within 10 min in 75% of women. After 10 min, risks of retained placenta, hemorrhage, and need for transfusion increase.
- If 3rd stage of labor is longer than 30 min, >40% will require manual placental extraction
- Preterm gestation, 2 or more previous abortions, induced or augmented labor, and nulliparity increase risk of prolonged 3rd stage of labor

PERIOPERATIVE RISKS

- Retained placenta places patient at ↑ risk of significant blood loss, need for transfusion, and need for D&C
- Uterine perforation is a risk with D&C

WORRY ABOUT

- Full stomach (airway, other forms of effective analgesia present—epidural)
- Volume status
- Need uterine relaxation?
- Risk of placenta accreta/percreta

OVERVIEW

- Obstetrician requires good analgesia ± uterine relaxation
- One cause of prolonged 3rd stage of labor is abnormal placental implantation

- Women with a previous cesarean delivery may be at greater risk of placenta accreta. Women with placenta accreta are at very high risk of post-partum hemorrhage and may require immediate hysterectomy to remove placental fragments and control bleeding.

ICD-9-CM Code: 666-0 (Retained placenta with hemorrhage)

INDICATIONS/USUAL TREATMENT

- Most obstetricians will attempt manual removal of placenta if 3rd stage of labor lasts beyond 30 min
- Some will intervene earlier, especially if lower uterine segment contracts and will not allow placenta to pass
- Usual treatment is manual exploration and extraction

ASSESSMENT POINTS

SYSTEM	EFFECT	ASSESSMENT BY HX	PE	TEST
AIRWAY	Pregnancy-related changes: ↑ vascularity, airway edema, ↑ risk of difficult intubation	Previous difficulties	Mouth opening, oropharyngeal structures, dentition	
CV (volume status)	Significant, rapid hemorrhage possible ↑ Blood volume with pregnancy	EBL	BP, HR, tissue turgor, mucous membranes	Tilt table test
GI	Delayed gastric emptying (worse with systemic or epidural opioids used for labor analgesia)	Last meal		

Key Reference: Combs CA, Laros RK Jr: Prolonged third stage of labor: morbidity and risk factors. Obstet Gynecol 1991; 77:863–867.

PERIOPERATIVE MANAGEMENT

Preoperative Preparation

- Prepare for IV resuscitation (if needed) including potential for blood transfusion

Anesthetic Technique

- Epidural: if present and functioning and volume status adequate
- MAC: if *minimal* sedation/analgesia required. Most appropriate if placenta separated but trapped by contracted lower uterine segment.
- GA: excessive bleeding, no epidural, need for uterine instrumentation, placenta accreta

Monitoring

- Consider arterial line, CVP, Foley catheter if significant blood loss

Airway

- Full stomach: rapid-sequence induction with cricoid pressure if GA
- Minimal sedation if MAC/regional anesthesia used (constant verbal contact). *Remember:* pregnancy increases sensitivity to both inhaled and intravenous agents and speeds uptake of inhaled anesthetics.
- Increased risk of difficult intubation: be prepared

Induction/Maintenance

- Regional requires T10 sensory level
- May require uterine relaxation if placenta trapped by firmly contracted lower uterine segment
  – Beta-adrenergic agonists (terbutaline): slow onset, significant hemodynamic effects
  – Amyl nitrate: explosive, difficult to titrate, headache
  – Potent anesthetic agent: effective, requires general ET anesthesia
  – NTG: rapid onset, short duration, minimal hemodynamic effects; IV: 50 μg: onset 60 sec, duration 60 sec (obstetrician must be ready, hands in vagina, traction on umbilical cord); sublingual spray NTG (Nitrolingual Spray, Rhone Poulenc Rorer Pharmaceuticals Inc., Collegeville, PA): 0.8 mg (2 sprays): onset 35–65 sec; minimal maternal side effects

SURGICAL STAGES

- Removal can be complete, partial, or unsuccessful
- Partial: may require manual exploration of uterus or curettage; will need more complete analgesia; very difficult with sedation alone; consider GA if no regional anesthesia
- Unsuccessful: if placenta accreta, will require laparotomy, possible hysterectomy (↑ blood loss due to changes associated with pregnancy)
- EBL (uncomplicated): 500 ml
- Postpartum hysterectomy: potential for severe hemorrhage 1–20 L

Postoperative Considerations

- Uncomplicated: minimal pain
- Hysterectomy: pain like that of C-section (neuraxial opioids if regional, PCA [24–48 h] if GA)

ANTICIPATED PROBLEMS/CONCERNS

- Amount of blood loss correlates with ease of extraction

RETINAL BUCKLE SURGERY

Nader El-Gamal, M.D.

RISK

- People within USA: 20,000–30,000/y
- Racial predominance: none

PERIOPERATIVE RISKS

- Morbidity and mortality: 0.1% mortality rate related to patient-associated diseases
- Airway management
- Intravitreal injection of gas (sulfur hexafluoride) and N_2O

WORRY ABOUT

- Oculocardiac reflex
- Intravitreal injection of gas
- Other associated diseases (diabetes mellitus, Htn)
- Postop N/V, pain

OVERVIEW

- Age and co-morbidity of patient: usually elderly with other associated diseases
- Scleral buckle then positioned over tears and sutured in place to cover every retinal tear

ICD-9-CM Code: 361.9 (Retinal detachment)

INDICATIONS AND USUAL TREATMENT

- Treatment of retinal detachment
- Cryotherapy over retinal tears

ASSESSMENT POINTS

SYSTEM	EFFECT	ASSESSMENT BY HX	PE	TEST
RESP	Associated diseases	SOB, exercise tolerance	Chest exam	O_2 sat
HEME	Bleeding disorder Retrobulbar hemorrhage	Hx of easy bruising		PTT PT
RENAL	Impairment 2° to age, DM			BUN, Cr, glucose

Key Reference: Wong DH: Regional anesthesia for intraocular surgery. Can J Anaesth 1993; 40:635–657.

PERIOPERATIVE MANAGEMENT

Anesthetic Technique

- Regional preferred over general
  - ↓ Incidence of oculocardiac reflex
  - ↓ Interference with body physiology
  - ↓ Incidence of postop N/V
- Contraindications to local retrobulbar block
  - Abnormal coagulation or bleeding profile
  - Infection at or near injection site
  - Inability to communicate (language barrier, deafness)
  - Inability to lie flat
  - Chronic cough or tremor
  - Patient refusal
  - Open globe

Monitoring

- Routine

Airway

- In sedation cases avoid oversedation that may obstruct the airway, since intraoperative access difficult
- If using heated instrument, ensure that drapes are such that oxygen is not directed to instrument and is diluted rapidly in air

SURGICAL STAGES

Induction

- Sedation: midazolam, fentanyl, propofol
- Retrobulbar block and then titrate sedation, but avoid oversedated, disoriented, uncooperative patient
- In GA: avoid any sudden bucking or coughing; muscle relaxation preferred

Surgery

- During isolation of muscles monitor for bradycardia, asystole

- In GA twitch monitor to make sure patient is completely paralyzed
- Near end of procedure, surgeon might inject air or SF_6, so N_2O should be discontinued 15–20 min before

Postoperative Considerations

- Pain score: 3–5
- EBL: minimal

ANTICIPATED PROBLEMS/CONCERNS

- Airway obstruction, respiratory depression from oversedation
- Oculocardiac reflex
- Inappropriate level of sedation (disoriented, confused, oversedated patient or anxious, hypertensive, lightly sedated patient)
- Postop N/V

RETROPHARYNGEAL AND PERITONSILLAR ABSCESS DRAINAGE IN ADULTS

Michael F. Roizen, M.D.

RISK

- Rare without other debilitating conditions, such as alcohol abuse, immune compromise, or dental disease

PERIOPERATIVE RISKS

- Losing airway—no perfect approach (see below): all have risks and benefits

WORRY ABOUT

- Airway compromise, esp if severe enough to cause patient to drool and lean forward

OVERVIEW

- Complications of acute tonsillitis in which the infection has spread deep to the tonsillar capsule. Pus forms between the tonsillar capsule and the superior constrictor of pharynx, and the tonsil is displaced medially. Uvula becomes edematous, marked trismus and pain occur (head usually tilted toward site of abscess).
- Local infection with systemic implications due to airway compromise and potential for sepsis. Usually a β-hemolytic strep or anaerobe.

ICD-9-CM Code: 478.24 (Retropharyngeal abscess)

INDICATIONS AND TREATMENT

- Depends on degree of airway compromise: goal is 48 h of antibiotic prior to incision and drainage

ASSESSMENT POINTS

SYSTEM	EFFECT	ASSESSMENT BY HX	PE	TEST
ENT	Can be massive swelling and edema that inhibits airway and mouth opening and access	Ability to lie flat Drooling	Airway exam	Lateral neck x-ray
CV	Sepsis Hypovolemia	Hx of symptoms of infection	HR BP Temperature	ECG ? CVP

Key Reference: Snow JB: Surgical disorders of the ears, nose, paranasal sinuses, pharynx and larynx. *In* Sabiston DC: Textbook of Surgery, 15th ed. Philadelphia, WB Saunders, 1997, p 1290.

PERIOPERATIVE MANAGEMENT

Anesthetic Technique

- Alternatives based on two factors:
  - Most important—how to secure airway
  - Presence of sepsis

Monitoring

- Without sepsis: usual
- With sepsis: CVP vs. PAC, and consider arterial line

Airway

- Difficult choices depending on severity and judgment of individual anatomy
- Topical and awake I & D if pt can tolerate is usual 1st choice
- Awake trach preferable if no other easy means and sepsis does not involve that area of neck
- Awake fiberoptic risks abscess contamination or accidental I & D and severe lung infection or losing airway

SURGICAL STAGES

Induction

- After airway secure

Surgery

- Usual I & D and return at another time for tonsillectomy, etc.
- Pus cavity and site of infection can be difficult to find
- Airway patency
- Lung infection
- Underlying problem
- Sepsis management usually easier after abscess drained

ANTICIPATED PROBLEMS/CONCERNS

- Airway compromise
- Underlying illness, including drug withdrawal

ROTATOR CUFF SURGERY

Noel Lee Chun, M.D.

RISK

- People within USA: ~ 50,000/y; almost all > 40 y; some younger athletes
- Fluoroscopic examination of 6061 random asymptomatic people revealed cuff calcification in 2.7%
- 20–30% incidence of rupture of supraspinatus tendon in cadavers > 60 y
- Males >> females (3:1)

PERIOPERATIVE RISKS

- Risks associated with interscalene block anesthesia include spinal, epidural, and IV injection of local anesthetic, recurrent laryngeal nerve block, and pneumothorax
- Infections in 1–5%
- Limitation of motion in 5%

- Nerve damage in 1–5%
- Mortality—minimal and related to preop conditions

WORRY ABOUT

- Whether to use regional or general anesthesia
- Airway management critical, as head is often only partially accessible

OVERVIEW

- Rotator cuff composed of subscapularis tendon anteriorly and supraspinatus, infraspinatus, and teres minor tendon insertions posteriorly
- Most common injury is tear of supraspinatus insertion; however, any of the tendons may be involved

- Associated surgical findings include biceps tendon rupture, glenohumeral arthritis, and labral fraying, resulting in shoulder pain and variable degrees of loss of function and ROM

ICD-9-CM Codes: 727.61 (Nontraumatic); 840.4 (Traumatic)

INDICATIONS AND USUAL TREATMENT

- Cuff tears are repaired primarily when possible; however, sometimes hardware and special techniques necessary owing to poor quality of tissue involved
- Arthroscopic evaluation and debridement often performed prior to repair

ASSESSMENT POINTS

(see Rheumatoid Arthritis if appropriate)

SYSTEM	EFFECT	ASSESSMENT BY HX	PE	TEST
HEENT	If RA or connective tissue disease, may have limited ROM of head/neck	Limited ROM head/neck or neck	Airway exam	C-spine x-ray
CV	If RA or connective tissue disease, may have valvular heart disease/conduction defects	Angina/PND/orthopnea Palpitations/CHF Exercise tolerance	Chest exam Exam of peripheral pulses and vital signs	ECG ECHO
RESP	If RA, may have pulm fibrosis or pleural effusion	SOB Exercise tolerance	Chest exam	CXR ABGs PFTs
HEME	Hx NSAID use—may affect coagulation	Hx medications, bleed/bruise	Inspection for evidence of same	
IMMUNO	If RA, may be immunocompromised	Hx medications, infectious disease		CBC and differential

Key References: Brown AR, et al: Interscalene block for shoulder arthroscopy: comparison with general anesthesia. Arthroscopy 1993; 9:295–300; McKee MD, Yoo DJ: The effect of surgery for rotator cuff disease on general health status: results of a prospective trial. J Bone Joint Surg Am 2000; 82:970–979.

PERIOPERATIVE MANAGEMENT

Monitoring
- Routine
- Precordial Doppler/end-tidal N_2 or TEE to monitor for venous air embolism in sitting position
- Pad pressure points, and protect eyes to avoid corneal abrasion

Airway
- Lateral decubitus or sitting position with restricted access to head
- Securing airway management crucial

Induction
- For GA, routine
- For interscalene block, 40 ml of local
  – 100% incidence of phrenic nerve paralysis, and significant incidence of recurrent laryngeal nerve paralysis and cervical plexus blockade
- Technique contraindicated if advanced pulm disease or contralateral vocal cord paralysis

- Field blocks or SQ local infiltration may be used for skin of shoulder (C3–C4) and medial upper arm (T2)
- Muscular relaxation important to help mobilize cuff; this can be provided by regional anesthesia or NMB

SURGICAL STAGES

Skin Incision
- Rotator cuff approached via oblique incision over acromion

Dissection
- Part of overlying deltoid muscle detached and then divided to reach rotator cuff. Care must be taken in reattaching deltoid to acromial bone edge to avoid avulsion and loss of function. If splitting of deltoid is carried more than 5 cm anteriorly, axillary nerve may be damaged with loss of function of all or part of deltoid.
- Supraspinatus tendon should not be dissected and elevated from contiguous bone floor for a distance exceeding 2 cm medial to superior glenoid rim; otherwise, suprascapu-

lar nerve injury with additional weakening of external rotator muscles may result

Definitive Surgery
- Ruptured tendons sewn together primarily if possible; sometimes necessary to dissect additional length of muscle and anchor it to head of humerus with suture or hardware

Closure and Postoperative Considerations
- Arm is placed in sling or abduction pillow prior to awakening; usually no active motion for several weeks to avoid possibility of disruption of repair
- Pain score: 3–8. Pain can be significantly mitigated by use of long-acting local anesthetics in an interscalene block.

ANTICIPATED PROBLEMS/CONCERNS

- Preop medical condition determines anticipated complications; majority of patients, even those in poor medical condition, tolerate this procedure well
- Postoperative pain management with IV PCA or interscalene block

SCOLIOSIS AND KYPHOSIS SURGERY
Ralph L. Bernstein, M.D.

RISK

- 1–3% of screened adolescents with curves >10°
- Females > males, 3.6:1

PERIOPERATIVE RISKS

- Pneumonia, atelectasis
- Neurologic damage—injury to spinal cord by excessive traction

WORRY ABOUT

- Extensive blood loss
- Postop atelectasis, pneumonia
- Superior mesenteric artery syndrome—when curve straightened, superior mesenteric artery occludes duodenum, may require nasogastric tube or surgery

OVERVIEW

- Thoracoabdominal approach to release vertebrae anteriorly, remove disks, apply instrumentation or bone grafts, followed by posterior spinal fusion at the same operation
- In kyphosis surgery, anterior release and grafting may be followed by posterior instrumentation and fusion during a subsequent operation
- Prepare for large blood loss

ICD-9-CM Code: 737.10 (Kyphoscoliotic, acquired)

INDICATIONS AND USUAL TREATMENT

- Scoliosis with increasing curve in growing child or severe deformity, or pain not controlled by conservative measures such as bracing
- In kyphotic curve that is progressing and curves causing severe back pain, in curves in which neurologic impairment is occurring from congenital, post-traumatic, or infectious causes

ASSESSMENT POINTS

SYSTEM	EFFECT	ASSESSMENT BY HX	PE	TEST
HEENT	Regurgitation, aspiration in neuromuscular patients	Parents' report		
CV	Cardiomyopathy in Friedreich's ataxia and muscular dystrophy	Exercise tolerance		ECG, ECHO, CXR
RESP	Restrictive pulm disease in patients with severe deformities of thorax Paralytic or neuromuscular scoliosis may cause severe resp impairment	Exercise tolerance		Vital capacity if curves >50–60°, ABGs
HEME	Preop autologous blood donation			Hgb, Hct
CNS	In neuromuscular and congenital scoliosis, evaluation of neurologic status		Neuro exam	Preop SSEP

Key Reference: Bernstein RL, Rosenberg AD: Scoliosis. *In* Manual of Orthopedic Anesthesia and Related Pain Syndromes. New York, Churchill Livingstone, 1994.

PERIOPERATIVE MANAGEMENT

Preoperative Preparation

- Instruct patient concerning possibility of wake-up test (shut off N_2O, relaxants reversed, naloxone given if needed)
- Tell patient to move the hands; if done, to move toes of both feet
- In anterior thoracolumbar approach, chest tube will be present
- Teach patient pulm toilet and how to use PCA devices

Monitoring

- Consider arterial line
- CVP line useful to assess blood volume status; urinary catheter
- SSEP
- Blood loss: measure suction canister contents, weigh sponges, use blood salvage device

Induction/Maintenance

- Consider administering β-blockers to control heart rate if hypotensive anesthesia is used
- Inhalation agents may interfere with SSEP monitoring
- ET intubation: secure tube (double-lumen tube not required)

SURGICAL STAGES

- For anterior approach—patient placed in lateral decubitus position. Recommend adequate padding and axillary roll on down side.
- Apply external warming device
- Thoracolumbar incision is made, diaphragm detached, vertebra approached
- Vascular compromise of spinal cord may occur if segmental vessels taken are major feeders to spinal cord. Disks removed, bone graft and instrumentation placed according to structural needs.
- Following closure, chest tube inserted, patient placed into prone position
- Surgeon may infiltrate incision with epinephrine 1:250,000–1:500,000 solution
- Blood loss can be brisk, esp as dissection is made down to bleeding bone, more in neuromuscular scoliosis. Instrumentation inserted, correction obtained, bone graft inserted.
- Consider hypotensive anesthesia with MAP at 60 mmHg in normotensive patients. During correction, pressure returned to normal levels. Sodium nitroprusside infusion or labetalol commonly used.
- Excessive crystalloids may cause postop edema

- Monitor SSEPs or NMEPs—if decrease in latency of 10% or decrease in amplitude of 60%. Check $ETCO_2$, pulse oximeter, body temp.
  - Tell surgeon to stop operation
  - Raise BP to above-normal levels to increase perfusion of cord
  - Prepare to perform wake-up test
- At conclusion, patient placed supine
- Consider not rushing to extubate until extubation criteria are met and patient is normothermic
- Blood loss may continue with wound drainage apparatus. Reinfusion of this blood has resulted in red-colored urine on occasion.
- Make certain chest tube is functioning
- Have patient awake enough for neurologic evaluation
- Consider pain relief by PCA

ANTICIPATED PROBLEMS/CONCERNS

- Pulm: atelectasis
- GI: ileus
- In patients with neuromuscular scoliosis, postoperative ventilatory support may be needed. Consider weaning these patients as soon as possible to avoid loss of muscle strength.

SEIZURE SURGERY

Barbara A. Dodson, M.D.

RISK

- 0.5–2% of general population with recurrent seizures (Szs)
- 25–30% of patients with epilepsy have > 1 Sz/mo
- ~ 300,000 patients have medically refractory Szs, with ~ 1% undergoing Sz surgery

PERIOPERATIVE RISKS

- ↑ or ↓ Sz threshold with anesthetics
- Adverse drug reactions from anticonvulsants themselves and interactions with anesthetic adjuvants

WORRY ABOUT

- Status epilepticus, loss of airway during conscious sedation, ↑ ICP in patients with mass lesions, movement during brain surgery; systemic, cardiovascular, or hypoxic complications 2° to Szs

OVERVIEW

- Szs, of both epileptic and nonepileptic origin, classified as partial or generalized. Partial Szs have focal origins (but may progress to bilateral). Simple partial Sz implies undetectable change in consciousness and limited EEG distribution. Sz focus spreads in complex partial Szs to multiple areas and alters consciousness. Generalized Szs simultaneously involve both hemispheres and are subdivided into inhibitory (absence and atonic) and excitatory (clonic, tonic, and myoclonic).

ICD-9-CM Code: 790.3

ETIOLOGY

- Szs may be secondary to multiple neurologic conditions, including post-traumatic injuries, tumors, AVMs, infections, and idiopathic epilepsy
- Other causes include psychiatric disorders, neurofibromatosis, tuberous sclerosis, drug and alcohol abuse

INDICATIONS

- Primary goal to render patient Sz-free with minimal toxicity using variety of anticonvulsants
- Szs arising from discrete foci may be amenable to surgical resection (e.g., temporal lobectomy, AVM resection)

ASSESSMENT POINTS

SYSTEM	EFFECT	ASSESSMENT BY HX	PE	TEST
HEENT	Gingival hyperplasia, facial trauma		Facial fracture, broken or missing teeth, gingival hyperplasia	
RESP	Aspiration during Szs	Hx of pneumonia	Rales, ↓ breath sounds	CXR
GI	Liver toxicity 2° to medications			LFTs
ENDO	Bone marrow suppression and thrombocytopenia 2° to medication	Bleeding, infection	Petechiae, ecchymoses	CBC, plt; PT, PTT
CNS	Szs, both partial and generalized Personality disorders	Preseizure auras, automations	Neurologic exam	CT, MRI, EEG telemetry, Wada test (to determine dominant hemisphere for memory and speech)
MS	Injury during Szs		Signs of trauma	

Key Reference: Kofke WA, Tempelhoff R, Dasheiff RM: Anesthetic implications of epilepsy, status epilepticus, and epilepsy surgery. J Neurosurg Anesthesiol 1997; 9:349–372.

PERIOPERATIVE IMPLICATIONS

Preoperative Preparation

- Determine baseline neurologic status
- Evaluate cooperativeness if conscious sedation planned
- Determine type and frequency of Szs; anticonvulsant medications, and whether tapered preop
- Review results of preop neurologic evaluation, esp hemispheric dominance and relationship of surgical field to speech, motor, and memory areas
- Avoid premedication with drugs such as benzodiazepines that could ablate seizure foci even temporarily

Monitoring

- Consider arterial catheter and Foley catheter
- End-tidal CO_2 via nasal cannula during conscious analgesia

Airway

- Obvious airway difficulties may preclude use of conscious analgesia technique

Maintenance

- NO_2-narcotic technique with low-dose isoflurane and/or propofol can be used for GA if electrocorticography (ECoG) is not planned. Anticonvulsant medications will ↑ both opioid and muscle relaxant requirements. Hyperventilation should be avoided. If ECoG is planned, NO_2-narcotic technique should be used and benzodiazepines, volatile anesthetics, and muscle paralysis should be meticulously avoided.
- Fentanyl and/or alfentanil infusion, droperidol, and benadryl can be used for conscious sedation. Effect of low-dose propofol on ECoG controversial.
- Be prepared to treat emergency intraoperative Szs

Extubation

- Facilitate rapid emergence and avoid Htn and coughing

Postoperative Period

- Anticonvulsant blood levels can both ↑ and ↓ postop

Adjuvants

- Low-dose methohexital and etomidate can be used to ↑ activity at Sz focus to aid in location and evaluation of area for resection during surgery
- Benzodiazepine and higher dose methohexital to ↓ Sz activity

ANTICIPATED PROBLEMS/CONCERNS

- New neurologic deficits, seizures, anticonvulsant toxicity, status epilepticus

SPINAL FUSION

Madelyn Kahana, M.D.

RISK

- Prevalence: 4/1000 in North America
- Female predominance: 8:1

PERIOPERATIVE RISKS

- Perioperative mortality rare (0–0.5%)
- Venous air embolism (VAE) can occur and produce CV collapse
- Postop neurologic deficit (0.7–5%)
- Massive blood loss possible (1–5%)
- Pneumothorax (1–5%)

WORRY ABOUT

- Etiology (? syndrome or tumor rather than idiopathic)
- Large intraoperative blood loss
- Potential for VAE
- Problems of prone position
- Postop resp insufficiency 2° to SIADH

OVERVIEW

- Scoliosis is rotational abnormality of spine and ribs
- Dx of idiopathic scoliosis one of exclusion
- May be significant restrictive lung disease
- Evoked potential monitoring can limit choice of anesthetic technique
- An intraoperative wake-up test may be requested by operating surgeon
- Intraoperative VAE is possible

ICD-9-CM Code: 737.30

INDICATIONS AND USUAL TREATMENT

- Surgical correction absolutely indicated if curve is >60° or if a lesser curve with resp compromise, pain, or likelihood of progression to 60°
- Most patients with curve <40° do not need surgical correction
- Medical management with proven efficacy includes a variety of bracing techniques but is generally used if curve is 20–45°
- Failure to correct significant curve results in a doubling of mortality for age, potential for progressive back pain, and progressive pulmonary dysfunction

ASSESSMENT POINTS

SYSTEM	EFFECT	ASSESSMENT BY HX	PE	TEST
CV	Cor pulmonale possible if significant lung disease	Exercise tolerance		ECG ECHO
RESP	Pulm dysfunction occurs with significant thoracic curves		Exercise tolerance testing	PFTs corrected for height
CNS	Preop neurologic dysfunction unusual; should lead to further assessment and diagnostic tests		Complete neurologic exam	?CT ?MRI
MS		Careful exam may lead to an alternative Dx, e.g., Marfan's, Ehlers-Danlos, Goldenhar's syndromes; syrinx		

Key Reference: Winkler M, Merker E, Hetz H: The peri-operative management of major orthopaedic procedures. Anaesthesia 1998; 53(suppl 2):37–41.

PERIOPERATIVE IMPLICATIONS

Anesthetic Technique

- Performed utilizing general ET anesthesia in prone position
- Controlled hypotension used to limit blood loss
  - Potential for interference with evoked potential monitoring influences anesthetic agent choice

Monitoring

- Arterial line useful
- Consider CVP line to monitor volume and perhaps to treat VAE
- Foley catheter may facilitate adequate volume resuscitation

Induction/Maintenance

- Narcotics do not interfere with SSEPs or MEPs
- <1 MAC inhalation agent exerts only minimal effect on potential monitoring
- Anticipate need for midprocedure wake-up test
- Controlled hypotension accomplished with β-blockade and IV vasodilators

Preoperative Management

- Large-bore IV lines because of anticipated blood loss

SURGICAL STAGES

Positioning

- Patient positioned prone on a frame that allows abdomen to be free from external compression to reduce venous pressure
- Pressure points padded carefully
- There must be no pressure on ocular structures or ear cartilage

Dissection/Definitive Surgery

- Prior to skin incision, surgical field is often infiltrated with dilute solution of epinephrine
- Steady bleeding during dissection
- Steady bleeding during decortication
- Hypotension may be due to blood loss or VAE
- After instrumentation in place, distraction is performed
- After distraction complete, a wake-up test is often performed
- Approximate duration: 4–8 h

Postoperative Considerations

- Pain score: 6–9
- Postop resp failure unusual but should be considered a possibility in patients with pre-existing restrictive lung disease
- New neurologic injury is an emergency and requires urgent removal of all hardware

ANTICIPATED PROBLEMS/CONCERNS

- Potential for massive blood loss and rapid development of hypotension
- Modest risk of VAE because of open epidural veins and prone position
- Perioperative neurologic injury in 0.7–5%; generally occurs during distraction
- Occasional reports of neurologic injury in spite of normal evoked responses support considering continued use of wake-up test
- Be confident that patient has idiopathic scoliosis (vs. neurologic/spine abn or other etiology)

SPLENECTOMY

Wendy K. Bernstein, M.D.
Lee A. Fleisher, M.D.

RISK

- No age or sex predilection

PERIOPERATIVE RISKS

- Mortality rate 0–3%
- Overall complication rate is 11.8% associated with pulm complications, DVT

WORRY ABOUT

- Potential for major blood loss requiring transfusion

OVERVIEW

- Spleen most commonly injured organ in blunt trauma
- Splenic trauma frequently associated with other intra-abdominal injuries

ICD-9-CM Codes: 865.10 (Splenic trauma); 289.4 (Hypersplenism)

ETIOLOGY

- S/P blunt or penetrating abdominal trauma requiring emergency operation (14%)
- Idiopathic thrombocytopenic purpura
- Hodgkin's lymphoma (27%)
- Hereditary spherocytosis
- Felty's syndrome
- Myeloid metaplasia
- Sickle cell disease
- Thalassemia
- Chronic leukemia

USUAL TREATMENT

- Depends upon indication
- Splenorrhaphy for splenic salvage after trauma

ASSESSMENT POINTS

SYSTEM	EFFECT	ASSESSMENT BY HX	TEST
CV	Cardiotoxicity Dysrhythmias, CHF	Chemotherapeutic agents— doxorubicin (dose > 550 mg/m^2)	ECG, ECHO, MUGA → determine LV function
RESP	Pleural effusions; left lower lobe atelectasis if splenomegaly; pulm fibrosis	Chemotherapeutic agents— bleomycin, methotrexate, cytarabine	CXR
GI	Hepatotoxicity	Chemotherapeutic agent— methotrexate	LFTs
HEME	Splenomegaly Cytopenia	Hematologic disease	CBC with differential Plt count Bleeding time
GU	Renal insufficiency	Chemotherapeutic agents— methotrexate, cisplatin	BUN, serum Cr UA, electrolytes
CNS	Neurologic deficits Peripheral neuropathies	Chemotherapeutic agents— vinblastine, cisplatin	

Key Reference: Pivalizza EG, Tjia IM, Juneja HS, Cohen AM, Duke JH Jr: Elective splenectomy in an anemic Jehovah's Witness patient with cirrhosis. Anesth Analg 1998; 87:529–530.

PERIOPERATIVE IMPLICATIONS

Preoperative Implications

- Polyvalent pneumococcal vaccine (7 days prior to surgery, if possible)
- Nasogastric decompression
- Stress steroids (100 mg IV hydrocortisone q8h), if received in past

Monitoring

- Routine
- Large-bore IV access

Airway

- Trauma patients: rule out cervical instability

Induction

- Routine

Maintenance

- Prevent hypothermia

Extubation

- Routine

Adjuvants

- Combined general/epidural (1.5–2% lidocaine with 1:200,000 epinephrine)
- Muscle relaxants required
- Minimize sedatives: ↑ likelihood of postop resp depression

Postoperative Period

- Postsplenectomy sepsis: due to encapsulated organisms (e.g., pneumococci)

ANTICIPATED PROBLEMS/CONCERNS

- Bleeding
- Atelectasis (left lower lobe)
- Complications related to underlying cause for splenectomy

SPLIT-THICKNESS SKIN GRAFT

Robert Gaiser, M.D.

USES

- To cover granulating wound:
  - Burns: 2 million people injured/y
  - Wounds: trauma, diabetic foot ulcers, postradiation skin breakdown, sacral decubitus, melanoma excision

PERIOPERATIVE RISKS

- Perioperative mortality: rare
- 40% BSA burns have 40% mortality in 60–75 y (90% survival in <45 y)
- Large areas may involve significant blood loss

WORRY ABOUT

- Airway involvement in burns that may make intubation difficult
- Blood loss if large areas to be debrided and grafted

- Hypotensive shock, electrolyte abn, sepsis, arrhythmias, myoglobinemia, ATN, compartment syndromes
- Nutritional status of patient
- Cleanliness of donor and recipient sites
- Suitable locations for application of monitors and IV access
- Loss of joint mobility due to scarring

OVERVIEW

- Split-thickness skin graft (STSG) consists of epidermis and only a portion of dermis. STSGs categorized as thin (0.005–0.012 in.), medium (0.012–0.018 in.), or thick (0.018–0.028 in.).
- Must consider both donor and recipient sites: addition of epinephrine will decrease bleeding at donor site without affecting survival of STSG

ICD-9-CM Codes: Procedure Code: 151.00; Diagnosis Code (dependent upon location): 707.00 (Decubitus ulcer); 707.10 (Ulcer on LE); 873.40 (Ulcer on face); 884.00 (Ulcer on UE); 941.00 (Burn on face); 942.00 (Burn on trunk); 944.00 (Burn on UE); 945.00 (Burn on LE)

INDICATIONS AND USUAL TREATMENT

- Used to cover granulating wound: tolerates less vascularity than full-thickness skin graft
- Disadvantage: lack of growth in children, abnormal pigmentation, contraction
- Donor site: any area of body including scalp and extremities; depends on resulting skin match and appearance of the donor scar

ASSESSMENT POINTS

SYSTEM	EFFECT	ASSESSMENT BY HX	PE	TEST
DERM	Donor/recipient site	Discussion with surgeon		
HEENT	Burns or radiation	Review medical record	Airway exam	
CV	Hypotensive shock, arrhythmias, myocardial contractile depression	Dyspnea, orthopnea, chest pain	Vital signs, chest exam	CXR, ECG, orthostatic vital signs
RESP	ARDS	Dyspnea, SOB, chest pain, mental status change	Chest exam	CXR ABGs
GI	Debilitated patient	Bed-bound		Albumin
HEME	Possible large blood loss			Hct
RENAL	ATN, myoglobinemia	Massive tissue destruction Prolonged hypotension	Oliguria, anuria	BUN, serum Cr Cr clearance; serum/urine myoglobin
NEURO	Paresis of lower extremity Compartment syndromes	Functional limitations Hx of circumferential extremity burns	Neuro exam Weak pulses	Transduce compartment pressures

Key Reference: Skouge JW: Techniques for split-thickness skin grafting. J Dermatol Surg Oncol 1987; 13:841–849.

PERIOPERATIVE MANAGEMENT

Preoperative Preparation

- Determine donor/recipient sites
- Stabilize hemodynamically first
- IV access: large-bore IVs if anticipate large blood loss
- Warm room and all fluids

Monitoring

- Donor/recipient sites limit locations available for application of monitors: secure leads and pulse oximeter to sites used
- May use lower extremity for BP monitoring
- Temp monitoring

Airway

- For burn or postradiation patient, determine if airway involved. Involvement of face may make intubation more difficult: consider fiberoptic intubation/consider consultative, collaborative airway management.

Induction/Maintenance

- Avoid succinylcholine, as may precipitate hyperkalemic response
- No generally accepted preferred agent or technique
- Regional anesthesia is an option
- Consider lateral femoral cutaneous nerve block if donor site is lateral thigh

- If using local anesthetic, keep amount within recommended limits
- Addition of epinephrine to local anesthetic is not contraindicated
- EMLA cream has been used for anesthesia for donor site
- Application of lidocaine spray to donor site ↓ postop pain
- Acute phase: anticipate hemostatic problems if large area is to be grafted; consider electrolyte abnormalities and volume status
- Chronic phase: scarring may cause loss of function and difficulty with positioning of the patient

SURGICAL STAGES

- Variety of dermatomes available to cut STSG. In general, air- or electric-powered dermatomes and free hand knife are used to cut lengthwise on extremity; drum dermatomes used sidewise across extremity.
- Width of graft determined by width setting on dermatome
- If Betadine is used to prep donor area, it must be washed off to prevent sticking
- Skin thoroughly lubricated with sterile mineral oil to facilitate graft cutting
- Advancing the dermatome flat across the skin with gentle downward pressure
- Wound cleaned with saline or Betadine solution

- Surgical debridement may cause bleeding; hemostasis important for graft survival
- Graft placed on the wound, sutured around the periphery, and dressed. Main object of the dressing is to ensure contact between graft and host bed. Dressing left in place for ~7 days, at which time sutures can be removed.
- Reasons for graft failure: inadequate graft bed (poor vascularity), hematoma, movement, infection, technical errors
- EBL: depends on extent of grafting, minimal to 250–500 ml

Postoperative Considerations

- Pain score: 4–6
- Application of lidocaine spray to donor site ↓ postop pain
- Activity level kept at a minimum for first 2 days after surgery
- Monitor CV status
- Heat loss in transfer to/from OR

ANTICIPATED PROBLEMS/CONCERNS

- Blood loss may be difficult to assess and may be high; assess Hct and volume status frequently
- Malnutrition may lead to unexpected amounts of edema
- Hypothermia common if not assiduously avoided pre- and intratransport

STRABISMUS SURGERY

Eric Weissend, M.D.
Ronald S. Litman, D.O.

RISK

- 5% of the population have malalignment of visual axes
- Strabismus repair is the most commonly performed pediatric ocular operation
- Gender/race predominance: none

PERIOPERATIVE RISKS

- Mortality: extremely rare
- Probably higher than average incidence of masseter muscle rigidity (MMR) and malignant hyperthermia (MH)

WORRY ABOUT

- Oculocardiac reflex (trigeminal-vagal)
- Postop nausea/vomiting
- Development of MH

OVERVIEW

- Can be congenital anomaly or acquired defect
- Congenital strabismus due to innervation abnormalities
- Acquired strabismus has multiple potential etiologies including restrictive disease (e.g., orbital mass), ocular myopathy, myasthenia gravis
- Strabismus can be sign of an as yet undiagnosed underlying myopathy
- High incidence of strabismus in patients with CNS disease (e.g., meningomyelocele with hydrocephalus, cerebral palsy, congenital myopathies)

ICD-9-CM Codes: 368.01 (Amblyopia); 378.60 (Mechanical)

INDICATIONS AND USUAL TREATMENT

- Surgical correction within the first 4 mo of life will help ensure proper development of stereoscopic vision
- Strabismus repair in the older child is performed for cosmetic reasons

ASSESSMENT POINTS

SYSTEM	EFFECT	ASSESSMENT BY HX	PE	TEST
CV	Myopathies (e.g., Duchenne) can cause conduction abn and myocardial dysfunction	Palpitations, exercise tolerance	S_3, irregular rhythm	ECG, ECHO if central myopathy exists
RESP	Cerebral palsy patients may have chronic lung disease Congenital myopathies may affect oropharyngeal and esophageal muscles	Prolonged intubation, reactive airway disease, frequent aspiration	Rhonchi, wheezing	Baseline SpO_2 Consider CXR if recent change in pulm status

Key Reference: Tramer M, Moore A, McQuay H: Prevention of vomiting after paediatric strabismus surgery: a systemic review using the numbers-needed-to-treat method. Br J Anaesth 1995; 75:556–561.

PERIOPERATIVE IMPLICATIONS

Preoperative Preparation

- IM atropine decreases incidence of oculocardiac reflex from 90% to 50%

Anesthetic Technique

- Possible masseter muscle rigidity with use of succinylcholine—use with caution
- Oral RAE tube required in most instances; may be performed with LMA
- Narcotics increase incidence of postop N/V
- Consider postop N/V prophylaxis
- Prophylaxis with droperidol or ondansetron decreases incidence of postop N/V from >50% to <25%
- Propofol has high incidence of oculocardiac reflex without any significant antiemetic effect

SURGICAL STAGES

- Oculocardiac reflex can be induced by traction on extraocular muscles, pressure on eyeball, eye pain
- Hypercapnia increases incidence of bradycardia
- First step in treatment is to stop surgical stimulation. If necessary, follow with IV atropine.

Postoperative Considerations

- Pain score: 2–3 (severe irritation rather than pain)
- Postop N/V occurs in 50–80% of patients

ANTICIPATED PROBLEMS/CONCERNS

- Higher than average incidence of MMR and MH
- Postop N/V

TESTICULAR TORSION SURGERY

Eric Weissend, M.D.
Ronald S. Litman, D.O.

RISK

- 1/160 males, most commonly around puberty but also in neonatal period
- 20% have antecedent trauma
- Racial predominance: none
- Left testicle affected twice as often as right

PERIOPERATIVE RISKS

- Pts are generally young and healthy—no special risks

WORRY ABOUT

- Full stomach
- Testicular ischemia
- Patient anxiety

OVERVIEW

- Manifested by acute scrotal pain and results from twisting of spermatic cord with vascular compromise of testicle
- Caused by high investment of tunica vaginalis on spermatic cord (bell-clapper deformity)
- If not surgically corrected in relatively short time (6–8 h), testicular ischemia can result
- Generally considered a surgical emergency
- Temporizing treatment involves manual detorsion by a urologist, which may alleviate ischemia, but orchidopexy still required
- Difficult to diagnose. Color Doppler US considered to be test of choice.

ICD-9-CM Code: 608.2

INDICATIONS/USUAL TREATMENT

- Emergency scrotal exploration usually indicated for any male with acute scrotal pain and swelling
- Differential Dx includes epididymitis, orchitis (testicular appendix torsion, hydrocele, inguinal hernia), Henoch-Schönlein purpura (abdominal pain, hematuria, nephritis). Studies show that color Doppler US reliable for Dx of testicular torsion, which may spare majority of children with acute testicular pain (from other causes) unnecessary surgery.

ASSESSMENT POINTS

Patients usually young and healthy. Testicular torsion not associated with and does not cause abnormalities in other organ systems.

Key Reference: Blavais M, Batts M, Lambert M: Ultrasonographic diagnosis of testicular torsion by emergency physicians. Am J Emerg Med 2000; 18:198–200.

PERIOPERATIVE IMPLICATIONS

Preoperative Preparation

- Patient should be considered to have full stomach (recent meal), pain/anxiety
- Treat with metoclopramide and oral sodium citrate
- IV opioids for preop pain and IV midazolam for anxiety and amnesia

Anesthetic Technique

- General endotracheal, spinal, epidural, or local infiltration—scrotum innervated by inferior pudendal branch (long scrotal nerve) of posterior femoral cutaneous nerve (from the sacral plexus), and the medial and lateral posterior scrotal branches of perineal nerve (from the pudendal nerve)

Monitoring

- Depends on physical condition

Airway

- No special considerations

Induction/Maintenance

- Rapid-sequence induction if GA and full stomach likely

SURGICAL STAGES

- Scrotal incision, detorsion, bilateral orchidopexy (to prevent recurrence). No special postop considerations.
- Blood /fluid losses—none, usually

ANTICIPATED PROBLEMS/CONCERNS

- Full stomach—risk of pulm aspiration with induction of GA
- Testicular ischemia if duration of torsion prolonged (>6–8 h)

TETRALOGY OF FALLOT, CORRECTION OF

Michael A. Seropian, M.D., F.R.C.P.C.
Wendell C. Stevens, M.D.
Henry Casson, M.D.

RISK

• Congenital heart disease incidence <1% of live births
• TOF accounts for 10–15% of total congenital heart disease

PERIOPERATIVE RISKS

• Operative mortality <5% for children without RV failure
• Major perioperative risk factors after repair: major pulmonary artery anomaly, other major cardiac defect, very young age, increased Hct, placement of outflow conduit
• 96% 10-year survival

WORRY ABOUT

• Degree of R → L shunt and hypercyanosis
• Arterial hypoxemia
• Venous air embolus and ↑ likelihood of paradoxical embolism
• Polycythemia and thrombotic events
• Other congenital anomalies

OVERVIEW

• Anatomic problems: VSD(s), dynamic RV outflow obstruction, aorta overriding RV and LV, RV hypertrophy
• Functional problems: bidirectional or R → L shunt, arterial hypoxemia, progressive RV dysfunction

• Symptoms and urgency of correction depend on degree of pulmonary obstruction with resultant RV failure, R → L shunt, and diminished pulmonary blood flow
• Challenge:
 – Avoid ↑ R → L shunt
 – Avoid ↓ SVR and/or ↑ RV outflow obstruction

ICD-9-CM Code: 745.2

INDICATIONS AND USUAL TREATMENT

• Severe cyanosis in first month of life may necessitate palliative systemic-to-pulmonary shunt
• Increase in severity of cyanosis and polycythemia leads to early correction of TOF
• Correction often done in first year of life to avoid progressive RV failure

ASSESSMENT POINTS

SYSTEM	EFFECT	ASSESSMENT BY HX	PE	TEST
CV	R → L shunt	"Cyanotic" spells, relation to crying or exercise	Observe for clubbing, squatting during "tet spell," and cyanosis	ECHO, catheterization Pulse oximetry (O₂ sat 80–90% room air)
	RV failure	Exercise intolerance, SOB, syncope	↑ JVP, tachypnea, hepatosplenomegaly (late)	ECG: RV hypertrophy, right axis deviation ECHO, CXR
	Polycythemia Prior palliative shunt	CVA (increased risk)	Neurologic exam Look for scars, absent peripheral pulses	Hct ECHO, catheterization, look at old operative reports
RESP	Decreased pulmonary blood flow	Exercise intolerance	Tachypnea, clubbing	Catheterization, ECHO, expect low oxygen saturation
OTHER	Developmental and growth delay	Developmental and growth delay	Small size, test for developmental delay	Variety of measures
	Associated congenital anomalies	Thorough Hx of all systems	Thorough exam of pertinent systems	Variety of tests

Key References: Samuelson PN, Lell WA: Tetralogy of Fallot. *In* Lake CL (ed): Pediatric Cardiac Anesthesia, 3rd ed. Stamford, Appleton & Lange, 1998, pp 303–314; Lake CL: Anesthesia for patients with congenital heart disease. *In* Kaplan JA (ed): Cardiac Anesthesia, 4th ed. Philadelphia, WB Saunders, 1999, pp 785–820.

PERIOPERATIVE MANAGEMENT

Monitoring

• Arterial catheter: consideration should be given to catheter location if patient has had a palliative systemic-to-pulmonary shunt
• Two large-bore IV catheters: scrupulous attention to avoid air bubbles in lines
• Central venous line
• Other standard anesthetic monitors

Airway

• Avoid excessive airway pressures and hyperventilation (may ↑ PVR)

Induction

• Premedication is important and may include (but is not limited to) midazolam, morphine, and ketamine
• Ketamine does not appear to ↑ PVR
• Halothane or sevoflurane is often used for inhalation induction; practitioners must use caution to avoid ↓ in SVR associated with inhaled agents
• Ensure adequate hydration: special risk in severely polycythemic children

Anesthetic Technique

• Choice of maintenance drugs should seek to avoid ↑ HR, ↑ myocardial contractility, and ↓ SVR
• A variety of anesthetic inhaled and IV drugs may achieve this goal; halothane and fentanyl are a common combination

SURGICAL STAGES

Pre-Cardiopulmonary Bypass

• Maintain adequate preload, cardiac output, and SVR
• Severe episodic "tet spells"
 – Goal is to ↓ R → L shunt
 – May require IV fluids to increase blood volume and decrease Hct
 – 100% O₂
 – Phenylephrine to increase SVR
 – Esmolol and deepening anesthetic level to decrease RV outflow obstruction
 – Avoid decrease in SVR while deepening anesthetic level

Cardiopulmonary Bypass

• Special consideration relating to age and size and if there is a pre-existing systemic-to-pulmonary shunt

Post-Cardiopulmonary Bypass

• Measure of successful repair will be RV pressure: ideally no more than ½ LV pressure
• If RV pressure remains high, consider residual VSD: TEE of great help
• Inotropic support and high filling pressures may be required 2° to postop RV dysfunction
• Arrhythmias are uncommon but may be present
• EBL: moderate

Postoperative

• Ensure adequate RV function and low PVR
• Early extubation if possible

ANTICIPATED PROBLEMS/CONCERNS

• Persistent RV dysfunction
• Persistent pulmonary outflow obstruction or high PVR
• Postop bleeding
• Persistent R → L shunt
• Most postop mortality found in patients with
 – Acute RV failure
 – Acute or chronic pulmonary dysfunction

THORACIC AORTIC REPAIR

Christopher C. Young, M.D.

RISK

- People within USA: 3.4% incidence of aortic aneurysm; 26% involve thoracic aorta
- ↑Incidence with Htn (?African-Americans)
- M:F, 2.9:1
- Peak incidence 50–70 y

PERIOPERATIVE RISKS

- Htn, coronary and carotid vascular disease
- Untreated dissection: 25–35% mortality within 24 h, 90% in 3 mo
- Surgical repair carries 10% mortality. Causes of postop death are hemorrhage (29%); cardiac events—ischemia, MI, CHF (26%); and multiorgan system failure (22%).
- Traumatic disruption immediately fatal in 85%

WORRY ABOUT

- Elevated HR and BP promote dissection
- Acute dissection can lead to compromised blood flow (coronary, renal, splanchnic, spinal cord), pericardial tamponade, acute aortic valvular insufficiency, or bleeding

- Associated injuries (lungs, heart, head, abdomen) with traumatic rupture
- Major blood loss; need for rapid transfusion intraoperatively
- Acute dissections frequently brought for repair with minimal preop preparation

OVERVIEW

- Primary risk factors are Htn and atherosclerosis
- Thoracic aortic aneurysms 2–3× more likely to dissect than abdominal
- Distribution of thoracic dissections: ascending aorta 60–70%; descending aorta 30–35%; aortic arch 5–10%

ICD-9-CM Code: 441.2 (Thoracic aortic aneurysm, descending)

ETIOLOGY

- Aneurysm develops as vascular wall weakens from hydraulic forces (Htn) coupled with degeneration (atherosclerosis). Involves all 3 layers of aortic wall. Usually becomes symptomatic by compression of adjacent structures.
- Dissection risk factors: Htn, syphilis, Marfan's, congenital anomalies (coarctation, AS), pregnancy, bacterial infection. Intimal tear al-

lows separation of intima from media and adventitia.

Location	DeBakey	Dailey
Ascending and descending aorta	Type I	Group A
Ascending aorta only	Type II	Group A
Distal to left subclavian	Type III	Group B

- Traumatic rupture occurs commonly at ligamentum arteriosum (aorta fixed at this point)

INDICATIONS AND USUAL TREATMENT

- Group A (types I and II) dissections are surgically repaired immediately via median sternotomy using CPB
- Group B (type III) dissections are medically managed; when operation is indicated (>10 cm diameter, progressive enlargement, or producing symptoms), left thoracotomy and one-lung ventilation employed
- Traumatic aortic dissections are treated surgically regardless of symptoms
- Endovascular aneurysm repair is gaining in popularity

ASSESSMENT POINTS

SYSTEM	EFFECT	ASSESSMENT BY HX	PE	TEST
HEENT	SVC syndrome Recurrent laryngeal nerve compression	Dyspnea Hoarseness	JVD Edema	Flow-volume loop Indirect laryngoscopy
CV	Myocardial ischemia LV dysfunction Valvular disease Venous compression	Angina Dyspnea	S_3 gallop Friction rub Muffled heart sounds Plethora	ECG ECHO Stress testing Coronary angio
RESP	Bronchial/tracheal compression Recurrent pneumonia Pulm compression	Dyspnea Cough	Wheezing Tracheal deviation Hemoptysis	ABGs Flow-volume loop CXR Chest CT or MRI
GI	Mesenteric ischemia	Abdominal pain Bloody diarrhea	Tenderness	Colonoscopy Angio
RENAL	↓ Renal perfusion	Oliguria		Cr, Cr clearance
CNS	Spinal cord ischemia Carotid stenosis	Weakness Paraplegia		Carotid duplex
MS		Back or chest pain		Chest CT or MRI

Key Reference: Elefteriades JA: Diseases of the aorta. Cardiol Clin 1999; 17:609–854.

PERIOPERATIVE IMPLICATIONS

Preoperative Preparation

- IV sodium nitroprusside with β-blockers
- Premedication to prevent anxiety and pain

Monitoring

- Invasive arterial BP—left radial for group A, right radial for group B, and femoral or dorsalis pedis for distal aortic pressure measurement during crossclamping
- PA catheter and/or TEE
- SSEPs not consistently reliable guide to spinal cord ischemia

Airway

- Difficult airway if compression or deviation of tracheobronchial tree
- May interfere with placement of double-lumen ET tube

Induction/Maintenance

- High-dose narcotic useful to blunt intubation response
- Inhalation agent useful to ↓ myocardial contractility, provide amnesia
- Avoid N_2O during one-lung ventilation and to prevent expansion of air emboli

Extubation

- Usually keep sedated and mechanically ventilated 12–24 h until warmed and stable
- Prevent hemodynamic response to extubation

Adjuvants

- β-blockers, nitroprusside, nitroglycerin continued perioperatively
- Maintain adequate hydration
- Consider mannitol 0.5 g/kg well prior to crossclamping; "renal dose" dopamine

- Maintenance of aortic pressure distal to crossclamp; mild hypothermia; CSF drainage; steroids, intrathecal papaverine may limit spinal cord ischemia (5–7% incidence)

ANTICIPATED PROBLEMS/CONCERNS

- Aortic crossclamping causes ↑LV afterload, LV wall tension, and O_2 consumption. Vasodilators useful, but distal hypotension may induce spinal cord ischemia. Vascular shunting or partial bypass during crossclamp may overcome these effects.
- Aortic unclamping results in ↑ stroke volume but profound ↓ in SVR and significant metabolic acidosis if no shunt used. Fluid management, α-agonists (phenylephrine), and sodium bicarbonate may be useful.

THYROIDECTOMY FOR HYPERTHYROIDISM

Michael F. Roizen, M.D.

RISK

- People within USA: 400,000/y develop hyperthyroidism + 5% of pregnant females
- 1/1000 females, 1/3000 males; ~200,000 thyroid operations/y (1985–1989 data)

PERIOPERATIVE RISKS

- ↑ Risk of thyroid storm, even if patient was made euthyroid prior to surgery
- Risk of postop airway compromise
- Occasionally late tetany (usually 2–3 days postop) due to removal of, or damage to, parathyroid glands
- Mortality < 0.3%
- Hypoparathyroidism 2–3%

WORRY ABOUT

- Assessing euthyroid state
- Securing airway if large goiter or displaced trachea
- Postop risks of nerve injury (immediate stridor requires immediate reintubation); surreptitious bleeding (examine wound prior to PACU discharge); thyroid storm (uncommon without acute illness or 3 days postop)

OVERVIEW

- Major goal is to avoid thyroid storm; if not euthyroid prior to surgery, try to delay operation
- If emergency operation, use β-blockers and iodides to ↓ perioperative effects of released thyroid hormones and ↓ further synthesis and release of hormones; keep in ICU until risk of storm has passed
- Done in young adults with hyperthyroidism, or normal thyroid function with a cold nodule, or with a goiter that is bothersome physiologically or psychologically
- Hyperthyroidism is an endocrinopathy with CV disease—tachycardia (commonly idiopathic if no prior Dx of hyperthyroidism), CHF, dysrhythmias (AFIB)—as major manifestation
- Other target systems of hyperthyroidism are resp and CNS (↓ drive to breathe, anxiety, psychoses) and metabolic
- If patient is made euthyroid prior to operation, risk of thyroid storm and perioperative CV problems diminished by > 90%

ICD-9-CM Codes: 242.9 (Hyperthyroidism [thyrotoxicosis]); 242.0 (Graves' disease); 245 (Thyroiditis); 193 (Malignant thyroid disease)

ETIOLOGY

- Multinodular diffuse enlargement (Graves' disease)
- Thyroid adenoma—toxic multinodular goiter (firm gland) later in life and almost never malignant; unilateral solitary nodule with autonomous function earlier in life almost always benign
- Cold nodules associated with radiation therapy of other diseases as well as idiopathic
- Goiter associated with iodine deficiency

ASSESSMENT POINTS

SYSTEM	EFFECT	ASSESSMENT BY HX	PE	TEST
HEENT	Weakened tracheal rings, distorted/displaced trachea Ophthalmopathy Large tongue if associated with goiter or amyloidosis	Snoring, hoarseness, neck pain	Ask to vocalize "e"; examine airway and neck Look at eyes	CXR (PA and lat) Lat neck films CT scan of neck
CV	CHF, cardiomyopathies Sinus tachycardia, mitral valve prolapse, AFIB	DOE, orthostatic SOB Palpitations; ↑ HR during sleep	Standard exam	Rhythm strip or full ECG
GI	Wt loss, diarrhea, dehydration	Dizziness on arising; Hx of diarrhea, constipation	Skin turgor, orthostatic VS	↑ Serum alkaline phosphatase
HEME		Mild anemia, thrombocytopenia Agranulocytosis 2° to propylthiouracil or methimazole	Skin/mucous membranes for infection/petechiae	CBC with plt count, differential
CNS		Shaking, anxiety, emotional lability Hypothyroid goiter associated with slow thought processes	Reflex speed, tremor, nervousness, mental status	
METAB	Need to assess if euthyroid Malnourished	Reflex speed, tremor, heat intolerance, fatigue, weakness; wt loss, anorexia, or ↑ appetite	Reflex speed, HR	Free T$_4$ estimate

Key Reference: Roizen MF: Implications of concurrent disease. *In* Miller RD: Anesthesia, 4th ed. New York, Churchill Livingstone, 2000, pp 927–930.

PERIOPERATIVE IMPLICATIONS

Anesthetic Technique
- No one best technique

Airway
- Occasionally distorted anatomy 2° to goiter, tracheal ring involvement, inflammation 2° to thyroiditis
- Consider awake fiberoptic intubation
- Consider armored tube or equivalent if tracheal rings are affected

Preinduction/Induction
- Prehydrate if CV status tolerates
- Routine unless abnormal airway or CV system or noneuthyroid condition

Monitoring
- Temp (also place cooling blanket on OR table to treat thyroid storm if it occurs)
- Consider invasive monitoring if CV system severely affected
- If considerable head-up position, consider air embolus monitoring and therapy strategies

Induction/Maintenance/Extubation
- Extubate with optimal conditions for reintubation

SURGICAL STAGES

Initial Dissection
- Transverse collar incision
- Thyroid lobe freed from strap muscles with securing of superior thyroid vessels; these are clamped after ensuring localization and preservation of recurrent laryngeal nerve and parathyroid glands

Thyroid Removal
- Following division of middle and inferior thyroid vessels, thyroid lobe is retracted medially and liberated

Adjuvants
- Usually no requirement for NMB
- Can be done with regional: superficial and deep cervical plexus blocks and infiltration

Postoperative Considerations
- EBL: 50–150 ml
- Pain score: 2–4
- Usually can be treated with NSAIDs or occasionally with PCA

ANTICIPATED PROBLEMS/CONCERNS

- Thyroid storm is life-threatening illness manifested by hyperpyrexia, tachycardia, striking alterations in consciousness
- Bleeding can compromise airway function
- Recurrent laryngeal nerve injuries damage abductor fibers, resulting in hoarseness. Bilateral injury results in fixed narrow opening to glottis with inspiratory airflow obstruction (stridor), inability to vocalize, aspiration risk, and immediate need for tracheal intubation.

TMJ ARTHROSCOPY

Stephen O. Heard, M.D.

RISK

- Up to 17% of population suffers from TMJ disorders
- Majority of patients aged 15–45 y
- Female: male—estimates vary from 3:1 to 9:1
- Initiating factors: trauma, adverse loading of masticatory system

PERIOPERATIVE RISKS

- Perioperative mortality exceedingly rare
- Epistaxis

WORRY ABOUT

- Co-existing diseases (e.g., rheumatoid arthritis)
- Establishing and maintaining airway
- Medications

OVERVIEW

- Used to evaluate and treat pain or lack of motion in TMJ
- TMJ anatomy: joint divided into superior and inferior articular cavities by articular disk
- Approaches: inferolateral, posterolateral, anterolateral
- Structures to watch: facial nerve, superficial temporal branch of auriculotemporal nerve, maxillary artery, superficial temporal artery and vein, parotid gland

ICD-9-CM Code: 524.6

INDICATIONS AND USUAL TREATMENT

- Diagnosis of TMJ pain
- Surgery
  - Biopsies
  - Debridement and lavage
  - Incision of adhesions
  - Restoration of disk mobility and position
  - Instillation of medication
  - Capsular or disk attachment scarification/plication
- Usual treatment
  - Behavior modification
  - Pharmacotherapy
  - Physical therapy
  - Appliance therapy
  - Occlusive therapy

ASSESSMENT POINTS

SYSTEM	EFFECT	ASSESSMENT BY HX	PE	TEST
HEENT	Epistaxis associated with nasotracheal intubation Mouth opening	Epistaxis; nasal polyps; occluded nostril Trismus Pain on opening mouth Headache	Airway exam including assessment of nostril patency Clicking of TMJ Muscle spasm	
CV/RESP	Arthritis can be systemic disease: restrictive pulmonary disease, cardiomyopathy	SOB Exercise tolerance	Auscultation of heart and lungs Inspection of legs	O_2 saturation, ECG or CXR (if suggested by Hx, PE)
MS	Look for other joint involvement	Arthralgias	Inspection Palpation	

Key Reference: Kryshtalskyj B, Weinberg S: Surgical arthroscopy of the temporomandibular joint. Ont Dent 1996; 73:40–42.

PERIOPERATIVE MANAGEMENT

Preoperative Preparation
- IV sedation if needed

Monitoring
- Standard

Induction/Maintenance
- After standard induction, prepare nostrils with 4% cocaine or phenylephrine and dilate with lubricated nasal airways of increasing diameter
- Nasotracheal intubation (soften NT tube in warm H_2O; may need Magill forceps)
- Cover eyes with moistened eye pads (possible laser use)
- Some surgeons request IV administration of dexamethasone (10 mg)

SURGICAL STAGES

- Injection of local anesthesia: usually 1% lidocaine with 1:100,000 epinephrine
- Incision over superior joint space, insertion of obturator/sheath, removal of obturator, camera attachment
- Use of helium or Nd:YAG laser
  - Protective eyewear for patient and staff
  - Wet towels surrounding operative area
  - Water readily available
- Complications (< 1%)
  - Hemorrhage (usually superficial temporal artery or vein)
  - Joint damage
  - Perforation into middle cranial fossa
  - Damage to middle ear ossicles
  - Injury to auriculotemporal nerve
- Minimal blood loss
- Some surgeons inject intra-articular steroids or local anesthetics (bupivacaine 0.5% with 1:200,000 epinephrine) for anti-inflammatory and analgesic effects

Postoperative Considerations

- Pain score: 0–5
- IV or PO narcotics/anti-inflammatory medications in PACU

ANTICIPATED PROBLEMS/CONCERNS

- Epistaxis with intubation or extubation
- Postextubation pulm edema reported
- IV injections of local anesthetic

TONSILLECTOMY AND ADENOIDECTOMY — Helen W. Karl, M.D.

RISK

- >340,000 procedures/y in USA
- Incidence ~ 120/100,000 (↓ by 23% from 1970)
- Racial/gender predominance: none

PERIOPERATIVE RISKS

- Estimates of 30-day mortality range from 1/4000 to 1/27,000, usually from hemorrhage (0.1–8% of tonsillectomies ± adenoidectomy)

WORRY ABOUT

- Indication for procedure: usually airway obstruction (81% of pts < 3 y) or recurrent tonsillitis
- Associated URI
- Perioperative fluid deficiency
- Bleeding, airway obstruction, or apnea postop
- Obstructive sleep apnea

OVERVIEW

- Adenoidectomy and tonsillectomy usually performed together, but consideration given to the specific risk-benefit ratio for each procedure
- Bleeding most common about 7 days postop, but may occur in first 8–24 h
- Age and co-morbidities of patients dictate postop care

ICD-9-CM Codes: 474.0 (Chronic tonsillitis); 474.1 (Hypertrophy of tonsils and adenoids)

INDICATIONS AND USUAL TREATMENT

- Obstruction of nasal or pharyngeal airway, especially when associated with anatomic or physiologic disturbances
- Chronic or recurrent infection of adenoids (also ears or sinuses) or tonsils despite adequate antibiotic therapy
- Acute peritonsillar abscess

ASSESSMENT POINTS

SYSTEM	EFFECT	ASSESSMENT BY HX	PE	TEST
HEENT	Chronic nasal obstruction associated with abnormal facial growth	Snoring, poor feeding, speech disorders	Adenoid facies, mouth breathing	Ask child to breathe with mouth closed
CV	Chronic airway obstruction may lead to pulm Htn and right heart failure		Cardiac exam	ECHO, ECG, CXR
RESP	Tonsillar hyperplasia may result in sleep apnea and CO_2 retention	Disturbed sleep, daytime sleepiness	Airway exam, tonsil size	Polysomnography O_2 saturation
HEME	Patients with pre-existing bleeding disorders are at greater risk of postoperative hemorrhage	Patient or family Hx of bleeding, bruising, or aspirin (check OTC meds)	Multiple bruises above the knees	PT, PTT, plt count, bleeding time *if positive history*
NEURO	Brainstem dysfunction may amplify sleep apnea with moderate tonsillar hyperplasia	Cerebral palsy, Arnold-Chiari malformation		Polysomnography O_2 saturation
SYSTEMIC	Children with craniofacial abnormalities (e.g., trisomy 21, Treacher Collins) may have pre-existing airway narrowing		General exam	

Key Reference: Ferrari LR, Vassalo SA: Anesthesia for otorhinolaryngology procedures. *In* Cote CJ, Ryan JF, Todres ID, Goudsouzian NG (eds): A Practice of Anesthesia for Infants and Children, 2nd ed. Philadelphia, WB Saunders, 1993.

PERIOPERATIVE MANAGEMENT

Perioperative Preparation

- Avoid preanesthetic sedatives if Hx of sleep apnea or very large tonsils
- Consider moderate dose of anxiolytic to ease induction
- Evaluate for bleeding abnormalities
- Consider COX-2 preop

Monitoring

- IV prior to induction if Hx of significant airway obstruction

Airway

- Preformed RAE endotracheal tubes fit best into groove of mouth gag

Induction

- Consider antisialagogue during induction

SURGICAL STAGES

- Placement or removal of mouth gag may dislodge ET tube

- Corticosteroid administration may decrease edema and postop N/V
- Local infiltration with epinephrine-containing local anesthetic decreases intraoperative blood loss but does not improve pain control
- Check that oropharynx is clear of blood packs and secretions before extubation
- Extubation and recovery in lateral position with head slightly down keeps blood away from larynx
- If trachea is extubated while patient is anesthetized, recovery personnel must be very experienced in management of airway obstruction in small children

Postoperative Considerations

- EBL: underestimated because blood may be swallowed during or after surgery
- Bleeding most common cause of morbidity; ketorolac might be avoided
- N/V in up to 60% of patients after tonsillectomy due to blood in stomach, inflammation of posterior pharynx, and/or early oral fluid intake may necessitate hospital admission
- If N/V is suppressed, patient may have swallowed large amounts of blood without overt evidence of bleeding. Be esp careful in such patients to gauge surreptitious blood loss.
- Pain score: 3–4 after adenoidectomy; managed with acetaminophen alone in some patients
- Pain score: 7–9 after tonsillectomy; may require IV and PO opioids
- Children with Hx of sleep apnea should receive greatly reduced doses of opioids and be admitted for overnight monitoring
- Admission for those < 3 y and with associated anatomic or physiologic abnormalities
- Most children may be discharged day of surgery if stable, no evidence of bleeding, and free of pain and vomiting

TOTAL ABDOMINAL HYSTERECTOMY

Ferne B. Sevarino, M.D.

RISK

- ~650,000/y in USA
- ~Half of women undergo hysterectomy
- Racial predominance: none
- Age: 30+ y

PERIOPERATIVE RISKS

- Overall mortality ~0.1%; lowest mortality in women <55 y, greatest mortality in women >75 y
- Perioperative morbidity rare; overall incidence of 7.5% (fever and wound infections most common)

WORRY ABOUT

- Femoral nerve injury
- Bladder/ureter injury
- Hemorrhage requiring transfusion

OVERVIEW

- Choice of TAH vs. total vaginal hysterectomy (TVH) made according to pelvic anatomy, uterine size, adnexal or other associated disease (i.e., malignant vs. benign)
- Technique for TAH varies according to indication for operation; may include oophorectomy, lymph node dissection, omentectomy, or tumor debulking
- Choice of anesthetic will vary with indication for surgery as well as presence of coexisting disease

ICD 10 Codes: 179 (Uterine neoplasm, malignant); 219.9 (Uterine neoplasm, benign); 218.9 (Uterine fibroid); 180.9 (Cervical neoplasm, malignant); 219.0 (Cervical neoplasm, benign); 220.x (Ovarian neoplasm, benign); 614.6 (Pelvic adhesions); 617.9 (Endometriosis)

INDICATIONS AND USUAL TREATMENT

- Indications for hysterectomy include
  - Uterine, cervical, ovarian cancer
  - Pelvic relaxation syndrome, fibroids, abnormal bleeding, endometriosis, or other benign disorders (usually via vaginal approach)
- Vaginal approach may be used unless uterine size, pelvic adhesions, or cancer requires abdominal approach
- Laparoscopic-assisted hysterectomy an option

ASSESSMENT POINTS

SYSTEM	EFFECT	ASSESSMENT BY HX	PE	TEST
CV	Dehydration 2° to bowel prep Blood loss from primary problem	Menorrhagia	Orthostasis	Hgb/Hct Lytes
RESP	Rule out effusion or metastases	SOB, bronchospasm	Auscultation	CXR ABGs ± PFTs as indicated

Key Reference: Vaida SJ, David BB, Somri M, Croitoru M, Sabo E, Gaitini L: The influence of preemptive spinal anesthesia on postoperative pain. J Clin Anesth 2000; 12:374–377.

PERIOPERATIVE MANAGEMENT

Anesthetic Technique

- Regional, general, or combined techniques are options. Regional/combined techniques allow for postoperative regional analgesia.

Monitoring

- Routine
- Consider arterial line, central monitoring for extensive oncologic procedure if indicated by surgical plan/skill or by co-existing disease

Induction/Maintenance

- GA—abdominal manipulation makes ET intubation preferable to LMA or mask airway
- Regional anesthesia—dense T3–T4 level necessary for patient comfort

SURGICAL STAGES

Incision

- Pfannenstiel or low transverse incision—limited access to upper abdomen
- Midline incision extending from ~4 cm above symphysis pubis to umbilicus offers greater exposure, important for oncologic procedure

Inspection

- Avoid excessive bowel manipulation
- Self-retaining retractor may be used

Dissection

- Extrafascial hysterectomy
- Intimate proximity of uterus to ureters makes ureteral identification and dissection important
- Bladder must be carefully advanced down off lower uterine segment
- EBL: 1500 ml

Postoperative Considerations

- Moderate–severe postop pain (VAS 5–7)
- Single-dose spinal opioid followed by IV PCA for 36–48 h (48–72 h for oncologic procedures)
- Nononcologic patients usually taking oral medication on postop day 1
- High incidence of postop N/V

ANTICIPATED PROBLEMS/CONCERNS

- Older patients and oncology patients at risk for DVT
- Bladder/ureteral damage may prolong Foley catheterization/hospitalization
- Recognition of femoral nerve injury may be delayed by use of regional anesthesia—consider epidural opioid analgesia without local anesthetic postop

TOTAL ANOMALOUS PULMONARY VENOUS RETURN CORRECTION

Kristin K. Galli, M.D.
William J. Greeley, M.D.

RISK

- 1–3% of all congenital heart disease
- Marked male predominance

PERIOPERATIVE RISKS

- Perioperative mortality rare (< 3%)
- Symptomatic arrhythmias infrequent
- Pulmonary venous obstruction
- Cyanosis, impaired systemic oxygen delivery
- Myocardial dysfunction

WORRY ABOUT

- Obstructed form typically presents in neonatal period with cyanosis, tachypnea, heart failure, and alveolar edema secondary to pulmonary venous hypertension

OVERVIEW

- All pulmonary veins drain abnormally to right atrium (RA), directly or indirectly, via remnants of cardinal or umbilical venous system
- Classification based on anatomic site of abnormal connection: type 1—supracardiac (45%), most commonly enters right innominate vein; type 2—cardiac (25%), connection to coronary sinus; type 3—infracardiac (25%), distal site of connection usually below diaphragm, connecting with vessel of portal system; type 4—mixed (5%), 2 or more sites of abnormal pulmonary venous connections
- Because venous return to RA is mixture of oxygenated (pulmonary veins) and deoxygenated (IVC, SVC) blood, R → L atrial shunt causes systemic desaturation; under most circumstances, this is not severe enough to cause significant hypoxemia or end-organ dysfunction

- Pulmonary venous obstruction results in pulmonary hypertension, diminished pulmonary blood flow, and significant R → L shunting, with severe hypoxemia and heart failure in the newborn period
- Degree of shunting and presence/degree of pulmonary venous obstruction determine age at presentation. Range is neonatal period up to adulthood, with majority presenting in childhood.

ICD-9-CM Code: 747.41

INDICATIONS AND USUAL TREATMENT

- All require surgery; anatomy, physiology, and clinical presentation dictate timing
- In severe cases of obstructed pulmonary veins, institution of ECMO is required as a temporary preoperative measure to ensure adequate oxgenation, promote systemic blood flow, and reduce myocardial oxygen demand

ASSESSMENT POINTS

SYSTEM	EFFECT	ASSESSMENT BY HX	PE	TEST
CV	CHF	Tachycardia, cyanosis	Flow murmur	ECHO
RESP	PV obstruction	Tachypnea	Pulmonary edema	CXR
RENAL	Renal insufficiency (prerenal)	↓ UO, acidosis		BUN, Cr

Key Reference: Juneja R, Saxena A, Kothari SS, Taneja K: Obstructed infracardiac total anomalous pulmonary venous connection in an adult. Pediatr Cardiol 1999: 20:152–154.

PERIOPERATIVE IMPLICATIONS

Anesthetic Technique

- Opioid, NMB, controlled ventilation

Monitoring

- IV, arterial line, CVP, or transthoracic atrial/PA line placed by surgeon intraoperatively
- TEE helpful (limited by patient size, potential for airway compression)
- Placement of temporary epicardial pacing wires for potential postoperative use

Airway

- No unique concerns

Induction and Maintenance

- IV induction with high-dose opioid, NMB, ± benzodiazepine
- Volatile anesthetics poorly tolerated by neonates with CHF, myocardial dysfunction

Extubation

- Usually deferred until after immediate postoperative period

SURGICAL STAGES

- Goals: (1) redirection of pulmonary venous drainage to left atrium, (2) ligation of abnormal connection to systemic venous system
- Pulmonary veins normally converge to a confluence posterior to LA; correction involves creation of unobstructed pathway from pulmonary veins to this confluence, and ultimately to LA. Anomalous ascending or descending venous connection is ligated.
- Surgery is performed with CPB, occasionally with deep hypothermic circulatory arrest

Postoperative Considerations

- Pulmonary Htn poses significant risk for perioperative morbidity. Strategies for management include controlled hyperventilation, inotropic support, liberal use of opioids, NMB, maintaining adequate Hct in immediate postop period. Inhaled nitric oxide as a selective pulmonary vasodilator can be effective in some cases; its potential to promote methemoglobinemia warrants frequent monitoring of methemoglobin levels.
- Agents most useful for inotropic support include dopamine (3–10 μ/kg/min), epinephrine (0.03–0.1 μg/kg/min), and milrinone (0.25–0.75 μg/kg/min)

- After immediate postop period, weaning of inotropic support, ventilation, and sedation are guided by atrial/PA pressure monitoring, ABGs

ANTICIPATED PROBLEMS/CONCERNS

- If patient has obstructed pulmonary veins, at higher risk for perioperative morbidity/mortality from pulmonary Htn and/or ventricular dysfunction
- Pulmonary Htn can result from volatile PVR, kinking at anastomotic site, impaired LV function
- RV dysfunction resulting directly from pulmonary Htn can lead to decreased pulmonary blood flow, diminished LA-LV filling, and dramatic reduction in systemic blood flow
- Etiology of LV dysfunction includes inadequate myocardial protection or inadequate LV preconditioning due to predominant L → R atrial shunt
- Arrhythmias are infrequent, but loss of AV synchrony worsens poor ventricular function. Sequential pacing via temporary epicardial leads and/or pharmacologic management of supraventricular tachycardia is indicated.

TOTAL HIP ARTHROPLASTY

Michael F. Roizen, M.D.

RISK

- People in USA: > 200,000/y
- Racial predilection: none

PERIOPERATIVE RISKS

- Risks: 2–3% 30-day mortality
- CV collapse ? 2° to pulm emboli, embolization of fat, marrow, bone, or cement
- Thromboembolism (peripheral venous thrombophlebitis in 60+% of patients w/o prophylaxis—50+% ↓ with prophylaxis)—pulm emboli in 2–4% of patients who do not receive prophylaxis

WORRY ABOUT

- Causes of Fx (? CV disease)
- Perioperative fluid deficiency
- Hypoxia/hypotension on cementing
- Pulm emboli perioperatively

OVERVIEW

- Associated with high immediate morbidity, mortality 2° to volume shifts, embolization
- 1–6-day mortality associated with pulm emboli
- Age, co-morbidities of patients dictate monitoring strategies
- Regional anesthesia and postop analgesia preferred by many to ↓ blood loss, risk of thromboembolism; to ↑ mobility

ICD-9-CM Code: 715.9 (Osteoarthritis)

INDICATIONS AND USUAL TREATMENT

- Replacement of hip socket (acetabulum) and/or femur with alloys of metals/plastic/porcelain for
  – Chronic osteoarthritis
  – Hip Fx (large amounts of blood can be sequestered around Fx site). Investigate cause.
  – Avascular necrosis 2° to steroids, infarction (e.g., sickle cell disease)
- Usual medical Rx includes NSAIDs, aspirin, chondroitin and glucosamine, exercise, calcium, vitamin D

ASSESSMENT POINTS

SYSTEM	EFFECT	ASSESSMENT BY HX	PE	TEST
HEENT	Arthritis can involve airway joints	Snoring	Airway exam	
CV	Impairment due to age; if Fx caused by CV problem—dysrhythmia, etc. Hypovolemia if Fx, bleed into leg	CV status Hx chest pain/SOB Hx palpitations Exercise tolerance	CV exam	ECG Orthostatic BP by tilt table test
RESP	Arthritis can be systemic restrictive pulmonary disease/fat emboli with Fx or with replacement of hip	SOB Exercise tolerance	Chest exam Leg exam	O₂ sat
HEME	Blood loss 2° to Fx	Orthostatic dizziness	Leg; tilt table BP	Hct
RENAL/ CNS	Impairment 2° to age; if Fx, investigate cause: CNS Hx if cause of Fx is CVA, dysrhythmia, etc.	CNS Hx	CNS exam	BUN/Cr

Key References: Merli GJ: Update: Deep venous thrombosis and pulmonary embolism prophylaxis in orthopedic surgery. Med Clin North Am 1993; 77:397–411; Stevens RD, Van Gessel E, Flory N, Fournier R, Gamulin Z: Lumbar plexus block reduces pain and blood loss associated with total hip arthroplasty. Anesthesiology 2000; 93: 115–121.

INTRAOPERATIVE MANAGEMENT

Monitoring

- Volume status monitoring of blood loss a major concern—blood loss ↓ with regional anesthesia or intentional hypotension
- Consider CVP or PA line, several large-bore IVs
- Check availability of predeposited autologous and/or homologous blood; irradiate directed donor blood
- UO, HR, BP not reliable signs of intravascular volume during anesthesia or with postop epidural pain relief
- Myocardial ischemia with ECG, ST segments, even PA cath or TEE if general anesthesia
- Patients' Sx of angina or CHF may be used but may be distorted if "high" regional anesthesia (need T6 level for regional)

Airway

- Side operated on is usually up, so securing airway after positioning may be difficult
- Airway involvement with arthritis possible
- Delayed gastric emptying of acute hip fracture with pain
- Positioning often uncomfortable after 1–2 h in patient with regional anesthesia due to

pressure on side, axilla; in GA patients, pay special attention to eye-ear position
- BP can be taken in up arm (but ↓)—down arm may have altered BP

SURGICAL STAGES

Induction

- CV instability 2° to volume status
- If regional, consider slow titration

Skin Incision

- Large incision over operated hip, leg
- Can observe wound for excessive bleeding

Dissection

- During dissection down to femur, acetabulum, major blood vessel can be accidentally injured, difficult to control—esp femoral, iliac vessels
- Reaming of acetabulum, then femur
- Major blood loss 2° to bone dissection
- High-pressure lavage occasionally used to prepare surfaces: embolization of fat possible
- Use of heparin during reaming of femur ↓ risk of thromboembolism

Definitive Surgery

- Some are cemented—methacrylate produces hypotension (within 30 min)
  - ↑ Pulmonary embolization (?fat, air, methylmethacrylate monomer) that results in ↑ ventilation-perfusion mismatch or shunt, ↓ O₂ sat, right heart dysfunction

- ↓ Myocardial contractility 2° to above
- Can anticipate, hydrate for 10–20 min prior to cementing, ↑ FIO₂, have ephedrine ready
- Duration: ~5 h
- Fluid shift can be sizable
- ↓ Emboli by cath removal of pressure on cement insertion

Closure/Postoperative Considerations

- Blood loss of 1–2 units continues—if autotransfusion used, may have reaction to nonwashed cells immediately and may not get as great a long-term boost in Hct as planned (Hcts of 30 desirable if CV disease)
- Keep warm to reduce complications and blood Tx
- Pain score: 6–9
- Pain relief via NSAIDs, PCA, or epidural (start epidural narcotics 1 h prior to end of surgery)
- Early ambulation reduces thromboemboli

ANTICIPATED PROBLEMS/CONCERNS

- Blood volume status and rapid changes due to position, onset of regional/general anesthesia
- Extreme age may make less able to tolerate resp insult and CV instability after cementing
- Thromboembolism and infection prophylaxis desirable
- Pain with early ambulation may be considerable

TOTAL KNEE ARTHROPLASTY
Michael Urban, M.D., Ph.D.

RISK

- 200,000 cases in USA/y
- Gender predominance: none

PERIOPERATIVE RISKS

- Mortality rare ($<1\%$)
- Despite prophylactic Rx, highest incidence ($>40\%$) of DVT of all orthopedic patients
- Pulmonary emboli in 1–5% of patients
- Fatal pulmonary embolism after tourniquet release rare
- Common orthopedic surgical procedure in morbidly obese patients with concomitant ↑ risk
- Age, co-morbidity ↑ risk, need for more invasive monitoring
- Postop bone-cement implantation syndrome, more common with simultaneous bilateral knee arthroplasty

WORRY ABOUT

- CV collapse with tourniquet deflation
- Postop bone-cement implantation syndrome
- Pulmonary emboli perioperatively
- Postoperative bleeding

OVERVIEW

- Replacement of both tibial, femoral components of knee joint, often with methylmethacrylate cemented implants

ICD-9-CM Codes: 715.26 (Osteoarthritis, knee); 714.0 (Rheumatoid arthritis)

INDICATIONS AND USUAL TREATMENT

- Chronic osteoarthritis
- Rheumatoid arthritis
- Seronegative spondyloarthropathies (ankylosing spondylitis)
- Post-traumatic arthritis
- Hemophilia arthropathy of knee

TREATMENT

- NSAIDs and COX-2 inhibitors
- Glucosamine and chondroitin sulfate
- Calcium and vitamin D
- Surgery

ASSESSMENT POINTS

SYSTEM	EFFECT	ASSESSMENT BY HX	PE	TEST
HEENT	Arthritis involving cervical spine, TMJ, cricoarytenoids Sleep apnea	Hoarseness, difficult intubation Pickwickian Sx	ROM of neck Morbid obesity	C-spine x-ray or CT scan
CV	Pericardial effusion, cardiac conduction abn, cardiac valve fibrosis	Dyspnea, palpitations		ECG, ECHO
RESP	Restrictive disease, pulmonary effusions	Dyspnea, cough	Lung auscultation	CXR, ABGs
GI	Obesity: full stomach	Weight gain Inability to lie flat	Observation, lying flat	
HEME	Hemophiliac arthropathy of knee	Hemophilia		PTT, PT
CNS	Cervical nerve root compression	Pain on movement, paresthesias	Extremity weakness, ↓ sensation	Lateral neck x-ray

Key References: Parmet JL, Horrow JC, Singer R, et al: Echogenic emboli upon tourniquet release during total knee arthroplasty: pulmonary hemodynamic changes and embolic composition. Anesth Analg 1994; 79:940–945; Parmet JL, Horrow JC, Berman AT, Miller F, Pharo G, Collins L: The incidence of large venous emboli during total knee arthroplasty without pneumatic tourniquet use. Anesth Analg 1998; 87:439–444.

PERIOPERATIVE MANAGEMENT

Preoperative Preparation

- Treat hemophilia if present
- Thromboembolism: Rx with DVT prophylaxis, stockings, early ambulation

Anesthetic Technique

- Although no clear advantage of regional over GA, regional eliminates manipulation of airway, provides vehicle for postop pain Rx; epidural anesthesia may be extremely difficult with severe arthritis, scoliosis, or ankylosing spondylitis. Consider paramedian approach.
- Consider GA if LMWH

Monitoring

- Consider arterial catheter for dramatic swings in BP with tourniquet inflation, deflation
- For patients with Hx of significant cardiac disease (LV dysfunction or ischemic disease) consider PA cath or TEE; embolization of fat, cement, bone marrow debris may result in significant ↑ in PA pressure without change in PAOP

SURGICAL STAGES

- Positioning may be difficult
- Prolonged tourniquet inflation may result in elevated BP, myocardial ischemia and/or elevated pulmonary artery pressure in patients with ASCVD, LV dysfunction
- Tourniquet deflation: hypotension, tachycardia, pulmonary emboli with hypoxia, possible cardiac arrest. Consider hydration, ephedrine before deflation.
- EBL: 100–200 ml
- Pain score: 7–10

Postoperative Considerations

- Significant blood loss over the 1st 24 h from surgical drain; if possible, consider autologous blood donation, erythropoietin preop
- Pain Rx with epidural infusion of narcotic, local anesthesia

ANTICIPATED PROBLEMS/CONCERNS

- Pulmonary emboli of cement, thrombi, bone marrow debris with tourniquet deflation
- Blood volume status postop
- DVT, thromboembolization
- Fat embolism syndrome: hypoxia, tachycardia, hyperpyrexia, thrombocytopenia, leukocytosis, mental status changes; if monitoring PA pressures, pulmonary artery diastolic to PAOP gradient present. Rx aimed at minimizing pulmonary edema while maintaining end-organ perfusion; judicious use of diuretics, O_2, blood transfusions; may progress to ARDS.

TRACHEOESOPHAGEAL FISTULA REPAIR   Michael J. Tobin, M.D.

RISK

- 1/3000 live births
- Dx confirmed by the inability to pass a soft suction cath into stomach

PERIOPERATIVE RISKS

- Perioperative mortality low in full-term, healthy newborns; almost 100% survival
- Perioperative mortality approaches 15–60% in infants less than 1800 g
- Tracheomalacia
- Esophageal stricture

WORRY ABOUT

- Difficult ventilation/hypoxemia

- Prematurity: up to 30% associated with TEF; consider possibility of retinopathy of prematurity
- VATER syndrome: vertebral anomalies, anal atresia, tracheoesophageal fistula, esophageal atresia, radial dysplasia
- Congenital heart disease to 25% associated with TEF (VSD, ASD, PDA, tetralogy of Fallot), causing CV instability
- CV collapse/hypotension due to gastric distention or surgical compression
- Hypothermia, consequent acidosis/metabolic dysfunction

OVERVIEW

- Primary repair including fistula ligation, esophageal anastomosis

- Staged repair includes placement of gastrostomy tube under local anesthesia, subsequent ligation of fistula, esophageal repair when more stable

ICD-9-CM Code: 750.3 (Congenital)

INDICATIONS AND USUAL TREATMENT

- Carefully define other congenital defects
- Unstable patients: consider staged procedure
- Premature infants: consider staged procedure
- Gastrostomy tube placement when gastric distention compromises ventilatory status
- Passage of Fogarty cath through gastrostomy into esophagus can occlude esophagus/fistula, thus promoting ventilation of lungs

ASSESSMENT POINTS

SYSTEM	EFFECT	ASSESSMENT BY HX	PE	TEST (IF INDICATED)
CV	CV decompensation, cyanosis, CHF	Cyanosis, tachypnea, resp distress	Murmur, cyanosis, enlarged liver, hypotension, bounding pulses	CXR, ECG, ECHO, cardiac cath
RESP	Pneumonia, subglottic stenosis	Resp distress, tachypnea, stridor	↓ Breath sounds, tachypnea, cyanosis	CXR, ABGs (if indicated), flexible fiberoptic bronchoscopy
GI	Gastric distention, associated anal atresia or bowel obstruction	Enlarged abdomen Resp distress	Tympanic abdomen, enlarged abdomen	KUB series
RENAL	Dysplastic/dysfunction	Anuria	Palpation for kidneys	Créde, cath, or collect urine by bag appliance BUN/Cr

Key Reference: Andropoulos DB, Rowe RW, Betts JM: Anaesthetic and surgical airway management during tracheo-oesophageal fistula repair. Paediatr Anaesth 1998; 8:313–319.

PERIOPERATIVE IMPLICATIONS

Anesthetic Technique

- GA for complete repair
- Local anesthesia for gastrostomy tube placement in staged repair

Monitoring

- Large, well-functioning IV for blood loss
- Consider art line if respiratory or CV problems
- Urinary catheter

Airway

- Awake intubation/careful rapid-sequence
- ET tube positioned just above carina to avoid ventilating fistula and to ensure ventilation of both lungs: intentional right main stem intubation with subsequent slow withdrawal of ET tube until breath sounds 1st heard on left usually ensures that ET tube optimally placed
- Consider facing bevel post during intubation to avoid direct intubation of fistula
- Monitor for kinking/obstruction of trachea/ET tube by surgical traction during dissection, repair
- Monitor for complete obstruction of ET tube by blood/secretions, necessitating suctioning/replacement
- Precordial stethoscope on left chest to monitor breath sounds intraoperatively; accidental advancement of ET tube into right main stem bronchus may then be detected
- Subglottic stenosis may necessitate placement of smaller diameter ET tube than usual

- Soft Silastic cath or esophageal stethoscope most easily placed in blind esophageal pouch before final positioning

Induction

- Healthy neonates may tolerate inhalation induction with spontaneous ventilation until chest opened when a muscle relaxant is given
- Premature infants or those with significant respiratory disease may require careful mechanical ventilation, use of muscle relaxant at induction

SURGICAL STAGES

Dissection

- Blood loss usually minimal, although large blood vessels may be transected
- Recurrent laryngeal nerve damage may occur

Definitive Surgery

- Hypercarbia/hypoxemia possible from these causes: compression/retraction of right lung, kinking of trachea/ET tube from surgical traction, plugging of the ET tube, its migration into right main stem bronchus or fistula, preferential ventilation of fistula
- Hypotension may result from cardiac compression, hypovolemia, or blood loss
- Hypothermia may result from administration of cold IV fluids, cool ambient room, anhydrous gas administration, heating pad malfunction. Metabolic acidosis may result from hypothermia.
- Blood loss can be steady; apparently small losses can be clinically significant in newborn

Postoperative Considerations

- Vigorous infants may be extubated at conclusion of surg: this preferred for maintenance of repair
- Premature infants and those with significant pulmonary disease may require continued mechanical ventilation
- Suction caths marked to point at which they will contact repair

Postoperative Complications

- Pulmonary aspiration, tracheomalacia, vocal cord paralysis
- At later date, patients at risk for intubation of tracheal diverticulum that may develop at site of fistula closure
- Esophageal stricture, esophageal foreign body entrapment relatively common following repair
- Regional anesthesia may be used as a supplement to general anesthesia and may improve management of postoperative pain. A single-dose caudal block may be administered. Alternatively, a caudal catheter may be placed and advanced to a thoracic level for intermittent dosing.

ANTICIPATED PROBLEMS/CONCERNS

- Pulmonary disease
- Difficulty sustaining airway, avoiding hypoxemia/hypercarbia
- CV compromise/congenital heart disease
- Hypovolemia/blood loss
- Hypothermia
- Prematurity

TRANSJUGULAR INTRAHEPATIC PORTOSYSTEMIC SHUNT (TIPS)

Zheng Xie, M.D., Ph.D.

RISK

- Occurs in 3–4/1000 adults in USA
- >60% with cirrhosis have portal Htn
- 33–98% with cirrhosis have GI varices
- Variceal bleeding occurs in 25–40%

PERIOPERATIVE RISKS

- Direct procedure mortality rate <2%
- 30-Day mortality rate ranges from 4 to 45%
- Rebleeding rate is 10–26% and usually associated with shunt stenosis or thrombosis
- Postprocedural encephalopathy: 5–55%
- Fever has been reported in 10% of patients

WORRY ABOUT

- Hypotension secondary to bleeding
- CHF, cardiac arrhythmias: HB, VF, AF
- Oxygen desaturation 2° to excessive sedation
- Aspiration
- Tension pneumothorax
- MS changes— ↑ encephalopathy postop
- Septic shock

OVERVIEW

- TIPS is a creation of a communication between hepatic and portal veins through the liver parenchyma with an expandable metallic stent to relieve portal hypertension (>12 mmHg)
- Portal Htn causes ↑ flow through the portosystemic collaterals that bypass the liver to the systemic circulation. Results in gastroesophageal varices, intestinal varices, and splenomegaly.
- Cirrhosis is the most common cause of portal Htn in USA. Others include portal vein obstruction, hepatic vein thrombosis (Budd-Chiari syndrome), hepatic veno-occlusive disease.
- Major clinical manifestations of portal Htn: hemorrhage from gastroesophageal varices, splenomegaly, encephalopathy, ascites, death
- Main periop complications of TIPS: intra-abdominal hemorrhage, aspiration, cardiopulmonary failure, arrhythmias, worsening encephalopathy, infection, fluid and lyte disturbance

ICD-9-CM Code: 572.3 (Portal hypertension); 571.5 (Portal cirrhosis)

INDICATIONS AND USUAL TREATMENT

Accepted Indications

- Acute variceal bleeding not successfully controlled with medical Rx
- Recurrent variceal bleeding refractory or intolerant to conventional medical Rx
- Particularly helpful when bleeding occurs from inaccessible intestinal or gastric varices or is the result of severe portal hypertensive gastropathy

Promising Uses

- Refractory ascites, refractory hepatic hydrothorax, hepatorenal syndrome, Budd-Chiari syndrome, and veno-occlusive disease
- Acute variceal bleed while awaiting Tx

Usual Treatments

- Pharmacologic Rx to ↓ portal pressure
- Endoscopic band ligation or sclerotherapy of the varices
- Balloon tamponade, then devascularization
- Surgical portosystemic shunting

Absolute Contraindications

- Right-sided heart failure
- Polycystic liver disease
- Severe hepatic failure, unless active variceal bleeding or fulminant Budd-Chiari syndrome is the inciting event
- Cavernous portal vein thrombosis

ASSESSMENT POINTS

SYSTEM	EFFECT	ASSESSMENT BY HX	PE	TEST
NEURO	Hepatic encephalopathy (from confusion to coma)	Disturbances of awareness and mentation, personality change	Asterixis (liver flap), rigidity, hyperreflexia	EEG, ammonia level
CV	Cardiomyopathy, CAD	ETOH abuse, smoking Hx	Tachycardia, S_3, edema	ECG, ECHO
RESP	Atelectasis, pulmonary shunting, hypoxemia, hyperventilation, pulmonary effusion	SOB, poor exercise tolerance		CXR, ABGs, PFTs
GI	Ascites, aspiration, variceal bleeding, gastritis, ulcer	↑ Abdominal girth, hematemesis	Fluid wave, bulging flanks, postural tachycardia	US, paracentesis, endoscopy
HEPATIC	Drug metabolism change			LFTs
RENAL	Hepatorenal syndrome			BUN, electrolytes
ENDO	Hypoglycemia			Glucose
HEME	Anemia, coagulopathy	GI bleed		CBC, plt, PT

Key Reference: Ong JP, Sands M, Younossi ZM: Transjugular intrahepatic portosystemic shunts (TIPS): a decade later. J Clin Gastroenterol 2000; 30:14–28.

PERIOPERATIVE MANAGEMENT

Preoperative Preparation

- Avoid excessive sedation aspiration risk
- Pre-existing LBBB may require a pacemaker pre-TIPS due to the risk of RBBB during TIPS
- PRBCs, FFP, and platelets available
- Some centers recommend correction of coagulopathy if platelets <60,000 and INR >1.8
- Monitor blood glu if hepatic failure

Monitoring

- Standard monitors; in selected cases, arterial line and central venous catheters can be added

Anesthetic Technique/Care

- Based on severity of liver disease and comorbidities and preference of institution
- Sedation and local anesthesia may suffice
- General anesthesia preferred if patient is agitated or uncooperative from encephalopathy

Induction/Maintenance

- Rapid-sequence induction is often required with encephalopathy, abdominal distention, and recent variceal bleed
- Broad-spectrum antibiotic for gram-negative organisms (e.g., 1 g ceftizoxime) at start
- May be sensitive to all agents

Emergence

- Extubation after protective laryngeal reflexes present

SURGICAL STAGES

- Ultrasound is performed to assess the size and patency of portal and hepatic venous systems
- Jugular and hepatic vein access and pressure measurement—right internal jugular vein approach is preferred because it provides a straight path into the infrahepatic IVC. An angiographic catheter is advanced to the infrahepatic IVC and pressures measured. Sheath is advanced into the right hepatic vein, and both free hepatic vein pressure and wedged hepatic vein pressure are measured.
- Identification of portal vein—wedged hepatic venogram is performed with either iodinated contrast or CO_2 for portal vein localization
- Dilation and stent placement—a puncture needle is advanced to access the portal vein. The needle is removed and a guidewire is advanced to the superior mesenteric vein or splenic vein. Portal pressures are measured and a portal venogram is obtained. An angioplasty balloon is advanced to dilate the transhepatic tract. A bridging expandable stent is deployed and then dilated to 8–12 mm. Ideally, the pressure gradient following shunting should be 6–12 mmHg.
- US within 24 h to assess patency of the stent
- EBL: 0–3000 ml

Postoperative Considerations

- Monitor in an ICU or step-down unit for 24–48 h due to potential for portal vein thrombus, worsening encephalopathy, sepsis, bleeding, pulmonary edema, and fluid and lyte disturbance
- Pain score is 7–8 in first few hours. Usually, IV opioid is needed for the first few hours only.

ANTICIPATED PROBLEMS/CONCERNS

- Portal vein rupture and perforation of liver capsule → intra-abdominal hemorrhage
- Cardiopulmonary failure from sudden hemodynamic changes
- Patients with pre-existing LBBB may need pacemaker pre-TIPS due to risk of RBBB
- Encephalopathy may worsen due to ↓ hepatic portal BF

TRANSPOSITION OF THE GREAT VESSELS (TGV), REPAIR OF

Irene B. O'Hara, M.D.
Alan Jay Schwartz, M.D., M.S.Ed.

RISK

• Incidence: 19.3–33.8/100,000 live births; 5–7% of all congenital cardiac defects
• M > F (2–3.1:1)

PERIOPERATIVE RISKS

• Associated cardiac anomalies: VSD, LV outflow obstruction
• Systemic or pulmonary ventricular failure
• Pulmonary Htn
• Polycythemia, associated coagulopathy in cyanotic patients
• Rhythm disturbances affecting CO
• Preop ductal patency may be maintained with PGE_1 infusion

WORRY ABOUT

• Neonates with CHF, cyanosis should be evaluated for presence of TGV. In presence of intact ventricular septum, PGE_1 infusion may maintain ductal patency, blood mixing until balloon atrial septostomy performed.

• Pulmonary and systemic resistance may need to be balanced to maintain optimal ratio of systemic-to-pulmonary blood flow
• In cyanotic patients, polycythemia may cause sludging; has been implicated in CVAs
• Thrombocytopenia, ↓ plasma clotting factors can be present

OVERVIEW

• Common cardiac defect rarely associated with other congenital anomalies; is second only to VSD in frequency
• Without intervention, 30% mortality in 1st wk, 45% in 1st mo, 90% in 1st y; anoxia, CHF primary causes of death
• Palliation vs. definitive surgery depends on associated presence of VSD or LV outflow obstruction
• Balloon septostomy, early corrective surgery have improved long-term outcome

ICD-9-CM Code: 745.10

ETIOLOGY

• Common congenital cardiac defect; accounts for 5–7% of congenital cardiac lesions
• Associated risks: possible maternal diabetes

USUAL TREATMENT

• PGE_1 infusion to maintain ductal patency
• Balloon (Rashkind-Miller) atrial septostomy
• Palliative surgery; if LV outflow obstruction, VSD present, systemic to PA shunt. If VSD and advanced pulm vascular occlusive disease present, atrial switch (Mustard) may be performed without VSD closure.
• Definitive repair: intra-atrial repair (Mustard or Senning) to connect systemic, pulm circuits at atrial level. Arterial switch (Jatene) with coronary artery reimplantation to anatomically correct circulation by anastomosing aorta to systemic ventricle and PA to pulm ventricle.

ASSESSMENT POINTS

SYSTEM	EFFECT	ASSESSMENT BY HX	PE	TEST
CV	CHF	Respiratory distress Poor perfusion	Rales, S_3, hypotension	ECHO
RESP	Pulmonary vascular occlusive disease	Dyspnea	Clubbing, cyanosis	CXR, cath
HEME	Polycythemia (if >6–9 mo) Coagulopathy, bleeding Thrombocytopenia	Bleeding		CBC Coag factor levels, plt studies
CNS	CVA	Associated with polycythemia	Focal deficit	CT or MRI

Key Reference: DiNardo JA: Transposition of the great vessels. *In* Lake CL (ed): Pediatric Cardiac Anesthesia, 3rd ed. Norwalk, CT, Appleton & Lange, 1998, pp 315–335.

PERIOPERATIVE IMPLICATIONS

Preoperative Preparation

• Maintain CO with adequate HR, contractility, preload
• Maintain ductal patency with PGE_1 (0.05–0.1 μg/kg/min)
• Atropine vs. sedative premedication (usually if >6 mo old)

Monitoring

• Arterial line may be placed after induction
• Consider right atrial line (for drug infusion, pressure monitoring)
• TEE

Airway

• Patient may already be intubated

Preinduction/Induction

• Avoid ↑ PVR—can ↓ PBF, intercirculatory mixing
• If pulmonary vascular occlusive disease present, use ventilatory interventions—i.e., ↑FIO_2, ↓ $PaCO_2$ to ↓ PVR

• If ventricular outflow tract obstruction present, ↑ ventilation can ↓ PVR, ↑ pulmonary blood flow and intercirculatory mixing
• Maintain SVR relative to PVR to maintain effective pulmonary blood flow and thus adequate SpO_2
• If CHF present with VSD, ventilatory manipulations may be deleterious, due to preexisting ↑ pulmonary blood flow, difficulty of maintaining systemic blood flow with failing heart
• Anesthetic induction may be accomplished with opioid if IV line in place; otherwise inhalation induction may be used

Maintenance

• Avoid agents that depress contractility; in infants with TGV, intact ventricular septum, O_2 delivery tenuous; with VSD, volume overload possible. Opioids preferred drugs for maintenance anesthesia (fentanyl up to 75 μg/kg or sufentanil 5–20 μg/kg); affords hemodynamic stability; does not depress myocardium; blunts reactive pulmonary Htn. Pancuronium usually relaxant of choice for vagolytic properties.

Extubation

• In ICU postop 24–48 h when pulmonary, hemodynamic stability present, patient awake
• EBL: 200–2000 ml
• Pain score: 6–9

ANTICIPATED PROBLEMS/CONCERNS

• Atrial switch
  – Interatrial baffle may result in venous obstruction (systemic or pulmonary) immediately postop with result of low CO or SVC syndrome; pulmonary venous obstruction may result in low CO, pulmonary edema
  – Dysrhythmias: sinus bradycardia may require atrial pacing; junctional rhythm may require AV sequential pacing; rapid AFIB may require cardioversion
  – RV (systemic) dysfunction may occur if right ventriculotomy used
• Arterial switch
  – Bleeding from suture lines
  – Myocardial ischemia due to coronary reimplantation (air or kinking)
  – Inadequate LV function due to insufficient mass, ischemia, or inadequate preservation during CPB—inotropic support

TRANSSPHENOIDAL SURGERY
Lauren Berkow, M.D.

RISK
- Pituitary adenoma: 14.7/100,000/y

PERIOPERATIVE RISKS
- Mortality $< 1\%$
- Morbidity $3-5\%$ (diabetes insipidus [DI], CSF leak, carotid artery injury, visual loss, meningitis, hemorrhage)

WORRY ABOUT
- Endocrine abnormalities (panhypopituitarism, Addison's, Cushing's, thyroid dysfunction)
- DI: increased urine output, hypernatremia, dehydration
- Acromegaly (potential difficult mask airway and intubation)
- Increased ICP
- Intracranial hemorrhage 2° to invasion into cavernous sinus

OVERVIEW
- Resection performed through nasal, sublabial incisions with aid of microscope
- Newer techniques often use fluoroscopic or MRI guidance, endoscopic approaches, intraoperative hormonal assays
- Tumors may secrete hormones (GH, ACTH, TSH, prolactin) or be nonfunctional
- Tumors may compress optic chiasm, causing visual field deficits, or may abut or invade cavernous sinus

ICD-9-CM Code: 227.3 (Benign pituitary adenoma)

INDICATIONS AND USUAL TREATMENT
- Pituitary tumor without extensive suprasellar extension or hypothalamic involvement (these usually require craniotomy)
- Other options include transcranial approach, radiation or radiosurgery, medical treatment with bromocriptine or somatostatin analogues (octreotide, simvastatin)
- Patients with acromegaly often receive preop bromocriptine

ASSESSMENT POINTS

SYSTEM	EFFECT	ASSESSMENT BY HX	PE	TEST
HEENT	Overgrowth of chin, tongue, vocal cord paralysis, subglottic stenosis (acromegaly)	Snoring, sleep apnea hoarseness	Airway exam Stridor, facial features	Lateral neck films FOB
CV	Htu, DM, CHF Obesity, ischemia	Chest pain, dyspnea Exercise tolerance	CV exam	ECG, CXR Stress thallium ECHO
ENDO	Panhypopituitarism Acromegaly (incl GH) Cushing's (incl ACTH) Hyperthyroidism (incl TSH)	Cold intolerance Weight gain Nervousness	Hemodynamic instability CV collapse Obesity	GH, TSH, glucose Cortisol level Dexamethasone suppression test
RENAL/ LYTES	↑ Aldosterone (ACTH) → ↑ Na$^+$, ↓ K$^+$, metab alkalosis ↑ ADH → DI	Oliguria Thirst, polyuria	Pulm/peripheral edema Orthostasis, hypotension Urine output	ABGs, lytes Urine lytes, Osm Serum Osm

Key Reference: Jho H, Park I, Alfieri A: The future of pituitary surgery. Clin Neurosurg 2000; 47:83–98.

PERIOPERATIVE IMPLICATIONS

Preoperative Preparation
- Assess and document neurologic deficits, evaluate endocrine function
- Avoid sedation, especially if concerns about increased ICP

Anesthetic Technique
- GA with controlled ventilation

Monitoring
- Routine monitoring plus Foley catheter to follow UO
- Consider arterial line to watch BP during local infiltration and to follow electrolytes perioperatively
- Consider precordial Doppler to detect VAE if head elevated $> 15°$

Airway
- Anticipate difficult airway if acromegaly present (may require awake FOB)
- Routine oral intubation if normal airway, consider oral RAE ETT to facilitate surgery

- Packs placed in oropharynx intraoperatively to prevent aspiration of blood and irrigating solution

Induction/Maintenance
- Similar to any craniotomy: balanced vapor/narcotic/relaxant
- Stress dose steroids, antibiotics to cover naso/oropharyngeal flora
- Minimal postop pain; avoid overdosing narcotics

SURGICAL STAGES

Incision
- Infiltration of nose and mouth with local anesthetic, cocaine may trigger Htn, tachycardia, arrhythmias

Definitive Surgery
- Watch for DI, hemorrhage from carotid artery or cavernous sinus
- Watch for venous air embolism; discontinue nitrous oxide if suspected

Postoperative Considerations
- Confirm oropharyngeal packing removed, potential for aspiration of blood from nasopharynx, extubate awake
- May need postop steroid replacement
- EBL variable, may be hard to quantitate
- Potential complications: CSF leak, epistaxis, sinusitis or meningitis, intracranial hemorrhage, nasal septum perforation

ANTICIPATED PROBLEMS/CONCERNS
- DI 2° to lack of ADH: increased UO, hypernatremia, increased osmolality, dehydration; treat with IVF, DDAVP as needed
- Hemorrhage from ICA or cavernous sinus can lead to herniation, CN dysfunction, death
- Watch closely for postop neurologic changes
- Addisonian crisis: hemodynamic instability, CV collapse; treat with steroids

TRANSURETHRAL RESECTION OF BLADDER TUMOR

Denis L. Bourke, M.D.

RISK

- USA incidence: 16.5/100,000; 50,000 new cases/y. Fourth most common cancer in men.
- Gender, race: male 2:1; Caucasian, 2:1
- Risk factors: chemical exposure, cigarettes, coffee, analgesics, artificial sweeteners

PERIOPERATIVE RISKS

- Perioperative mortality low (< 1%)
- Ureteral obstruction from tumor or tumor resection
- Less risk of absorption syndromes than during TURP

WORRY ABOUT

- Bladder perforation
- Occult blood loss
- Nerve injury in lithotomy position
- Obturator nerve stimulation

OVERVIEW

- Usually relatively simple, brief (15–45 min) procedure
- 70% of patients achieve 5-y survival with simple transurethral resection/fulguration
- Median age at Dx: 67–70; suggests probability of co-morbidities
- Metastases in order of frequency: regional nodes, liver, lung, bone, adrenal, intestine
- Usually minimal postop pain

ICD-9-CM Code: 188.0

INDICATIONS AND USUAL TREATMENT

- Usual presenting symptom: painless hematuria
- Dx tests include cytology of bladder washings, excretory urography, cystoscopy
- Procedure for diagnosis, tumor staging, definitive Rx
- Tumor recurrence, repetitive procedures common
- Other Rx includes intravesical chemotherapy, intravesical immunotherapy, systemic chemotherapy, photoradiation therapy, laser therapy, vitamins, cystectomy

ASSESSMENT POINTS

SYSTEM	EFFECT	ASSESSMENT BY HX	PE	TEST
CV	↓ Reserve primarily due to age	Hx of chest pain, SOB, palpitations, etc.	CV exam, auscultation	ECG, CXR
RESP	Age effects, associated with cigarettes, pulmonary metastases	Smoking, SOB, cough, sputum, hemoptysis	Auscultation	CXR, CT scan, PFTs
GU	Age, obstructive effects	Hematuria, oliguria		BUN, Cr

Key Reference: Ansari MZ, Costello AJ, Ackland MJ, Carson N, McDonald IG: In-hospital mortality after transurethral resection of the prostate in victorian public hospitals. Aust N Z J Surg 2000; 70:204–208.

INTRAOPERATIVE MANAGEMENT

Anesthetic Technique

- Either GA or regional can be used

Monitoring

- Routine
- CVP may be considered because UO cannot be measured

Airway

- Lithotomy position: airway can be managed by mask or ET tube

Induction

- GA dictated by general health status. Resection of lateral bladder wall tumors may stimulate obturator nerve, cause leg to jump, can cause bladder perforation; in these cases, profound muscle relaxation required, or change in electrocautery settings.
- Spinal anesthesia: T10 sensory level sufficient, higher level masks Sx of perforation of bladder. Spinal anesthesia will not prevent obturator n. stimulation during resection of lateral wall tumors. Obturator n. block below pubic ramus if resection at lateral wall to be performed.

SURGICAL STAGES

- Stimulation can begin and end suddenly, unexpectedly
- Moderate pain
- Large veins or artery rare, IV absorption of irrigating solution rare
- Actual resection time usually < 30 min
- Blood loss is usually minimal
- Bladder wall perforation rare

Postoperative Considerations

- Pain score: 2–5
- Upper abdominal, precordial, shoulder, or back pain may indicate bladder perforation
- Observe for ureteral obstruction if resection near ureteral orifice
- Peroneal nerve injury can be caused by lithotomy position

ANTICIPATED PROBLEMS/CONCERNS

- Patient age–related CV, pulmonary complications
- Occult blood loss
- Obturator nerve stimulation during lateral wall resections

TRANSURETHRAL RESECTION OF PROSTATE (TURP)

Dorene A. O'Hara, M.D., M.S.E.

RISK

- 11–12% of male population >65 y
- Racial predominance: none; but African-American patients have higher co-morbidity (stroke, COPD, DM, preop infection)

PERIOPERATIVE RISKS

- 30-Day mortality 0.1–0.3% (higher in patients >90 y, 2.6%)
- Morbidity 7–20%; TURP syndrome 2% (hyponatremia, headache, confusion, visual changes, nausea, twitching, hypotension, bradycardia), due to intravascular absorption of irrigating fluid
- Blood loss requiring transfusion, 2.5% (0.2–0.3 ml blood loss/g tissue/min resection)
- Capsule perforation 1%

WORRY ABOUT

- Concomitant CV disease
- Volume of irrigant absorbed
- Time of resection (limit to 60 min if poss)
- Sudden perforation
- Hypothermia
- Rx of benign bothersome (Sx) disease; other Rx aimed at shrinking size of prostate (drugs) or watchful waiting (tolerating Sx)

OVERVIEW

- Common procedure in males >65 y
- High incidence of cardiopulmonary disease in this population
- Preop renal insufficiency associated with poorer outcome

- Bacteremia common perioperatively
- Significant benefits with use of regional anesthesia

ICD-9-CM Code: 600 (Benign prostatic hypertrophy)

INDICATIONS AND USUAL TREATMENT

- Enlarged prostate → urinary retention
- Urodynamic studies may be performed
- Size of gland estimated at <80 g (>80 g: consider open prostatectomy)
- Tissue may be benign or malignant
- Medical Rx include α-blocker, androgen-blocking agents

ASSESSMENT POINTS

SYSTEM	EFFECT	ASSESSMENT BY HX	PE	TEST
CV	Risk of MI, arrhythmias, hypovolemia	Htn, stroke, angina, CHF, SOB	BP, HR, cardiac exam	ECG, Holter ECHO
RESP	Resp difficulty during regional, cough	Smoking, cough, sputum, SOB	Chest exam	PFTs (only if Sx severe)
GI	Risk of GI bleeding, anemia	Ulcer, GI bleeding, melena		Hemoccult, Hct
HEME	Added intraoperative blood loss; regional risks	Weakness, fatigue, anticoagulant Rx	VS, pallor	Hct PT, PTT
GU	Concomitant renal failure	Hx of chronic renal failure, kidney stones		UA, BUN, Cr
CNS	Mental status and regional anesthesia, stroke risk	Visual, general CNS	Neuro, carotids	
MS	Osteoarthritis, difficult spinal/epidural	Arthritis, back problems	Back	

Key Reference: Malhotra V: Transurethral resection of the prostate. Anesthesiol Clin North Am 2000; 18:883–897.

PERIOPERATIVE MANAGEMENT

Preoperative Preparation

- As indicated by assessment above

Anesthetic Technique

- Regional (esp spinal) preferred for monitoring of CNS, early recognition of perforation, poss EBL
- General may be chosen if spinal osteoarthritis, contraindications to regional, or patient preference

Monitoring

- Routine
- Light/minimal sedation to communicate with patient, monitor CNS
- Temperature (risk of hypothermia)
- Time of resection, surgeon estimate of gland size; vascularity, volume of irrigant
- Consider CVP/PA if severe co-existing disease
- Serum Na$^+$ postop, if CNS changes develop

Airway

- Coughing/straining must be prevented during resection

Induction/Maintenance

- Regional requires levels T8–T10; higher level may mask Sx of bladder perforation, impede respiration
- High sympathetic block may cause undesirable bradycardia, hypotension

SURGICAL STAGES

- Preparation, positioning (lithotomy)
- Via resectoscope, excision of prostate with electrically charged wire loop; coagulation used to control bleeding (to limit blood loss, improve surgical view)
- Continuous irrigation required; water clearest but if absorbed can cause hyponatremia, RBC hemolysis, CNS effects. Lyte solutions disperse current; nonelectrolyte solutions generally used: sorbitol, mannitol, glycine. Fluid absorption = 10–30 ml/min resection time (glycine metabolized to NH_3).

- Postresection: supine position; observe for hypotension with legs again dependent
- Blood loss can be 2 units or more
- Volume overload major risk due to irrigant
- Hyponatremia: Lasix 40–120 mg, consider hypertonic saline 3%

Postoperative Considerations

- Postop pain generally minimal, mainly due to indwelling catheter maintained with traction, continuous irrigation

ANTICIPATED PROBLEMS/CONCERNS

- BP changes due to onset of regional anesthesia, positioning
- Development of CNS changes, esp double vision, confusion, headache (TURP syndrome)
- Sudden pain, hypotension, loss of returning irrigant (perforation)
- Transient blindness (possible glycine toxicity)

TRAUMA
Alexander W. Gotta, M.D.

RISK

- 2.5 million hospital discharges (1998) in USA
- 146,400 deaths (1998) in USA
- Leading cause of death ages 1–35 y

PERIOPERATIVE RISKS

- Perioperative morbidity, mortality dependent on extent of injury
- Hemorrhage, hypovolemia, hypotension
- Specific organ damage, i.e., blunt or penetrating trauma to vital organs, brain, lungs, kidney
- Difficult airway 2° to injury to face, neck, chest
- Full stomach
- Recent drug and/or alcohol use

WORRY ABOUT

- Replacing blood volume
- Securing airway
- Ventilating traumatized lungs

OVERVIEW

- Loss of 3.5 million y of potential life (1995); 5th leading cause of death in USA
- Cost: $160 billion/y
- Morbidity and mortality: hemorrhage, head injury, airway disruption, fractures

ICD-9-CM Code: 959.9

ETIOLOGY

- Alcohol as a factor in traffic fatalities is declining. The 16,189 (39%) alcohol-related traffic fatalities in 1997 represent a 32% reduction from the 23,641 alcohol-related fatalities in 1987.
- Drug use other than alcohol; cocaine leads to manic behavior; heroin creates need for money to support habit
- Absence of gun control legislation; guns in home not protective; marker for suicide; homicide rates highest in countries without gun control legislation

USUAL TREATMENT

- Blood, fluid resuscitation, correction of acid-base abnormalities
- Mnemonic: "WOVCATH":
  - Wonder if can tolerate anesthesia
  - O_2
  - Vecuronium or pancuronium
  - Coagulation
  - Acid-base
  - Temperature
  - Hemodynamics

ASSESSMENT POINTS

SYSTEM	EFFECT	ASSESSMENT BY HX	PE	TEST
HEENT	TMJ dysfunction; basal skull fracture	Nature of trauma; location; ability to open jaw; CSF rhinorrhea	Often misleading; skeletal fracture often not related to soft tissue trauma	CT, X-rays of face, base of skull, neck
CV	Hypotension, myocardial depression due to hypovolemia; cardiac tamponade Cardiac contusion	Nature of injury; reported and observed blood loss Blunt trauma to thorax	Hypotension, tachycardia, cold, sweaty, cyanotic; ↓ heart sounds with tamponade	Hgb, Hct (of little value early in course) ECG, ECHO
RESP	Hyperpnea to counter metab acidosis; labored ventilation with airway injury	Nature, location of injury	↓ Breath sounds with hemo- or pneumothorax; subcutaneous emphysema with penetrating injury of airway	CXR
GI	Ruptured viscus; torn spleen, liver; bowel disruption	Location of injury, tenseness of abdomen	Sx of shock, sepsis	CT scan; minilaparotomy
RENAL	Hypoperfusion ↓ UO	Amount of blood loss	Sx of shock, hypotension, tachycardia	UO, Na^+ IVP
CNS	Confusion, obtundation	Location of injury, amount of blood loss	Cranial injury, paresis, paralysis, dilated pupils	X-rays of skull, cervical spine CT scan

Key Reference: Gotta AW (ed): Trauma. Anesthesiol Clin North Am. 1996; 14.

PERIOPERATIVE IMPLICATIONS

Preoperative Preparation

- Large-bore (16-gauge or larger) IV lines, Foley, adequate blood and components for transfusion
- Consider pulmonary arterial catheter introducer or CVP

Monitoring

- Consider arterial line, CVP
- Pulmonary arterial catheter rarely acutely indicated
- Consider TEE for volume status

Airway

- May be disrupted by direct trauma; consider tracheotomy or cricothyrotomy
- In-line traction if C-spine not cleared

Preinduction/Induction

- May become hypotensive with anesthesia induction
- Attempt to correct hypovolemia as quickly as possible
- Ketamine offers no advantages if catecholamine depleted

Maintenance

- Treat severe metabolic acidosis
- Beware hyperkalemia due to tissue injury and/or acidosis
- Maintain normothermia since hypothermia associated with morbidity/mortality

Extubation

- Consider prolonged intubation, mechanical ventilation postop

- Facial edema must subside before extubation

Postoperative Period

- Pain Rx not a problem until patient resuscitated, responsive
- EBL: depends on procedure

Adjuvants

- Inotropes, blood components

ANTICIPATED PROBLEMS/CONCERNS

- Hypovolemia leads to shock, inadequate organ perfusion, multiorgan failure
- Hypotension and/or release of tissue factor (especially in neurotrauma) may lead to DIC
- Hypothermia leads to coagulopathies, cardiac arrhythmias, death

TUBAL LIGATION

Gilbert J. Grant, M.D.

RISK

- 500,000 performed in 1992
- Performed post partum (minilaparotomy) or as interval procedure (laparoscopy)

PERIOPERATIVE RISKS

- Risk for serious complication <2%: hemorrhage, sepsis, embolism, cardiac arrest (2/1000)

WORRY ABOUT

- Post partum: aspiration risk; hypovolemia (hemorrhage, uterine atony)
- Interval: complications of laparoscopy: hypercarbia, adverse hemodynamics, pneumoperitoneum, Trendelenburg position
- Peripheral nerve injury from malpositioning; embolism (gas); trauma to vessel or viscus (trocar, cautery)

OVERVIEW

- Usually, choice technique for isolating uterus from ovary (sterilization) by interrupting tube with rings or by cutting tube (surgically with laser) into 2 separate sections
- With either minilaparotomy or laparoscopy, peritoneal traction painful
- Regional technique preferred post partum to reduce aspiration risk (local technique can also be used—i.e., direct injection of local anesthetic into wound, onto mesosalpinx)
- For laparoscopy, GA with controlled ventilation avoids hypercarbia from peritoneal insufflation. Laparoscopy may be contraindicated if Hx of abdominal surgery.

ICD-9-CM Codes: V25.2 (Elective sterilization); 659.4 (For multiparity)

INDICATIONS AND USUAL TREATMENT

- Multiparity
- Medical contraindication to pregnancy (appropriate advance consent must be obtained with reaffirmation)

ASSESSMENT POINTS

(Post partum)

SYSTEM	EFFECT	ASSESSMENT BY HX	PE	TEST
HEENT	Airway edema		Airway exam	
CV	Hypovolemia	Hemorrhage	HR, BP (orthostatics)	Hct
GI	↑ Gastric vol, ↓ gastric pH, ↓ lower esophageal sphincter tone	Heartburn		
GU	Uterine atony, chorioamnionitis	Postpartum hemorrhage, fever, diaphoresis	HR, BP (orthostatics), foul lochia	Hct, ↑ WBC, temp

Key Reference: Hawkins J: Postpartum tubal sterilization. *In* Chestnut DH (ed): Obstetric Anesthesia. St Louis, Mosby–Year Book, 1994, pp 443–454.

PERIOPERATIVE MANAGEMENT

Preoperative Preparation

- If post partum, assess volume status, replace as necessary

Anesthetic Technique

- Can be performed using local, regional, or GA

Monitoring

- Routine

Airway

- If post partum, may have upper airway edema

Induction

- If post partum, use nonparticulate antacid ± H_2 antagonist, metoclopramide; induce with rapid-sequence technique
- For spinal or epidural, T6 level required; if epidural already in place, inspect catheter site; administer test dose to confirm proper position
- If laparoscopic, suction stomach before trocar insertion; use large-bore IV, hyperventilate to maintain normocarbia; reassess ventilatory variables after insufflation (peak airway pressure, minute volume)

SURGICAL STAGES

- Post partum: small periumbilical incision
- Interval: introduction of trocar to peritoneal cavity; insufflation of CO_2 (or N_2O); insertion of laparoscope, instruments
- Interval/post partum (both): fallopian tubes identified, incised, ligated, or cauterized

Postoperative Considerations

- EBL: minimal
- Time <30 min
- Pain minimal (score 1–3)
- Consider local infiltration by surgeon (mesosalpinx, wound)

URETERAL REIMPLANTATION
Constance L. Monitto, M.D.

RISK
- Gender predominance: female
- Racial predilection: Caucasian
- Age: Dx antenatally or in childhood, with majority of surgical procedures performed by 5–6 y

PERIOPERATIVE RISKS
- Mortality extremely rare
- Minimal perioperative blood loss
- Postoperative ureteral obstruction (caused by edema, bleeding or blood clots, bladder spasms, or ureteral ischemia) can occur; usually asymptomatic and resolves spontaneously
- Symptomatic obstruction can present with abdominal pain, nausea, and vomiting but is usually diagnosed on postop follow-up renal US

WORRY ABOUT
- Most patients are healthy children (ASA I–II)
- Some patients will have significant congenital anomalies (e.g., spinal dysraphism) or GU anomalies (e.g., UPJ obstruction, ureteral duplication, bladder diverticula, posterior urethral valves, bladder or cloacal exstrophy)

OVERVIEW
- Ureteral reimplantation is usually performed to treat high-grade (grade III–V) vesicoureteral reflux (VUR)
- 1° VUR is a congenital anomaly resulting in development of an inadequate valvular mechanism at the ureterovesical junction
- 2° VUR is caused by anatomic (e.g., posterior urethral valves or ureteroceles) or functional (e.g., neuropathic bladder or bladder instability) bladder outlet obstruction
- Untreated VUR can result in chronic/recurrent UTIs, renal scarring, renal insufficiency, Htn, and impaired somatic growth; renal failure is uncommon (estimated risk <1%)

ICD-9-CM Code: 593.7 (Vesicoureteral reflux)

INDICATIONS AND USUAL TREATMENT
- Most initially managed medically (low-dose prophylactic antibiotics), as 70–90% of low-grade reflux will resolve spontaneously as patient grows
- Indications for surgery include breakthrough UTIs while on antibiotics, noncompliance, severe reflux (grades IV and V), deteriorating renal function, persistent reflux in females approaching puberty, associated congenital anomalies of the ureterovesical junction
- Goal of surgery (ureteroneocystostomy) is the creation of a submucosal valvular mechanism that allows ureteral compression with bladder filling and contraction
- >95% success rate of surgical correction

ASSESSMENT POINTS

SYSTEM	EFFECT	ASSESSMENT BY HX	PE	TEST
HEENT/RESP	Generally uninvolved	Snoring Exercise tolerance	Routine airway exam and lung auscultation	
CV	Hypertension		Measure BP	
IMMUNO	Possible latex allergy in patients with spinal dysraphism or exstrophy	History of rash, hives, or anaphylaxis with latex exposure		
RENAL	Possible renal insufficiency or RTA			Electrolytes, BUN/Cr
CNS	Weakness or paralysis with spinal dysraphism	CNS Hx, including Hx of bladder or bowel dysfunction	CNS exam Sacral dimple or hair tuft	MRI of spine

Key Reference: Atala A, Keating MA: Vesicoureteral reflux and megaureter. *In* Walsh PC, Retik AB, Vaughan ED, Wein A (eds): Campbell's Urology, 7th ed. Philadelphia, WB Saunders, 1998, pp 1859–1897.

PERIOPERATIVE MANAGEMENT

Preoperative Preparation
- Appropriate fasting interval and premedication (e.g., rectal, oral, IM, or IV midazolam), given patient age and level of preoperative anxiety

Monitoring
- Routine

Anesthetic Technique
- Mask or intravenous induction depending on patient age, preference, and risk factors (e.g., GERD)
- General endotracheal anesthesia alone or a combined technique (caudal or lumbar epidural catheter inserted following induction)
- Regional anesthesia alone is not generally advocated given patient age

- Combined techniques are not employed in patients with associated spinal dysraphism

SURGICAL STAGES
- Attempts to treat endoscopically (by injecting material behind the ureter) and lap-aroscopically; most procedures are open
- Surgical techniques can be extravesical, intravesical, or combined depending on the approach to the ureter, and suprahiatal or infrahiatal depending on the position of the new submucosal tunnel in relation to the original hiatus
- Extravesical repairs leave the bladder intact, lessening the risk of urinary contamination, bladder spasms, and hematuria, but concerns exist about disrupting bladder innervation and causing urinary retention with bilateral reimplantation

Postoperative Considerations
- Postop pain can be incisional or related to bladder spasms; treated with IV opioids, anticholinergics, and bladder smooth muscle relaxants (e.g., oxybutynin and valium), and/or epidural local anesthetic/opioid infusions
- Ketorolac has ↓ frequency and severity of bladder spasms following ureteroneocystostomy
- Complications of postoperative pain management include ileus, respiratory depression, sedation, emesis, and urinary retention
- Postop pain/bladder spasms may persist after discharge and require treatment with oral opioids, acetaminophen, NSAIDs, valium, and/or oxybutymin

URETERAL STENT PLACEMENT

Denis L. Bourke, M.D.

RISK

- Common procedure performed for variety of reasons
- Gender/racial predominance: M more common; no racial predilection
- Risk factors: related to co-existing disease; etiologic need for procedure

PERIOPERATIVE RISKS

- Perioperative mortality very low (≪1%)
- Ureteral perforation

WORRY ABOUT

- Nerve injury in lithotomy position
- Some urologists prefer "one leg down" position, which ↑ potential for hip dislocation or fracture, especially in debilitated patients
- Occasionally immediate open repair performed if ureter is perforated during procedure
- Occult blood loss (rare)

OVERVIEW

- Usually relatively straightforward, minimally painful, brief (5–25 min) procedure
- Usually 2° or temporizing procedure
- Patient profiles span extremes from young, healthy to old, moribund
- Procedure → minimal physiologic disturbance
- Many different types of stents can be used (see Key Reference)
- Usually minimal postop pain
- Fluoroscopy may be required

INDICATIONS AND USUAL TREATMENT

- Prophylactic for potential ureteral obstruction after ureteral instrumentation
- Bypass intrinsic obstruction—e.g., stones (especially during pregnancy) or strictures
- Bypass fistulas—e.g., ureterovaginal, ureteroenteric, or ureterocutaneous
- Bypass extrinsic obstructions—e.g., tumors, hematoma, or post-traumatic (surgical or other) edema
- For ureteral identification during gynecologic or pelvic cancer surgery
- To maintain reimplantation site patency following transplant

ASSESSMENT POINTS

SYSTEM	EFFECT	ASSESSMENT BY HX	TEST
CV	Depends on patient's age, diseases		
ENDO	Depends on nature of stone		Ca^{2+}
GU	Age, obstructive effects	Hematuria, oliguria	BUN, Cr

Key Reference: Saltzman B: Ureteral stents: indications, variations, and complications. Urol Clin North Am 1988; 15:481–491.

INTRAOPERATIVE MANAGEMENT

Anesthetic Technique

- Usually monitored anesthesia care with IV sedation adequate
- Occasionally, GA or regional anesthesia required

Monitoring

- Routine monitoring
- Age, co-existing diseases may dictate more extensive monitoring
- CVP occasionally indicated if UO cannot be measured

Airway

- Patient usually awake with minimal sedation required
- Patient in lithotomy position if GA required; airway can be managed by mask or ET tube

Induction

- Commonly, no specific induction required; sedation/analgesia used
- Spinal anesthesia: T12 level usually sufficient: discomfort confined to urethra

SURGICAL STAGES

- Like other endoscopic procedures, ureteral stent placement stimulation can begin and end suddenly, unexpectedly
- Surgically painful stimulation minimal
- Large veins or arteries rarely encountered; IV absorption of irrigating solution rare
- Placement time usually < 15 min
- Blood loss often small

ANTICIPATED PROBLEMS/CONCERNS

- Ureteral perforation rare, seldom of any immediate consequence to anesthetist unless immediate open repair required
- Nerve injury in lithotomy position

VAGINAL DELIVERY, NORMAL

Mukesh C. Sarna, M.D.
Nancy E. Oriol, M.D.

RISK

- ~4 million live births in USA y

PERIPARTUM RISKS

- Maternal mortality ↓: 7.8/100,000 live births in 1985 compared with 582/100,000 in 1935
- Perinatal mortality rate also ↓: 14.7/1000 live births in 1985
- Thromboembolism, hemorrhage, Htn disorders, infection remain common causes of maternal mortality, morbidity
- Decline in anesthetic-related causes noted (UK data)

WORRY ABOUT

- Supine hypotension syndrome
- Difficult airway
- Co-morbid conditions: preeclampsia, DM, ante-postpartum hemorrhage, multiple gestation, vaginal delivery after C-section
- Fetal well-being

OVERVIEW

- Effects of maternal interventions on fetus
- Effects of maternal interventions on course of labor
- Role of anesthesiologist
  - Labor analgesia
  - Anesthetic for operative delivery
  - High-risk obstetrics
  - Newborn resuscitation
  - Maternal resuscitation

ICD-9-CM Code: V22.2

INDICATIONS AND USUAL TREATMENT

- Labor analgesia
  - Lumbar epidural
  - Spinal
  - Combined spinal/epidural
  - Parenteral opioids
  - Others: psychoprophylaxis, parenteral, TENS, hypnosis/inhalational analgesia
- Operative delivery
  - Spinal anesthesia
  - Epidural anesthesia
  - Continuous spinal analgesia
  - GA
  - Local anesthesia
  - Bilateral pudendal nerve block
- Spinal/epidural anesthesia
- Neonatal resuscitation, especially in situations of nonreassuring fetal heart tracings, meconium-stained amniotic fluid

ASSESSMENT POINTS

SYSTEM	EFFECT	ASSESSMENT BY HX	PE	TEST
CV	↑ CO, ↓ SVR		BP, HR	
RESP	Edema, ↑ soft tissue	Previous GA	Airway exam	None
HEME	↑ Plasma vol > ↑ RBC mass	Sx of easy fatigability with significant anemia	None specific	CBC: occasional ↓ plt in normal preg
HEPATIC/ RENAL	Significant changes if pregnancy complicated by PIH	Epigastric pain, N/V, headache	Epigastric tenderness, hyperreflexia	BUN, Cr, LFTs, UA

Key Reference: Glosten B: Anesthesia for obstetrics. *In* Miller RD (ed): Anesthesia, 5th ed. New York, Churchill Livingstone, 2000, pp 2024–2068.

INTRAPARTUM MANAGEMENT

- Parturients in active labor should consider brief interview with anesthesiologist; emphasis on airway exam, previous anesthesia experience, co-morbid conditions
- Establish fetal status by cardiotocography, relevant prenatal test
- Antacid prophylaxis before any anesthetic intervention
- Establish IV access; consider preload before regional procedure; maintain left uterine displacement at all times

Monitoring

- Baseline pulse, BP, temp
- Following regional technique, monitor hemodynamics aggressively for the 1st 30 min; then at ½-h to 1-h intervals
- Equal attention to fetal status at induction, during maintenance of regional analgesia for labor

LABOR ANALGESIA

Lumbar Epidural

- Drugs
  - Local anesthetics, opioids alone or in combination; low-dose, ultra low dose (0.04% bupivacaine) solutions; latter allow for consideration of ambulation during labor as incidence of motor blockade is low
- Complications
  - Hypotension
  - Inadequate analgesia
  - Dural puncture headache
  - Subarachnoid block
  - Subdural block
  - Nerve damage (rare)
- Contraindications
  - Coagulopathy
  - Infection
  - Patient refusal

Spinal

- Intrathecal drugs
- Opioids: sufentanil/fentanyl/morphine commonly used; addition of bupivacaine 2.5 mg may improve quality, duration of analgesia
- Much ↓ incidence of spinal headache since introduction of pencil-point needles

Parenteral Opioids

- Maternal N/V, sedation
- ↓ Beat-to-beat variability in FHR
- Risk of neonatal depression
- Despite low efficacy, remain commonest form of labor analgesia

ANTICIPATED PROBLEMS/CONCERNS

- Airway: ↑ incidence of difficult/failed intubation with resultant hypoxemia, aspiration
- Aortocaval compression
- Peripartum hemorrhage
- Effect of interventions on fetus
- Postpartum neuropathy
- 20–25% of all planned normal spontaneous vaginal deliveries go to cesarean section

VENOUS AIR EMBOLISM

Thomas J. Toung, M.D.

RISK

• Patients with operative right heart gradient of >5 cm
• Probe patent foramen ovale in 25% of adult population
• Patients for laparoscopic surgery
• Incidence of VAE in children same as adults

PERIOPERATIVE RISKS

• Perioperative mortality <1%, but depends on early detection
• VAE: 40–80% in sitting, 10% in prone, 15% in supine, and 8% in lateral position
• Paradoxical air embolism (as high as 12%)
• Children suffer greater hemodynamic derangements

WORRY ABOUT

• Pulmonary venous outflow obstruction
• CV collapse
• Paradoxical air embolism

OVERVIEW

• Lethal volume of venous air in adult: 100–300 ml
• Entrained venous air can cause
  – Right ventricle outflow obstruction
  – Paradoxical arterial embolism (coronary embolism, stroke)
• Multiorifice catheter is preferable; the tip must be placed 2 cm below the SVC-atrial junction
• 75% N_2O can increase air bubble size about 3-fold
• Sensitivity for detection of VAE: TEE > precordial Doppler > PAP and end-tidal CO_2 > CVP > BP > ECG
• Mill-wheel murmurs late, catastrophic sign
• PA catheter may provide prognostic information

ICD-9-CM Codes: 958.0; 673.0 (Obstetrical)

INDICATIONS AND USUAL TREATMENT

• Operative site elevated to gain better exposure, blood drainage
• When VAE occurs
  – Notify surgeon of episode
  – Turn off N_2O
  – Gently apply bilateral jugular vein compression
  – Inflate MAST
  – Aspirate air from central catheter
  – CV support
  – Left decubitus position (Durant's maneuver)

ASSESSMENT POINTS

SYSTEM	EFFECT	ASSESSMENT BY HX	PE	TEST
CV	Patent foramen ovale	SOB	Auscultation	CXR, cath

Key Reference: Albin MS, Carroll RG, Maroon JC: Clinical considerations concerning detection of venous air embolism. Neurosurgery 1978; 3:380–384.

INTRAOPERATIVE MANAGEMENT

Monitoring

• Direct arterial pressure
• Precordial Doppler
• End-tidal CO_2
• Consider CVP or PAP catheter

SURGICAL STAGES

Dissection

• VAE mostly in beginning, closure

Definitive Surgery

• Depends on pathology
• When VAE occurs
  – Notify surgeon of episode
  – Turn off N_2O
  – Gently apply bilateral jugular vein compression
  – Inflate MAST
  – Aspirate air from central catheter
  – CV support
  – Left decubitus position (Durant's maneuver)

Postoperative Considerations

• Possible hypoxemia from pulmonary infarction
• Possible stroke from parodoxical air embolism
• Possible cardiac arrest from massive venous air or paradoxical air embolism

ANTICIPATED PROBLEMS/CONCERNS

• Hypoxemia, ARDS (late sequelae of massive air embolism and resuscitation)
• Stroke
• MI

VENTRICULAR SEPTAL DEFECT, REPAIR OF Cindy Hughes, M.D.

RISK

- Incidence: 2/1000 live births
- Isolated defect in 23% with CHD
- In combination with other cardiac anomalies 26% of time
- High incidence in premature births; most close spontaneously

PERIOPERATIVE RISKS

- Endocarditis: antibiotic prophylaxis required for any medical/dental procedure
- Worsening L → R shunting in infant with pain, hypoxia, hypothermia
- ↑Risk of perioperative CHF, arrhythmia, shunting, paradoxical air embolism
- High surgical mortality (20%) if VSD repair necessitated before age 6 mo

WORRY ABOUT

- Paradoxical air embolism
- Poor tolerance of induction if CHF (unable to feed, sweating while feeding, FTT, irritability)

- Residual or unrecognized VSD causing failure to separate from CPB, CHF, or failure to wean from mechanical ventilation
- Arrhythmia or heart block due to damage of conducting system post repair
- Ventricular outflow obstruction post repair
- Aortic regurgitation 2° to prolapse of aortic valve leaflet post repair

OVERVIEW

- Most common congenital heart defect
- 30–40% of all small membranous VSDs close spontaneously by 1st y
- 80% of those that do not spontaneously close develop CHF by 4 mo if untreated
- Pulmonary vascular Htn can be seen by 1 y if large VSD, multiple VSDs, or PDA exists; Eisenmenger's syndrome seen in 2nd decade of life
- Factors determining time of repair include
    - Degree of L → R shunting
    - CHF unresponsive to medical Rx
    - FTT
    - Sx of ↑pulmonary vascular Htn

ICD-9-CM Code: 745.4

ETIOLOGY

- Interventricular septum divided into 3 parts:
    - Membranous septum (part of endocardial cushion)
    - Muscular septum
    - Bulbus cordis (divides outflow tract into right, left ventricles)
- Type I (8%), supracristal VSD: close to pulmonary valve, right coronary cusp of aortic valve may lack support
- Type II (75%), membranous VSD: failure of septum to grow up to cushion
- Type III (4%), endocardial cushion VSD or complete AV canal: associated with ostium primum (ASD); lies very high in septum
- Type IV (12%), muscular VSD: frequently multiple VSDs; caused by excessive absorption of septal tissue

INDICATIONS AND USUAL TREATMENT

- Medical Rx for control of CHF: digoxin, diuretics
- High surgical mortality (20%) if VSD repair required before age 6 mo; closure of associated PDA or palliative procedure—e.g., banding—may precede definitive repair
- Surgical mortality in children ≥2 y with slight elevations in PVR: <2%

ASSESSMENT POINTS

SYSTEM	EFFECT	ASSESSMENT BY HX	PE	TEST
CV				
Small defect	Trivial L → R shunting	Incidental murmur found by pediatrician	Left parasternal holosystolic murmur	CXR normal, ECG may show mild LVH
Large defect	Significant L → R shunting, ↑ PAP	FTT, dyspnea, feeding difficulties, recurrent pulmonary infections	Harsh pansystolic murmur, systolic thrill	CXR: cardiomegaly, pulmonary congestion ECG: biventricular hypertrophy, notched P waves

Key Reference: Kambam J: Ventricular septal defects. *In* Kambam J (ed): Cardiac Anesthesia for Infants and Children. St. Louis, Mosby–Year Book, 1993, pp 193–202.

PERIOPERATIVE IMPLICATIONS

Preoperative Preparation

- Optimal control of CHF
    - Child should be feeding, growing
- Adequate premedication for hemodynamic stability
- Antibiotic prophylaxis

Monitoring

- Arterial, central venous monitoring for tight control of hemodynamics
- Consider TEE or color flow Doppler to assist with postop Dx of residual VSD

Preinduction/Induction

- Heavy premedication, ↓ SVR to limit L → R shunting

Airway

- PPV may limit degree of L → R shunting

Maintenance

- Choice based on preference

Extubation

- If repair of VSD, extubate in ICU when hemodynamically stable (weaned from inotropes, free of arrhythmias, normothermic, etc.)
- If patient with unrepaired VSD is undergoing noncardiac surgery, extubate at end of procedure if overall condition good. Avoid worsening L → R shunting (hypoxia, pain, shivering) or worsening CHF (excess fluid administration).

Adjuvants

- Oxygen, furosemide, digoxin for continued CHF

Postoperative Period

- Pain management critical

ANTICIPATED PROBLEMS/CONCERNS

- If large VSDs, CHF, or FTT, at greatest risk and difficult to wean from bypass

VENTRICULOPERITONEAL SHUNT

Aaron Lloyd, M.D.

RISK

- Elevated ICP
  - Congenital (e.g., meningomyelocele, Chiari malformations)
    - Aqueductal stenosis
    - Traumatic
    - Post fossa tumors
    - Overproduction of CSF
- Normal ICP
  - Associated dementia, gait disorders in elderly
- Gender predominance: none

PERIOPERATIVE RISKS

- Perioperative mortality rare
- Intracranial bleeding may occur with placement of proximal tubing

WORRY ABOUT

- Prevent further elevations in ICP, which can lead to herniation syndromes
- Ventricular dysrhythmias associated with rapid removal of CSF
- Associated pathology

OVERVIEW

- Procedure to divert CSF from ventricles to peritoneum
- Proximal catheter passed into lateral ventricle through burr hole, preferably on the right to reduce risk of dominant hemisphere injury
- Distal catheter tunneled subcutaneously; multiorificed tip placed in peritoneum
- Patients typically present signs of shunt malfunction or elevated ICP

ICD-9-CM Code: 331.4 (Hydrocephalus: acquired)

INDICATIONS AND USUAL TREATMENT

- Clinical and radiographic evidence of elevated ICP and/or shunt malfunction
- Hx of previous shunts
- Pseudotumor cerebri
- Normal-pressure hydrocephalus with demonstrated improvement in Sx with large-volume lumbar puncture
- If multiple failed ventriculoperitoneal shunts, ventriculojugular, atrial, or pleural shunt may be placed

ASSESSMENT POINTS

SYSTEM	EFFECT	ASSESSMENT BY HX	PE	TEST
CV	Htn, bradycardia			VS
RESP	Aspiration	Vomiting	Auscultation	CXR
CNS	Herniation, seizures	Obtundation	Shunt tap by neurosurgeon	CT, EEG

Key Reference: Ruge JR, McLone DG: Cerebrospinal fluid diversion procedures. *In* Apuzzo MLJ (ed): Brain Surgery: Complications, Avoidance and Management. New York, Churchill Livingstone, 1993, pp 1463–1494.

PERIOPERATIVE IMPLICATIONS

Anesthetic Technique

- GA usual

Monitoring

- Routine
- Consider arterial line in cases of uncontrolled ICP, hemodynamic instability

Airway/Induction

- Normal ICP: IV or mask induction adequate
- Elevated ICP: atropine (in children), preoxygenate, cricoid pressure, thiobarbiturate, narcotic, lidocaine, rapid-acting nondepolarizing muscle relaxant followed by hyperventilation

Maintenance

- Hyperventilate to maintain $PaCO_2$ at 24–30 mmHg in patients with elevated ICP
- If used, maintain low levels of inhaled agent to avoid ↑ CBF, blood volume, and ICP

SURGICAL STAGES

Positioning

- Table turned 90°, head to surgeon
- Head turned 30° from neutral, bump placed under shoulder ipsilateral to shunt

Dissection

- Small flap turned in parietal region with subsequent burr hole
- Small abdominal incision, enters peritoneum
- Subcutaneous tunnel tracked to pull distal catheter through; can be stimulating, associated with ↑ anesthetic needs

Definitive Surgery

- EBL: minimal
- Rapid decompression can be associated with tachydysrhythmias, hypotension
- Ventriculoatrial shunts can be complicated by air embolism

Postoperative Considerations

- Patient remains flat to avoid overdrainage of CSF
- Associated with minimal pain (pain score: 2)

ANTICIPATED PROBLEMS/CONCERNS

- Elevated ICP with associated hemodynamic changes

WHIPPLE PROCEDURE (PANCREATICO-DUODENECTOMY)

Edward J. Norris, M.D., M.B.A.

RISK

- 30,000 cases of cancer of exocrine pancreas diagnosed annually (5th leading cause of cancer death in USA)
- Mean: 60 y
- Male:female ratio, 1.5:1
- Racial predominance: none

PERIOPERATIVE RISKS

- Perioperative mortality rate (30 days) <5%; may be as low as 1% in centers of excellence
- Major morbidity most often 2° to underlying cardiopulmonary disease, pancreatic or biliary fistula, hemorrhage, or infection
- Leak or fistula from pancreatic anastomosis is leading cause of morbidity (incidence 5–25%)

WORRY ABOUT

- Massive blood loss (superior mesenteric vessels, portal vein, or vena cava injury)
- Significant fluid shifts
- Venous air embolism with injury to vena cava

OVERVIEW

- Most commonly performed cancer-directed operation for pancreatic cancer
- Distal stomach, gallbladder, common bile duct, head of pancreas, proximal jejunum, duodenum, regional lymphatics removed
- Requires pancreaticojejunostomy, choledochojejunostomy, gastrojejunostomy
- Risk factors include diabetes, cigarette smoking, alcohol ingestion
- Age, co-morbidities of patient will dictate perioperative monitoring strategies
- Significant blood loss, fluid shifts with extended Whipple resections (more extensive soft tissue, lymphatic dissections, resection of superior mesenteric vessels, portal vein if necessary)
- ~70% of tumors of head of pancreas unresectable at time of exploratory laparotomy

ICD-9-CM Code: 157.0 (Cancer of pancreas)

INDICATIONS AND USUAL TREATMENT

- Following conditions should be met:
  - All evidence of gross tumor can be resected with standard resection
  - No evidence of distant metastatic disease or extensive vascular or retroperitoneal involvement by work-up
  - Good general health
- Palliative operations directed to relief of obstructive jaundice (cholecystojejunostomy, choledochojejunostomy), gastric outlet obstruction (gastrojejunostomy), pain (celiac plexus injection with ethanol)
- 5-y survival ~20%
- Combined radiotherapy and chemotherapy have been shown to ↑ survival in patients with resectable, unresectable disease

ASSESSMENT POINTS

SYSTEM	EFFECT	ASSESSMENT BY HX	PE	TEST
GI	Gastric outlet obstruction	Vomiting	Abdominal mass	CT scan
HEPATIC	Liver metastases		Hepatomegaly	CT scan Laparoscopy
	Bile duct obstruction		Jaundice, hepatomegaly	CT scan Bilirubin level
NUTRITION	Tumor Malnutrition	Wt loss		Total protein, albumin
ENDO	Tumor			Blood glucose

Key Reference: Sosa JA, Bowman HM, Gordon TA, Bass EB, Yeo CJ, Lillemoe KD, Pitt HA, Tielsch JM, Cameron JL: Importance of hospital volume in the overall management of pancreatic cancer. Ann Surg 1998; 228:429–438.

PERIOPERATIVE IMPLICATIONS

Preoperative Preparation

- Bowel prep routine, requiring rehydration
- Consider referral to "large-volume" hospital

Anesthetic Technique

- General
- Combined
  - General/lumbar epidural (narcotics)
  - General/low-thoracic epidural (local anesthesia/narcotics)
  - General/intrathecal narcotics
- Technique needs to allow for unresectability (open, close)

Monitoring

- Large-bore IV access for fluid requirements, blood loss
- Consider central venous, arterial pressure monitoring

Airway

- None

Induction

- Cricoid pressure if gastric outlet obstruction suspected
- Combined technique with low-thoracic epidural requires only moderate volume of local anesthetic (6–8 ml)

SURGICAL STAGES

Dissection

- Small-to-moderate amount of blood loss
- Moderate ongoing fluid requirements
- Resectability determined by absence of distant metastases, extent of major vascular involvement

Definitive Surgery

- Significant volume requirements; consider colloid
- Blood loss can be massive with portal vein or vena cava injury

Postoperative Considerations

- Pain score: 5–9
- Usual hospital stay: 8–12 days
- Combined technique with neuraxial narcotics
- May develop significant fluid shifts
- May require postop ventilation

ANTICIPATED PROBLEMS/CONCERNS

- Risk of significant fluid shifts, blood loss
- Malnutrition
- Ileus

SECTION III

DRUGS

ACE INHIBITORS

Thai Nguyen, M.D.

USES

- Treatment of Htn and CHF
- ↓ Mortality after myocardial infarction

PERIOPERATIVE RISKS

- Severe hypotension on induction

WORRY ABOUT

- Acute renal failure in patients with renal artery stenosis
- Angioedema including swelling of lips, tongue, mouth, throat, nose, or other parts of the face
- Fetal anomalies and fetal and neonatal death

OVERVIEW/PHARMACOLOGY/DOSE

- Enalaprilat is the only ACE inhibitor available in IV dosage (onset 5–10 min, off-set 12–24 h)
- Lisinopril offers once-a-day dosing

CHARACTERISTIC	CAPTOPRIL	ENALAPRIL	LISINOPRIL	BENAZEPRIL	FOSINOPRIL	QUINAPRIL	RAMIPRIL
Elimination	Renal	Renal	Renal	Renal	50% Renal 50% Hepatic	61% Renal 37% Hepatic	Renal
Onset of hypotensive action (h)	0.25	1	1	1	1	1	1–2
Peak hypotensive effects (h)	1–1.5	4–6	6	2–4	2–6	2	3–6
Duration of hypotensive effects (h)	Dose related	24 (18–30)	24 (18–30)	24	24	24	>24 (24–60)
Dose (mg)	25–150, max 450	5–40, max 40	10–40, max 80	20–80, max 80	10–40, max 80	10–80, max 80	2.5–20, max 20

DRUG CLASS

- Affects the renin-angiotensin system by blocking angiotensin II formation and delaying bradykinin breakdown and associated prostaglandins

DRUG EFFECTS

SYSTEM	EFFECT	ASSESSMENT BY HX	PE	TEST
HEENT	Angioedema	Swelling of face, neck, tongue Dyspnea	Difficulty speaking, swallowing	Airway exam
	Bronchospasm		Wheezing	
CV	Hypotension	Assess CV response to Rx		
GU	Renal failure Hyperkalemia	Orthopnea, dyspnea	Edema	BUN, Cr, lytes
HEME	Leukopenia, agranulocytosis	Fever		CBC with diff

Key Reference: Brabant SM, Eyraud D, Bertrand M, Coriat P: Refractory hypotension after induction of anesthesia in a patient chronically treated with angiotensin receptor antagonists. Anesth Analg 1999; 89:887–888.

DRUG INTERACTIONS

Preoperative Period

- Assess for evidence of renal insufficiency
- Monitor for hyperkalemia
- Consider holding morning dose to avoid severe hypotension

Induction/Maintenance

- Severe hypotension
- Use of succinylcholine with elevated K^+ may be associated with cardiac arrhythmia

Adjuvant/Regional Anesthesia/Reversal

- Hypotensive episodes may be associated with spinal and epidural anesthesia

Postoperative Period

- Monitor for hypotension

ACETAMINOPHEN

Matthew K. Miller, M.D.

USES

- Effective alternative to aspirin as an analgesic for low- to moderate-intensity pain, and as an antipyretic
- Especially useful if aspirin contraindicated (e.g., those with PUD) or when prolongation of bleeding time, inhibition of platelet aggregation, or impairment of excretion of uric acid is disadvantageous
- Often used in combination with an opiate for more potent analgesia

PERIOPERATIVE RISK

- In recommended therapeutic doses, usually well tolerated
- In cases of acute or chronic overdose, acetaminophen is associated with hepatotoxicity, nephrotoxicity, metabolic acidosis, and hypoglycemic coma

OVERVIEW/PHARMACOLOGY

- Acetaminophen acts as a prostaglandin (PG) synthesis inhibitor, with more pronounced effects centrally than peripherally
- Strong central inhibition of PG synthesis confers analgesic and antipyretic activity, but modest peripheral inhibition of PG synthesis results in weak anti-inflammatory activity
- Systemic absorption after oral administration is nearly complete, mostly absorbed by passive diffusion in the small intestine (rate of absorption dependent on rate of gastric emptying)
- May also be administered rectally
- Peak plasma concentration occurs in 30–60 min, plasma half-life is approximately 2 h
- At therapeutic doses, minimal protein binding occurs
- 90–100% of drug can be recovered from urine within the first day
- Metabolism is primarily by hepatic conjugation with glucuronic acid, sulfuric acid, or cysteine
- Small portion undergoes cytochrome P450-mediated N-hydroxylation to form N-acetyl-p-benzoquinone, a highly reactive intermediate

MECHANISM OF ACTION/USUAL DOSE

- Central inhibition of the enzyme cyclooxygenase (COX) results in inhibition of PG synthesis
- PG may ↑ the excitability of neurons receiving ongoing afferent input; thus, inhibition of PG synthesis results in ↓ excitability of neurons to afferent input (i.e., painful stimuli)
- Inhibition of PG synthesis in the hypothalamus is thought to be responsible for antipyretic activity
- Weak peripheral inhibition of PG synthesis results in minimal anti-inflammatory effects
- Usual adult dosage is 325–1000 mg administered orally q 4–6 h (total daily dose not to exceed 4000 mg)
- In children, recommended oral dosage is 10–18 mg/kg q 4 h or a rectal dosage of 25–30 mg/kg q 4 h

TOXIC EFFECTS

- Occasionally associated with skin rash and other allergic reactions
- Patients with hypersensitivity to salicylates rarely exhibit hypersensitivity to acetaminophen
- Isolated cases of neutropenia, thrombocytopenia, and pancytopenia have been reported
- Most serious toxic effects are seen in overdose and include potentially fatal hepatic necrosis as well as renal tubular necrosis, metabolic acidosis, and hypoglycemic coma
- In adults, hepatotoxicity may occur after ingestion of a single dose of 10–15 g (150–250 mg/kg); doses >20–25 g are potentially lethal
- In children, doses up to 150 mg/kg usually do not require treatment
- With overdose, the reactive intermediate (N-acetyl-p-benzoquinone) is formed in amounts sufficient to deplete hepatic stores of glutathione. N-acetyl-p-benzoquinone then reacts with hepatocellular proteins, and hepatic necrosis can result
- Symptoms within the first 48 h after overdose are relatively mild (e.g., nausea, vomiting, anorexia, and abdominal pain)

- Clinical indications of hepatic damage do not occur until 2–4 days after ingestion (elevated transaminases, hyperbilirubinemia, prolonged PT time)
- Severe cases result in acute hepatic necrosis, which can progress to fulminant liver failure and death
- Hepatic tissue reveals centrilobular necrosis; in nonfatal cases, the hepatocellular damage is reversible over a period of weeks to months
- Rumack-Matthew's nomogram is used to determine the need for antidotal treatment, as well as to evaluate risk for hepatic failure
- Plasma concentration of acetaminophen at 4 h >300 μg/ml predicts severe liver damage; <120 μg/ml predicts minimal liver damage

TREATMENT OF OVERDOSE

- Early diagnosis is vital in treatment; treatment should not be delayed while awaiting laboratory results if Hx indicates significant overdose
- Gastric lavage if within 4 h of ingestion
- N-acetyl-L-cysteine (NAC) should be administered as guided by Rumack-Matthew's nomogram
- NAC most effective within 8 h of ingestion; can be effective up to 36 h after ingestion
- NAC replenishes hepatic glutathione and prevents drug-induced hepatic necrosis
- Initial oral dosage of NAC is 140 mg/kg, followed by 70 mg/kg q 4 h for 17 doses (72-hour regime)
- Administration of NAC within 8 h is associated with excellent prognosis; after 8 h prognosis becomes increasingly poorer

SPECIAL CONSIDERATIONS

- Hepatotoxicity is less common in children after overdose, probably due to ↓ glucuronidation and a greater ability to regenerate depleted glutathione
- Patients taking agents that induce the P450 system (e.g., ethanol, phenobarbital) may be at greater risk for hepatotoxicity

DRUG EFFECTS (TOXICITY)

SYSTEM	EFFECT	ASSESSMENT BY HX	TEST
CNS	Encephalopathy	Coma with overdose	
GI	Hepatic dysfunction	Nausea, vomiting, anorexia with overdose	Liver enzymes PT Bilirubin
RENAL	Nephrotoxicity with overdose or chronic abuse		Cr
METAB	Metabolic acidosis		ABGs

Key Reference: Insel PA: Analgesic-antipyretic and antiinflammatory agents and drugs employed in the treatment of gout. *In* Hardman JG, Limbird LE (eds): Goodman and Gilman's The Pharmacological Basis of Therapeutics, 9th ed. New York, McGraw-Hill Professional Publishing, 1996, pp 617–657.

PERIOPERATIVE IMPLICATIONS

- In patients with known or suspected overdose or chronic abuse, surgery should be delayed until acetaminophen levels are determined and appropriate therapy is instituted

- After overdose, elective surgery should be postponed until hepatic function returns to baseline or has been optimized

- Avoidance of drugs and techniques that impair hepatic and renal blood flow should be considered

ALKYLATING AGENTS

Mark J. Lema, M.D., Ph.D.

USES

- Hodgkin's disease, lymphoma
- Breast and bladder cancers
- Lung, pancreas, brain, ovarian, testicular cancers
- Sarcomas, multiple myeloma, leukemias
- Bone marrow transplants, melanoma

PERIOPERATIVE RISKS

- Increased risk of infection
- Aspiration (subsequent to N/V)
- Prolonged succinylcholine action (CTX)
- Fluid retention (HN_2)

WORRY ABOUT

- Extravasation if given by IV infusion
- Prolonged bleeding (thrombocytopenia)
- Aspiration during intubation

OVERVIEW/PHARMACOLOGY

- Structurally diverse compounds; first chemotherapy agents (1940s)
- Generate reactive, electron-deficient intermediates
- Covalently bind to DNA bases (guanine), especially during mitosis
- Disrupt DNA replication, transcription
- High incidence of cytotoxicity to normal, rapidly dividing cells

SIDE EFFECTS (ACUTE): 1–3 WEEKS AFTER THERAPY

- Myelosuppression (pancytopenia)
- N/V
- Sterility
- ↑ Risk of secondary malignancies (leukemia)
- Alopecia
- Bladder toxicity (hemorrhagic cystitis)
- Phlebitis

DRUG EFFECTS

CLASS	NAME	ABBREV	SPECIAL INDICATION*	ADVERSE EFFECTS
Nitrogen Mustards				
Mechlorethamine	Mustargen	HN_2	LM	N/V, phlebitis
Cyclophosphamide	Cytoxan	CTX	LM, Brt, Bl, Lu, Ov	Decreases pseudo-ChE; myocardial toxicity, hemorrhagic cystitis, pulmonary toxicity
Ifosfamide	Ifex		LM, Ov, Te, Sa	Bladder toxicity, CNS toxicity
L-Phenylalanine	Alkeran (melphalan)	L–PAM	MM	Mild N/V
Chlorambucil	Leukeran	CLR	CLL, LM	N/V
Triethylene-thiophosphoramide	Thiotepa	T-TEPA	BMT	Can ↓ pseudo-ChE
Alkyl Sulfonates				
Busulfan	Myleran	MYL	CML	Pulmonary toxicity
Nitrosoureas				
Chloroethyl-cyclohexyl-nitrosourea	Lomustine	CCNU	LM, Brn	N/V
Bis-chloroethyl-nitrosourea	Carmustine	BCNU	LM, Brn	N/V, phlebitis
Streptozocin	Zanosar	STZ	Pa	N/V
Triazenes				
Dimethyltriazenoimidazole carboxamide	Dacarbazine	DTIC	HD, Sa, Me	N/V, anaphylaxis, phlebitis

*CLL, CML: leukemias; Bl: bladder; BMT: bone marrow transplant; Brn: brain; Brt: breast; HD: Hodgkin's; LM: lymphoma; Lu: lung; Me: melanoma; MM: multiple myeloma; Ov: ovarian; Pa: pancreas; Sa: sarcoma; Te: testicular

Key Reference: Selvin BL: Cancer chemotherapy: implications for the anesthesiologist. Anesth Analg 1981; 60:425.

PERIOPERATIVE IMPLICATIONS

Preoperative Preparation

- Full-stomach precautions
- Risk of infection (leukopenia)
- Adequate hydration (bladder toxicity)
- Check plt count (thrombocytopenia)
- PFT (busulfan, cyclophosphamide)
- MUGA (cyclophosphamide)

Intraoperative

- Risk of aspiration during induction
- Prolonged bleeding
- Plan for RBC transfusion (anemia)
- Maintain UO
- Reduced dose of succinylcholine (CTX, thiotepa)

POSTOPERATIVE CONCERNS

- Risk of N/V (most agents)
- Continued fluid hydration
- Monitor cardiac/pulmonary dysfunction (CTX, busulfan)

ALPHA$_2$-ADRENERGIC AGONISTS — Ramon Núñez-Hernandez, M.D.

USES

- Management of hypertension
- Nonapproved indications
  - Management of narcotic, alcohol, tobacco withdrawal manifestations
  - Hemodynamic stability with less BP and HR fluctuations
  - ↓ In inhalation, narcotic anesthetic requirements (30–90% MAC reduction)
  - Sedative/anxiolytic with no or minimal respiratory depression
  - Postop analgesia with ↓ in narcotic requirements and no addiction liability
  - Reduction of postop shivering
  - ↓ Cardiac toxicity of IV bupivacaine
  - Attenuation of sympathetically mediated hyperperfusion phase after focal ischemia
  - For intrathecal/epidural anesthesia with prolongation of motor and sensory blockade by local anesthesia

PERIOPERATIVE RISKS

- Bradycardia requiring Rx with atropine/ephedrine when hemodynamically unstable
- ↓ In BP potentiated by other antihypertensive drugs
- Severe rebound tachycardia, Htn associated with withdrawal
- Larger BP reduction with blood losses less than 20% of blood volume
- Drug interactions (cimetidine ↑ CNS toxicity)
- High concentrations may ↓ uterine blood flow 2° to direct vascular effect
- Associated with LFT abnormalities (methyldopa)
- Xerostomia most common complaint

WORRY ABOUT

- Severe bradycardia, cardiac arrest
- May produce positive Coombs' test (10–20% of patients in chronic Rx with methyldopa)
- Hemolytic anemia (methyldopa)
- Potentiation of lithium toxicity (methyldopa)

OVERVIEW/PHARMACOLOGY

- Clonidine, dexmedetomidine are imidazoline deriv with antihypertensive properties; BP effect central by binding to imidazoline receptor, resulting in ↓ sympathetic outflow from vasomotor center to heart, vessels; → ↓ HR, ↓ PVR
- Effect at presynaptic α_2-adrenergic receptor of preganglionic sympathetic fibers; → predominantly parasympathetic tone; direct peripheral, postsynaptic activation by the α_2 agonist causes vasoconstriction
- Activation of α_2 receptors induces ↓ in production of cAMP by inhibitory G protein (Gi), resulting in changes in protein kinase activity; protein phosphorylation determines extent of inhibition of voltage-sensitive Ca^{2+} channels or activation of K^+ channels in neuronal inhibition
- Physiologic effects depend on specificity for α_2 receptor type, subtype
- Dexmedetomidine, guanfacine, clonidine, oxymetazoline arranged in order of selectivity for the α_2- vs. α_1-adrenergic receptor
- Dexmedetomidine $\alpha_2:\alpha_1$ ratio is 2000:1, whereas clonidine selectivity $\alpha_2:\alpha_1$ is 300:1
- Physiologic effects also depend on lipid solubility; clonidine similar to fentanyl, whereas oxymetazoline is poorly lipid soluble, lacks sedative and BP effects of clonidine; dexmedetomidine most lipid soluble

- Clonidine concentration ↓ in biexponential fashion, with β phase of 5–10 min, slow β phase of 8–12 h; guanfacine has a faster elimination (6–8 h); dexmedetomidine even faster (4–5 h)
- After PO intake of clonidine, BP ↓ in 30–50 min, peak effect at 1–3 h and plasma $T_{1/2}$ of 6–24 h; ~50% of absorbed dose metabolized by microsomal enzymes of liver, finally is excreted by kidney; in chronic renal insufficiency, $T_{1/2}$ may be ↑ up to 40 h

DRUG CLASS/MECH OF ACTION/USUAL DOSE

Clonidine

- Imidazoline deriv; central-acting antihypertensive agent
  - Usual dosage: PO 0.1 mg, 0.2 mg, 0.3 mg bid; transdermal (patch) delivery of 0.1, 0.2, 0.3 mg/d for 1 wk

Guanfacine

- Central-acting antihypertensive agent
  - Usual dosage 1–2 mg PO/d

Guanabenz

- Aminoguanidine deriv; central-acting antihypertensive agent
  - Usual dose 4–8 mg PO/d

Dexmedetomidine

- Imidazoline deriv; highly selective α_2 agonist in clinical trials in the USA, given IV

DRUG EFFECTS

SYSTEM	EFFECT	ASSESSMENT BY HX	PE	TEST
HEENT	Nasal decongestant	Nasal breathing improvement		
	Antisialagogue	Xerostomia	Dry mouth	
CV	Reduces HR	Bradycardia	↓ HR	ECG
	BP control	Htn controlled	Normal BP	
Vessels	↑ SVR	Htn	↑ BP	SVR
	↑ BP			
Heart	Slowed conduction		HR	ECG
	Temporary fall in CO			
CNS	Sedation	Mental status/responsiveness	Tension/anxiety relief	EEG changes
	Cerebral vasoconstriction			VAS
	Analgesia/anesthesia			
	Fatigue/asthenia	↓ Anesthetic requirements		
	Attenuates ↑ in CBF to inhalation agents	Weakness	Reduced strength	
	↓ ICP, IOP			
GU	Urinary retention/diuretic			
	Impotence/↓ libido			
	Impaired insulin secretion	No evidence of hyperglycemia		
	↓ Uterine blood flow (high conc)	in acute or chronic Rx		

Key Reference: Kamibayashi T, Maze M: Clinical uses of alpha2-adrenergic agonists. Anesthesiology 2000; 93:1345–1349.

PERIOPERATIVE IMPLICATIONS

- If patient is on chronic Rx with α_2 agonist, continue medication in the perioperative period to avoid withdrawal
- Cimetidine may be associated with CNS dysfunction when combined with clonidine by reduction in hepatic P450 clearance or by reduction in hepatic blood flow and potential for clonidine toxicity; also, cimetidine, an imidazo-

line deriv without α_2-adrenergic activity, can produce CV depression by interacting centrally with midazoline receptor
- Administration of preop CNS depressants adjusted in patients on Rx with α_2 agonist

Induction/Maintenance

- Interaction with induction agent may produce hypotension

- Maintenance doses of anesthetics reduced to avoid severe hypotension or delayed awakening

Postoperative Period

- Avoid withdrawal by continuing management with α_2 agonist in patients on chronic Rx
- In single preop use of clonidine, follow HR, adjust analgesic requirements

AMINOPHYLLINE

USES

- Acute and chronic Rx for asthma, COPD
- Rx for neonatal apnea
- Occasionally for CHF
- As 2° agent in CPR settings
- Potential for life-threatening CNS, cardiac toxicity
- Administered IV, PO, or rectally

PERIOPERATIVE RISKS

- Toxic levels from overaggressive use or coadministration of cimetidine/propranolol
- ↑ Arrhythmogenicity with halothane or pancuronium
- ↑ CNS toxicity (lower seizure threshold) with ketamine

WORRY ABOUT

- Prolonged clearance in presence of cimetidine, erythromycin, propranolol, or in patients receiving influenza vaccines
- Enhanced clearance in smokers and patients taking dilantin, barbiturates
- Narrow therapeutic/toxic ratio

OVERVIEW/PHARMACOLOGY

- Methylated xanthine
- Bronchodilatory and anti-inflammatory effects
- Onset of effect within 1 h from IV dose
- Biotransformed by demethylation in liver; renally excreted
- 7–15% excreted unchanged in urine
- Crosses placenta, found in breast milk

DRUG CLASS/MECH OF ACTION/USUAL DOSE

- Methylated xanthine
- Proposed mechanisms of action include inhibiting phosphodiesterase, antagonizing the effect of adenosine, causing catecholamine release, inhibiting cellular immune function
- Usual dosage: 4 mg/kg q 8–12 h PO; 5–6 mg/kg IV load followed by 0.2–0.75 mg/kg/h IV

DRUG EFFECTS

SYSTEM	EFFECT	ASSESSMENT BY HX	PE	TEST
CV	Inotropy and chronotropy; ↓ in SVR, PCWP, BP	Predisposes to ventricular arrhythmia	Auscultation of heart sounds	ECG
RESP	Bronchodilation, suppression of cellular immune response	Relief of dyspnea, improvement of bronchospastic symptoms	Auscultation of chest	Peak flow, PFTs
CNS	Nonspecific CNS stimulation; stimulates central respiratory drive	N/V, irritability, insomnia, delirium, convulsions, stupor, coma		

Key References: Perouansky M, Shamir M, Hershkowitz E, Donchin Y: Successful resuscitation using aminophylline in refractory cardiac arrest with asystole. Resuscitation 1998; 38:39–41; Stirt JA, Sullivan SF: Aminophylline. Anesth Analg 1981; 60:587–602.

PERIOPERATIVE IMPLICATIONS

Preoperative Concerns

- Toxic preoperative blood level 2° to overadministration or coadministration of drugs that affect clearance (cimetidine, erythromycin, propranolol, verapamil, phenytoin [Dilantin])
- Potential for seizures or malignant arrhythmias if toxic levels
- Presence of underlying bronchospastic disease
- Administration via peripheral vein to avoid cardiotoxicity

Induction/Maintenance

- Can interact with halothane or pancuronium to cause ventricular arrhythmias
- Can interact with ketamine to lower seizure threshold
- Continue infusion if carefully monitoring for toxicity
- No proven effectiveness in treating intraoperative bronchospasm in humans
- Reduction of NMB

Postoperative Period

- Check plasma levels before restarting infusion if toxicity is suspected
- May be used as central respiratory stimulant in neonates recovering from general anesthesia

ANTICIPATED PROBLEMS/CONCERNS

- Most common problems are from narrow therapeutic/toxic window, potential for severe CNS, cardiac toxicity
- Patients taking aminophylline often have severe bronchospastic disease
- Dialysis or charcoal hemoperfusion can acutely lower blood levels

AMPHETAMINES

Earl S. Ransom, Jr., M.D.

USES

- Major medical uses include treatment of attention-deficit hyperactivity disorder (ADHD) and narcolepsy
- Uses as anorexiants and to allay fatigue are not recommended
- Usually administered orally; IV form ("crystal") found in substance abuse settings
- Use on the increase during the past decade, especially in western USA and among young adults

PERIOPERATIVE RISKS

- High risk of abuse resulting in changes in MAC (chronic use, MAC ↓; acute use, MAC ↑)
- Risk of hypertension when used with other sympathomimetics and MAOIs
- Risk of arrhythmias/cardiac arrest when used with thyroid hormones, K⁺-losing diuretics, laxatives, phenylpropanolamine, and acute ingestion of alcohol. Methamphetamine alone has been documented to cause myocardial ischemia/infarction or death, even after GA induction.

- Risk of acute lead poisoning from the use of lead acetate as a reagent during production of methamphetamine
- Large acute doses may result in hyperthermia

WORRY ABOUT

- Severe hypertension and generalized SNS stimulation worrisome in pts with ischemic heart disease, pre-existing hypertension, hyperthyroidism, advanced arteriosclerosis

OVERVIEW/PHARMACOLOGY

- Indirect-acting sympathomimetic
- Schedule II drug
- Acute administration results in ↑ in cortical alertness, ↓ appetite, profound anxiety, paranoia, mydriasis, hyperreflexia, chest pain; ↑ in cardiac output, peripheral vascular resistance, dysrhythmias, and possible myocardial infarction/ischemia
- Chronic use results in depletion of body stores of catecholamines, tolerance, psychological dependence, weight loss, cerebrovascular disease, and cardiac toxicity (e.g., car-

diomyopathy). There is an ↑ risk of perinatal complications (premature delivery, congenital deformities, altered neonatal behavioral patterns). Seizures may occur on abrupt withdrawal.
- Use of EPI controversial during cardiac arrest. Sodium bicarbonate may be useful.
- May enhance opioid analgesia
- Metabolized slowly by hepatic enzymes
- Overdosage treated with supportive therapy, sedation, possible gastric lavage, urine acidification, and combined α and β blockade, if needed

DRUG CLASS/MECH OF ACTION/USUAL DOSE

- Phenethylamine derivative
- Mechanism of action via displacement of neurotransmitter (centrally and peripherally) from storage sites in SNS/PNS and/or blockade of re-uptake
- Usual dosages (oral)
  - Obesity, 5–10 mg of amphetamine 30–60 min before meals
  - Narcolepsy, 10 mg initial dose/d
  - ADHD, 0.1–0.5 mg/kg/d in children

DRUG EFFECTS

SYSTEM	EFFECT	ASSESSMENT BY HX	PE	TEST
CV	Increases in CO, HR, BP, SVR, dysrhythmias	Hx of recent or chronic ingestion	Monitoring of variables	
RESP	Mild respiratory stimulation	Hx of recent or chronic ingestion	Pulmonary exam	ABGs
CNS	Increased cortical alertness and electrical activity (generalized); overdosage results in anxiety, psychoses, hyperactivity, possible seizures	Hx of recent or chronic ingestion	CNS exam	
METAB	Dehydration, lactic acidosis, ketosis	Hx of overusage or abuse	Vital signs, general PE	ABGs; electrolytes
OTHER	Decreased GI motility, mydriasis, diaphoresis, hyperthermia	Hx of overusage or abuse	Vital signs, general PE	

Key Reference: AMA Drug Evaluations, 1993, pp 8, 290, 322–323, 2251.

PERIOPERATIVE IMPLICATIONS

Preoperative Concerns

- Recent, acute ingestion
- Hx of polysubstance abuse
- Current medications, particularly MAO inhibitors
- Monitor BP for hypertension, ECG for possible ischemia
- If suspicious and if time allows, cardiology consult regarding cardiomyopathy may be appropriate

Induction/Maintenance

- With acute ingestion, may have severe hypertension; α/β-adrenergic blocker and receptor drugs and vasodilators may be necessary

- If necessary to treat hypotension, use sympathomimetics cautiously
- With chronic use, anesthetic requirements will be lower
- Anticipate potentiation of opioid analgesic effects

Adjuvants/Regional Anesthesia/Reversal

- Drug interactions noted are the major concerns

Postoperative Period

- Look for continued signs of CV, CNS hyperactivity
- Withdrawal symptoms not life threatening

ANTICIPATED PROBLEMS/CONCERNS

- Look for a history of substance abuse. These drugs have a high potential for abuse and are frequently combined with other addictive substances.
- Inquire as to recent drug usage, as this will alter anesthetic requirements and possibly monitoring
- Possible drug interactions

ANGIOTENSIN II RECEPTOR ANTAGONISTS Vidya T. Raman, M.D.

USES

- Only 25% of patients taking antihypertensives have adequately controlled BP
- New class of antihypertensives that are relatively safe and efficacious
- Alternative for patients not tolerating ACE inhibitors 2° to cough and angioedema

PERIOPERATIVE RISKS

- Rebound Htn if drug acutely withdrawn esp with longer-acting agents

WORRY ABOUT

- Refractory hypotension in patients undergoing general anesthesia. BP responds to vasopressin agonists.

OVERVIEW/PHARMOCOLOGY

- Renin-angiotensin cascade begins with the cleavage of angiotensin by renin
- This forms the inactive angiotensin I
- Angiotensin I converted by ACE to angiotensin II
- Angiotensin II receptors activated by binding of angiotensin II
- Two clinically important receptor subtypes are types 1 and 2
- Clinical effects of angiotensin II (vasoconstriction, sodium/water retention, renin suppression, etc.) are mediated by the angiotensin receptor 1 (AT1)
- Excreted mainly in bile and by kidneys
- Contraindicated in pregnancy

DRUG CLASS/USUAL DOSE

- Like ACE inhibitors, much more effective when coupled with diuretic. Thiazide diuretics used in combination.
- Available in once-a-day dosing
  - Candesartan (Atacand)
  - Irbesartan (Avapro)
  - Losartan (Cozaar)
  - Telmisartan (Micardis)
  - Valsartan (Diovan)

CHRONIC RX USES

- Antihypertensive, especially in those not tolerating ACE inhibitors
- CHF

ACUTE RX

- ACE inhibitors may be more efficacious initially
- Does not have first-dose hypotension effect in susceptible patient population

DRUG EFFECTS

SYSTEM	EFFECT	ASSESSMENT BY HX	PE	TEST
CV	Lowers BP	Assess response to Rx	BP	Monitor BP, can also have tachycardia and bradycardia with lowering BP Careful when D/C
GI	↑ in LFTs Rare reversible hepatotoxicity reported			Watch for rebound Htn, LFTs
METAB	Hyperkalemia			K^+
DERM	Angioedema reported	Ask patients for clinical Hx		
HEME	Microcytic anemia			CBC
RENAL	Can cause ARF if patients with renal artery stenosis or diffuse infrarenal stenosis			BUN/Cr
CNS		Rare headache, dizziness, fatigue Insomnia		

Key Reference: Burnier M: Angiotensin II receptor antagonists. Lancet 2000; 355:637–645.

POSSIBLE DRUG INTERACTIONS

Perioperative Period
- Assess BP and overall cardiac function

Induction/Maintenance
- Watch for refractory hypotension, which needs treatment with vasopressin agonist

Adjuvants/Regional Anesthesia/Reversal

- No known interactions

Postoperative Concerns
- Resumption of preop drugs for BP control
- Be aware of potential for rebound Htn in acute withdrawal
- Only available in PO forms

ANTICIPATED PROBLEMS

- Watch for hypotension with general anesthesia

APROTININ (TRASYLOL)

Frank W. Dupont, M.D.

USES

- To reduce periop blood loss
- Indications
  – Repeat CABG surgery and selected cases of primary CABG if risk of bleeding is especially high (e.g., preop NSAID use) or if transfusion is unacceptable or unavailable (orphan drug designation by FDA)
  – Complex primary and repeat operations, including aortic procedures
  – In repeat heart transplantation and in transplant candidates who require an LVAD
  – Role in pediatric cardiac surgery needs further definition
- Administered IV through a central line

PERIOPERATIVE RISKS

- Aprotinin, tranexamic acid, aminocaproic acid, desmopressin, and/or cell salvage are used in over 70% of cardiac surgery centers worldwide
- Side effects: anaphylactic and anaphylactoid reactions with repeated administration
- Adverse events such as myocardial infarction, graft closure, stroke, and renal failure are not more frequent with aprotinin Rx

WORRY ABOUT

- Increases ACT as measured by celite surface activation in the presence of heparin

OVERVIEW AND PHARMACOLOGY

- Modulates the systemic inflammatory response syndrome (SIRS) associated with CPB
- Rapid dispersion into extracellular space is followed by glomerular filtration and reabsorption into the proximal tubules where proteolytic degradation slowly inactivates it
- Biphasic elimination: initial $T_{1/2}$ of about 65 min followed by a terminal elimination $T_{1/2}$ of 12 h
- Reduced clearance and prolonged $T_{1/2}$ in patients with renal function impairment; alterations unnecessary if creatinine clearance is > 50 ml/min
- Insufficient pharmacokinetic data for hepatic disease

DRUG CLASS/MECH OF ACTION/USUAL DOSE

- Serine protease inhibitor obtained from bovine lung
- Precise mechanisms of action unclear, but inhibition of multiple mediators (kallikrein-kinin system, plasmin) results in attenuation of SIRS (↓ thrombin generation, fibrinolysis, and platelet glycoprotein loss)
- Dosing (do not administer with other drug in same line)
  – 1 ml (1.4 mg or 10,000 KIU) IV test dose 10 min before loading dose
  – Full dose: loading dose of 200 ml IV given over 20–30 min; constant infusion of 50 ml/h until the patient leaves the OR; pump priming dose of 200 ml
  – Half dose: loading dose of 100 ml IV given over 20–30 min; constant infusion of 25 ml/h until the patient leaves the OR; pump priming dose of 100 ml
- In patients with severe renal dysfunction, consider a reduction of the infusion rate to 25 ml/h after a full loading dose but elimination of the pump priming dose

ASSESSMENT POINTS

SYSTEM	EFFECT	ASSESSMENT BY HX	PE	TEST
CV	Anaphylactic shock	Prior exposure	Vital signs	
GU	Transient rise in creatinine concentration in postop period		Oliguria	BUN/Cr
DERM	Hypersensitivity reaction	Prior exposure	Pruritus, urticaria, erythema	

Key Reference: Segal H, Hunt BJ: Aprotinin: pharmacological reduction of perioperative bleeding. Lancet 2000; 355:1289–1290.

PERIOPERATIVE IMPLICATIONS/POSSIBLE DRUG INTERACTIONS

Preoperative Concerns

- Assess risk for hypersensitivity incidence: 5% within 6 mo, 0.9% after 6 mo, < 0.1% without prior exposure
- Test dose; patients who had hypersensitivity reaction to aprotinin should not be rechallanged
- In patients with a history of prior exposure to aprotinin
  – Availability of equipment and medications to manage anaphylaxis
  – Administration of test dose and loading dose only when able to rapidly cannulate

– Delay the addition of aprotinin into the pump priming solution of the cardiopulmonary bypass circuit until after both the test dose and the loading dose have been safely administered; H_1- and H_2-antagonists can be administered before the test dose
- Benefits in uncomplicated primary operations should be balanced against cost-benefit ratio and possibility of anaphylaxis should aprotinin be needed for repeat operation

Maintenance

- Maintain adequate anticoagulation by measurement of kaolin ACT, determination of free heparin levels (Hepcon/HMS), or fixed heparin dosing

- Base protamine dose not on ACT but on the actual amount of heparin administered
- Consider transfusion of platelets, FFP, and cryoprecipitate in the presence of bleeding not caused by hyperfibrinolysis

Postoperative Period

- Continue assessment of bleeding and monitoring of coagulation profiles after discontinuation of aprotinin Rx

ANTICIPATED PROBLEMS/CONCERNS

- Risk of serious or even fatal allergic reactions in patients re-exposed to aprotinin

ASPIRIN (ACETYLSALICYLIC ACID)

Christopher D. Beatie, M.D.

USES

- People within USA consume 10,000–20,000 tons annually
- Rx for mild/moderate pain, fever, arthritis, prevention of myocardial infarction

PERIOPERATIVE RISKS

- Peptic ulcer disease
- Plt dysfunction
- Hemorrhage
- Stroke
- Interstitial nephritis
- Reye's syndrome

WORRY ABOUT

- Displacement of protein-bound drugs: e.g., warfarin, sulfonylureas, thiopental, methotrexate
- Potentiation of anticoagulants

OVERVIEW/PHARMACOLOGY

- Cyclooxygenase inhibition prevents plt aggregation and vasoconstriction
- Plt inhibition irreversible for the life of the plt
- Aspirin
  - Metabolized by liver, excreted by kidney
  - Mildly antagonizes antihypertensive medications (β-blockers, vasodilators, diuretics)
  - Displaces protein-bound drugs, increasing their effects

DRUG CLASS/MECH OF ACTION/USUAL DOSE

- NSAID
- Cyclooxygenase inhibitor
- Chronically taken for
  - Musculoskeletal pain (e.g., arthritis, neuralgia)
  - Prevention of myocardial infarction
  - Claudication
- Acutely taken for
  - Acute, mild to moderate pain (e.g., headache, myalgia)
  - Fever
  - Dysmenorrhea
- Usual dose, 325–1000 mg q 3–4 h for acute illnesses and pain
- 62.5–325 mg for plt inhibitor effects
- Alternatives: acetaminophen, other NSAIDs (ibuprofen, naproxen), steroids, opioids, gold, ticlopidine, dipyridamole, pentoxifylline

DRUG EFFECTS

SYSTEM	EFFECT	ASSESSMENT BY HX	PE	TEST
RESP	Hyperventilation, respiratory alkalosis		Tachypnea	ABGs
GI	Gastritis PUD	Dyspepsia Nausea, vomiting, hematemesis, melena		Endoscopy Upper GI x-rays, stool heme, Hgb
ENDO	Hyperglycemia, corticosteroid release			Glucose
HEME	Plt dysfunction	Bleeding, bruising	Hematomata, petechiae	Bleeding time
HEPATIC	Hepatocellular damage	Nausea, anorexia	Hepatomegaly, jaundice	SGOT, SGPT, alk phos
TOXICITY				
CV	Vasomotor paralysis		Hypotension	
RESP	Hypoventilation, respiratory acidosis		Hypopnea	ABGs
DERM	Eruptions	Pruritus	Acneiform, erythematous, pruritic, eczematoid, or desquamative lesions	
RENAL	Renal failure due to analgesic nephropathy	Oliguria, anuria	Edema, rales	BUN/Cr, UA, CXR
CNS	Headache, tinnitus, drowsiness, dizziness, diminished vision and hearing		Sweating, confusion, convulsions, coma	
ACID-BASE	Metabolic acidosis			ABGs

Key Reference: Urmey WF, Rowlingson J: Do antiplatelet agents contribute to the development of perioperative spinal hematoma? Reg Anesth Pain Med 1998; 23:146–181.

PERIOPERATIVE IMPLICATIONS

Preoperative Concerns

- Discontinued 1 wk prior to surgery for full reversal of plt inhibition (need only 1/7 of normally functioning platelets, so if no dilution effect expected, need only 48 h off low-dose ASA; can be switched to shorter-acting antithrombotic agents (e.g., heparin) until just before surgery if desired
- May potentiate the effects of protein-bound drugs

Induction/Maintenance

- Possible mildly exaggerated effects of thiopental

Adjuvants/Regional Anesthesia/Reversal

- May increase the risk of hemorrhagic complications of regional anesthesia. Aspirin does not contraindicate regional anesthesia, but those techniques with low potential for bleeding are preferable (e.g., spinal may be preferred over epidural).
- May increase the risk of hemorrhagic complications of invasive monitoring

SPECIAL CONSIDERATIONS

- A potent inhibitor of plt aggregation that can seriously impair surgical hemostasis. Most surgeons request discontinuation of aspirin 1 wk prior to surgery. However, if CAD or other vascular occlusive disease will be left untreated, consult with surgeon, pt's primary physician, and pt about advisability of discontinuing aspirin.
- Risks of regional anesthesia and invasive monitoring may be increased
- May displace protein-bound drugs (e.g., warfarin, sulfonylureas, thiopental, methotrexate), thus augmenting their effects
- Associated with gastritis, PUD, GI bleeding, and increased risk for aspiration of gastric contents
- Associated with Reye's syndrome and contraindicated in febrile viral illness in children

ASTHMA DRUGS, NEW— ORAL ANTILEUKOTRIENE DRUGS
(ACCOLATE [ZAFIRLUKAST], SINGULAIR [MONTELUKAST], ZYFLO [ZILEUTON])

Michael J. Bishop, M.D.

USES

• Recent advances in asthma therapy have resulted from the recognition that it is primarily an inflammatory disease
• No major changes in the last 5 y in treatment of acute asthma
• Changes in the treatment of chronic asthma include
  − ↑ Use of inhaled corticosteroids
  − Introduction of the inhaled anti-inflammatory nedocromil
  − Introduction of oral antileukotriene drugs zileuton, montelukast, and zafirlukast
• Drugs for chronic treatment have no place in the treatment of an acute asthma attack

RISKS

• All three drugs are taken orally
• As of now, these drugs are recommended for use in mild persistent asthma. Their ultimate place in therapy remains to be determined.
• Effects of antileukotriene antagonists are modest. Do not rely on these to prevent asthma attack in the presence of airway stimulation.
• Zafirlukast and zileuton inhibit warfarin metabolism and can affect liver function
• Zileuton can inhibit metabolism of theophylline
• Zileuton can result in liver enzyme elevation in some

OVERVIEW AND PHARMACOLOGY

• Antileukotriene inhibitors target the lipoxygenase pathway, which converts arachidonic acid to leukotrienes whose effects include chemotaxis, bronchoconstriction, mucus secretion, edema, and eosinophilia
• Zileuton inhibits the first step of the pathway—conversion of arachidonic acid to leukotriene A4 by the enzyme 5-lipoxygenase
• Zafirlukast and montelukast act as receptor antagonists for the cysteinyl leukotrienes, leukotrienes C4, D4, and E4
• Related enzyme and receptor inhibitors are under development. Other drugs that act on leukotriene synthesis and receptors are under investigation, including drugs that act on 5-lipoxygenase activating protein and LTB_4 receptor antagonists.
• Based on responses to existing drugs, however, it is not anticipated that any of these approaches will provide monotherapy

DRUG EFFECTS

SYSTEM	EFFECT	ASSESSMENT BY HX	PE	TEST
HEPATIC	Dysfunction	N/V, itching, bleeding	Excoriations, jaundice, hemarthrosis	LFTs

Key Reference: Georgitis JW: The 1997 asthma management guidelines and therapeutic issues relating to the treatment of asthma. Chest 1999; 115:210−217.

PERIOPERATIVE IMPLICATIONS

• Drug interactions with warfarin and theophylline
• Patients requiring these drugs are asthmatic; these drugs will not necessarily prevent bronchoconstriction to an acute stimulus

• Prophylactic β-adrenergic agonists prior to surgery

• These drugs are sometimes used in an effort to lower doses of oral steroids. If recent steroid usage, may be at risk of adrenal suppression.

ATORVASTATIN (LIPITOR)

Lori Heller, M.D.

USES

- Synthetic lipid-lowering agent
- Evidence widely shows lowering cholesterol reduces the incidence of CAD and results in ↓ in morbidity and mortality
- Selective, competitive HMG CoA reductase inhibitor (the rate-limiting enzyme of cholesterol synthesis)
- Statins also modify endothelial function, inflammatory responses, plaque stability, and thrombogenicity
- Also been shown to ↓ risk of first major coronary event in patients with no known risk factors for CAD and normal LDL cholesterol levels

PERIOPERATIVE RISKS

- Clinically important side effects of all statins include myositis and liver dysfunction
- Incidence of ↑ transaminase levels of more than 3× normal is <2%
- LFT elevations completely reversible and resolve within few weeks on discontinuation of the drug
- Severe hepatic dysfunction or cirrhosis not reported
- Associated rarely with rhabdomyolysis in the periop period of major surgeries
- Myositis rarely seen with monotherapy. ↑ Significantly (to nearly 30%) when used in combination with immunosuppressives (cyclosporine, tacrolimus), azole antifungal agents (ketoconazole, itraconazole), fibrinic acid derivatives (gemfibrozil), niacin, erythromycin, clarithromycin, and fluvoxamine. Greater risk with those on higher doses of statins, >age 70 y, and with baseline renal insufficiency.

PHARMACOKINETICS/PHARMACODYNAMICS

- Antilipemic drug: interferes with production and enhances uptake of cholesterol and its lipoprotein complexes
- Orally administered and rapidly absorbed
- Hepatic first-pass metabolism causes a low systemic bioavailability
- Undergoes extensive metabolism to active metabolites
- Elimination of parent drug and metabolites occurs primarily in bile after hepatic and/or extrahepatic metabolism
- <2% of a dose recovered in urine
- Mean plasma elimination $T_{1/2}$ 14 h, but $T_{1/2}$ of HMG CoA reductase inhibitory activity is 20–30 h due to the active metabolites. As a result, drug has greater efficacy than other statins.

DRUG CLASS/MECH OF ACTION/USUAL DOSE

- Inhibition of HMG CoA reductase results in decreased synthesis of hepatic cholesterol
- Compensatory ↑ in hepatic LDL receptor production then results in an ↑ in uptake of LDL cholesterol from the circulation
- Reduces elevated total cholesterol, LDL-C, apo B, triglyceride levels and ↑HDL-C
- Usual initial dosage 10 mg once daily. Maintenance dosage 10–80 mg once daily.
- No dosage modifications needed for renal insufficiency

DRUG EFFECTS

SYSTEM	EFFECT	ASSESSMENT BY HX	PE	TEST
HEPATIC	Transaminitis	Asymptomatic		LFTs
GI	Bloating, dyspepsia	Abdominal pain	Abdominal exam	
MS	Myalgias, myositis, arthralgias, rhabdomyolysis	Muscle aches, tenderness or weakness; malaise, fever	Musculoskeletal exam/palpation	CPK
DERM	Rash		Inspection of skin	

Key Reference: Rosenberg AD, Neuwirth MG, Kagen LJ, Singh K, Fischer HD, Bernstein RL: Intraoperative rhabdomyolysis in a patient receiving pravastatin, a 3-hydroxy-3-methylglutaryl coenzyme A (HMG CoA) reductase inhibitor. Anesth Analg 1995; 81:1089–1091.

PERIOPERATIVE IMPLICATIONS

Preoperative Concerns

- Assess for CAD and other associated conditions such as Htn, diabetes, atherosclerotic CVD
- When possible, HMG CoA reductase inhibitors should be discontinued preoperatively, esp for surgery that may result in significant skeletal muscle damage
- Based on a $T_{1/2}$ of 30 h for its active metabolites, the drug should be discontinued 3–5 days preoperatively
- Should also be discontinued in patients with symptoms suggestive of a myopathy or with other risk factors predisposing to the development of renal failure 2° to rhabdomyolysis such as hypotension, trauma, and severe acute infection
- No known concern about rebound or side effects from short-term discontinuation

Induction/Maintenance

- No reported cases of atorvastatin associated intraop/periop events, although other statins have been associated with adverse events such as rhabdomyolysis and concomitant myoglobinuria and renal failure

Adjuvants/Regional Anesthesia/Reversal

- No interactions known

Postoperative Concerns

- Relatively long elimination $T_{1/2}$ makes resumption of drug in immediate postop period unnecessary
- May be at ↑risk for cardiac event given known risk factor

DRUG INTERACTIONS

- Risk of myopathy ↑ with concurrent administration of cyclosporine and erythromycin
- Antacids ↓ plasma concentrations by 35%
- Digoxin levels can ↑ by 20%

ANTICIPATED PROBLEMS/CONCERNS

- Assess for CAD, discontinue 3–5 days before major surgery

ATROPINE

Nishan G. Goudsouzian, M.D.

USES

- Major use: treatment for sinus bradycardia
- Decrease perioperative oral and tracheobronchial secretions
- Counteract muscarinic effects of cholinergic agents during reversal of muscle relaxants
- Symptomatic type I second degree AV block
- Bradycardia with hypotension during resuscitation
- Treatment of organophosphate poisoning

PERIOPERATIVE RISKS

- Tachycardia that may aggravate cardiac ischemia or CHF

WORRY ABOUT

- ?Increase in intraocular tension in patients with acute angle glaucoma
- Inhibition of mucus secretion in respiratory tract
- Dry mouth
- Blurred vision
- Flushing (occasionally in infants)

OVERVIEW/PHARMACOLOGY

- Competitive inhibition of the action of acetylcholine at autonomic cholinergic receptors (parasympatholytic)
- Plasma $T_{1/2}$ 4 h
- Metabolized by liver, excreted by kidneys

DRUG CLASS/MECH OF ACTION/USUAL DOSE

- Inhibits action of acetylcholine on autonomic effectors innervated by postganglionic cholinergic nerves (antimuscarinic effect)
- At high doses produces partial block of autonomic ganglia (nicotinic receptors)

USUAL DOSE (70 KG ADULT)

- 0.4–0.5 mg IV for intraoperative bradycardia
- 1–2 mg IV before reversal of muscle relaxants
- 1–2 mg IV for intrinsic sinus node dysfunction
- 1–2 mg IV initial treatment of organophosphate poisoning repeated prn
- 0.4–0.5 mg SQ, IM for control of secretions
- 0.01–0.02 mg/kg in infants and children (minimum 0.1 mg)

DRUG EFFECTS

SYSTEM	EFFECT	RX ASSESSMENT	PE	TEST
HEENT	Diminished secretions	Dry mouth and upper airways	Dry mucosa, difficulty in swallowing	
	Blocking of the sphincteric and ciliary muscles	Mydriasis	Dilated pupils	? ↑ Intraocular tension in acute angle glaucoma
CV	Blocking vagal effects of M2 receptors on SA node	Tachycardia	Palpitation	ECG, sinus tachycardia, marked in young people with ↑ vagal tone
RESP	Dry airways	Thick secretions	? ↓ Air entry (rare)	CXR
GI	Some ↓ in gastric acid secretions	Large doses ↓ peristalsis	Decrease in gastric residual volume	Mild decrease in acidity
GU	Blocking of the sphincteric muscles	Pain in lower abdomen	Enlarged bladder	Urine output Percussion on US of bladder
CNS	Toxic doses	Restlessness, disorientation, delirium		
DERM	Flushing (rarely, in infants after large doses)	Red body, dry skin	? ↑ Body temp	

Key Reference: Brown JH, Taylor P: Muscarinic receptor agonists and antagonists. *In* Hardman JG, Limbird LE (eds): Goodman & Gilman's The Pharmacological Basis of Therapeutics, 9th ed. New York, McGraw-Hill Professional Publishing, 1996, pp 148–154.

PERIOPERATIVE COMPLICATIONS

- Dry mouth (consider mouthwash)
- Thick pulmonary secretions (humidity)
- Aggravate CHF or angina (slow HR by cholinergic drugs or β-blockers)

Induction/Maintenance

- Rarely used routinely

Adjuvants/Regional Anesthesia/Reversal

- Effect cleared within few hours
- In emergency, consider cholinergic drugs or β-blockers

SPECIAL CONSIDERATIONS

- For resuscitation, larger doses are required
- In the absence of IV, 2–4 mg/70 kg diluted in 10 ml NS can be given via an endotracheal tube

BENZODIAZEPINES
(MIDAZOLAM, LORAZEPAM, DIAZEPAM)

Harry J.M. Lemmens, M.D., Ph.D.

USES
- Prescribed for the treatment of anxiety
- Used for conscious sedation and premedication

PERIOPERATIVE RISKS
- High levels associated with hypnosis, unconsciousness, respiratory depression, apnea

WORRY ABOUT
- Combination with opioids or other CNS depressants may result in severe respiratory depression, apnea, hypotension

OVERVIEW/PHARMACOLOGY
- Anxiolysis, sedation, hypnosis, muscle relaxation, anterograde amnesia, anticonvulsant
- Midazolam: short-elimination $T_{1/2}$ (2.5 h)
- Lorazepam: intermediate-elimination $T_{1/2}$ (15 h)
- Diazepam: long-elimination $T_{1/2}$ (30 h)
- Metabolized by hepatic microsomal oxidation and glucuronide conjugation
- Diazepam has active metabolites

- Midazolam IV: peak effect in 2–4 min
  IM: peak effect in 30–60 min
- Lorazepam IV: peak effect in 5–15 min, painful injection, thrombophlebitis
  IM: peak effect in 60–90 min
  Oral: peak effect in 2 h
- Diazepam IV: peak effect in 1–2 min, painful injection, thrombophlebitis
  IM: painful, unpredictable absorption, do not use
  Oral: peak effect in 30–60 min, well absorbed; food, aluminum-containing antacids delay absorption
- No clear difference in speed of recovery from diazepam and midazolam drug effect after low dose for sedation in short procedures; faster recovery from midazolam drug effect becomes more prominent after larger dose/prolonged administration

- Lorazepam provides long duration (> 4 h) of sedation and amnesia by any route of administration; do not use when rapid recovery from drug effect desired
- Prolonged use can lead to tolerance

DRUG CLASS/MECH OF ACTION/USUAL DOSE
- Anxiolytic, sedative, hypnotic
- Potentiation of gamma-aminobutyric acid–mediated neural inhibition
- Safe use involves careful titration to the desired effect
- Usual dosage for premedication and conscious sedation:
  - Midazolam IV: 0.5–1 mg, repeated; maintenance infusion: 0.04–0.10 mg/kg/h
    IM: 0.07 mg/kg
    Oral: 15 mg (not available in USA)
  - Lorazepam IV: 0.25 mg, repeated
    IM: 0.05 mg/kg, max 4 mg
    Oral: 0.5–4 mg
  - Diazepam IV: 1–2 mg, repeated
    Oral: 5–10 mg

DRUG EFFECTS

SYSTEM	EFFECT	PE	TEST
CV	Decreased systemic vascular resistance and cardiac output	Arterial BP	
RESP	Central respiratory depression Apnea	Resp rate	Tidal volume Minute volume, capnography, oximetry
CNS	Anxiolysis Sedation Hypnosis Amnesia Anticonvulsant ↓ Cerebral metabolic rate and cerebral blood flow	Slurred speech, drowsiness, ataxia Unresponsiveness	

Key Reference: Reves JG, Glass PSA, Lubarsky DA: Nonbarbiturate intravenous anesthetics. *In* Miller RD (ed): Anesthesia, 5th ed. Philadelphia, Churchill Livingstone, 2000, pp 228–272.

PERIOPERATIVE IMPLICATIONS / POSSIBLE DRUG INTERACTIONS

Preoperative Concerns
- Elderly: Reduce dose up to 5-fold (5–10%/decade reduction)
- Cimetidine, ranitidine (microsomal cytochrome P450 inhibitors), and liver cirrhosis ↓ clearance; enhanced effect may be seen

- Smoking and enzyme-inducing drugs ↑ diazepam clearance
- Renal failure ↑ diazepam $T_{1/2}$
- Monitor ventilation

Induction/Maintenance
- Synergistic interaction with anesthesia induction agents, opioids

Regional Anesthesia
- Possibly exacerbated respiratory depression during spinal anesthesia (mechanism unknown)

ANTICIPATED PROBLEMS/CONCERNS
- Combination with opioids or other CNS depressants may result in severe respiratory depression, apnea, hypotension
- Large doses result in prolonged drowsiness and respiratory depression, especially in the elderly
- Undesirable degree of amnesia

BETA-ADRENERGIC RECEPTOR ANTAGONISTS (BLOCKERS)

Roberta Hines, M.D.

USES

- 10 Million in USA receive routinely
- Used in management of essential Htn
- Effective in decreasing infarct size
- Used to ↓ HR
- Available as oral and IV preparations
- Used to suppress cardiac dysrhythmias
- Value in prevention of excess SNS activity
- Should certainly be continued periop in patients who have been taking them
- Reduced CV morbidity and mortality in patients with ischemic heart disease for major surgery with periop use of β-blockers
- Traditional use of β-blockers may be overestimated in this population
- Whether one should give β-blockers perioperatively to patients with cardiac risk factors alone remains unclear

PERIOPERATIVE RISKS

- Nonselective blocker may precipitate bronchospasm
- May worsen or precipitate CHF in patients with ↓ LV function
- May cause hypotension, bradycardia

WORRY ABOUT

- ↓ Ventricular performance especially with underlying cardiac dysfunction
- Can worsen lung disease, especially with nonspecific blockers and Hx of COPD or bronchospasm

OVERVIEW/PHARMACOLOGY

- All β-blockers are derivatives of isoproterenol
- β-adrenergic receptor agonists classified as partial or pure agonists on basis or absence of intrinsic sympathomimetic activity
- Partial antagonists often better tolerated than pure antagonists in patients with ↓ LV function
- β-blocker may produce varying degrees of membrane stabilization in heart (detectable only at extremely high plasma concentration)
- Effective in both acute, chronic management

DRUG CLASS/MECH OF ACTION/USUAL DOSE

- All β-blockers bind selectively to β-receptors
- β-blockers interfere with ability of other drugs/substances with sympathomimetic activity to activate β-receptors
- Action of β-blockers negates effect of catecholamines, other sympathomimetics on heart and smooth muscle of airways, blood vessels
- Bind to β-receptor by competitive inhibition
- Exhibit selective affinity for β-adrenergic receptors
- Binding of agonists to the β-receptor is reversible
- Chronic administration is associated with ↑ in number of β-adrenergic receptors
- Principal method of clearance hepatic, renal, or plasma hydrolysis (esmolol)
- Elimination $T_{1/2}$ specific to individual agents, depends on dose, protein binding, route of administration (oral/IV)

DRUG EFFECTS

SYSTEM	EFFECT	ASSESSMENT BY HX	PE	TEST
CV	↓ HR ↓ CO ↓ LV function ↑ Coronary vascular resistance ↓ Myocardial O_2 consumption	Relief of angina ↓ BP ↓ HR	HR BP	ECG; stress ECG
RESP	↑ Airway resistance (especially nonselective agents)	↑ Wheezing ↑ Bronchospasm		FEV_1 ↑ Peak airway pressure
ENDO	Hyperglycemia Hypokalemia			Laboratory measurements of K^+ and glucose
CNS	Fatigue, lethargy, peripheral paresthesia, withdrawal hypersensitivity			
OB	All cross placenta, fetal effect: bradycardia, hypotension, hypoglycemia			

Key Reference: Poldermans D, Boersma E, Bax JJ, et al: The effect of bisoprolol on perioperative mortality and myocardial infarction in high-risk patients undergoing vascular surgery. Dutch Echocardiographic Cardiac Risk Evaluation Applying Stress Echocardiography Study Group. N Engl J Med 1999; 341:1789–1794.

PERIOPERATIVE IMPLICATIONS / POSSIBLE DRUG INTERACTIONS

Preoperative Concerns

- β-blocker should be continued in periop period
- Acute discontinuation can result in excess SNS activity that manifests in 24–48 h

Induction/Maintenance

- Myocardial depression observed with inhaled or injected anesthetic is worsened with addition of β-blocker

- Esolol has been associated with profound bradycardia in presence of inhaled anesthetics

Adjuvants/Regional Anesthesia/Reversal

- Bradycardic effects often can be reversed by atropine
- Isoproterenol most effective at reversing negative cardiac (both dromotropic and inotropic) effects; but need to administer 1 dose of isoproterenol (2–25 $\mu g/min^{-1}$) to reverse negative cardiac effect

- $CaCl_2$ (250–1000 mg) or glucagon (1–5 mg) administered IV (adult) effectively reverses myocardial depression
- Life-threatening bradycardia may require insertion of transvenous pacemaker

SPECIAL PROBLEMS/CONSIDERATIONS

- When β-blockers are administered in presence of anesthetic drugs they may unmask direct negative inotropic effects of concomitantly administered anesthetic; this effect results in profound ↓ in BP, CO

BICARBONATE SODIUM

Randy H. Steadman, M.D.

INDICATIONS

- IV Rx for moderate to severe acidemia most commonly due to cardiac arrest, also to non-arrest-related lactic or ketoacidosis
- May be given orally in renal tubular acidosis
- To treat hyperkalemia

PERIOPERATIVE RISKS

- Administration results in rapid generation of CO_2, a potent negative inotrope; also intramyocardial acidosis worsened by CO_2 generated as it rapidly diffuses intracellularly.
- Ability to defibrillate VFIB successfully correlates more with tissue P_{CO_2} than extracellular pH: thus the change in recommendations for restraint in use. Used only after more definitive and better substantiated Rx—defibrillation, chest compression, adequate ventilation, and other drugs such as vasopressors and antiarrhythmics.

WORRY ABOUT

- CSF acidosis due to rapid diffusion of bicarbonate-generated CO_2
- ↑ Affinity of hemoglobin for O_2, limiting O_2 release to tissues
- Hypernatremia, hyperosmolality associated with ↓ survival

OVERVIEW/PHARMACOLOGY

- During cardiopulmonary arrest, hypoxia-caused anaerobic metabolism results in lactic acidosis; ventilatory failure results in hypercarbic respiratory acidosis; prompt ventilation necessary for oxygenation, elimination of CO_2
- Acts as H^+ ion acceptor or base to buffer metabolic acidosis; after reacting with H^+ ion, carbonic acid and then ultimately CO_2, H_2O formed; CO_2 eliminated by lungs under conditions of normal ventilation and perfusion
- During CPR (CO 25% of normal) results in accumulation of CO_2, which diffuses readily, causing intracellular hypercarbic acidosis

DRUG CLASS/MECH OF ACTION/USUAL DOSE

- Clinically the most widely used buffer
- Acutely used to correct moderate to severe metabolic acidosis of any cause
  - To treat hyperkalemia
  - To treat tricyclic overdose
  - Alkaline diuresis promotes excretion of phenobarbital and salicylate
- Chronically used orally to correct metabolic acidosis of any cause
- Usual dose: 0.5–1 mEq/kg
  - Alternatives: *Tham:* rapidly crosses cell membranes to work intracellularly (bicarbonate works predominantly extracellularly); however, its vasodilatory action reduces aortic and coronary perfusion pressures, which adversely affects outcome; *sodium carbonate:* works extracellularly; very alkaline pH may induce local tissue injury and cardiac dysrhythmias; *carbicarb* (Na bicarbonate plus Na carbonate): ↓ in coronary perfusion pressure due to vasodilator effect; *tribonate* (Na bicarbonate plus Tham plus phosphate plus acetate): may be more effective in treating intracellular acidosis, but documentation of effectiveness in outcome during human CPR not available

DRUG EFFECTS

SYSTEM	EFFECT	TEST
CV	Although metabolic acidosis lowers threshold for VFIB, bicarb *has no effect on the defibrillation threshold; no change in survival in cardiac arrest*	
RESP	CO_2 produced requires ↑ ventilation	ABGs (P_{CO_2}, pH, P_{O_2}, HCO_3)
HEME	Alkalemia shifts oxyhemoglobin dissociation curve to the left with less O_2 release to tissue	ABGs
GU	Alkaline diuresis aids in excretion of phenobarbital and salicylate after toxic ingestions	Urine pH > 7
CNS	CSF acidosis possibly associated with post-CPR cerebral depression; hyperosmolar state may be associated with ↓ survival, intraventricular hemorrhage, alkalemia, ↑ CVR, ↓ CBF	

Key Reference: Levy M: An evidence-based evaluation of the use of sodium bicarbonate during cardiopulmonary resuscitation. Crit Care Clin 1998; 14:457–483.

PERIOPERATIVE IMPLICATIONS/POSSIBLE DRUG INTERACTIONS

- In the presence of bicarbonate, Ca^{2+} salts precipitate as carbonates

Preoperative Concerns

- Bicarbonate shift of K^+ from extra- to intracellular (digoxin toxicity may be worsened)

Induction/Maintenance

- With alkalemia, basic drugs (opioids, local anesthetics) ↑ activity due to higher non-ionized fraction crossing membranes

Adjuvants/Regional Anesthesia/Reversal

- Metabolic alkalosis associated with difficulty antagonizing NMB
- Inhibitory effect of metabolic acidosis on catecholamines not documented at pH values encountered during cardiac arrest

SPECIAL CONSIDERATIONS

- Effective ventilation, oxygenation, and circulation during CPR are the primary means of prevention and treatment of acidemia associated with cardiac arrest. Bicarbonate has not been shown to change survival in cardiac arrest.

BLEOMYCIN

Mark J. Lema, M.D., Ph.D.

RISK

- 10% incidence of interstitial pneumonitis
- 1% mortality from pulm fibrosis
- Pulm toxicity both dose-related (>250 U total dose) and age-related (>65 y)
- Idiosyncratic reactions have occurred at lower doses (20 U)
- Pts having previous radiation Rx to lungs or with a Hx of COPD are at ↑risk
- Anaphylaxis known to occur idiosyncratically

PERIOPERATIVE RISKS

- Rapidly progressive interstitial pneumonitis known to occur after general anesthesia using O_2 conc >30%, overhydrating pt
- Pts who received ≥250 U or additional antineoplastic drugs are at ↑ risk of pulm toxicity

WORRY ABOUT

- Sustained O_2 conc >30%
- Liberal use of maintenance fluids

OVERVIEW/PHARMACOLOGY

- 1 U bleomycin = 1 mg activity of bleomycin
- $T_{1/2}\beta$ 2 h, but Cr <35 ml/min exponentially ↑ $T_{1/2}$; 70% is recovered in urine as active bleomycin
- For squamous cell carcinoma (head and neck, skin, genitals; lymphomas; testicular carcinomas)

DRUG CLASS/MECH OF ACTION

- Mixture of cytotoxic antibiotics isolated from *Streptomyces verticillus*
- Cytotoxic action caused by inhibition of DNA synthesis
- Usual dose: 0.25–0.5 U/kg (10–20 U/m^2) to 400 U (total dose)

DRUG EFFECTS

SYSTEM	EFFECT	ASSESSMENT BY HX	PE	TEST
CV	Raynaud's (rare)	Color changes in fingers	Observation	
RESP	Interstitial pneumonitis (10%) Pulmonary fibrosis (1%)	Dose (>250 U), age (>65 y) Previous lung disease	Dyspnea, fine rales and cough, fever	PFTs ($\downarrow$ TLC, $\downarrow$ VC)
GI	N/V			
HEME	(Not associated with pancytopenia)			
DERM	Mucocutaneous toxicity (50%)	1–3 wk after start of Rx (dose 150–200 U)	Urticaria, hyperpigmentation, hyperkeratosis, alopecia	

Key Reference: McEvoy GK (ed): AHRS 95 Drug Information. Bethesda, MD, pp 600–602.

PERIOPERATIVE IMPLICATIONS

Preoperative Period

- Assess bleomycin cumulative dose (>250 U)
- Assess age (>65 y)
- Assess previous lung disease Hx
- Ask about previous radiation to thorax
- Obtain PFTs, CXR, ABGs

Interoperative Period

- Limit delivered O_2 to <30% if adequate for O_2 sat >89%
- Limit fluids and avoid fluid overload
- Consider CVP or PA monitoring
- Consider arterial monitoring and sampling
- Use upper limit alarm for % O_2 delivery

Postoperative Period

- Keep delivered O_2 to <30% if adequate for O_2 sat >89%
- Limit fluids
- Corticosteroid use for pulm toxicity controversial

SPECIAL CONSIDERATIONS

- Cyclophosphamide, radiation Rx (thorax) potentiates pulmonary toxicity
- Cisplatin potentiates renal insufficiency
- Vinca alkaloids (vincristine, vinblastine, VP-16) potentiate Raynaud's phenomenon
- Mitomycin C exhibits similar properties to those of bleomycin but with milder effects

BRETYLIUM TOSYLATE

K. Gage Parr, M.D.
George S. Leisure, M.D.
Roger A. Johns, M.D.

INDICATIONS

- Rx for
  – IV admin in VFIB or life-threatening VTach unresponsive to conventional antiarrhythmic Rx
  – May be useful in the treatment of ventricular tachyarrhythmias induced by accidental IV injection of bupivacaine

WORRY ABOUT

- Tricyclic antidepressants, guanethidine may interfere with bretylium's actions
- Electrophysiologic effects possibly antagonized by concomitant use of quinidine
- Concomitant use of catecholamines can lead to increased BP due to sympathetic denervation

OVERVIEW/PHARMACOLOGY

- Class III antiarrhythmic agent
- Cleared by renal excretion, found unchanged in urine
- $T_{1/2}$ of 6–14 h
- GFR 10–50 ml/min: reduce dose by 25–50%
- GFR < 10 ml/min; avoid bretylium
- Dialysis removes bretylium
- Negligible protein binding, 1–6%
- Large V_d

DRUG CLASS/MECH OF ACTION/USUAL DOSE

- Class III antiarrhythmic agent with anti-adrenergic, direct electrophysiologic actions
- Prolongs action potential duration without altering conduction velocity, upstroke, membrane responsiveness
- Delays conduction of premature electrical impulses
- Seldom prolongs QT interval sufficiently to induce torsades de pointes
- Biphasic hemodynamic response; initial transient tachycardia, Htn lasting ~ 15 min, reflecting catecholamine release; thereafter HR, BP, and vascular resistance fall
- ↓ The energy required to defibrillate heart; improves success rate for countershock
- May lead to spontaneous cardioversion
- Dose: IV bolus of 5–10 mg/kg, repeated 15–30 min later if needed to max 30 mg/kg; continuous infusion of 1–2 mg/min

DRUG EFFECTS

SYSTEM	EFFECT	ASSESSMENT BY HX	PE	TEST
HEENT	Congestion, parotitis			
CV	Initial transient ↑ BP, ↑ HR, inevitable ↓ BP, rare bradycardia, rare proarrhythmia	Syncope, dizziness	Orthostasis	
GI	N/V, diarrhea			
ENDO	Hyperthermia			
GU	Renal dysfunction (rare)			↑ BUN, Cr
CNS	Confusion (rare due to poor CNS penetration), lethargy, anxiety			

Key Reference: Gallagher JD: Class III antiarrhythmic agents: Bretylium, sotalol, amiodarone. *In* Lynch C III (ed): Clinical Cardiac Electrophysiology. Philadelphia, JB Lippincott, 1994, p 113.

PERIOPERATIVE IMPLICATIONS/POSSIBLE DRUG INTERACTIONS

- Only used when defibrillation, epinephrine, lidocaine have failed to correct VFIB, or defibrillation, lidocaine, procainamide have failed to control VTach associated with a pulse
- Usually considered to be contraindicated in Rx of arrhythmias induced by cardiac glycosides

- Initial release of norepinephrine by bretylium may worsen these arrhythmias; some animal, human studies showed benefit in Rx for cardiac glycoside–induced ventricular arrhythmias

SPECIAL CONSIDERATIONS

- Admin with extreme caution to those with fixed cardiac output (severe pulm hypertension, aortic stenosis) since ↓ BP, peripheral resistance may not be accompanied by ↑ in cardiac output
- Orthostatic hypotension common
- Severe N/V can occur
- Hyperthermia: body temp may reach 108°F within 30 min of admin

CALCIUM-CHANNEL BLOCKERS Carol L. Lake, M.D., M.B.A., M.P.H.

INDICATIONS

- Prescribed to treat Htn, arrhythmias, heart failure, angina, cerebral vasospasm, atherosclerosis, and HCM

PERIOPERATIVE RISKS

- Many patients receive Ca^{2+}-channel blockers because of their systemic, cerebral, and coronary vasodilator properties, antiarrhythmic properties through slowed conduction velocity and prolonged refractoriness of nodal tissues, antiatherogenic effects, and reduced platelet aggregation in coronary and systemic vasculature

WORRY ABOUT

- Hypotension, decreasing coronary perfusion pressures
- Excessive myocardial depression in patients with depressed myocardial function
- AV nodal block, bradycardia, asystole
- Worsening heart failure
- Physiologic effects of Ca^{2+}-channel blockers may be additive with volatile anesthetic agents
- Acute withdrawal may precipitate acute coronary ischemia

OVERVIEW AND PHARMACOLOGY

- Ca^{2+} channels—functional pores in cardiac and smooth muscle cell membranes—allow calcium to flow down an electrochemical gradient. Channels are also present in sarcoplasmic reticulum and mitochondria. Calcium is a primary generator of the cardiac action potential and intracellular second messenger regulating many intracellular events.
- Calcium enters through voltage-dependent or receptor-operated channels. There are 3 types of voltage-dependent channels: N (neuronal), T (transient), and L (long lasting).
- Nifedipine: 90% absorbed PO, 65–76% bioavailability, PO onset of action 20 min and peak effect 1–2 h, elimination by first-pass hepatic metabolism with $T_{1/2}$ of 2–5 h
- Verapamil: 90% absorbed PO, 20–35% bioavailability, IV onset of action in 2 min, PO onset of action 2 h, peak effect IV 3–5 min, PO peak effect 3–4 h, 85% eliminated by first-pass hepatic metabolism with elimination $T_{1/2}$ of 3–7 h.
- Diltiazem: 89–90% PO absorption, 40–70% bioavailability, PO onset of action <15 min, peak effect 30 min, 60% metabolized by liver, remainder excreted by kidneys, $T_{1/2}$ 3.5–6.0 h

- Bepridil: >90% absorption, >80% bioavailability, PO onset of action 2–3 h, peak effect 8 h, hepatic elimination with $T_{1/2}$ 26–64 h
- Hepatic disease may necessitate decreased dosing of verapamil and other Ca^{2+}-channel blockers

DRUG CLASS/MECH OF ACTION/USUAL DOSE

- Four different classes of Ca blockers: (1) 1,4 dihydropyridine (e.g., nifedipine, nicardipine, nimodipine), (2) phenylalkyl-amines (e.g., verapamil), (3) benzothiazepines (e.g., diltiazem), (4) diarylaminopropranolamine ether (e.g., bepridil)
- Mechanisms of action: (1) Nifedipine—blockade of voltage-dependent L-type inactive Ca^{2+}-channel receptor that has recently undergone activation and cannot open; (2) Verapamil—binding to active or open L-type channels, (3) Diltiazem—binding to specific receptor on L-type Ca^{2+} channel, (4) Bepridil—binding to specific receptors on L-type Ca^{2+} channel
- Usual dosages: (1) Nifedipine PO or SL 10–30 mg tid or qid; (2) Verapamil IV 0.075–0.15 mg/kg, PO 80–120 mg tid or qid; (3) Diltiazem IV .025 mg/kg bolus then 0.15 mg/kg/h, PO 30–90 mg tid or qid; (4) Bepridil PO 200–400 mg/d

ASSESSMENT POINTS

SYSTEM	EFFECT	ASSESSMENT BY HX	PE	TEST
CV	Myocardial depression, vasodilation, reflex activation of the autonomic nervous system, $\downarrow$ Mvo_2, $\downarrow/\rightarrow$ HR and AV nodal conduction	Dose and type of Ca^{2+}-channel blockers determines effects	Hypotension, bradycardia	BP measurement, ECG, ECHO for ventricular contractility
RESP	$\downarrow$ Airway smooth muscle response to histamine, exercise-induced bronchospasm	$\downarrow$ Episodes of bronchospasm in patients prone to wheezing	Reduced wheezing in patients with asthma or COPD	Chest auscultation
CEREBRAL	Cerebral vasodilation and $\downarrow$ vasospasm, cerebral ischemia, and neuronal death	Ongoing assessment of neurologic status in patients at risk for vasospasm	Changes in neurologic assessment	Cranial Doppler or angiogram
HEME	Inhibition of plt aggregation	$\downarrow$ Hemostasis		Tests of plt aggregation
ENDO	Nifedipine delays insulin release and $\downarrow$ serum glucose in DM; diltiazem has no effect on insulin, glucagon, growth hormone, cortisol levels	Better glucose control in DM patients on nifedipine		Blood glucose

Key Reference: Royster RL, Zvara DA: Anti-ischemic drug therapy. *In* Kaplan JA (ed): Cardiac Anesthesia. Philadelphia, WB Saunders, 1999, pp 114–123.

PERIOPERATIVE IMPLICATIONS/POSSIBLE DRUG INTERACTIONS

Preoperative Concerns

- Need for continuation of Ca^{2+}-channel blockers throughout the periop period to minimize Htn, hypercontractility, or heart failure
- Careful assessment of baseline hemodynamic variables
- Drug interactions—verapamil $\uparrow$ digoxin levels; cimetidine and ranitidine $\uparrow$ serum levels of Ca^{2+}-channel blockers through $\downarrow$ hepatic blood flow

Monitoring

- Routine
- PA catheter with pacing capability if associated heart failure or AV block
- Intra-arterial catheter if BP instability likely

Airway

- No special concerns

Preinduction/Induction

- Assess hemodynamics and ECG before induction
- $\downarrow$ Volatile anesthetic doses to avoid undesired myocardial depression/vasodilation

Maintenance

- Fluid requirements may be $\uparrow$ owing to vasodilation
- Negative inotropic effects in conjunction with volatile anesthetics
- Effects of Ca^{2+}-channel blockers can be antagonized by administration of calcium to raise the extracellular calcium and increase the influx gradient across the remaining unblocked channels or by administration of epinephrine

Extubation

- No special concerns

Adjuvants

- Potentiation of neuromuscular blockers (succinylcholine, pancuronium, D-tubocurarine, atracurium, vecuronium) described in vitro

Postoperative Period

- Potential for incomplete reversal of neuromuscular blockers owing to interaction with Ca^{2+}-channel blockers on the postsynaptic membrane and blockade of Ca^{2+} channels in skeletal muscle

ANTICIPATED PROBLEMS/CONCERNS

- Hypotension
- Heart failure
- Bradycardia/asystole
- AV nodal block
- Paradoxical aggravation of myocardial ischemia resulting from associated hypotension of $\uparrow$ Mvo_2 resulting from reflex sympathetic stimulation and tachycardia

CAPSAICIN

Martin Hautkappe, M.D.

INDICATIONS

- People within USA: ?unknown
- Rx for RA, OA, diabetic neuropathy, herpes zoster neuralgia, pruritus, psoriasis, cluster headache, trigeminal neuralgia, reflex sympathetic dystrophy syndrome, fibromyalgia, myofascial pain syndrome
- Beneficial effect of intravesical capsaicin in patients with detrusor hyperreflexia

PERIOPERATIVE RISKS

- Erythema

WORRY ABOUT

- Hepatotoxicity
- Irritation, burning sensation of skin, especially at beginning of Rx
- Contact with eyes, broken or irritated skin may cause painful irritation

OVERVIEW/PHARMACOLOGY

- Local anesthetic creme with clinical effects on small fiber function
- Interacts with xenobiotic metabolizing enzymes, particularly microsomal cytochrome P450–dependent mono-oxygenases (involved in activation, detoxification of various chemical carcinogens, mutagens)
- Hepatic cytochrome P450 2E1 catalyzes conversion of capsaicin to reactive species—e.g., phenoxy radical intermediate capable of covalently binding to active site of enzyme and tissue macromolecules

DRUG CLASS/MECH OF ACTION/USUAL DOSE

- Local anesthetic creme: a primary pungent, irritating agent present in red peppers believed to
  - Exert pharmacologic actions by interacting at recognition site, depleting stores of substance P from sensory neurons
- Systemic and topical applications block C-fiber conduction and inactivate neuropeptide release from peripheral nerve endings
- Repetitive administration produces desensitization, inactivation of neurons caused by receptor-dependent block of Ca^{2+} channels, subsequent accumulation of intracellular ions
- Causes localized antinociception, reduction of neurogenic inflammation
- Usual dose: adults, children 2 y and older: apply Zostrix (or Zostrix-HP) to affected area $3-4\times$/d; transient burning may occur on application; generally disappears in several days
- Application schedules of less than $3\times$/d may not provide optimum pain relief, burning sensation may persist

DRUG EFFECTS

SYSTEM	EFFECT
GI/HEPATIC	Increase of microsomal xenobiotic metabolizing enzyme activity
CNS	Good penetration to CNS after administration: amplification of pain relief

Key Reference: Hautkappe M, Roizen MF, Toledano A, Roth S, Jeffries JA, Ostermeier AM: Review of the effectiveness of capsaicin for painful cutaneous disorders and neural dysfunction. Clin J Pain 1998; 14:97–106.

POSSIBLE DRUG INTERACTIONS

- ↓ Clearance of drugs using P450 2E1—e.g., phenothiazines, phenytoin, theophylline, oral contraceptives

SPECIAL CONSIDERATIONS

- Some recommend a combination of capsaicin with other local anesthetics for reduction of the initial burning pain

- Competitive antagonist: capsazepine
- Block of capsaicin-induced effects: ruthenium red (cationic dye) blocks capsaicin-activated ion channels

CARBAMAZEPINE (TEGRETOL) Leslie Newberg Milde, M.D.

USES

- Indications
  - Single treatment for psychomotor epilepsy
  - Adjunct treatment for partial epilepsies including simple partial seizures and complex partial seizures
    - Rx for trigeminal neuralgia
    - Rx for glossopharyngeal neuralgia
    - Rx of acute mania in combination with lithium or neuroleptics and/or prophylactic Rx of bipolar disease
- Administration: oral in 100-, 200-, or 400-mg tablets
- Patients receiving carbamazepine in USA: 360,000–450,000

ADVERSE REACTIONS

- Acute intoxication: stupor, coma, hyperirritability, convulsions, respiratory depression
- CV: may suppress both AV conduction and ventricular automaticity due to its membrane depressant effect similar to that of quinidine or procainamide. Bradycardia or AV block can occur at therapeutic levels; CHF, vasculitis (rare).
- CNS: vertigo, drowsiness, unsteadiness, dizziness (common); headache, slurred speech, confusion, depression with agitation, psychosis, paresthesias, worsening tics, and dystonic reactions such as dyskinesias and myoclonus. Exacerbation of absence seizures can occur in children.
- Derm: rash, urticaria (common); dermatitis, Stevens-Johnson syndrome, alterations in pigmentation (rare)

- EENT systems: blurred vision, transient diplopia, nystagmus (common); lens opacifications, conjunctivitis, oculogyric crisis (rare); auditory disturbances including tinnitus and hearing loss
- Endo: decreased thyroid function tests and SIADH; development of nonhereditary acute porphyria; hyperthermia (one case report), neuroleptic malignant syndrome (one case report)
- GI: N/V (common); hepatitis, cholangitis, cholestatic and hepatocellular jaundice, and abnormal LFTs (rare)
- GU: urinary frequency, acute urinary retention, acute renal failure (rare)
- Hematologic: aplastic anemia or agranulocytosis (occurs 5–8 times greater than in general population); leukopenia; thrombocytopenia (rare)
- MS: aching joints, muscle cramps, connective tissue disorders such as systemic lupus erythematosus; osteomalacia
- Hypersensitivity reaction: dyspnea, rash, lymphadenopathy, eosinophilia, or pneumonia

WORRY ABOUT

- Chronic use of carbamazepine induces the drug-metabolizing enzymes in P450 system. Carbamazepine therefore induces its own metabolism and that of other drugs metabolized by P450 and will increase the degree of heart block in patients with heart block or taking drugs whose mechanism of action decreases conduction through the AV node; CNS depression with relative overdose.

- *Contraindications:* hypersensitivity to carbamazepine or other tricyclic antidepressants; history of bone marrow depression; concomitant use of MAO inhibitors; history of severe hepatic disease; AV block

OVERVIEW/PHARMACOLOGY

- An iminostilbene related to tricyclic antidepressants
- Moderate anticholinergic action
- Absorption and distribution: the oral tablet form is 70–79% absorbed
- Protein binding: 76%
- Volume of distribution: 0.8–2 L/kg
- Metabolism: 98% by the liver via cytochrome P450 3A4; 50% to 10,11-epoxide, an active metabolite; further metabolism to inactive metabolites by conjugation and hydroxylation
- Excretion: 72% renal excretion as glucuronide; fecal excretion 28%; ↓ clearance by 70% in patients > 70 y; elimination $T_{1/2}$ is 12–17 h, prolonged in patients receiving only one dose; shortened in patients receiving other metabolism-inducing drugs such as phenobarbital or phenytoin

DRUG CLASS/MECH OF ACTION/USUAL DOSE

- Reduces the propagation of abnormal impulses by blocking sodium channels, thereby inhibiting the generation of repetitive action epileptic foci. An antiepileptic.
- Usual dose: 300–600 mg bid
- Alternatives: phenytoin, phenobarbital, valproate

DRUG EFFECTS

SYSTEM	EFFECT	ASSESSMENT BY HX	PE	TEST
CV	AV block			ECG
	LV failure	SOB, orthopnea		ECHO
ENDO	ADH	Water retention	Oliguria	
RENAL	Urinary failure			BUN, Cr
				UA
HEME	Aplastic anemia			CBC
	Agranulocytosis			
	Thrombocytopenia			

Key Reference: Spacek A, Neiger FX, Krenn CG, Hoerauf K, Kress HG: Rocuronium-induced neuromuscular block is affected by chronic carbamazepine therapy. Anesthesiology 1999; 90:109–112.

PERIOPERATIVE IMPLICATIONS/ DRUG INTERACTIONS

- Patients on carbamazepine may require ↑ dosages of anesthetic drugs (etomidate, midazolam, propofol, thiopental), muscle relaxants (pancuronium, vecuronium, rocuronium, atracurium, cisatracurium) metabolized by the liver

- Carbamazepine causes ↓ effect of droperidol or haloperidol
- Carbamazepine will ↑ the degree of heart block produced by other agents such as adenosine
- Diltiazem and verapamil may ↑ carbamazepine levels, causing toxicity
- Concomitant use of carbamazepine and ketorolac may cause seizures

ANTICIPATED PROBLEMS/CONCERNS

- AV block
- CNS depression with relative overdose
- Use of ↑ dosages of drugs metabolized by the liver

CHEMOTHERAPEUTIC AGENTS

Margaret G. Pratila, M.D.
Vasilios Pratilas, M.D.

Best available therapy for malignant diseases but requires complete destruction of cancer cells for cure. Combination therapy on an intermittent basis works well, but a level of toxicity far greater than with other drugs has to be accepted.

CATEGORIES

Alkylating Agents
- Busulfan (Myleran)
- Melphalan (Alkeran)
- Cyclophosphamide (Cytoxan)
- Chlorambucil (Leukeran)
- Ifosfamide
- Thiotepa
- Nitrogen mustard (HN_2)
- Altretamine (Hexalen)
- DTIC (dacarbazine)

Antimetabolites
- Methotrexate (MTX)
- 6-Mercaptopurine
- Thioguanine
- 5-Fluorouracil (5FU)
- Cytosine arabinoside (ara-C)
- Floxuridine (FUDR)

Plant Alkaloids
- Vincristine (Oncovin)
- Vinblastine (Velban)
- Paclitaxel (Taxol)
- Vindesine
- L-Asparaginase (enzyme)

Antibiotics
- Doxorubicin (Adriamycin)
- Daunorubicin
- Dactinomycin
- Bleomycin
- Mithramycin
- Mitomycin-C
- Idarubicin
- Actinomycin-D
- Mitoxantrone
- Streptozocin

Miscellaneous
- BCNU (carmustine)
- CCNU (lomustine)
- Procarbazine (Matulane)
- Carboplatinum
- Cisplatin
- Hydroxyurea
- Teniposide (VM-26)
- Etoposide (VP-16)
- Mitotane

MODE OF ACTION

Alkylating Agents: Alkylation of nucleic acids; DNA cross-linking. Activation by microsomal liver enzymes (Cytoxan).

Antimetabolites: Inhibit synthesis of DNA. Interact with specific enzymes to give unusable metabolites

Plant Alkaloids: Bind with microtubular proteins to cause arrest at metaphase stage

Antibiotics: Inhibit DNA synthesis. Anthracyclines bind to nucleic acids and prevent their synthesis.

Miscellaneous: Alkylation of DNA and RNA or inhibition of key enzymes for DNA synthesis

USED TO TREAT

Alkylating Agents:
- Leukemia: CLL, CGL, AML, ALL
- Lymphoma
- Carcinoma—breast, ovary
- Melanoma
- Multiple myeloma
- Neuroblastoma
- Retinoblastoma
- Malignant pleural effusions (HN_2)

Antimetabolites:
- Carcinoma—GI, pulmonary, breast, H & N, epidermoid
- Advanced NHL
- Sarcoma
- Leukemia—ALL
- Gestational choriocarcinoma
- Hydatidiform mole
- Osteogenic sarcoma (MTX and leucovorin)
- Hepatic metastases from GI cancer
- Primary hepatic cancer (FUDR)

Plant Alkaloids:
- Acute leukemia
- Lymphoma
- Rhabdomyosarcoma
- Neuroblastoma
- Wilms' tumor
- Histiocytosis X
- Karposi's sarcoma

Antibiotics:
- Carcinoma—testicular, breast, lung, ovary, thyroid
- Squamous cell of H & N
- Streptozocin used to treat metastatic islet cell tumors of pancreas
- Reticulum cell sarcoma
- Lymphosarcoma

Miscellaneous:
- Hodgkin's lymphoma (procarbazine, carboplatin)
- Carcinoma—testicular, ovary, bladder, H & N (cisplatin)
- Brain tumors (BCNU) (VM-26)
- Multiple myeloma, lymphomas (CCNU)
- Melanoma
- CML
- Ovarian CA, H & N + radiation Rx (hydroxyurea) (DTIC)
- Adrenocortical CA (mitotane)

ADVERSE EFFECTS

Alkylating Agents: *Severe bone marrow depression. Pulmonary toxicity* with busulfan, chlorambucil, and melphalan. *Cardiac toxicity* with high-dose Cytoxan and busulfan; rapid destruction of tumor mass causes ↑ purine and pyrimidine breakdown products with resultant *uric acid nephropathy.* Cytoxan and ifosfamide cause *hemorrhagic cystitis, inappropriate water retention. Secondary malignancies.*

Antimetabolites: *Bone marrow suppression. Pulmonary infiltrates. Diarrhea, nausea, vomiting. Hemorrhagic enteritis. Acute and chronic hepatitis.* Renal tubular necrosis with MTX. *Acute cerebellar syndrome* with 5FU. *Leukoencephalopathy* with MTX following craniospinal R/T. *Neurotoxic—*(ara-C).

Plant Alkaloids: *Bone marrow suppression* with vinblastine and Taxol. *Neurotoxicity* with loss of deep tendon reflexes, peripheral paresthesia, and muscle wasting. Vincristine: *Severe bronchospasm. Hypo- or hypertension,* tachycardia (ventricular), AV block with Taxol. *Idiosyncratic reactions* may occur but may be due to Cremophor EL used as a diluent.
- Serious hypersensitivity reactions (L-asparaginase).

Antibiotics: *Acute cardiac toxicity,* not dose-related, with the anthracyclines. *Chronic cardiac toxicity,* biventricular failure (dose-related). Majority irreversible > 550 mg/m^2. Bleomycin, 10% *pulmonary toxicity* ↑ with dose and age. Serial estimation of DLCO may give early warning. *Idiosyncratic:* hypotension, fever, wheezing. *Hyperkeratosis:* streptozocin, *renal toxicity, abnormal glucose tolerance test. Hypoinsulinism* due to destruction of β cells.

Miscellaneous: *Myelosuppression. Nephrotoxicity,* coagulation necrosis of distal renal tubules, collecting ducts. ↑ By use of aminoglycoside antibiotics. *Pulmonary toxicity:* BCNU and CCNU dose-related; late-onset pulmonary fibrosis (> 15 y). *Hepatotoxicity: GI toxicity* Promethazine: *hypotension, tachycardia, and syncope.* High-dose cisplatin: *Ocular toxicity. Neuropathies:* stocking/glove distribution of paresthesia, areflexia, loss of proprioceptive and vibratory senses.

Key Reference: Dorr RT, Von Hoff DD: Cancer Chemotherapy Handbook, 2nd ed. Norwalk, CT, Appleton & Lange, 1994.

ANESTHETIC IMPLICATIONS

Alkylating Agents:
- Prolonged response to succinylcholine due to cholinesterase inhibition (Cytoxan)
- Thiotepa—neuromuscular block due to pancuronium

Antimetabolites:
- NSAIDs elevate MTX levels and ↑ toxicity
- ↑ Neuromuscular block with nondepolarizing muscle relaxants (6-mercaptopurine)

Plant Alkaloids:
- Risk of elevated K^+ levels with vincristine due to muscle wasting; avoid or use care with succinylcholine
- Isolated cranial nerve paresis may occur, including laryngeal muscles

Antibiotics:
- Lung damage may occur in patients treated with bleomycin
- Maintain FIO_2 at 28% or less perioperatively if possible
- Careful fluid monitoring; colloid vs. crystalloid

Miscellaneous:
- To minimize CNS depression, use CNS-acting drugs with caution in those on procarbazine. Procarbazine has MAOI activity; avoid meperidine and sympathomimetics.
- ↑ Myelosuppression with BCNU with cimetidine

ADJUVANT AGENTS

IFN α-2a, -2b, recombinant
- Antiproliferative effects when bind to specific cell membrane receptors and modulate host immune response; used for hairy cell leukemia and AIDS-related Kaposi's sarcoma. Adverse reactions are those on CV system: hypotension, arrhythmias, tachycardias > 150 bpm, and a transient reversible cardiomyopathy.

Proleukin—human recombinant IL-2
- Actions like native IL-2: enhancement of lymphocyte mitogenesis and cytotoxicity; induction of killer cell activity and of interferon-γ production; used to treat metastatic renal cell carcinoma and malignant melanoma. Adverse reactions include capillary leak syndrome with hypotension; hypoperfusion; edema and effusions; arrhythmias; cardiac ischemia/infarction; and pulmonary, hepatic, and renal insufficiency. Delayed reactions to contrast media may occur (1–4 h).

Tamoxifen (Nolvadex)
- Estrogen agonist-antagonist, binds to cytoplasmic receptors and affects nucleic acid function; used to treat breast and endometrial carcinomas. Adverse reactions are N/V, skin rashes, pruritus, rare myelosuppression.

CHLORAMPHENICOL (CHLOROMYCETIN)   Helmut F. Cascorbi, M.D., Ph.D.

USES
- Infections such as typhoid fever, *Haemophilus influenzae* meningitis, rickettsiosis not treatable with other antibiotics

RISKS
- Bone marrow depression, blood dyscrasia
- P450 inhibition

WORRY ABOUT
- Increased $T_{1/2}$ of dicumarol, warfarin sodium, chlorpropamide, phenytoin, tolbutamide

OVERVIEW/PHARMACOLOGY
- Inhibition of protein synthesis by interfering with the incorporation of amino acids into ribosomes
- Active against gram-positive and gram-negative bacteria, including *Salmonella typhi, Proteus, Rickettsiae;* some large viruses (ornithosis, lymphopathia venereum) susceptible
- Decreases P450 activity, thus changing $T_{1/2}$ of P450-dependent drugs, such as dicumarol (see above)

DRUG CLASS/USUAL DOSE
- Antibiotic for otherwise intractable gram-negative infections, e.g., salmonellosis, *Haemophilus influenzae* meningitis
- Usual dosage: 50 mg/kg/d IV in divided doses

DRUG EFFECTS
- Newborns who cannot glucuronide-conjugate chloramphenicol may develop abdominal distention, cyanosis, vascular collapse, death (rare)

DRUG EFFECTS

SYSTEM	EFFECT	TEST
GI	Nausea, vomiting	
HEME	Agranulocytosis, aplastic anemia	CBC

Key Reference: Kapusnik-Uner JE, Sande MA, Chambers HF: Antimicrobial agents: tetracyclines, chloramphenicol, erythromycin, and miscellaneous antibacterial agents. *In* Hardman JG, Limbird LE (eds): Goodman & Gilman's The Pharmacological Basis of Therapeutics, 9th ed. New York, McGraw-Hill Professional Publishing, 1996, pp 1130–1135.

PERIOPERATIVE IMPLICATIONS/POSSIBLE DRUG INTERACTIONS
- Acute prolongation of action of dicumarol, chlorpropamide
- Action: assess clotting status
- Chronic use: assess status of bone marrow

SPECIAL CONSIDERATIONS
- Expect prolonged/increased action of drugs predominantly cleared via P450 biotransformation

CIMETIDINE

Michael F. Roizen, M.D.

INDICATIONS/USES

- People in USA: > 1,000,000 plus
- Rx for ulcers, gastric reflux, gastric hypersecretion
- High levels associated with confusional states in elderly

PERIOPERATIVE RISKS

- Drug interactions esp with local anesthetics (↑ toxicity), Aldomet, clonidine (CNS toxicity)

WORRY ABOUT

- Decreased hepatic P450 clearance of drugs, ↓ hepatic blood flow, ↑ fentanyl, phenothiazine, β-blocker drug, lidocaine, with ↑ potential for toxicity

OVERVIEW/PHARMACOLOGY

- H_2 antagonist
- Cleared by renal excretion; ↓ dosage intervals to 12 h with Cr clearance of 0–20 mL/min/1.73 m^2
- ↓ Hepatic metab of drugs requiring specific cytochrome P450 (β-blocking agents, Ca^{2+}-channel blockers, theophylline, phenothiazines) or drugs requiring liver for 1st pass metab (by ↓ hepatic blood flow—lidocaine, β-blocking agents)

DRUG CLASS/MECH OF ACTION/USUAL DOSE

- H_2 antagonist
- Chronically taken for
  - Ulcer Rx, prophylaxis
  - Raise gastric pH for prophylaxis or Rx of gastric reflux
- Acutely taken for
  - Prophylaxis against pulm aspiration
  - Part of prophylaxis against immune or nonimmune CV effects from immune or nonimmune release of H_2
- Usual dose: 100–300 mg bid
- Alternatives
  - Other H_2 antagonists
  - Antibiotics to ↓ *Helicobacter pylori* (tetracycline + metronidazole + bismuth)

DRUG EFFECTS

SYSTEM	EFFECT	PE	TEST
HEPATIC	↓ Hepatic drug metab ↓ Hepatic blood flow		
GI	↓ Gastric acid secretion		
ENDO	Weak antiandrogenic effect; gynecomastia (men)		
GU	Renal Placenta—crosses placental barrier, excreted in milk	Gynecomastia	BUN, Cr
CNS	Poor penetration to CNS; with high doses in pts, esp with impaired renal function, assoc with disorientation to coma	CNS exam	

Key Reference: Lam AM, Parkin JA: Cimetidine and prolonged post-operative somnolence. Can J Anaesth 1981; 28:450.

PERIOPERATIVE IMPLICATIONS/POSSIBLE DRUG INTERACTIONS

Preoperative Concerns

- Cimetidine + clonidine or Aldomet assoc with CNS dysfunction
- ↓ Clearance of phenothiazines, phenytoin, theophylline

Induction/Maintenance

- Fentanyl $T_{1/2}$ may be prolonged 2° to direct or indirect ↓ in hepatic BF by cimetidine

Adjuvants/Regional Anesthesia/Reversal

- ↑ Biologic availability of lidocaine and other local anesthetics and thus toxicity
- ↑ NMB agent requirements anecdotally reported (mechanism unknown)

SPECIAL CONSIDERATIONS

- ↓ Hepatic P450 clearance of drugs, ↓ hepatic blood flow: ↑ fentanyl, phenothiazine, β-blocking drug, lidocaine potential for toxicity
- CNS dysfunction by itself (esp in aged and those with ↓ renal function) or with clonidine and Aldomet

CISPLATIN

Joseph F. Foss, M.D.

USES (SEE ALSO CHEMOTHERAPEUTIC AGENTS)

• Patients undergoing chemotherapy for testicular, ovarian, or bladder cancer

PERIOPERATIVE RISKS

• End-organ damage, especially renal

WORRY ABOUT

• ↓ Clearance of renally excreted drugs if previous damage
• Avoid aminoglycosides (increased toxicity)

OVERVIEW/PHARMACOLOGY

• Inorganic platinum-containing compound (cis-diamminedichloroplatinum [cis-DDP])
• Renal toxicity prominent, seen in 28–36% of patients after 1 dose: effect cumulative, minimized by aggressive hydration, allowing renal function to return to baseline between treatments
• Decrease in renal tubular function is dose-related, typically occurs during 2nd wk of administration

• Hyperuricemia, hypomagnesemia, hypocalcemia, hyponatremia, hypokalemia, hypophosphatemia have been reported and are related to renal tubular damage. Allopurinol Rx reduces uric acid levels.
• Reaches site of action by diffusion
• High concentrations in kidneys, liver, prostate, intestines, testes; low CNS penetration
• $T_{1/2}$ 20–30 min following bolus administration or infusion of 50 or 100 mg/m^2; clearance is 15–16 L/h/m^2; vol of distribution, 11–12 L/m^2
• Highly protein-bound, poorly dialyzable
• Cleared renally at rate greater than that of Cr; 13–17% of parent compound excreted within 1 h after administration

DRUG CLASS/MECH OF ACTION/USUAL DOSE

• Disrupts DNA helix, preventing duplication
• In chemotherapy of metastatic ovarian and testicular CA and advanced bladder CA, often used in combination with other drugs, particularly cyclophosphamide (Cytoxan)

• Contraindicated (relatively) in patients with pre-existing renal disease, hearing loss, myelosuppression; use of other nephrotoxic or ototoxic agents (e.g., aminoglycosides) may increase toxicity
• Must be administered intravenously (See the current oncology literature for dosage, administration guidelines, and protocols. Has been used in doses of 20 mg/m^2 for 5 days for testicular cancer, 75–100 mg/m^2 once every 4 wk for ovarian tumors in combination with other agents, 50–70 mg/m^2 for advanced bladder CA.)
• Pretreatment hydration of 1–2 L over 12 h before administration and infusion of cis-DDP in a dilute vol with mannitol recommended. Repeat courses usually not given until renal function returns to baseline, circulating blood elements are at acceptable levels, and audiometric and hepatic function monitoring have been completed.

DRUG EFFECTS

SYSTEM	EFFECT	ASSESSMENT OF HX	PE	TEST
HEENT	Ototoxicity (31% of patients) manifested as tinnitus or loss of hearing; more pronounced in children	Total exposure		Audiometry
CV	Anaphylactic-like reactions with edema, bronchospasm reported Cardiac dysrhythmias reported	SOB after administration, palpitations	CV exam	ECG
HEPATIC	Transient elevations in liver enzymes reported with use of cis-DDP			Hepatic transaminases
GI	N/V severe, triggered by action at chemoreceptor trigger zone of medulla	N/V within 1–4 h up to 24 h		
HEME	Mild–moderate myelosuppression (25–30%)			CBC
GU	Renal toxicity			BUN, Cr, electrolytes, Mg^{2+}
CNS	Seizures with high acute doses			
MS	Peripheral neuropathies in a stocking/glove distribution with prolonged Rx of 4–7 mo	Total exposure	Neuro exam	Pinprick vibration

Key Reference: Tomioka S, Kurio T, Takaishi K, Nakajo N: Propofol is effective in chemotherapy-induced nausea and vomiting: a case report with quantitative analysis. Anesth Analg 1999; 89:798–799.

POSSIBLE DRUG INTERACTIONS

Adjuvants/Regional Anesthesia/Reversal

• Plasma levels of anticonvulsants may become subtherapeutic with the use of cisplatin

SPECIAL CONSIDERATIONS

• Should not be administered through needles or IV sets containing aluminum, which reacts with cisplatin, causing precipitation
• Cis-DDP and equipment used for administration should be handled as potentially carcinogenic

• May be irritating to the skin; if extravasated may cause local soft tissue toxicity

CLOPIDOGREL BISULFATE

Ann M. Cartarius, R.N.
Lee A. Fleisher, M.D.

USES

- Indicated for reduction of atherosclerotic events in patients with known atherosclerosis confirmed by a history of stroke, TIAs, MI, or peripheral vascular disease; after coronary stent procedures

PERIOPERATIVE RISKS

- ↑ Risk of bleeding if not discontinued 7 days before surgery

WORRY ABOUT

- Hypersensitivity reactions (rare): bronchospasms, angioedema, and anaphylactoid reactions
- ↑ Bleeding intra- and postop
- Elective surgery undertaken < 14 days from coronary stent placement demonstrated a high occurrence of stent thrombosis. It is recommended to postpone elective noncardiac surgery until the course of antiplatelet treatment is completed, thus reducing the risk of bleeding complications and stent thrombosis.

OVERVIEW/PHARMACOLOGY

- Inhibitor of platelet aggregation. Irreversibly modifies the platelet ADP receptor, affecting the platelet for its entire lifespan after exposure.
- Platelet inhibition can be seen within 2 h of single dose of clopidogrel bisulfate with steady-state of inhibition reached between days 3 and 7 with a 75 mg/d dose
- Bleeding time and platelet aggregation returned to baseline in 5–7 days
- Metabolized: liver
- Excretion: urine, feces, and breast milk

DRUG CLASS/USUAL DOSE

- Antiplatelet
- 75 mg PO daily (no effect whether taken with meals or not)

CONTRAINDICATIONS

- Hypersensitivity to the drug or components of it
- Active pathologic bleeding such as intracranial bleeding or peptic ulcers

DRUG EFFECTS

SYSTEM	EFFECT	ASSESSMENT BY HX	PE	TEST
CV	Edema, Htn, cardiac failure, and AFIB	MI, stroke, established PVD	Pulse, rales	ECG, BP
CNS	Headache, dizziness, depression, and fatigue Intracranial bleeding	Intracranial bleeding	↑ LOC	CT scan (if indicated)
GI	Abdominal pain, dyspepsia, diarrhea, nausea, GI hemorrhage	GI bleeding	Stool guaiac	Bleeding time
HEME	Purpura, epistaxis, bleeding disorders, neutropenia	TTP (rare, ~ 4 cases/1 million exposed)		Bleeding time
RESP	Upper resp infections, rhinitis, coughing, bronchitis		Lung auscultation	
ENDO/METAB	Hypercholesterolemia			Cholesterol level
DERM	Rash, pruritus, purpura	Rash, pruritus, purpura	Rash, pruritus	
MS	Back pain and arthralgia	Back pain and arthralgia		

Key Reference: Gachet C: Platelet activation by ADP: the role of ADP antagonists. Ann Med 2000; 32:515–520.

POSSIBLE DRUG INTERACTIONS/ PERIOPERATIVE IMPLICATIONS

- Markedly ↑ risk of surgical bleeding if D/C < 7 days
- When used in conjunction with Integrilin (eptifibatide) could produce enhanced anticoagulation and an ↑ risk of hemorrhage
- Minimal data on any other drug interactions

RISK

- Prevalence: 3 million regular users; 35 million in USA have tried drug
- Abuse in the OB population 7.5 to 45%

PERIOPERATIVE RISKS

- Hemodynamic instability, ↑ sympathetic discharge
- Myocardial ischemia, MI

WORRY ABOUT

- CV: hypertension, tachycardia, dysrhythmias, MI
- Neurologic: intracerebral bleed, seizures
- Pulmonary: pneumomediastinum, cocaine-induced asthma, hypersensitivity pneumonitis, chronic cough, pulmonary edema, diffusing capacity abnormalities
- OB: placenta previa, abruptio placentae, premature labor, fetal distress

OVERVIEW/PHARMACOLOGY

- Cocaine is an ester local anesthetic that prevents rapid ↑ in cell membrane permeability to Na$^+$ during depolarization; blocks propagation of action potential
- Interferes with presynaptic catecholamine uptake and results in activation of SNS
- May produce neg inotropic, chronotropic effects on heart muscle
- Impairs reuptake in brain of dopamine, serotonin, tryptophan
- Accumulation of dopamine in synaptic cleft may lead to acute euphoria, increased alertness

ICD-9-CM Codes: 305.6 (Nondependent); 364.2 (Dependent)

ETIOLOGY

- Cocaine abuse
- OD during HEENT surgery; ER use (part of tetracaine, epinephrine, cocaine mix)

USUAL TREATMENT

- Supportive
- Myocardial ischemia induced by cocaine should be treated initially with oxygen, aspirin, and benzodiazepines. If there is continuing ischemia, use of additional vasodilators such as nitrates or phentolamine to reverse residual coronary spasm may be necessary.
- β-Blockers may worsen coronary vasoconstriction and should be used with caution if patient presents with signs of ischemia
- In management of short-lived arrhythmias, drug treatment should be avoided if possible, as antiarrhythmic agents and cocaine may have a synergistic depression of contractile function
- For sustained hemodynamically tolerated SVT associated with AV nodal re-entry, adenosine is safe and free of major side effects. If adenosine is unsuccessful, administration of an α-antagonist and a β-blocker in combination is likely to be both safe and effective. No reliable information on the safety and efficacy of other antiarrhythmic drugs.
- *Supraventricular or ventricular tachyarrhythmias* associated with hemodynamic compromise require urgent DC cardioversion

DRUG EFFECTS

SYSTEM	EFFECT	ASSESSMENT BY HX	PE	TEST
CV	Hypertension, MI, dysrhythmias, myocarditis	Exposure		BP/HR ECG
RESP	Pneumomediastinum, asthma, chronic cough, pulmonary edema		Wheezing	CXR
HEME	Thrombocytopenia	Bleeding problems		Plt
OB	Preterm labor Premature rupture of membranes Abruptio placentae Spontaneous abortion Meconium-stained amniotic fluid	Uterine contractions		US
CNS	Subarachnoid hemorrhage Intracerebral bleed Seizures	Headache	Neuro exam	

Key Reference: Ghuran A, Nolan J: Recreational drug misuse: issues for the cardiologist. Heart 2000; 83:627–633.

PERIOPERATIVE IMPLICATIONS

Preoperative Concerns

- Self-reporting of drug abuse unreliable, 35–55% deny cocaine use but have at least 1 pos urine assay
- Hx of smoking, alcohol use, pos syphilis serology, and use of other illicit drugs should alert to possibility of cocaine abuse
- Chronic sinusitis, ulceration of nasal mucosa may suggest cocaine use; sclerosis of peripheral veins, needle marks from IV injection possibly seen. Recent injection sites have characteristic look of multiple ecchymoses.
- Consider urine screen (reliable for only 14–60 h after use)

Monitoring

- Routine
- Consider arterial line if Hx of acute intoxication, recent exposure

Airway

- No special precautions

Preinduction/Induction

- Control hemodynamics before induction
- ↑ Anesthetic requirements possibly from acute cocaine exposure
- Usage of succinylcholine in acutely intoxicated patient may be assoc with prolonged paralysis
- Use ketamine with caution; it potentiates CV toxicity of cocaine
- Spinal anesthesia possibly assoc with more frequent episodes of hypotension

Maintenance

- Myocardial ischemia may manifest as CV instability, ECG changes
- ↑ Catecholamine levels due to inadequate anesthesia, cocaine in blood may result in cardiac dysrhythmias
- Temp rise, sympathomimetic effects assoc with cocaine can mimic malignant hyperthermia

Extubation

- No special issues

Adjuvants

- Ester local anesthetics, which undergo metabolism by plasma ChE, may compete with cocaine, resulting in ↓ metabolism of both
- Cocaine ↓ seizure threshold, enhances convulsant effect of other local anesthetics

Postoperative Period

- Myocardial ischemia possible in postop period
- Pain medication requirements in chronic abusers are same as for nonabusers

CROMOLYN SODIUM

USES

- First prophylactic nonsteroidal drug available for treatment of chronic asthma
- Not effective in acute episodes of bronchospasm
- May be beneficial in allergic rhinitis and atopic diseases of eye
- Adverse effects infrequent; include
  - Direct irritant reactions: e.g., wheezing, coughing
    - Dizziness, nausea, rash
    - Rarely anaphylaxis

OVERVIEW/PHARMACOLOGY

- Inhibits antigen-induced degranulation of pulmonary mast cells
- Prevents release of histamine, other autacoids
- Ineffective when administered orally (only 1% absorbed systemically)
- Administered by inhalation route (nebulizer or special turbo inhaler)
- 10% of inhaled dose absorbed systemically; $T_{1/2}$ = 80 min
- Absorbed portion excreted unchanged in urine (50%), bile (50%)

DRUG CLASS/MECHANISM OF ACTION

- Cromolyn sodium (disodium cromoglycate) is a derivative of 2–chromone–carboxylic acid
- Mechanism of action poorly defined; one proposed explanation is ↓ in accumulation of intracellular Ca^{2+} in sensitized mast cells
- Used primarily in the prophylactic treatment of bronchial asthma
- Effective in preventing degranulation of mast cells only if given prior to antigenic challenge
- Beneficial effects may take several weeks or even months to become evident
- Can be taken prophylactically shortly before exercise or exposure to known allergen to prevent bronchospasm

USUAL DOSE

- Available as cromolyn sodium for inhalation (Intal) to be inhaled qid using a special turbo inhaler
- Available as 4% liquid nasal spray (Nasalcrom), 1 spray each nostril 3–6 times/d for treatment of allergic rhinitis
- Opticrom (4% ophthalmic solution) for treating atopic eye conditions (1–2 drops each eye 4–6 times/d)

DRUG EFFECTS

SYSTEM	EFFECT	ASSESSMENT BY HX	TEST
RESP	Inhibition of pulmonary mast cell degranulation; ↓ release of histamine and autacoids	↓ Episodes of exercise- or antigen-induced bronchospasm after chronic use of drug over 2–3 mo	↓ Bronchial hyperactivity as measured by histamine or methacholine challenge

Key Reference: Serafin WE: Drugs used in the treatment of asthma. *In* Hardman JG, Limbird LE (eds): Goodman & Gilman's The Pharmacological Basis of Therapeutics, 9th ed. New York, McGraw-Hill Professional Publishing, 1996, pp 659–682.

PERIOPERATIVE IMPLICATIONS/POSSIBLE DRUG INTERACTIONS

- Continue administration preoperatively
- Cromolyn sodium is of no benefit in treating an acute perioperative exacerbation of asthma
- Rare possibility of potential serious side effects, including laryngeal edema, angioedema, urticaria, anaphylaxis

DIGITALIS

Robert G. Merin, M.D.

USES

- Dosing: PO, IV—digoxin most common drug
- Indications: CHF, AFIB/AFLT
- Ambulatory side effects: cardiac arrhythmia, CNS disturbances

PERIOPERATIVE RISKS

- Cardiac arrhythmia (especially associated with hypokalemia); AV block (especially associated with administration of β-adrenergic and Ca^{2+}-channel blocking drugs)

WORRY ABOUT

- Hypokalemia, renal insufficiency (producing ↓ digoxin excretion and need for dose alteration)

OVERVIEW/PHARMACOLOGY

- General pharmacologic effect: positive inotropic, anticholinergic, antiarrhythmic

Dosing/Pharmacokinetics

DRUG	ONSET	PEAK	$T_{1/2}$	DOSE INITIAL	DOSE MAINTENANCE
Digoxin: IV	5–30 min	1–3 h	34 h	0.5–1.0 mg	0.25 mg/d
PO	1–3 h	4–6 h	34 h	0.75–1.2 mg	0.125–0.5 mg/d
Digitoxin: PO	3–6 h	6–12 h	7 d	0.8–1.2 mg	0.05–0.3 mg/d

Excretion

- Digoxin: renal, mostly unchanged; ↓ dose for ↑ Cr
- Digitoxin: hepatic degradation

Drug Interactions

- Quinidine: ↓ excretion, ↑ serum levels
- Diuretics: ↓ serum K^+, ↑ toxicity

Treatment for Toxicity

- Digoxin immune Fab

DRUG CLASS/MECHANISM OF ACTION

- Mechanism of action: positive inotropic effect; from inhibition of Na^+,K^+-ATPase, producing ↑ intracellular Ca^{2+} concentration, leading to ↑ cardiac contractility
- Chronotropic and antiarrhythmic effect: ↑ vagal activity; ↑ SA, AV nodal response to acetylcholine; inhibits afferent baroreceptor traffic, ↓ AV conduction

DRUG EFFECTS

SYSTEM	EFFECT	ASSESSMENT BY HX	PE	TEST
HEENT			↓ JVD	
CV	↓ HR, ↑ CO Arrhythmia from toxicity	↓ SOB, orthopnea Palpitations	↓ Heart rate, size Irregular pulse	CXR: ↓ heart size ECG: any arrhythmia except AFIB
RESP	↓ Congestion	↓ SOB, orthopnea	↓ Rales	CXR: ↓ pulmonary edema
GI	Anorexia from toxicity			Serum digoxin > 2 ng/ml
CNS	Headache, confusion from toxicity			Serum digoxin > 2 ng/ml
MS	Fatigue from toxicity			Serum digoxin > 2 ng/ml

Key Reference: Hood WB, Dans A, Guyatt GH, Jaeschke R, McMurray J: Digitalis for treatment of congestive heart failure in patients in sinus rhythm (Cochrane Review). Cochrane Database Syst Rev 2001; CD002901.

PERIOPERATIVE IMPLICATIONS

Preoperative Concerns

- Do not discontinue digitalis preoperatively
- Correct and maintain serum K^+
- ↓ Dose with ↑ serum Cr

Possible Drug Interactions

- ↑ AV block with β-adrenergic and Ca^{2+}-channel blocking drugs
- ↓ Dose with concurrent quinidine therapy

ANTICIPATED PROBLEMS/CONCERNS

- Ventricular rate with AFIB/AFLT is a rough bioassay for digoxin level; fast ventricular rate with AFIB indicates inadequate serum level of digoxin
- Digoxin is the only positive inotropic, antiarrhythmic (for AFIB/AFLT) drug available; drug of choice for this arrhythmia in patient with a failing heart
- Digoxin may depress CNS function in elderly more than it decreases AV nodal conduction
- Treatment of digoxin toxicity

DIURETICS

Nikolaus Gravenstein, M.D.

INDICATIONS

- Prescribed for patients with Htn, CHF, elevated ICP, edema, hemoglobinuria, low intraop UO
- Mannitol may function as renal preservative by free-radical scavenging, toxin dilution mechanisms
- Fenoldopam is a selective dopamine-1 agonist. As a vasodilator it lowers BP and augments renal blood flow 50% and improves UO and CFR. It is emerging as a renal protectorant. Usual dose begins at 0.03 μg/kg/min titrated to effect.

PERIOPERATIVE RISKS

- Hypokalemia
- Hypovolemia, hypotension
- Hyperkalemia with aldosterone antagonists
- Hypomagnesemia

WORRY ABOUT

- Hypokalemia, hypovolemia
- Hypokalemia provoking/ aggravating digitalis toxicity
- Cross-sensitivity: furosemide, sulfonamides
- Deafness with ECA (ethacrynic acid)
- Nephrotoxicity of cephaloridine is enhanced by furosemide
- End result of diuretic use is ↑ UO with net loss of H_2O, solute
- Onset of diuresis within 10 min after IV administration
- With exception of aldosterone antagonist, K^+-sparing diuretics, all others cause K^+ loss
- Serum K^+ <3.5 mEq/L in 15% of patients, <3.0 mEq/L in 10% of diuretic-treated patients
- Chronic diuretic-induced hypokalemia less arrhythmogenic than acute, but serum K^+ <3.0 mEq/L associated with 2-fold greater incidence of ventricular arrhythmias than K^+ >3.0 mEq/L
- Site-specific action associated with additional effect if diuretics from 2 classes used

DRUG CLASS/MECH OF ACTION/USUAL DOSE

- Diuretics belong to osmotic, carbonic anhydrase inhibition, benzothiadiazide, high-ceiling (loop), K^+-sparing, or aldosterone antagonist class of drugs, based on mechanism of action
- Only osmotic and loop diuretics used intraoperatively
- Osmotic diuretic: mannitol—ascending loop, limits H_2O reabsorption; onset of action 5–15 min after IV dose—renal clearance
  - Usual dose: mannitol 0.25–2.0 g/kg
- Loop diuretics—ascending loop, limit NaCl reabsorption; onset of action 5 min after IV dose; $T_{1/2}$ 1–2 h; duration of action 3–6 h to renal clearance
  - Usual dose: furosemide: 5–40 mg (0.1–1.0 mg/kg); ECA: 50 mg (0.5–1.0 mg/kg); bumetanide: 0.5–1.0 mg q 2–3 h; max 10 mg/d

DRUG EFFECTS

SYSTEM	EFFECT
HEENT	Transient (<24 h) deafness or vertigo may follow IV rapid bolus ECA; less common after furosemide or bumetanide; rarely permanent Furosemide administration rate <4 mg/min advised by some
CV	Transient ↑ in venous capacitance with IV loop diuretic administration Acute transient ↑ in intravascular vol precedes diuresis with mannitol, vasodilation with fenoldopam
GI	Diarrhea may follow ECA use
ENDO	Hypokalemia, metabolic alkalosis, hyperkalemia may follow K^+-sparing diuretic use
GU	Diuresis
CNS	Mannitol ↓ ICP

Key References: Greenberg A: Diuretic complications. Am J Med Sci 2000; 39:10–24; Willcox CS: Metabolic and adverse effects of diuretics. Semin Nephrol 1999; 19:557–568.

PERIOPERATIVE IMPLICATIONS/POSSIBLE DRUG INTERACTIONS

Preoperative Concerns

- In chronic hypertensive patients treated with diuretics a significant intravascular volume contraction may exist, which renders them more prone to hypotension following induction of anesthesia
- Enhanced digitalis toxicity from hypokalemia
- Enhanced oto- and nephrotoxicity of loop diuretics is associated with rapid administration of large intravenous doses and concurrent use of another nephro/ototoxic drug, e.g., aminoglycoside antibiotic, another loop diuretic, and some cephalosporins, e.g., cephaloridine

- Probably best to continue chronic dose through the perioperative period, including day of surgery. (UO will decline if diuretic not given on day of surgery.)

Induction/Maintenance

- Intraoperative loop diuretic use may significantly decrease serum K^+ level following a brisk diuresis

Adjuvants

- Enhancement of renal clearance of other drugs, e.g., neuromuscular blocking agents, provoked by diuresis is not clinically problematic

SPECIAL CONSIDERATIONS

- Patients receiving diuretics preoperatively should be considered volume contracted until proven otherwise
- Hypokalemia associated with diuresis will be aggravated by hyperventilation, which imposes an additional 0.5 mEq/L decrease in serum K^+ for each 10 mmHg decrease in $Paco_2$
- Catecholamine β effect (endogenous and/or exogenous) further lowers K^+

DOBUTAMINE

Anil Aggarwal, M.D.
David C. Warltier, M.D., Ph.D.

INDICATIONS

- Prescribed for patients with low cardiac output (CO) 2° to decreased right or left ventricular function associated with CHF, MI, or cardiac surgery
- Used for treatment of pulmonary hypertension with right ventricular dysfunction
- Provocative test for diagnosis of coronary artery disease (e.g., dobutamine stress-echocardiography)
- Administered as an intravenous infusion

PERIOPERATIVE RISKS

- Risk of tachyarrhythmias

WORRY ABOUT

- Tachycardia and tachyarrhythmias, worse at high doses
- Ventricular ectopy
- Rarely, hypotension or Htn may be observed
- Hypokalemia may occur

OVERVIEW/PHARMACOLOGY

- Inotrope used for increasing CO simultaneous with a decrease in systemic and pulmonary vascular resistance
- Was considered to have relatively greater inotropic than chronotropic actions, but recent investigation does not support this contention
- β_1-agonist with lesser effect at β_2-receptors and minimal effects at α-receptors
- Increases intracellular Ca^{2+} by elevating cAMP through effects on β_1-receptors
- Increases SA-node automaticity and AV nodal and intraventricular conduction
- May cause systemic and pulmonary vasodilation through β_2-receptor stimulation
- Quick onset (within 2 min) and short duration (approximately 2–6 min)

DRUG CLASS/MECH OF ACTION/USUAL DOSE

- Synthetic catecholamine
- β-adrenergic action increases adenylyl cyclase activity
- Increases CO by increasing SV and HR and decreasing SVR
- Usual dosage: 1–10 μg/kg/min IV
- Combined use with other agents increases cardiac output via different mechanisms (e.g., milrinone, sodium nitroprusside)
- Concurrent use of dobutamine with epinephrine may reduce efficacy of epinephrine

DRUG EFFECTS

SYSTEM	EFFECT	ASSESSMENT BY HX	PE	TEST
CV	↑ HR ↑ CO ↓ PVR ↓ SVR	Relief of dyspnea	Capillary perfusion, JVD, UO, rales	Mixed venous O_2 saturation, CO, PVR, SVR data

Key Reference: Kelly RA, Smith TW: Pharmacological treatment of heart failure. *In* Hardman JG, Limbird LE (eds): Goodman & Gilman's The Pharmacological Basis of Therapeutics, 9th ed. New York, McGraw-Hill Professional Publishing, 1996, pp 809–838.

PERIOPERATIVE IMPLICATIONS/DRUG INTERACTIONS

Preoperative Concerns

- Assess systemic perfusion
- Monitor BP, CO, PCWP
- PA catheter essential for adequate drug titration

Induction/Maintenance

- Despite adequate CO and BP before induction, there may be a decrease in these values during induction of anesthesia
- Therapy should be guided by measures of adequacy of systemic perfusion such as CO, mixed venous O_2 saturation, and ABG tensions

Adjuvant/Regional Anesthesia/Reversal

- Combining therapy with inotropes that are not β_1-agonists such as milrinone may provide greater than additive effects
- Improvement in cardiac output may also be achieved by adding sodium nitroprusside if SVR is high
- Excessive effect can be reversed with β-adrenergic antagonists such as esmolol
- Consider using digoxin prior to dobutamine in patients with AFIB and rapid ventricular response
- May be ineffective or larger doses required in patients receiving β-blockers

Postoperative Period

- Duration of treatment determined by assessment of cardiac function with PA catheter

ANTICIPATED PROBLEMS/CONCERNS

- Sinus tachycardia can occur, and in patients with AFIB, the ventricular rate may increase 2° to enhanced AV conduction
- Pulmonary V/Q mismatch 2° to pulmonary vasodilation and loss of hypoxic pulmonary vasoconstriction may lead to a decrease in Pao_2
- In patients with myocardial ischemia, there may be occurrence or exacerbation of ventricular arrhythmias
- Contraindicated in IHSS
- Prolonged use associated with β-receptor downregulation and theoretically reduced effectiveness

DOPAMINE

Richard C. Prielipp, M.D., F.C.C.M.

INDICATIONS

- Hypotension
- Cardiac failure/shock with low-to-normal SVR
- Oliguria or periods of renal "stress" such as vascular surgery, sepsis, cardiopulmonary bypass, and concurrent use of other vasopressors
- Bradycardia

PERIOPERATIVE RISKS

- Tachycardia, angina, arrhythmias
- N/V
- Vasoconstriction and hypertension (possible gangrene of extremities)
- Skin sloughing and necrosis if infiltrated in subcutaneous tissue
- Impairs T-lymphocyte function (hypoprolactinemia)
- Depression of hypoxic ventilatory drive
- Increases intraocular pressure
- Potentiates other chronotropes

PHARMACOLOGY

- Preparations: 200-, 400-, 800-mg ampules (must be diluted before IV administration)
- Endogenous central and peripheral neurotransmitter

OVERVIEW/MECH OF ACTION

- Mixed indirect and direct sympathomimetic effects, by activating dopamine (DA_2 and DA_1), β- and α-adrenergic receptors in dose-dependent fashion
- Presynaptic DA_2 receptors (0.2–0.4 μg/kg/min) inhibit endogenous norepinephrine and prolactin release
- Postsynaptic DA_1 receptors (0.5–3.0 μg/kg/min) produce vasodilation in renal, mesenteric, coronary, cerebral arteries
- β-Adrenergic receptors (4–10 μg/kg/min) activate adenylyl cyclase and ↑ myocardial cAMP concentration, ↑ myocardial contractility, inotropy
- α-Adrenergic receptors (>10–20 μg/kg/min) produce progressive vasoconstriction
- Metabolism: substrate for both MAO and COMT

- $T_{1/2}$: 6–9 min (recent evidence suggests attainment of steady-state plasma concentrations may require 70–125 min)
- Marked interpatient variability in plasma concentrations

CLINICAL APPLICATIONS

- Renal dose dopamine
  - DA_1 (1.5–3.0 μg/kg/min) selectively increases renal blood flow and inhibits tubular reabsorption (increases urinary output)
  - Induces diuresis, usually without changing creatinine clearance
  - Low-dose dopamine may also improve splanchnic blood flow
- Inotropic dose dopamine
  - (~4–10 μg/kg/min) Induces release of endogenous norepinephrine (~50% of total activity)
  - β_1-Adrenergic adenylyl cyclase activation increases myocardial cAMP
- Higher dose dopamine
  - In addition to effects noted above, α_1-adrenergic receptors (>10–20 μg/kg/min) are activated with progressive vasoconstriction

DRUG EFFECTS

SYSTEM	EFFECT	ASSESSMENT BY HX	PE	TEST
CV	↑ Cardiac inotropy; vasoconstrictor activity	Improved mental status, perfusion	Pulses, BP Capillary refill	↑ Cardiac output; urinary output
RESP	↓ Hypoxic drive ↑ Pulmonary artery pressure (PAP)	Hypoventilation	Resp rate, depth	ABGs Pulse oximetry Monitor PAP
RENAL	↑ Renal blood flow: ↓ renal Na^+, water reabsorption	Urinary output	Urine volume	Urine volume, electrolytes Cr, CrCl

Key Reference: Smit AJ: Dopamine in heart failure and critical care. Clin Exp Hypertens 2000; 22:269–276.

PERIOPERATIVE IMPLICATIONS

Dopamine Infusion Issues

- Ensure adequate intravascular volume
- Consider invasive monitoring
  - Continuous arterial and PAP catheters; central venous and pulmonary artery occlusion pressure ("filling pressures"); thermodilution cardiac output
  - Urinary output and Cr clearance

Adjuvants

- Additional inotropes—other β-agonists (dobutamine, epinephrine, etc.) or phosphodiesterase inhibitors (milrinone or amrinone) may be needed to ↑ cardiac contractility

Cautions

- Watch for arrhythmias
- May increase heart rate and LV wall stress excessively (dopamine >10 μg/kg/min frequently causes progressive tachycardia and ↑ diastolic ventricular filling pressure)
- Diminished response in patients with chronic CHF or active sepsis
- In cardiogenic shock, myocardial lactate may ↑
- Long-term infusions may suppress immune (T-cell) function with ↓ prolactin
- May exacerbate glaucoma

Related Agent: Dopexamine

- Dopexamine, a synthetic analogue of dopamine, lacks any direct α-adrenergic agonist activity, expressing only β_2-adrenergic and dopaminergic (DA_1) agonist action
  - DA_1 and β_2 arterial vasodilation reduces cardiac afterload while simultaneously increasing blood flow to the kidneys, intestines, liver, spleen

  - Dopexamine (doses between 1 and 4 μg/kg/min) significantly ↑ cardiac index while decreasing systemic and pulmonary vascular resistances after cardiac surgery
  - HR ↑, but not SV index; thus, dopexamine combines positive inotropic, chronotropic, vasodilatory, diuretic, natriuretic properties
- Fenoldopam mesylate (Corlopam) is a pure D_1-receptor agonist inducing selective coronary, renal, mesenteric, and peripheral arterial vasodilation. It causes a linear, dose-dependent reduction in systolic and diastolic BP (pharmacokinetic $T_{1/2}$ = 5 min); produces potent renal vasodilation and natriuretic actions (similar to dopamine), and ↑ UO even in the setting of ↓ BP. May replace "renal dose dopamine." No known drug interactions with β-blockers, α-blockers, Ca^{2+}-channel blockers, or ACE inhibitors.

DOXORUBICIN (ADRIAMYCIN)
DAUNORUBICIN (CERUBIDINE)

Richard I. Cook, M.D.

TOXICITY

- Two phases of toxicity, acute and chronic
- Acute toxicity: cardiac (may be from direct effects of histamine)
  - ECG changes and conduction disturbances: ↓ QRS voltage; nonspecific ST changes; T wave flattening
  - Rhythm disturbances: supraventricular tachyarrhythmias; PVCs
  - ↓ EF
- Acute toxicity: other
  - Nausea, vomiting, alopecia, diarrhea, mucositis
  - Bone marrow suppression (may limit dose acutely); counts lowest about 2 wk after beginning therapy
  - Infiltrated drug with IV delivery may cause extensive tissue necrosis, requiring wide debridement
- Late toxicity: cardiac
  - Most acute toxic cardiac effects (except ↓ QRS voltage) diminish with time
  - Late toxicity occurs weeks to months after administration; reports of onset up to 5 y after dosing
  - Effects are permanent (some indication that children may recover with time)
  - CHF unresponsive to inotropic drugs
  - Increased risk of CHF with higher doses but heart failure can occur after 1st dose
  - Risk 0.1–7% up to 550 mg/m^2
  - Risk rises sharply after 550 mg/m^2 to 50% at 1000 mg/m^2
  - Risk increased by radiation of LV, other cardiotoxic drugs, prior LV dysfunction
  - Risk greater in young children
  - Risk of CHF ↓ by divided dosing (e.g., weekly)
- Myocardial function evaluation requires measurement of EF by ECHO or MUGA (serial CXR, ECGs, systolic time intervals, and other clinical signs not reliable)
- Myocardial biopsy but not myocardial function shows characteristic changes

PERIOPERATIVE RISKS

- Acute: anemia, thrombocytopenia, cardiac arrythmias, and conduction disturbances
- Late: cardiac contractile dysfunction (variable; may be severe)

OVERVIEW/PHARMACOLOGY

- Intravenous chemotherapeutic agents used for wide variety of tumors
- Sensitizes tissues to the effects of radiation; used in combined chemo/radiation therapy protocols
- Excretion primarily by liver

DRUG CLASS/MECH OF ACTION/USUAL DOSE

- Anthracycline antibiotic chemotherapeutic agents
- Works by binding to DNA and interfering with DNA-directed DNA and RNA synthesis
- Variety of dosing regimens: often given weekly until maximum dose is reached
- Maximum dosage ~ 550 mg/m^2 BSA; dose decreased when used in combination with other cardiotoxic drugs (e.g., cyclophosphamide) or radiation (see under Toxicity)

DRUG EFFECTS

SYSTEM	EFFECT	ASSESSMENT BY HX	PE	TEST
CV	Conduction		Unreliable CHF signs;	ECG
	Contractile force	Exercise tolerance	orthopnea, DOE, etc.	ECHO, MUGA
GI	Mucositis, diarrhea		Volume indicators	
HEME	Marrow suppression	Bleeding	Unreliable	CBC with platelet count

Key Reference: Allen A: The cardiotoxicity of chemotherapeutic drugs. Semin Oncol 1992; 19:529–542.

PERIOPERATIVE IMPLICATIONS

Preoperative Concerns
- Some authorities insist on preop echocardiogram for any child who has received these drugs at any time in the past, although history assists in determining need
- Evaluation for signs and symptoms of CHF
- Expected nature of surgical trespass

Induction/Maintenance
- Issues dominated by cardiac condition

ANTICIPATED PROBLEMS/CONCERNS

- LV dysfunction perioperatively with pulmonary edema
- Risk of infection in acute toxicity

RELATED DRUGS

- Epirubicin (Ellence) is a newer derivative of doxorubicin, with similar anesthetic-related features. It may be found as part of breast cancer chemotherapy. It *may* be slightly less cardiotoxic on a milligram basis.
- Idarubicin (Idamycin, Idamycin PFS) is a newer derivative of daunorubicin, with similar anesthetic-related features. It may be found as part of acute myelogenous leukemia chemotherapy. An oral form of idarubicin has been tested as part of long-term chemotherapy regimens.

EPHEDRINE

Eric Jacobsohn, M.B., Ch.B., F.R.C.P.C.
Charl de Wet, M.B., Ch.B.

INDICATIONS

- Intraoperatively for treatment of hypotension from central neuraxial blockade, IV/inhalational anesthesia
- IV as emergency Rx for acute hypotension, shock of still-undetermined cause
- Orally for treatment of asthma, symptomatic treatment of coryza
- Nasally for treatment of coryza

PERIOPERATIVE RISKS

- Hypertensive crisis if administered to patients taking MAO-inhibitor antidepressants
- May precipitate dysrhythmias, if myocardium sensitized to catecholamines (e.g., due to inhalational agents)
- May precipitate ischemia in some ischemic heart disease patients

OVERVIEW/PHARMACOLOGY

- Nonselective indirect-acting sympathomimetic at both α and β receptors (structurally similar to amphetamine but less blood-brain barrier penetration)
- Absorbed by norepinephrine pump in postganglionic nerve endings and displaces norepinephrine from the storage granules (indirect effect); also has some direct effects at adrenergic receptors
- Tachyphylaxis develops. Exact mechanism is unclear; may be due in part to depletion of norepinephrine stores and persistent blockade of adrenergic receptors.
- No catecholamine nucleus, therefore not metabolized by COMT
- Conjugated and deaminated slowly by MAO in liver; slow inactivation accounts for prolonged effect ($10\times$ longer than epinephrine)
- 40% of dose recovered unchanged in urine

DRUG CLASS/USUAL DOSE

- Nonselective, noncatecholamine adrenergic stimulant with mainly indirect, but some direct, activity
- Dosage: mix 50 mg in 10 ml (5 mg/ml) IV, titrated to desired effect
- Starting doses from 5–10 mg in adults
- Can also be given IM, SQ
- Adult dose: 15–50 mg

DRUG EFFECTS

SYSTEM	EFFECT	ASSESSMENT BY HX	PE	TEST
RECEPTORS	α: ++ β_1: ++ β_2: +			
CV	HR: ++ Contractility: ++ Automaticity: ++ Peripheral resistance: + CO: ++ Mean BP: ++ PAP: ++		HR PR Mean BP	SV SVR CO PAP
RESP	Airway resistance:–– Resp stimulant: +			Airway resistance Min ventilation
VASC BED FLOW	Skin/viscera:– Muscle: + Kidney:–– Coronary: + Cerebral: +		Skin perfusion	
ENDO	Oxygen consumption: + Blood glucose: + Blood lactic acid: NC			O_2 consumption Blood glucose Blood lactate
GU	Uterine relaxation; restores uterine BF in hypotension from epidural/spinal			
CNS	Mild stimulant Mild mydriasis	Anxiety, agitation		

+ minimal increase; ++ moderate increase; – minimal decrease; –– moderate decrease; NC = no change

Key Reference: Kee WD, Khaw KS, Lee BB, Lau TK, Gin T: A dose-response study of prophylactic intravenous ephedrine for the prevention of hypotension during spinal anesthesia for cesarean delivery. Anesth Analg 2000; 90:1390–1395.

POSSIBLE DRUG INTERACTIONS

Preoperative Concerns

- Hypertensive crisis with MAO inhibitors
- Response to ephedrine ↑ 2–10× in patients taking tricyclic antidepressants
- ↑ Risk of arrhythmias if taking digoxin
- ↑ Response in cocaine users
- Response may be reduced if taking reserpine or guanethidine (depletion of norepinephrine stores in nerve endings)
- ↑ Response in patients receiving β-blockers

Induction/Maintenance

- As in Preoperative Concerns

ANTICIPATED PROBLEMS

- Myocardium sensitized to catecholamines by some inhalational agents
- Tachyphylaxis with repeated doses
- Possibility of interactions with other drugs that affect ANS
- Precipitates ischemia in some patients

EPINEPHRINE

Charl de Wet, M.B., Ch.B.
Eric Jacobsohn, M.B., Ch.B., F.R.C.P.C.

INDICATIONS

- Intraoperatively: systolic dysfunction—weaning from CPB, in critical care for CV collapse from many causes: cardiogenic (including RV failure), distributive (including anaphylaxis—stabilizes mast cells), obstructive shock
- Addition to local anesthesia to prolong action (1:200,000) and for hemostasis (field block)
- Nebulized racemic epinephrine for airway edema: postop stridor or laryngotracheobronchitis in children, usually not for angioneurotic edema
- Inhalational forms for mild asthma
- Topical solutions for vasoconstriction (nasal, ophthalmic)
- Large repeated doses in cardiac arrest

PERIOPERATIVE RISKS

- Increased risk of arrhythmias (limit to 1 μg/kg with halothane, 2–3 μg/kg with isoflurane, enflurane)
- May precipitate myocardial ischemia
- Severe hypertension/stroke if dosed incorrectly
- Large doses may precipitate pulmonary edema

OVERVIEW/PHARMACOLOGY

- Potent β_1, β_2, α stimulant. More potent at both α- and β-receptors than norepinephrine.
- Water soluble—no blood-brain barrier penetration
- ↑Pulse pressure at low doses because of β_2 effect
- β Stimulation causes ↑ intracellular cAMP
- α_1 Stimulation causes ↑ intracellular Ca^{2+} by G protein interaction as well as ↑ turnover of phosphoinositol
- α_2 Stimulation inhibits adenylyl cyclase
- Metabolized by MAO, COMT; conjugated and excreted in urine
- Biologic activity terminated principally by uptake in postganglionic sympathetic nerve terminals

DRUG CLASS/USUAL DOSE

- Naturally occurring sympathomimetic
- Dosage: depends on route and clinical situation—low, moderate, high doses.
  - IV: mix 1 mg in 250 mL (4 μg/mL); adult bolus doses for ↓BP from anaphylaxis: 10–20 μg as starting dose, ↑ as needed
- Infusion, mainly β at 0.01–0.03 μg/kg/min, increasing α at 0.03–0.15 μg/kg/min, predominant α at 0.15–0.3 μg/kg/min. Cardiac arrest dose: 0.5–1 mg q5 min.
  - Subcutaneous: 10 μg/kg for mild to moderate allergic reactions, severe asthma

DRUG EFFECTS

SYSTEM	EFFECT	ASSESSMENT BY HX	PE	TEST
RECEPTORS	α: ++ (dose-dependent)			
	β_1: ++			
	β_2: ++			
CV	HR: ++	Palpitations	HR	SV
	Contractility: ++			
	Automaticity: ++		Pulse	
	SVR ± (dose-dependent)		Perfusion	SVR
	CO: ++			CO
	Mean BP: + (dose-dependent)		Mean BP	BP
	PAP: +			PAP
RESP	Airway resistance: −		Wheezing	Airway resistance
	Resp stimulant: +		TV	Minute ventilation
VASC BED FLOW	Skin/viscera: −−		Skin perfusion	
	Muscle: ++			
	Kidney: −−			
	Coronary: +			
	Cerebral: +			
ENDO	O_2 consumption: ++			O_2 consumption
	Blood glucose: ++			Blood glucose
	Blood lactic acid: ++			Blood lactate
	(with infusion)			
	Hypokalemia			Serum K^+
	Serum FFA: ++			FFA
GU	Relaxation of uterus			
CNS	Mild stimulant	Anxiety, agitation, headache		
	Mild mydriasis	Mydriasis, arousal		

+ minimal increase; ++ moderate increase; +++ marked increase; − minimal decrease; −− moderate decrease

Key Reference: Andrzejowski J, Sleigh JW, Johnson IA, Sikiotis L: The effect of intravenous epinephrine on the bispectral index and sedation. Anaesthesia 2000; 55:761–763.

PERIOPERATIVE IMPLICATIONS/POSSIBLE DRUG INTERACTIONS

Preoperative Concerns

- Hypertensive crisis with MAO inhibitors
- May precipitate malignant arrhythmias
- ↑Risk of arrhythmias if taking digoxin
- Response exaggerated if taking reserpine, guanethidine
- ↑Sensitivity if taking cocaine, tricyclic antidepressants
- ↓Response with β-blockers

- Hypertensive, hyperthyroid pts more susceptible to pressor response
- Hypokalemia

Induction/Maintenance

- Arrhythmias with halothane

ANTICIPATED PROBLEMS

- Myocardium sensitized to catecholamines by inhalational agents—possibility of malignant arrhythmias
- Severe hypertension, possible stroke if dosed incorrectly
- Aggravates symptoms in psychoneurotic pts on emergence
- Hypokalemia, hyperglycemia
- Possibility of pulm edema

EPSILON-AMINOCAPROIC ACID (EACA) (AMICAR)

Frank W. Dupont, M.D.

USES

- Treatment of bleeding associated with hyperfibrinolysis
- Indications: hyperfibrinolysis; surgical bleeding prophylaxis and Rx; reduction of surgical bleeding associated with CPB[†], dental bleeding[†], hemorrhagic cystitis[†], hereditary hemorrhagic telangiectasia (Osler-Weber-Rendu disease), traumatic hyphema[†], subarachnoid hemorrhage[†]
- Methods of administration: oral solution, IV solution, topical[†], intravesical[†]

[†]Non–FDA approved

PERIOPERATIVE RISKS

- Aprotinin, tranexamic acid, aminocaproic acid, desmopressin, and/or cell salvage used in over 70% of cardiac surgery centers worldwide
- Side effects: hypotension, sinus bradycardia, GI symptoms, CNS effects, anaphylactic reactions (paraben hypersensitivity), agranulocytosis, rhabdomyolysis (rare)

WORRY ABOUT

- Potentiation of hypercoaguable state if receiving estrogens or oral contraceptives
- ↑ Risk of developing thrombosis in hemophiliac patients treated with human factor IX complex or anti-inhibitor coagulant complex

OVERVIEW AND PHARMACOLOGY

- Inhibits fibrinolysis and enhances hemostasis when fibrinolysis contributes to bleeding
- Prevents formation of excessive plasmin, thus inhibiting fibrinolysis
- Elimination $T_{1/2}$ is approximately 2 h
- Primarily excretion in the urine, with 40–65% eliminated unchanged within 12 h, ~11% is metabolized
- Plasma concentrations are ↑ in patients with severe renal dysfunction, but no quantitative recommendations for dosing adjustments are available

DRUG CLASS/MECH OF ACTION/USUAL DOSE

- An antifibrinolytic agent of the lysine analogue class
- Binds competitively to lysine-binding sites within the plasminogen/plasmin molecule to interfere with ability of plasmin to lyse fibrin clots
- Optimal dosage in the setting of CPB is undefined, but the following are commonly used regimens
  - Adults: initial loading dose is 4–5 g IV over 1 h, followed by a continuous infusion at 1 g/h; maximum recommended daily dosage is 30 g
  - Children: 100 mg/kg IV as a loading dose, followed by continuous infusions of 33.3 mg/kg/h; total dosage should not exceed 18 g/m^2/d
- Anti-inflammatory effect may be mechanism of most benefit

ASSESSMENT POINTS

SYSTEM	EFFECT	ASSESSMENT BY HX	PE	TEST
CNS	Dizziness, headache, tinnitus, delirium		Neuro exam	
CV	Hypotension, bradycardia		Vital signs	ECG
GI	Nausea, vomiting, diarrhea			Lytes
HEME	Thrombosis	Potential causes for DIC	Evidence for paradox of simultaneous thrombosis and bleeding	CBC, PT/PTT, DIC profile
MS	Rhabdomyolysis	Myalgia, malaise, fatigue	Muscle weakness	CPK

Key Reference: Mannucci PM: Hemostatic drugs. N Engl J Med 1998; 339:245–253.

PERIOPERATIVE IMPLICATIONS/POSSIBLE DRUG INTERACTIONS

Preoperative concerns

- Patients with DIC at ↑ risk for thrombotic events
- If hematuria originating in the upper urinary tract, can cause intrarenal obstruction due to clot retention
- Paraben hypersensitivity sought

Drug interaction

- Contraindicated in hemophilic patients treated with factor IX concentrates or anti-inhibitor coagulant unless the risk of thrombosis is outweighed by the potential benefit

Induction/Maintenance

- Close hemodynamic monitoring because of risk of hypotension and sinus bradycardia, particularly with rapid IV administration and in hypovolemia
- Monitor renal function if renal dysfunction and consider dosage adjustments
- Consider transfusion of platelets, FFP, and cryoprecipitate in the presence of bleeding not caused by hyperfibrinolysis

Postoperative Period

- Continue assessment of bleeding and monitoring of coagulation profiles after discontinuation of EACA therapy

ANTICIPATED PROBLEMS/CONCERNS

- Potential for thrombotic complications if has DIC or underlying hypercoaguable states
- Concern for potential of thrombosis in key vessels not totally disproven by current high usage

FLUOXETINE (PROZAC)

Donald D. Koblin, M.D., Ph.D.

USES

- Taken by 5 million Americans
- Rx for depression, obsessive-compulsive disorder, bulimia nervosa

PERIOPERATIVE RISKS

- May be associated with perioperative anxiety
- Drug interactions with β-blockers, phenytoin, benzodiazepines, antipsychotics (may increase levels by inhibition of metabolism)

WORRY ABOUT

- Psychotic or extrapyramidal reactions (rare)
- Serotonin syndrome with concomitant administration of MAO inhibitors, tricyclic antidepressants, antipsychotics (?), or meperidine (?)

OVERVIEW/PHARMACOLOGY

- Selective inhibitor of serotonin reuptake
- Administered as racemic mixture of R- and S-enantiomers
- S-enantiomer more potent than R-enantiomer
- Active metabolites, R- and S-norfluoxetine, formed by demethylation
- Eliminated mainly through oxidative metabolism and conjugation
- Long elimination $T_{1/2}$: 1–10 days for fluoxetine; 3–20 days for norfluoxetine
- Fluoxetine inhibits (and probably metabolized by) liver cytochrome P450 enzymes CYP2D6 and possibly CYP3A4: may inhibit metabolism, ↑ levels of β-blockers, benzodiazepines, antipsychotics
- Difficult to establish relationship between plasma conc of fluoxetine and effect, probably because these are 4 active compounds (R- and S-fluoxetine and R- and S-norfluoxetine) that require separate measurements

DRUG CLASS/MECH OF ACTION/USUAL DOSE

- Selective inhibitor of serotonin reuptake chronically taken for depression, obsessive-compulsive disorder, bulimia nervosa
- Not useful for acute administration, since full antidepressant effect may be delayed until 4 wk of treatment or longer
- Initial PO dose, 20 mg/d
- Maximal dose, 80 mg/d
- Alternatives: other antidepressant medications

DRUG EFFECTS

SYSTEM	EFFECT	ASSESSMENT BY HX	PE	TEST
CV	Bradycardia, dysrhythmia in elderly patients (rare)		Pulse	ECG
CNS	Extrapyramidal symptoms (rare), mania (rare), serotonin syndrome (rare)	Headache, anxiety, tremor		
ENDO	SIADH secretion (rare)			Urine specific gravity
GI	Nausea, weight loss			
MS	Serotonin syndrome (rare)	Arthritic complaints (infrequent), muscle rigidity		

Key Reference: Gram LF: Fluoxetine. N Engl J Med 1994; 3:1354–1361.

PERIOPERATIVE IMPLICATIONS/POSSIBLE DRUG INTERACTIONS

- Headache, anxiety, nausea are common symptoms
- May inhibit cytochrome P450 enzymes and ↑ the serum concentrations of other drugs (β-blockers, phenytoin, benzodiazepines, antipsychotics) and potentiate their effects

SPECIAL CONSIDERATIONS

- Approximately 7% of Caucasians lack the cytochrome P450 (CYP2D6) that probably metabolizes fluoxetine; these individuals may develop higher serum concentrations of fluoxetine and be more prone to side effects
- Serotonin syndrome, characterized by agitation, confusion, diaphoresis, and muscle rigidity, may develop in patients who receive a combination of fluoxetine and MAO inhibitors

FOLIC ACID

John P. Lawrence, M.D.

USES

- Folic acid deficiency
- Megaloblastic anemia
- Prevents neural tube defects in fetuses
- Reduces risk of atherosclerosis (coronary and peripheral), stroke, and venous thrombosis by reducing homocysteine levels. Effect present if folic acid given with or without vitamin B_{12}.
- Malnutrition due to alcoholism or malabsorption syndromes—e.g., sprue (tropical and nontropical)
- Folinic acid (leucovorin calcium) for leucovorin rescue but not vitamin replacement

PERIOPERATIVE RISKS

- Rare patient may experience folate deficiency after repeated exposure to N_2O
- At high doses (> 15 mg/d), ↓ seizure threshold in epileptics on phenobarbital, phenytoin, primidone

WORRY ABOUT

- At high doses (15 mg/d), may precipitate seizures in epileptics
- Rare reaction to parenteral form
- Rare deficiency after repeated exposure to N_2O

OVERVIEW/PHARMACOLOGY

- Vitamin, responsible for transferring 1-carbon molecules to other organic molecules
- Absorbed in proximal intestine, undergoes extensive enterohepatic recirculation
- Nonmethylated forms of folate are protein-bound
- Excreted fecally
- Interferes with levels of antiepileptic drugs
- Alcohol directly decreases blood levels by blocking enterohepatic recirculation

DRUG CLASS/MECH OF ACTION/USUAL DOSE

- Vitamin
- Converts homocysteine to methionine, serine to glycine (reduces risk of atherosclerosis)
- Assists synthesis of thymidylate and purines, metabolism of histidine
- Oral and parenteral forms
- Usual dosage (normal requirements): 0.4−0.5 mg/d (found in multivitamin)
- Higher requirements (hemolytic anemia, pregnancy, or antifolate drug therapy): 1 mg 1−3×/d (PO, IM, IV)
- Give with vitamin B_{12}, or can precipitate neurologic component of combined system disease

DRUG EFFECTS

SYSTEM	EFFECT	ASSESSMENT BY HX	PE	TEST
CV	Improves O_2 delivery	Better exercise tolerance		Hgb
GI		Less nausea/diarrhea	Better hydration	
ENDO/METAB	Nucleic acid/ protein synthesis		Weight gain	Folate level
HEME	RBC synthesis	Better exercise tolerance		Hgb

Key Reference: Pancharuniti N, Lewis CA, Sauberlich HE, et al: Plasma homocyst(e)ine, folate, and vitamin B-12 concentrations and risk for early-onset coronary artery disease. Am J Clin Nutr 1994; 59:940−948.

PERIOPERATIVE IMPLICATIONS

Preoperative Concerns

- Anemia (rarely pancytopenia)
- Consider overall nutritional status
- Consider co-existing diseases: alcoholism, malignancy, malabsorptive syndromes, hydration status
- Continue supplements perioperatively

Induction/Maintenance

- Avoid repeated use of N_2O

Adjuvants/Regional Anesthesia/Reversal

- Same as Preoperative Concerns

Postoperative Period

- Same as Preoperative Concerns

ANTICIPATED PROBLEMS/CONCERNS

- May precipitate seizures at high doses (> 15 mg/d) in epileptics on chronic antiepileptic therapy
- Folinic acid (leucovorin calcium) not used for repleting folic acid deficiency

GLYBURIDE, ORAL HYPOGLYCEMIC AGENTS

Sean M. Berenholtz, M.D.
Todd Dorman, M.D.

USES

- Oral hypoglycemic agent (2nd-generation sulfonylurea) for treatment of type II DM

PERIOPERATIVE RISKS

- Hypoglycemia can occur with glyburide or oral hypoglycemic agent therapy; hyperglycemia, ketoacidosis, or hyperosmolar non-ketotic coma can occur if medication held, requiring frequent periop glucose monitoring
- Routine therapy is recommended if hypoglycemia or hyperglycemia occurs

WORRY ABOUT

- Hypoglycemia: estimated incidence of serious hypoglycemia 16.6% (95% CI 13.2–19.9); risk factors include erratic eating habits, intense or prolonged exercise, alcohol ingestion, renal or hepatic disease, age >85 y, and concomitant medication use; case reports of death exist with sulfonylurea overdose
- ↑ Risk of hypoglycemia reported with concomitant antacids (magnesium type), MAO inhibitors, aspirin, pindolol or propranolol, chlorpropamide, cimetidine, ranitidine, ciprofloxacin, clofibrate, cotrimoxazole, enalapril, erythromycin, fluconazole, itraconazole, ethanol

OVERVIEW/PHARMACOLOGY

- First generation sulfonlyurea agents: tolazamide, chlorpropamide, tolbutamide, acetohexamide; 2nd generation: glyburide, glipizide
- Maximal hypoglycemic effects similar with all agents: 2–4 h
- Duration of action (hours): glyburide 12–24, glipizide 12–24, tolazamide 12–24, chlorpropamide 60, tolbutamide 6–12, acetohexamide 12–18
- Sulfonylureas are excreted primarily via the kidney. Glyburide is excreted in both urine and bile, 50% by each route.

DRUG CLASS/USUAL DOSE

- Sulfonylurea agents stimulate pancreatic insulin production, ↓ hepatic glucose production, and ↑ tissue responsiveness to insulin, resulting in lower blood glucose levels
- Usual daily dosage: glyburide 2.5–20 mg, glipizide 5–20 mg, tolazamide 100–1000 mg, chlorpropamide 100–500 mg, tolbutamide 500–2500, acetohexamide 250–1500 mg

DRUG EFFECTS

SYSTEM	EFFECT	ASSESSMENT BY HX	PE	TEST
GI	Nausea, heartburn, rare cholestasis, rare hepatitis	Fatigue, malaise	Jaundice, dark urine, pale stools	Bilirubin, alkaline phosphatase, transaminases
HEME	Rare eosinophilia, neutropenia, thrombocytopenia, hemolytic anemia, ↑ prothromboplastin times		Jaundice, purpuric rash	CBC
DERM	Alcohol-induced flushing	Alcohol ingestion, headache, lightheadedness		

GU
  Glyburide
  Other sulfonylureas
	Mild diuresis
	Antidiuresis			

ENDO	Hypoglycemia	Palpitations, tremor, headache, confusion, visual disturbances, seizures	Tachycardia, diaphoresis, agitation, combativeness	Glucose

Key Reference: DeFronzo RA: Pharmacologic therapy for type 2 diabetes mellitus. Ann Intern Med 1999; 131:281–303.

POSSIBLE DRUG INTERACTIONS

Preoperative Period

- General recommendation is to hold sulfonylurea agents on the day of surgery while patients are NPO to ↓ risk of periop hypoglycemia
- Concomitant β-blocker therapy may mask signs and symptoms of hypoglycemia

Induction/Maintenance

- Frequent blood glucose monitoring; standard treatment of hypoglycemia/hyperglycemia as indicated
- Most sulfonylurea agents possess antidiuretic properties; glyburide may induce diuresis

Adjuvants/Regional Anesthesia/Reversal

- No known contraindications or interactions

Postoperative Concerns

- Sulfonylureas can be restarted when the patient has resumed oral intake, provided renal function has remained normal

ANTICIPATED PROBLEMS/CONCERNS

- Sulfonylurea agents can cause serious hypoglycemia
- ↑ Risk of hypoglycemia reported with several common periop drugs

GOLD (AURANOFIN, AUROTHIOGLUCOSE, AUROTHIOMALATE)

Martin D. Sokoll, M.D.

USES

- ~500,000 patients/y receive gold Rx
- Rx for RA patients who do not respond to aspirin, NSAIDs

RISKS OF ADMINISTRATION

- Cutaneous reactions from erythema to exfoliative dermatitis
- Mucous membrane lesions—stomatitis, pharyngitis, gastritis, colitis
- Chrysiasis (gray-to-blue pigmentation of skin) poss; effect of transcutaneous Hgb saturation measurement unknown
- Potential problems—hepatic, renal dysfunction and pulmonary fibrosis, which is difficult to distinguish from rheumatoid pulmonary disease. Resolves with discontinuance of Rx.
- Severe hematologic problems—thrombocytopenia (usually reverses with cessation of Rx) to aplastic anemia (usually fatal)
- Not usually administered to pregnant patients or those given antimalarials, phenylbutazone, or oxyphenylbutazone because of concomitant blood dyscrasias
- Not well tolerated by elderly

OVERVIEW/PHARMACOLOGY

- Usually administered IM; a few patients take drug PO
- Au compounds have anti-inflammatory activity
- Aurothioglucose, aurothiomalate administered IM
- Auranofin is oral prep
- Oral prep has lower incidence of side effects
- $T^{1/2}$ of single 50-mg dose IM ~ 7 days
- After full dose, blood levels return to normal in 40–80 days; 60–90% of a given dose is eliminated renally, remainder by fecal excretion
- Renal disease delays excretion and is a contraindication to gold administration

DRUG CLASS/MECH OF ACTION/USUAL DOSE

- Anti-inflammatory
- Gold compounds sequestered in organs, areas having high mononuclear phagocyte concentrations
- Gold concentrates in phagocytes and synovial membranes; suppresses phagocyte migration and has general anti-inflammatory effect
- Administered in progressive doses (10–50 mg/wk, total dose not to exceed 1 g)
- Continuing Rx 50 mg every 2–4 wk

DRUG EFFECTS

SYSTEM	EFFECT	PE	TEST
HEENT	Glossitis, pharyngitis		
RESP	Tracheitis, pneumonitis, pulm fibrosis		CXR
GI	Hepatitis		LFTs
GU	Proteinuria, hematuria, membranous glomerulonephritis (contraindicated during pregnancy, breast feeding)		Renal function, pregnancy
CNS	Encephalitis, peripheral neuritis	CNS exam	

Key Reference: Insel PA: Gold. *In* Hardman JG, Limbird LE (eds): Goodman and Gilman's The Pharmacological Basis of Therapeutics, 9th ed. New York, McGraw-Hill Professional Publishing, 1996, pp 644–646.

PERIOPERATIVE IMPLICATIONS/POSSIBLE DRUG INTERACTIONS

- Severe RA; difficulty positioning on operating table
- Airway: laryngeal arthritis, cervical instability, and pulm fibrosis; other problems of arthritis may be encountered
- Stomatitis, pharyngitis, tracheitis may make mucous membranes fragile

Drug Interactions

- None during anesthesia, but chrysiasis may interfere with pulse oximeter function

ANTICIPATED PROBLEMS

- Beware of hepatic, renal, and pulm dysfunction
- Lesions of skin, mucous membranes may make these tissues friable
- Investigate cervical instability in all severe arthritides
- Condition may mandate fiberoptic, blind oral, or nasal intubation of trachea
- Hematologic problems (thrombocytopenia, leukopenia) may manifest as bleeding or postop infection

HALOPERIDOL (HALDOL)

Donald D. Koblin, M.D., Ph.D.

USES

- Rx for
  - Psychotic disorders in ambulatory population (PO)
  - Agitation caused by delirium in ICU patients (IV or IM)

PERIOPERATIVE RISKS

- Laryngospasm
- Extrapyramidal symptoms
- Neuroleptic malignant syndrome
- Cardiac arrest at high doses

WORRY ABOUT

- May exacerbate symptoms in pts with Parkinson's disease
- Potential concern for neurotoxic metabolites
- Extrapyramidal symptoms less common with IV than PO doses

OVERVIEW/PHARMACOLOGY

- Dopaminergic antagonist
- Precise mechanism of action unknown
- Onset time: 5–20 min for IV; 30–60 min for PO
- Long (and variable) serum $T_{1/2}$ (13–60 h)
- 90–94% bound to serum proteins
- Therapeutic plasma concentration in range of 4–40 μg/L, but large variability among pts
- Clearance by hepatic metabolism
- Metabolized to reduced haloperidol, which has ~10% of activity of parent drug; reduced haloperidol may be oxidized and reconverted to haloperidol
- Renal excretion of parent drug is negligible

DRUG CLASS/MECH OF ACTION/USUAL DOSE

- Dopaminergic antagonist
- Chronically taken for
  - Management of psychotic disorders
  - Control of tics and vocal utterances of Tourette's disorder
- Acutely taken to control agitation caused by delirium
- Usual PO dose 1–6 mg/d
- Usual IV or IM dose
  - 0.5–2 mg for mild agitation
  - 5 mg for moderate agitation
  - 10 mg for severe agitation (+10 mg/h infusion)
- Alternatives
  - Other antipsychotic medications
  - Other antidelirium medications (e.g., physostigmine)
  - Usually for agitation caused by delirium; agitation caused by anxiety/pain can be treated with benzodiazepines/narcotics

DRUG EFFECTS

SYSTEM	EFFECT	TEST
HEENT	Laryngospasm (infrequent side effect)	
CV	Hypotension or hypertension, cardiac arrest (high doses)	
HEPATIC	↓ metabolism and ↑ serum concentration with hepatic disease	Monitoring of haloperidol concentrations is indicated only in pts with poor response at high doses or with hepatic disease
GI	Nausea	
ENDO	Gynecomastia	
GU	Urinary retention	
CNS	Extrapyramidal symptoms (akathisia, dystonia, tardive dyskinesia)	
MS	Neuroleptic malignant syndrome (NMS)	

Key References: Riker RR, Fraser GL, Cox PM: Continuous infusion of haloperidol controls agitation in critically ill patients. Crit Care Med 1994; 22:433–440.

PERIOPERATIVE IMPLICATIONS/POSSIBLE DRUG INTERACTIONS

- Encephalopathic syndrome with combined use of lithium and haloperidol
- May potentiate effects of general anesthetics and narcotics

SPECIAL CONSIDERATIONS

- Laryngospasm infrequent but life-threatening
- Cardiac arrests reported with high (~10 mg) doses
- IV haloperidol is not approved by the FDA for routine use
- NMS may develop 1–3 days after haloperidol administration and is characterized by muscle rigidity, hyperthermia, tachycardia, altered consciousness, and elevated serum creatine kinase concentrations. A mild form of NMS may occur in as many as 1% of pts given haloperidol.

HORMONE REPLACEMENT THERAPY Mitzi K. Hemstreet, M.D., Ph.D.

USES

- To prevent or treat physical and psychologic signs and symptoms associated with surgical or age-related menopause in women: osteoporosis, hyperlipidemia, cardiovascular disease, cerebrovascular disease, vaginal dryness, irritability, mood swings, "hot flashes," and sleeplessness
- Available in oral or injectable forms, transdermal patches, creams, or vaginal inserts
- Many formulations, including estrogen alone or combined estrogen-progestin therapies

PERIOPERATIVE RISKS

- Potential for coagulopathy (either prothrombotic or profibrinolytic)
- Early in the course of estrogen replacement therapy, there is an increased risk of thromboembolism
- With combined estrogen-progestin replacement therapy, many (but not all) studies suggest a shift toward increased fibrinolytic activity and prolonged bleeding
- Risk of hypertension in older patients

WORRY ABOUT

- ↑ Risk of DVT, pulmonary embolism, stroke, and myocardial infarction with estrogen replacement therapy
- ↑ Risk of prolonged bleeding or hemorrhage with combined estrogen-progestin therapy
- Alterations in drug metabolism and serum protein binding due to ↑ hepatic synthetic activity
- Potential for hypercalcemia with history of bone metastases from breast cancer

OVERVIEW/PHARMACOLOGY

- Hormone replacement therapy uses a mixture of conjugated estrogens derived from natural sources, often combined with synthetic progestins (similar to oral contraceptives), in either a continuous or cyclic dosing regimen
- Estrogens: a family of 18-carbon steroids that includes the ovarian products estradiol and estrone and the placental estrogen estriol. Via both membrane-receptor–mediated and intranuclear DNA-binding effects, estrogens stimulate growth and maintenance of the female sexual organs, urogenital structures, and bone and modulate activity of the liver, brain, and hypothalamic-pituitary axis. Estrogen has been shown to potentiate the activity of excitatory amino acids in the brain and enhance dopaminergic transmission.
- Progestins: a group of 21-carbon steroids, with progesterone being the principal natural hormone. Secreted by the corpus luteum, progesterone modulates secretory activity of the endometrium, stimulates glandular activity in the breast, and inhibits uterine contractions. It has also been shown to mimic the action of GABA in the central nervous system, with inhibition of synaptic activity.

DRUG CLASS/USUAL DOSE

- Conjugated estrogens: the typical daily oral dosage is 0.625 mg but may be 0.3, 0.625, 0.9, 1.25, or 2.5 mg, depending on response
- Synthetic progestins: medroxyprogesterone, alone or combined with conjugated estrogens, is given as 2.5 or 5.0 mg orally/d. Other synthetic progestins are prescribed for oral contraception rather than hormone replacement therapy.

DRUG EFFECTS

SYSTEM	EFFECT	ASSESSMENT BY HX	PE	TEST
HEENT	↑ Corneal curvature	Intolerance of contact lenses		Exam by ophthalmologist
CV	Fluid retention Htn	Weight gain	Edema Htn	BP
GI	Cholelithiases, pancreatitis Glucose intolerance	Intolerance of fatty foods	RUQ or epigastric tenderness	Total bilirubin, LDH, alk phos, amylase, lipase Serum glucose
HEME	Prothrombotic	Hx DVT, pulm embolus	Asymmetric LE edema	PT/PTT, D-dimer
	Profibrinolytic	Prolonged bleeding, hemorrhage		PT/PTT, fibrinogen, antithrombin III, activated protein C
DERM	Rashes, alopecia, hirsutism, pigment changes	Changes in skin or hair	Erythema, nodules, hair change	Exam by dermatologist
GU	Irregular vaginal bleeding, enlargement of fibroids, vaginal yeast	"Spotting," ↑ abdominal girth, vaginal candidiasis		Exam by gynecologist
CNS	Headaches, depression, dizziness, chorea	Headaches, mood change, imbalance, abnormal movements	Movement disorder	Exam by neurologist
IMMUNO	None at physiologic doses			

Key Reference: Demirol A, Baykal C, Kirazlis, Ayhan A: Effects of hormone replacement on hemostasis in spontaneous menopause. Menopause 2001; 8:135–140.

POSSIBLE DRUG INTERACTIONS

- Due to ↑ hepatic synthetic activity by estrogens, dosage of hepatically cleared drugs may need adjustment
- Some individuals on estrogens show a resistance to barbiturates, requiring higher induction dosages
- Many individuals on hormone replacement therapy develop impaired glucose tolerance and blunting of the metyropone test of the hypothalamic-pituitary-adrenal axis

ANTICIPATED PROBLEMS/CONCERNS

- Estrogen-progestin combinations have variably been shown to alter a number of laboratory values, including prolonged PT and PTT; ↑ factors VII, VIII, IX, and X; elevated fibrinogen; ↑ or ↓ antithrombin III; ↓ platelet aggregation; ↑ thyroid binding globulin; and ↓ serum folate level
- Rigorous prophylaxis of DVT must be observed, as well as a heightened suspicion for postop DVT, pulmonary embolus, stroke, myocardial infarction, gallbladder disease, and glucose intolerance
- Discontinuation of oral hormone replacement therapy in the periop period may lead to withdrawal uterine bleeding

INSULIN RECEPTOR MODIFIERS
Maneesh Sharma, M.D.

USES

- New class of oral antidiabetic agents for treatment of type II diabetes mellitus—thiazolidinediones (Actos [ploglitazone], Avandia [rosiglitazone], Rezulin [troglitazone] off market 2000). AKA insulin sensitizers.

PERIOPERATIVE RISKS

- Hypoglycemia: risk is elevated when used with other hypoglycemic agents. As monotherapy, the risk is low as the drugs are designed to not lower blood glucose levels below euglycemia.
- Cardiovascular: volume expansion, preload-induced cardiac hypertrophy, edema
  - Ongoing studies indicate no deleterious alterations in cardiac structure or function
  - Used in caution with pre-existing mild to moderate edema, pts of NYHA class III or worse
- Hepatic: no evidence of hepatotoxicity to date; however, the chemically/structurally related first-generation troglitazone was noted to have potentially fatal drug-induced hepatotoxicity. That drug was removed from the market. LFTs are monitored for potential manifestations of hepatotoxicity.

WORRY ABOUT

- ↑ Plasma volume leading to decline in Hgb by 2–4%
- Hypoglycemia: ↑ risk potentiated by concomitant use of other oral hypoglycemics, insulin
- Hyperglycemia: risk potentiated by concomitant use of thiazide and loop diuretics

OVERVIEW/PHARMACOLOGY

- ↑ Sensitivity to insulin, and therefore ↓ its resistance in tissues. Enhances cellular responsiveness to insulin, ↑ insulin-dependent glucose disposal, improves hepatic sensitivity to insulin, ↓ glucose output, and improves dysfunctional insulin homeostasis.
- Mechanism of action: highly selective agonist for PPAR the gamma receptor, ↑ transcription of insulin-responsive genes in many tissues, thus ↑ insulin sensitivity
- Does not stimulate insulin secretion; therefore, it depends on the presence of insulin for its mechanism of action
- Absorption: oral administration, absorbed from GI system
  - Pioglitazone—peak in 2 h
  - Rosiglitazone—peak in 1 h
- Distribution: drug and metabolites are extensively protein bound
- Clearance: metabolized by cytochrome P450. Each of the two drugs, pioglitazone and rosiglitazone, is metabolized by different P450 isoenzymes; therefore, their drug interaction profiles are slightly different. Interactive pharmacokinetic studies with drugs metabolized by the respective P450 isozymes have not been performed yet.
- Excretion: primarily excreted in bile, eliminated in feces
  - Pioglitazone metabolized by hydroxylation and oxidation
  - Rosiglitazone metabolized by hydroxylation and N-demethylation

DRUG CLASS/USUAL DOSE

- Oral antidiabetic agent: thiazolidinediones class. Acting primarily by ↓ insulin resistance.
- Usual daily dosage
  - Pioglitazone 15–45 mg/d
  - Rosiglitazone 4–8 mg/d PO

DRUG EFFECTS

SYSTEM	EFFECT	ASSESSMENT BY HX	PE	TEST
GENERAL	Weight gain			
HEENT	Pharyngitis, sinusitis, URI, headache, myalgia	Cough, sneeze, rhinorrhea	Injected mucous membrane, productive cough, thick sputum	
CV	Plasma volume expansion, fluid retention Preload-induced cardiac hypertrophy	SOB, DOE, fatigue	Wheeze, pulmonary crackles, edema	↑ BUN, Cr, liver enzymes Hyponatremia CXR, ECHO ECG
HEME	Anemia	Fatigue, pallor		At most Hgb ↓ by 2–4%
ENDO	Hypoglycemia	Headache, vision changes, tremor, palpitations, Sz Concurrent hypoglycemic use	Diaphoresis, tachycardia, combativeness	Glucose level
	↑ Risk of pregnancy	Use of OCs or anovulatory females with insulin resistance (PCO disease)		Pregnancy test
GI/GU	1st generation (troglitazone) was related to idiosyncratic hepatotoxicity; no evidence of this in the 2nd-generation newer agents	N/V, fatigue, anorexia	Abd pain, Jaundice, dark urine	Liver enzymes

Key Reference: Mudalias S, Henry RR: New oral therapies for type 2 diabetes: the glitazones or insulin sensitizers. Annu Rev Med 2001; 52:239–257.

PERIOPERATIVE IMPLICATIONS

Preoperative Period
- Recommend to withhold antidiabetic agent on the day of surgery to ↓ chances of hypoglycemia that may occur with concurrent NPO requirements
- Although the risk is low, one should especially pay attention to CV, hematologic, and hepatic effects

Induction/Maintenance
- Serum glucose monitoring for hyper- or hypoglycemia with treatment as needed
- No known drug interactions

Postoperative
- Disturbances in glucose regulation (both hyper- and hypoglycemia) have been noted with several postop drugs: large doses of ASA, salicylates, quinolones
- Resume therapy with antidiabetic drug when patient has restarted PO intake, provided hepatic function is normal

ANTICIPATED PROBLEMS/CONCERNS
- Use of β-blockers can promote hyperglycemia (by ↑ insulin secretion and ↓ insulin sensitivity) and prolong hypoglycemia (by blocking compensatory action to epinephrine). Can mask the signs of hypoglycemia.

ISOPROTERENOL (ISUPREL)

Eric Jacobsohn, M.B., Ch.B., F.R.C.P.C.
Charl de Wet, M.B., Ch.B.

INDICATIONS

- IV in heart block (Stokes-Adams), atropine-resistant sinus bradycardia, AV block due to β-blocker overdose (glucagon preferred). IV infusion for pulmonary hypertension and in right heart failure.
- Bronchodilator in status asthmaticus (nebulized or as aerosol)
- Potent inotrope (shock, β-blocker overdose)

PERIOPERATIVE RISKS

- ↑ Risk of arrhythmias
- Multiple possible drug interactions: ↓ effect if taking guanethidine, reserpine; ↑ sensitivity if taking TCAs, and in cocaine users
- Can precipitate myocardial ischemia in susceptible patients

OVERVIEW/PHARMACOLOGY

- Potent synthetic direct-acting, pure β_1, β_2 stimulant
- No α-adrenergic effects
- β-Adrenergic stimulation causes ↑ intracellular cAMP (2nd messenger), → change in cellular function by causing enzyme or protein phosphorylation
- Short $T_{1/2}$ of 2 min; 60% excreted unchanged in urine, conjugated in liver; reuptake < that of epinephrine, norepinephrine; metabolized by MAO, COMT

DRUG CLASS/USUAL DOSE

- Direct-acting, synthetic catecholamine
- IV dose: mix 1–2 mg in 250 ml IV solution (4–8 μg/ml); infuse at 0.01–0.5 μg/kg/min
- Aerosol: 0.25% inhaler
- Nebulized: 0.25–1% solution, 0.5 ml in 2.5 ml H_2O over 10–20 min

DRUG EFFECTS

SYSTEM	EFFECT	ASSESSMENT BY HX	PE	TEST
RECEPTORS	α: 0 β_1: +++ β_2: +++			
CV	HR: +++ Contractility: +++ Automaticity: +++ Total peripheral resistance: − CO: +++ Mean BP: ± PAP: −	Palpitations, angina	HR Pulse Perfusion Mean BP	SV SVR CO BP PAP
RESP	Airway resistance: −−− Resp stimulant: +	Wheezing	Wheezing	Airway resistance Minute ventilation
VASC BED FLOW	Skin/viscera: + Muscle: ++ Kidney: − in normotensive patients, ++ in cardiogenic shock Coronary: + Cerebral: +	 Mentation	Skin perfusion	 Urine output
CNS	Mild stimulant Mild mydriasis	Anxiety, agitation, headache Mydriasis		
GU	Relaxation of uterus			
ENDO	O_2 consumption: ++ Blood glucose: ++ Blood lactic acid: ++ Hypokalemia Serum FFA: ++			O_2 consumption Blood glucose Blood lactate Serum K^+ Serum FFA

0: none; + minimal ↑ ; ++ moderate ↑ ; +++ marked ↑ ; − minimal ↓ ; −− moderate ↓ ; −−− marked ↓

Key Reference: Kondo V, Kim SO, Nakayama M, Murray PA: Pulmonary vascular effects of propofol at baseline, during elevated vasomotor tone, and in response to sympathetic alpha- and beta-adrenoreceptor activation. Anesthesiology 2001; 94:815–823.

POSSIBLE DRUG INTERACTIONS

Preoperative Concerns

- Interactions with MAO inhibitors
- ↑ Risk of arrhythmias. Response exaggerated in presence of cocaine and TCAs.
- ↓ Response in taking β-blockers, reserpine, or guanethidine
- Hypertensive, hyperthyroid patients are more susceptible to effects
- Hypokalemia can occur

Induction/Maintenance

- As in Preoperative Concerns

ANTICIPATED PROBLEMS/CONCERNS

- Hypotension from unopposed β-adrenergic activity
- Myocardium sensitized to catecholamines by some inhalational agents
- Risk of malignant arrhythmias, esp if dosed incorrectly
- Aggravates symptoms in psychoneurotic patients on emergence
- Hypokalemia, hyperglycemia
- Pulm edema can occur with infusions

LITHIUM CARBONATE

Charl de Wet, M.B., Ch.B.
Eric Jacobsohn, M.B., Ch.B., F.R.C.P.C.

INDICATIONS

• For acute manic states, as maintenance therapy for bipolar and some schizoaffective disorders
• For neutropenia associated with HIV antiviral therapy (may also ↑ platelet count)
• Measurement of cardiac output (small IV dose—no need for PA catheter)

PERIOPERATIVE RISKS

• Response to depolarizing, nondepolarizing muscle relaxants prolonged
• ↓ Dose requirement for IV and inhalational anesthetic
• Low therapeutic index and therefore requires vigilance and monitoring of serum levels. Toxicity is heralded by nausea/vomiting/diarrhea, thirst, neuromuscular weakness, hand tremors → gross tremors, dysarthria, ↓ level of consciousness, seizures, and death. CV problems include AV block, dysrhythmias, and hypotension.

OVERVIEW/PHARMACOLOGY

• At cellular level, acts as imperfect substitute for Na^+, intracellular accumulation of lithium ↓ phosphatidylinositides by interfering with hydrolysis of myoinositol-1-phosphate in the brain
• ↓ Availability of norepinephrine at central adrenergic synaptic clefts because of increased reabsorption into storage granules. Also interferes with Ca^{2+} depolarization–mediated release of norepinephrine and dopamine centrally.
• May also inhibit ability of some hormones to activate adenylyl cyclase
• Almost complete absorption from GI tract; peak levels 2–4 h after oral dose
• Initial distribution in extracellular fluid, subsequent accumulation in tissues
• No plasma protein binding
• Excreted via kidney; $1/3$–$2/3$ acute dose excreted in 6–12 h; 80% filtered lithium reabsorbed in proximal convoluted tubule

• Lithium clearance is 20% of creatinine clearance
• Na^+ depletion causes retention of lithium; ↑ lithium levels from thiazide diuretics, ECA, furosemide; Na^+ loading causes ↑ excretion of lithium
• Has low therapeutic index; therapeutic range: 0.8–1.25 mEq/L, toxic at levels >1.5 mEq/L

DRUG CLASS/USUAL DOSE

• Lithium salt
• Daily dose individualized; determined by regular monitoring of lithium levels. Usual adult dose varies: 750–1500 mg/d, in divided doses.

DRUG EFFECTS

SYSTEM	EFFECT	ASSESSMENT BY HX	PE	TEST
CV	Therapeutic levels cause benign ST interval/T wave changes Toxicity: malignant arrhythmias, heart block, hypotension	Dose, intercurrent illness, drugs precipitating toxicity	CVS exam	ECG
ENDO	Enlarged tender thyroid; hypothyroidism rare	Neck pain, hypothyroid symptoms	Thyroid	FT₄E/TSH
GU	Nephrogenic diabetes insipidus	Polyuria, polydipsia		Urine/serum lytes/osmolality
CNS	Toxicity: tremor, drowsiness, coma, convulsions Therapeutic: may cause drowsiness, EEG slowing	Dose, concomitant therapy, illnesses	CNS exam	Lithium level
DERM	Dermatitis			

Key Reference: Hill GE, Wong KC: Lithium carbonate and neuromuscular blocking agents. Anesthesiology 1977; 46:122–126.

POSSIBLE DRUG INTERACTIONS

Preoperative Concerns

• ↑ Linithium with risk of toxicity; thiazide diuretics, ECA, furosemide, ACE inhibitors, carbamazepine
• ↑ Risk of neurotoxicity: verapamil, diltiazem, metronidazole
• ↑ Risk of serotonin syndrome with fluoxetine

Induction/Maintenance

• Concerns same as Preoperative Concerns
• May have reduced requirement for inhaled and injected anesthesia
• Delayed recovery from barbiturates reported
• ↑ Response to depolarizing, nondepolarizing muscle relaxants

ANTICIPATED PROBLEMS/CONCERNS

• Be aware of signs and symptoms of toxicity. Toxic levels can be ↓ with *osmotic* diuretics (do *not* use furosemide), administration of saline, or dialysis.
• Severe CV collapse; arrhythmias, heart block possible with toxicity
• Nephrogenic diabetes insipidus occurs commonly and can be managed with KCl (preferred) or thiazide diuretics (risk of lithium toxicity). Other electrolyte abnormalities also can occur and may include hypocalcemia.
• Prolongs both types of NMB
• Avoid using haloperidol

MAGNESIUM SULFATE

Brett B. Gutsche, M.D.

INDICATIONS

- Primary use in obstetrics for
  – Tocolysis (treatment of preterm labor)
  – Treatment of preeclampsia-eclampsia for its anticonvulsant, tocolytic, vasodilator properties. It also has bronchial dilator properties and has been used to treat acute asthmatic attacks.
- Usually given by the IV route (IM rarely used in modern obstetrics)
- Orally as a cathartic or laxative (minimal absorption from the gut)

PERIOPERATIVE RISKS

- Skeletal muscle weakness
- Hypotension

WORRY ABOUT

- Increased sensitivity to all muscle relaxants, but especially to nondepolarizing muscle relaxants. Recent data suggest that initial intubation dose of succinylcholine is not reduced; it may be somewhat antagonized in patients receiving magnesium sulfate.
- Severe hypotension with potent inhalation anesthetics, sympathetic block, antihypertensive drugs
- Attenuation of pressor substance effects

OVERVIEW/PHARMACOLOGY

- Tocolytic, ↓ uterine activity associated with preterm labor and preeclampsia-eclampsia
- Anticonvulsant, direct CNS depression (central hippocampus)
- Skeletal muscle relaxant acting at myoneural junction; may antagonize nondepolarizing muscle relaxant reversal by anti-ChEs
- 90% renal excretion, $T_{1/2}$ of 4 h
- Appears to produce sedation that is not associated with amnesia or analgesia

DRUG CLASS/MECH OF ACTION/USUAL DOSE

- Mg^{2+} is a major intracellular ion
- Depresses release of acetylcholine (ACh) and sensitivity of receptor to ACh; causes increased levels of both AMP and cGMP. Interferes with action of Ca^{2+} required for both muscle contraction and neuromuscular transmission.
- Usually administered intravenously
  – Therapeutic blood levels 4–8 mEq/L (5–10 mg/dl)
- Usual dosage
  – 4% IV solution (40 mg/L)
  – Initial bolus 4–6 g over 20 min, then 1–3 g/h by continuous infusion
  – 10% IV solutions (100 g/L) as above
  – 50% Solution (500 mg/ml) for IM use only; 10 g IM initially; 5 g q 4 h maintenance doses

DRUG EFFECTS

SYSTEM	EFFECT	ASSESSMENT BY HX	PE	TEST
CV	Vasodilation	Flushing, ↓ BP	↓ BP
Signs of shock, depressed CO	Blood level
	Myocardial depression
Pulmonary edema	Bradycardia
Asystole		ECG
PA catheter
RESP	Muscle weakness
Bronchial dilatation
Upper airway edema	Dyspnea	Obstruction
Hypoxia	ABGs, pulse oximetry, capnography
CNS	Depression	Cessation of convulsion	Somnolence	Blood level of Mg^{2+}
MS	Weakness, ↑ sensitivity to nondepolarizing muscle relaxants	Respiratory obstruction, exaggerated response to small doses of muscle relaxants	Lethargy, weakness, depressed or absent deep tendon reflexes (DTR)	↓ or absent DTR; high levels serum Mg^{2+} (should be <8 mEq/L); nerve stimulator
OB	↓ Strength and frequency of contractions	↓ Pain, hemorrhage, failure to contract following delivery	Abdominal palpation of uterine activity	External or internal monitoring of uterine contractions

Key Reference: Muir HA, McGrath JM, Chestnut DH: Preterm labor and delivery; Gambling DR, Writer D: Hypertensive disorders. *In* Chestnut DH (ed), Obstetric Anesthesia: Principles and Practice, 2nd ed, St. Louis, Mosby, 1999, pp 680–684 and pp 891–892 and 899–901, respectively.

PERIOPERATIVE IMPLICATIONS

Preoperative Concerns

- Assess respiratory adequacy, muscle strength before major conduction analgesia
- Avoid nondepolarizing muscle relaxant if possible
- Renal dysfunction may lead to accumulation and overdose with continued administration
- Pulmonary edema is possible

Monitoring

- Routine
- Nerve stimulator

Induction/Maintenance

- Intubate with full dose of succinylcholine (1 mg/kg)
- Avoid or use in very small doses the rapid-acting nondepolarizing muscle relaxants, being guided by a nerve stimulator
- Continue during labor, delivery, post partum in preeclampsia-eclampsia; discontinue in preterm labor when delivery is to occur
- Hypotension requiring therapy is common after both regional and general anesthesia

Adjuvants/Regional Anesthesia/Reversal

- May attenuate response to vasopressors
- Ca^{2+} may partially reverse CNS and CV effects, but not NM effects. Do not give Ca^{2+} in preeclampsia or eclampsia unless required for CV reasons.

Postoperative/Postpartum Periods

- Preterm labor patients may develop pulmonary edema, especially if general anesthesia is used
- Continue for delivery and post partum in preeclampsia-eclampsia
- Assess respiratory adequacy before extubation

Anticipated Problems/Concerns

- Development of pulmonary edema
- Incomplete NM reversal of nondepolarizing muscle relaxant
- Postpartum hemorrhage
- Exaggerated hypotensive response to major conduction anesthesia, potent inhalation anesthetics, and other antihypertensives
- MAC may be decreased

MARIJUANA

James P. Zacny, Ph.D.

USES

• In smoked form or as the resin (hashish), which is ingested, a DEA Schedule I drug indicative of high abuse liability and no putative medical indication; however, a recent Institute of Medicine report (1999) recommends urgent need for carefully controlled clinical trials to determine if smoked marijuana has medical indications (e.g., AIDS wasting syndrome, glaucoma)
• In oral form as delta-9-tetrahydrocannabinol, or nabilone, a DEA Schedule II drug for chemotherapy-induced N/V

PERIOPERATIVE RISKS

• Overdose of marijuana can induce a paranoid state

WORRY ABOUT

• Acute effects include tachycardia and ↑ systolic BP
• Chronic effects can include asthma or bronchitis and ↓ transport of secretions

OVERVIEW/PHARMACOLOGY

• Major active constituent is delta-9-tetrahydrocannabinol (THC), although contains other active cannabinoids
• Bioavailability of smoked and oral THC is 2–50% and 4–12%, respectively
• $T_{1/2}$ of THC is 30 h because of its high lipid solubility
• Most of THC is metabolized; only a small fraction is excreted unchanged
• When smoked, produces a rapid onset of intoxication lasting 2–3 h; when ingested, duration of effect is 6 h
• With low to moderate doses, acute intoxication includes ↑ sense of well-being (euphoria), short-term memory and complex psychomotor impairment, depersonalization, time distortion (i.e., overestimation), ↑ sensation and perception of surrounding stimuli, ↑ hunger
• Physiologic changes include dry mouth and throat, marked reddening of the conjunctivae, ↓ IOP, ↑ HR, ↑ BP when supine, ↑ myocardial O_2 demand
• Overdosage may produce hallucinations, delusions, paranoid feelings
• In predisposed people, seizures can develop

DRUG CLASS/MECH OF ACTION/USUAL DOSE

• Cannabinoid: a cannabinoid receptor, as well as a ligand for it, anandomide, has been isolated in the CNS, indicative of endogenous cannabinoids
• Dosage depends on route of administration, especially with smoked marijuana
• Average THC content of marijuana in USA ranges from 0.5–11%

DRUG EFFECTS

SYSTEM	EFFECT	ASSESSMENT BY HX	PE	TEST
CV	Tachycardia, Htn	Chronicity and acuity of exposure	Vital signs	Urine toxicology screen
	Occasional orthostatic hypotension			
CNS	Intoxication, psychosis; ↓ IOP, antiemesis			

Key Reference: O'Brien CP: Drug addiction and drug abuse. *In* Hardman JG, Limbird LE (eds): Goodman and Gilman's The Pharmacological Basis of Therapeutics, 9th ed. New York, McGraw-Hill Professional Publishers, 1996, pp 572–573.

PERIOPERATIVE IMPLICATIONS/POSSIBLE DRUG INTERACTIONS

Preoperative Concerns

• Chronic use of smoked marijuana can cause bronchitis or asthma
• Tachycardia and drowsiness/sedation
• Ventilatory depression by opioids accentuated

Induction/Maintenance

• ↓ Anesthetic requirement (in animals) while intoxicated
• Barbiturate- and ketamine-induced sleep times may be prolonged
• Tachycardia and hypertension

Postoperative Period

• Pt may awaken in a state of agitation or psychosis
• Withdrawal usually mild

SPECIAL CONSIDERATIONS/CONCERNS

• Chronic use can lead to resp diseases, even in young adults
• Heavy use (7+ times/wk) is associated with impaired learning and memory; may predispose to inadequate compliance with perioperative instructions

METFORMIN (GLUCOPHAGE)

Sean M. Berenholtz, M.D.
Todd Dorman, M.D.

USES

- Oral hypoglycemic agent (biguanide class) for treatment of type II diabetes mellitus
- Second most prescribed oral glucose lowering agent in Europe
- Currently available in USA as Glucophage and Glocovan (glyburide/metformin)

PERIOPERATIVE RISKS

- Metformin-associated lactic acidosis (MALA): incidence about 3 cases/100,000 patient years
- Hypoglycemia rarely occurs with metformin therapy; hyperglycemia can occur if medication withheld, requiring frequent perioperative glucose monitoring
- Routine therapy is recommended if hyperglycemia occurs

WORRY ABOUT

- MALA-type 2 (not due to tissue ischemia); mechanism thought to be due to a shift in the intracellular redox potential away from aerobic to anaerobic metabolism, leading to an increase in cellular lactate production
- MALA has been reported almost exclusively in patients with one or more risk factors, including perioperative renal impairment, radiocontrast dye, hypoperfusion state (septic or cardiogenic shock), hepatic impairment, or hypoxemia
- 50% mortality with biguanide-induced lactic acidosis includes phenformin use; mortality of MALA is unclear but thought to be 33–56%

OVERVIEW/PHARMACOLOGY

- Oral hypoglycemic agent: biguanide class includes metformin, phenformin, and buformin

- Exact mechanism of biguanides is unclear but may involve inhibition of glycogenolysis and hepatic glucose production and/or increasing sensitivity of peripheral tissues to insulin, resulting in tighter glucose control
- Absorption 0.9–2.6 h; maximal plasma concentration 1–2 h after oral dose; plasma $T_{1/2}$ 1.5–4.9 h; negligible binding to plasma proteins
- Not measurably metabolized; 90% is eliminated in urine in 12 h
- Hemodialysis effectively removes lactate and metformin

DRUG CLASS/USUAL DOSE

- Oral hypoglycemic: two main biguanides, phenformin and metformin, introduced in the late 1950s; phenformin withdrawn from clinical use in the USA in 1976 because of association with fatal lactic acidosis
- Usual start dose of metformin is 500 mg bid and increased slowly to a maximum of 2550 mg/d

DRUG EFFECTS

SYSTEM	EFFECT	ASSESSMENT BY HX	PE	TEST
CV	MALA	Presence of risk factors		Serum bicarbonate or ABGs
GI	Diarrhea, abdominal discomfort, nausea; hepatotoxicity (rare)			
HEME	Anemia (rare)			Hemoglobin
CNS	Headache, agitation, dizziness, fatigue (rare)			
ENDO	Hypoglycemia	Concurrent hypoglycemic agents		Serum glucose

Key Reference: Chan NN, Brain HPS, Feher MD: Metformin-associated lactic acidosis: a rare or very rare clinical entity? Diabet Med 1999; 16:273–281.

POSSIBLE DRUG INTERACTIONS

Preoperative Period

- Recommendations vary; metformin should be withheld for a minimum of 8 h preoperatively; PDR Recommendations: withhold metformin for at least 1 or 2 $T_{1/2}$ preoperatively

Induction

- No known drug interactions
- Hypotension, hypovolemia, and hypoxia are risk factors for MALA

Maintenance

- No known drug interactions

Adjuvants/Regional Anesthesia/Reversal

- No known contraindications or interactions

Postoperative Concerns

- Metformin can be restarted when the patient has resumed oral intake, provided that renal function has remained normal and is expected to remain normal, and no risk factors for MALA are present
- Metformin should be withheld for 48 h after radiocontrast dye and restarted only if renal function has remained normal and unchanged

ANTICIPATED PROBLEMS/CONCERNS

- Assess for MALA or risk factors for MALA (hypovolemia, hypotension, hypoxemia)
- Monitor for hyperglycemia if medication withheld

MONOAMINE OXIDASE INHIBITORS; REVERSIBLE INHIBITORS OF MONOAMINE OXIDASE

Kent Z. Ozkum, M.D.

USES

- Oral agents (Nardil [phenelzine], Marplan [isocarboxazid], Eutonyl [pargyline], Parnate [tranylcypromine], and others) prescribed primarily for patients with depression refractory to other antidepressant agents
- Newer, reversible agents may widen use in treating depression, related disorders

PERIOPERATIVE RISKS

- Hepatotoxicity
- Peripheral sympathetic overactivation (Htn, tachycardia, hallucinations, agitation, hyperthermia, seizures, coma)
- Orthostatic hypotension; mechanism unclear, possibly 2° to sympathetic *under*activity
- Central hyperpyrexia

WORRY ABOUT

- Sympathetic crisis
- Multiple drug interactions, including
  - Foods: high tyramine- and dopamine-containing products often produced by aging, fermentation, pickling, smoking; broad (fava) beans (NB: tyramine acts as indirect sympathomimetic with release of norepinephrine at postganglionic sympathetic nerve endings); L-tryptophan, phenylalanine, tyrosine
  - Indirect sympathomimetics, such as ephedrine
  - Direct sympathomimetics (epinephrine, norepinephrine, amphetamines, cocaine) may produce prolonged effect
  - Uncommonly, *opioids*, especially dextromethorphan, pethidine, meperidine; 3 types of interactions: excitatory—2° to serotonin overactivity; depressive—inhibition of hepatic microsomal enzymes, leading to accumulation of excess narcotic; febrile → coma
    - Serotonin-uptake inhibitors (Prozac)
    - Buspirone (Buspar)
    - Bupropion (Wellbutrin)
    - Excessive caffeine
  - Antiparkinsonian agents (methyldopa, L-dopa)
  - Numerous OTC formulations

OVERVIEW/PHARMACOLOGY

- Readily absorbed PO
- Widely distributed enzyme system
- Traditional agents bind covalently, produce max enzyme inhibition 5–10 days; reversible agents have rapid onset (<1 h), short $T_{1/2}$ (~4 h)
- Large vol of distribution
- Clearance primarily hepatic; caution with concomitant cimetidine administration or hepatic dysfunction
- Most appear to have no clinically significant active metabolites
- Contraindications: known hypersensitivity, pheochromocytoma, liver dysfunction/disease, advanced HD, cerebrovascular disease; pts receiving antiparkinsonian agents, potent hypotensive agents, sedatives/CNS depressants

DRUG CLASS/MECH OF ACTION/USUAL DOSE

- Block oxidative deamination of amine-based neurotransmitters such as serotonin, dopamine, norepinephrine (A enzyme), and/or tyramine, phenethylamine (B enzyme) into VMA
- Antidepressant effects appear related to ↑CNS neurotransmitter levels
- May be
  - Hydrazine vs. nonhydrazine
  - A or B enzyme specificity: type A preferentially deaminates norepinephrine, epinephrine, serotonin; type B preferentially deaminates phenylethylamine. "Specific" agents appear to lack many side effects traditionally attributed to nonspecific MAO inhibitors, even in overdosage
  - Reversible vs. irreversible inhibitor; reversible agents bind noncovalently, have shorter duration of action; may be called RIMAs
  - Traditional nonselective MAO inhibitors, bind covalently to enzyme, require up to 2 wk for new enzyme biosynthesis
- There may be down-regulation of α and/or β postsynaptic receptors
- No direct sedative, arrhythmogenic effects
- Overdosage Rx includes α-blocker, β-blocker, ganglionic-blockers, direct vasodilators, supportive care, mech ventilation, cooling, etc.

DRUG EFFECTS

SYSTEM	EFFECT	ASSESSMENT BY HX	PE	TEST
CV	Sympathetic under-, overactivation	Duration Rx Discontinuation?	Orthostatics Vital signs stable	
CNS	Hyperthermia, agitation?, dizziness, headache, myoclonus		Normothermia?	
GI/HEPATIC	Constipation, dry mouth Low incidence of hepatotoxicity			LFTs

Key Reference: Nemeroff CB: The neurobiology of depression. Sci Am 1998; 278 (June): 42–49.

PERIOPERATIVE IMPLICATIONS

Preoperative Concerns

- Check liver enzymes/LFTs
- Discontinue Rx?
  - Enzyme inhibition may be either reversible or irreversible; if *irreversible* enzyme inhibition, discontinue drug 14–21 days before elective surgery—biosynthesis of new enzyme may take weeks. *Reversible* inhibition may not require discontinuation before anesthesia.
  - Specificity of agent in use: type A enzyme–specific agents appear to have fewer side effects, drug interactions of clinical significance
- Urgency of surgery
- Sx of toxicity?

Induction/Maintenance

- Avoid meperidine, H_2 release
- Possible accentuation of CNS/resp depression
- May have prolonged response to succinylcholine 2° to ↓ serum ChE levels
- Anesthetic requirements may be ↑ by SNS hyperactivity
- Avoid SNS activation (anxiety, pain) when possible
- Avoid indirect-acting sympathomimetics
- Use direct-acting sympathomimetics cautiously; response may be exaggerated.
- Consider regional anesthesia techniques
- MAO inhibitors may produce nonspecific hepatic microsomal inhibition, leading to ↓ clearance of anesthetic agents such as barbiturates; potentially ↑ risk of toxic (reductive) metabolites
- Avoid
  - Ketamine 2° to potential for postop delirium/excitation/sympathetic activation
  - Pancuronium 2° to mild epinephrine-releasing activity
  - Anticholinergics may produce clinical Sx similar to those from MAO inhibitor toxicity
  - All local anesthetics appear safe except *cocaine*

Adjuvants/Regional Anesthesia/Reversal

- Regional anesthesia possibly helpful
- Antihypertensive agents should be readily available: consider α-blocker as first-line agents (vs. β-blocker) to avoid unopposed α activity in combination with β-blockade

Postoperative Period

- Regional technique in use?
- Use narcotics very cautiously

ANTICIPATED PROBLEMS/CONCERNS

- Sympathetic crisis
- Hepatotoxicity

NICOTINE (TOBACCO, CIGARETTES, SNUFF, SPIT TOBACCO) AND NICOTINE REPLACEMENT THERAPIES (GUM, INHALER, NASAL SPRAY, PATCH)

James P. Zacny, Ph.D.
Christopher J. Young, M.D.

RISK

- Inhalation of tobacco smoke (28% of USA citizens directly smoke, with 10+% exposed and absorb significant amounts via second-hand smoke); other sources of nicotine include nicotine gum, chewing tobacco, pipe smoking, nicotine inhaler (absorption through buccal cavity), snuff, nicotine nasal spray (absorption through nasal mucosa), transdermal patch (absorption through dermis)
- Nicotine gum, inhaler, nasal spray, and patch are FDA-approved devices for the treatment of tobacco dependence

PERIOPERATIVE RISKS

- Adverse CV and resp effects

WORRY ABOUT

- Whether to advise patients to stop smoking for several days before surgery; short-term abstinence (<1–2 mos) may actually increase airway secretions and induce a bronchospastic state and is associated with increased postoperative complications

OVERVIEW/PHARMACOLOGY

- $T_{1/2}$ of nicotine via inhaled tobacco smoke = 2 h
- 80–90% of nicotine is altered in liver and to lesser extent in kidneys and lungs
- Significant fraction of nicotine is metabolized in the lungs to cotinine and nicotine-1'-N-oxide
- Nicotine and its metabolites are rapidly eliminated by the kidneys
- Nicotine stimulates hepatic enzyme induction; results in faster metabolism of some anesthetics, sedatives, analgesics
- Drug has subtle subjective effects, including (depending on circumstances and individual) stimulation or relaxation
- Withdrawal syndrome includes irritability and restlessness that can last up to 72 h; craving can last for months after cessation of smoking

DRUG CLASS/MECH OF ACTION/USUAL DOSE

- A natural alkaloid that stimulates autonomic ganglia
- Acts at the nicotinic cholinergic receptor as an agonist
- Dose used by a dependent smoker is 10–40 mg/d

DRUG EFFECTS

SYSTEM	EFFECT	ASSESSMENT BY HX	PE	TEST
CV	Tachycardia, Htn	Magnitude and duration of smoking	Clubbing, cyanosis	O_2 saturation
RESP	Hypersecretion of mucus	Presence of cough, degree of sputum production, co-existing cardiac disease, reversible pulm disease assessment	Sputum characteristics, retractions or resp compromise, bronchospasm	PFTs with bronchodilation
CNS	Stimulatory			
IMMUNO	↓ Neutrophil and NK cell activity, immunoglobulin conc			

Key References: Bluman LG, Mosca L, Newman N, Simon DG: Preoperative smoking habits and postoperative pulmonary complications. Chest 1998; 113:883–889; Warner MA, Offord KP, Warner ME: Role of preoperative cessation of smoking and other factors in postoperative pulmonary complications: a blinded prospective study of coronary artery bypass patients. Mayo Clin Proc 1989; 64:609–616.

PERIOPERATIVE IMPLICATIONS/POSSIBLE DRUG INTERACTIONS

Preoperative Concerns

- Long-term abstinence (8 wk) should be encouraged, especially for thoracic surgery; it leads to improvement in mucociliary transport and small airway function and ↓ in airway secretions and reactivity, but perioperative morbidity may transiently ↑ as mucociliary transport returns
- Short-term abstinence (24–48 h) has benefits including ↑ in hemoglobin available for O_2 transport and availability of O_2 to tissues, and ↓ in nicotine-induced tachycardia
- In some pts, excessive anxiety may occur in nicotine withdrawal

Induction/Maintenance

- Hypersecretion of mucus

POSTOPERATIVE PERIOD

- ↑ Risk of bronchospasm, purulent sputum with pyrexia, pleural effusion or pneumothorax requiring drainage, segmental pulmonary collapse, atelectasis, pneumonia
- ↑ Use of respiratory therapy care services (vigorous pulmonary toilet)
- Postop agitation/anxiety from nicotine withdrawal

SPECIAL CONSIDERATIONS

- Pts should be advised to quit smoking as early as possible
- For pts with increased anxiety, an anxiolytic can be prescribed, or consider nicotine supplementation (transdermal patch)
- ↑ Risk of perioperative hypersecretion from short-term smoking abstinence can be countered by use of bronchodilators
- ↑ Risk of perioperative deep vein thrombosis from short-term smoking abstinence can be countered by anticoagulants, including aspirin, 325 mg/d

NITRIC OXIDE, INHALED

Warren M. Zapol, M.D.

INDICATIONS

• Children: persistent pulm Htn of newborn, congenital diaphragmatic hernia, meconium aspiration, before or after surgery for congenital heart disease, acute or chronic pulm Htn
• Adults: ARDS, pulm embolism, acute or chronic pulm Htn

PERIOPERATIVE RISKS

• Methemoglobinemia (esp breathing > 20 ppm NO)
• NO_2 and peroxynitrite formation

WORRY ABOUT

• Methemoglobinemia; measure metHb esp for infants, within 6 h, then every 24 h
• Measure NO and NO_2 levels continuously
• Do not give high NO_2 levels (> 2 ppm)
• Do not leave NO in ventilator or anesthesia machine; it slowly converts to toxic NO_2 gas

• High inhaled NO levels may inhibit platelet aggregation
• In severe heart failure, reducing PVR with NO may raise LAP
• Rebound pulm Htn during NO withdrawal

OVERVIEW/PHARMACOLOGY

• Inhaled NO activates guanylate cyclase in lung vessels, airways ↑ cGMP levels, causes pulm vasodilation, bronchodilation
• Very rapid reaction and acid binding with Hgb inactivates NO, prevents systemic vasodilation
• Inhaled NO becomes nitrate and nitrite, is excreted in urine
• Supplied as stock gas of ≤ 1,000 ppm by vol NO in nitrogen or other inert gas
• Mixed with O_2-containing gas immediately before breathing
• Gas inhaled via ventilator, mask, nasal prongs, intratracheal catheter

MECHANISM OF ACTION/DRUG/CLASS

• $N{=}O^{\cdot}$ is a free radical with short $T_{1/2}$ in aqueous solutions (~ 17 sec)
• It combines with ferrous-heme ring of guanylate cyclase, activating it, thereby converting GTP to cyclic GMP; cGMP reduces intracellular Ca^{2+}, causing smooth muscle relaxation; cGMP broken down by phosphodiesterases
• Usual inhaled NO dose is 0.1 to 20 ppm by vol

DRUG EFFECTS

SYSTEM	EFFECT	PE	TEST
RESP	↓ PVR		↓ PAP ↑ CO
	↑ Gas exchange	Skin color	↑ PaO_2 ↑ SaO_2 ↓ $PaCO_2$

Key Reference: Clark RH, Kueser TJ, Walker MW, Southgate WM, Huckaby JL, Perez JA, Roy BJ, Keszler M, Kinsella JP, for the Clinical Inhaled Nitric Oxide Research Group. Low-dose nitric oxide therapy for persistent pulmonary hypertension of the newborn. N Engl J Med 2000; 342:469–474.

PERIOPERATIVE IMPLICATIONS

• Check for heart failure; do not use in severe heart failure (e.g., PCWP > 25 mmHg)

Monitoring

• Consider monitoring
  – PA pressure
  – RV ECHO
  – ABGs, SpO_2
• Must monitor
  – Inhaled NO, NO_2 levels
• metHb levels

Induction/Maintenance

• Inhale 0.1–20 ppm in ARDS (usual dose: 5–15 ppm)
• In persistent pulm Htn of newborn, begin near 20–40 ppm, slowly reduce to 5 ppm or less
• Ideal doses need better definition
• Give as little NO as possible to reduce oxidant burden of lung

Adjuvants

• Phosphodiesterase inhibitors (e.g., dipyridamole, zaprinast) increase sensitivity to NO, duration of dilatory effect

Postoperative Period

• Slowly wean from NO over hours if possible

ANTICIPATED PROBLEMS/CONCERNS

• Beware rapid discontinuation of inhaled NO; reactive pulm vasoconstriction, RHF may ensue
• Do not allow NO stock tanks to run low
• Provide NO in gas for manual ventilation
• If inhaled NO does not reverse hypoxemia despite mechanical ventilation with PEEP, high-frequency oscillatory ventilation, etc., ECMO may be required

NITROGLYCERIN

Lee A. Fleisher, M.D.

INDICATIONS

- Rx for patients with angina
- CHF
- In MI, ↓ infarct size
- Prinzmetal's angina
- Can be given as patch, paste, PO, sublingually prn
- Uterine relaxation

PERIOPERATIVE RISKS

- Development of hypotension
- Drug rash (rare)

WORRY ABOUT

- Severe hypotension, especially with regional anesthesia

OVERVIEW/PHARMACOLOGY

- Used for both chronic Rx and acute management
- Prophylactic nitroglycerin not shown to ↓ incidence of intraoperative myocardial infarction
- Tolerance to drug from prolonged IV infusion or continuous patch can occur
- Metabolized by reductive hydrolysis in liver
- Rapidity of onset, duration of action directly related to method of administration
  - SL: onset 1–2 min, duration < 1 h
  - Oral: peak effect 60–90 min, duration 3–6 h
  - Paste: onset 60 min, duration 4–8 h
  - Patch: duration up to 24 h
- Prolonged use can → tolerance (↓ effectiveness)
- Nitroglycerin paste/patch may have uneven absorption intraoperatively

DRUG CLASS/MECH OF ACTION/USUAL DOSE

- Organic nitrate
- Activates guanylate cyclase; ↑ cGMP levels in smooth muscle, other tissues; increases nitric oxide
- Usual dosage:
  - SL: 0.4 mg prn
  - Paste: $\frac{1}{2}''$–1″
  - Patch: 1/d
  - Isordil: 5–30 mg q 6 h
  - IV: 0.5–2.0 μg/kg/min
- Bolus for uterine relaxation (slow 50 μg; may repeat × 1 with caution if has regional anesthesia actively causing sympathectomy)

DRUG EFFECTS

SYSTEM	EFFECT	ASSESSMENT BY HX	PE	TEST
CV	Vasodilation of veins > arteries Redistribution of coronary blood flow	Relief of angina	BP	PCWP
RESP	Decreased pulmonary vascular resistance			PCWP
GU	Uterine (smooth muscle) relaxation			
CNS	Dilation of meningeal arterial vessels	Headache		

Key Reference: Zvara DA, Groban L, Rogers AT, et al: Prophylactic nitroglycerin did not reduce myocardial ischemia during accelerated recovery management of coronary artery bypass graft surgery patients. J Cardiothorac Vasc Anesth 2000, 14:571–575.

PERIOPERATIVE IMPLICATIONS

Preoperative Concerns

- Assess volume status
- Consider monitoring:
  - BP (arterial catheter)
  - PA catheter (may give useful information if nitroglycerin infusion used)

Induction/Maintenance

- May interact with other induction agents to cause hypotension
- Ideally should be given IV because of uneven absorption intraoperatively (binding sites on tubing)
- Effective means of alleviating myocardial ischemia intraoperatively
- Has been used prophylactically as bolus during induction
- Anesthetic agents may mimic beneficial effects of nitroglycerin

Adjuvants/Regional Anesthesia/Reversal

- Agents that can result in hypotension may be exacerbated by nitroglycerin

Postoperative Period

- Patients on chronic nitroglycerin may benefit by resumption of agent
- Can give as patch or paste after rewarming of patient

ANTICIPATED PROBLEMS/CONCERNS

- Tolerance to nitroglycerin manifests by ↓ hemodynamic effects; a function of dose, frequency of administration
- Many inhalational agents and opiates have some aspect of hemodynamic effects of nitroglycerin—e.g., venodilation, ↓ O_2 demand

NONSTEROIDAL ANTI-INFLAMMATORY DRUGS (NSAIDS)

Peter L. Bailey, M.D.

INDICATIONS

- 100 million USA prescriptions/y; many additional taken through OTC route
- Taken orally for rheumatic disorders, pain states
- Given IM/IV for periop pain

PERIOPERATIVE RISKS

- 10% of all patients take NSAIDs
- Most common risks = gastric bleeding, renal dysfunction, impaired platelet function
- Drug interactions: NSAIDs displace albumin-bound drugs and/or ↓ drug elimination (e.g., warfarin, methotrexate)
- NSAIDs may ↓ antihypertensive agent efficacy

WORRY ABOUT

- Decreased NSAID clearance in elderly may ↑ adverse effects and drug interactions: especially warfarin, methotrexate; also lithium, phenytoin, digoxin, aminoglycosides, sulfonylurea hypoglycemic agents
- NSAIDs may ↓ antihypertensive agent efficacy

OVERVIEW/PHARMACOLOGY

- Weak organic acid compounds (non-ionized) of diverse chemical structure and half-lives
- Well absorbed by GI tract, highly protein-bound (albumin mostly)
- Cyclooxygenase inhibition and ↓ prostaglandin synthesis lead to ↓ inflammatory response and ↓ nociception (peripheral and central action) and ↓ fever
- Clearance by hepatic metabolism and renal excretion, can accumulate with liver disease, age
- Displaces albumin-bound drugs (e.g., warfarin), increasing drug effect

Ketorolac tromethamine (Toradol)

DRUG CLASS/MECH OF ACTION/USUAL DOSE

- NSAIDs are cylooxygenase and prostaglandin synthesis inhibitors
- > 12 NSAIDs available in the USA
- Ketorolac (Toradol) available for parenteral use; maximum loading dose = 1 mg/kg up to 60 mg; usual dose is 30 mg; ↓ dose in elderly; maintenance dose, $\frac{1}{2}$ loading dose q 6 h, up to 5 days

Ibuprofen (Advil, Nuprin)

Acetylsalicylic acid (aspirin)

DRUG EFFECTS

SYSTEM	EFFECT	ASSESSMENT BY HX	PE	TEST
CV	Hypertension may be more difficult to control		BP	
RESP	Nasal polyps, rhinitis, dyspnea, bronchospasm	In asthmatics		
HEPATIC	Hepatitis			LFTs
GI	Gastropathy (can be asymptomatic) can develop in days to weeks, GI bleeding, esophageal disease, diarrhea, pancreatitis	Hx ulcers, heartburn		↑ Transaminase
ENDO	Angioedema, anaphylactoid reactions			
HEME	↑ Bleeding	Hx easy bruising/bleeding		Bleeding time, eosinophilia; rarely, aplastic anemia
DERM	Urticaria, erythema multiforme, rash			
GU	Renal insufficiency, hyperkalemia, sodium/H_2O retention		BP	↑ K^+, BUN, Cr, ↓ UO, biopsy
CNS	Headache, aseptic meningitis, hearing disorders	Cognitive dysfunction, somnolence, confusion		CSF

Key Reference: Pavy TJ, Paech MJ, Evans SF: The effect of intravenous ketorolac on opioid requirement and pain after Cesarean delivery. Anesth Anal, 2001; 92:1010–1014.

PERIOPERATIVE IMPLICATIONS/DRUG INTERACTIONS

Preoperative Concerns
- GI bleeding, renal function, hemostasis

Monitoring
- Hct/Hgb, Cr/BUN/K^+, bleeding time

Drug Interactions
- Warfarin, sulfonylureas, phenytoin, valproic acid, digoxin, aminoglycosides, albumin-bound drugs (benzodiazepines)

Precautions
- ↓ Above drug doses, monitor blood levels, NSAIDs may ↓ antihypertensive drug efficacy

Resumption of Agent
- NSAIDs should be resumed cautiously with monitoring for GI bleeding, renal dysfunction. Avoid resumption in seriously ill patients.

SPECIAL PROBLEMS/CONSIDERATIONS
- Gastropathy: occult bleeding
- Renal dysfunction: ↑ K^+
- Drug interactions, especially coumadin
- Hemostasis: bleeding time
- Miscellaneous and rare: hepatic dysfunction, pancreatitis, cutaneous reactions

NUTRITIONAL SUPPORT

Terrence H. Liu, M.D.
Jerome H. Abrams, M.D.

RISK

• 3–5% of patients malnourished preop; elderly at greater risk (20% of patients >85 y malnourished)

PERIOPERATIVE RISKS OF MALNUTRITION

• ↓ Resp, cardiac, skeletal muscle mass, strength
• ↓ Visceral protein mass, altered GI mucosal barrier
• Altered humoral, cell-mediated immunity
• Altered neutrophil function
• ↑ Pulm, thromboembolic complications
• Patients with protein-calorie malnutrition have ↑ risk for postop cardiac, noncardiac complications

WORRY ABOUT

• Hypo- or hyperglycemia, depending on additives to TPN

OVERVIEW

• Nutritional risk index (NRI) = $1.519 \times$ serum albumin (g/L) + $[0.417 \times$ (current wt/usual wt) $\times 100]$. (Malnutrition defined as NRI <100; severe malnutrition defined as NRI <83.5.)
• Preop nutritional support for 5–7 days may result in ↓ in infectious complications in severely malnourished patients

TPN Composition

• Fluid: 30 ml/kg/d, additional losses
• Calories: 25–30 Kcal/kg/d
  – Glucose: 3.0–5.0 g/kg/d
  – Fat: 1.0–1.5 g/kg/d
  – Protein: 1.5–2.0 g/kg/d
• Additives:
  – Multivitamins in the form of balanced formula should be provided daily
  – IV formula requires addition of vitamin K, 2 mg/d
  – Trace elements should be given daily to patients with GFR >20 ml/d; magnesium: 15–20 mg/d; zinc: 15–20 mg/d. (Requirement for replacement is based on serum level.)

ICD-9-CM Code: 261 (Malnutrition)

Special Formulas

• Modified amino acid formula is more efficient in restoring positive nitrogen balance, ↓ ureagenesis, and ↑ support of protein synthesis

---

ASSESSMENT POINTS

SYSTEM	EFFECT	ASSESSMENT BY HX	PE	TEST
MS	>10% loss of body wt over 6 mo	Hx of renal, hepatic dysfunction Hx of short gut	Muscle wasting ↓ Triceps and skinfold thickness	Alb <3.0 g/dl Total lymphocyte count <1500 cells/mm³

Key References: The VA Total Parenteral Nutrition Cooperative Study Group: Perioperative total parenteral nutrition in surgical patients. N Engl J Med 1991; 325, 8:525; Barton RG: Nutritional support in critical illness. Nutr Clin Pract 1994; 9:127–139.

PREOPERATIVE CONCERNS

Monitoring

• Monitoring is essential to maximize benefit and to minimize complications
• Weight: daily
• Electrolytes: daily initially
• Zinc: weekly
• Magnesium: daily
• Liver function test: weekly
• PT/PTT: weekly
• Nutritional variable: albumin, prealbumin, transferrin. Failure to improve or maintain adequate levels usually represents inadequate nutritional support, intercurrent systemic inflammatory response, or advanced organ failure.

INDUCTION/MAINTENANCE

• TPN is usually continued intraoperatively
• Monitor glucose

ADJUVANTS

• For morbidly obese patients use ideal wt for calculation of TPN requirement
• For severely underweight patients use $\frac{1}{2}$ difference between patient's ideal weight and actual weight

ANTICIPATED PROBLEMS/CONCERNS

• Caloric and glucose overload can result in hyperglycemia and hepatic dysfunction
• Fat overload can result in WBC dysfunction and infectious complication

OKT3 (MUROMONAB-CD3)

Steven Roth, M.D.

- Patients undergoing solid organ transplantation, especially kidney

RISKS

- OKT3 (muromonab-CD3) causes (often after 1st dose) fever and chills, headache, N/V, tachycardia, hypertension, seizures, dyspnea
- Patients most likely to develop intraoperative reactions are those with hypovolemia; patients receiving volatile anesthetic agents, therapy with β- or Ca^{2+}-channel antagonists, or phenytoin; or receiving increased OKT3 dose (recommended dose, 5 mg IV)
- Rate of administration does not affect incidence of reactions
- Steroids, antihistamines, acetaminophen do not alter incidence of reactions

WORRY ABOUT

- With intraoperative administration, usual signs may be masked, instead manifest as hypotension and bradycardia, acute pulm edema, cardiac arrest

OVERVIEW/PHARMACOLOGY

- Used to prevent, treat rejection; T cells react with OKT3 and are removed from circulation in liver or spleen
- Effect on immune system lasts 24–48 h
- T cells mediate rejection of transplanted kidneys; OKT3 about 95% effective in treating allograft rejection
- Actual incidence of intraoperative reactions unknown
- Adverse responses = result of immune reactions; T cells stimulated by binding of OKT3 to produce cytokines, which cause WBCs to release leukotrienes with CV responses and ↑pulm vascular permeability
- Destruction of T cells after OKT3 binding releases prostaglandins

USUAL TREATMENT

- Depends on reaction
- Treat pulm edema with fluid restriction, PEEP, diuretics; hypotension, bradycardia with vasopressors, inotropes
- Other antirejection drugs are more commonly used now (FK-506)

DRUG EFFECTS

SYSTEM	EFFECT	ASSESSMENT BY HX/PE	TREATMENT
CV	Bradycardia, hypotension	ECG, BP	Inotropes, vasopressors
RESP	Pulm edema, wheezing	Clinical exam SaO_2	Diuretics, PEEP Bronchodilators
CNS	Seizures	Clinical exam	Prevention: phenytoin Rx: Support airway, benzodiazepines

Key Reference: Roth S, Kupferberg JP: Adverse responses following intraoperative administration of orthoclone OKT3. Anesth Analg 1989; 69:822–825.

POSSIBLE DRUG INTERACTIONS

- Watch for
  - Particular attention to SaO_2 and hemodynamics after IV administration
  - Reaction may occur immediately or within 1 h after OKT3 given
  - Arterial catheter helpful for rapid detection of reaction
  - Especially watch patient receiving the 1st dose of OKT3 intraoperatively
- Administer
  - Phenytoin prophylaxis preoperatively to prevent seizures
- Avoid
  - Fluid overload
  - High concentration of inhalational anesthetic agent

ORAL CONTRACEPTIVES

Tracey L. Stierer, M.D.

USES

- 25–33% premenopausal women in USA
- For desired infertility
- To attenuate dysmenorrhea
- Administered PO

PERIOPERATIVE RISKS

- ↑ In venous thrombosis (especially if blood group A+)
- Drug interactions may increase theophylline levels by 30%

WORRY ABOUT

- Although these agents are highly effective in preventing pregnancy, β-hCG assay should be considered in sexually active patient preoperatively

OVERVIEW/PHARMACOLOGY

- Synthetic estrogen (ethinyl estradiol or mestranol) combined with a progestin (norethindrone, ethynodiol diacetate, norgestrel, levonorgestrel): e.g., Ortho-Novum, Triphasil
- Progestin alone (norgestrel): e.g., Ovrette, Micronor
- For prevention of pregnancy, and to ↓ incidence and severity of dysmenorrhea
- Oral preparations of synthetic estrogen, progestin generally well absorbed with variable bioavailability
- Primarily metabolized in liver, excreted in urine and feces as glucuronides

DRUG CLASS/MECH OF ACTION/USUAL DOSE

- Combination synthetic estrogen with progestin; progestin alone
- Combination oral contraceptives inhibit ovulation by negative feedback effect on hypothalamus, altering normal pattern of gonadotropin secretion by anterior pituitary; cervical mucus thickens, is unfavorable to sperm even if ovulation occurs. Progestin-only oral contraceptive may act by directly inhibiting ovulation or creating thick cervical mucus that is impenetrable to sperm.
- Combination oral contraceptives taken for 21 days of cycle followed by 1 wk without medication; most contain 7 inactive pills, so medication can be taken daily
- Combination oral contraceptives are available in low-dose (<50 μg) estrogen or high-dose (50 μg) estrogen
- Low-dose combination preparations may have constant (monophasic) or variable (biphasic, triphasic) doses of estrogen, progestin, depending on number of dosing regimens within cycle

DRUG EFFECTS

SYSTEM	EFFECT	ASSESSMENT BY HX	PE	TEST
CV	↑ Thromboembolic phenomena, including DVT, pulmonary emboli Slight ↑ in systolic and/or diastolic BP	Prior Hx of DVT	Deep vein exam	
GI/HEPATIC	May excerbate gallbladder disease ↑ Incidence of hepatic adenomas ↑ Incidence of hepatocellular cancer	Hx of jaundice/cholestasis during pregnancy		↑ Cholesterol
ENDO	May ↑ serum glucose levels ↑ Thyroxine-binding globulin			↑ Glucose ↑ T_4 ↓ T_3 resin uptake

Key Reference: Manley S, de Kelaita G, Joseph NJ, Salem MR, Heyman HJ: Preoperative pregnancy testing in ambulatory surgery: incidence and impact of positive results. Anesthesiology 1995; 83:690–693.

PERIOPERATIVE IMPLICATIONS

- Consider discontinuing oral contraceptives within 1 mo before or after major elective surgery or immediately preoperatively because of ↑ risk of thromboembolism or administration of prophylaxis for DVT

- Consider low-dose heparin Rx when cannot discontinue oral contraceptives before surgery

- Oral contraceptives may ↓ theophylline elimination by up to 30%, thus increasing serum concentrations

ORAL HYPOGLYCEMICS

Christopher D. Beatie, M.D.

USES

- Two classes of agents: sulfonylureas and biguanides (metformin)
- Rx for non−insulin-dependent diabetes mellitus (NIDDM) not controlled by diet or weight loss (~ 14 million patients in USA)
- ~ \$1 billion spent on oral hypoglycemics (>6 million persons received prescriptions) in 2000

PERIOPERATIVE RISKS

Sulfonylureas

- Hypoglycemia
- N/V
- Cholestatic jaundice
- Agranulocytosis
- Aplastic, hemolytic anemias
- Alcohol-induced flushing (as with disulfiram) especially with chlorpropamide (in 10–15% of patients)
- Enhanced ADH actions—reduction in urine vol, hyponatremia especially with chlorpropamide, tolbutamide—in up to 5% of patients

Metformin

- Lactic acidosis
- N/V
- Anorexia
- Diarrhea

WORRY ABOUT

Sulfonylureas

- May be potentiated by the following agents: sulfonamides, chloramphenicol, propranolol, clofibrate, warfarin, salicylates, phenylbutazone, probenecid, MAO inhibitors, ethanol

Metformin

- Concentration may be ↑ by cimetidine
- Can ↓ absorption of vit B_{12}, folate, resulting in deficiency

OVERVIEW/PHARMACOLOGY

- **Sulfonylureas:** 1st generation: tolbutamide, acetohexamide, tolazamide, chlorpropamide; 2nd generation: glyburide, glipizide
  - *Clearance:* various metabolic pathways followed by renal excretion; chlorpropamide is only partially metabolized (20% excreted unchanged in urine)

- **Biguanides:** metformin, phenformin (latter taken off market, 1976—high incidence of lactic acidosis)
  - *Clearance:* renal excretion; no metabolism; metformin can also cause lactic acidosis when concentrations are ↑ as in renal insufficiency (see also Glyburide in Drugs section)

DRUG CLASS/MECH OF ACTION/USUAL DOSE

- **Sulfonylureas** lower blood glucose by stimulating islet cells to secrete insulin, ↑ insulin sensitivity of peripheral tissues
  - Usual daily dose: acetohexamide, 500–750 mg; chlorpropamide, 250–375 mg; tolazamide, 250–500 mg; tolbutamide, 1000–2000 mg, glipizide, 10–20 mg; glyburide, 5–20 mg
- **Metformin** ↓ hepatic glucose production, ↑ glucose uptake, does not cause clinical hypoglycemia, has no effect on pancreatic insulin secretion, requires presence of insulin to be effective. Metformin can be used concurrently with a sulfonylurea. When endogenous secretion of insulin adequate, can be used alone to overcome insulin resistance.
  - Usual daily dose: 1700 mg

DRUG EFFECTS

SYSTEM	EFFECT	ASSESSMENT BY HX	PE	TEST
OVERALL (Metformin)	Lactic acidosis		Tachypnea	Lactate
ENDO (Sulfonylureas)	Hypoglycemia	Altered mental status, convulsions, coma	Sweating, tachycardia	Glucose
DERM (Sulfonylureas)	Alcohol-induced flushing			
GU (Sulfonylureas)	Antidiuresis	↓ Urine volume	Edema	Na^+
TOXICITY				
GI (All) (Sulfonylureas) (Metformin)	N/V Cholestasis Diarrhea, anorexia		Jaundice	Electrolytes Bilirubin
HEME (Sulfonylureas) (Metformin)	Agranulocytosis; aplastic, hemolytic anemias Megaloblastic anemia	Fatigue, weakness	Pallor	CBC Vit B_{12}, folate

Key Reference: Metformin for non-insulin-dependent diabetes mellitus. Med Lett Drugs Ther 1995; 37:41–42.

PERIOPERATIVE IMPLICATIONS

Preoperative Concerns

- Generally withhold sulfonylureas day of surgery while patients NPO, to avoid hypoglycemia
- Patients with NIDDM usually do not have fasting hyperglycemia and are not ketosis-prone
- Hold metformin before major surgery to ↓ risk of lactic acidosis

Induction/Maintenance

- Blood sugar measurements required frequently in periop period; use regular insulin to control hyperglycemia as needed until patient able to resume oral agent

SPECIAL CONSIDERATIONS

- Sulfonylureas can cause significant hypoglycemia if administered to NPO patients not receiving dextrose-containing IV solutions; NIDDM patients do not usually have fasting hyperglycemia and are not ketosis-prone, so little risk in holding these agents day of surgery
- Metformin does not cause clinical hypoglycemia, so can be given safely while patients NPO. However, because major surgery may be associated with acidotic states and periop renal dysfunction, withhold metformin before major surgery to ↓ risk of lactic acidosis.
- Sulfonylureas potentiated by variety of other drugs as noted

PENICILLINS

Lucy Waskell, M.D., Ph.D.

USES

- Prescribed for patients with infections by sensitive organisms, primarily pneumococci and those in genera *Streptococcus*, *Staphylococcus*, *Neisseria*, *Pseudomonas*, *Proteus*, *Haemophilus*, etc; used as prophylaxis for subacute bacterial endocarditis (penicillin G benzathine)
- Can be administered PO, IM as regular or slow-release repository form, or IV

WORRY ABOUT

- Hypersensitivity reactions: rash, fever, bronchospasm, vasculitis, angioedema, anaphylaxis
- Hyperkalemia when penicillin G potassium is administered IV (1.7 mEq K^+/MU penicillin G)
- Platelet dysfunction, defective hemostasis after carbenicillin, ticarcillin, and penicillin G
- Headaches, seizures after 1 dose of 5 MU of penicillin G procaine

OVERVIEW/PHARMACOLOGY

- Used to treat wide spectrum of infectious diseases
- Many penicillins are acid-labile; not administered orally
- Actively, rapidly excreted by renal tubule
- $T_{1/2}$ of penicillin markedly increased in anuria
- Dosage should be ↓ in renal failure
- Other organic acids, e.g., probenecid, can compete at the renal tubule for excretion, prolonging the $T_{1/2}$ of the antibiotic

DRUG CLASS/MECH OF ACTION/USUAL DOSE

- Penicillins are organic acids consisting of a β-lactam ring to which is attached a side chain and a thiazolidine ring; they prevent bacterial cell wall synthesis by inhibiting the transpeptidase reaction that is essential for cell wall synthesis
- Dose, route of administration depend on penicillin used and severity of disease treated

DRUG EFFECTS

DRUG	ABSORPTION AFTER ORAL DOSE	RESISTANCE TO PENICILLINASE	DOSE IV	ANTIMICROBIAL SPECTRUM	SPECIFIC SIDE EFFECTS
Penicillin G	Poor: ~$\frac{1}{3}$ of dose	No	1–10 MU	*Streptococcus, Neisseria*	Hyperkalemia 1.7 mEq K^+/MU Pen G; >20 MU/day can cause seizures; inhibits platelet aggregation
Methicillin	Poor	Yes	1.5–3 g q6h	*Staphylococcus aureus*	
Oxacillin	Good	Yes	0.5–3 g q6h		
Cloxacillin	Good	Yes	250–500 mg po q6h	*Staphylococcus aureus*	
Dicloxacillin	Good	Yes	250–500 mg po q6h		
Nafcillin	Variable	Yes	6–9 g q4h	*Staphylococcus aureus*	
Ampicillin	Good	No	1–2 g q6h	*Listeria monocytogenes*	
Amoxicillin	Good	No	0.75–1.5 g po q8h	*P. mirabilis, E. coli*	
Carbenicillin	Poor	No	7.5–10 g q6h	Same as ampicillin plus *Pseudomonas*, *Enterobacter*, and indole-positive *Proteus*	CHF 2° to Na^+ overload; 5 mEq Na^+/g; low K^+ 2° to obligatory cation excretion with anion; ↓ in platelet aggregation
Ticarcillin	Poor	No	50–75 mg/kg q6h	Same as carbenicillin	Same as carbenicillin 5 mEq Na^+/g
Piperacillin	Poor	No	2–6 g q8h	*Pseudomonas*, *Enterobacter*, some *Klebsiella spp.*	Same as carbenicillin 2 mEq Na^+/g
Mezlocillin	Poor	No	1.5–4.5 g q6h	*Pseudomonas*, *Enterobacter*, *Klebsiella spp.*	2 mEq Na^+/g

Key Reference: Mandell GL, Petri WA: Antimicrobial agents: penicilins, cephalosporins, and other β-lactam antibiotics. *In* Hardman JG, Limbird LE (eds): Goodman & Gilman's The Pharmacological Basis of Therapeutics, 9th ed. New York, McGraw-Hill Professional Publishing, 1996, pp 1073–1101.

PERIOPERATIVE IMPLICATIONS

Preoperative Concerns

- Is patient allergic to any penicillins? What exactly happens when the drug is taken (rash vs. anaphylaxis)?
- If patient on large doses of penicillin G, carbenicillin, ticarcillin, or piperacillin, are serum electrolytes normal?
- Hemostasis, especially platelet aggregation, may be inhibited by the antibiotics
- If patient has renal insufficiency or failure, dose of antibiotic should be q12 h or less frequently

Induction/Maintenance/Postoperative Period

- Penicillins should have no effect on induction or maintenance unless allergic reaction occurs; no known interactions with any anesthetic agents

ANTICIPATED PROBLEMS/CONCERNS

- Relate to administration of large amounts of Na^+, K^+, and organic anions (acids). Possible bleeding problems due to platelet dysfunction.

PHENCYCLIDINE (PCP)

James P. Zacny, Ph.D.

RISK

- DEA Schedule I drug of abuse with no medical indications
- In past used as anesthetic in humans and animals (Sernylan)
- Common routes of administration: snorting, smoking (often laced in marijuana cigarettes), oral ingestion; less common is IV injection
- More severe symptoms found with oral and injected routes

PERIOPERATIVE RISKS

- Acute intoxication, including aggressive and/or psychotic behavior, may require premedication with sedative or antipsychotic

WORRY ABOUT

- High doses can produce anesthesia, coma, convulsions

OVERVIEW/PHARMACOLOGY

- Effects due to parent compound, although metabolites are active
- $T_{1/2}$ 3 days
- Highly lipid soluble, pK_a of 8.6
- Metabolized in the liver; urinary excretion of metabolites at low doses, excretion of free drug at high doses
- Only small fraction of the drug excreted unchanged
- Produces an acute state of intoxication lasting 4–6 h, may produce a chronic state of psychosis that can last for up to several weeks
- With low-moderate doses, acute intoxication includes staggering gait, slurred speech, nystagmus, numbness of extremities, sweating, catatonic muscular rigidity, blank stare, changes in body image, disorganized thought, drowsiness, apathy, anterograde amnesia, possibly aggressive behavior

- With moderate-high doses, Sx can include elevated HR and BP, hypersalivation, sweating, fever, repetitive movements, muscle rigidity on stimulation
- With high doses, anesthesia, stupor, coma, convulsions can occur

DRUG CLASS/MECH OF ACTION/USUAL DOSE

- Arylcyclohexylamine
- Acts at the N-methyl-D-aspartate receptor as a noncompetitive antagonist
- Chronic user dose may be up to 1 g/d

DRUG EFFECTS

SYSTEM	EFFECT	ASSESSMENT BY HX	PE	TEST
CV	Tachycardia, Htn	Quantification, chronicity, acuity of drug exposure	Vital signs	Blood, urine toxicology screens
RESP	Depression	Concurrent drug exposure (e.g., alcohol)	Resp rate	
CNS	Intoxication, psychosis, coma, convulsions, ↓ anesthetic requirement			
ANS	Hypersalivation Fever		Observation, temp	

Key Reference: O'Brien CP: Drug addiction and drug abuse. *In* Hardman JG, Limbird LE (eds): Goodman & Gilman's The Pharmacological Basis of Therapeutics, 9th ed. New York, McGraw-Hill Professional Publishing, 1996, pp 574–575.

PERIOPERATIVE IMPLICATIONS/POSSIBLE DRUG INTERACTIONS

Preoperative Concerns

- No elective cases if patient is intoxicated or has potentially taken PCP as a self-premedication
- Concern about psychosis, hypersalivation, respiratory depression, fever, convulsions
- Steps to increase elimination of PCP from body
  - Acidification of urine (tripled excretion rate)
  - Interrupt considerable gastroenteric recirculation by continuous gastric suction
- Adequate sedation of patient

Induction/Maintenance

- Ketamine contraindicated as part of anesthetic regimen (cross-tolerance)
- Level of intoxication may lessen anesthetic, analgesic requirement

Postoperative Period

- Patient may awaken in state of intoxication, agitation, or psychosis

SPECIAL CONSIDERATIONS/CONCERNS

- Significant rhabdomyolysis, myoglobinuria may induce renal failure, can be exacerbated by continuous gastric suction, acidification of urine
- Tolerance, withdrawal

PHENOTHIAZINES

Jeffrey K. Lu, M.D.
Theodore H. Stanley, M.D.

USES

- Prescribed for patients with acute and chronic psychiatric disorders, most commonly, but not exclusively, schizophrenia, mania, psychoses
- Prescribed in low doses for patients as antiemetic drug
- Prescribed for acutely agitated and possibly violent patients

PERIOPERATIVE RISKS

- ↓ Cerebral blood flow; does not affect cerebral metabolic rate
- Dysphoria: patients receiving antipsychotic drugs may outwardly appear calm and sedated when inwardly they are experiencing overwhelming fear
- Chlorpromazine can cause hypothermia and glucose intolerance

WORRY ABOUT

- Exaggerated sedation or ventilatory depression in patients receiving opioids or ethanol
- Patients on phenothiazines may also be resistant to exogenous dopamine

OVERVIEW/PHARMACOLOGY

- Strongly protein-bound
- β elimination $T_{1/2}$: 20–30 h
- Metabolized by oxidation in liver
- Metabolites inactive except for 7-hydroxychlorpromazine
- Related drug classes include butyrophenones (droperidol, haloperidol), thioxanthenes

DRUG CLASS/MECH OF ACTION/USUAL DOSE

- Perphenazine 5 mg IV (or 70 μ/kg in children) is as effective as ondansetron 4 mg IV or droperidol 1.25 mg IV and is not associated with hypotension or sedation
- Droperidol (a butyrophenone) has been reported to cause hypertension in patients with pheochromocytoma
- Causes dopamine receptor blockade in limbic region and basal ganglia of brain
- Erratic, unpredictable absorption from oral administration
- Highly lipid-soluble, accumulates in well-perfused tissues such as brain

DRUG EFFECTS

SYSTEM	EFFECT	ASSESSMENT BY HX	PE	TEST
HEENT	Acute dystonia	Acute administration of phenothiazines	Muscle rigidity and cramping of neck, eyes, tongue, face, back, larynx	Relieved by diphenhydramine, 25–50 mg IV
CV	α-Adrenergic blockade; prolonged P-R and QT intervals, ST-segment depression		Orthostatic hypotension; hypotension	ECG orthostatic blood pressure
GI	Allergy-induced obstructive jaundice	Usually 2–4 wk of use	Scleral icterus	Elevated direct bilirubin
ENDO	↑ Prolactin production ↓ Corticosteroid synthesis ↓ Insulin production		Gynecomastia	
CNS	Tardive dyskinesia, sedation, altered temperature regulation, lowered seizure threshold	Long-term use	Purposeless, involuntary movements (lip smacking, choreiform movements) that disappear during sleep	Temperature

Key Reference: Stoelting RK: Pharmacology and Physiology in Anesthetic Practice, 3rd ed. Philadelphia, JB Lippincott, 1991, pp 369–376.

PERIOPERATIVE IMPLICATIONS/DRUG INTERACTIONS

Preoperative Preparation

- Phenothiazines, other antipsychotic drugs may interact with narcotic to cause respiratory depression

Induction/Maintenance

- Does not enhance narcotic-induced analgesia but prolongs it

Postoperative Period

- Neuroleptic malignant syndrome occurs rarely, typically develops in young males over 24–72 h. Symptoms include hyperthermia, generalized hypertonicity of skeletal muscles (relieved with nondepolarizing muscle relaxants).
- Autonomic nervous system instability (tachycardia, BP changes, cardiac dysrhythmias, fluctuating LOC, respiratory failure, ↑ liver transaminases. Dantrolene, bromocriptine, and amantadine can reverse neuroleptic malignant syndrome.

PHENOXYBENZAMINE
Michael F. Roizen, M.D.

USES

- People within USA: ?3,000/y
- Rx for preop pheochromocytoma; occasionally, chronic Rx of pheochromocytoma, sympathetic hyperactivity states, carcinoid syndrome, benign prostatic hypertrophy (BPH)

PERIOPERATIVE RISKS

- Drug interactions: sometimes requires very high doses of α-adrenergic agents to produce vasoconstriction
- Vasodilation, orthostatic hypotension accentuated in hypovolemic patients

WORRY ABOUT

- Occasionally associated with confusional states
- Associated with fatigue and prolonged sedation
- Drop attacks on preop standing to urinate

OVERVIEW/PHARMACOLOGY

- α_1-Blocker (relatively selective $\alpha_1 \gg \alpha_2$) by covalent (irreversible) binding to a receptor; compensatory response calls for production or availability of more (spare) receptors
- Effect develops slowly; peak effect not attained for 2 h after IV or 4 h after oral administration
- Absorption from GI tract incomplete
- Renal excretion of 50% in 12 h, 80% in 24 h
- $T_{1/2}$ of effect over 24 h, effects accumulate for at least 4–6 days
- High lipid solubility at body pH

DRUG CLASS/MECH OF ACTION

- α_1-Blocker agent (a haloalkylamine)
- Chronically taken:
  - $\downarrow \alpha_1$-Blocker effects in pheochromocytoma
  - High doses inhibit release of H_2, serotonin (occasionally used in carcinoid syndrome)
  - Ameliorate or prevent Raynaud's phenomenon
  - Vasodilator for chronic treatment of CHF (occasionally)

DRUG EFFECTS

SYSTEM	EFFECT	ASSESSMENT BY HX	PE	TEST
HEENT	Vasodilation of mucous membranes of nasopharynx; miosis	Nasal congestion	Mouth breathing	
CV	Antihypertensive agent Postural hypotension, reflex tachycardia $\uparrow$ CO	Orthostatic dizziness	Orthostatic VS	Hct ECG
GI	$\uparrow$ Intestinal motility, causes diarrhea	Orthostatic hypotension		
ENDO	Stimulates insulin release $\uparrow$ Presynaptic norepinephrine release (blockade of presynaptic α_2 receptors inhibiting release of norepinephrine)			
GU	$\uparrow$ Blood volume, Na^+ retention Inhibits contraction of vas deferens	Impairs ejaculation		BUN, Cr Electrolytes
CNS	Depression, sedation, fatigue Extrapyramidal symptoms rarely N/V, motor excitability rare		CNS exam	

Key Reference: Hoffman BB, Lefkowitz RJ: Catecholamines, sympathomimetic drugs, and adrenergic receptor antagonists. *In* Hardman JG, Limbird LE (eds): Goodman & Gilman's The Pharmacological Basis of Therapeutics, 9th ed. New York, McGraw-Hill Professional Publishing, 1996, pp 222–229.

PERIOPERATIVE IMPLICATIONS/POSSIBLE DRUG INTERACTIONS

(See also Pheochromocytoma in Diseases section and Adrenalectomy for Pheochromocytoma in Procedures section)

Preoperative Period

- Ensure not hypovolemic
- Interaction with methyldopa (Aldomet): urinary incontinence
- Preop treatment: major goal to avoid pheochromocytoma crisis; pre- and intraoperative goals of management of extra-adrenal surgery same as for adrenal surgery. If patient not on α-blocker before surgery, try to delay until appropriate de-

gree of α-blockade. $\uparrow$ Dose of phenoxybenzamine by 10 mg bid to qid every 3rd day until "appropriately blocked." Judge "appropriate" level of blockade by:

1. No BP readings higher than 165/90 mmHg (even during psychologic stress) for 48 h before surgery
2. Orthostatic hypotension present, but BP on standing should not be lower than 80/45 mmHg
3. ECG free of ST-T changes due to cardiomyopathy
4. Absence of other signs of catecholamine excess and presence of blockade effects such as nasal stuffiness

Induction/Maintenance

- Can produce $\uparrow$ sedation, $\downarrow$ anesthetic requirements by $1/3$ (not studied but anecdotally reported)

Muscle Relaxants

- No interactions known

Regional Anesthesia/Reversal

- No interactions known

ANTICIPATED PROBLEMS/CONCERNS

- May need very high doses of vasopressors to $\uparrow$ vascular resistance, BP in patient taking large doses
- CNS dysfunction by itself

PHENYLEPHRINE (NEO-SYNEPHRINE)

Edelberto Perez, M.D.
Kenneth J. Tuman, M.D.

USES

- Prescribed mainly as nasal decongestant or ophthalmically for mydriasis Rx, capillary decongestion
- Reliable vasopressor in treatment of hypotension
- Prolongs local anesthetic duration in regional anesthesia
- Available as parenteral IM and various ophthalmic/nasal preparations

PERIOPERATIVE RISKS

- Risk of hypertension increases left heart work; may precipitate myocardial ischemia, MI
- Infusions to augment systolic BP ↑ incidence of myocardial ischemia in patients undergoing carotid endarterectomy
- ↑ Pulmonary vascular resistance, right heart work
- Bradycardia may occur (usually not severe)
- ↓ Renal, splanchnic blood flow
- May ↑ uterine artery vascular resistance, ↓ uterine artery blood flow in pregnant patients
- Systemic absorption of topical preparations may cause hypertension, headache, tremulousness, myocardial ischemia

WORRY ABOUT

- ↑ Preload, afterload may worsen LV failure in patients with LV dysfunction
- ↑ PA pressures may worsen RV dysfunction
- May ↓ renal blood flow

OVERVIEW/PHARMACOLOGY

- Direct α_1-agonist activity causes systemic and PA vasoconstriction, resulting in ↑ impedance to forward flow, ↑ BP
- Rapidly metabolized by MAO
- IV duration less than 5 min
- May terminate supraventricular tachycardia by vagal reflex from baroreceptor stimulation
- ↑ SVR during CPB
- ↑ Perfusion pressure to vital organs in hypovolemic patients until vol restored, CPR
- May be used in conjunction with nitroglycerin to elevate coronary perfusion pressure in hypotensive patients with myocardial ischemia
- ↓ R → L shunts in patients with cyanotic spells (tetralogy of Fallot)

- Vasopressor of choice in hypertrophic cardiomyopathy and aortic stenosis, when ↑ inotropy or tachycardia undesirable
- Advantageous in catecholamine-depleted patients (chronic cocaine or amphetamine abuse), or in patients on tricyclic antidepressants or MAO inhibitors, when indirect vasopressors are unpredictable

DRUG CLASS/MECH OF ACTION/USUAL DOSE

- Synthetic noncatecholamine activates predominantly α_1-adrenergic receptors (postsynaptic, heart, iris), triggers release of intracellular Ca^{2+}, resulting in smooth muscle contraction
- Differs structurally from epinephrine only in lacking 4-hydroxyl group on benzene ring
- Usual adult dosage:
  - IV bolus: 50–100 μg
  - IV infusion: 20–50 μg/min
  - Ophthalmic solutions: 2.5–10%
  - Supraventricular tachycardia dose: 150–800 μg titrated to ↑ BP

DRUG EFFECTS

SYSTEM	EFFECT	PE	TEST
HEENT	Mydriasis without cycloplegia ↓ Production of aqueous humor		
CV	Vasoconstriction of veins and arteries ↑ Systolic and diastolic BP ↓ HR	BP HR	PCWP ECG
RESP	↑ PVR		PCWP, PAP
RENAL	↓ Renal blood flow	Urine output	BUN, Cr

Key Reference: Hoffman BB, Lefkowitz RJ: Catecholamines, sympathomimetic drugs, and adrenergic receptor antagonists. *In* Hardman JG, Limbird LE (eds): Goodman & Gilman's The Pharmacological Basis of Therapeutics, 9th ed. New York, McGraw-Hill Professional Publishing, 1996, pp 222–229.

PERIOPERATIVE IMPLICATIONS

Preoperative Concerns

- Assess LV function and history of CAD
- Consider arterial catheter if phenylephrine infusion anticipated (carotid endarterectomy, relative hypovolemia)
- Assess renal function (Cr)
- For nasal intubations, phenylephrine can be used as a nasal vasoconstrictor in a mixture with 3–4% lidocaine

Induction/Maintenance

- Stimulation of cardiac α_1 receptors may interact with halothane and cause dysrhythmias
- Monitor ECG for signs of ischemia due to increased ventricular work or coronary artery spasm
- May ↓ hepatic blood flow due to α-adrenergic–mediated vasoconstriction of portal venous vasculature

Adjuvants/Regional Anesthesia/Reversal

- Duration may be prolonged in patients on MAO inhibitors
- Side effects with ophthalmic use occur within 20 min; usually self-limited
- 2.5% nasal, ophthalmic solutions recommended in infant and elderly populations or in patients with CAD

ANTICIPATED PROBLEMS/CONCERNS

- Small doses can be titrated in a parturient when a β-adrenergic agonist is undesirable
- Can be titrated slowly to avoid overshoot (with resultant hypertension)
- Can be used when severe hypotension presents immediate danger to compromised myocardium or other end-organ (e.g., brain)
- With a failing heart, increasing afterload and preload may ↑ left-sided filling pressures enough to cause pulm edema

PHENYTOIN

Vandana Kulkarni, M.D.

INDICATIONS

- Rx focal, grand mal seizures
- Rx ventricular arrhythmias; especially related to digitalis, tricyclic antidepressant toxicity
- Occasional Rx for chronic pain states—e.g., trigeminal neuralgia
- Can be administered IV or PO

PERIOPERATIVE RISKS

- Interaction with muscle relaxants ($\downarrow$ efficacy)
- Hypotension, bradycardia with IV administration faster than 50 mg/min (believed related to vehicle, propylene glycol)

WORRY ABOUT

- $\uparrow$ P450 clearance causing $\downarrow$ effectiveness of quinidine, procainamide, oral anticoagulants, oral contraceptives, some antibiotics
- Phenytoin toxicity in patients with uremia, liver disease, hypoalbuminemia

OVERVIEW/PHARMACOLOGY

- Drug of choice for control of status epilepticus
- Rx for acute, chronic seizures
- >90% protein bound to albumin
- 98% hydroxylated, then conjugated in liver with glucuronic acid for renal elimination
- Elimination $T_{1/2}$ 24 h
- Therapeutic range 10–20 μg/ml

DRUG CLASS/MECH OF ACTION/USUAL DOSE

- Hydantoin derivative
- $\downarrow$ Na$^+$ influx during action potential; $\downarrow$ presynaptic Ca^{2+} prelease, limiting spread of seizure activity to seizure focus
- Extracellular K$^+$ $\uparrow$ during seizures, functions to propagate seizure; extracellular K$^+$ concentrations $\downarrow$ by phenytoin, limiting spread of seizure activity
- Raises seizure threshold selectively in cerebral cortex
- In heart
  - Depresses spontaneous depolarization of ventricular tissue, limiting re-entrant arrhythmias
  - AV nodal conduction not $\downarrow$ (may be slightly $\uparrow$)
  - SA nodal conduction particularly depressed in presence of volatile agents
- Usual dose: IV, PO doses are same
  - Seizures: adult: 1 g for loading dose, then 5 mg/kg/d in 2–3 divided doses; pediatric: 15 mg/kg loading dose, then 5 mg/kg/d in divided doses
  - Cardiac: 1.5 mg/kg IV $\uparrow$ 5 min for max dose of 15 mg/kg or 1.5 g
  - GI absorption variable (30–97%)

DRUG EFFECTS

SYSTEM	EFFECT	ASSESSMENT BY HX	PE	TEST
HEENT	Nystagmus seen in acute toxicity		Gingival hyperplasia with chronic use	
CV	Hypotension with rapid admin (>50 mg/min)		BP	
GI/HEPATIC	$\uparrow$ Hepatic drug metabolism Toxicity in hypoalbuminemia/ hyperbilirubinemia Variable absorption	GI irritation if not taken with food		Albumin
ENDO	Megaloblastic anemia			CBC
RENAL	Toxicity in uremic patients			BUN/Cr
CNS	Acute toxicity—ataxia, nystagmus, lethargy		CNS exam	

Key Reference: Soriano SG, Kaus SJ, Sullivan LJ, Martyn JA: Onset and duration of action of rocuronium in children receiving chronic anticonvulsant therapy. Paediatr Anaesth 2000; 10:133–136.

PERIOPERATIVE IMPLICATIONS/POSSIBLE DRUG INTERACTIONS

Preoperative Concerns

- Renal, liver disease, nutritional state can $\uparrow$ level of free phenytoin, active form of drug

Induction/Maintenance

- Resistance to nondepolarizing muscle relaxants
- Shorter duration of nondepolarizing muscle relaxants
- IV administration at a rate not greater than 25–50 mg/kg/min to avoid hypotension, bradycardia

Contraindications

- Pregnancy—crosses placenta and causes fetal hydantoin syndrome (wide-set eyes, broad mandible, finger deformities)

SPECIAL PROBLEMS/CONSIDERATIONS

- Associated with phenytoin syndrome—fever, rash, lymphadenopathy, hepatitis; may progress to interstitial nephritis, pulmonary infiltrates, anemia, thrombocytopenia, eosinophilia, DIC
- Also associated with Stevens-Johnson syndrome

PHYSOSTIGMINE SALICYLATE (ESERINE, ANTILIRIUM)   Hassan H. Ali, M.D.

USES

- Rx for
  - Glaucoma: ointment or eye drops
  - Central anticholinergic syndrome
  - Less than optimal reversal agent of NMB

PERIOPERATIVE RISKS

- Risk of muscarinic stimulation if given IV rapidly
- Risk of tachycardia, hypertension due to central hemodynamic stimulation

WORRY ABOUT

- N/V, salivation, ↑ peristalsis
- Tachycardia, hypertension in hypertensive patients (esp if given IV rapidly, but risk even if slow IV or IM)
- Convulsions in patients with closed craniocerebral injuries, barbiturate intox due to high level of ACh in brain tissue
- Withheld from patients with myotonic dystrophy, cholinergic intox

OVERVIEW/PHARMACOLOGY

- A tertiary amine alkaloid from calabar beans
- Reversibly inhibits AChE
- Potent inhibitor of phosphodiesterase enzyme, regulating transmitter ACh release at many synapses in the CNS
- Crosses BBB, exerts cholinergic effects in CNS
- In large doses → cholinergic crisis (fasciculation followed by muscle paralysis)
- Peak effect 7–11 min after slow IV administration
- $T_{1/2}\alpha$ about 2–3 min, $T_{1/2}\beta$ 22 min
- Because of its rapid $T_{1/2}\alpha$, slow injection associated with much lower incidence of intestinal, cardiac side effects

DRUG CLASS/MECH OF ACTION/USUAL DOSE

- Tertiary amine alkaloid inhibits reversible anti-ChE peripherally and at CNS
- For glaucoma:
  - Physostigmine sulfate ointment, 0.25%
  - Physostigmine salicylate solution, 0.25%, 0.5%
- For central anticholinergic syndrome:
  - Physostigmine salicylate (Antilirium), 1 mg/ml; dose 0.04 mg/kg or 1–2 mg IM or IV

DRUG EFFECTS

SYSTEM	EFFECT	ASSESSMENT BY HX	PE	TEST
HEENT	Pupillary constriction	Glaucoma		↓ IOP
CV	Tachycardia and hypertension		High BP	BP, ECG
RESP	Reversal of respiratory depressant effect of opiates Can produce bronchoconstriction			Restore sensitivity for CO_2
GI	Nausea, salivation, abd cramps			
CNS	Reversal of anticholinergic syndrome			Alert, improved vigilance and memory in ACS, possibly in Alzheimer's disease

Key Reference: Taylor P: Anticholinesterase agents. *In* Hardman JG, Limbird LE (eds): Goodman & Gilman's The Pharmacological Basis of Therapeutics, 9th ed. New York, McGraw-Hill Professional Publishing, 1996, pp 161–172.

PERIOPERATIVE CONCERNS

- Interaction with pressors (significant ↑ BP)
- Very poor reversal of nondepolarizing relaxants at doses recommended as Rx for central anticholinergic syndrome

ANTICIPATED PROBLEMS/CONCERNS

- Significant tachycardia, hypertensive response in pts with Hx of high BP
- Convulsions in pts with closed head injuries, barbiturate poisoning

- Can → cholinergic crisis in presence of other anti-ChEs. Atropine effective antidote for physostigmine OD centrally, glycopyrrolate peripherally

PRILOCAINE (CITANEST)

Stanley W. Stead, M.D.

INDICATIONS

• Infrequently used local anesthetic in USA, still used extensively in Germany
• Administered either as an injection local anesthetic 4% (with or without epinephrine) or topically as EMLA, a mixture of 2.5% prilocaine and 2.5% lidocaine
• Widely used for anesthesia and analgesia during circumcision. Newborns at higher risk for toxicity and methemoglobinemia.

PERIOPERATIVE RISKS

• Toxicity from excessive dose
• Hypersensitivity reaction
• Methemoglobinemia

WORRY ABOUT

• Metabolism to o-toluidine, which causes Hgb to be reduced to methemoglobin

OVERVIEW/PHARMACOLOGY

• 2-Propylamino-o-propionotoluidide
• Pharmacokinetics: $T_{1/2}\alpha$ 0.5 min; $T_{1/2}\beta$ 5 min, Vd_{ss} 261 L; $T_{1/2}\gamma$ 1.5 h; clearance rate 2.84 L/min (distributed at rapid rate from blood to tissue)

DRUG CLASS/MECH OF ACTION/USUAL DOSE

• Amide local anesthetic (less readily metabolized than esters); this ↓ in metabolism ↑ risk of adverse reactions
• Permeates nerve's axon membranes and equilibrates there and in axoplasm, depending on drug's pK_a (8.0), hydrophobicity of base and cation specificity, and concentration. Hydrophobicity measured by octanol:buffer partition coefficient of base:129, making it moderately hydrophobic.

• Binds to local anesthetic sites on voltage-gated Na^+ channels. A conformational change of receptor prevents opening of channel during activation; axon potentials cease to be propagated. Onset, recovery from blockade limited by diffusion of local anesthetic molecules into/out of nerve membrane and axoplasm.
• Prilocaine is dealkylated in the liver by mixed-function oxidases. About 75% in liver; the most rapidly metabolized of amides.
• Excreted in kidney; perhaps some kidney metabolism
• Low protein-binding capacity leads to ↑ clearance rate

DRUG EFFECTS

• Addition of epinephrine does not affect block duration, a result of vasodilating action of prilocaine
• Contraindicated in patients with G6PD deficiency

Methemoglobinemia

• Dose-response relationship exists between amount of prilocaine and methemoglobinemia (occurs with ≥600 mg). Occurrence related to chemical structure: prilocaine has one less methyl group in benzene ring than lidocaine; metabolism in liver results in formation of o-toluidine, which oxidizes Hgb to methemoglobin.
• Methemoglobinemia significant when methemoglobin 10% of total Hgb (shift to left with less release of O_2). Cyanosis observed; methemoglobinemia of concern if anemic or pregnant (when maternal transfer leads to methemoglobinemia of fetus).
• Treatment, if spontaneous reversal does not occur, or IV injection with 1–2 mg/kg of 1% methylene blue solution (tetramethylthionine chloride)
• Other toxicity may involve CNS, CV systems; generally 4–7× the amount producing convulsions → CV collapse
• Toxicity associated with >400 mg
• Intercostal injection → higher blood levels than with epidural

INDICATION	CONC	DRUG DOSE	ONSET	DURATION
Minor nerve block	1%	50–200 mg	10–20 min	60–120 min, up to 180 with epinephrine
Major nerve block	1–2%	400–600 mg	10–20 min	180–300 min
Epidural	1–3%	150–600 mg	5–15 min	120–180 min

DRUG EFFECTS

SYSTEM	EFFECT	ASSESSMENT BY HX	PE	TEST
HEENT	Toxicity	Metallic taste, tinnitus		
CV	Pulm vasoconstriction			↑ PAP ↑ PVR
	Systemic vasodilator Neg inotrope Neg chronotrope			↓ SVR ↓ CO ECG: ↑ P-R, ↓ QRS
CNS	Toxicity: more sensitive than CV	Shivering, twitching, tremors in face, extremities, progressing to tonic-clonic seizure	Twitching, hyperreflexia possible Resp depression	
PNS	Block nerve transmissions		Loss of sensation and motor function	
MS	IV may augment NM blocker (both depolarizing and nondepolarizing)			Nerve stimulator: ↓ twitch height

Key Reference: Arthur GR, Scott DHT, Boyes RN, Scott DB: Pharmacokinetic and clinical pharmacologic studies with mepivacaine and prilocaine. Br J Anaesth 1979; 51:481–485.

POSSIBLE DRUG INTERACTIONS

• In large doses, blocks NM transmission; in smaller doses, enhances NMB from nondepolarizing and depolarizing NM blockers
• Acidosis, hypercarbia, hypoxia may potentiate neg chronotropic, inotropic actions

Preoperative Considerations/Induction/Maintenance

• Routine

ANTICIPATED PROBLEMS/CONCERNS

• EMLA cream = eutectic mix of 5% lidocaine + prilocaine base for topical cutaneous anesthesia. EMLA applied under occlusive bandage for 45–60 min to obtain effective cutaneous anesthesia.
• EMLA → methemoglobinemia when large amounts used in children, particularly in newborns
• Methemoglobinemia if >600 mg given or given to anemic or pregnant patients

PROCAINAMIDE

Philippe Housmans, M.D.

USES

- Supraventricular, ventricular antiarrhythmic effect: most commonly used for management of ventricular dysrhythmias
- Useful for chronic suppression of PVCs, yet newer class IB agents—e.g., tocainide, mexiletine—may supplant procainamide

PERIOPERATIVE RISKS

- Acute cardiac toxicity heralded by significant hypotension and/or 50% QRS prolongation
- A lupus-like syndrome (fever, serositis, arthritis) may be seen in $1/3$ of patients during chronic therapy; this syndrome usually spares kidneys, abates when drug stopped
- Positive ANAs develop in 75% of patients during chronic admin but not an indication to discontinue unless Sx of drug-induced lupus develop
- Other reactions include fever, rash, N/V, diarrhea, confusion, agranulocytosis
- Since NAPA and procainamide toxicities are additive, serum levels of both can be monitored during therapy

WORRY ABOUT

- Convulsions
- Systemic toxicity due to accidental intravascular injection

OVERVIEW/PHARMACOLOGY

- ↓ In V_{max}, action potential amplitude during phase 0; ↓ in rate of phase 4 depolarization
- Prolonged refractory period, action potential duration (similar to effects of quinidine)
- Prolongs conduction, ↓ effective refractory period in atrial, His-Purkinje portions of conduction system
- Prolongs QT interval less than does quinidine
- AV nodal effective refractory period may ↓ by indirect anticholinergic effects
- When used for supraventricular dysrhythmias, esp AFIB or atrial flutter, ventricular rate usually ↑, unless AV nodal conduction slowed by other means
- Procainamide and quinidine reported to reduce frequency of short coupling-interval PVCs (< 400 ms), ↓ frequency of VTach or fibrillation caused by R-on-T phenomenon
- Absorption of PO dose rapid; initial effects seen within 20–30 min after PO admin, immediately after IV admin
- Peak serum concentrations observed 1 h after PO ingestion
- 15% of drug is protein bound
- IV: 100 mg or 1.5 mg/kg, given at 5-min intervals until therapeutic effect observed, to total dose of lesser of 1 g or 15 mg/kg
- Arterial pressure and ECG monitored, admin stopped if hypotension and/or a > 50% QRS prolongation

- Maintenance infusion 20–80 μg/kg/min for therapeutic plasma conc of 4–8 μg/ml
- PO: 50 μg/kg/h or 500–600 mg q 3–4 h; absorption 75–95%
- Plasma levels peak after 1–2 h
- Elimination $T_{1/2}$ = 3–4 h
- 50–60% excreted unchanged by kidneys; remainder metabolized by liver
- Principal metabolite NAPA has antiarrhythmic effects, is excreted by kidneys, accumulates when renal function is impaired
- Major metabolic pathway is hepatic acetylation to NAPA metabolite that prolongs repolarization
- Rate of acetylation may vary genetically (fast or slow acetylators)
- NAPA has a serum $T_{1/2}$ of 6–8 h, but possibly as long as 60 h in patients with severe renal dysfunction
- Elimination of procainamide ↓ in patients with impaired liver or kidney function (serum $T_{1/2}$ as long as 60 h) and in patients in CHF (serum $T_{1/2}$ of 5 h) (in such patients, loading dose of 12 mg/kg over 1 h and maintenance infusion of 1.4 mg/kg/h have been recommended)

DRUG CLASS/MECH OF ACTION

- Class IA antiarrhythmic: class I drugs are membrane stabilizers that cause pharmacologic blockade of the Na⁺ channel with ↓V_{max} rate, max rate of depolarization of AP during phase 0

DRUG EFFECTS

SYSTEM	EFFECT	ASSESSMENT BY HX
CV	Myocardial depression and peripheral arterial dilation	Suppression of ventricular arrhythmias. Higher doses cause enhanced vasodilation, depression of myocardial contractility, and depression of peripheral vascular resistance, resulting in profound hypotension
CNS	Crosses blood-brain barrier, causing CNS excitation followed by CNS depression	Excitation evidenced as restlessness and tremor. Higher plasma concentrations result in convulsions, coma, and cardiorespiratory arrest
PNS	Inhibition of propagation of action potential	Loss of sensation and motor ability in area of blockade
NMJ	Transmission may be inhibited	Potentiation of muscle relaxants

Key Reference: Naccarelli GV, Dell'Orfano JT, Wolbrette DL, Patel HM, Luck JC: Cost-effective management of acute atrial fibrillation: role of rate control, spontaneous conversion, medical and direct current cardioversion, transesophageal echocardiography, and antiembolic therapy. Am J Cardiol 2000; 85: 36D–45D.

PROPYLTHIOURACIL— ANTITHYROID DRUGS

Michael F. Roizen, M.D.

USES

- In USA: in addition to 5% of pregnant women, ?400,000/y develop hyperthyroidism
- Rx for hyperthyroidism, goiter associated with hyperthyroidism
- Definitive Rx to control hyperthyroidism in anticipation of spontaneous remission
- Rx for hyperthyroidism in conjunction with ^{131}I or ^{125}I to hasten recovery while awaiting effects of radiation therapy
- Rx for hyperthyroidism to control disorder in preparation for surgery

PERIOPERATIVE RISKS

- Side effects of drug: hypothyroidism (see Hyperthyroidism or Hypothyroidism in Diseases section)

WORRY ABOUT

- Agranulocytosis (less than 0.5% of treated patients develop this side effect)

OVERVIEW/PHARMACOLOGY

- Antithyroid drug: absorbed within 20–30 min; effect begins to ↓ in 2–3 h (methimazole $T_{1/2}$ estimated to be 6–13 h)
- Drug and metabolites cleared by renal excretion
- Antithyroid drugs cross placenta, can be found in breast milk

DRUG CLASS/USUAL DOSE

- Antithyroid drug: interferes directly with synthesis of thyroid hormones by preventing incorporation of iodine into tyrosyl residual thyroglobulin; inhibits coupling of iodotyrosyl residues to form iodothyronines by inhibiting peroxidase enzyme
- Depletes preformed hormone over time; only then do clinical effects become noticeable ($T_{1/2}$ of thyroid hormones is >3 days in circulation)

- Other useful antithyroid Rx drugs include those inhibiting conversion of less active T_4 into more active T_3, such as propranolol; methimazole, carbimazole do not appear to do so with anti–β-blocker effects—e.g., propranolol and others; those that inhibit release of preformed thyroid hormone—e.g., iodine (also temporarily inhibits synthesis and ↓ vascularity of thyroid glands)
- A thioureylene

Chronic Rx Uses

- ↓ Hyperthyroidism and thyrotoxicosis
- ↓ Goiter size in hyperthyroidism

Acute Rx Uses

- Relieves symptoms of hyperthyroidism while waiting for ^{131}I or ^{125}I to take effect

DRUG EFFECTS

SYSTEM	EFFECT	ASSESSMENT BY HX	PE	TEST
HEENT	Goiter shrinkage; occasionally goiter develops if hypothyroidism occurs	Snoring, hoarseness, neck pain	Ask patient to vocalize "e"; examine airway, neck	Check CXR (PA, lat), lat neck films; if needed, CT scan of neck
CV		Assess CV response to Rx		Rhythm strip or full ECG if CV system is involved by either Hx or PE
GI	Rare hepatotoxicity			SGPT, SGOT
HEME	Mild anemia, thrombocytopenia; agranulocytosis as toxic reaction to propylthiouracil or methimazole (0.05–0.12% of patients)	Hx of sore throat or fever often heralds agranulocytosis	Skin/mucous membranes for infection/petechiae; purpura if at risk	CBC with platelet count; differential leukocyte count
DERM		Rare depigmentation of hair		
MS		Pain/stiffness in joints (rare side effect)		
GU	Placenta—crosses placental barrier and is excreted in breast milk			
CNS		Headache, paresthesia rare side effects Shaking, anxiety, emotional instability are signs that hyperthyroidism not yet controlled	Reflex speed, tremor, nervousness, mental status	
ENDO	Need to assess if euthyroid	Refer to all other systems: especially reflex speed, tremor, heat intolerance, wt loss, fatigue, weakness, anorexia, ↑ appetite	Reflex speed; HR	Free T_4 estimate needed; unable to assess if euthyroid by Hx, PE

Key Reference: Earling PA: Thyroid disease. Br J Anaesthesia 2000; 85:15–28.

POSSIBLE DRUG INTERACTIONS

Preoperative Period

- Assess euthyroid state (see table)
- Fairly certain sign that remission may have occurred is ↓ in size of goiter

Induction/Maintenance

- No interactions known

Adjuvants/Regional Anesthesia/Reversal

- No interactions known

Postoperative Concerns

- Resumption not necessary if surgery to correct hyperthyroidism successful

- Short $T_{1/2}$ makes resumption in nonthyroid surgery necessary ASAP, or give medication IV

ANTICIPATED PROBLEMS/CONCERNS

- Assess for hyperthyroidism, agranulocytosis

PYRIDOSTIGMINE BROMIDE

Hassan H. Ali, M.D.

- Rx for myasthenia gravis
- Reversal of nondepolarizing NMB

PERIOPERATIVE RISKS

- Can produce significant muscarinic stimulation if admin IV without adequate protection with anticholinergic drug (e.g., atropine or glycopyrrolate)
- Can precipitate a cholinergic crisis in myasthenics receiving high doses of AChEs
- Prolonged response to succinylcholine if administered shortly after reversal with either pyridostigmine or neostigmine (inhibition of plasma ChE)

WORRY ABOUT

- Cardiac arrhythmias; muscarinic, nicotinic activation (cholinergic crisis); prolonged admin may → myopathic changes in postsynaptic region consistent with accumulation of Ca^{2+}, nuclear alterations
- Changes have been reversed with Ca^{2+}-channel blockers (diltiazem)

OVERVIEW/PHARMACOLOGY

- A quaternary nitrogen reversible AChE; is analogue of neostigmine
- Incorporates N in ring structure to form dimethylcarbamic ester of 3-hydroxy 1-methylpyridinium bromide
- May possess less muscarinic agonist effects than neostigmine
- Peak effect of pyridostigmine is at 12–17 min, compared with 7–11 min for neostigmine

- Distribution $T_{1/2}$ ($T_{1/2}\alpha$) 6.8 min; $T_{1/2}\beta$ 112 min in pts with normal kidney function with clearance of 9.0 ml/kg/min
- Anephric pts have a longer $T_{1/2}\beta$ of 379 min, reduced clearance of 2 ml/kg/min
- 25% metabolized, 75% dependent on renal elimination
- Anticholinergic glycopyrrolate matches better onset, duration of pyridostigmine

DRUG CLASS/MECH OF ACTION/USUAL DOSE

- Quaternary amine AChE
- For reversal of nondepolarizing relaxants at dose of 0.2–0.25 mg/kg (12.5–15 mg) IV
- For Rx of myasthenia gravis: generally PO, 60-mg tablets (5 or 6 times/d) with a slow-release tablet 180 mg (qhs)

DRUG EFFECTS

SYSTEM	EFFECT	TEST
CV	Bradyarrhythmia	ECG
RESP	Improved NM transmission, resp mechanics	PFTs
GI	Less nausea, salivation than with neostigmine	
CNS	Reversal of NMB, postsynaptic dysfunction	Normal evoked muscle responses

Key Reference: Bevan DR, Donati F, Kopman AF: Reversal of neuromuscular blockade. Anesthesiology 1992; 77:785–805.

PERIOPERATIVE CONCERNS

- High doses preoperatively in myasthenics may ↑ requirements of nondepolarizing relaxants; response to succinylcholine can be prolonged

ANTICIPATED PROBLEMS/CONCERNS

- Use as a reversal agent in high doses may precipitate a cholinergic crisis in myasthenics

- Prolonged use may → short-lived myopathy; can be resolved with Ca^{2+}-channel blockers

QUINIDINE

(Michael B. Howie, M.D.

See also Procainamide

USES

• Rx for supraventricular arrhythmias (AFIB/flutter, PAT, WPW syndrome—associated arrhythmias) for conversion, maintenance of sinus rhythm

PERIOPERATIVE RISKS

• High plasma levels associated with QT and QRS prolongation, life-threatening ventricular arrhythmias (torsades de pointes); acidosis, hypomagnesemia, hypokalemia increase risk

WORRY ABOUT

• Quinidine accumulation with concurrent hepatic disease, renal failure, cimetidine administration
• ↓ Concentrations in association with rifampin, phenytoin, barbiturates
• Serious side effects with amiodarone
• Raising serum levels of digoxin to toxic levels
• Caution in incomplete AV block because quinidine may produce complete block or asystole

OVERVIEW/PHARMACOLOGY

• Well absorbed from GI tract (80% bioavailability)
• 90% plasma protein bound
• Elimination through kidneys, 20% unchanged, 80% after hepatic metabolism; $T_{1/2}$ 4–8 h
• Interactions with drugs that alter hepatic enzyme function, other highly protein-bound drugs
• Serum conc should be monitored to fit therapeutic range: 1.5–4 μg/ml
• The effect lasts 6–8 h; PO takes 1–3 h to onset
• Urine alkalinization ↓ excretion
• Affects both resistance and capacitance vessels, causing ↓ in system pressure and preload (especially IV)
• Quinidine blocks the fast inward sodium channel
• It has anticholinergic properties
• Used with digoxin or other drugs that slow AV node conduction (anticholinergic may be vagolytic)
• Principal products of metabolism are antiarrhythmic

DRUG CLASS/MECH OF ACTION/USUAL DOSE

• Class IA antiarrhythmic; use-dependent Na^+-channel block (local anesthetic–like action) responsible for effectiveness in tachyarrhythmias
• Dosage
  – Conversion: quinidine polygalacturonate tabs 275 mg (×2 if necessary) q 3–4 h for 3–4 doses; dose can be ↑ by 275 mg every 3rd or 4th dose until rhythm restored; quinidine gluconate injection 600 mg IM, then up to 400 mg q 2 h if necessary
  – Maintenance: quinidine polygalacturonate 275 mg bid/tid, as needed
• Alternatives: other class IA drugs (e.g., procainamide, disopyramide, cibenzoline, pirmenol)
• Slow IV infusion 0.25 mg/kg/min

DRUG EFFECTS

SYSTEM	EFFECT	ASSESSMENT BY HX	PE	TEST
CV	↑ QRS duration, vagolytic cardiac/peripheral α blockade, negative inotropic, ↓ conduction velocity	↑ HR	↑ HR, ↓ BP, JVD, abnormal S_3	ECG CXR
		Dyspnea	Bradycardia, asystole	ECG (3° AV block)
GI	Diarrhea (18%), nausea (18%)	α blockade		
HEME	Thrombocytopenia		Mucosal bleeding	Platelet count
CNS	Headache (13%), dizziness (8%), tinnitus, blurred vision			Quinidine serum conc
MISC	Anaphylactoid reactions, aggravation of asthma (caution)		CV collapse	

Key Reference: Nappi I, Mason JW: Quinidine. *In* Messerli F (ed): Cardiovascular Therapy, 2nd ed. Philadelphia, WB Saunders, 1996, pp 1362–1369.

PERIOPERATIVE IMPLICATIONS/POSSIBLE DRUG INTERACTIONS

Preoperative Preparation

• Serial measurements of QRS duration and QT interval on the ECG to prevent arrhythmias; QRS should be < 140 ms
• Digoxin, warfarin plasma levels ↑ displacement from storage sites, hepatic interaction, respectively; ↓ dosage to prevent toxicity
• ↓ Dose in hypoproteinemia

Induction/Maintenance

• Possible ↓ in hepatic metabolism of halogenated agents
• ↓ Levels of plasma proteins after CPB augment free fraction of drug

Adjuvants/Regional Anesthesia/Reversal

• Quinidine may ↑ muscle weakness in patients with myasthenia gravis, ↓ effect of anticholinesterases, enhances NMB
• Quinidine can enhance the effects of vasodilating, negative inotropic, sinus node depressant agents (e.g., β-blockers, verapamil, rauwolfia alkaloids, bretylium)
• Concurrent administration of other class IA drugs, amiodarone, or phenothiazines ↑ risk of torsades de pointes
• Quinidine has additive effect with anticholinergic drugs

SPECIAL CONSIDERATIONS

• Quinidine contraindicated when ventricular arrhythmias associated with or caused by QT prolongation (risk of torsades)
• IM injection very painful; IV routes cause vasodilation and myocardial depression
• In patients with AFIB/flutter, quinidine can ↑ AV transmission (1:1) and cause ↑ in ventricular rate; prevent by administering verapamil or digoxin before cardioversion
• In patients with severe AV block, quinidine can aggravate block or cause asystole; this applies to patients with SSS

RIBOFLAVIN (VITAMIN B₂)

John K. Stene, M.D., Ph.D.

INDICATIONS

- For common deficiency with general nutritional deficiency (e.g., malnutrition, starvation, chronic alcoholism)
  - Associated with causes of malnutrition, general vitamin deficiency
  - Isolated deficiency rare or nonexistent in USA

PERIOPERATIVE RISKS

- Excessive intake ↑ urinary excretion of unchanged riboflavin
- Deficiency causes anemia, neuropathy

OVERVIEW/PHARMACOLOGY

- Component of electron transfer chain in mitochondria, oxidative metabolic coenzymes
- Absorbed from upper GI tract by specific transport mechanism involving phosphorylation of enzyme to FMN by enzyme flavokinase
- Distributed to all tissues, but little stored

DRUG CLASS/MECH OF ACTION/USUAL DOSE

- Water-soluble B-complex vitamin
- Phosphorylated to FMN by flavokinase, ATP
- FMN reacts with phosphate bond to adenine monophosphate to form FAD
- FMN, FAD are electron transfer cofactors in mitochondrial electron transfer chain, oxidative metabolism (e.g., xanthine oxidase)
- 0.6 mg/1000 kcal/d (RDA)

ASSESSMENT POINTS

SYSTEM	EFFECT OF DEFICIENCY	ASSESSMENT BY HX	PE	TEST
HEENT	Sore throat, cheilosis, glossitis, corneal vascularization, cataracts	Burning tongue, soreness in mouth and throat	Red, fissured lips; blue-red tongue with edematous surface—"cobblestone tongue"	Urinary excretum of <50 μg/24 h of riboflavin
HEME	Anemia			Reticulocytopenia, normochromic-normocytic anemia
DERM	Seborrheic dermatitis of face, dermatitis of arms and trunk	Burning, itching eyes	Rough, sharkskin appearance of nose	
PNS	Neuropathy		PNS function exam	

Key Reference: Marcus R, Coulston AM: Water-soluble vitamins. *In* Hardman JG, Limbird LE (eds): Goodman & Gilman's The Pharmacological Basis of Therapeutics, 9th ed. New York, McGraw-Hill Professional Publishing, 1996, pp 1555–1572.

PERIOPERATIVE IMPLICATIONS/POSSIBLE DRUG INTERACTIONS

- Absorption depends on flavokinase activity; it in turn depends on thyroid hormone status and is inhibited by tricyclic antidepressants, chlorpromazine
- Peripheral neuropathy of potential concern with regional anesthesia
- Preop normochromic-normocytic anemia in nutritionally depleted patient responds to riboflavin administration
- See also under Malnutrition in Diseases section for interactions, abnormalities of malnutrition
- Boric acid poisoning induces riboflavin deficiency

ANTICIPATED PROBLEMS/CONCERNS

- Adequate phosphorus must be given along with riboflavin and other vitamins when refeeding starved patients to prevent ↑ phosphorylation from depleting phosphate stores, energy of cells

USES

- Antibiotic therapy for TB (incidence 9.4/100,000/y) and *Neisseria meningitidis* infection (incidence 4.6–10/100,000/y)
- May be administered PO or IV
- 10% of patients receiving rifampin develop chemical hepatitis; 16 deaths/500,000 receiving drug
- 20% of patients receiving rifampin with isoniazid develop ↑ liver enzymes

PERIOPERATIVE RISKS

- Hepatic dysfunction most likely in patients receiving isoniazid with pre-existing liver disease
- Decreased duration of action of narcotics and barbiturates
- Patients on antiarrhythmic therapy, digoxin, theophylline, phenytoin, or glucocorticoid therapy may need ↑ doses of these drugs

WORRY ABOUT

- Induces hepatic microsomal (P450) activity, ↓ $T_{1/2}$ of hepatically metabolized drugs
- Hepatotoxicity caused by ↑ metabolism of isoniazid to acetylhydrazine
- Theoretical ↑ risk of halothane hepatitis
- Hemolytic anemia, thrombocytopenia (rare)

OVERVIEW/PHARMACOLOGY

- Complex macrocyclic antibiotic
- H_2O-soluble at acidic pH; inhibits gram-positive and many gram-negative organisms, including *Escherichia coli, Pseudomonas, Proteus, Klebsiella, N. meningitidis, Haemophilus influenzae, Mycobacterium tuberculosis*
- Increases in vitro activity of streptomycin and isoniazid
- Eliminated by biliary clearance with significant enterohepatic circulation
- $T_{1/2}$ 1.5–5 h, ↑ with hepatic dysfunction

DRUG CLASS/MECH OF ACTION/USUAL DOSE

- Rifamycin antibiotic family
- Inhibits DNA-dependent RNA polymerase in bacteria and mycobacteria; nuclear eukaryotic RNA polymerase not affected
- Administered for chemoprophylaxis of meningococcal infections, with β-lactams for *Staphylococcus* endocarditis, osteomyelitis; for methicillin-resistant *S. aureus* infections; and in conjunction with isoniazid and streptomycin for active TB
- Usual dose: 600 mg/d, pediatric dose 10 mg/kg/d, PO or IV
- Should be administered 1 h before or 2 h after meals, PO

DRUG EFFECTS

SYSTEM	EFFECT	ASSESSMENT BY HX	PE	TEST
OVERALL		Fatigue, drowsiness, dizziness, ataxia, confusion, weakness		
HEENT	Secreted in saliva, tears		Orange sputum, tears, conjunctivae	
GI	Hepatic dysfunction (rare with normal pre-Rx hepatic function)	N/V	Jaundice	Elevated transaminases
HEME	Thrombocytopenia, hemolytic anemia	Bruising/bleeding		Platelet count, Hgb/Hct, microscopic exam
RENAL	Interstitial nephritis, ATN, renal failure (with high doses)			Cr clearance, light-chain proteinuria

Key Reference: Venkatesan K: Pharmacokinetic drug interactions with rifampicin. Clin Pharmacokin 1992; 22:47–65.

PERIOPERATIVE IMPLICATIONS/POSSIBLE DRUG INTERACTIONS

Preoperative Concerns

- ↓ Duration of action of benzodiazepines, narcotics, barbiturates due to hepatic enzyme induction
- Adequacy of pre-existing drug regimens should be verified (see Special Considerations)

Induction/Maintenance

- Decreased narcotic and analgesic efficacy: barbiturates, methadone, diazepam, midazolam; β-blockers have ↑ clearance, ↓ duration of action
- Halothane metabolism ↑ with ↑ risk of hepatotoxicity

Adjuvants/Reversal

- Mycobacteria quickly develop resistance when rifampin used alone; administer with isoniazid and/or streptomycin

Special Considerations

- Risk of hepatic dysfunction perioperatively ↑ by pre-existing hepatic disease
- Delays oral absorption of ASA
- ↓ $T_{1/2}$, requiring ↑ doses to maintain adequate therapeutic levels: digoxin, digitoxin, quinidine, propranolol, metoprolol, verapamil, warfarin, theophylline, phenytoin, prednisone, cortisol, prednisolone, cyclosporine, oral hypoglycemic agents, ketoconazole, fluconazole, protease inhibitors
- Should be avoided in patients taking protease inhibitors for HIV
- Risk of a false-positive urine opiate screen

ANTICIPATED PROBLEMS/CONCERNS

- 10% on therapy may develop hepatitis; patients with pre-existing liver disease are at higher risk
- Rifampin induces microsomal enzyme activity in liver, results in ↓ efficacy, duration of action of hepatically metabolized drugs

SEROTONIN: AGONISTS, ANTAGONISTS, AND REUPTAKE INHIBITORS

David F. Stowe, M.D., Ph.D.

INDICATIONS

- Serotonin (5-HT) not given as a drug
- Partially selective receptor *agonists* (used for Rx of acute migraine headaches)
  - Sumatriptan (Imitrex) 4–6 mg SQ
  - Naratriptan (Amerge) 2.5 mg/d PO
  - Rizatriptan (Maxalt) 5 mg/d PO
  - Zolmitriptan (Zomig) 2.5 mg/d PO, and
  - Metoclopramide (Reglan) 5–15 mg qid PO, 2–10 mg IV (Rx for GERD, gastroparesis, N/V)
- Partially selective receptor 5-HT₃ antagonists *antagonists*
  - Dolasetron (Anzemet) 12.5 mg IV 1 h before emergence to prevent postop N/V
  - Ondansetron (Zofran) 4–8 mg tid PO for prevention of N/V due to emetogenic chemotherapy treatment
  - Granisetron (Kytril) 10 μg/kg IV for prevention of N/V due to chemoRx; for postop N/V (not FDA-approved)
  - Clozapine (Clozaril) 12.5–50 mg PO/d for severe schizophrenia refractory to standard antipsychotic drug Rx
- Selective serotonin reuptake inhibitors (SSRIs) (all used for Rx of major depressive episodes)
  - Fluoxetine (Prozac) 20–80 mg/d
  - Paroxetine (Paxil) 20–50 mg/d
  - Sertraline (Zoloft) 50–200 mg/d
  - Fluvoxamine (Luvox) 25–50 mg/d PO
  - Citalopram (Celexa) 20–40 mg/d PO

PERIOPERATIVE RISKS

- Sumatriptan: not for pts with IHD, angina, Prinzmetal's angina, severe Htn
- Metoclopramide: not for pts with pheochromocytoma, on MAOIs; may worsen mental depression; effect antagonized by narcotics
- Clozapine: can cause orthostatic hypotension; may ↑ incidence of Szs; like other antipsychotic drugs, can → tardive dyskinesia; NMS
- SSRIs can cause "serotonin syndrome" (hyperthermia, muscle rigidity, myoclonus, rapid mental change) if given in the presence of MAOIs; may ↑ warfarin, digitalis effects by ↓ plasma protein binding

WORRY ABOUT

- Sumatriptan and other 5-HT agonists: pts taking these may have exacerbation of anginal Sx
- Ondansetron, granisetron: chemoRx pts may exhibit ↑ N/V during anesthesia
- Clozapine: pt may have drug-induced agranulocytosis
- SSRIs: concomitant use of MAOIs, displacement of other drugs highly bound to plasma protein increased bleeding with warfarin, so monitor prothrombin time

OVERVIEW/PHARMACOLOGY

- Serotonin secreted 90% by enterochromaffin cells of GI tract; released into plasma by unclear mech, neuronal stimuli; some taken up, much is stored in platelets; 5-HT receptors on vasc endothelium stimulate release of NO to promote vasodilation, but receptors on vasc smooth muscle promote vasoconstriction. Excess release involved in "carcinoid syndrome," due to enterochromaffin cell neoplasm. As an amine neurotransmitter, serotonin also secreted, stored, released by raphe nuclei in brainstem (serotonergic neurons).
- Serotonergic neurons diffusely innervate most regions of CNS; with other neurotransmitters is involved in modulating mood, depression, anxiety, migraine headache, sleep, appetite, temp regulation, perception of pain and itch, regulation of BP
- Abnormalities in secretion or receptor activation likely underlie mental depression, migraine headache, sensitivity to pain, sleep pattern, and central BP control. In CNS, 5-HT receptor activation increases K⁺ conductance to promote membrane hyperpolarization, → mostly inhibitory action. As CNS neurotransmitter, 5-HT modulates effects of other monoamine transmitters—e.g., norepinephrine, dopamine, and other transmitters such as ACh, glycine, GABA. Inhibition of 5-HT reuptake elevates mood, normalizes behavior.

DRUG EFFECTS

SYSTEM	EFFECT	ASSESSMENT BY HX	PE	TEST
CV	Hypertension, IHD (agonists)		BP	
	ECG: longer P-R and QT$_c$ intervals (antagonists)			
	Hypotension (SSRIs)			
	Serotonin syndrome (SSRIs)	MAO drug interaction	BP, CNS	
	Altered drug levels (SSRIs)	Dysrhythmias, bleeding	Bleeding	Drug levels
ENDO	Carcinoid syndrome (↑ 5-HT)	Diarrhea, abd pain, asthma, flushing, hyperglycemia, PAT, SVT		5-HT, kallikreins
HEME	Leukopenia (antagonists)			CBC
CNS	Psychosis, depression, altered mood, Sz disorder	Mental disorder	CNS evaluation	Drug levels

Key Reference: Katzung BG (ed): Basic and Clinical Pharmacology, 6th ed. East Norwalk, CT, Appleton & Lange, 1995.

PERIOPERATIVE IMPLICATIONS

- Avoid narcotics in pts with carcinoid syndrome (surgery or 5-HT antagonists usual Rx for carcinoid tumor)

- Use caution in giving metoclopramide; pt must not be taking MAOIs—e.g., isocarboxazid (Marplan), phenelzine (Nardil), or tranylcypromine (Parnate)
- Check pt's drug profile if Hx of migraine; ↑ risk of coronary vasoconstriction with sumatriptan

- Check pt's drug profile if Hx of schizophrenia; may have low WBC count if taking clozapine
- Check pt's drug profile if Hx of major depression; if taking coumadin or digitalis, levels may be ↑

SILDENAFIL CITRATE (VIAGRA)

Lee A. Fleisher, M.D.
Mohammad Naqibuddin, M.B., B.S., M.P.H.

INDICATIONS

- Treatment of erectile dysfunction

PERIOPERATIVE RISKS

- None for elective surgery based on $T_{1/2}$
- Drug may still be present in emergent surgery

WORRY ABOUT

- Potentiation of vasodilating agents
- History of coronary ischemia or congestive heart failure
- Severe hepatic impairment

OVERVIEW/PHAMACOLOGY

- Sildenafil citrate was discovered by accident during testing as a treatment for heart disease
- Terminal $T_{1/2}$ 4–6 h
- Total protein binding 96%, also distributed in tissues
- Bioavailability 41%
- Metabolized in liver via the cytochrome P450 isoenzymes, 3A4 (major route) and 2C9 (minor route)
- Active N-desmethyl metabolite
- Peak plasma concentration 60 min
- Excreted via feces (80%), kidney (13%), and semen ($<0.001\%$ of a dose)
- Metabolism may be delayed after a high-fat meal and in patients with liver disease
- Contraindicated in patients with hypersensitivity to sildenafil products and patients taking nitroglycerin or other organic nitrates
- Precautions: anatomic deformities of the penis, conditions predisposing patients to priapism, bleeding disorders or active peptic ulceration, retinitis pigmentosa or other retinal abnormalities, coronary ischemia or congestive heart failure, multidrug antihypertensive regimens
- Excretion in breast milk is unknown

DRUG CLASS/MECH OF ACTION

- Potent and selective inhibitor of phosphodiesterase type V (PDE V)
- PDE V isoform is responsible for breaking down cyclic guanosine monophosphate (cGMP) in corpus cavernosum. cGMP relaxes smooth muscle to cause local vasodilatation and swelling of corpora as they fill with blood.
- With sexual arousal, nitric oxide (NO) is produced in cavernosal tissue to stimulate the secretion of cGMP
- Sildenafil inhibits PDE V, causing 35% increase in cGMP levels

USUAL DOSE

- Supplied in 100-mg, 50-mg, 25-mg tablets
- May be taken 0.5–4 h prior to sexual activity
- Dose ranges from 25 to 100 mg, with a maximum frequency of once-a-day orally
- Dose adjustments required in patients with severe renal and hepatic impairment
- For geriatric patients (>65 y), starting dose should be 25 mg

DRUG EFFECTS

SYSTEM	EFFECT	ASSESSMENT BY HX	PE
HEENT	Activity on PDE VI (PDE VI is important for phototransduction in the retina)	Transient disturbance of blue-green color discrimination	
CV	Dilatation of systemic blood vessels	Transient drop in BP, flushing, Hx of nitrates	Low BP
GI	Relaxation of lower esophageal sphincter	Dyspepsia, diarrhea	
CNS		Headache, dizziness	
RESP	Mucosal vasodilatation	Nasal congestion	

Key Reference: Carvalho B, Smith M: Viagra: are anaesthetists rising to the challenge? Anaesthesia 2001; 56:91–93.

PERIOPERATIVE IMPLICATIONS

- Risk primarily related to emergent cases based on $T_{1/2}$
- Caution with the concomitant use of hypotensive agents
- Precautions to prevent reflux and regurgitation

DRUG INTERACTIONS

- Concurrent use of nitrates may cause hypotension
- Drug interactions with cytochrome P450 inhibitors (e.g., ketoconazole, erythromycin, and cimetidine) can be expected, and during concomitant therapy a lower dose is suggested

STATINS

Mohammad Naqibuddin, M.B., B.S., M.P.H.

INDICATIONS

- Treatment of hypercholesterolemia
- Treatment of hyperlipoproteinemia

PERIOPERATIVE RISKS

- ↑ In hepatic transaminase; in selected patients this may be associated with alcohol intake
- Myopathy

WORRY ABOUT

- Underlying diseases without CAD

OVERVIEW/PHARMACOLOGY

- Used to reduce LDL cholesterol levels by 25–45% in a dose-dependent manner
- Effective in a variety of patients including those with heterozygous familial hypercholesterolemia, polygenic hypercholesterolemia, or other form of hypercholesterolemia, and individuals with low HDL levels
- Also work with patients with diabetes and with nephrotic syndrome
- Well absorbed, highly protein bound
- Liver is the major route of excretion; also excreted via urine and feces
- Peak plasma concentration is achieved within 1–2 h for atorvastatin, 2.5 h for cerivastatin, 0.6 h for fluvastatin, 2–4 h for lovastatin, 1–1.5 h with pravastatin, and 1–2 h with simvastatin
- In randomized trials, shown to decrease both primary and secondary cardiac morbid events

DRUG CLASS/MECH OF ACTION

- hMG CoA reductase inhibitors
- Block synthesis of cholesterol in the liver by competitively inhibiting hMG CoA reductase activity
- Deplete critical intracellular pools of sterols
- Increase transcription of LDL receptors, leading to enhanced removal of LDL and LDL precursors from plasma
- VLDL removal from plasma may also be increased
- Triglyceride concentrations also decline
- HDL cholesterol level may rise 8–10%

USUAL DOSE

- Atorvastatin 10 to 80 mg/d PO
- Cerivastatin 0.4 to 0.8 mg/d PO
- Fluvastatin 20 to 80 mg/d PO
- Fluvastatin XL 80 mg/d PO
- Lovastatin 20 to 80 mg/d PO
- Pravastatin 10 to 40 mg/d PO
- Simvastatin 10 to 40 mg/d PO
- Lower dose may be required for patients treated with cyclosporine, fibrates, or niacin and for patients with renal insufficiency
- Not recommended for use during pregnancy or during breast feeding

DRUG EFFECTS

SYSTEM	EFFECT	ASSESSMENT BY HX	TEST
HEPATIC	Elevated hepatic transaminase	Alcohol abuse in some patients	LFTs
MS	Increase in hMG CoA reductase synthesis Myopathy	Followed by treatment with statins Rhabdomyolysis, renal failure ↑ in patients taking nicotinic acid or fibrates or erythromycin	CK measurement
CVS	Used in patients with CAD or risk factors	Angina, MI, exercise tolerance	ECG, stress test

Key References: LaRosa JC, He J, Vupputuri S: Effect of statins on risk of coronary disease: a meta-analysis of randomized controlled trials. JAMA 1999; 282:2340–2346.

PERIOPERATIVE IMPLICATIONS

- May reduce risk of ischemia
- In conscious dogs, found to increase coronary endothelial NO production, which enhances NO-dependent coronary vasodilation and NO-mediated regulation of in vivo myocardial oxygen consumption

STEROIDS

Tommy Symreng, M.D., Ph.D.

USES

- Patients with arthritis, asthma, immunologic diseases, allergies, malignancies, transplantation

PERIOPERATIVE RISKS

- Unique problems with disease requiring steroid medication
- Inadequate stress response

WORRY ABOUT

- Preop correction of fluid, electrolyte balance
- Htn
- Adrenal insufficiency

OVERVIEW

- Mineralocorticoids: aldosterone
  – Hyperaldosteronism: hypokalemic alkalosis, hypernatremia, Htn, renal tubular malfunction
  – Hypoaldosteronism: hypovolemia, hyperkalemic acidosis
- Glucocorticoids: cortisol
  – Cushing's syndrome: hypokalemic alkalosis, hypernatremia, fluid retention, Htn, hyperglycemia
  – Glucocorticoid deficiency: hyponatremia, hyperkalemia, hypotension, nausea, abd pain
- Sex hormones: less important acutely

CAUSES

- Mineralocorticoid excess: adrenal adenoma or hyperplasia
- Glucocorticoid excess: glucocorticoid Rx, overproduction of ACTH (pituitary/ectopic), adrenal tumor
- Mineralocorticoid deficiency: congenital, post adrenalectomy, renal failure
- Glucocorticoid deficiency: withdrawal of long-term steroid med, pituitary/hypothalamic tumor, adrenal destruction (both mineralo-, glucocorticoid decreased) by autoimmune disease, tumor, infection, or hemorrhage, congenital, post adrenalectomy

USUAL TREATMENT

- Mineralocorticoid excess: spironolactone, surgery
- Glucocorticoid excess: ↓ glucocorticoid med, surgery
- Mineralocorticoid deficiency: fludrocortisone
- Glucocorticoid deficiency: maintenance dose 25–30 mg hydrocortisone/d, stress dose 100–200 mg hydrocortisone/d
- Perioperative coverage: if steroid treated in last year: 25–100 mg/70 kg/d

DRUG EFFECTS

SYSTEM	EFFECT	ASSESSMENT BY HX	PE	TEST
CV	Hypotension	Orthostatic	BP supine, standing	ECG
	Htn	Angina, CHF, exercise tolerance	Chest pain	CXR
GI	Addison's	N/V, wt loss, abd pain	Buccal hyperpigmentation	Na$^+$, K$^+$
		Diarrhea		
	Cushing's	Thirst, peptic ulcer		
ENDO	Insulin resistance	Glucose intolerance		Glucose—blood/urine
		Oligo/amenorrhea		Hormone levels
HEME	Steroid effect	PMN leukocytes ↑,		CBC,
		leukocytes ↓		differential
DERM	Addison's		Hyperpigmentation	
	Cushing's		Centripetal obesity, thin skin, acne, striae, hirsutism, edema	
RENAL	Nephropathy			BUN/Cr
				K$^+$, Na$^+$, Ca^{2+}, acid-base
CNS		Psychiatric changes		
MS	Muscle	Addison's—fatigue, weakness		
		Cushing's—wasting	Muscle wasting	

Key Reference: Salem M, Tainsh RE, Bromberg J, Lorraux DL, Chernow B: Perioperative glucocorticoid coverage. A reassessment 42 years after emergence of a problem. Ann Surg 1994; 219:416–425.

PERIOPERATIVE IMPLICATIONS

Preoperative Preparation
- Assess volume, electrolyte, metabolic status

Monitoring
- Routine plus consider UO

Airway
- Dependent on underlying disorder

Induction
- Routine if pt normovolemic and underlying disease controlled

Maintenance
- Consider stress steroid coverage if steroid used any time in last year:
  – Minor surgery: 25 mg IV at induction/70 kg
  – Major surgery: 100 mg hydrocortisone/24 h/70 kg
  – If regular steroid dose is given in the morning, supplementation can be decreased

Adjuvants
- Etomidate blocks adrenal corticosteroid production for 5–8 h; steroids can prolong effects of steroid NMBs

Postoperative Period
- Most likely time for adrenal insufficiency to develop if hydrocortisone omitted
- Continue steroid supplementation in ↓ doses until patient mobilized
- If septic problems: continue supplementation 100–200 mg/24 h until hemodynamically stable

COMPARISON OF CORTICOSTEROIDS

Compound	Anti-inflamatory Potency	Na$^+$-Retaining Potency	Duration (h)
Cortisol	1	1	Short (8–12)
Prednisone	4	0.8	Intermediate
Dexamethasone	25	0	Long (36–72)
Fludrocortisone	10	125	Short
Aldosterone	0	500	Short

ANTICIPATED PROBLEMS/CONCERNS

- Problems with disease as cause for steroid med
- Inadequate stress response
- Fluid, electrolyte balance and metabolic problems

TACROLIMUS (FK-506)

Aisling Conran, M.D.

INDICATIONS

- Rescue of primary immunosuppressant Rx following liver, lung, heart, pancreas transplant
- Approx candidates: 3000 liver and 9000 kidney transplants in USA; 15,000 living liver, 50,000 kidney transplant recipients chronically receiving immunosuppressants

PREOPERATIVE RISKS

- Htn: Ca^{2+}-channel blockers may be effective in treating tacrolimus-associated Htn, but care required—interference with tacrolimus metabolism may necessitate a dosing reduction
- Nephrotoxicity: do not administer concurrently with cyclosporine; administer cautiously with other potentially nephrotoxic drugs—e.g., aminoglycoside antibiotics
- Hypersensitivity may occur with IV formulation; patients should be monitored for 30 min after injection

WORRY ABOUT

- Drug is metabolized by cytochrome P450 (3A) enzyme system. Other medications that inhibit or induce this enzyme may affect tacrolimus drug levels.

OVERVIEW/PHARMACOLOGY

- General effect: macrolide antibiotic with potent immunosuppressive properties, often used for rescue therapy in liver transplant patients with rejection refractory to other immunosuppressants
- Tacrolimus metabolized by liver; metabolites primarily excreted in bile; elimination $T_{1/2}$ of 8.5 h prolonged with hepatic dysfunction
- Ca^{2+}-channel blockers, cyclosporine, erythromycin, antifungal agents, metoclopramide may ↑ blood levels of tacrolimus as function of P450 inhibition
- Anticonvulsants (carbamazepine, phenobarbital, phenytoin), rifampin may ↓ blood levels of tacrolimus 2° to induction of cytochrome P450 system

- Adverse effects requiring dose adjustments include nephrotoxicity, neurotoxicity, alterations in glucose metabolism, infection, or susceptibility to malignancy

DRUG CLASS/MECH OF ACTION/USUAL DOSE

- Macrolide antibiotic, highly protein bound (>75%), binds primarily to albumin and/or α_1-glycoprotein
- Tacrolimus binds to calcineurin, blocking production of interleukin-2, thereby inhibiting further T-lymphocyte proliferation, immunosuppression
- Dosing: IV 0.05–0.1 mg/kg/d; PO 0.15–0.3 mg/kg/d in 2 divided doses

DRUG EFFECTS

SYSTEM	EFFECT	ASSESSMENT BY HX	PE	TEST
GENERAL	Hypersensitivity, rash	Observe ½ h; have epinephrine 1:1000 available		
CV	Htn		BP/HR	
RESP	Pleural effusion, dyspnea			
GI	Diarrhea, N/V, constipation, abn liver function, anorexia, abd pain			LFTs
RENAL	Abn kidney function, oliguria			BUN, Cr
ENDO	Hyperkalemia, hypokalemia, hyperglycemia			K^+, glucose
HEME	Anemia, leukocytosis, thrombocytopenia			CBC
CNS	Headache, tremor, insomnia, paresthesias, mental status changes, circumoral numbness		Preop neuro exam	

Key Reference: Chakrabarti P, Wong HY, Scantlebury VP, Jordan ML, Vivas C, Ellis D, Lombardozzi-Lane S, Hakala TR, Fung JJ, Simmons RL, Starzl TE, Shapiro R: Outcome after steroid withdrawal in pediatric renal transplant patients receiving tacrolimus-based immunosuppression. Transplantation 2000; 70:760–764.

PERIOPERATIVE IMPLICATIONS

Preoperative Preparation

- Continue all immunosuppressants through perioperative period
- Monitor levels: therapeutic range 5–30 ng/ml; maintenance level 5–10 ng/ml

Monitoring

- Consider frequent NIBP or arterial catheter

Induction/Maintenance

- Inducers of P450 system include phenobarbital, phenytoin, isoniazid; some volatile anesthetics may result in ↑ metabolism of tacrolimus

Possible Drug Interactions

- Ca^{2+}-channel blockers, cyclosporine, erythromycin, antifungal agents, metoclopramide may ↑ blood levels of tacrolimus as function of P450 inhibition

- Anticonvulsants (carbamazepine, phenobarbital, phenytoin), rifampin may ↓ blood levels of tacrolimus 2° to induction of cytochrome P450 system
- Adverse effects requiring dose adjustments include nephrotoxicity, neurotoxicity, alterations in glucose metabolism, infection, and susceptibility to malignancy

ANTICIPATED PROBLEMS/CONCERNS

- Hypersensitivity may occur with IV formulation

TERBUTALINE

P. Allan Klock, M.D.

USES

- Prescribed for pts with bronchospasm
- Effective for acute asthmatic attacks, COPD
- Used as tocolytic for preterm labor (not FDA-approved for this use)

PERIOPERATIVE RISKS

- Complications of tachyarrhythmias, hypokalemia, hyperglycemia

WORRY ABOUT

- Tachycardia, surreptitious adrenergic cardiomyopathy
- Hyperglycemia
- Hypokalemia
- Pulm edema (from surreptitious adrenergic cardiomyopathy)

OVERVIEW/PHARMACOLOGY

- Used for both acute bronchospasm, chronic management of COPD
- Tachyphylaxis poss with prolonged use
- 7–14% of delivered aerosol reaches circulation
- $\frac{1}{3}$ SQ dose metabolized in liver to inactive sulfate conjugates
- Metabolites I and II, unchanged drug excreted in urine

Onset/Duration

- SQ
  - Onset: significant $\uparrow$ in FEV_1 in 15 min, peak 30–60 min
  - Duration: 1.5–4 h; $T_{1/2}$ 3–4 h
- IV (not FDA-approved route)
  - Onset: immediate; $T_{1/2}$ 3–4 h
- PO
  - Onset: significant improvement in FEV_1 in 60–120 min
  - Duration: at least 4 h
- Metered dose inhaler/nebulizer
  - Onset: 5 min; peak, 1–2 h
  - Duration: 3–4 h

DRUG CLASS/MECH OF ACTION/USUAL DOSE

- β_2-agonist (found to be β_2-selective in animals but selectivity not seen in humans)
- β_2 stimulation $\uparrow$ adenylyl cyclase conversion of ATP to cAMP; this effect $\rightarrow$ cell hyperpolarization, $\uparrow$ inward Ca^{2+} flux, $\rightarrow$ relaxation of bronchial, uterine, vasc smooth muscle

Usual Dose

- SQ: 0.005–0.01 mg/kg to a max 0.25 mg/dose; inject every 15–20 min as needed
- PO: 5 mg tid
- Metered dose inhaler: 2 inhalations every 4–6 h (200 μg/actuation)
- Nebulizer: 0.01–0.03 ml/kg (1 ml = 1 mg); minimum = 0.1 ml, maximum = 2.5 ml; dilute in 1–2 ml N/S

DRUG EFFECTS

SYSTEM	EFFECT	ASSESSMENT BY HX	PE	TEST
CV	Tachycardia, Htn, hypotension, arrhythmias, $\downarrow$ SVR	Palpitations	$\uparrow$ HR; irregular rhythm, BP; rales	ECG
RESP	Bronchodilation	$\downarrow$ Dyspnea	$\downarrow$ Wheezing	O_2 saturation, PFT, PEF
GI	Nausea	Nausea		
ENDO	Hyperglycemia, hypokalemia*	Polydipsia, polyuria	Dehydration	Blood glucose, serum K^+
CNS	CNS stimulation	Insomnia, anxiety, hyperactivity, drowsiness, headache	Tremor	

*Plasma hypokalemia is due to intracellular transport of K^+. Hypokalemia is seen most often with IV terbutaline Rx for preterm labor. K^+ supplementation rarely required, serum levels usually normalize within 3 h of discontinuation of infusion.

Key Reference: Wagner JM, Morton MJ, Johnson KA, O'Grady JP, Speroff L: Terbutaline and maternal cardiac function. JAMA 1981; 246:2697–2701.

PERIOPERATIVE IMPLICATIONS

Preoperative Concerns

- Evaluate disease being treated: asthma, preterm labor
- For asthmatic pts, consider administering inhaled β_2-agonist before inducing anesthesia
- For pts in preterm labor, assess fetal well-being: FHR, wt, indices of lung maturity, etc.
- Evaluate VS, especially HR, BP; rule out CHF
- Assess volume status
- Lab studies to check: glucose, K^+

Induction/Maintenance

- $\uparrow$ CO may prolong inhalation induction
- Theoretical concern of $\uparrow$ ventricular irritability with halothane
- Intraoperative bronchospasm possible with inhaled or IV terbutaline; absorption after SQ injection possibly unreliable
- Tachycardia possible owing to drug effect, not light anesthesia

ANTICIPATED PROBLEMS/CONCERNS

- $\uparrow$ HR, $\downarrow$ SVR possibly not tolerated well by pts with CAD, mitral or aortic stenosis
- CHF may be surreptitious

TETRACYCLINES

Thomas F. Boerner, M.D.
W. David Watkins, M.D., Ph.D.

USES

- Administered PO (most common), IV (fewer side effects), IM (rare, painful), topical (eyes only)
- Original broad-spectrum antibiotic for gram-pos, gram-neg aerobes, anaerobes. One of few agents active against organisms without cell walls. Resistance ↑ worldwide.
- Rx for STDs, other GU infections, dental infections, periodontal diseases, Lyme disease, OA, sclerotherapy, chemoRx, antidiarrheal prophylaxis
- 20 million doses/y in USA

PERIOPERATIVE RISKS

- Barbiturates may ↓ $T_{1/2}\beta$; tetracycline will ↑ conc of digoxin, warfarin. Pts may exhibit GI distress, even *Clostridium difficile* colitis.
- IV tetracycline frequently → thrombophlebitis, lessens efficacy of oral contraceptives
- ↓ Dose with age, poor renal/hepatic functions

WORRY ABOUT

- Tetracycline (esp 1st generation) absorbed poorly if given within 3 h of di-/trivalent cations (Ca^{2+}, Al^{3+}, Mg^{2+}, Fe^{2+}, Bi^{3+})

OVERVIEW/PHARMACOLOGY

- Classified as bacteriostatic (newest ones possibly bactericidal)
- 2 generations: 1st (e.g., tetracycline); 2nd (e.g., doxycycline)
- PO uptake in duodenum (esp 1st generation); peak level, 2 h; IV peak level, 1 h
- 1st generation $T_{1/2}\beta$ 6–12 h; excreted in urine, feces; 2nd generation more lipophilic, greater V_d, recirculation, $T_{1/2}\beta$ 16–18 h; doxycycline excreted 90%+ in feces; safe for anephric pts
- Adjust dose with age, impaired renal/hepatic functions

DRUG CLASS/MECH OF ACTION/USUAL DOSE

- Original broad-spectrum antibiotic
- Nml dose: impairs bacterial protein synthesis; binds via a Mg^{2+} bridge to single active site of 30 S subunit of bacterial ribosome; prevents binding of aminoacyl tRNA to the mRNA-ribosome complex. Without this codon–anticodon interaction, peptide chain formation cannot proceed.
- Effective against *Rickettsia, Mycoplasma, Chlamydia, Borrelia,* spirochetes, some fungi
- Inhibit collagenase (osteoarthritis), tumor-induced angiogenesis (chemoRx)
- Local irritant (sclerotherapy)
- Usual dose: doxycycline, 100 mg PO bid

DRUG EFFECTS

SYSTEM	EFFECT	ASSESSMENT BY HX	TEST
HEENT	Children: brown teeth; risk greatest from second trimester to age 8 y		
CV	Frequently causes thrombophlebitis ↓ Tumor-mediated angiogenesis		
HEPATIC	Rare toxicity, esp with ↑ dose, IV route, preg Usually reversible with drug cessation	Hepatitis	LFTs
GI	Irritation, distress, especially PO, ↑ dose may → superinfection (*C. difficile* colitis)		
HEME	May inhibit/suppress antibody production, leukotaxis, complement system		
GU	May aggravate uremia in susceptible pt; crosses placenta, excreted in breast milk		BUN
CNS	Penetrates CNS; may ↑ ICP during Rx, esp in infants Minocycline: vestibular problems, esp in women	Vision change, headache Dizziness, nausea	
DERM	Phototoxic skin reaction, esp 1st generation		
MS	↓ Bone growth in preemies, ↓ collagenase in joints		

Key Reference: Chopra I, Hawkey PM, Hinton M: Review: Tetracyclines, molecular and clinical aspects. J Antimicrob Chemother 1992; 29:245–277.

PERIOPERATIVE IMPLICATIONS

Preoperative Concerns

- May ↑ digoxin levels, higher prothrombin time if patient on warfarin

Possible Drug Interactions

- Barbiturates may ↓ $T_{1/2}\beta$
- Methoxyflurane, tetracycline may → renal failure

Reversal

- May augment nondepolarizing NM blocker

SPECIAL CONSIDERATIONS

- Although resistance is rising, drugs remain useful antibiotics, with nonantibiotic indications increasing
- Contraindicated in preg, childhood

John M. Murkin, M.D., F.R.C.P.

INDICATIONS

- >3 million chronic users in USA
- T_4 prescribed for patients with chronic hypothyroidism
- T_3 used in myxedema coma
- Not currently indicated but somewhat successfully used for cardiogenic shock post-CPB
- T_3 also favorably administered to brain-dead donors before organ harvesting for heart, heart-lung transplantation
- T_4 generally administered PO; T_4 and T_3 can be administered IV

PERIOPERATIVE RISKS

- Drugs (amiodarone, catecholamines, radiopaque contrast media), cirrhosis, renal failure, sepsis, operation (CPB) can induce "euthyroid sick syndrome" (reduced peripheral conversion of T_4 to T_3); may precipitate myxedema coma

WORRY ABOUT

- T_4 or T_3 can aggravate Sx of myocardial ischemia

OVERVIEW/PHARMACOLOGY

- Hypothyroidism (overt) estimated at 0.5%–0.8% of adults, ↑ with age
- Post-thyroidectomy <30% of patients euthyroid at 10 y due to inadequacy or discontinuation of therapy
- Reversal of clinical Sx of chronic hypothyroidism, including myocardial effusions, requires 2–4 mo Rx
- $T_{1/2}$ for T_4: 7 days, T_3: 1.5 days
- T_4 relatively inactive prohormone undergoing monodeiodination in liver, kidney to biologically active T_3

ICD-9-CM Code: 244.9

DRUG CLASS/MECH OF ACTION/USUAL DOSE

- Thyroid hormone replacement Rx
- T_3 binding to specific membrane receptor proteins augments membrane transport activity, mitochondrial oxidative phosphorylation, protein synthesis
- Extranuclear effects of T_3 occur in minutes, ↑myocardial mitochondrial and transmembrane transport activity
- Nuclear effects of T_3 occur within 0.5–1.0 h, involve transcription, translation of myocardial enzymes, contractile proteins
- Direct effect of T_3 ↓ arterial smooth muscle tone
- Usual dosage of T_4 is 0.15 mg/d PO
- Acute Rx: T_4, 0.3–0.5 mg by slow IV infusion followed by 0.1–0.15 mg/d, or T_3, 0.005–0.01 mg IV

DRUG EFFECTS

SYSTEM	EFFECT	ASSESSMENT BY HX	PE	TEST
CV	Chronotropy, inotropy, ↓ SVR Arrhythmogenesis	Less fatigue Palpitations	HR, reflexes	FT_4E, TSH, ECG
RESP	Restoration of hypoxic, hypercapnic ventilatory drive			
GI	↑ Protein synthesis; enhanced hepatic, renal clearance/ excretion functions		Normal skin turgor	
ENDO	Thermogenesis	Reversal of cold intolerance	Skin warm to touch	

Key Reference: Bennett-Guerrero E, Kramer DC, Schwinn DA: Effect of chronic and acute thyroid hormone reduction on perioperative outcome. Anesth Analg 1997; 85:30–36.

PERIOPERATIVE IMPLICATIONS/POSSIBLE DRUG INTERACTIONS

Preoperative Concerns

- Thyroid hormones ↑ breakdown of vit K–dependent clotting factors—can alter coag status

Induction/Maintenance

- Exaggerated Htn, tachycardia can occur with agents such as ketamine, exogenous catecholamines including ephedrine, epinephrine; in patients on both acute and chronic thyroid hormone replacement

Adjuvants/Regional Anesthesia/Reversal

- Anticholinergics with minimal CV effects, e.g., glycopyrrolate, preferred over atropine
- Caution in the presence of spinal anesthesia; T_3 administration may produce aggravated hypotension

Postoperative Period

- Cirrhosis, sepsis, renal failure, surgery may all ↓ peripheral conversion of T_4 to T_3 (euthyroid sick syndrome), precipitate hypothyroidism

ANTICIPATED PROBLEMS/CONCERNS

- In critically ill patients, T_3 replacement can produce detrimental increases in O_2 requirements (esp myocardial), protein catabolism without improving mortality rates

TISSUE PLASMINOGEN ACTIVATOR

J. Christopher Sill, M.D.

USES

- Patients with acute myocardial infarction
- Best used within 1–2 h of onset of symptoms, but benefit continues until at least 12 h
- Rapid clot lysis by t-PA offers advantages in comparison with streptokinase
- Used with heparin and aspirin and often also with β-blockers, morphine, nitroglycerin, and platelet IIb/IIIa blockers
- Sometimes indicated for acute ischemic stroke, severe deep vein thrombosis, pulmonary embolism, and obstructive vascular disease and to clear thrombi from venous catheters

PERIOPERATIVE RISKS

- Increased bleeding during surgery; if severe, possible need for blood transfusion, fresh frozen plasma, cryoprecipitate, and platelet infusion therapy
- Risk of intracranial hemorrhage (about 1%) can be increased by Htn in the perioperative period
- Incomplete restoration of coronary flow and persisting thrombogenicity may lead to cardiac instability and risk for perioperative infarction

WORRY ABOUT

- Invasive procedures; damage to blood vessels during vascular access procedures can cause severe bleeding—especially at noncompressible sites—e.g., subclavian vein. Consequences of catheter-induced PA damage can be dire.
- Minor bleeding at venipuncture sites

OVERVIEW/PHARMACOLOGY

- Thrombolytic agent; natural t-PA is produced by vascular endothelial cells and accelerates the conversion of plasminogen to plasmin, with consequent clot fibrinolysis
- t-PA (alteplase) is commercially produced using cDNA for natural t-PA, transfected into a mammalian cell line
- Initial thrombolytic response is seen within 30 min when given intravenously. $T_{1/2}$ ~5 min; elimination $T_{1/2}$ ~30–50 min. Eighty percent cleared from plasma within 10 min of stopping a standard infusion.
- Plasminogen activator inhibitors, also released by endothelial cells, oppose t-PA action. Their concentrations are insufficient to be a major consequence during t-PA therapy.
- Clearance is by proteolytic breakdown in the liver

- Reteplase and tenecteplase are recombinantly modified t-PA but have not shown improved clinical efficiency

DRUG CLASS/MECH OF ACTION/USUAL DOSE

- Thrombolytic agent. Fibrin-dependent serine protease. t-PA binds to newly deposited fibrin, where it becomes active in converting plasminogen to plasmin, with subsequent clot lysis. For this reason, unlike streptokinase, t-PA can be considered fibrin specific; t-PA lacks effect on circulating plasminogen.
- In myocardial infarction, usual dose for patients 70 kg or more is a front-loading protocol, with 100 mg t-PA being given IV by bolus and infusion over 90 min, with heparin
- Amount of salvaged myocardium is directly related to the time until the occluded artery is reopened. GUSTO I investigators showed 84% patency within 6 h of front-loaded t-PA.
- More rapid lysis, less systemic fibrinolysis, and few if any anaphylactic reactions when compared to streptokinases—but t-PA is more expensive
- In ischemic stroke, IV t-PA dose is lower; heparin is not used

DRUG EFFECTS

SYSTEM	EFFECT	ASSESSMENT	CHECK	TREATMENT
CV	Bleeding from vascular puncture sites	Hematoma Check for retroperitoneal bleed in presence of femoral puncture	Hgb	Manual compression at puncture sites Blood transfusion may be necessary
	Severe bleeding during surgery	Check if heparin or platelet IIb/IIIa blockers are being given	Hgb Platelets APTT	Blood transfusion Fresh frozen plasma, cryoprecipitate to provide fibrinogen, and factor VIII and platelets may be needed—but increased risk of reocclusion
	Effects of ancillary treatment	Check for ongoing β-blocker, nitroglycerin, or morphine treatment		Discontinue if necessary; however, β-blockade has considerable benefit with little risk in most patients
	Reperfusion arrhythmias	Can occur on restoration of blood flow to ischemic myocardium	Cardiovascular stability	Antiarrhythmics
CNS	Intracranial hemorrhage	Signs of stroke or raised intracranial pressure	Neurologic assessment Urgent CT, MRI	Supportive BP control (risk is increased in presence of heparin)

Key Reference: GUSTO Investigators: An international randomized trial comparing four thrombolytic strategies for acute myocardial infarction. N Engl J Med 1993; 329:673–682.

PERIOPERATIVE IMPLICATIONS

- Danger of bleeding with central line placement
- Risk of hypotension on anesthetic induction with adjuvant nitroglycerin infusion

- Severe Htn may predispose to hemorrhagic stroke
- In absence of optimal recanalization, myocardial ischemia may persist

- Residual thrombus is highly thrombogenic, posing risk of rethrombosis
- Regional anesthesia should not be used

TRANEXAMIC ACID

William B. Weems, M.D.

INDICATIONS

- For short-term use (2–8 days) in hemophilia patients to reduce or prevent hemorrhage and to reduce the need for replacement therapy during and following tooth extraction
- To prevent bleeding after surgery or trauma (e.g., tonsillectomy and adenoidectomy, prostatic surgery, or cervical conization) and to prevent rebleeding of subarachnoid hemorrhage
- To treat primary menorrhagia, gastric and intestinal hemorrhage, recurrent epistaxis, and hereditary angioneurotic edema. The drug also inhibits induced hyperfibrinolysis during thrombolytic treatment with plasminogen activators.

PERIOPERATIVE RISKS

- Side effects of drug: nausea, diarrhea, vomiting, and abdominal pain are the most common adverse effects
- Giddiness has been reported
- Hypotension (if the drug is injected too rapidly)

WORRY ABOUT

- Potential for thrombotic complications 2° to the inhibition of fibrinolysis

OVERVIEW/DRUG CLASS

- A competitive inhibitor of plasminogen activation, and at much higher concentrations a noncompetitive inhibitor of plasmin
- Suppresses fibrinolysis by inhibiting activation of plasminogen
- Contains lysine-binding sites important for plasminogen-fibrin interaction
- Has a structure similar to that of lysine, and reversibly binds to lysine-binding sites on plasminogen, thereby blocking the binding of plasminogen to fibrin and its activation and transformation to plasmin
- Because fibrinolysis requires plasminogen (and plasmin) binding to fibrin, fibrinolysis is inhibited
- Another useful antifibrinolytic drug is aminocaproic acid, which acts according to the same mechanism as tranexamic acid but is 6 to 10 times less potent

PHARMACOLOGY/USUAL DOSE

- Administered either PO 25 mg/kg every 6–8 h or IV 10 mg/kg every 6–8 h beginning the day prior to surgery
- Absorption after oral use is 30–50%; bioavailability is not affected by food
- An antifibrinolytic concentration of drug remains in serum up to 7–8 h
- The protein binding to plasminogen is approximately 3% at therapeutic plasma levels; it does not bind to serum albumin
- The $T_{1/2}$ of elimination when administered orally is 120 min
- Volume of distribution equals 9 to 12 L
- Urinary excretion is the main route of elimination via glomerular filtration
- Overall renal clearance is equal to overall plasma clearance, and >95% of the dose is excreted unchanged in the urine
- Only a small fraction of tranexamic acid is metabolized

DRUG EFFECTS

SYSTEM	EFFECT	ASSESSMENT BY HX	PE	TEST
HEENT	Retinal degeneration is associated with prolonged use; incidence 25–100% and dose-dependent	Visual changes	Ophthalmologic examination in patients receiving tranexamic acid >4 or 5 days	Visual acuity Visual field Color vision Eyeground
CV	Hypotension	Mental status changes, nausea	BP monitoring, heart rate, ECG	
RENAL	Reduce dose in patients with renal insufficiency			BUN/Cr, CrCl
GI	Nausea, diarrhea, vomiting, abdominal discomfort			
OB	Category B There are no well-controlled studies in pregnant females	Crosses placenta and appears in cord blood at concentration equal to that in maternal blood		
IMMUNO	Male mice receiving tranexamic acid up to 5 g/kg/d have been found to develop leukemia			

Key Reference: Zohar E, Fredman B, Ellis M, Luban I, Stern A, Jedeikin R: A comparative study of the postoperative allogenic blood-sparing effect of tranexamic acid versus normovolemic hemodilution after total knee replacement. Anesth Analg 1999; 89:1382–1387.

PERIOPERATIVE IMPLICATIONS

Airway
- No interactions known

Preinduction/Induction
- If given IV, inject slowly to avoid hypotention

Maintenance
- No interactions known

Emergence
- No interactions known

Adjuvant/Regional Anesthesia/Reversal
- No interactions known

Anticipated Problems/Concerns
- Potential for increased thrombotic events

Contraindications
- Acquired defective color vision: prohibits measuring one end point of toxicity
- Subarachnoid hemorrhage: cerebral edema and cerebral infarction may be caused by tranexamic acid in patients with subarachnoid hemorrhage

TRIMETHAPHAN

Lorna L. Im, M.D.

USES

- Production of controlled hypotension during surgery
- Acute control of BP in Htn emergencies, autonomic hyperreflexia, dissecting aortic aneurysm
- Emergency Rx of pulmonary edema in pulmonary Htn assoc with systemic Htn
- Given only IV

PERIOPERATIVE RISKS

- Risk of severe hypotension
- Incompatible with thiopental or other alkaline solutions of iodides and bromides; avoid trimethaphan infusion as vehicle for simultaneous administration of any other drug
- Produces mydriasis, so pupillary dilation may confuse CNS exam
- Histamine release at high doses

WORRY ABOUT

- Severe hypotension, especially with regional anesthesia, state of hypovolemia, or use of other antihypertensive drugs
- Not available readily in the USA, but available in rest of world and in the USA by special import for a specific patient

OVERVIEW/PHARMACOLOGY

- Ganglionic blocking agent, direct peripheral arterial and venous vasodilator
- Rapid onset (1–3 min), short duration of action (5–15 min) after single IV dose
- Partial clearance by plasma ChE hydrolysis, partly by renal elimination (therefore if BP so low that GFR is decreased, ↓ in renal excretion can prolong duration of action)
- Tachyphylaxis may result after continuous IV infusion
- Autoregulation is preserved in cerebral and possibly coronary vascular beds; vasodilation can ↑ total blood flow to a region; autoregulation can then distribute flow to ischemic areas, therefore steal is less likely

DRUG CLASS/MECH OF ACTION/USUAL DOSE

- Autonomic ganglion blocker
- Binds to receptors on autonomic ganglion cells, stabilizes postsynaptic membranes against action of ACh released from presynaptic cell
- Lowers BP by lowering SVR. At high doses, CO ↓ due to venous pooling in capacitance vessels with fall in venous return.
- Used to produce controlled hypotension; also used to improve perfusion during, after cardiac surgery
- Usual dose
  - Intermittent IV bolus of 1–20 mg; may start with a 1 mg IV bolus, then double dose every few min until desired fall in BP produced
  - Continuous IV infusion of 0.5–6.0 mg/min; may dilute 500 mg of drug in 500 ml of D_5, N/S, or lactated Ringer's to a 0.1% soln, start rate at 60 drops/min (3–4 ml); titrate to desired BP
  - Infants more resistant to drug: infuse 0.2% soln
  - Elderly: dilute to < 0.1% soln

DRUG EFFECTS

Adverse reactions due to its nonselective blockade of autonomic nervous system (sympathetic and parasympathetic), predominant tone at effector sites

SYSTEM	PREDOMINANT TONE	EFFECT	ASSESSMENT OF HX	PE
HEENT	Parasympathetic	Cycloplegia, mydriasis, difficulty in accommodation	Blurred vision	
CV		Tachycardia		
Arterioles	Sympathetic	Vasodilation, ↑ peripheral blood flow, hypotension, ↓ SVR		
Veins	Sympathetic	Dilation, peripheral pooling of blood, ↓ preload	Syncope	Postural hypotension
RESP		Rare respiratory arrest of uncertain mechanism with high doses		
GI	Parasympathetic	↓ Secretions, ↓ tone/motility	Dry mouth, paralytic ileus, abd discomfort, N/V/diarrhea, reflux	
GU	Parasympathetic	Bladder atony ↓ Potency	Urinary hesitancy, incomplete voiding Impaired erection, ejaculation	
CNS		↑ in ICP during controlled hypotension is less than with other direct vasodilators (nitroprusside); does not cross blood-brain barrier		
OB		Does cross placenta; ↓ fetal GI motility results in meconium ileus		

Key Reference: Nagata N, Takasaki M, Ibusuki S, Taniguchi M, Kondo O: Intravenous trimethaphan during epidural plus general anesthesia decreases the direct radial artery pressure lower than the brachial artery pressure. J Clin Anesth 1996; 8:180–187.

PERIOPERATIVE IMPLICATIONS

Preoperative Concerns

- Assess volume status
- Monitor arterial BP continuously

Induction/Maintenance

- May interact with other induction agents to cause hypotension
- May be given prophylactically as bolus during induction before laryngoscopy
- Trimethaphan has pH of 5.2 and is incompatible with alkaline solutions, e.g., thiopental

- Anesthesia can modify dose of trimethaphan—e.g., the deeper the plane of anesthesia, the smaller the dose of trimethaphan required to produce hypotension

Adjuvants/Regional Anesthesia/Reversal

- Possible delay in onset, prolonged duration of action of NM blockers, especially succinylcholine, by this ganglionic blocking drug, because of (1) ↓ skeletal muscle blood flow, (2) inhibition of plasma ChE activity, (3) ↓ sensitivity of postjunctional membranes
- Interaction with aminoglycoside antibiotics at NMJ may prolong blockade

SPECIAL CONSIDERATIONS

- Potential problems with continuous administration include
  - Tachyphylaxis
  - Persistently low BP up to 30 min after discontinuance of drug
- H_2 release may precipitate catecholamine "surge" in patients with pheochromocytoma
- May not be available (see Worry About)

VITAMIN B$_{12}$ (CYANOCOBALAMIN)

John K. Stene, M.D., Ph.D.

INDICATIONS

- Prevalence of deficiency: 13 million in USA, especially in elderly
- Prescribed for pernicious anemia
- Lack of gastric secretion of intrinsic factor → malabsorption of vit B$_{12}$; therefore IM route preferred. Strict vegetarian diet–induced deficiency state; responds to oral supplementation.

WORRY ABOUT

- Permanent neurologic injury in long-term deficiency states
- Interactions and neurologic injury with folate, methionine synthetase inhibitors, N$_2$O

OVERVIEW/PHARMACOLOGY

- Vit B$_{12}$ binds to intrinsic factor (gastric glycoprotein from parietal cells) in GI tract, is absorbed from ileum, bound to transcobalamin II in plasma for transport to tissues. Approximately 3 μg of cobalamin secreted into bile/d.
- Excess vit B$_{12}$ admin ↑ urinary excretion
- Vit B$_{12}$ enzymatically converted to 2 active forms: deoxyadenosylcobalamin, methylcobalamin
  – Deoxyadenosylcobalamin is a cofactor for mitochondrial mutase enzyme that catalyzes L-methylmalonyl CoA to succinyl CoA
  – Methylcobalamin is cofactor in methionine synthetase reaction (a methyl group is transferred from 5-methyltetrahydrofolate to homocysteine to form methionine and tetrahydrofolate), pivotal in normal synthesis of purines, pyrimidines, and a number of methylation reactions through formation of N-adenosylmethionine

DRUG CLASS/MECH OF ACTION/USUAL DOSE

- H$_2$O-soluble B vit complex
- Cyanocobalamin administered IM or deep SQ route in doses of 1–1000 μg
- Oral dose to 80 μg can be administered with purified intrinsic factor; 1 U binds 15 μg of cyanocobalamin
- Need glycoprotein (intrinsic factor 60,000 MW) produced by gastric parietal cells for its absorption
- RDA: 2 μg/d for adults
- Therapeutic 100 μg SQ every month

ASSESSMENT POINTS

SYSTEM	EFFECT	ASSESSMENT BY HX	PE	TEST
GI	Achlorhydric or gastrectomy patients at risk; associated with atrophic glossitis	Burning and tingling of mouth	Small, slick, glistening tongue	Schilling test (for vit B$_{12}$ absorption)
HEME	Megaloblastic anemia	Apathy, lassitude, fatigue	Pale skin, mucous membranes, esp nailbeds, palmar surfaces	Peripheral blood smear: macrocytic hyperchromic RBCs Bone marrow: megaloblasts, ↓ megakaryocytes ↓ Platelet count
CNS	Degeneration of dorsal, lateral columns of spinal cord	Numbness, tingling in extremities, difficulty walking	Loss of vibration, vibration, position sense; ataxia, Romberg's sign, muscle flaccidity	Plasma B$_{12}$ < 150 pM suggests B$_{12}$ deficiency
PNS	Neuropathy	Paresthesias, dysesthesias of lower extremities		

Key Reference: Hillman RS: Hematopoietic agents: growth factors, minerals, and vitamins. *In* Hardman JG, Limbird LE (eds): Goodman & Gilman's The Pharmacological Basis of Therapeutics, 9th ed. New York, McGraw-Hill Professional Publishing, 1996, pp 1311–1340.

PERIOPERATIVE IMPLICATIONS/POSSIBLE DRUG INTERACTIONS

- Folate admin reverses megaloblastic anemia but does not prevent (may precipitate) spinal cord degeneration
- N$_2$O oxidizes vit B$_{12}$, reduces activity of methionine synthetase
- Effect of N$_2$O can be reversed by large doses of folic acid

ANTICIPATED PROBLEMS/CONCERNS

- Scavenging waste anesthetic gas prevents OR personnel from developing vit B$_{12}$ deficiency states due to prolonged exposure to N$_2$O
- Extensive interaction between folate and vit B$_{12}$ makes it imperative that pernicious anemia be treated with B$_{12}$ at same time as folate to prevent CNS degeneration

WARFARIN (COUMADIN)

Charise T. Petrovitch, M.D.

INDICATIONS

- Management of thromboembolic disorders: for prophylaxis, Rx, and prevention of recurrence of thromboembolic event including DVT, pulm embolism, thrombosis of grafts. Prevention of arterial emboli associated with prosthetic heart valves, nonvalvular AFIB, acute MI. Prevention of MI, stroke, and recurrent MI. Rx for antithrombin III, protein C, protein S deficiency.
- Newer indications: after angioplasty, for patients who have had coronary graft thrombosis when taking only ASA or ASA and dipyridamole
- Number of individuals receiving the drug: unknown

PERIOPERATIVE RISKS

- Hemorrhage (minor to major life risk)
- "Purple-toe" syndrome, or warfarin necrosis
- Teratogenicity in pregnancy (↓ synthesis of vit K–dependent clotting factors by fetus)

WORRY ABOUT

- Major drug interactions
  – Multiplicity of drugs affecting action of warfarin. List extensive, continually expanding (see later). Be concerned with other drugs that potentiate bleeding—e.g., antiplatelet agents, ASA, NSAIDs; drugs that displace warfarin from protein-binding sites or ↑ or ↓ vit K levels.

OVERVIEW/PHARMACOLOGY

- General effect: anticoagulant with dose-dependent effect on coagulation

PHARMACOKINETICS/PHARMACODYNAMICS

- Warfarin is a racemic mixture of R and S isomers (R-warfarin; S-warfarin)
- Racemic warfarin absorbed rapidly from GI tract, reaches max plasma conc in 90 min, has $T_{1/2}$ of 36–42 h; time to peak effect 36–72 h; duration after discontinuing 2–5 days at least
- In circulation, bound to plasma proteins, accumulates in liver. R-warfarin metabolites excreted in urine; S-warfarins eliminated in bile.
- "Warfarin resistance" or ↓ warfarin effect: when warfarin absorption from GI tract impaired from malabsorption syndromes, concurrent use of liquid paraffin laxatives, cholestyramine resin, or excessive amts of certain antacids—e.g., Mg trisilicate
  – Vit K intake ↑ through diet or administration of vit K IM or IV
  – With induction of hepatic enzymes, increasing metabolism of warfarin. Enzyme inducers include anticonvulsants, barbiturates, primidone, carbamazepine, antimicrobials—e.g., griseofulvin, rifampin, nafcillin, ethanol—and smoking
- ↑ Warfarin effect, or "warfarin sensitivity":
  – Drugs displacing warfarin from albumin ↑ its bioavailability (NSAIDs, ASA, phenytoin sodium, oral hypoglycemic agents, sulfa drugs, nalidixic acid, estrogen, miconazole)
  – Deficiency of vit K enhances; occurs with malabsorption syndromes and during administration of liquid paraffin laxatives, and clofibrate; after long-term use of oral antimicrobials that deplete intestinal bacterial source of vit K. Large doses of vit E antagonize action of vit K; anabolic steroids, danazol impair synthesis of vit K–dependent clotting factors; Olestra removes vit K.
  – Metabolism blocked by phenytoin, chloramphenicol, erythromycin, clofibrate, TCAs,

cimetidine, sulfinpyrazone, sulfamethoxazole-trimethoprim, thus increasing warfarin effect. Disulfiram (Antabuse) significantly slows metabolism.
  – Certain cephalosporins have a warfarin effect themselves—thus contraindicated
  – Elderly, febrile, debilitated patients and those with hepatic dysfunction, hyperthyroidism, or heart failure may have increased warfarin effect

DRUG CLASS/MECH OF ACTION/USUAL DOSE

- Interferes with synthesis of 6 vit K–dependent proteins involved in coagulation sequence: factors II, VII, IX, X; proteins C and S. Before these proteins are released into circulation, they undergo reactions converting glutamic acid residues to carboxyglutamic acid residues and require presence of reduced form of vit K.
- Inhibits cyclic interconversion between reduced form of vit K and its 2,3-epoxide (vit K epoxide)
- Defective clotting factors lacking "carboxyl tail" are produced, impairing coagulation
- Factor II has $T_{1/2}$ of 48 h; requires 3–4 days before drops to level when PT significantly prolonged
- Usual dose
  – Nonurgent need for anticoagulation: adult with average body mass, 5 mg/d PO prolongs PT to 1.5 × control value in 36–48 h; if not achieved by 3rd day, daily dose may be adjusted by ↑ or ↓ of 2.5 mg; goal: PT = 1.5–2 × control. ↑ bleeding complications when PT is 2.5× control. Once anticoagulation stabilized, warfarin dose should be adjusted to maintain INR of 2–3 for all indications, except mech prosthetic cardiac valves, which require higher level of anticoagulation.
  – More urgent need: heparin anticoagulation 1st; start warfarin, 10 mg for 2 days

DRUG EFFECTS

SYSTEM	EFFECT	ASSESSMENT BY HX	PE	TEST
GI	Vit K deficiency may result from a poor diet, extrahepatic biliary obstruction, malabsorption, sterile gut	GI bleeding Tarry stools Hematemesis	Wt:height ratio (BMI)	Hct Fecal occult blood
ENDO	Vit K deficiency Hyperthyroidism, hypermetabolism potentiate warfarin effect		Malnourished	PT/PTT INR
GU	Diuresis, pregnancy ↓ effect; warfarin teratogenic			PT/PTT INR
MS	Arthritis pain medications that affect plts—e.g., ASA, NSAIDs—potentiate bleeding			

Key Reference: Enneking FK, Benzon H: Oral anticoagulants and regional anesthesia: a perspective. Reg Anesth Pain Med 1998; 23:140–145.

PERIOPERATIVE IMPLICATIONS/POSSIBLE DRUG INTERACTIONS

Preoperative Concerns

- Anticoag: consider Rx with vit K (oral, IM, IV, SQ: 2.5–5 mg/70 kg) or FFP (15–20 ml/kg)
- Monitor this drug: PT, INR

Possible Drug Interactions

- Regional: risk of spinal or epidural hematoma when performing a regional when patient is anticoagulated. Risk theoretically ↑ with anticoagulant. Epidural catheter thought to be associated with greater risk of spinal or epidural hematoma if no "measurable" anticoagulant effect from warfarin (i.e., PT nml), but if receiving warfarin, not known if risks of spinal or epidural hematoma significant.

ANTICIPATED PROBLEMS/CONCERNS

- Bleeding most likely complication due to further depletion of clotting factors during surgery; factor depletion may follow massive transfusions or with development of DIC
- If anticoagulation reversed preop with large doses of vit K, warfarin resistance possible initially; thrombosis a risk in this setting

- If anticoagulation reversed with administration of FFP, anticoagulation more easily achieved postop, but infectious risks are a concern
- Preoperative dose of warfarin can be restarted with oral fluids; when risk of thromboembolism is considered esp high (as in patients with recurrent pulm emboli undergoing pelvic surgery) or delay of more than 48 h anticipated before warfarin can be restarted, postop heparin infusion appropriate.

SECTION IV

ALTERNATIVE MEDICINE

ANDROSTENEDIONE

Amr R. Hegazi, M.D.
Alan D. Kaye, M.D., Ph.D.
Adam D. Kaye, Pharm.D., F.A.S.C.P.

USES

- Used to ↑ endogenous testosterone production to enhance athletic performance and recovery from exercise, to keep red blood cells healthy, and to heighten sexual arousal and function

PERIOPERATIVE RISKS

- Coagulopathy
- Polycythemia

OVERVIEW/PHARMACOLOGY

- Testosterone enters the cell by passive diffusion and is converted by 5α-reductase to 5α-dihydrotestosterone, which binds to intracellular androgen receptors
- It ↑ protein anabolism and ↓ protein catabolism. Nitrogen balance is improved only when there is sufficient intake of calories and protein.
- It stimulates the production of red blood cells by enhancing the production of erythropoietic stimulating factor

MECH OF ACTION/USUAL DOSE

- Androstenedione is a direct precursor of testosterone and estrone in both males and females; it might ↑ testosterone levels
- 50–100 mg twice daily taken 1 h before exercise or upon awakening

CONTRAINDICATIONS

- Males with carcinoma of the breast, prostate gland
- Women who are or may become pregnant
- Patient with serious cardiac, hepatic, or renal disease

DRUG EFFECTS

SYSTEM	EFFECT	ASSESSMENT BY HX	TESTS
CV	↓ HDL, atherosclerosis	Angina	ECG, cholesterol
GI	Cholestasis, hepatocellular tumors, hepatitis, nausea		Liver enzymes, bilirubin
HEME	Polycythemia Chronic usage: suppression of clotting factors, sodium and water retention	Easy bruising	PT, PTT Lytes
CNS	Depression, anxiety, behavioral changes, headache		

Key Reference: Leder BZ, Catlin DH, Longscope C, et al: Metabolism of orally administered androstenedione in young men. J Clin Endocrinol Metab 2001; 86:3654–3658.

PERIOPERATIVE IMPLICATIONS

- Retention of sodium, chloride, potassium, calcium, inorganic phosphate, and water
- Nausea, vomiting, rarely hepatocellular neoplasms and hepatitis
- Suppression of clotting factors II, V, VII and X; bleeding in patients on concomitant anticoagulant therapy
- Polycythemia
- ↑ Serum cholesterol, ↓ HDL
- Patients with osteolytic lesions or who are semi-ambulatory may develop nephrocalcinosis
- In geriatric patients, high risk of prostate hypertrophy and prostate carcinoma

POSSIBLE DRUG INTERACTIONS

- Metabolic effects of androgens may ↓ blood glucose level and insulin requirements
- Androgens ↓ levels of thyroxin-binding globulin, resulting in ↓ total T_4 serum levels and ↑ resin uptake of T_3 and T_4
- Might interfere with androgenic or estrogenic drug therapy

β-SITOSTEROL

Alan D. Kaye, M.D., Ph.D.

USES

- Coronary heart disease and hypercholesterolemia
- Benign prostatic hyperplasia and prostatitis
- Gallstones
- Enhances sexual activity
- Prevents colon cancer
- Boosts immune system
- Migraine headache, chronic fatigue syndrome, and symptoms of menopause
- Asthma, bronchitis, systemic lupus erythematosus, and alopecia

OVERVIEW

- β-Sitosterol is a plant sterol with a chemical structure similar to that of cholesterol with an ethyl group added at position 24
- It inhibits intestinal absorption of cholesterol by competing for limited space with cholesterol in mixed micelles and also accelerates the esterification rate of the lecithin-cholesterol acyltransferase (LCAT) enzyme
- In benign prostatic hyperplasia, it binds to prostatic tissue, inhibits prostaglandin synthesis in the prostate, and has anti-inflammatory activity
- Enhances proliferative responses of T cells in vitro
- Inhibits colon cancer growth in vitro

USUAL DOSE

- For hypercholesterolemia, usual dosage is 800 mg–6 g before meals; for severe cases up to 15 g
- For benign prostatic hyperplasia and prostatitis, 60–130 mg tid
- About 175–200 mg is consumed daily in diet

CONTRAINDICATIONS

- Sitosterolemia, which is an inherited lipid storage disease with ↑ absorption of cholesterol and β-sitosterol from diet. Elevated liver β-sitosterol competitively inhibits cholesterol catabolism, which will lead to hypercholesterolemia.

ASSESSMENT POINTS

SYSTEM	EFFECT	ASSESSMENT BY HX	PE	TEST
CV	CAD	Angina MI		ECG
RESP	Asthma	Wheezing	Wheezing	

Key Reference: Wong NC: The beneficial effects of plant sterols on serum cholesterol. Can J Cardiol 2001; 17:715–721.

PERIOPERATIVE IMPLICATIONS

- Obtain adequate Hx to determine indication, since may have significant co-morbidity
- No known perioperative implications

SIDE EFFECTS

- May cause nausea, vomiting, indigestion, gas, diarrhea, or constipation
- Interactions
- Antihyperlipidemic drugs such as atorvastatin (Lipitor), cholestyramine, and gemfibrozil have additive effects in lowering cholesterol level
- Pravastatin (Pravachol) can lower the blood level of β-sitosterol
- β-Sitosterol may reduce absorption and blood level of α- and β-carotene and vitamin E

BLUE COHOSH *(CAULOPHYLLUM THALICTROIDES)* — Jane M. Murphy, R.N., M.S.

USES

- Emmenagogue
- Inducing labor
- Abortifacient
- Antispasmodic

RISK

- When used orally it is unsafe and may cause serious toxicity
- Poisonings have occurred after ingestion of the leaf or seeds
- Case of life-threatening toxicity to newborn when mother consumed blue cohosh near term
- Reports of stroke and aplastic anemia in infants following maternal use
- Not for use with diabetes, in women with hormone-sensitive conditions or cancers, and in patients with diarrhea

PERIOPERATIVE RISKS

- Constricts coronary arteries and appears to decrease the flow of oxygen to the heart

WORRY ABOUT

- Differs from black cohosh
- Safety and efficacy of products differ among manufacturers
- OB: use to facilitate delivery
- Peds: may cause birth defects, hyperglycemia in fetus, neonatal acute myocardial infarction, congestive heart failure, and shock

OVERVIEW/PHARMACOLOGY

- Contains alkaloids and saponins as well as other constituents. Several alkaloid constituents and *N*-methylcystosine may be teratogenic.
- Can ↑ effects of nicotine
- Toxic quantities may result in tachycardia, Htn, and coronary vasoconstriction

ETIOLOGY

- Berberidaceae family
- Typically the dried rhizome/root parts are used
- Listed in the *United States Pharmacopeia* 1882–1905 as a labor inducer

DRUG EFFECTS

SYSTEM	EFFECT	ASSESSMENT BY HX	PE	TEST
HEENT	Mucous membrane irritation		Irritation	
OB/GYN	Stimulates uterus Probable estrogenic effects	Uterus stimulation Changes in menstruation Miscarriage	Abdominal palpation	
GI	Stomach upset, diarrhea, cramping, ↑ gastric motility	GI changes, intestinal spasms		
CV	Angina, Htn	Chest pain, Htn, tachycardia	Cardiac assessment	ECG ECHO
ENDO	Hyperglycemia			Blood glucose

Key References: Jones TK, Lawson BM: Profound neonatal congestive heart failure caused by maternal consumption of blue cohosh herbal medication. J Pediatr 1998; 132:550–552.

PERIOPERATIVE IMPLICATIONS

Preoperative Concerns

- Unclear if safe in pediatrics, during pregnancy and lactation
- Reliable self-reporting of use
- Use in conjunction with nicotine is dangerous
- Can be associated with coronary vasoconstriction

Monitoring

- Routine plus ECHO if cardiac involvement is a concern
- Blood sugar

Airway

- No known effects

Preinduction/Induction

- Coronary constriction

Maintenance

- Evaluate for hyperglycemia, cardiac changes, Htn

Adjuvant

- May accentuate effects of other vasoactive drugs

Postoperative Period

- Monitor blood pressure, blood sugar, and cardiac status

CARNITINE

Mitzi K. Hemstreet, M.D., Ph.D.

USES

- Dietary supplement for individuals with primary or secondary L-carnitine deficiency
- Adjunctive treatment of the hepatotoxic effects of valproic acid, to reduce mitochondrial stress from this anticonvulsant
- Anecdotal treatment to improve cardiac function in cardiomyopathy of childhood, to enhance the efficacy of erythropoietin therapy, and to treat peripheral vascular disease, ischemic cardiomyopathies, congestive heart failure, chronic cardiac dysrhythmias, and the cardiotoxic effects of anthracycline. Most of these uses are of unproven benefit, however.

PERIOPERATIVE RISKS

- None. The only known side effects are transient nausea and vomiting, and body odor. However, if carnitine is taken for L-carnitine deficiency, individuals should be advised to continue this medication as scheduled up to the time of surgery to avoid acute hypoglycemia, lactic acidosis, hepatic failure, cardiomyopathy, and myopathy associated with primary carnitine deficiency.
- If severe vomiting or diarrhea is present, intravenous L-carnitine may be administered in place of oral supplementation

WORRY ABOUT

- Need for dextrose-containing IV solutions in the preop, intraop, and postop periods (while fasting) for individuals with primary L-carnitine deficiencies

OVERVIEW/PHARMACOLOGY

- L-Carnitine is a trimethylated amino acid similar in structure to choline and is an essential cofactor of fatty acid metabolism. It facilitates transport of long-chain fatty acids into the mitochondrial matrix for β-oxidation and cellular energy production, and promotes intramitochondrial glucose and amino acid catabolism. It thus plays an essential role in cellular energy production, primarily in skeletal and cardiac muscle and hepatocytes.
- Found primarily in liver, striated muscle, and cardiac muscle, it is derived from dietary intake of preformed carnitine and is formed de novo in the liver and kidney from the metabolism of methionine and lysine
- L-Carnitine is stored mainly in skeletal muscle and is excreted in urine
- Benefits are not proven by rigorous study

DRUG CLASS/USUAL DOSE

- Carnitine is a naturally occuring substance required for mammalian cellular energy production
- Pregnancy: category B. No adequate studies of the effects on human reproduction have been performed, so L-carnitine should be used with caution in pregnant women.
- Oral dosing: for adults, the usual dose is 990 mg bid to tid. For infants and children, recommended dosage is between 50 and 100 mg/kg/d in divided doses, max 3 g/d.
- Intravenous dosing: for acute treatment of lactic acidosis and cardiomyopathy in primary L-carnitine deficiency, the recommended dosage is a 50 mg/kg bolus injection over 2–3 min, followed by an equivalent dosage over the next 24 h (divided every 3–4 h). Further dosage depends on response. Daily intravenous dosing (divided q 3–4 h) as high as 300 mg/kg/d has been used.
- Overdosage: the only known toxicity of high doses of L-carnitine in humans is diarrhea. The MLD for L-carnitine in mice is 19.2 g/kg.

DRUG EFFECTS

SYSTEM	EFFECT	ASSESSMENT BY HX	PE	TEST
GI	Nausea, vomiting, diarrhea	May be related to acute Sx of L-carnitine deficiency rather than medication	Muscle weakness, lethargy, stupor, petechiae, rapid resp	Serum glucose, PT/PTT LFTs, lactic acid, NH_3
DERM	Body odor	Relation to use of drug	Odor	

Key Reference: Physicians' Desk Reference, 50th ed. Montvale, NJ, Medical Economics Company, Inc., 1996.

POSSIBLE DRUG INTERACTIONS

- There are no known drug-drug interactions with L-carnitine

ANTICIPATED PROBLEMS/CONCERNS

- None related to L-carnitine. For patients with primary L-carnitine deficiency, concerns include hypoglycemia with fasting, lactic acidosis, hepatic failure, coagulopathy, cardiomyopathy, and myopathy.

CHITOSAN

Jane M. Murphy, R.N., M.S.

USES

- Orally used for weight loss (not effective)
- Orally used for reducing high cholesterol by patients with renal failure on chronic hemodialysis
- Topically used for treating periodontitis

RISK

- Clinical trials show no effect on weight loss
- Mixed clinical results related to effect on serum lipids

- Chitosan appears to interact with erythrocyte cell membranes
- Protects periodontal tissue by acting as a surgical cement

PERIOPERATIVE RISKS

- No known interactions with drugs
- No known perioperative risks

WORRY ABOUT

- Insufficient data about safety in pediatrics, pregnancy, and lactation
- Patients with allergies to shellfish should not take this supplement

OVERVIEW/PHARMACOLOGY

- A cationic polysaccharide component of crustacean skeletons
- Not hydrolyzable and differs from other fibers because it contains an amino group

ETIOLOGY

- Chitosan is a derivative of chitin, which is found in the tough shells of crab, lobster, and shrimp

DRUG EFFECTS

SYSTEM	EFFECT	TEST
CARDIAC	Possible reduction of serum cholesterol in patients with renal failure on chronic hemodialysis	Cholesterol (LDL and HDL)
HEME	Possible improvement in serum hemoglobin levels in patients with renal failure on chronic hemodialysis	Hgb
RENAL	Possible reduction in urea and creatinine levels in patients with renal failure on chronic hemodialysis	Urea/Cr

Key References: Jing SB, Li L, Ji D, Takiguchi Y, Yamaguchi T: Effect of chitosan on renal function in patients with chronic renal failure. J Pharm Pharmacol 1997; 49:721–723; Pittler MH, Abbot NC, Harkness EF, Ernst: Randomized, double-blind trial of chitosan for body weight reduction. Eur J Clin Nutr 1999; 53:379–381.

PERIOPERATIVE IMPLICATIONS

Preoperative Concerns

- Unknown effects in pediatrics, pregnancy, and lactation
- Reliable self-reporting of use

Monitoring

- Routine

Airway

- No known concerns

Preinduction/Induction

- No known concerns

Postoperative Period

- Routine

CHOLESTIN

Shuomin Zhu, M.D., Ph.D.

USES

- Related to red yeast rice. Prepared by growing red yeast (*Monascus purpureus*) on rice to produce a red-colored product.
- Prevalence: red yeast rice is very popular in many Asian countries, with consumption ranging from 14 to 55 g/person/d (0.5–2 oz). Consumption in USA is unknown.
- Dietary supplement marketed to maintain healthy cholesterol levels and prevent coronary artery disease
- Cholestin costs slightly less than the traditional commercially available cholesterol-lowering drugs ($20–40/mo vs. $40–60/mo).

PERIOPERATIVE RISKS

- Unknown

WORRY ABOUT

- Liver and skeletal muscle diseases

OVERVIEW/PHARMACOLOGY

- Cholestin (Pharmanex, Simi Valley, Ca) contains starch, protein, fiber, and at least eight statin compounds (about 4% by weight). Differs from the traditional red yeast rice in containing larger amount of lovastatin or other statins.
- Significantly reduces total cholesterol, LDL-C, and total triacylglycerol concentrations if patient is hypercholesterolemic
- Excreted via liver metabolism

DRUG CLASS/MECH OF ACTION/USUAL DOSE

- Functions as hMG CoA reductase inhibitor to reduce cholesterol biosynthesis
- Recommend not taking more than 2 capsules bid (2.4 g)

DRUG EFFECTS

SYSTEM	EFFECT	ASSESSMENT BY HX	PE	TESTS
CV	Reduces total cholesterol, LDL, and total triacylglycerol		Xanthomas	HDL LDL VLDL
GI	Rare hepatitis and cholestasis	Itching Skin color change Fatigue	Jaundice, excoriations, enlarged and tender liver	Transaminase and bilirubin levels
MS	Rare myositis, rhabdomyolysis	Myalgia Myoglobinuria	Tender muscles	CK
IMMUNO	Anaphylactic reactions	Rashes or other allergic Sx Pruritus	Urticaria Angioedema Dyspnea	Positive RAST to Chinese red yeast rice and/or *M. purpureus*
CNS	Psychiatric disorders including depression if too great ↓ in LDL and HDL levels	Mood changes		

Key Reference: Heber D, Yip I, Ashley JM, Elashoff DA, Elashoff RM, Go VLW: Cholesterol-lowering effects of a proprietary Chinese red yeast rice dietary supplement. Am J Clin Nutr 1999; 69:231–236.

PERIOPERATIVE IMPLICATIONS

Preoperative Concerns

- Hx of arterial-aging diseases: hypercholesterolemia, atherosclerosis, ischemic heart disease, stroke or occlusive peripheral vascular disease
- ↑ Incidence of Htn, DM, obesity, and cigarette smoking

Induction/Maintenance

- Consider invasive monitoring if patient has CAD
- No drug interactions known with general and local anesthetics

Postoperative Concerns

- Immediate resumption not necessary

ANTICIPATED PROBLEMS/CONCERNS

- Assess for diseases associated with hypercholesterolemia, hepatic function, and myopathy

CHONDROITIN SULFATE

Keith K. Lee, D.O.

USES

- Osteoarthritis (OA) is the most prevalent form of joint disease in USA, affecting >20 million people and expected to rise with the aging population
- Europeans used chondroitin sulfate (CS) for decades before acceptance in the USA
- CS is relatively free of adverse reactions or side effects and thus offers an attractive alternative to traditional treatments mainly consisting of nonsteroidal anti-inflammatories
- As CS has gained in popularity, researchers have recognized the need to conduct more scientific studies to validate or refute its efficacy, as well as its safety
- To date, most trials testing the efficacy of CS have demonstrated significant improvement of patients' OA, although the level of improvement continues to be debated

PERIOPERATIVE RISKS

- Side effects of drug and adverse events: poorly documented in published literature, although side effects and adverse reactions seem to approximate those of placebo

WORRY ABOUT

- No known significant complications of CS and no known anesthetic implications

OVERVIEW/PHARMACOLOGY

- Nutritional supplement for the treatment of OA
- Shown to have activity and capable of ↑ proteoglycan synthesis in articular cartilage; mechanism of action may be related to local inhibition of interleukin 1β
- CS usually takes 1 mo to exert any effect, with maximum benefits seen after 4 wk of therapy; conversely, benefits are sustained for 1–2 mo after discontinuation of therapy

DRUG CLASS/USUAL DOSE

- CS is a glycosaminoglycan found in the proteoglycans of articular cartilage
- Derived from animal sources (e.g., shark cartilage)
- Sold as Osteo Bi-Flex manufactured by Rexall Sundown, Inc.; regular-strength tablets contain 250 mg glucosamine HCl and 200 mg CS; also manufactured as maximum-strength tablets containing double the active ingredients
- Dose: manufacturer of Osteo Bi-Flex recommends 6 regular-strength tablets daily for the first 60 days and 3–6 regular-strength tablets daily thereafter
- Most studies have tested doses of 1–2 g CS daily, although a higher dose has not clearly been linked to a greater effect

ASSESSMENT POINTS

SYSTEM	DRUG EFFECT	ASSESSMENT BY HX	PE	TEST
MS	Anti-inflammatory effect, slows joint degeneration	Patient assessment of pain scores	Joint tenderness and function	Joint narrowing on x-rays
GI	Low incidence of nausea and diarrhea	Subjective reports of nausea and diarrhea		

Key Reference: Mazieres B, Combe B, Phan Von A, Tondut J, Grynfeltt M: Chondroitin sulfate in osteoarthritis of the knee: a prospective, double blind placebo controlled multicenter clinical study. J Rheumatol 2001; 28:173–181.

PERIOPERATIVE IMPLICATIONS/DRUG INTERACTIONS

- None

CHROMIUM

Lee A. Fleisher, M.D.

USES

- Body building (ineffective)
- May aid in glycemic control of type II DM and gestational DM
- Hyperlipidemia
- Hypoglycemia—reactive
- Obesity

PERIOPERATIVE RISK

- Risks minimal
- Chronic ingestion associated in one case with thrombocytopenia, hepatic dysfunction, renal dysfunction

WORRY ABOUT

- Nephrotoxicity

OVERVIEW

- A trace mineral
- Improves glucose tolerance in type II DM and gestational DM (in some studies)
- Shown to ↑ insulin sensitivity and ↓ serum triglycerides
- Shown to alleviate symptoms of reactive hypoglycemia
- Popular as weight loss and body building supplement, but effect not supported in clinical trials

DRUG CLASS/MECH OF ACTION/USUAL DOSE

- Hypothesis: in normal functioning, it ↑ circulating insulin, results in binding of chromium to peripheral, insulin-sensitive tissue; ↑ insulin receptor number and activates insulin receptor kinase
- Usual dosage recommended: 50–200 μg/d
  – Available orally or IV
  – Taken as supplement of 200–1000 μg/d
- Not effective in randomized clinical tests

DRUG EFFECTS

SYSTEM	EFFECT	TEST
RENAL	Nephrotoxicity	Cr
ENDO	Insulin sensitivity	Glucose

Key Reference: Anderson RA: Chromium in the prevention and control of diabetes. Diabetes Metab 2000; 26:22–27.

PERIOPERATIVE IMPLICATIONS

- No known interactions

CRANBERRY

Shuomin Zhu, M.D., Ph.D.

USES

- Prevalence: ~40% of patients use herbal medicines including cranberry; 47% of cranberry juice consumers are aware of a link between cranberry juice and urinary tract health
- Most common as alternative prophylactic antibacterial agent
- Native Americans use cranberries for treating wounds and blood poisoning and the plant leaves for urinary disorder, diarrhea, and diabetes

PERIOPERATIVE RISKS

- Unknown

WORRY ABOUT

- Urinary stone formation (if > 2.5 quarts of cranberry juice consumed daily)

OVERVIEW/PHARMACOLOGY

- Cranberries are a fruit native to New England and belong to the *Vaccinium* genus
- The most popular cranberry beverage today is the cranberry-juice cocktail, containing about 27% cranberry juice, sweetener, water, and vitamin C
- Cranberry tablets are also available

DRUG CLASS/MECH OF ACTION/USUAL DOSE

- ↑ Concentration of hippuric acid and ↑ acidification of urine (current studies do not substantiate this mechanism)
- Inhibits bacterial adherence to mucosal surface by at least 2 kinds of inhibitors: fructose and proanthocyanidins
- Fructose and proanthocyanidins in cranberries inhibit type I–fimbriated *Escherichia coli* adhesion
- Prophylaxis effect found in females taking 300–400 ml cranberry juice per day

ASSESSMENT POINTS

SYSTEM	DRUG EFFECT	ASSESSMENT BY HX	PE	TEST
HEENT	Reduces dental plaque and periodontal and gum disease	Toothache	Dental examination	
CV	Improves ability of LDL to resist oxidative stress (antioxidation)			ECHO of arteries
GU	Prevents UTI; stone formation	Frequency and urgency and painfulness of urination	Cloudy urine Low back pain	UA Culture of urine

Key Reference: Harkins KJ: What's the use of cranberry juice? Age Ageing 2000; 29:9–12.

PERIOPERATIVE IMPLICATIONS

Preoperative Concerns

- Hx of UTI, urolithiasis, antibiotic usage

Induction/Maintenance

- Routine monitoring
- Consider antibiotic coverage if UTI is present

Postoperative Concerns

- Immediate resumption not necessary

ANTICIPATED PROBLEMS/CONCERNS

- Assess for UTI, antibiotic use, and urolithiasis

CREATINE

R. Blaine Easley, M.D.

USES

- Medical: historically used to lower cholesterol and treat rare conditions of heart failure due to creatine deficiencies
- Fitness: ↑ usage over past decade to ↑ muscle mass and enhance physical performance. Initially used by professional athletes, now used as nutritional supplement in almost all areas of exercise fitness (in both casual and competitive athletes).
- Incidence: unknown incidence in population

PERIOPERATIVE RISKS

- Unknown. Theoretical problems in patients with impaired renal function. Potential for drug interactions, though no definitive studies (see Possible Drug Interactions).

WORRY ABOUT

- Hypovolemia/dehydration if inadequate nutrition

OVERVIEW/PHARMACOLOGY

- Commercially available as creatine citrate, creatine monohydrate, and creatine phosphate
- Creatine exists intracellularly in skeletal muscle, cardiac muscle, brain, and testes as creatine phosphate, otherwise called phosphocreatine. Phosphocreatine contains a high-energy phosphate bond, used for short, intense muscle activity via the phosphagen energy system.
- Studies in animal and human subjects have demonstrated ↑ of cellular phosphocreatine levels in skeletal muscle following creatine ingestion. Few studies demonstrating ↑ in muscle strength or endurance.
- Recent randomized trials have shown neither increased strength nor increased stamina

- ↑ In muscle mass is thought related to ↑ in intracellular H_2O content brought about by influx of phosphocreatine into myocyte
- Creatine is eliminated from the body by renal excretion as creatinine, the anhydrous form of creatine
- Creatine is usually ingested dissolved in fluid
- Use creatine to ↑ muscle mass and performance. (Special concern should be paid to athletes desiring weight loss, i.e., wrestlers, gymnasts, body builders, football players.)

DRUG CLASS/USUAL DOSE

- Creatine is classified as a nutritional or dietary supplement; therefore, it is unregulated by the FDA
- Typical usage: initially 20–25 g ingested daily for 5–7 days, followed by 5–10 g daily for 10–12 wk. However, some individuals take higher dosages continually.

DRUG EFFECT

SYSTEM	EFFECT	ASSESSMENT BY HX	PE	TEST
CV	Hypovolemia/hypotension	Exposure	BP/HR	Lytes

Key Reference: Juhn MS, Tarnopolsky M: Potential side effects of oral creatine supplementation: a critical review. Clin J Sport Med 1998; 8:298–304.

POSSIBLE DRUG INTERACTIONS

Preoperative Period

- Because of the associated risk of hypovolemia/dehydration in patients using creatine, there are theoretical problems when used with the following classes of medications: diuretics, H_2 antagonists (e.g., cimetidine), NSAIDs, probenecid, and trimethoprim, or when taken near the time of exercise

Induction/Maintenance

- No known interactions. May need bolus of intravascular fluids and careful attention to BP at time of induction.

Adjuvants/Regional Anesthesia/Reversal

- No known interactions. Consider pro/cons of NSAID usage intraoperatively, especially if no assessment of renal function.

DANDELION

Kimberly M. King, M.D.

USES

- Rx for liver congestion, bile duct inflammation, hepatitis, gallstones, and jaundice
- Rx for fluid retention
- Rx for diabetes with specific hypoglycemic effects
- Less commonly used for mastitis, heartburn, boils, and fevers, among other uses
- Dietary supplement as a source of vitamins and minerals (leaves contain the highest concentration of vitamin A at 14,000 IU/100 g raw) in addition to vitamin D, vitamin B complex, vitamin C, iron, silicon, Mg, Na, K, zinc, manganese, copper, and phosphorus

PERIOPERATIVE RISKS

- Hemodynamic instability 2° to ↓ in circulating blood volume from diuretic effect

WORRY ABOUT

- If used in combination with prescription diuretic drugs, effects of either or both drugs may be enhanced, leading to a hypovolemic state
- Multiple minerals in dandelion may ↓ systemic absorption of PO-administered drugs

OVERVIEW/PHARMACOLOGY

- Primary digestive therapeutic effects thought to be 2° to the bitter principle, taraxacin, which acts to produce a reflexive ↑ in saliva and digestive juice secretion
- Stimulation of bile release by the liver and gallbladder, hence improving both bile flow (choleretic effect) and release (cholagogue effect)
- Diuretic activity comparable to that of furosemide has been demonstrated in mice; however, because dandelion replaces potassium lost through diuresis, metabolic complications occur only rarely
- Inulin, a polysaccharide fiber composed of long chains of fructose-containing molecules contained in the plant, may act to buffer fluctuations in blood sugar levels

USUAL DOSE

- Root used for general tonic and mild liver remedy up to tid
  - Dried root: 2–8 g by boiling, steeping, or decoction
  - Fluid extract: 4–8 ml
  - Tincture, alcohol based: not recommended 2° to high dosage required
  - Juice of fresh root: 4–8 ml
  - Powdered solid extract: 250–500 mg
- Leaf preparations used for diuretic effects tid
  - Dried leaf by infusion: 4–10 g
  - Fluid extract: 4–10 ml

TOXICITY

- Generally considered one of the safest medicinal plants used
- Concern includes possible role as an allergen in atopic individuals—most allergenic is the plant's pollen

DRUG EFFECTS

SYSTEM	EFFECT	ASSESSMENT BY HX	PE	TEST
CV	Hypovolemia	Orthostasis, polyurea, polydipsia	↓ Skin turgor Hypotension, tachycardia, orthostasis	Orthostatic BP, HR
GI	↑ Gastric secretion	Diarrhea		
RENAL	Prerenal failure	Polyurea, polydipsia	As for CV	BUN/Cr
METAB	Hypoglycemia	Lightheaded, clammy, shaky	Sweaty	Blood glucose

Key Reference: Pizzorno JE Jr, Murray M: *Taraxacum officinale* (dandelion). *In* A Textbook of Natural Medicine, 2nd ed. London, Churchill Livingstone, 1999, pp 979–982.

PERIOPERATIVE IMPLICATIONS

Preoperative Concerns

- Patients often fail to report herbal use as a medication—ask specifically if patient is taking any herbal, alternative, or folk remedies

Induction/Maintenance

- Assess volume status before induction; may need additional fluid bolus to account for hypovolemia and lessen likelihood of hypotension often observed with induction agents
- Follow urine output closely for extended procedures

Adjuvants/Regional Anesthetics/Reversal

- No interactions known

Emergence/Extubation

- No known complications

Postoperative Period

- Continue to assess volume status and treat accordingly
- Due to the numerous physiologic compounds found within plant substances such as dandelion (both water and fat soluble), a specific duration of action cannot be stated; each compound has its own effect—none of which are documented well in the literature at this time

DEHYDROEPIANDROSTERONE (DHEA)

Carol Norred, C.R.N.A., M.H.S.
Bracken J. De Witt, M.D., Ph.D.

USES

- Unconfirmed benefit for, but sold for Rx or prevention of
  - Depression
  - Cardiovascular disease
  - Erectile dysfunction
  - SLE
  - Memory aid
  - Immune system stimulation
  - Athletic performance enhancement
  - Menopause

PERIOPERATIVE RISKS

- Single case report associated DHEA with cardiac arrhythmias
- May induce insulin resistance
- Unknown effects on perioperative stress response, adrenal and cardiac function

WORRY ABOUT

- Cardiac arrhythmias occur rarely, esp with large doses
- Hyperglycemia if used by diabetics
- Unknown effects on coagulation

PHARMACODYNAMICS

- Steroid hormone produced by adrenals, interconverted to testosterone, estrone, estradiol, androsterone
- Effects similar to those of anabolic steroids
- ↑ Protein synthesis in skeletal muscle
- Several studies report no increase in serum testosterone or enhancement of strength in resistance training
- Inhibits glucose-6-phosphate, which supposedly accounts for postulated antiatherogenic properties
- DHEA levels ↓ with CHF, oxidative stress, aging, and cancer
- May stimulate hormone-producing tumors

OVERVIEW

- Came on scene due to New England Journal report that high levels correlated with fewer cardiac events (Rancho-Bernardo study); later, not found so in larger Rancho-Bernardo study
- FDA categorized DHEA as unapproved drug in 1985; reclassified as dietary supplement by 1994
- Banned by NFL and Olympics
- Contraindicated in breast, ovarian, and prostate cancers
- May cause hirsutism, acne, headache, insomnia, weight gain, alopecia; deepening of voice and abnormal menses in women, or gynecomastia in men
- No data indicate benefit greater than long-term risk

USUAL DOSE

- 25–50 mg/d for angioedema
- 50 mg tid for cardiovascular disease
- 30–90 mg/d for depression, memory improvement, or cognition
- 200 mg/d for SLE

DRUG EFFECTS

SYSTEM	EFFECT	ASSESSMENT BY HX	PE	TEST
HEENT	Hirsutism			
CV	Anabolic steroids associated with sudden cardiac arrest, Htn; DHEA rarely causes arrhythmias	Determine chronic and acute dose and duration of self-administration Palpitations	HR	Preop ECG for chronic or excessive use
GI	Anabolic steroids associated with hepatitis, cholestatic jaundice			
HEME	Inhibits platelet aggregation in vivo Antiglucocorticoid actions		Ecchymoses	?Bleeding time Preop glucose for diabetics
DERM	Increased acneiform dermatitis			
GU	Hypogonadism with anabolic steroids Prostate tumor growth		Prostate exam	PSA
CNS	Anabolic steroids may cause aggressiveness; DHEA binds to NMDA, sigma, GABA receptors	↑ Pituitary tumor growth		ACTH

Key Reference: Gaby AR: Dehydroepiandrosterone: biological and clinical significance. Altern Med Rev 1996; 1:60–69.

POSSIBLE DRUG INTERACTIONS

Preoperative Period

- Insulin resistance
- Synergism with corticosteroids

Induction/Maintenance

- Unknown effects of inhibition of steroid synthesis if combined with etomidate, or immunosuppressives for transplantation

Postoperative Concerns

- Unknown effects on stress response

ANTICIPATED PROBLEMS

- Unpredictable cardiovascular effects

ECHINACEA *(ECHINACEA ANGUSTIFOLIA, E. PALLIDA, OR E. PURPUREA)*

Carol Norred, C.R.N.A., M.H.S.

USES

- Immune system stimulant
- Anti-inflammatory
- Treatment of bacterial, viral, and fungal urinary and upper respiratory infection
- Promotes tissue granulation and healing when used locally

PERIOPERATIVE RISKS

- No cardiovascular, coagulation, sedative, or electrolyte effects that may interact with anesthetics
- No known side effects, drug interactions, or toxicities

WORRY ABOUT

- Concern that echinacea might counteract immunosuppressive drugs in transplant patients
- Speculations that echinacea exacerbates toxicity of anesthetic drugs
- Although it contains flavonoids, unknown if echinacea inhibits P450 3A4 and sulfotransferase

PHARMACODYNAMICS

- No direct bactericidal or bacteriostatic effects to directly destroy or prevent the growth of bacteria
- Antiviral activity postulated
- Promotes the release of tumor necrosis factor by lymphocytes
- Inhibits bacterial hyaluronidase
- Enhances WBC phagocytosis

OVERVIEW

- Allergies infrequently, especially if pt allergic to sunflowers and ragweed (Asteraceae)
- Contraindicated for systemic diseases such as AIDS, TB, collagen vascular, leukosis, or autoimmune disorders such as MS, but no adverse effects noted in clinical studies
- Speculation of tachyphylaxis with prolonged use
- Echinacea pyrrolizidine alkaloids lack unsaturated necine structure associated with hepatotoxicity
- No acute or chronic toxicity reported with oral doses. Slight potential toxicity with IV administration.

USUAL DOSE

- Expressed juice: 8–9 ml/d
- Capsules: 1–3 g tid
- Tinctures: 3–5 ml/d

DRUG EFFECTS

SYSTEM	EFFECT
IMMUNO	Stimulant (see Overview)

Key Reference: Chavez MI, Chavez PI: Monographs on alternative therapies: echinacea. Hosp Pharm 1998; 33:180–188.

POSSIBLE DRUG INTERACTIONS

- Speculated hepatotoxicity with methotrexate, ketoconazole, cyclosporine, phenytoin, amiodarone

Induction/Maintenance

- Speculated hepatotoxicity with barbiturates

Adjuvants/Regional Anesthesia/Reversal

- No interactions known

Postoperative Concerns

- No interactions known

ANTICIPATED PROBLEMS

- Liver dysfunction

EPHEDRA (MA-HUANG)

Bracken J. De Witt, M.D., Ph.D.

USES

• Ephedra is a plant that contains a variety of ephedrine alkaloids, including ephedrine and pseudoephedrine
• Dietary supplements containing ephedra are marketed in USA as agents that may aid in weight reduction and energy enhancement
• Over 3 billion servings of ephedra-containing dietary supplements were sold in 1999
• Several governmental agencies have inquired into the safety of ephedra and regulated the use of dietary supplements containing ephedra in response to reported patient adverse reactions
• Ephedra is also commonly known as ma-huang, Mormon tea, squaw tea, and herbal ecstasy

PERIOPERATIVE RISKS

• Risks associated with an ↑ in the sympathetic nervous system

WORRY ABOUT

• Lethal cardiac arrhythmias, Htn, myocarditis, MI, angina
• Hemorrhagic/ischemic stroke, subarachnoid hemorrhage, cerebral vasculitis, seizures
• Acute hepatitis
• Preterm labor

OVERVIEW/PHARMACOLOGY

• Mechanism of action is via ↑ in sympathetic stimulation
• Ephedrine is an indirect-acting sympathomimetic that exerts its effects mainly by stimulating release of norepinephrine
• Other ephedrine alkaloids in ephedra have direct-acting effects on both α- and β-adrenoceptors
• Ephedra is often packaged with guarana-derived caffeine, which may add to the sympathetic stimulation

DRUG CLASS/MECH OF ACTION

• Works via stimulation of sympathetic nervous system

DRUG EFFECTS

SYSTEM	EFFECT	ASSESSMENT BY HX	PE	TEST
CV	Arrhythmias, Htn, myocarditis, MI, angina	Chest pain	BP	BP/HR ECG Cardiac enzymes
GU	Acute hepatitis			LFTs
CNS	Stroke, subarachnoid hemorrhage, vasculitis, seizure	Decreased mental status Headache	Neuro exam	CT Vascular biopsy EEG

Key Reference: Haller CA, Benowitz NL: Adverse cardiovascular and central nervous system events associated with dietary supplements containing ephedra alkaloids. N Engl J Med 2000; 343:1833–1838.

POSSIBLE DRUG INTERACTIONS

Preoperative Period

• Ephedra may produce adverse patient reactions with medications such as MAO inhibitors, digoxin, cold medications containing ephedrine, diuretics, and antihypertensives
• Assess preop BP, HR, and ECG
• Consider as a potential cause of preterm labor

Preinduction/Induction Period

• Control hemodynamics before induction
• Observe ECG for arrhythmias

Maintenance Period

• Response to ephedrine may be hampered 2° to tachyphylaxis; therefore, control hypotension with direct-acting adrenergic agonists, like phenylephrine
• Ephedra may interact with volatile anesthetics (e.g., enflurane) to promote dysrhythmias

Postoperative Period

• Assess postop BP, HR, and ECG for CV changes

EVENING PRIMROSE

Leila L. Reduque, M.D.

USES

• Evening primrose oil (EPO) is obtained from the seed of the plant species *Oenothera biennis*
• EPO is also known as fever plant, huile d'onagre, king's cureall, night willow-herb, scabish, and sundrops
• EPO may be used as a food supplement for the essential fatty acids: linoleic acid (LA) and γ-linolenic acid (GLA)
• Infusion of the whole plant has been used for asthma, gastrointestinal disorders, whooping cough, and as a sedative pain killer
• Poultices of the plant have been used externally for bruises and to facilitate wound healing
• EPO is licensed for treatment of atopic eczema and cyclic and noncyclic mastalgia
• Other uses for EPO include PMS, psoriasis, multiple sclerosis, hypercholesterolemia, rheumatoid arthritis, Raynaud's phenomenon, Sjögren's syndrome, postviral fatigue syndrome, asthma, and diabetic neuropathy

PERIOPERATIVE RISKS

• EPO may cause an ↑ risk of temporal lobe epilepsy in schizophrenic patients being treated with epileptogenic drugs (e.g., phenothiazines)

WORRY ABOUT

• Obstetrics: orally administered EPO may be associated with an ↑ in the incidence of prolonged rupture of membranes, oxytocin augmentation, arrest of descent, and vacuum extraction

OVERVIEW/PHARMACOLOGY

• EPO is a rich source of the essential fatty acids LA and GLA. These essential fatty acids are involved in prostaglandin biosynthetic pathways.
• DGLA, a metabolite of GLA, is a precursor of both the inflammatory prostaglandin series (PGE_2), via arachidonic acid (AA), and the less inflammatory series (PGE_1)
• Actions of PGE_1 include anti-inflammatory, immunoregulatory, and vasodilatory properties, inhibition of platelet aggregation and cholesterol biosynthesis, hypotension, and elevation of cyclic AMP
• GLA has been shown to have a favorable effect on the DGLA:AA ratio. The ↑ in AA is smaller and less consistent when compared with the ↑ in DGLA. This is beneficial since DGLA leads to the less inflammatory prostaglandin series PGE_1.

• GLA is not normally obtained from the diet. The body relies on the metabolic conversion of LA to GLA. This conversion is rate limiting in the production of GLA. It has been shown that there is a reduced rate of conversion of LA to GLA in several clinical situations including aging, diabetes, cardiovascular disorders and high cholesterol concentrations, high alcohol intake, viral infections, cancer, nutritional deficits, atopic eczema, and premenstrual syndrome. Dietary supplementation of GLA, via EPO, bypasses the rate-limiting conversion step and has a beneficial effect on the ratio of inflammatory to less inflammatory prostaglandin synthesis.

DRUG CLASS/USUAL DOSE

• Dose of EPO is specific for each condition being treated, e.g., the EPO dose for atopic eczema is 6–8 g for adults or 2–4 g for children. Treatment for cyclic and noncyclic mastalgia is 3–4 g of EPO daily. These doses of EPO are based on standardized products containing 8% GLA. EPO may be swallowed directly, mixed with milk or another liquid, or taken with food. The clinical response is usually seen after 3–4 mo of continuous use.

DRUG EFFECTS

EPO studies are in a preliminary phase; its effects have been proved only in animal models. Many of the effects mentioned here have yet to be proved in humans.

SYSTEM	EFFECT
CV	Inhibits the ↑ of serum total cholesterol + VLDL + IDL + LDL cholesterol concentrations in the presence of excess cholesterol in the diet Serves as an antioxidant in hyperlipemic states. Reduces oxidative stress by inhibiting lipid peroxidation and reinforcing the glutathione-dependent antioxidant defense system.
GI	Has anti-ulcer and cytoprotective effects on experimentally induced gastric lesions
HEME	Reduces platelet aggregation when subject fed an atherogenic diet
DERM	May be used for Rx of atopic eczema. Patients with this disorder have impaired conversion of LA to GLA resulting in deficits of DGLA and AA, both of which are required for normal skin structure and function. Dietary supplementation of GLA bypasses the rate-limiting step of LA to GLA, resulting in improved relief of itchiness. Treatment of atopic eczema with EPO is controversial. Clinical studies have been equivocal on whether symptoms of atopic eczema benefit from EPO.
GU	Has been used for PMS and to help reduce frequency of nighttime hot flashes during menopause. Treatment is controversial because clinical studies have not shown a clear benefit of EPO for PMS and menopause. Has been shown to be a little better than placebo for treatment of mastalgia Has been used by many midwives to hasten cervical ripening in an effort to shorten labor and ↓ incidence of postdate pregnancies. One retrospective study showed that EPO does not shorten gestation or ↓ length of labor. Moreover, it was found that EPO may be associated with the above-mentioned adverse effects on labor.
CNS	Significantly reduced headache in women with PMS. Patients given both EPO and fish oil had fewer symptoms associated with headache, such as depression and fatigue.
IMMUNO	In patients with mild RA, EPO has been shown to improve morning stiffness, and there was also improvement in the Ritchie articular index for each patient. Patients with severe RA did not exhibit improvement. Although not scientifically proved, EPO has been taken by asthmatics to gain the anti-inflammatory effects of PGE_1.

Key Reference: Hardy ML: Herbs of special interest to women. J Am Pharm Assoc 2000; 40:234–242.

PERIOPERATIVE IMPLICATIONS

Preoperative Concerns

• EPO may cause an ↑ risk of developing temporal lobe epilepsy, specifically in patients taking known epileptogenic drugs

such as phenothiazines. Seizures have not been seen in patients not taking phenothiazines.

Preinduction/Induction

• No interactions known

Maintenance

• No interactions known

Postoperative Period

• No interactions known

FISH OIL

Omega-3 fatty acids: eicosapentaenoic acid (EPA) and docosahexaenoic acid (DHA)
Dietary supplements available in capsules or oil by brand names: Cardi-Omega 3, Marine 500, Marine 1000, MaxEPA, Promega, Proto-Chol, Sea-Omega
Fish oil supplements are not regarded as drugs and are not regulated by the FDA

USES

• To ↓ plasma concentrations of triglycerides. Reduces elevated VLDL and chylomicrons, causes slight ↑ in HDL. To ↓ risk of death from CAD and to ↓ risk of stroke.
• Beneficial antithrombogenic and anti-inflammatory effects
• Management of collagen vascular diseases (lupus, psoriasis, Raynaud's phenomenon). Symptomatic improvement in rheumatic disease.
• To prevent immunologic injury in patients with IgA nephropathy; to retard renal function loss. May benefit renal transplant recipients treated with cyclosporine. Significant beneficial effects on diabetic nephropathy and macroangiopathy.
• Beneficial in chronic and severe mental disorders (bipolar disorder, depression)
• To reduce inflammatory Sx associated with inflammatory bowel diseases
• Diet enhancement
• Other uses: dysmenorrhea, kidney stones, diabetic neuropathy, gout, migraine headaches, male infertility, osteoporosis, multiple sclerosis

PERIOPERATIVE RISKS

• Risks of long-term use not known. Variable ↑ in bleeding time.

WORRY ABOUT

• Coagulation disorders
• Reduced platelet aggregability

OVERVIEW/PHARMACOLOGY

• Fish oils produce biologic effects on prostaglandins, thromboxanes, and leukotrienes; ↑ TXA_3 levels and ↓ TXA_2 levels stimulate the formation of prostaglandin I_3, moderately reduce formation of TXB_2 in platelets, inhibiting aggregation and adhesion
• Results in reduced platelet aggregation and vasoconstriction
• Improves large artery endothelium-dependent dilation of hypercholesterolemics without affecting endothelium-independent dilation
• Reduces blood viscosity by ↑ RBC deformability
• Substantial ↓ of triglyceride levels; variable effects on cholesterol levels

DRUG CLASS/USUAL DOSE

• Not clear: usual dosage is 2–9 g/d

DRUG EFFECTS

SYSTEM	EFFECT	ASSESSMENT BY HX	PE	TEST
GI	Abdominal distention, belching, halitosis, heartburn, flatulence, diarrhea			
HEME	Prolongs bleeding time, inhibits platelet aggregation	Anticoagulant Rx, fatigue, weakness, bleeding problems	VS	Bleeding time, Hct
ENDO	Mild glucose intolerance in patients with NIDDM			FBS

Key Reference: Miller LG, Wallace JM: Herbal Medicinals: A Clinician's Guide. Pharmaceutical Products Press, 1998.

PERIOPERATIVE IMPLICATIONS

Preoperative Concerns
• May reduce blood clotting

Induction/Maintenance
• No interactions known

Adjuvants/Possible Drug Interactions
• Caution if receiving heparin, warfarin, dipyridamole, ticlopidine, sulfinpyrazone, or aspirin

ANTICIPATED PROBLEMS/CONCERNS

• Assess for possible adverse effects on the coagulation system
• May reduce reclosure of arteries after angioplasty

GARLIC *(ALLIUM SATIVUM)*

Lara Bonasera, M.D.

USES

- Administered orally and topically as a powder, oil, tablet, and raw clove. Allicin is pharmacologically active component.
- Potential beneficial activity as an antihyperlipidemic, antimicrobial (*Microsporum canis,* sporotrichosis, tinea pedis), antiplatelet (via ↑ thromboxane levels), fibrinolytic, antioxidant (↑ catalase and glutathione peroxidase), antidiabetic, and vasoprotective agent (i.e., antihypertensive and agents to protect elastic properties of the aorta)

   – *Note:* These indications are not FDA approved, but garlic is generally recognized as safe (GRAS). Interpretation of data must take into account publication bias (preferential publication of positive findings).

PERIOPERATIVE RISKS

- ↑ Bleeding diathesis

WORRY ABOUT

- Major drug interactions: anticoagulants, antidiabetic agents, ASA, NSAIDs, platelet inhibitors, herbs (danshen, dong quai, feverfew, ginger, ginkgo biloba, ginseng, horse chestnut), thrombolytic agents

OVERVIEW/PHARMACOLOGY

- Intact cells of garlic bulbs contain allinin, an odorless, sulfur-containing amino acid. Crushed garlic causes the enzyme allinase to convert allinin to allicin—a potent antibacterial agent that is odoriferous and unstable. Ajoenes, a self-condensation product of allicin, has antithrombotic activity. Fresh garlic releases allicin in the mouth during the chewing process. Dried garlic preparations lack allicin but contain allinin and allinase; they should be enteric-coated so they pass through the stomach into the small intestine where allinin can be enzymatically converted to allicin. Allicin is unstable in oil. Allinase is inactivated by heat (cooking) and acid.

- Potency can vary substantially among manufacturers
- Dosage: no clear consensus, but dosage varies with reason for use. Hypercholesterolemia/arteriosclerosis: German Commission E recommends 4 g/d (5–20 average-sized garlic cloves) fresh garlic; or at least 5000 μg of allicin or chewing one garlic clove daily. Extract standardized to 1.3% allicin is recommended.
- Treatment should be evaluated over a 3–6-mo period to determine efficacy. *M. canis,* sporotrichosis, tinea pedis, oral dosage: 2–5 mg of allicin extract/d; topical dosage: sliced cloves or garlic extract (ajoenes) 2–3 times/d to lesion for 1–2 wk.
- Usual dosage is 300 mg, 2–3 times/d, standardized to at least 1.3% allicin (equivalent to approximately 3 g or 1 fresh clove daily

DRUG EFFECTS

Moderate daily consumption has no effects on normal individuals. Effects not seen with cooked garlic.

SYSTEM	EFFECT	ASSESS BY HX	PE	TEST
CV	Reduced BP			BP
	Reduced cholesterol			Lipid profile
RESP		Halitosis; sulfuric odor		
ENDO	Hypoglycemia	Insulin, oral hypoglycemic use		FSBG
HEME	Bleeding	Anticoagulant use, coagulopathy, dysfunctional platelets, bleeding disorders	Hematomas; poor surgical hemostasis	Prolonged PT (INR) Plt Hgb/Hct
GU		>5 cloves/d		
Low dose	Enhanced peristalsis	Dyspepsia, eructation, pyrosis (heartburn), flatulence		
Large doses	Inhibited peristalsis; possible reduction in stomach cancer	Constipation		
CNS	Spontaneous spinal epidural hematoma	Headache		
		Paralysis	Neuro exam	CT scan
ALLERGY/ IMMUNO	Allergic reaction	Garlic oil contact dermatitis	Facial/tongue swelling	

Key Reference: Blumenthal M, et al (eds): The Complete German Commission E Monographs: Therapeutic Guide to Herbal Medicines. Boston, American Botanical Council & Integrative Medicine Communications, 1998.

PERIOPERATIVE IMPLICATIONS

Perioperative Concerns/Possible Drug Interactions

- High consumption may cause significant antiplatelet activity; ASA, NSAIDs, other platelet inhibitors, thrombolytic agents, or certain herbs may cause risk of bleeding, but no clinical data are available
- Hypoglycemia may be ↑ for individuals receiving antidiabetic agents

Monitoring

- Preop PT (INR), blood glucose levels

Airway

- Malodorous breath and skin

Preinduction/Induction

- No special concerns

Maintenance

- Monitor blood glucose levels

Extubation

- No special risks

Adjuvants

- No special risks

Postoperative Period

- Theoretical ↑ risk of bleeding and hypoglycemia

ANTICIPATED PROBLEMS/CONCERNS

- See Postoperative Period
- Patients who are avid garlic consumers should not double up doses to make up for missed doses while undergoing surgery
- If on coumadin postop, should be warned against heavy consumption

GINGER *(ZINGIBER OFFICINALE)*

Wei Pan, M.D.

- Ginger ranked as no. 18 in herb supplement sales
- Rx for loss of appetite
- Popular remedy for prevention of motion sickness
- Rx for nausea and vomiting

PERIOPERATIVE RISKS

- No toxic or unpleasant side effects reported in human studies with therapeutic amounts
- May prolong bleeding time due to inhibition of thromboxane synthetase and stimulation of prostacyclin

WORRY ABOUT

- Potential additive or synergistic effects with antiplatelet agents, heparin, or warfarin, with ↑ bleeding risks

OVERVIEW/PHARMACOLOGY

- Pungent constituents: shogaol, gingerol, gingerdiols, and diarylheptanoids
- Inhibits thromboxane synthetase and acts as a prostacyclin agonist
- Possible mutagenesis in *Escherichia coli*
- Onset of antiemetic effect in motion sickness is 25 min with a duration of 4 h

USUAL DOSAGE/TREATMENTS

- Dosage: the total daily dose of the drug is 2–4 g. The antiemetic dose is 2 g of the freshly powdered drug taken with some liquid.
- Indications
  – Prevents motion sickness by a gastrointestinal mechanism
  – Used for Rx of dyspepsia to promote salivary and gastric secretion
  – Rx for loss of appetite
  – Possible effects on postop or ChemoRx-induced nausea and vomiting
- Contraindications
  – Not used in morning sickness
  – Not to be taken in the presence of gallstone conditions

DRUG EFFECTS

SYSTEM	EFFECTS	ASSESSMENT BY HX	PE

CV	Animal studies
	   Hypotension and bradycardia
	   Positive inotropic effect
	   Arrhythmias with overdose
			BP/HR

GI	↑ Gastric and intestinal motility Promotes secretion of saliva and gastric secretion Antiemetic Cholagogic		
HEME	Inhibits thromboxane synthetase Acts as a prostacyclin agonist	Hx of herb use Antiplatelet agents or warfarin Symptoms of bleeding	

CNS	Animal studies
	   Prolonged duration of anesthesia
	   Induced by sodium hexobarbital
	   Anticonvulsive effect
	   CNS suppression with overdose		

Key References: Blumenthal M, et al (eds): The Complete German Commission E Monographs: Therapeutic Guide to Herbal Medicines. Boston, American Botanical Council & Integrative Medicine Communications, 1998; Miller LG: Herbal medicinals: selected clinical considerations focusing on known or potential drug-herb interactions. Arch Intern Med 1998; 158:2200.

POSSIBLE DRUG INTERACTIONS

Preoperative Period

- Possible interaction with antiplatelet agents or warfarin

Induction/Maintenance

- May potentiate anesthesia agents, e.g., barbiturate

Adjuvants/Regional/Anesthesia/Reversal

- May prolong sleep time

Postoperative Concerns

- May ↑ bleeding complications

ANTICIPATED PROBLEMS/CONCERNS

- May ↑ bleeding complications when used with warfarin, antiplatelet agents, or heparin

GINKGO

Mary L. Chavez, Pharm.D.

USES

- Available as capsules, tablets, extract, liquids, tinctures, bars, colas, homeopathic preparations, and sublingual sprays

PERIOPERATIVE RISKS

- Side effects of drug: nausea, vomiting, increased salivation, seizures, bleeding

WORRY ABOUT

- Unexpected spontaneous bleeding
- Due to inhibition of platelet activating factor, may interact with antiplatelet and antithrombotic drugs (aspirin, NSAIDs, clopidogrel, cilostazol, dipyridamole, ticlopidine), and anticoagulant drugs (dalteparin, enoxaparin, heparin, warfarin)
- May potentiate MAO inhibitors (phenelzine, selegiline, tranylcypromine)
- Rx of dementia, intermittent claudication, impotence, macular degeneration, PMS, tinnitus, and vertigo
- Rigid quality control standards are not required for dietary supplements

OVERVIEW/PHARMACOLOGY

- Activity attributed to several chemical constituents including ginkgo, flavonoid, glycosides, and terpene lactones
- Proposed effects: antioxidant activity, ↓ blood viscosity and elasticity, platelet-activating factor antagonism, ↑ uptake and utilization of oxygen and glucose, calcium membrane stabilization, modulation of neurotransmitters
- In vitro MAO-inhibiting activity (MAO-A and MAO-B)
- Ginkgolic acid (mainly found in fruit pulp) may be responsible for allergic reactions

DRUG CLASS/USUAL DOSE

- Dietary supplement
- Most commercial formulations are standardized to contain 22–27% flavonoids and 6% terpenes
- 40–80 mg tid of standardized extract

DRUG EFFECTS

SYSTEM	EFFECT	ASSESSMENT BY HX	PE	TEST
HEENT	↑ Ocular blood flow Hypema	Bleeding	Mucosal bleeding	
CV	Vasodilation of arteries, capillaries, veins			BP/HR
HEME	Inhibition of plt aggregation	Bleeding, bruising	Mucosal bleeding Petechiae	Plt count, bleeding time

GU	Leaf extract
	   Nausea/vomiting, diarrhea,
	   GI upset, flatulence
	Fruit
	   Tenesmus, rectal burning, pruritus ani			

CNS	↑ CBF Headache Subdural hematoma Seizures	Headache Seizures	Localized CNS dysfunction	CT scan
DERM	Contact dermatitis	Exposure	Rash	

Key References: The Hartford Group 1999; Chavez ML, Chavez PI: Ginkgo (Part I and Part II). Hosp Pharm 1998; 33:658–672, and 33:1076–1095.

PERIOPERATIVE IMPLICATIONS

- Use of dietary supplements is underreported; up to 75% of users do not report self-use

Preoperative Concerns

- Interferes with platelets and blood clotting; ginkgo might be discontinued 2–3 wk before surgery

Monitoring

- Routine

Airway

- Avoid nasal intubation

Preinduction/Induction

- Control hemodynamics before induction
- May ↓ effect of antiepileptic drugs
- May shorten hexobarbital sleeping time

Maintenance

- May potentiate CNS depressants and hypotensive effect of inhalation GA, sedative-hypnotics, antidepressants, β_1-blockers, opiate agonists, skeletal muscle relaxants, phenothiazines, barbiturates, and benzodiazepines
- Monitor for ↑ ICP

Extubation

- None

Adjuvants

- Due to potential MAO-inhibiting activity, may produce Htn with local anesthetics containing epinephrine or norepinephrine

Postoperative Period

- Avoid in patients with bleeding disorders or coagulopathy
- Avoid with active bleeding (GI, intracranial, retinal, retroperitoneal)
- Avoid with risk factors for intracranial bleeding (DM, amyloid senile plaques, severe Htn)
- Avoid in combination with anticoagulant drugs, antiplatelet drugs, SSRIs, meperidine, OTC cold products

GINSENG *(PANAX GINSENG, PANAX QUINQUEFOLIUS)*

Michael K. Lee, M.D.
Chun-Su Yuan, M.D., Ph.D.

USES

- 3.2% of *all* presurgical patients report using ginseng
- Originally labeled an "adaptogen"—a drug that helps to ↑ resistance to stress and restore homeostasis
- Taken for many reasons—general health and vitality, fatigue, immune function, cancer, endocrine function (DM), CV disease, impotence, cognitive function, viral infections (HIV), and enhancing athletic performance
- Usefulness in treating specific diseases still needs to be proved in randomized, controlled studies

WORRY ABOUT

- Inhibition of platelet function and bleeding
- Possible reduction in anticoagulant effects of warfarin
- Possible ↓ analgesic effects of opiates
- Possible Htn, tachycardia, CNS stimulation at high doses
- Possible hypoglycemia, especially in patients taking oral hypoglycemics/insulin
- Adulterants such as ephedrine and germanium (associated with hepatitis) in commercial preparations

OVERVIEW/PHARMACOLOGY

- Herbal drug derived from the root of the ginseng (*Panax* genus) plant; at least a dozen varieties of ginseng exist; the most common are Asian ginseng (*P. ginseng*) and American ginseng (*P. quinquefolius*)
- Siberian ginseng (*Eleintherococcus senticosus*) and Brazilian ginseng (*Pfaffia paniculata*) are different plants from the *Panax* species and are easily confused by consumers
- Classified as a dietary supplement and not subject to FDA drug regulation; pharmacologic activity can be unpredictable and highly variable in different preparations
- Contains a variety of complex chemicals, but the ginsenosides (steroid class of compounds) are responsible for many of the pharmacologic effects
- Exerts complex pharmacologic actions: inhibition of platelet aggregation, lowering of blood glucose, estrogen-like effects, antioxidant effects, possible antineoplastic and immunomodulatory effects

- Has nonopioid receptor–mediated analgesic properties while reducing the analgesic effects of opiates (in animal studies)
- No significant CV or CNS effects at normal doses but can cause Htn, tachycardia, restlessness, agitation at high doses

MECH OF ACTION/USUAL DOSE

- Mechanism(s) of action not completely understood; probably exerts some effects via classic genomic steroid mechanism
- Reversibly inhibits platelet function through an action on calcium, inhibition of platelet activating factor, or inhibition of ATP release
- CV and antioxidant effects partly mediated through increasing endogenous nitric oxide release
- CNS effects may be mediated by neuronal calcium channels and/or GABA
- Usual dosage is 1–2 g/d of dried root or 200–400 mg/d of root extract

DRUG EFFECTS

SYSTEM	EFFECT	ASSESSMENT BY HX	PE	TEST
CV	Htn, tachycardia possible at high doses or with CNS stimulants	Dosage and duration taken	BP/HR	ECG
GI	Rarely diarrhea			Lytes
HEME	Inhibits plt aggregation	Bleeding problems		?Bleeding time
CNS	Restlessness, agitation possible at high doses	Dosage and duration taken		
ENDO	Hypoglycemia Mastalgia and postmenopausal bleeding from estrogen-like effects			Blood glucose Hct

Key Reference: Flemming T (ed): PDR for Herbal Medicines, 2nd ed. Montvale, NJ, Medical Economics Company, 2000, pp 346–351.

PERIOPERATIVE IMPLICATIONS

Preoperative Period

- History can include dose, duration, and preparation taken and the reasons for their use
- No accepted guidelines on whether to discontinue preoperatively
- Due to the risk of ↑ bleeding, consider discontinuing ginseng ~2 wk before surgery
- May also see a ↓ effect of warfarin given preoperatively for thrombosis prophylaxis in high-risk (orthopedic) surgery; consider alternatives to warfarin
- May need to follow blood glucose, especially if taking oral hypoglycemics/insulin and fasting

Induction/Maintenance

- Not known

Adjuvants/Regional Anesthesia/Reversal

- If taking ginseng up until the time of surgery, may want to avoid epidural/spinal due to bleeding risk

Postoperative Concerns

- Postop pain control because ginseng may reduce the analgesic effects of opiates; may need higher than average doses of opiates; consider adjuvant nonopiate analgesics

ANTICIPATED PROBLEMS/CONCERNS

- Bleeding risk
- Possible ↓ analgesic effects of opiates
- Possible reduction in anticoagulant effects of warfarin
- Possible Htn, tachycardia, CNS stimulation at high doses
- Possible hypoglycemia

GLUCOSAMINE SULFATE

Roy Mongkolpradit, M.D.

USES

- Oral administration to people with osteoarthritis. Glucosamine sulfate alleviates pain, improves mobility, and aids in cartilage repair.
- Unknown usage patterns: estimates at 30 million in USA

INDICATIONS

- Rx osteoarthritis or DJD: reportedly aids in repair of cartilage (onset of efficacy 1–3 mo) and relieves pain and inflammation
- Rx kidney stones: helps reduce urinary oxalate levels

SIDE EFFECTS

- No demonstrated side effects > those of NSAIDs
- Rare side effect limited to minor GI symptoms (stomach upset), which is reduced by taking the drug with meals and/or digestive enzymes

WORRY ABOUT

- No drug interactions known
- If taking diuretics, may need to take slightly higher dosage because of urinary excretion

OVERVIEW/PHARMACOLOGY

- Naturally produced in body and commercially produced from chitin (from exoskeleton of shrimp, lobster, and crabs)
- Pharmacokinetics and pharmacodynamics (mech of clearance, how excreted, what delays excretions, interactions)
  – PO absorption as high as 98%, incorporated into tissue matrix of cartilage, ligaments, and tendons
  – After PO, IV, IM administration, it is broken down into D-glucosamine and sulfate
  – When orally absorbed, first goes to liver, where a large portion gets broken down into carbon dioxide, urea, and water
  – Excreted mainly in urine after parenteral administration; equally excreted in urine and feces after oral administration

DRUG CLASS/MECH ACTION/USUAL DOSE

- Aminosaccharide that serves as a constituent of glycoprotein, proteoglycans, glycosaminoglycans, and other building blocks of connective tissue
- Reportedly stimulates cartilage cells to synthesize glycosaminoglycans and proteoglycans by providing body with the needed raw material
- Reportedly promotes incorporation of sulfur in the cartilage
- Free radical scavenging effect
- Therapeutic effects of glucosamine reportedly potentiated by sulfate
- ≤ 200 lb (91 kg): 1500 mg/d in divided doses (500 mg tid)
- > 200 lb: 2000–2250 mg/d
- Wide variation in actual amounts found in packages with similar labeled content

DRUG EFFECTS

SYSTEM	EFFECT	ASSESSMENT BY HX	PE	TEST
GI	Stomach irritation, upset	N/V GI distress		
ENDO	Insulin resistance			Glucose
HEMO	Inhibition of platelet adhesion	Mucosal bleeding	Petechiae	Tourniquet bleeding test

Key Reference: Delafuente J: Glucosamine in the treatment of osteoarthritis. Rheum Dis Clin North Am 2000; 26:1–11.

PERIOPERATIVE IMPLICATIONS/POSSIBLE DRUG INTERACTIONS

Perioperative Concerns/Monitoring

- ↑ Bleeding diathesis reported—similar to usual NSAIDs

Induction/Maintenance Interactions

- No interactions known

Adjuvant/Regional Anesthesia/Reversal Interactions

- No interactions known other than bleeding diathesis

Postoperative Resumption

- Patients need to resume taking their daily regimen following surgery, but no urgency. When patients stop taking glucosamine, the benefits often continue for another 6–12 wk.

ANTICIPATED PROBLEMS/CONCERNS

- No data published regarding long-term safety/efficacy of glucosamine

GLYCINE

Lisa F. Miller, M.D.

USES

• Nutritional supplement sold as a natural sugar substitute, a sedative, a gastric antacid; for relief of BPH; and to ↓ the negative Sx of schizophrenia
• Intrathecal glycine investigated for Rx of chronic pain
• Used as an irrigant during TURP
• Used as a vehicle for some pharmaceuticals
• Glycine site antagonists (felbamate) used to treat epilepsy and investigated to ↓ infarct size in acute stroke
• Glycine/NMDA receptor antagonists HA966 used to treat chronic pain associated with less locomotor impairment than other NMDA receptor antagonists

PERIOPERATIVE RISKS

• As a nutritional supplement, minimal adverse effects; when initiated, it may cause fatigue and nausea
• Remifentanil/glycine combination may cause a dose-dependent reversible motor impairment

WORRY ABOUT

• TURP syndrome: 10–15% incidence. May occur within 15 min after resection, up to 24 h later. Bradycardia, acute arterial hypotension, and nausea most common. Other Sx include pulm edema, seizure, headache, visual changes, weakness, and encephalopathy. Glycine toxicity manifests at an infusion of 3.5 mg/kg/min (in a 70-kg man, 1.5% glycine solution absorbed at a rate of 54 ml/min would be a toxic dose).
• Glycine site antagonists associated with aplastic anemia, dysphoria, paranoia, hallucinations, Htn, motor retardation, and N/V

OVERVIEW/PHARMACOLOGY

• Smallest amino acid. It is glycogenic and a major inhibitory neurotransmitter.
• Two subtypes of glycine receptor: one is linked to a Cl^- ionophore and sensitive to the antagonist strychnine; the other is a strychnine-insensitive modulatory site on the NMDA receptor complex antagonized by HA966
• Glycine metabolism: liver, kidney, and portal beds metabolize glycine via oxidative deamination. Leads to formation of two potentially toxic metabolites: glyoxylic acid and ammonia. The brain also contains a glycine enzyme cleavage system that splits glycine into CO_2, a one-carbon fragment, and NH_3. $T_{1/2}$ 85 min.

DRUG CLASS/USUAL DOSE

• Used as an irrigant during TURP surgery. Usually found in 1.5% glycine solution.
• Homeopathic Rx for BPH at 780 mg/d × 2 wk and then 390 mg for the next 3 mo
• Glycine 0.4–0.8 mg/kg/d combined with haloperidol ↓ the negative Sx of schizophrenia. Rx based on NMDA receptor hypofunction hypothesis of schizophrenia.
• NMDA receptor allows influx of Na^+ and Ca^{2+}. Overstimulation of this channel leads to Ca^{2+} overload in neurons, which has been shown to be neurotoxic. Glycine antagonists at the NMDA receptor potentiate GABA receptor–mediated events, resulting in ↑ Cl^- conductance, leading to membrane hyperpolarization and neuroprotection. Glycine site antagonists ↓ the release of excitatory amino acids, such as glutamate, which are known to potentiate cerebral ischemic injury.

DRUG EFFECTS

SYSTEM	EFFECT	ASSESSMENT BY HX	PE	TEST
CV	Htn and bradycardia via Cushing reflex Hypotension, dysrhythmia	Exposure		BP, HR, ECG
HEME	Antagonists associated with aplastic anemia	Hx of schizophrenia or intractable epilepsy	Skin/mucous membranes for infection/petechiae	CBC w/plts, peripheral smear, bone marrow Bx
GU	Brisk osmotic diuresis Metabolism into oxalate and glycolate may produce renal failure ↓ BPH	TURP BPH		Serum Na, elevated BUN/Cr
GI	Gastric antacid			
CNS	Glycine accumulates in cells, which ↑ cerebral edema Hyponatremia and direct toxicity and metabolism of glycine account for neurologic Sxs in TURP syndrome Intrathecal glycine antinociceptive Glycine antagonists ↓ infarct size in acute stroke and traumatic brain injury and ↓ negative Sxs of schizophrenia	Headache, N/V, visual changes, Sz, weakness, encephalopathy, lethargy Spasticity, paranoia, agitation, seizure	Mental status, visual acuity, strength	Serum Na Serum osmolality
PULM	Pulm edema	TURP		CXR

Key References: Gravenstein D: Transurethral resection of the prostate (TURP) syndrome: a review of the pathophysiology and management. Anesth Analg 1997; 84:438–446; Muir K, Lees K: Clinical experience with excitatory amino acid antagonist drugs. Stroke 1995; 26:503–513.

POSSIBLE DRUG INTERACTIONS

• Glycine synergistically acts with haloperidol to ↓ the negative Sx of schizophrenia
• Glycine receptor sensitive to inhaled anesthetics and alcohol, resulting in enhanced receptor function

PERIOPERATIVE IMPLICATIONS

Preoperative Period

• Hx of schizophrenia or intractable epilepsy signals poss of glycine antagonist therapy

Induction/Maintenance

• No known interactions with homeopathic doses of glycine

• If pt is using glycine antagonist therapy, control hemodynamics before induction. Pt affect/mental status may be problematic given underlying disease and side effect profile of drug.
• Glycine shown to have higher risk of TURP syndrome than mannitol. Awareness of degree of blood loss and amount of irrigant used. If regional anesthetic used, monitor for signs of glycine toxicity: N/V, visual changes, weakness. Monitor for hemodynamic instability; bradycardia, hypo- or hypertension.

Postoperative Concerns

• TURP syndrome may occur within 15 min of resection or as late as 24 h postop. Monitor for signs of changing mental status, hemodynamic instability, seizures.
• Seizures associated with glycine are theoretically best treated with NMDA receptor antagonists or glycine antagonists. May also check Mg^{2+} level post-TURP. (Low Mg^{2+} ↓ the threshold for seizure.)

GOLDENSEAL (HYDRASTIS CANADENSIS)

Hong Li, M.D.

OTHER NAMES

• Orange root, yellow root, yellow puccoon, ground raspberry, wild *Curcuma,* turmeric root, Indian paint, Indian dye, eye root, eye balm, jaundice root, warnera, and Indian plant

USES

• Parts used: rhizome and root
• Represented ~5% of the total herbal sales in 1997 in USA
• Sold as an antidiarrheal, anti-inflammatory, antibacterial, diuretic, and hemostatic agent
• Rx for digestive problems, peptic ulcers, and colitis
• Used externally on wounds, herpes labialis, eczema, ringworm, itching, earache, and conjunctivitis
• Investigational uses: antineoplastic and anti-HIV

PERIOPERATIVE RISKS

• Side effects of drug (large doses): mucocutaneous irritation, GI tract upset, cardiac and uterine contractility, vasoconstriction, CNS stimulation, neonatal jaundice

WORRY ABOUT

• Not to be used by pregnant or lactating women, neonates, or patients with CV disease, epilepsy, or coagulation problems

OVERVIEW/PHARMACOLOGY

• Compounds: isoquinoline alkaloids—chief alkaloids hydrastine, berberine, (-)-canadine
• One of its main bioactive constituents, berberine, is thought to act intraluminally; exerts antimicrobial activity against numerous bacteria, fungi, and protozoa to block adhesion of bacteria to epithelial cells to inhibit the intestinal secretory responses of cholera and *Escherichia coli* toxins
• May ↑ effectiveness of insulin
• May act as a vasoconstrictor to ↓ uterine bleeding

DRUG CLASS/USUAL DOSE

• Native to North America: used extensively by Native Americans as an herbal medication and clothing dye
• Dosage
  – Infusion: 1 cup/d for 1 wk
  – Tincture: 1 ml of the tincture tid for 1 week
  – Berberine sulfate: 5–10 mg/kg for 6 days

DRUG EFFECTS

SYSTEM	EFFECT	ASSESSMENT BY HX	PE	TEST
CV	Hypertension Hypotension Inotropic effect Bradycardia	Assess CV response to Rx		BP, HR ECG
RESP	Respiratory failure	SOB	Wheezing	CXR
GI	Mucosal irritation Laxative Displaces bilirubin	N/V Diarrhea Neonatal jaundice	Jaundice	LFTs Lytes Bilirubin
GU	Oxytocic Diuretic	Abortion Free water excretion		US U-lytes
CNS	CNS stimulation Central paralysis	Muscle spasm Excitatory state Hallucinations Seizures Occasionally delirium		EMG EEG
ENDO	Increase the effectiveness of insulin	Hypoglycemia	Tachycardia Hypotension	Glucose
HEME	Hemostatic	Oppose anticoagulation		PT, PTT

Key Reference: O'Hara M, Kiefer D, Farrell K, Kemper K: A review of 12 commonly used medicinal herbs. Arch Fam Med 1998; 7:523–536.

POSSIBLE DRUG INTERACTIONS

• It may oppose heparin or coumadin anticoagulation

PERIOPERATIVE IMPLICATIONS

• Huge dose can cause labile BP, cardiac inotropy, CNS stimulation, muscle spasm, ↓ seizure threshold, and respiratory failure

LICORICE *(GLYCYRRHIZA GLABRA)*   R. Blaine Easley, M.D.

USES

• Incidence: Licorice is one of the "top ten" herbal medications used in the USA
• Medical: historically used to improve immune function and treat a variety of conditions including PUD, duodenal ulcers, cough/bronchitis, atherosclerosis, chronic fatigue syndrome, various cancers, AIDS, and Addison's disease

PERIOPERATIVE RISKS

• Unknown. Theoretical problems in patients with impaired renal function, Htn, chronic liver disease, cardiac arrhythmias, and hypertonia. Potential for drug interactions. Pseudohyperaldosteronism has been produced experimentally in healthy subjects taking >100 g/wk.

WORRY ABOUT

• Pseudohyperaldosteronism: documented mineralocorticoid effects that result in fluid retention, hypernatremia, hypokalemia, and edema
• Hypertension: direct effects on vascular smooth muscle tone independent of mineralocorticoid properties
• Vasospasm/headache: case reports of cerebral artery spasm causing severe headache, visual disturbances, and potential ischemia have recently been published

• Hypokalemia/muscle weakness: chronic usage related to hypokalemic myopathies, muscle cramps, and skeletal muscle spasms
• Arrhythmias: rare side effect, but more worrisome in patients with history of arrhythmias requiring medication (i.e., digoxin)
• Paresthesias: numbness in extremities may be a sign of licorice toxicity

OVERVIEW/PHARMACOLOGY

• Licorice is the common name given to various substances derived from the plant root *Glycyrrhiza glabra* (Spanish licorice). This plant is a perennial that grows 3–7 ft high and originated from parts of Europe and Asia. Also called sweet root and licorice root.
• Glycyrrhizin/glycyrrhizic acid (the glucoside form) and glycyrrhetininic acid (the glycoside form) are the most important substances/ metabolites found in licorice. The roots also contain coumarins, flavonoids, volatile oils, and plant sterols.
• Licorice and its components are metabolized and excreted by the liver and kidneys.
• Mineralocorticoid effects of licorice, via glycyrrhetininic acid, result from the inhibition of 11-β-hydroxysteroid dehydrogenase (an enzyme that normally inactivates cortisol by converting its C11 alcohol to a ketone). Excess glucocorticoids then bind to mineralocorticoid receptors and produce a mineralocorticoid response, as

evidenced by ↑ sodium retention and Htn. Thereby, licorice ingestion creates a syndrome of hyperaldosteronism characterized by hypernatremia, hypertension, hypokalemia, and suppression of the renin-angiotensin system.
• Glycyrrhetinic acid also inhibits 15-hydroxyprostaglandin dehydrogenase and prostaglandin reductase. These two enzymes are important in the metabolism of prostaglandin E and F_2, perhaps explaining licorice's immunologic benefits, effects on reducing cough/bronchospasm, protection of gastric mucosa, and benefit by decreased platelet aggregation.

DRUG CLASS/USUAL DOSE

• Made from peeled and unpeeled dried root compounded and sold as powders, dry extracts, and liquid extracts. Some preparations such as deglycyrrhized licorice (DGL) have removed "harmful" compounds. Unfortunately, preparation and advertising of these compounds is unregulated by the FDA.
• Licorice is taken in the following manner
  – Dried root: 1–5 g PO tid, up to 6 wk (indication: general use)
  – Extract: (1:1 preparation) 2–5 ml PO tid, up to 6 wk (indication: general use)
  – DGL extract: 1.5–3 g/d for peptic ulcer
  – DGL extract: 380–760 mg PO 20 min before meals for peptic ulcer

DRUG EFFECT

SYSTEM	EFFECT	ASSESSMENT BY HX	PE	TEST
CNS	Headache Visual changes Paresthesia	Exposure/use of licorice	Visual acuity Sensory exam	Neuro consult, possible MRI
CV	Hypovolemia Hypervolemia Hypertension Arrhythmia	Exposure/use of licorice	BP/HR, consider orthostatics	ECG rhythm strip
GI	Black stools (rare) Laxative effect	Report of loose, dark stool	Abdominal exam	Stool guaiac
HEME	↓ Clotting (rare)	Bleeding problems		Platelets PT/PTT
ENDO	Hyperglycemia Hypernatremia Hypokalemia	Exposure/use of licorice Weight gain ↑ Urination		Serum chemistries

Key Reference: Farese RV Jr, Biglieri EG, Shackleton CH, Irony I, Gomez-Fontes R: Licorice-induced hypermineralocorticoidism. N Engl J Med 1991; 325:1223–1227.

POSSIBLE DRUG INTERACTIONS

Preoperative Period

• Multiple adverse drug interactions reported in the literature in patients using licorice preparations and prescription medications. Licorice can interfere with the function of hormone supplements (i.e., birth control pills), oral hypoglycemic agents, and corticosteroids. Electrolyte imbalances and GI symptoms can be worsened by usage of licorice with diuretics and laxatives. Digoxin usage and licorice-induced hypokalemia can be potentially arrhythmiagenic.
• Electrolyte abnormalities of hypokalemia, hypernatremia, and metabolic alkalosis should be sought and corrected before surgery
• Patient should be instructed to discontinue use of the herbal medicine approximately 2 wk before elective surgery

Induction/Maintenance

• No known interactions with licorice metabolites. However, pseudohyperaldosteronism should be considered and anesthetic management directed at the problems of hypokalemia, Htn, and fluid status. Placement of an arterial line and/or central venous line should be considered in symptomatic patients. (See Hyperaldosteronism [Secondary] in Diseases section.)

Adjuvants/Regional Anesthesia/Reversal

• No known interactions. Consider pros/cons of NSAID use intraop, esp if no assessment of renal function. Careful attention to neurologic exam/paresthesias before initiation of regional technique.

Emergence/Extubation

• No known interactions. However, hypokalemia with or without a history of muscle weakness could potentially modify nondepolarizing muscle relaxant response.

Postoperative Concerns

• Failure of resolution of preop symptoms attributed to licorice use with discontinuation of licorice-containing compound should prompt investigation of other causes
• Continued monitoring of fluid and electrolyte status. If problems with hypokalemia continue, despite potassium supplementation, then consider potassium-sparing diuretics (i.e., triamterene), a competitive aldosterone antagonist (i.e., spironolactone), and investigating other causes.

MELATONIN (N-ACETYL-5-METHOXYTRYPTAMINE, BEVITAMEL, VITAMIST, MELATONEX)

Ori Gottlieb, M.D.

USES

- Regulates sleep-wake cycles
- Rx for jet lag, shift work, depression
- Use as antineoplastic, antioxidant, and anticonvulsant is under investigation
- Questionable benefit in treating breast cancer and migraines
- Currently categorized as a nutraceutical

ENDOGENOUS ACTIONS

- Secreted by the pineal gland in response to the absence of photic stimuli
- Reduces the body's core temperature in preparation for sleep
- Secretion peaks during the pediatric years and decreases with age
- In some way, melatonin is involved in reproductive function. Receptors found in reproductive tissues.

EXOGENOUS ACTIONS

- Resets the body to the environmental clock and allows patients to normalize physiologic and behavioral sleep patterns
- Useful in individuals with poor circadian synchrony such as the visually impaired
- May be helpful in autism or Rett's syndrome

RISKS

- May interact with other CNS-acting medications such as hypnotics, sedatives, or psychotropics
- Contraindicated during pregnancy and when breast feeding
- May cause excessive somnolence
- Not recommended in infants and children due to insufficient data
- Not FDA controlled—quality/potency may vary
- The use of animal-source melatonin products is not recommended due to the risk of viral contamination or infection

OVERVIEW/PHARMACOLOGY

- Secretion modulated by enzymes secreted by hypothalamus in response to dark
- Exogenous routes of administration: oral tablets, capsules, lozenges, teas, sprays
- Unlike endogenous melatonin, oral doses undergo first-pass hepatic metabolism with a bioavailability of 30–50%
- Crosses the blood-brain barrier
- The mean elimination $T_{1/2}$ is 45 min. Only 0.01% of melatonin is excreted unchanged in urine.
- To date, pharmacologic tolerance to melatonin has not been described
- Alcohol may potentiate side effects

USUAL DOSE

- Taken 1–2 h before usual sleep time
- Significant individual dose variation
  - Insomnia: 0.3–3 mg PO q.p.m.
  - Insomnia with depression: 5–10 mg PO q.p.m.
  - Jet lag: 3–6 mg PO q.p.m.—on the destination's sleep schedule; may require up to 5 nights
  - Tinnitus: 3 mg PO q.p.m.
  - Circadian disruption/blindness/autism: Adults—5–7 mg PO q.p.m. Children—2.5–7.5 mg PO q.p.m.

DRUG EFFECTS

SYSTEM	EFFECT	ASSESSMENT BY HX	TEST
CNS	Drowsiness Prolonged sedation	Hx of sleepiness	
CV	Palpitations SOB		ECG

Key Reference: Naguib M, Samarkandi AH: The comparative dose-response effects of melatonin and midazolam for premedication of adult patients: a double-blinded, placebo-controlled study. Anesth Analg 2000; 91:473–479.

PERIOPERATIVE IMPLICATIONS

- Melatonin ↑ benzodiazepine binding to receptor sites, enhancing activity
- Methamphetamine users may also be taking melatonin to offset the insomnia brought on by the drug
- Preop use for anxiolysis sedation rivals effectiveness and safety of midazolam

NUTRACEUTICALS

Jessie A. Leak, M.D.

See also specific nutraceuticals

RISKS

- Prevalence: 49% of adult Americans have used an herbal product during the last year. 24% used herbs regularly. 31% use herbal drugs in combination with prescription medications, and 48% use them with OTC drugs. Unknown prevalence of megavitamin use. 60% of patients do not inform the physician about use of these products. There are multiple anecdotal reports of herb/supplement/possible anesthetic/surgical interactions.

PERIOPERATIVE RISKS

- Hemodynamic/cardiovascular instability or collapse
- Enhanced bleeding
- Potential for prolongation of anesthetic
- Electrolyte imbalance and/or renal dysfunction
- Abnormal thyroid function

WORRY ABOUT

- Unexplainable and possibly untreatable bleeding, particularly in patients on anticoagulants and/or antifibrinolytics
- Profound hypo- or hypertension
- Bradycardia or tachycardia
- Myocardial infarction, stroke

OVERVIEW/PHARMACOLOGY

- Particular concern regarding specific herbs/supplements

PERIOPERATIVE MANAGEMENT

- Prudence suggests (no data to support) discontinuing nutraceuticals 2 wk before elective surgery. If ephedra, patient may need to be managed as a cocaine user with either ↑ or ↓ catecholamine levels, depending on the duration, dose, and concurrency of use.

DRUG EFFECTS

NAME	COMMON USES	POTENTIAL SIDE EFFECTS OR DRUG INTERACTIONS
Creatine	Endurance/strength, bodybuilding	Exacerbation of pre-existing renal dysfunction
Echinacea	Common colds, coughs	May cause hepatotoxicity
Ephedra (Ma-Huang)	OTC diet aids	Severe intraop hypotension; arrhythmias; enhanced sympathomimetic effects with MAOI; Htn with oxytocin
Feverfew	Migraine prophylactic	Inhibition of plt activity with ↑ bleeding
Garlic	To ↓ BP and lipids; antioxidant and antithrombolytic	May potentiate warfarin; will see increased INR (PT)
GBL/GHB	Bodybuilding, sleep inducement, weight loss	GHB is "date rape" drug; may cause death, seizures, vomiting, bradycardia, slowed breathing, prolonged anesthetic
Ginger	Antinauseant	May ↑ bleeding time
Ginkgo biloba	Circulatory stimulant	May enhance bleeding with anticoagulants or antithrombotics
Ginseng	Energy-level enhancer, antioxidant	Tachycardia, Htn, mastalgia, postmenopausal bleeding, potential for ↑ bleeding with warfarin
Goldenseal	Diuretic	Works as an aquaretic (no sodium excreted); may worsen edema/Htn
Kava-Kava	Anxiolytic	Potentiates barbiturates and benzodiazepines
Licorice	Gastric/duodenal ulcers	May cause ↑ BP, hypokalemia, edema; contraindicated with chronic liver conditions, renal insufficiency
St. John's Wort	Mild/moderate depression	May prolong anesthesia (anecdotal)
Triax metabolic accelerator (Triax)	Weight loss aid	Contains potent thyroid hormone; may cause heart attacks, strokes; altered thyroid function
Valerian	Mild sedative or anxiolytic	May potentiate barbiturates
Vitamin E	Antioxidant, anticlotting agent	↑ BP in Htn patients with too high a daily dosage (400 IU/d); ↑ bleeding; may worsen vitamin K deficiency; may ↓ thyroid hormone levels

Key Reference: Miller LG: Herbal medicinals: selected clinical considerations focusing on known or potential drug-herb interactions. Arch Intern Med 1998; 158:2200–2211.

PHYTOSTEROLS

Lee A. Fleisher, M.D.

USES

- Naturally occurring in human diet
- Used as a supplement, especially in margarines, to reduce cholesterol levels
- May also possess anti-inflammatory, antipyretic, antineoplastic, and immune-modulating properties

PERIOPERATIVE RISKS

- None known

WORRY ABOUT

- Patients may be taking phytosterols because of hypercholesterolemia and occult CAD

OVERVIEW/PHARMACOLOGY

- Phytosterols (including plant sterols and stanols) are natural components of edible vegetable oils such as sunflower seed oil and, as such, are natural constituents of the human diet
- It is difficult to incorporate free sterols into edible fats/oils because of their insolubility, whereas sterols esterified to fatty acids are more fat soluble
- In the intestine, most sterol esters are hydrolyzed to free sterols as part of the normal digestive process
- Plant stanols are hydrogenation products of the respective plant sterols, e.g., campestanol/campesterol and sitostanol/sitosterol, and are found in nature at very low levels
- Enrichment of foods such as margarines with plant sterols and stanols is one of the recent developments in functional foods to enhance the cholesterol-lowering ability of traditional food products
- May reduce the absorption of some fat-soluble vitamins. Randomized trials have shown that plant sterols and stanols lower blood concentrations of β-carotene by about 25%, concentrations of α-carotene by 10%, and concentrations of vitamin E by 8%.

DRUG CLASS/USUAL DOSE

- Consumption of plant sterols and plant stanols lowers blood cholesterol levels by inhibiting the absorption of dietary and endogenously produced cholesterol from the small intestine, and the plant sterols/stanols are only very poorly absorbed themselves
- This inhibition is related to the similarity in physicochemical properties of plant sterols and stanols and cholesterol and may be related to two mechanisms:
  – The greater the amount of plant sterols/stanols, the lower the solubility and perhaps the greater the amount of cholesterol precipitated. Cholesterol in the crystalline form cannot be absorbed.
  – Competition for space in mixed micelles
- Currently being marketed in new margarine formulations

DRUG EFFECTS

SYSTEM	EFFECT	ASSESSMENT BY HX	PE	TEST
CV	Hypercholesterolemia	CAD, angina	Chest pain	ECG
GI	Malabsorption of some vitamins			

Key Reference: Miettinen TA, Puska P, Gylling H, Vanhanen H, Vartiainen E: Reduction of serum cholesterol with sitostanol-ester margarine in a mildly hypercholesterolemic population. N Engl J Med 1995; 333:1308–1312.

POSSIBLE DRUG INTERACTIONS

- No known drug interactions

ANTICIPATED PROBLEMS/CONCERNS

- None known

ALTERNATIVE MEDICINE   **603**

PSEUDOEPHEDRINE

Lori B. Heller, M.D.

USES

- An OTC sympathomimetic commonly used as a nasal decongestant or for opening obstructed eustachian ostia
- Used in the symptomatic treatment of reactive airway disease; however, appears to be ineffective as a bronchodilator

PERIOPERATIVE RISK

- Concern about the coadministration of other sympathomimetic agents because of the possibility of additive effects and increased toxicity
- Pressor effects of pseudoephedrine are more pronounced in
  - Hypertensive patients
  - Those taking β-adrenergic blocking drugs
- May ↑ heart irritability
- MAO inhibitors, by increasing the quantity of NE, potentiate pseudoephedrine's indirect pressor effects; infrequently, a hypertensive crisis may result
- May also reduce the antihypertensive effects of reserpine and methyldopa

ADDITIONAL INFORMATION

- Abuse and addiction to OTC stimulants does occur, particularly in those with eating disorders or erratic work hours such as truck drivers. Associated with myocardial injury and withdrawal symptoms in this setting.

OVERVIEW/PHARMACOLOGY

- Acts directly on α- and, to a lesser degree, β-adrenergic receptors. Has an indirect effect by releasing NE from its storage sites.
- α-Adrenergic effects result from the inhibition of the production of cAMP by inhibition of the enzyme adenylyl cyclase, whereas β-adrenergic effects result from stimulation of adenylyl cyclase activity
- Acts directly on α-receptors in the mucosa of the respiratory tract producing vasoconstriction, therefore shrinking mucous membranes, reducing edema and congestion

- May relax bronchial smooth muscle by stimulation of β-adrenergic receptors, but this effect is not consistent
- Readily and completely absorbed; elimination is predominantly renal and pH dependent

DRUG CLASS/DOSE

- Direct and indirect sympathomimetic
- $T_{1/2}$ 6 h for standard preparation and 12 h for extended release
- Adults and children > 12 y of age: 60 mg q 4–6 h with a maximum dosage of 240 mg/d
- Children 6–11 y of age: 30 mg q 4–6 h with a maximum dosage of 120 mg/d
- Children 2–5 y of age: 15 mg q 4–6 h with maximum dosage of 60 mg/d

DRUG EFFECTS

SYSTEM	EFFECT	ASSESSMENT BY HX	PE	TEST
CV	Htn, dysrhythmias, cardiac irritability	Palpitations	BP/HR	ECG
HEENT	Mucosal vasoconstriction Reduction of vol of nasal mucosa Drainage of sinus secretions, opening of obstructed ostia	Nasal congestion Head stuffiness	Absence of hyperemia of nasal mucosa	
NEURO	Nervousness, excitability, restlessness, dizziness, weakness, insomnia, headaches, drowsiness		Tremors, anxiousness	
GU/RENAL	Urinary retention	Difficulty voiding, emptying bladder completely	Tachycardia, Htn	Bladder US, postvoid residuals
GI	Nausea/vomiting		Abdominal tenderness	

Key Reference: Kanfer I: Pharmacokinetics of oral decongestants. Pharmacotherapy 1993; 13:116S–128S.

PERIOPERATIVE IMPLICATIONS

Preoperative Concerns

- Oral administration of usual doses to normotensive patients usually produces minimal effects
- Htn, tachycardia in those sensitive
- Those with concomitant hyperthyroidism, ischemic heart disease, or prostatic hypertrophy may be more at risk
- May ↑ the irritability of the heart muscle and result in multifocal PVCs
- Geriatric patients may be especially sensitive
- Overdose may cause hallucinations, CNS depression, seizures, and death

Monitoring

- Routine

Induction

- ↑ Absorption of pseudoephedrine with antacid administration

Airway

- Improvement of airway edema and congestion related to mucosal hyperemia is often seen

Maintenance

- Careful administration of other sympathomimetic drugs

Regional Anesthesia

- Patients may be more prone to urinary retention with regional techniques that block sacral roots

Postoperative Concerns

- Resumption of drug should not pose particular problems once vital signs are stable

ANTICIPATED PROBLEMS/CONCERNS

- Caution in administering other sympathomimetic agents
- β-Adrenergic blocking drugs may ↑ pressor effect
- Antihypertensive effects of reserpine, methyldopa may be diminished

PSYLLIUM, BULK-FORMING LAXATIVES (PLANTAGO ISPHAGULA, PLANTAGO OVATA)

Amar Setty, M.D.
Abraham C. Gaupp, M.D.

OTHER NAMES

- Trade names: Metamucil, Hydrocil, Fiberall, Citrucel
- Herbal names: psyllium seed, black; psyllium seed, blonde

USES

- Chronic constipation (requires adequate hydration)
- Diarrhea (bulk-forming agent)
- Irritable bowel syndrome
- Management of hemorrhoids
- Regulates the effluent for patients with colostomies
- Cholesterol-lowering agent for mild hypercholesterolemia

PERIOPERATIVE RISKS

- Allergic reaction (rare) from ingested or inhaled powder
- Do not use if vomiting, intestinal obstruction, abdominal pain, nausea, or fecal impaction is present
- Do not give other oral drugs for 2 h before or after psyllium

WORRY ABOUT

- Stenosis or obstruction of esophagus or GI tract
- Constipation, impaction, or obstruction can result without adequate hydration
- Loss of diabetic control (use sugar-free preparations in diabetics)
- ↓ Absorption of oral medications

OVERVIEW/PHARMACOLOGY

- Psyllium causes retention of water, which ↑ fecal bulk (expands 8–14 times normal size in water). This provides a mechanical stimulus for peristalsis and the rate of bowel transit.
- Effective within 12–24 h
- Maximum effect after several days
- May stabilize postprandial glucose levels in NIDDM

DRUG CLASS/USUAL DOSE

- Daily dose 10–30 g total in divided doses PO
- Available in powder, wafer, cereal, capsules, chewable pieces
- Must be taken with adequate fluid

DRUG EFFECTS

SYSTEM	EFFECT	PE	TEST
ENDO	Altered blood sugar	Symptoms of hyperglycemia/hypoglycemia	Glucose
GI	If not consumed with adequate fluid, esophageal/intestinal impaction and obstruction	Dysphagia, odynophagia, inability to swallow, abdominal pain and distention	Imaging studies
CV	↓ Cholesterol levels		Cholesterol profile
RESP	Inhalation-induced allergy/asthma	Exposure	Wheezing, skin rash, itching, hives
GU	Unknown effect on pregnancy and lactation		
DERM	Emollient		Dermatitis, pruritus

Key Reference: Blumenthal M, et al (eds): The Complete German Commission E Monographs: Therapeutic Guide to Herbal Medicines. Boston, American Botanical Council & Integrative Medicine Communications, 1998.

PERIOPERATIVE IMPLICATIONS

Preoperative Concerns

- Underreported due to impression that agent is not a drug
- Inquire into use of other herbal drugs
- Possible ↓ in absorption of oral drugs
- Concern with hypovolemia

Monitoring

- Routine
- Consider NG tube

Airway

- None

Induction

- Hypotension a concern if hypovolemic

Maintenance

- Hypotension a concern if hypovolemic

Extubation

- None

Postoperative Period

- Worry about constipation postoperatively if chronic use is not continued postoperatively

PYRUVATE

Marc B. Freeman, M.D.

RISKS

- Available OTC
- Used by athletic and obese persons as weight loss supplement
- Prevalence is difficult to determine; likely millions have tried
- May cause diarrhea and hypovolemia preop

WORRY ABOUT

- May potentiate the inotropic effects of isoproterenol on heart muscle
- Potential for hypoglycemia via ↑ insulin sensitivity

OVERVIEW/PHARMACOLOGY

- 3-Carbon compound that produces metabolic effects when infused directly into the bloodstream or when taken orally
- Converted to lactic acid with anaerobic exercise and enhances loss of fat mass and body weight via ↑ loss of calories as heat at expense of storage fat
- Greater reduction in body fat in overweight adults consuming low-fat diets
- Converted to H_2O and CO_2 via metabolism via citric acid cycle
- Present in red apples, red wine, cheese, and dark beer
- Advertised on 30-min infomercial (starring Steve Garvey) as miracle drug whose efficacy has been misrepresented, resulting in $10 million settlement against one company who touted that users of this dietary supplement could eat what they wanted and "never, ever, ever have to diet again"

DRUG CLASS/MECH OF ACTION/USUAL DOSE

- Studies showed positive effects of pyruvate on weight loss and fat loss with 6–30 g/d PO with exercise; however, actual use may vary per individual

DRUG EFFECTS

SYSTEM	EFFECT	ASSESSMENT BY HX	PE	TEST
CV	May potentiate inotropic effect of isoproterenol		HR	ECG
ENDO	May ↑ insulin sensitivity	Anxiety	HR	ECG, lytes

Key Reference: Hermann HP, Zeitz O, Keweloh B, Hasenfuss G, Janssen PM: Pyruvate potentiates inotropic effects of isoproterenol and Ca(2+) in rabbit cardiac muscle preparations. Am J Physiol Heart Circ Physiol 2000; 279:H702–H708.

PERIOPERATIVE IMPLICATIONS/POSSIBLE DRUG INTERACTIONS

- Obtain Hx of drug use and amount
- Check labs for glucose level

Monitoring

- Routine

Airway

- No special considerations

Preinduction/Induction

- No special concerns outside of other co-morbidities

Maintenance

- No special concerns outside of other co-morbidities

Extubation

- No special considerations

Adjuvants

- No special considerations

Postoperative

- No special considerations

S-ADENOSYL-L-METHIONINE (SAMe)

Alan D. Kaye, M.D., Ph.D.

USES

- Depression
- Heart disease, liver disease, cirrhosis, intrahepatic cholestasis
- Osteoarthritis, tendinitis, bursitis, chronic low back pain
- Dementia, Alzheimer's disease, Parkinson's disease
- Multiple sclerosis, migraine, seizure, spinal cord injury
- Chronic lead poisoning
- Disorder of porphyrin and bilirubin metabolism

PERIOPERATIVE RISKS

- Nausea, vomiting, flatulence, diarrhea
- Anxiety

OVERVIEW/PHARMACOLOGY

- SAMe is produced endogenously from methionine and adenosine triphosphate
- Exogenously administered SAMe has a low bioavailability due to rapid first-pass metabolism by the liver
- Peak plasma concentration in 3–5 h
- $T_{1/2}$ 100 min
- Excreted in urine and feces
- Crosses the blood-brain barrier
- Metabolized to homocysteine, which is remethylated to form methionine, which can form more SAMe
- Tosylate salt has 1% oral bioavailability
- Butane disulfonate salt has 5% oral bioavailability

MECHANISM OF ACTION

- Contributes to the synthesis, activation, and metabolism of hormones, neurotransmitters, nucleic acid, proteins, phospholipids, and some drugs
- Stimulates articular cartilage growth
- Antidepressant effect is probably due to ↑ serotonin turnover and elevated dopamine and norepinephrine levels or due to alteration of cellular membrane fluidity, which facilitates signal transduction across membranes and ↑ the efficiency of receptor-effector coupling
- In liver disease, it restores the biochemical factors that are depleted
- In AIDS myelopathy, it replenishes depleted endogenous SAMe

USUAL DOSE

- For depression, 400–1600 mg PO/d or 200–400 mg IV/d to speed the onset of tricyclic antidepressants
- For osteoarthritis, 200 mg tid PO or 400 mg IV
- For alcoholic liver disease, cirrhosis, or intrahepatic cholestasis, 1200–1600 mg PO or 800 mg IV/d
- For AIDS myelopathy, 800 mg IV/d for 14 days
- For fibromyalgia, 800 mg PO/d

DRUG EFFECTS

SYSTEM	EFFECT	ASSESSMENT BY HX	PE	TEST
GI	N/V, diarrhea	GI complaints		KUB
MS	Osteoarthritis	Stiff joints	ROM	

INTERACTIONS

- Additive serotonergic effects and serotonin syndrome–like effects with antidepressants
- Protect against hepatotoxic effect of certain drugs (e.g., alcohol, acetaminophen, phenobarbital, and steroids)
- Additive side effects like hyperthermia, agitation, confusion, coma when used with MAO inhibitors

CONTRAINDICATIONS

- Patients taking MAO inhibitors or within 2 wk of their discontinuation

SAW PALMETTO (SERENOA REPENS, SABAL BERRY, SERENOA REPENTIS FRUCTUS, SABAL SERRULATA BERRY)

Chadwick T. Dybowski, M.D.

USES

• Primary use: to ↓ symptoms of benign prostatic hypertrophy (BPH) stages 1 and 2 by reducing nocturia, dysuria, and residual urine volumes
• Sixth most popular herbal, representing 4.5% of the total herbal market
• Oral administration most common, and also a tea
• Tried as a mild diuretic and as therapy for chronic cystitis in the early 1900s
• Used by women as an aphrodisiac

WORRY ABOUT

• No health hazards or drug interactions known if taken at proper therapeutic dosages

OVERVIEW/PHARMACOLOGY

• Inhibits type 1 and 2 isoenzymes of 5α-reductase, responsible for the conversion of testosterone to dihydrotestosterone (DHT). Ultimately diminishes morphologic changes associated with BPH.
• May alter the estrogen/androgen balance
• Time to achieve peak concentration was 1.5 h after oral administration ($T_{1/2}$ estimated to be 1.9 h)
• Varied absorption from GI tract causes wide ranges of bioavailability
• Contraindicated in pregnant patients and those on hormone therapy
• Anti-inflammatory, antiexudative, anti-edema, anti–growth hormone, and antiestrogen properties demonstrated

DRUG CLASS/USUAL DOSE

• Inhibits 5α-reductase and ↓ transcription of messenger RNA for cytokines such as fibroblast growth factor and transforming growth factor β, thus reducing the autocrine effect of growing prostatic epithelial and stromal tissue
• The following mechanisms of action have also been observed
  – Displacement of DHT from nuclear and cytosolic receptors
  – Inhibition of leukotriene B_4 and thromboxane B_2
  – ↓ In smooth muscle tone by inhibiting calcium channels
  – Inhibition of cyclooxygenase and 5-lipoxygenase
• Inhibits hypertrophic growth of the periurethral region
• Daily doses of 1–2 g of Sabal berry or more commonly as 320-mg N-hexane lipophilic dried berry extract

CHRONIC USE

• Can cause gynecomastia

Acute Use

• Can cause minor GI problems, including stomach upset, abdominal pain, diarrhea, constipation, and nausea

DRUG EFFECTS

SYSTEM	ASSESSMENT BY HX	PE	TEST
DERM		Gynecomastia	
GI	Stomach upset		
GU	↓ Nocturia, dysuria	↓ Prostate size	↓ PSA

Key Reference: Drugs and Aging, *Serenoa repens A review of its pharmacology and therapeutic efficacy in BPH*; Adis Drug Evaluation, 1997

PERIOPERATIVE IMPLICATIONS

• None known

ANTICIPATED PROBLEMS/CONCERNS

• Urinary retention if anticholinergic used

SOY

Sasha M. Demos, M.D., Ph.D.

USES

- Important nutrient in traditional diets, especially vegetarian diets, of many regions
- Can be consumed as soy milk, soy flour, tofu, miso, whole green edible soybeans, edemame, isolated soy proteins
- Yearly soy food sales in the USA now exceed $1 billion
- Largest consumption occurs in Asian countries

PERIOPERATIVE RISKS

- None known
- May be ↑ risk of peripheral venous thromboembolism

WORRY ABOUT

- Vegetarians who consume large quantities of soy products, especially women, may be at risk of iron-deficiency anemia

OVERVIEW/PHARMACOLOGY/PHYSIOLOGY

- Concentrated source of isoflavones, specifically genistein, daidzein, and glycitein; naturally occurring plant chemicals of phytoestrogen class
- Isoflavones are a subclass of flavonoids, with a flavone nucleus composed of two benzene rings linked through a heterocyclic pyran C ring
- Isoflavones have potent antioxidant effects and weakly mimic estrogen (isoflavones have 1×10^{-4}–1×10^{-3} the activity of estradiol-17β)
- Genistein is a potent inhibitor of protein-tyrosine kinase, which may attenuate growth of cancer
- Soybeans and soy products contain 1–3 mg of isoflavones/g of protein. One serving provides approximately 25–40 mg of isoflavones.
- Soy is high in protein, low in saturated fat, and an excellent source of folate. High in iron but with poor bioavailability. Zinc bioavailability is moderate.

DRUG EFFECTS

SYSTEM	EFFECT	ASSESSMENT BY HX	PE	TEST
CV	Prevent oxidation of LDL, ↓ LDL and HDL cholesterol			LDL HDL
METAB	Dietary fiber includes glycemic control and enhances sensitivity to insulin	Anxiety		Glucose
RENAL	May ↓ RBF, GFR			BUN/Cr
GU Women	↓ Vaginal dryness and hot flashes			
GU Men	Cancer cells may be attenuating genistein		Prostate exam	PSA
MS	↑ Bone mass			Bone density

Key References: Anderson JW, Smith BM, Washnock CS: Cardiovascular and renal benefits of dry bean and soybean intake. Am J Clin Nutr 1999; 70:464S–474S; Messina MJ: Legumes and soybeans: overview of their nutritional profiles and health effects. Am J Clin Nutr 1999; 70:439S–450S.

PERIOPERATIVE IMPLICATIONS

Possible Drug Interactions

- No interactions known

Induction/Maintenance

- Propofol should be avoided in patients with a soy allergy since soybean oil is a component of propofol emulsion

Adjuvants/Regional Anesthesia/Reversal

- No interactions known

ST. JOHN'S WORT *(HYPERICUM PERFORATUM)*

Michael K. Lee, M.D.
Chun-Su Yuan, M.D., Ph.D.

USES

- 3.3% of *all* presurgical patients report using St. John's Wort
- Taken mainly for depression, although patients may take for a variety of reasons including anxiety, viral and bacterial infections, menstrual cramps, cancer, chest congestion, and skin wounds
- May be as effective as low-dose first-generation tricyclic antidepressant for treating mild depression

WORRY ABOUT

- Induction of cytochrome P450 enzymes; ↑ metabolism and ↓ effect of certain drugs—warfarin, benzodiazepines, cyclosporine, β-blockers, Ca^{2+}-channel blockers, steroids
- Can ↓ digoxin levels
- Possible serotonin-like syndrome (Htn, tachycardia, agitation, restlessness)
- May prolong the sedative effects of anesthetics
- Unpredictable effects due to lack of strict regulation

OVERVIEW/PHARMACOLOGY

- Classified as a dietary supplement and not subject to FDA drug regulation; pharmacologic activity can be unpredictable and highly variable in different preparations
- Contains many complex chemicals, but hypericin and hyperforin are responsible for the antidepressant effects
- Absorbed within 40 min of oral administration
- Mainly metabolized by the liver and cleared by renal excretion; elimination $T_{1/2}$ 43 h

MECHANISM OF ACTION/USUAL DOSE

- Seems to act as a nonspecific reuptake inhibitor of serotonin, norepinephrine, and dopamine
- Appears to work differently from conventional antidepressants
- Does not inhibit MAO to a clinically significant degree
- Usually taken as a capsule consisting of the plant extract; typical dosage is 300–500 mg of extract tid

DRUG EFFECTS

SYSTEM	EFFECT	ASSESSMENT BY HX	PE	TEST
HEENT	Rarely, photosensitivity			
CV	Rarely, Htn, tachycardia with serotonin-like syndrome	Dosage taken; also taking SSRI	BP/HR	ECG
GI	Nausea			
DERM	Rarely, rash			
CNS	Restlessness, fatigue, antidepression			

Key Reference: Flemming T (ed): PDR for Herbal Medicines, 2nd ed. Montvale, NJ, Medical Economics Company, 2000, pp 719–725.

PERIOPERATIVE IMPLICATIONS

Preoperative Period

- History can include dose, duration, and preparation taken and the reasons for its use
- No accepted guidelines on whether to discontinue preoperatively
- May see as much as a 50% ↓ effect of warfarin given preoperatively for thrombosis prophylaxis in high-risk (orthopedic) surgery; consider alternatives to warfarin
- Can ↓ digoxin levels, possibly by induction of a P-glycoprotein transporter
- Possible serotonin-like syndrome, especially when combined with an SSRI or MAO inhibitor (unproven)
- If discontinued preoperatively, probably stop at least 1 wk in advance for the drug to be cleared from body

INDUCTION/MAINTENANCE

- May prolong anesthesia via potentiation of central effects of sedatives and opioids

ADJUVANTS/REGIONAL ANESTHESIA/REVERSAL

- May see ↓ effect of drugs metabolized by cytochrome P450—warfarin, benzodiazepines, cyclosporine, β-blockers, Ca^{2+}-channel blockers, steroids; may need to ↑ doses of these drugs and titrate to effect

ANTICIPATED PROBLEMS/CONCERNS

- Effects may be variable among different preparations due to lack of standardization
- Anticipate ↑ metabolism and ↓ effect of certain drugs such as warfarin, benzodiazepines, cyclosporine, β-blockers, Ca^{2+}-channel blockers, steroids, digoxin
- May prolong the sedative effects of anesthetics
- Watch for serotonin-like syndrome (Htn, tachycardia, agitation, restlessness)

VALERIAN *(VALERIANA OFFICINALIS L.)*

Carol Norred, C.R.N.A., M.H.S.

USES

- Insomnia
- Anxiety
- Muscle spasms
- Benzodiazepine withdrawal
- Epilepsy

PERIOPERATIVE RISKS

- Chronic use of high-dose valerian associated with cardiac failure and delirium during emergence from GA

WORRY ABOUT

- Prolonged emergence from GA if taken preoperatively
- Synergistic effects with sedation
- Withdrawal reactions possible with high-dose chronic use

PHARMACODYNAMICS

- CNS depressant effects are more profound than muscle relaxant or neuroleptic effects
- Valerenic acid component given interperitoneally (IP) in mice comparable in potency to diazepam, chlorpromazine, and pentobarbital
- Valerenic acid (IP) resulted in prolonged sleep time when combined with pentobarbital
- Ethanolic extracts displace melatonin CNS receptors, but valerenic acid and aqueous components do not
- Sesquiterpenes and valepotriate components weakly bind to benzodiazepine receptors and displace miscumol from GABA-A sites
- Hydroalcoholic extract inhibits binding to adenosine receptors
- Aqueous extracts of valerian stimulate release of GABA

OVERVIEW

- Lipophillic fractions have affinity for barbiturate receptors, lesser affinity for benzodiazepine receptors
- Valepotriate components show toxicity in vitro, but no toxicity found with average oral consumption
- Significant efficacy as treatment for insomnia with ↓ sleep latency time and improved sleep quality
- Excessive doses may cause blurred vision, heart rate changes, excitability, restlessness, headache, stupor

USUAL DOSE

- 2–3 g dried root/d
- 2–6 ml 1:2 liquid extract/d
- 5–15 ml 1:5 tincture/d

DRUG EFFECTS

SYSTEM	EFFECT	ASSESSMENT BY HX	PE	TEST
CV	Heart rate changes with excessive doses Cardiac failure noted on emergence with chronic excessive use	Determine chronic and acute doses and duration of self-administration		Preop ECG for chronic or excessive use
CNS	CNS depressant Avoid sedatives with acute use	Determine chronic and acute doses and duration of self-administration		Pulse oximetry

Key Reference: Mills S, Bone K: Principles and Practice of Phytotherapy: Modern Herbal Medicine. Edinburgh, Churchill Livingstone, 2000, pp 581–589.

POSSIBLE DRUG INTERACTIONS

Preoperative Period

- Possible synergistic sedative effects if combined with benzodiazepines or narcotics

Induction/Maintenance

- Possible synergistic or unpredictable effects if combined with barbiturates, hypnotics

ADJUVANTS/REGIONAL ANESTHESIA REVERSAL

- Unknown

Postoperative Concerns

- Delayed emergence
- Sedative effects with narcotics

ANTICIPATED PROBLEMS

- Unpredictable sedative effects

SECTION V

TESTS

AUTONOMIC FUNCTION

Thomas J. Ebert, M.D., Ph.D.
Brian J. Robinson, Ph.D.

COST

- Depends on tests performed: those requiring BP, HR responses are inexpensive; tests measuring plasma hormone responses are more expensive
- Multiple tests are usually performed; presence of 2 or more abnormal results indicates some degree of autonomic dysfunction

RISK

- No risks assoc with most tests
- IV atropine is mildly unpleasant; arrhythmias may occur

OVERVIEW

- Simple bedside tests give valuable information on autonomic function
- Very sensitive quantitative tests to delineate severity of disorder, system (e.g., cardiovagal, vasomotor, sudomotor), distribution (pre- vs. postganglionic), and level affected
- Autonomic dysfunction is assoc with malignant arrhythmias, cardiac arrest, spontaneous cardiac ischemia, ↑ periop CV and cardiorespiratory instability

ICD-9-CM Codes: 337.0 (Autonomic nervous system disorder); 337.1

INDICATIONS

- Patients with symptoms of autonomic failure (e.g., intolerance to standing, bladder/sphincter disturbances, impaired sweating) may have autonomic failure due to primary causes—e.g., multiple system atrophy (Shy-Drager syndrome)—or from disorders such as diabetes mellitus, chronic alcoholism, chronic renal failure, advanced age, vit deficiency (e.g., B_{12}), HIV infection, or due to prescribed drugs (e.g., TCAs)

ADDITIONAL TESTS

- Additional tests include plasma catecholamines, atrial vasopressor protein, pancreatic polypeptide determinations in response to standing or other maneuvers to resolve site of lesion; responses to α_2-adrenoceptor agonist for peripheral denervation supersensitivity

ASSESSMENT POINTS

TEST	METHOD	SYSTEM	ABNORMAL RESPONSE
Orthostasis	Patient supine 10 min; then stands or tilted 80° head up; BP measured at 2 min	Sympathetic	↓ in SBP by >30 mmHg ↓ in DBP by >10 mmHg
30:15 Ratio	From continuous ECG strip; ratio of longest R-R interval (~30th beat) to shortest R-R interval (~15th beat) after assuming standing position	Parasympathetic	<1.03 (<1.01 if >65 y)
Deep breathing	Difference between mean HR at max inspiration, mean HR at max expiration for 6 breaths over 1 min	Parasympathetic	<15 bpm (<10 if >65 y)
Valsalva maneuver	Patient blows into manometer to maintain intrathoracic pressure at 40 mmHg for 15 sec; ratio of longest R-R interval after release of maneuver to shortest R-R interval during maneuver if arterial BP measured directly	Parasympathetic Sympathetic	<1.2 (<1.15 if >65 y) BP does not exceed baseline after release of blowing
Atropine	1.8 mg IV over 3 min	Parasympathetic	HR does not change by >20 bpm
Cold pressor	Immerse hand in ice water for 1 min	Sympathetic	SBP and DBP ↑ by <10 mmHg after 1 min
Isometric handgrip	Isometric contraction at 30% max strength for 3 min	Sympathetic	↑ DBP by <10 mmHg after 3 min

Key Reference: Ebert TJ: Preoperative evaluation of the autonomic nervous system. Adv Anes 1993; 10:49–68.

PERIOPERATIVE IMPLICATIONS

Preoperative Preparation

- Gastroparesis: consider premedication with agents to ↑ gastric motility (e.g., metoclopramide), and ↓ consequence of aspiration (e.g., antacids, H_2 blockers)
- Abnormal sensitivity to anesthetic agents and apneic tendencies: minimize narcotics or benzodiazepines as premedication; monitor intensively perioperatively
- Orthostatic hypotension treated by vol expansion, which may cause supine Htn

Monitoring

- Consider arterial line

Induction

- Consider rapid-sequence induction
- Consider etomidate
- Titrate agents with CV, resp effects

Maintenance

- Aggressively treat blood loss, keep well hydrated
- Denervation supersensitivity: unexpected Htn responses to adrenoceptor agonists used for Rx hypotension; if vasopressors required, use direct-acting agents; indirect-acting agents have unpredictable effects

- Impaired temp regulation may require active warming
- Consider controlled ventilation

Postoperative Care

- ↑ Risk of hypotension, hypothermia, apnea
- Peripheral neuropathy may be associated with requirement of less analgesic; use narcotics with caution

CHEST X-RAY

L. Reuven Pasternak, M.D., M.P.H.

COST

- $15–$40 for CXR
- $20–$75 for radiologist's interpretation

RISK

- No risk in isolated x-ray
- Risk from misinterpretation

OVERVIEW

- Test to assess presence of acute progressive or chronic changes of cardiac and/or pulm disease
- Presence of ↑ perihilar markings may be indication of fluid overload from noncardiac origin—e.g., renal failure, fluid overload, or acute ("flash") pulm edema from severe respiratory obstruction
- Presence of cardiomegaly on the CXR indicated by cardiothoracic ratio > 0.5 and/or presence of ↑ perihilar markings distinguishing pulm fluid congestion
- COPD characterized by hyperinflation with flattened diaphragm, ↑ radiolucency, ↑ AP diameter ("barrel chest")

INDICATIONS

- Thoracic procedures
- Otherwise, only if reason to believe there is acute or rapidly progressive deterioration of patient's clinical condition. Hx, PE usually sufficiently sensitive to determine appropriate level of patient's disease and adequately plan for peri-postoperative care. No indication for performance of CXRs based on age, exposure to tobacco products without associated positive findings on Hx and/or PE
- PFTs
- ECG (cardiac disease, pulm Htn)

ASSESSMENT POINTS

ASPECT OF TEST	POSITIVE RESULT	CONFOUNDING FACTORS	DX INFORMATION
Cardiothoracic ratio > 0.5		When associated with ↑ perihilar markings, cardiac silhouette may be difficult to determine	Cardiomegaly, indicating CHF
Diaphragmatic placement	Flattened hemidiaphragms	Patient not properly positioned in erect stance Splinting due to pain or other factors	Extent of COPD Extent of air trapping from acute reactive airway disease
AP diameter	"Barrel chest" with marked ↑ in this dimension		Extent of COPD
Perihilar markings	↑ Markings in area and/or in general lung fields	Improper penetration may cause this finding to be overlooked (overpenetration) or overdiagnosed (underpenetration) May be confused with interstitial scarring from other chronic diseases	Fluid overload, e.g., from excess fluid administration, renal failure, or other noncardiopulmonary cause Primary CHF CHF 2° to pulmonary Htn

Key Reference: Silvestri L, Maffessanti M, Gregori D, Berlot G, Gullo A: Usefulness of routine pre-operative chest radiography for anaesthetic management: a prospective multicentre pilot study. Eur J Anaesthesiol 1999; 16:749–760.

PERIOPERATIVE IMPLICATIONS

- CHF: must ensure optimal myocardial function, conservative fluid management; invasive monitoring for CVP indicated for procedures in which fluid shifts and/or blood loss anticipated, PA cath for measurement of CO, optimization of myocardial performance in patients in whom significant blood loss, other physiologic stress anticipated

- Reactive airway disease: must guarantee that airway management, especially intubation, is done with appropriate level of anesthesia to suppress bronchospasm. Consider chronic medication and steroid coverage before surgery; consider postponing surgery in those with acute episodes
- COPD: often associated in its advanced stages with pulm Htn, right-sided heart failure

SPECIAL CONSIDERATIONS

- If patient is debilitated or requires supplemental O$_2$, consider ICU during postop period, understanding that prolonged ventilatory support may be necessary
- When possible, consider anesthetic techniques to avoid stimulation of airway, compromise of the patient's intrinsic respiratory drive

DIAGNOSTIC 12-LEAD ECG

Martin J. London, M.D.

COST

- $15–$50 with physician charges

RISK

- None except misinterpretation

SENSITIVITY/SPECIFICITY

- Varies accord to specific clinical indication, population. For rhythm and conduction disorders, 100% sensitive. Sensitivity of Q waves for autopsy-proven MI is 33–62%, with a specificity of 88–98%. Sensitivity, specificity of ST-T changes on resting ECG for myocardial ischemia in absence of clinical Sx are low.

OVERVIEW

- ECG assesses myocardial ischemia, MI, rhythm and conduction disorders (intrinsic myocardial disease), electrolyte and metabolic disorders, and medical effects (extrinsic disorders)
- Appropriate, cost-effective starting point for more extensive, costly evaluation of cardiac diseases
- Predictive value, cost-effectiveness of preop 12-lead ECG are controversial. Incidence of ECG abnormality ↑ with age, concurrent medical illness (especially Htn, CAD, diabetes).

INDICATIONS

- Known or suspected (i.e., multiple risk factors or abnormalities on Hx or PE) CAD
- "Major" surgery regardless of clinical Hx
- Males over 40, females over 50

ADDITIONAL/ALTERNATIVE TESTS

- Exercise treadmill testing with or without thallium imaging, static or stress ECHO, dipyridamole or adenosine thallium imaging, coronary angiography to diagnose CAD, ischemia
- Holter monitoring for arrhythmias, conduction defect, ischemia

ASSESSMENT POINTS

DISORDER	POSITIVE RESULT	CONFOUNDING FACTORS	DX INFORMATION
Myocardial ischemia	ST-segment depression > 1 mm Deep T-wave inversion	Baseline ST-T wave changes BBB (esp LBBB) Digoxin/drug effects Abnormal autonomic tone Q waves ↑ ST segment due to pericarditis Intracranial pathology	ST-segment changes correlate poorly with site of CAD Magnitude of depression weakly related to severity
Myocardial infarction	New Q waves ≥40 msec, ampl > 25% of R wave ↑ ST during acute stage Poor R wave progression	Q waves in V_1 and aVL or isolated inferior leads may be normal BBB (esp LBBB)	Q waves are sensitive and specific indicators
Rhythm disorders	Abnormal timing of P wave, QRS or absence of normal P wave and P-R interval		Depends on chronicity, Rx, hemodynamic consequences Atrial dysrhythmias usually benign
Conduction disorders	Axis deviation PR > 120 msec QRS > 100 msec	Body habitus Digoxin Hypothermia Antiarrhythmics	LAFB—usually benign LPFB—likely myocardial or conduction damage RBBB—usually benign LBBB—associated with CAD and impaired ventricular function
Metabolic disorders	Hypokalemia—flattened T waves, ST ↓ Hyperkalemia—peaking T waves, wide QRS Hypocalcemia—lengthen QT_c interval Hypercalcemia—shorten QT_c interval	Other nonspecific changes	Chemistry Laboratory
LV hypertrophy	Multiple criteria Sum $V_1 + V_5 \geq 35$ mm	Body habitus, age, and race influence specificity	Associated with severe Htn or aortic stenosis

Key Reference: Guidelines for Electrocardiography: A report of the American College of Cardiology/American Heart Association Task Force for assessment of diagnostic and therapeutic cardiovascular procedures (Committee on Electrocardiography). Circulation 1992; 85:1221–1228.

PERIOPERATIVE IMPLICATIONS

- Q waves diagnostic of prior MI associated with elevated risk of postop cardiac morbidity
- Number of Q waves on ECG tracing negatively correlated with the ejection fraction

- LBBB more likely associated with significant CAD and impaired ventricular function than RBBB. However, "intraventricular conduction delay," with very wide and bizarre QRS morphology, may have similar significance as LBBB.
- Nonspecific ST-T–wave changes, T-wave flattening/inversion, and QT-interval prolongation markedly influenced by autonomic tone and common in the early postoperative period

SPECIAL CONSIDERATIONS

- Accuracy of computerized interpretation varies among manufacturers
- Sensitivity and specificity of ECG are poor following cardiac surgery
- Newer forms: these include computerized vectorcardiography and late- and mid-QRS signal-averaged electrocardiography utilizing a different lead system (the Frank-Lewis XYZ leads) and signal-averaging techniques. Their perioperative value is currently unknown.

DIBUCAINE NUMBER (ATYPICAL CHOLINESTERASE)

James E. Heavner, D.V.M., Ph.D.

COST

• Approximately $50

RISKS

• Requires a serum sample for in vitro testing. Risks associated with blood sample collection (i.e., venipuncture) include pain, bruising, infection, and/or syncope.
• Periop risks of not receiving the test or misinterpretation of test: prolonged muscle paralysis and apnea following succinylcholine (SCH) or mivacurium (MIV). Possible ↑ risk of toxicity of ester-linked local anesthetics.

OVERVIEW

• Dibucaine number is used to determine if a patient has a genetically determined form of "atypical" cholinesterase (ChE; plasma ChE, pseudo-ChE, serum ChE) that is resistant to dibucaine inhibition. There are a number of phenotypes and genotypes of serum ChE, including the "normal" gene, dibucaine-resistant genes, fluoride-resistant genes, and the silent gene. The silent gene has no ChE activity when in the homozygous state; the dibucaine and fluoride-resistant forms have reduced ChE activity.

• Dibucaine number usually is done to determine the etiology of prolonged muscle paralysis and apnea after SCH or MIV administration. It is indicated before SCH, MIV, or ester-linked local anesthetic administration to patients with confirmed or suspected familial history of atypical ChE or prior to readministration of SCH to patients who had prolonged apnea after SCH. ChE rapidly hydrolyzes SCH, MIV, and ester-linked local anesthetics at rates depending on the agent (procaine, rapidly; tetracaine, 25% the rate of procaine).
• A multitude of alternative methods for determination of dibucaine numbers have been developed since 1957, when the original test was reported. Distinction between normal and heterozygous enzyme may be difficult by some tests.
• If serum ChE activity is measured and is normal, there is no indication to check for dibucaine or fluoride-resistant forms of ChE
• Dibucaine and fluoride sensitivity testing confirm or rules out a genetic cause of low ChE activity

PATHOPHYSIOLOGY

• Normal ChE is sensitive to inhibition by dibucaine, whereas the dibucaine-sensitive homozygous variant is resistant
• Only patients homozygous for the atypical ChE variant will have a significant prolongation of muscle paralysis and apnea
• Inherited forms of abnormal ChE are present in ~4% of the general population
• Homozygous atypical variant occurs in < 1/1500 humans

ASSESSMENT POINTS

VARIANT	APPROX DURATION OF SCH-INDUCED NMB	DIBUCAINE NUMBER (% INHIBITION OF ENZYME ACTIVITY)	INCIDENCE
Homozygous	5–10 min	70–80	
Heterozygous	20 min	40–60	1/480
Homozygous atypical	60–180 min	20–30	1/3200

Key References: Holownia P, Newman DJ, Bruno C, LaGamba P, Gerrits M, Salamink G, Ossani M, Price CP: Automated dibucaine number measurement with DuPont Dimensions ES and AR analyzers. Clin Chem 1995; 41:664–667; Savarese JJ, Caldwell JE, Lien CA, Miller RD: Pharmacology of muscle relaxants and their antagonists. *In* Miller RD (ed): Anesthesia, 5th ed. Philadelphia, Churchill Livingstone, 2000, pp 420–421.

PERIOPERATIVE IMPLICATIONS

• Avoid use of, or use cautiously, SCH, MIV, or ester-linked local anesthetics in patients confirmed or suspected to be homozygous for atypical ChE

DIPYRIDAMOLE THALLIUM IMAGING

Lee A. Fleisher, M.D.

COST

- $1200–$1500, depending on laboratory

RISK

- In patients with CAD, risk of MI and death 1/100,000

SENSITIVITY AND SPECIFICITY

- Sensitivity: 70–80%
- Specificity: 80–90%
- Pos predictive value: 20–50%
- Neg predictive value: 85–99%

OVERVIEW

- Test to assess presence of coronary artery stenosis in patients unable to exercise
- Dipyridamole used to dilate normal coronary arteries, resulting in flow heterogeneity
- Thallium taken up by viable myocardial cells
- Obtain stress and at-rest images
- Areas of myocardial necrosis demonstrate fixed defect
- Areas at risk demonstrate reversible defect
- Able to quantify area at risk

INDICATIONS

- Dx of CAD in patients unable to exercise
- Quantification of area at risk for ischemia

ADDITIONAL/ALTERNATIVE TESTS

- Holter monitoring for silent ischemia
- Dobutamine thallium imaging
- Dobutamine stress ECHO
- Coronary angiography

ASSESSMENT POINTS

ASPECT OF TEST	POSITIVE RESULT	CONFOUNDING FACTORS	DX INFORMATION
CV thallium imaging	Reversible defect Fixed defect	Breast artifact Delayed imaging or reinjection needed to determine if severe ischemia or scar present	Area of myocardium at risk Area of old scar or severe ischemia
	LV dilation		LV dysfunction
Lung imaging	↑ Lung uptake		LV dysfunction
ECG	ST-segment changes	Baseline abnormalities	Indicates dipyridamole results in myocardial ischemia— ↑ risk
Sx during test	Chest pain	Multiple causes	May be ischemia or nonspecific cause

Key Reference: Fleisher LA, Rosenbaum SH, Nelson AH, Jain D, Wackers FJ, Zaret BL: Preoperative dipyridamole thallium imaging and ambulatory electrocardiographic monitoring as a predictor of perioperative cardiac events and long-term outcome. Anesthesiology 1995; 83:906–917.

PERIOPERATIVE IMPLICATIONS

- A reversible defect suggests the presence of a critical coronary artery stenosis; larger defects are associated with a greater area at risk and a higher incidence of perioperative cardiac morbidity
- Increased lung uptake or LV dilation identifies those patients at risk for LV dysfunction with ischemia
- Fixed defects represent old scar and are associated with reduced function and increased long-term risk

SPECIAL CONSIDERATIONS

- Patients with fixed defects may require reinjection or 24-h delayed imaging to differentiate scar from severe ischemia

DOBUTAMINE STRESS ECHOCARDIOGRAPHY

Thomas Ryan, M.D.

COST

- $600–$900

RISK

- Induction of ischemia can lead to MI or death (1 in 3000)
- Arrhythmias due to dobutamine include PVCs, AFIB, nonsustained VTach; sustained VTach or VFIB vary rarely

SENSITIVITY/SPECIFICITY

- Sensitivity for detection of CAD: 85–90%
- Specificity for detection of CAD: 80–85%
- Pos predictive value (for *any* perioperative event): 20–40%
- Pos predictive value (for a *hard* event): 15–25%
- Neg predictive value: 95–100%

OVERVIEW

- Dobutamine infused in incremental doses to ↑ HR, contractility (i.e., myocardial O_2 demand)
- 2D ECHO assesses wall motion, myocardial thickening at each stage
- *Nml* response is dose-dependent development of uniform hyperdynamic wall motion
- *Resting* wall motion abnormality suggests prior infarction
- *Induced* wall motion abnormality indicates ischemia
- Multiple wall motion abnormalities identify multivessel disease

INDICATIONS

- To detect presence and extent of coronary disease in patients unable to undergo adequate exercise; to distinguish prior MI from inducible ischemia
- For preop risk stratification, by identifying patients with evidence of inducible ischemia (esp patients with PVD)
- Most predictive in intermediate and high clinical risk patients

ALTERNATIVE TESTS

- Exercise testing
- Dipyridamole thallium imaging
- Dipyridamole stress ECHO
- Coronary angiogram

ASSESSMENT POINTS

TEST	POSITIVE RESULT	CONFOUNDING FACTORS	DIAGNOSTIC INFORMATION
Wall motion analysis	Resting abnormality	Cardiomyopathy, LBBB	Prior MI
	Induced abnormality	β-blockers; image quality	Ischemia
	Multiple abnormality	Cardiomyopathy	Multivessel disease
ECG	ST-segment depression	Baseline abnormality	Ischemia
		Low sensitivity	
Symptoms	Chest pain	Nonspecific; multiple causes	Angina or other causes

Key Reference: Boersma E, Poldermans D, Bax JJ, Steyerberg EW, Thomson IR, Banga JD, van De Ven LL, van Urk H, Roclandt JR: Predictors of cardiac events after major vascular surgery: role of clinical characteristics, dobutamine echocardiography, and beta-blocker therapy. JAMA 2001; 285:1865–1873.

PERIOPERATIVE IMPLICATIONS

- A normal stress ECHO confers favorable prognosis, very low risk of perioperative morbidity (*high* negative predictive accuracy)
- Inducible wall motion abnormality identifies patients at ↑ risk for perioperative event; but many patients with positive test can still undergo surgery without serious complications—e.g., MI or death (*low* positive predictive accuracy)
- Identifying *high risk* depends on extent, severity of abnormal wall motion, dose at which the abnormality develops, clinical factors (e.g., Hx of MI, CHF, diabetes)
- Patients with resting wall motion abnormality (i.e., prior MI) but no signs of inducible ischemia at *intermediate risk*

EXERCISE STRESS TESTING

Bernard R. Chaitman, M.D.

Key Reference: Chaitman BR: Exercise stress testing in heart disease. *In* Braunwald E (ed): Heart Disease: A Textbook of Cardiovascular Medicine, 4th ed. Philadelphia, WB Saunders, 1992, pp 161–179.

COST

- $100–$300, depending on lab

RISK

- Mortality < 0.01%, morbidity < 0.05% in nonselect patient populations

SENSITIVITY/SPECIFICITY

	Overall	Multivessel Disease
Sensitivity	68%	81%
Specificity	77%	66%
Sensitivity ↓ when exercise workload submax		

OVERVIEW

- Dx, prognostic estimate of presence, extent of coronary disease
- Assessment of functional capacity
- Determine effect of Rx
- Determine exercise prescription for cardiac rehabilitation
- Exercise-induced ST-segment elevation in noninfarct territory, profound ST-segment depression, fall in exercise systolic BP, or low exercise capacity associated with adverse prognosis, multivessel coronary disease

ICD-9-CM Code: 414.0

INDICATIONS

- Prognostic estimate of perioperative long-term cardiac risk
- Objective estimate of functional capacity

ADDITIONAL/ALTERNATIVE TESTS

- Exercise myocardial perfusion imaging
- IV dipyridamole/adenosine myocardial perfusion imaging
- Dobutamine stress ECHO
- Exercise stress ECHO
- Holter monitoring
- Coronary angiography

ASSESSMENT POINTS

ASPECT OF TEST	POSITIVE RESULT	CONFOUNDING FACTORS	DIAGNOSTIC INFO
ECG	Horizontal or downsloping ST-segment depression ≥1 mm Exercise-induced slow upsloping ST-segment depression ≥1.5 mm at 80 msec after J point ST-segment elevation ≥1 mm in noninfarct lead	LVH, digitalis Rx, glucose load, MVP	ST-segment depression ≥2 mm, downsloping ST-segment depression, ≥5 leads abn, persistent ischemic response ≥5 min postexercise, ischemic ST-segment depression onset < Bruce stage II
BP response	Inability to ↑ systolic BP ≥120 mmHg Sustained ↓ ≥10 mmHg repeatable within 15 sec Fall in systolic BP below standing rest values	Cardioactive drug Rx; women Dx information from test in patients with high pretest risk of disease; abn response indicates adverse prognosis, multivessel coronary disease	↑ Risk of perioperative events in patients with known or high pretest likelihood of CAD
Exercise capacity	< 4 METs	Pt motivation, cardioactive drug Rx, orthopedic limitations	Risk gradient according to level of METs achieved; < 4 METs, high risk; ≥10 METs, low risk
Sx during test	Chest pain	Character of chest pain	Presence of exercise-induced definite angina may be only ischemic marker in absence of exercise-induced ST-segment changes

MET, metabolic equivalent; 1 MET = 3.5 ml/kg/min VO_2; 1 MET = energy expenditure sitting quietly in a chair.

PERIOPERATIVE IMPLICATIONS

- Profound ST-segment changes, poor exercise capacity (< 4 METs), abn exercise-induced BP changes, exercise-induced angina associated with ↑ incidence of perioperative cardiac morbidity, mortality
- Absence of preceding associated with very low perioperative cardiac morbidity

- Intermediate exercise results may require additional noninvasive testing (exercise myocardial perfusion imaging or stress ECHO) to more accurately estimate prognosis

SPECIAL CONSIDERATIONS

- Patients with submax test (< 85% of age-predicted maximum) have reduced test accuracy
- Dx accuracy of test depends on pretest clinical risk estimate
- Optimal use of test results requires integration of all information acquired during test, not simply yes/no based on exercise ECG results

FLOW-VOLUME LOOPS

Peter Rock, M.D.

COST

- Variable: $20–$199 in survey of 5 hospitals

RISK

- Virtually no risks associated with flow-volume loops (PFTs)
- Risk from bronchodilator use and misinterpreting data

SENSITIVITY/SPECIFICITY

- Flows depend on patient factors, including body size (ht, wt); habitus; gender; age; ethnicity. The 95% confidence interval includes values 20–30% above and below mean for given healthy population. This wide range of normal values limits interpretation of PFTs; interpretation of PFTs critically depends on prior probability of disease. The Dx of COPD does not usually require PFTs; it is based on clinical criteria. Results within given patient reproducible to within 5% or less in cooperative subjects. Repeated measurements of PFTs over time are sensitive to changes in health or disease status. Some patients with confusing history and physical findings may need PFTs to diagnose lung disease.

OVERVIEW

- Flow-volume loops show relationship between airflow, with max effort starting from position of either max inspiration or exhalation, and volume (exhaled or inspired, respectively)
- Accuracy, interpretation of PFTs highly dependent on patient cooperation, patient effort; results must be reproducible to be valid

INDICATIONS

- Confirm Dx of suspected obstructive lung disease
- Suggest presence of restrictive lung disease
- Intra- vs. extrathoracic obstructions

ADDITIONAL/ALTERNATIVE TESTS

- CT images of sites of airway obstruction

ASSESSMENT POINTS

TEST	POSITIVE RESULT	CONFOUNDING FACTORS	DX INFORMATION
Measurements suggest OLD (obstructive lung disease)	Flow-volume loops show exaggerated upward concavity of descending limb of flow-volume curve with ↓ peak flows, ↓ volume; inspiratory flows relatively preserved		Causes of OLD: acute (asthma), chronic (bronchitis, emphysema), or related to upper airway lesions
Measurements suggest RLD (restrictive lung disease)	Flow-volume loops show preservation or ↑ of peak expiratory flow but ↓ volume; flow-volume curve has normal shape but reduced in all dimensions; inspiratory flows relatively preserved		Suggest RLD
Measurements suggest central airway obstruction (flow-volume loops)	Predominant ↓ in expiratory flow with relatively normal inspiratory flow; expiratory flow curve often has plateau (same flow at all lung volumes) rather than downward bowing normally seen Predominant ↓ in inspiratory flow with relatively normal expiratory flow Proportional ↓ in inspiratory and expiratory flows	Flow-volume loops have role in screening, but confirmation of location, size of lesion may be obtained from imaging studies—e.g., CT of chest	Variable intrathoracic obstruction; pleural pressure variations during inspiration, exhalation influence magnitude of obstruction so it is less during inspiration, indicating that site of lesion is in thorax (e.g., tracheal tumor) Variable extrathoracic obstruction: pleural pressure variations during inspiration and exhalation influence magnitude of obstruction so that it is less during exhalation, indicating that site of lesion is in upper airway (e.g., laryngeal tumor) Fixed central obstruction (e.g., tracheal stenosis): pleural pressure variations during inspiration and exhalation do not influence magnitude of obstruction

Key Reference: Gold WM: Pulmonary function testing. *In* Murray JF, Nadel JA (eds): Textbook of Respiratory Medicine. Philadelphia, WB Saunders, 1994, pp 798–900.

PERIOPERATIVE IMPLICATIONS

- Flow-volume loops can distinguish intrathoracic from extrathoracic lesions: see Mediastinal Masses in Diseases section for intrathoracic lesions

HIV TESTING

Barbara S. Gold, M.D.

COMMON TESTS

- HIV antibody
  - ELISA
  - Western blot
- HIV antigen
  - PCR
  - p24 antigen
- CD4$^+$ lymphocyte count

RISKS

- No known medical risk from test itself
- Risk is in false pos and false neg and lack of counseling and retroviral Rx for true pos patients

OVERVIEW

- Tests for presence of HIV infection, progression to AIDS; monitors exposed health care workers
- ELISA is the most commonly used screening test; positive results are confirmed by Western blot analysis. Both tests measure antibodies to HIV proteins and are extremely sensitive ($\sim 99\%$).
- Time from infection to detection of seropositivity is ~ 3 wk
- PCR amplifies HIV nucleic acid; is used to clarify discrepant ELISA and Western blot results, to detect HIV in high-risk patients who have not yet seroconverted, and to screen neonates
- HIV infects helper T cells, which have high concentration of CD4 antigen. These lymphocytes also orchestrate immune response; thus HIV infects, destroys cells that normally eliminate virus. In HIV infection, T4 lymphocyte, CD4 levels decline; CD4$^+$ counts of < 200 cells/μl correlate with significant morbidity.

INDICATIONS

- Dx infection with HIV in high-risk individuals or those with Sx compatible with AIDS
- CD4 used to follow response to therapy and measure disease progression

ASSESSMENT POINTS

TEST	REPORTED RESULT	CONFOUNDING FACTORS	DX INFORMATION
ELISA	Pos/Neg	Seroconversion takes 4–8 wk	Indicates presence or absence of antibodies to HIV; most common screening test
Western blot	Pos/Neg	Indeterminate at early stages	Confirms ELISA
p24 antigen	Pos/Neg	Asymptomatic patients may test neg	Detects presence of HIV antigen before antibodies are produced; screens blood donors
PCR	Pos/Neg	Extremely sensitive; subject to false pos from contamination	Clarifies positive ELISA and indeterminate Western blot; positive before seroconversion; monitor progression and response to Rx
CD4$^+$ count	< 200 cells/μl associated with significant morbidity		Monitor progression of AIDS, response to Rx

Key Reference: Mylonakis E, Paliou M, Lally M, Flanigan TP, Rich JD: Laboratory testing for infection with the human immunodeficiency virus: established and novel approaches. Am J Med 2000; 109:568–576.

PERIOPERATIVE IMPLICATIONS

- Patients testing pos for HIV may be asymptomatic or have acute illness
- Patients infected with HIV have neg screening tests for ~ 3 wk
- Health care provider should employ universal precautions with all patients, regardless of status of HIV testing

LIVER FUNCTION TESTS

Edward J. Frink, Jr., M.D.

COST

- AST (SGOT) $15–$45
- Alk phos $35–$45
- ALT (SGPT) $15–$45
- PT $15–$30
- Serum alb $15–$50
- GGTP $25–$40
- Total bilirubin $15–$40
- NTP $30–50$
- Direct bilirubin $15–$60
- AST, ALT, alk phos, serum alb, total bilirubin generally available as single test (SMA-20) $8–$35

RISK

- Not evaluating, or misinterpreting tests: potential risk if surgery, anesthesia performed in patient with early-stage hepatitis; risk low in healthy population
- Performing test: false pos, false neg
- Misdiagnosis of liver disease, or liver disease not found if tests incorrectly applied or misinterpreted
- Specificity:
  – AST, ALT: also present (listed in ↓ order) in cardiac muscle, skeletal muscle, kidney, brain, pancreas, and lungs
  – GGTP: typically rises with alcohol-related liver disease, may also ↑ with other hepatobiliary disease; drug injury—e.g., barbiturates or phenytoin. May ↑ in patients with many clinical conditions including pancreatic disease, myocardial infarction, COPD, and diabetes.
  – Alk phos: assoc ↑ with cholestatic disease, but ↑ with bone turnover; may be differentiated by isozyme fractionation, more commonly by NTP. May also ↑ normally during third trimester of pregnancy.

OVERVIEW

- Tests establish presence or absence of liver injury, degree of hepatic reserve in disease states
- AST, ALT
  – Transaminases located in liver cells; elevations may be indicative of hepatocellular damage
  – ALT generally more specific to liver than AST
  – Highest elevations with acute hepatitis or hepatic ischemia
  – May be low or only modestly elevated with chronic liver disease states
  – Elevated AST/ALT ratio >2:1 (if ALT <500 IU) suggestive of alcohol-induced liver injury; >3:1 highly suggestive
- Alk phos
  – Enzyme assoc with canalicular, sinusoidal membranes; other major source, release from bone
  – Highest levels occur in patients with cholestasis (biliary obstructive disease) or hepatic carcinoma
  – Source is likely from liver if NTP and GGTP are also elevated
  – If NTP and GGTP are normal, likely source is bone
- GGTP
  – Hepatocellular enzyme
  – High sensitivity, but low specificity (i.e., normal test result favors lack of hepatobiliary disease, positive test of little Dx value)
  – If ↑, helps confirm alk phos is not of bone origin

- NTP
  – ↑ With alk phos (source of elevation in alk phos is liver)
- Serum albumin
  – ↓ In chronic liver disease states
  – Low levels generally indicate poor synthetic function
- PT
  – If elevated in conjunction with liver disease, indicates poor synthetic function
- Bilirubin
  – Elevated with many hepatobiliary diseases
  – Highest levels with biliary obstruction
  – Direct bilirubin (conjugated) level may be subtracted from total bilirubin level to obtain indirect bilirubin level, defines where excess load or conjugation, excretion at issue

INDICATIONS

- To aid recognition of liver disease states

ADDITIONAL/ALTERNATIVE TESTS

- Urine bilirubin: presence in urine indicates hepatobiliary disease; only conjugated bilirubin enters urine; therefore, it will not be elevated with hemolysis, etc.
- ^{14}G aminopyrine breath test: ↓ $^{14}CO_2$ appearance indicates ↓ metabolic ability
- Viral hepatitis serologies: identify viral illnesses
- Liver biopsy: useful for histologic identification
- CT, US: detect tumor, blood vessel, biliary obstruction
- Antimitochondrial antibodies: ↑ is highly suggestive of primary biliary cirrhosis

ASSESSMENT POINTS

TEST	POSITIVE RESULT*	CONFOUNDING FACTORS	DX INFORMATION
AST (SGOT)	>30–40 IU/L	Possibly from sources other than liver (e.g., cardiac and skeletal muscle, kidneys, brain, pancreas, lungs)	Hepatocellular injury if markedly elevated (acute hepatic injury)
ALT (SGPT)	>30–40 IU/L	More specific to hepatocellular origin than AST, may be ↑ with muscle injury, but high levels only in liver	Hepatocellular injury if elevated (acute hepatic injury)
Total bilirubin	>1.2 mg/dl	Elevation may be due to excess bilirubin load (e.g., hemolysis)	Elevation with many disease states; greatest with cholestatic or parenchymal disease
Indirect bilirubin	>0.8 mg/dl (derive from total–direct level)	N/A	Determine unconjugated hyperbilirubinemia (e.g., Gilbert's syndrome, intravascular hemolysis)
Alk phos	>107 IU/L	Sources other than liver—notably bone, intestine, placenta	High elevations generally indicate biliary obstructive disease, especially in absence of high transaminase elevation
NTP	>15 IU/L	Possibly ↑ in late pregnancy	In nonpregnant patient, ↑ NTP suggests liver origin
GGTP	>66 IU/L	Possibly ↑ by dilantin or barbiturate use; also present in kidney, cardiac muscle	Confirms source of ↑ alk phos in liver
Serum alb	<3.6 g/dl	Possibly ↓ with poor nutrition, chronic infection, or nephrotic syndrome	Identifies chronic liver disease; low levels indicate poor hepatic function
PT	>13 sec Elevation of >2 sec above reported normal usually significant	Possibly prolonged by congenital coagulation factor deficiency, drugs affecting prothrombin complex, vit K deficiency	In chronic liver states, ↑ PT indicates poorer prognosis; in acute hepatocellular injury, prolonged PT may signal onset of fulminant hepatic failure

*Varies by laboratory: check specific laboratory reference ranges; values are for adults.

Key Reference: Herrera JL: Abnormal liver enzyme levels. The spectrum of causes. Postgrad Med 1993; 93:113–132.

PERIOPERATIVE IMPLICATIONS

- Acute liver disease (e.g., acute viral or drug-induced hepatitis)—tests aid in recognition of possibly important anesthetic/surgical risk
- Chronic liver disease (e.g., cirrhosis)—tests, especially of hepatic synthetic function, help evaluate mortality risk

PREGNANCY TESTING

Rebecca Twersky, M.D.
Fayez Kotob, M.D.

COST

- Numerous tests available; cost varies, both to patient and to institution
- Average cost to patient:
  - Urine hCG $18–$30
  - Serum hCG $20–$75

RISK

- Risk to patient is false positive or false negative test or misinterpretation; ↑ risk in anesthesia, surgery in pregnant women

OVERVIEW

- hCG is a glycoprotein secreted by developing placenta shortly after fertilization; hCG mole-

cule comprises 2 noncovalently bonded, dissimilar subunits, namely, α, β. The α subunit is structurally similar to α subunit of FSH, LH, TSH. Therefore, there is a high degree of cross-reactivity with these hormones. In contrast, the β subunit of hCG is structurally distinct, displaying differing immunologic specificities.
- Tests for detecting hCG include RIA, ELISA, agglutination immunoassay, IRMA, ICMA
- β hCG detectable in maternal blood and urine 8–9 days post conception
- Pos test can be analyzed as follows:

Week after LMP	Concentration (in mIU)
3	0–50
4	3–426
5	19–7,340
6	1,080–56,500
7–8	7,650–229,000
9–12	25,060–228,000
17–24	4,060–65,400
25–40	3,640–117,000

TEST INDICATION

- To diagnose pregnancy in perioperative period; to quantify gestation; can assess need for perioperative interventions before elective surgery

ADDITIONAL/ALTERNATIVE TESTS

- For borderline results, repeat test in 48 h (hCG doubles in 48 h); correlate hCG results with LMP, PE, pelvic US

ASSESSMENT POINTS

PREGNANCY TEST TECHNIQUE	SENSITIVITY	SPECIFICITY	POSITIVE RESULT	CONFOUNDING FACTORS	DX INFO
ICGA (immunochromatographic assay) Qualitative β hCG in serum or urine (e.g., genzyme DIAGNOSTICS)	2.0 mIU/ml	No cross-reactivity to LH, FSH, or TSH	Strong positive: 20 mIU/ml serum: in 5 min, urine: in 4 min Weak positive: 10 mIU/ml serum: read in 7 min	Molar preg, ectopic preg, choriocarcinoma, hydatidiform mole, delivery, or abortion within a few wk	For borderline results, repeat test in 48 h (hCG doubles in 48 h); correlate hCG with LMP, PE, US
IRMA (immunoradiometric assay) Total β hCG	2.0 mIU/ml	No cross-reactivity with LH	>25 mIU/ml; borderline result 2–25 mIU/ml	Same as above	Same as above
Whole-molecule hCG	1.5 mIU/ml	0.24% cross-reactivity with LH, no cross-reactivity with FSH, TSH	>25 mIU/ml; borderline result 2–25 mIU/ml	Same as above	Same as above
ELISA (enzyme-linked immunosorbent assay) (e.g., Abbott)	5 mIU/ml	Min cross-reactivity with LH, FSH, TSH @ 432, 500, 500 mIU/ml, respectively	>25 mIU/ml; color change indicates pos result, borderline result 5–25 mIU/ml	Same as above	Same as above
ICMA (immunochemiluminometric assay: change is a positive result) Whole hCG: quantitative serum or urine; qualitative serum or urine	3–200 mIU/ml 25 mIU/ml	0.015% cross-reactivity with 20,000 mIU/ml LH 0.03% cross-reactivity with 10,000 mIU/ml FSH 0.3% cross-reactivity with 1,000 mIU/ml TSH	>25 mIU/ml; chemiluminescence indicates pos result, borderline result 5–25 mIU/ml	Same as above	Same as above
RIA (radioimmunoassay) Quantitative serum β hCG (e.g., Tandam)	5 mIU/ml	Cross-reactivity with LH (0.5%), FSH (0.2%)	>25 mIU/ml; fluorescence indicates pos result, borderline result 5–25 mIU/ml	Pos result obtained with seminoma, teratoma, embryonic CA, hepatoblastoma, bronchogenic CA, prostate CA, breast CA	Same as above
Latex Agglutination Qualitative urine, β hCG (e.g., Organon Teknika)	500 mIU/ml	No interference with abn amount of protein, erythrocytes, Hgb	Granular clump indicates pos result, smooth suspension indicates neg result	Conditions other than nml preg that produce hCG Very high levels of hCG can produce neg result	Consider more sensitive test

Key Reference: Mazze RI, Kaller B: Reproductive outcome after anesthesia and operations during pregnancy: a registry study of 5405 cases. Am J Obstet Gynecol 1989;161:1178–1185.

PERIOPERATIVE IMPLICATIONS

- 2% of pregnant women undergo surgery for reasons unrelated to parturition
- Anesthetic considerations are related to possible teratogenicity of anesthetic agents, effect of anesthesia on uteroplacental BF, potential for spontaneous abortions, premature delivery, alteration in maternal physiology
- Numerous studies on fetal outcome post surgery, post anesthesia demonstrate ↑ incidence of spontaneous abortions, LBW, esp if surgery performed in 1st trimester
- No ↑ incidence of congenital anomalies even if N_2O used
- No specific anesthetic agent or technique
- If possible, local or regional anesthesia used in 1st trimester
- During 1st trimester, thiopental, muscle relaxants, narcotics safely used
- Use of benzodiazepines, N_2O, inhalation agents more controversial
- Because many diagnostic and therapeutic modalities may pose a direct or indirect risk to an embryo, need specific procedures applicable to all services for identifying unsuspected pregnancies in women of reproductive age who are undergoing surgery and anesthesia. A menstrual hx helpful. If suspect pregnancy, a pregnancy test should be done. Institution medicolegal policies should be followed.

RENAL FUNCTION TESTING

Solomon Aronson, M.D.

COST

- Urine indices
  - Basic analysis (SG, pH) $6–$12
  - Lytes (Na$^+$) $8–$56 (32)
  - Cr $10–$29
  - Osm $16–$46
- Serum chemistries
  - BUN $8–$29
  - Cr $8–$29
  - Lytes (Na$^+$) $8–$56 (29)
  - Osm $16–$46
- Combination indices
  - Cr clearance $60–$75
  - Free water clearance $90
  - Fe Na$^+$ $120

RISK

- No risk assoc with serum- or urine-derived renal function testing save inappropriate Rx based on misleading data or data misinterpretation

OVERVIEW

- Test to predict perioperative renal function reserve, predict or Dx renal morbidity during high-risk surg (trauma, vasc, cardiothoracic) in pts at high risk for renal failure (preoperative renal insufficiency, low CO syndrome, etc.)

TEST INDICATIONS

- Dx, evaluate extent of renal tubular function, GFR in pts to assess perioperative risk and/or morbidity

ADDITIONAL/ALTERNATIVE TESTS

- A plain KUB film may be used to identify renal disease with hematuria, pain, and/or fever to rule out trauma
- US to discriminate renal masses (cyst vs. mass), locate obstructive nephropathy source
- Doppler US can facilitate finding cause of allograph dysfunction when evaluating renal flow following transplant
- Renal flow scan (^{99m}Tc-DTPA) also useful for RBF analysis esp when comparing one kidney with the other
- Renal angio can be used to visualize medium/small artery anatomy
- Alternatives to above may include MRI and contrast US

ASSESSMENT POINTS

TEST	POSITIVE RESULT	CONFOUNDING FACTORS	DX INFORMATION
Urinalysis	Hematuria (>1–2 RBC) Pyuria (>4 WBC) Cellular cast Proteinuria (>3+)	Multiple causes	Glomerular disease, free Hgb or myoglobinuria, UTI, interstitial nephritis, pyelonephritis, glomerular disease
Urine Na$^+$	<20 mEq >40 mEq	Hormonal secretion (ADH, aldosterone), Na$^+$-avid states (CHF, cirrhosis), saline infusion, diuretics, dopamine	Prerenal azotemia sensitivity 50% (PPV 50%) ATN sensitivity 55% (PPV 50%)
Urine Osm	>500 mOsm/kg H$_2$O <350 mOsm/kg H$_2$O	Proteins, glucose, mannitol, dextran, diuretics, advanced age, Temperature extremes	Prerenal azotemia sensitivity 30% (PPV 60–90%), ATN sensitivity 80% (PPV 65–95%)
Serum Cr	>2 mg/dl >20% increase postoperative	↑ N balance, tissue breakdown, basal metabolism, diet, activity, hepatic disease, hematoma, GI bleeding, drugs	Associated with ↑ risk of postop renal insufficiency, LOS, and cost of care after CABG surgery when >1.4 mg/dl Nml variant or ↓ renal function reserve GFR ↓ by >50%
Fe Na$^+$ Urine$_{Na}$Plasma$_{Cr}$/ Urine$_{Cr}$Plasma$_{Na}$	<1% >1%	Vol depletion Diuretic, ATN, CHF, cirrhosis, high salt intake, saline infusion	Only helpful after ATN Does not allow prediction
Free water clearance: Urine vol (Urine Osm × Urine vol/Plasma Osm)	> −20 ml/h	See Urine Osm	Indicator if pending renal dysfunction not predictive
Cr clearance: Urine$_{Cr}$/Plasma$_{Cr}$	<25 ml/min	Changing hydration states, inaccurate vol collection, nml day-to-day variation	Predicts ↑ perioperative renal morbidity, renal failure

PPV = positive predictive value.

Key Reference: Garwood S, Aronson S: Renal protection in vascular surgery. Probl Anesth 1999; 11:247–265.

PERIOPERATIVE IMPLICATIONS

- Perioperative renal failure following high-risk procedures has a reported incidence of 0.1–50% depending on population analyzed and methods used to define renal failure; is associated with a reported mortality of 20–90%
- Perioperative renal failure accounts for half of all pts requiring acute renal dialysis

- No simple, inexpensive test adequately determines renal function
- Cr clearance appears to be most efficient test to estimate renal function reserve at this time
- Isolated changes in serum Cr have been shown to be predictive of ↑ morbidity and cost of care after CABG surgery

SPECIAL CONSIDERATIONS

- ATN accounts for nearly 70% of cases of perioperative renal failure
- Inadequate RBF is most common underlying cause for perioperative renal morbidity
- Serial determination of Cr clearance currently most sensitive test for predicting onset of perioperative renal dysfunction

SPIROMETRY

Peter Rock, M.D.

COST

- Variable: $20–$199 in survey of 5 hospitals

RISK

- Virtually no risks associated with spirometry PFTs; risk can occur with use of bronchodilators or misinterpretation of data

SENSITIVITY/SPECIFICITY

- Lung volumes, flows depend on patient factors, incl body size (ht, wt); habitus; gender; age; ethnicity; 95% confidence interval includes values 20–30% above and below mean for given healthy population; this wide range of normal values limits interpretation of PFTs
- Interpretation of PFTs critically depends on prior probability of disease
- Dx of COPD does not require PFTs and is based on clinical criteria but PFTs may be necessary in some patients with unclear H&P. Results within a given patient reproducible to within 5% or less in cooperative subjects.
- Repeated measurements of PFTs over time sensitive to changes in health or disease status

OVERVIEW

- Spirometry is relationship between exhaled volume (starting from position of maximum inspiration) with maximum effort (as forceful as possible—i.e., "forced") and time. Quotient of FEV in 1st sec of exhalation (FEV_1) and FVC (known as $FEV_1\%$) may be used to define obstructive lung disease and to suggest restrictive lung disease (see table following)
- PFTs reflect airway resistance, elastic properties of lungs, chest wall
- Airway resistance *not* measured by PFTs; presence of ↑ airway resistance inferred from ↓ expiratory airflow; assumes max effort was made by patient
- Accuracy, interpretation of PFTs highly dependent on patient cooperation, patient effort. Results must be reproducible to be valid.
- FEV_1, FVC expressed as percentage of predicted "normal" values, which may not be appropriate at extremes of wt
- Max midexpiratory flow rate (forced expiratory flow between 25% and 75% of FVC) is most sensitive to airflow obstruction in peripheral airways, where chronic diseases of airflow originate

- Peak flow determinations are inexpensive and noninvasive and can be used to assess changes in baseline in patients with bronchospasm

INDICATIONS

- Confirm Dx of suspected obstructive lung disease
- Dx reversible component of obstructive lung disease
- Dx change from baseline status in patients with asthma
- Dx unsuspected or occult bronchospasm or response to Rx of bronchospasm
- Suggest presence of restrictive lung disease
- Dx respiratory cause of SOB

ADDITIONAL/ALTERNATIVE TESTS

- Helium gas dilution measures total lung capacity
- Body plethysmography measures airway resistance, absolute lung vol
- Diffusing capacity for CO (DL_{CO}) measures ↓ surface area for transfer of gases from alveoli to pulm capillaries
- Exercise testing used to define relative contributions of respiratory, CV systems to development of dyspnea
- CT images sites of airway obstruction

ASSESSMENT POINTS

TEST	POSITIVE RESULT	CONFOUNDING FACTORS	DX INFORMATION
Measurements suggestive of OLD	$FEV_1/FVC \sim 0.8$	Requires patient's cooperation, max effort, measurements must be reproducible	Normal ratio
	1) $FEV_1/FVC = 0.66–0.8$ 2) FVC < predicted		Mild OLD
	1) $FEV_1/FVC = 0.5–0.65$ 2) FVC < predicted		Moderate OLD
	1) $FEV_1/FVC < 0.5$ 2) FVC < predicted		Severe OLD
			Causes of OLD: acute (asthma), chronic (bronchitis, emphysema), or related to upper airway lesions
Measurements suggestive of *reversible* OLD	↑ in FEV_1 *and* FVC of at least 15% with administration of inhaled bronchodilator		Lack of response to inhaled bronchodilator does not exclude reversible airway obstruction in patients with severe obstruction
Measurements suggestive of RLD	$FEV_1/FVC > 0.85$ *and* FVC < predicted	Requires lung vol measurement to confirm	Suggests RLD, including NM disease; chest wall disease (kyphoscoliosis); infiltrative or destructive interstitial diseases (interstitial fibrosis, ARDS); space-occupying lesions; or pleural disease
Measurements suggestive of mixed OLD/RLD	$FEV_1/FVC \sim 0.8$ *and* FVC < predicted or significantly ↓ VC assoc with ↓ FEV_1/FVC ratio	When mixed defect considered, lung volume determination must be made	Suggests presence of 2 processes—e.g., COPD and NM disease, or COPD and tumor; sarcoidosis

Key Reference: Gold WM: Pulmonary function testing. *In* Murray JF, Nadel JA (eds): Textbook of Respiratory Medicine. Philadelphia, WB Saunders, 1994, pp 798–900.

PERIOPERATIVE IMPLICATIONS

- Routine use of PFTs *not* indicated; consider PFTs if Dx of obstructive lung disease not possible on clinical basis

- Peak flow during max exhalation useful as simple bedside test to follow response of bronchospasm to Rx. Peak flow determined primarily by diameter of large airways; is ↓ in moderate-to-severe obstruction.

TRANSESOPHAGEAL ECHOCARDIOGRAPHY (TEE)

Daniel M. Thys, M.D.

COST

- $300–$500/pt use

RISK

- Esophageal injury or bleeding, vocal cord paralysis, dysrhythmias, hypotension, seizures, cardiac arrest (occur in less than 3% of exams)
- Minor injuries: lip injuries (13%), hoarseness (12%), dysphagia (1.8%), ET intubation (0.3%), bradycardia (0.2%), dental injuries (0.1%)
- Erroneous interpretation, distraction from other anesthetic duties (unknown incidence)

OVERVIEW

- Imaging technique utilizing ultrasound to examine structure, function of heart, great vessels, to gain information on blood flow within these structures
- Ultrasound crystals mounted on gastroscope inserted into esophagus/stomach; placed behind heart
- Tomographic images constructed from intensity of reflected signals, analyzed electronically, converted to image by echoscanner
- Flow from frequency shift between emitted and reflected ultrasound using Doppler equation

EQUIPMENT

- Esophageal probe: single-plane, transverse images; biplane, transverse, longitudinal images; multiplane, transverse to longitudinal to transverse images (180°)
- Echoscanner: analyzes reflected echoes, generates images or flow tracings
- Recorders: hard copy, videotape, or digital

INDICATIONS

- Cardiac function: especially useful to assess preload, systolic, diastolic function
- Ischemia: regional wall motion abnormalities, defined as changes in wall thickening, wall motion, indicative of ischemia
- Valvular function: valvular abnormalities identified using imaging, Doppler exam; intraoperative assessment allows ↑ use of valve repairs rather than replacements
- Aortic disease: TEE is the gold standard for Dx of aortic disease dissection; used by some to select cannulation site for A-cannulae to ↓ risk of emboli
- CHD: TEE allows assessment of adequacy of valve repairs intraoperatively
- Cardiac devices: placement of intracardiac devices and monitoring of their position during port access and other cardiac surgical interventions

CONTRAINDICATIONS

- Absolute: extensive esophageal or gastric disease
- Relative: esophageal varices, Zenker's diverticulum, Barrett's esophagus, postradiation therapy

TRAINING

- Development of competence in TEE requires acquisition of numerous cognitive and technical skills; a period dedicated to intensive training under direct supervision of expert is highly recommended

Key Reference: American Society of Anesthesiologists/Society of Cardiovascular Anesthesiologists Task Force on Guidelines for Transesophageal Echocardiography and Perioperative Care. Anesthesiology 1996; 84:986–1006.

V/Q SCAN (SPLIT LUNG FUNCTION)

Roger S. Wilson, M.D.

COST

- Variable, ~ $650–$1500

RISK

- Radiation exposure; risk to organs other than lung ↑ in presence of anatomic R → L shunt
- Pulmonary vascular occlusion (perfusion scan) by macroaggregated albumin or serum albumin microspheres; 0.1% of pulm arterioles/pulm capillaries blocked during routine clinical studies using ~ $2-5 \times 10^5$ particles, of 10–30 μm. Risk ↑ in presence of severe pulmonary Htn and/or pre-existing vascular injury secondary to co-existing disease.
- Transient, minimal ↓ in arterial O_2 sat

SENSITIVITY/SPECIFICITY

- Sensitivity: >90% for pulmonary embolism
- Specificity: 80–95% for pulmonary embolism

OVERVIEW

- Test to rule out pulmonary embolism, predict post-thoracotomy pulmonary function
- Methodology for perfusion scans standard, but wide variability in methodology for ventilation scans
- Interpretation can be difficult with co-existing pulmonary disease and influenced by sequence of tests. Pulmonary diseases (pneumonia, CA, obstructive pulmonary disease, etc.) produce perfusion defects.
- V scans optimally performed in sitting posture, perfusion scans in supine posture
- V studies may use 1 planar (posterior) view; perfusion studies use 6 standard views (anterior, posterior, right/left lateral, RPO, LPO); 2 additional views (RAO, LAO) optional
- V scans use single breath, equilibration, washout techniques; washout images (^{133}Xe) ↑ sensitivity for regional V abnormalities; equilibration images differ with tracer (e.g., ^{133}Xe vs. ^{81m}Kr) due to radioactive properties
- Sequence for scans determined by Dx implications and techniques used

INDICATIONS

- Dx of pulmonary embolism
- Prediction of post-thoracotomy pulmonary function

ADDITIONAL/ALTERNATIVE TESTS

- Pulmonary emboli: pulmonary artery angiogram and spiral CT
- Post-thoracotomy pulmonary function: bronchospirometry, lateral position test, temporary unilateral pulmonary artery balloon occlusion

ASSESSMENT POINTS

TEST	METHOD	CONFOUNDING FACTORS	DX INFORMATION
V scan	Radioactive gases ^{133}Xe ^{127}Xe ^{81m}Kr	Low cost/low energy; $T_{1/2}$ = 5.2 days Mod cost/med energy; $T_{1/2}$ = 36.4 days High cost/high resolution Low exposure; $T_{1/2}$ = 13 sec	Dx criteria for PE based on perfusion with or without V scan; results reported as nml, low, intermediate, or high probability
	Radioactive aerosols ^{99m}Tc (plus) DTPA Pyrophosphate Sulfur colloid Serum albumin Technegas	Droplet size ~ 0.2 μm Simple systems to produce aerosol; all provide good resolution with multiple views possible, $T_{1/2}$ = ~6 h ^{99m}Tc monodispersed aerosol; 1/3 size of generated aerosols	Post-thoracotomy pulmonary function is predicted using periop PFT value (e.g., FEV) and V/Q scan, as noted below
Perfusion scan	Microemboli Macroaggregated albumin Serum albumin microspheres	$T_{1/2}$ = 4.7 h $T_{1/2}$ = 6.5 days	

Key Reference: Loken MK: Pulmonary Nuclear Medicine. Norwalk, CT, Appleton & Lange, 1987, pp 1–142.

PERIOPERATIVE IMPLICATIONS

- Dx implications determine use of V and Q scans. Abnormal Q scan alone often adequate for Dx of pulmonary embolism; normal Q scan obviates need for V scan.

- Pulmonary embolism usually causes a perfusion defect with persistent ventilation while other diseases usually show matched defects
- Prediction of postop pulmonary function (FEV_1) possible using V or Q scan (predicted postop FEV_1 = preop $FEV_1 \times$ % perfusion [or V] in nonresected [remaining] lung). Predicted postop FEV_1 = 0.8–1.0 L identifies acceptable candidate for proposed surgical procedure.

- Prediction of FEV_1 following pneumonectomy similar with V or Q scans; Q scans possibly better predictors after lobectomy

Arthritis, 244
  chondroitin sulfate for, 583
  glucosamine sulfate for, 597
  rheumatoid, 288
    gold therapy for, 529
Arthroplasty
  hip, 472
  knee, 473
  methylmethacrylate cementing in, 421
Arthroscopy
  knee, 424
  temporomandibular joint, 468
Asphyxiating thoracic dystrophy (Jeune syndrome), 201
Aspiration
  foreign body, 144
  perioperative, prevention and management of, 32
Aspirin (acetylsalicylic acid), 499
Asthma
  acute, 33
  cromolyn sodium for, 517
  oral antileukotriene drugs for, 500
Ataxia, Friedreich's, 145
Atherosclerotic disease, 34, 94
Atopic eczema, evening primrose oil for, 591
Atorvastatin (Lipitor), 501
Atresia
  biliary, Kasai procedure for, 422
  duodenal, 128
  pulmonary, 275
  tricuspid, 325
Atrial fibrillation, 35
  in Wolff-Parkinson-White syndrome, 347
Atrial flutter, 36
Atrial septal defect
  ostium primum, 37
  ostium secundum, 38
  repair of, 361
Atrial tachycardia, paroxysmal. See Tachycardia, paroxysmal supraventricular (paroxysmal atrial).
Atrioventricular (AV) block, 41
  second-degree, 223, 224
Atropine, 502
Atypical cholinesterase, 618
Auranofin, 529
Aurothioglucose, 529
Aurothiomalate, 529
Autoimmune disease
  adrenal, 8
  cold, 39
Autonomic function, tests of, 615
Autonomic hyperreflexia, 40
AV (atrioventricular) block, 41
  second-degree, 223, 224
AV (arteriovenous) graft, for hemodialysis, 362
AVM (arteriovenous malformation), cerebral, 75
  surgery for, 381

B

Balloon counterpulsation, intra-aortic, 419
Bariatric surgery, 402
Beckwith-Wiedemann syndrome, 42
Below-knee amputation, 356
Benazepril, 491
Benign prostatic hypertrophy (BPH), 479
  saw palmetto for, 608
Benzodiazepines, 503
Bepridil, 508
Beta thalassemia, 319
Beta-adrenergic receptor antagonists, 504
Beta-sitosterol, 578
Bevitamel (melatonin), 601
Bicarbonate sodium, 505
  for acidosis, 5, 505
Bicuspid aortic valve, 27

Bifascicular heart block, 41
Biguanide hypoglycemic agents, 537, 546
Biliary atresia, Kasai procedure for, 422
Bilirubinemia, neonatal, 43
Bladder tumor, malignant, 59
  transurethral resection of, 478
Blalock-Taussig (BT) shunt, 363
Blebs, pleural, 44
Bleomycin, 45, 506
  toxicity of, 45, 506
Blindness
  as complication of anesthesia and surgery, 46
  as complication of glaucoma, 149
Blood components. See Transfusion.
Blood pressure. See Hypertension.
Blowout orbital fracture, 365
Blue cohosh (Caulophyllum thalictroides), 579
BO (bronchiolitis obliterans), 50
Body temperature
  dangerous increase in, 213
  mild decrease in, 189
Body weight. See Obesity.
Bone
  fractures of. See Fracture(s).
  loss of, 245
Bone marrow transplantation, harvest procedure in, 366
Bordetella pertussis infection, 257
Borrelia burgdorferi infection, 211
Botulism, 47
Bowel disease
  aganglionic, 168
  diverticular, 121
  inflammatory, 99, 329
  necrotizing, 239
Bowel surgery, 367, 389, 414
  for imperforate anus, 415
  for intussusception, 420
  for obstruction, 418
BPD (bronchopulmonary dysplasia), 52
BPH (benign prostatic hypertrophy), 479
  saw palmetto for, 608
Bradyarrhythmias, 354
Brain. See also Cerebral entries; Encephalopathy.
  Alzheimer's disease of, 109
  aneurysm in, clipping of, 380
  Arnold-Chiari deformity of, 30
  arteriovenous malformation of, 75
    surgery for, 381
  cortex of, resection of, for epilepsy, 368
  death of, 48
  infection of, 133
  inflammation of, 133
  ischemic vascular disease of, 77
  occlusive vascular disease of, 226, 242
  toxic injury to. See Encephalopathy.
  trauma to, 371
  tumors of, 195, 311
    hyperventilation associated with, 73
    surgery for, craniotomy in, with patient in sitting position, 392
  ventricles of
    excess cerebrospinal fluid in, 170
    shunt of cerebrospinal fluid from, 487
Brain death, 48
Breast cancer, 60
Breast pain, evening primrose oil for, 591
Bretylium tosylate, 507
Bronchial cancer, 61
Bronchiectasis, 49
  Kartagener's syndrome and, 202
Bronchiolitis obliterans (BO), 50
Bronchitis
  chronic, 51
  laryngotracheal, 100
  vs. epiglottitis, 100, 139

Bronchogenic cyst, congenital, 87
Bronchopulmonary dysplasia (BPD), 52
Bronchoscopy
  fiberoptic, 369
  rigid, 370
BT (Blalock-Taussig) shunt, 363
Buckle, scleral, in retinal surgery, 455
Buerger's disease, 53
Bulimia, 54
  vs. anorexia nervosa, 23
Bulk-forming laxatives, 605
Bullae, pulmonary, 44
Bundle branch block, 41
Burn injury
  chemical, 55
  electrical, 56
  flame, 57
Burr hole, 371
Bypass
  coronary artery, 390
  femoral-femoral, 372
  gastric, for morbid obesity, 402
  infrainguinal, 373
Bypass machine, cardiopulmonary, 375

C

Calcium
  diminished serum levels of, 58
  elevated serum levels of, 172
    hyperparathyroidism and, 179
Calcium-channel blockers, 508
Calculi
  gallbladder, 384, 385
    surgery for, 384, 385
  urinary, 331
    extracorporeal shock wave therapy for, 398
Cancer
  bladder, 59
    transurethral surgery for, 478
  breast, 60
  bronchial, 61
  chemotherapeutic agents for, 493, 511, 514, 522
  esophageal, 62, 396
    surgery for, 396
  gastric, 401
    surgery for, 401
  head and neck, surgery for, 451
  liver, surgery for, 430
  lung
    bronchi as site of, 61
    parenchymal, 63
    surgery for, 448
  neck and head, surgery for, 451
  pancreatic, 488
    surgery for, 488
  prostate, 64
    surgery for, 64, 452
  radiotherapy for, 453
  rectal, abdominoperineal resection for, 352
  renal, 438
    surgery for, 438
Candidiasis, 65
Cannabinoids, 536
Capsaicin, 509
Captopril, 491
Carbamazepine (Tegretol), 510
Carbenicillin, 547
Carbon monoxide (CO) poisoning, 66
Carcinoid syndrome, 67
Carcinoid tumor, 67, 374
  excision of, 374
Cardiac life support, advanced, 354
Cardiac pacemaker(s), 247
  implantation of, for sick sinus syndrome, 443

Nutrients, insufficient intake of, 214
Nutritional support, 543

O

Obesity, 225
  gastric bypass stapling for, 402
  Pickwickian syndrome associated with, 260
  Prader-Willi syndrome and, 267
Obstructive lung disease
  flow-volume loops in, 622
  spirometric findings in, 627
Obstructive sleep apnea, 307
Occlusive cerebrovascular disease, 226, 242
Office-based anesthesia, 439
OKT3 (muromonab-CD3), 544
Omphalocele, surgery for, 440
Open cholecystectomy, 385
Open reduction and internal fixation (ORIF), of fractured hip, 442
Open-angle glaucoma, 149
Opitz-Frias syndrome (G syndrome), 243
Oral antileukotriene drugs, 500
Oral contraceptives, 545
Oral hypoglycemic agents, 528, 537, 546
Orbital fracture, 365
Orchiopexy, 441
Organ failure, lung dysfunction in, 231
ORIF (open reduction and internal fixation), of fractured hip, 442
Osler-Weber-Rendu disease (hereditary hemorrhagic telangiectasia), 164
Osmotic diuretics, 519
Osteoarthritis, 244
  chondroitin sulfate for, 583
  glucosamine sulfate for, 597
Osteogenic sarcoma, 291
Osteoporosis, 245
Osteosarcoma, 291
Ostium primum atrial septal defect, 37
Ostium secundum atrial septal defect, 38
Otitis media, 246
Overdose. See Drug abuse; Poisoning.
Overweight patient. See Obesity.
Oxacillin, 547
Oxygenation, extracorporeal membrane, 397

P

Pacemaker(s), 247
  implantation of, for sick sinus syndrome, 443
Pain syndrome, peripheral, complex, 282
Palate, cleft, 83
  repair of, 388
Palmetto (saw palmetto), 608
Palsy, cerebral, 76
Panax species (ginseng), 596
Pancreas
  cancer of, 488
    surgery for, 488
  defective insulin production by. See Diabetes mellitus.
  gastrin-secreting tumor of, 146
  head of, resection of, for cancer, 488
  inflammation of
    acute, 248
    chronic, 249
  insulin-secreting tumor of, 196
  resection of head of, for cancer, 488
  transplantation of, 444
    kidney transplantation combined with, 444
Pancreaticoduodenectomy, 488
Pancreatitis
  acute, 248
  chronic, 249
Paralysis, periodic, familial, 141, 142
Paralysis agitans (Parkinson's disease), 250
Parathyroid excess, 179, 445

Parathyroidectomy, 445
Parenteral nutrition, 543
Parkinson's disease (paralysis agitans), 250
Paroxysmal supraventricular tachycardia (paroxysmal atrial tachycardia), 251, 312, 354
  in Wolff-Parkinson-White syndrome, 336, 347
Partial anomalous pulmonary venous drainage, 22
Patent ductus arteriosus, 252
  ligation of, 446
PCP (phencyclidine), 548
PCP (*Pneumocystis carinii* pneumonia), 264
Pediatric patient
  abdominal wall defects in, surgery for, 403, 440
  absence seizures (petit mal seizures) in, 298
  anemia in, 259
  anhidrotic ectodermal dysplasia in, 20
  anomalous pulmonary venous return in, 22, 471
    surgery for, 471
  aortopulmonary window in, 359
  apnea in, 28
  Arnold-Chiari syndrome in, 30
  atrial septal defect in, 37, 38
    surgery for, 361
  Beckwith-Wiedemann syndrome in, 42
  biliary atresia in, Kasai procedure for, 422
  bilirubinemia in, 43
  Blalock-Taussig shunt surgery in, 363
  botulism in, 47
  brain tumors in, 195
  bronchopulmonary dysplasia in, 52
  cardiac anomalies in. *See specific types, e.g.,* Pediatric patient, atrial septal defect in.
  cherubism in, 80
  circumcision in, 386
  cleft lip repair in, 387
  cleft palate in, 83
    surgery for, 388
  computed tomography in, 453
  craniosynostosis in, 96
  cri du chat syndrome in, 98
  croup in, 100
    vs. epiglottitis, 100, 139
  diaphragmatic hernia in, 116
  double aortic arch in, 123
  Down syndrome in, 124
  duodenal atresia in, 128
  dysautonomia in, 140
  emphysema in, 87
  endocardial cushion defect in, 137
  epiglottitis in, 139
    vs. croup, 100, 139
  esophagogastroduodenoscopy in, 405
  extracorporeal membrane oxygenation in, 397
  foreign body aspiration in, 144
  gastroesophageal reflux in, 147
  gastrointestinal endoscopy in, 405
  gastroschisis surgery in, 403
  heart transplantation in, 408
  hepatitis in, 161
  Hirschsprung's disease in, 168
  hyperbilirubinemia in, 43
  hypoplastic left heart syndrome in, 305
    transplantation for, 408
  hypospadias repair in, 411
  imperforate anus repair in, 415
  infratentorial brain tumors in, 195
  intussuscepted bowel repair in, 420
  Jeune syndrome in, 201

Pediatric patient *(Continued)*
  Leigh syndrome in, 206
  Lesch-Nyhan syndrome in, 207
  liver transplantation in, 432
  meningomyelocele in, 435
    Arnold-Chiari syndrome associated with, 30
    surgery for, 435
  methemoglobinemia in, 88
  moyamoya disease in, 226
  mucopolysaccharidoses in, 227
  muscular dystrophy in, 127
  myelomeningocele in, 435
    Arnold-Chiari syndrome associated with, 30
    surgery for, 435
  myringotomy in, 437
  necrotizing enterocolitis in, 239
  omphalocele surgery in, 440
  Opitz-Frias syndrome in, 243
  orchiopexy in, 441
  otitis media in, 246
  patent ductus arteriosus in, 252
    surgery for, 446
  pertussis in, 257
  physiologic anemia in, 259
  Pierre Robin syndrome in, 261
  Prader-Willi syndrome in, 267
  preterm, 273
    anemia in, 259
  5P$^-$-syndrome in, 98
  pulmonary atresia in, 275
  pulmonary cyst in, 87
  pyloric stenosis in, 279
    surgery for, 450
  radiotherapy in, 453
  Rett syndrome in, 286
  Reye's syndrome in, 287
  Riley-Day syndrome in, 140
  scoliosis in, 294
  strabismus surgery in, 463
  tetralogy of Fallot in, 318
  tracheoesophageal fistula repair in, 474
  transposition of great vessels in, 476
    surgery for, 476
  Treacher Collins syndrome in, 324
  tricuspid atresia in, 325
  truncus arteriosus in, 327
  tympanoplasty in, 437
  upper respiratory tract infection in, 330
  ventricular septal defect in, 337, 486
    surgery for, 486
  whooping cough in, 257
  Wilms' tumor in, 346
Pemphigus, 253
Penicillin(s), 547
Penicillin G, 547
Penis
  erectile dysfunction of, sildenafil for, 562
  removal of foreskin from, 386
  surgery of, for hypospadias and chordee, 411
Pericardial effusion, 254
Pericarditis, constrictive, 255
Periodic paralysis, familial, 141, 142
Peripheral nerve blocks, for labor, 426
Peripheral pain syndrome, complex, 282
Peripheral vascular disease, 256
Peritoneum, shunt of cerebrospinal fluid to, 487
Peritonsillar abscess, drainage of, 456
Pertussis, 257
Petit mal seizures (absence seizures), 298
Phencyclidine (PCP), 548
Phenothiazines, 549
Phenoxybenzamine, 550
Phenylephrine (Neo-Synephrine), 551
Phenytoin, 552
Phenytoin syndrome, 552

Tachycardia. *See also* Tachyarrhythmias.
  paroxysmal supraventricular (paroxysmal atrial), 251, 312, 354
    in Wolff-Parkinson-White syndrome, 336, 347
  supraventricular, 312
    paroxysmal. *See* Tachycardia, paroxysmal supraventricular (paroxysmal atrial).
  ventricular, 340, 354
Tacrolimus (FK-506), 565
Takayasu's arteritis, 31
Tamoxifen (Nolvadex), 511
TAO (thromboangiitis obliterans), 53
TB (tuberculosis), 328
TEE (transesophageal echocardiography), 628
Tegretol (carbamazepine), 510
Telangiectasia, hereditary hemorrhagic, 164
Temperature
  dangerous increase in, 213
  mild decrease in, 189
Temporomandibular joint (TMJ) arthroscopy, 468
Terbutaline, 566
Testis
  torsion of, surgery for, 464
  undescended, surgery for, 441
Tetanus, 317
Tetracyclines, 567
Tetralogy of Fallot, 318
TGV (transposition of great vessels), 476
  repair of, 476
Thalassemia, 319
Thallium imaging, after administration of dipyridamole, 619
Thoracic aorta, repair of aneurysm or dissection in, 466
Thoracic dystrophy, asphyxiating, 201
Thoracic spine, disk degeneration or herniation in, 107
Thromboangiitis obliterans (TAO), 53
Thrombocytopenia, 320
Thrombocytopenic purpura
  immune, 277
  thrombotic, 278
Thrombolytic therapy, for myocardial infarction, 569
Thrombosis, deep venous, 106
Thrombotic thrombocytopenic purpura (TTP), 278
Thyroid deficiency, 154, 190, 568
  treatment of, 568
Thyroid excess, 154, 182, 467, 556
  pharmacotherapy for, 556
  surgery for, 467
Thyroid neoplasms, 321
Thyroid storm, 182
Thyroid supplements, 568
Thyroidectomy, 467
Thyroiditis, Hashimoto's, 154
TIA (transient ischemic attack), 77
Tic douloureux (trigeminal neuralgia), 326
Ticarcillin, 547
TIPS (transjugular intrahepatic portosystemic shunt), 475
Tissue plasminogen activator (t-PA), 569
TMJ (temporomandibular joint) arthroscopy, 468
Tobacco use, 81
  cessation of, 82
    nicotine replacement therapies in, 539
Tomography, computed, 453
Tonic-clonic seizures (grand mal seizures), 296
Tonsillectomy, 469
Tonsillitis, abscess formation as complication of, 456

Torsion, testicular, surgery for, 464
Torticollis, spasmodic, 308
Total abdominal hysterectomy, 470
Total anomalous pulmonary venous drainage, 22, 471
  correction of, 471
Total hip arthroplasty, 472
Total knee arthroplasty, 473
Total parenteral nutrition (TPN), 543
  t-PA (tissue plasminogen activator), 569
TPN (total parenteral nutrition), 543
Trachea, vascular ring around, 123
Tracheoesophageal fistula, repair of, 474
Traffic fatalities, alcohol abuse and, 480
Tranexamic acid, 570
Transesophageal echocardiography (TEE), 628
Transfusion, 364
  hepatitis in recipients of, 163
  platelet, 320, 364
  religious objections to, 200
Transfusion-related lung injury, 322
Transient ischemic attack (TIA), 77
Transjugular intrahepatic portosystemic shunt (TIPS), 475
Transplantation
  bone marrow, harvest procedure in, 366
  heart, 407
    in pediatric patient, 408
  kidney, 423
    combined with pancreatic transplantation, 444
  liver, 431
    in pediatric patient, 446
  lymphoproliferative disease following, 265
  pancreatic, 444
    kidney transplantation combined with, 444
  rejection following
    OKT3 for, 544
    tacrolimus for, 565
Transposition of great vessels (TGV), 476
  repair of, 476
Transsphenoidal surgery, 447, 477
Transurethral resection
  of bladder tumor, 478
  of prostate, 479
Transverse myelitis, 323
Trasylol (aprotinin), 498
Trauma, 480. *See also specific types, e.g.,* Burn injury; Fracture(s).
  cerebral, 371
  chest, and myocardial contusion, 234
  head, 371
  ocular, as complication of anesthesia and surgery, 46
  orbital, 365
  spinal cord, and autonomic hyperreflexia, 40
  splenic, 461
Treacher Collins syndrome, 324
Triazenes, 494
Tricuspid atresia, 325
Trigeminal neuralgia (tic douloureux), 326
Triglycerides, elevated serum levels of, 183. *See also* Hyperlipidemia.
Triiodothyronine supplementation, 568
Trimethaphan, 571
Truncus arteriosus, 327
Trypanosomiasis, 79
TTP (thrombotic thrombocytopenic purpura), 278
Tubal ligation, 481
Tubal pregnancy, 269
Tuberculosis (TB), 328
Tumor(s)
  adrenal, catecholamine-secreting. *See* Pheochromocytoma.

Tumor(s) *(Continued)*
  bladder, malignant, 59
    transurethral resection of, 478
  brain, 195, 311
    hyperventilation associated with, 73
    surgery for, craniotomy in, with patient in sitting position, 392
  breast, malignant, 60
  bronchial, malignant, 61
  carcinoid, 67, 374
    excision of, 374
  cardiac, myxoma as, 237
  catecholamine-secreting. *See* Pheochromocytoma.
  chemotherapeutic agents for, 493, 511, 514, 522
  endocrine, multiple, 146, 228
  esophageal, malignant, 62, 396
    surgery for, 396
  gastric, malignant, 401
    surgery for, 401
  gastrin-secreting, 146
  glomus jugulare, 150
  head and neck, 150, 451
  infratentorial, 195
    surgery for, craniotomy in, with patient in sitting position, 392
  insulin-secreting, 196
  liver, 430
    surgery for, 430
  lung, malignant, 63
    bronchi as site of, 61
    surgery for, 448
  mediastinal, 217
    lymphoma as, 212, 217
  multiple endocrine, 146, 228
  neck and head, 150, 451
  pancreatic
    gastrin-secreting, 146
    insulin-secreting, 196
    malignant, 488
      surgery for, 488
  pituitary, 188, 262, 447, 477
    acromegaly due to, 6
    excision of, 447, 477
  prostate, malignant, surgery for, 64, 452
  radiotherapy for, 453
  rectal, malignant, abdominoperineal resection for, 352
  renal, malignant, 438
    surgery for, 438
  screening for, in child with Beckwith-Wiedemann syndrome, 42
  supratentorial, 311
  thyroid, 321
  Wilms', 346
TURP (transurethral resection of prostate), 479
Twelve-lead ECG, 617
Tympanoplasty, 437
Type I diabetes mellitus (insulin-dependent diabetes mellitus), 111
  ketoacidosis in, 115
  pancreatic transplantation for, 444
Type I herpes simplex virus infection, 166
Type I multiple endocrine neoplasia (MEN I, Werner's syndrome), 146, 228
Type II diabetes mellitus (non−insulin-dependent diabetes mellitus), 112
  hyperosmolar nonketotic coma in, 178
  insulin receptor modifiers for, 532
  oral hypoglycemic agents for, 528, 537, 546
Type II herpes simplex virus infection, 167
Type IIa multiple endocrine neoplasia (MEN IIa, Sipple's syndrome), 228
Type IIb multiple endocrine neoplasia (MEN IIb), 228

Type III diabetes mellitus (gestational diabetes mellitus), 113

U

Ulcerative colitis, chronic, 329
Ultrasonography, cardiac
    after infusion of dobutamine, 620
    transesophageal, 628
Undescended testis, surgery for, 441
Unipolar depression, 110. *See also* Depression.
Upper respiratory tract infection, 330
Ureteral reimplantation, 482
Ureteral stent placement, 483
Urinalysis, 626
Urolithiasis, 331
    extracorporeal shock wave therapy for, 398
Urticaria, cold, 332
Uterus
    endoscopic evaluation of, 413
    removal of, 412, 470
    rupture of, 333

V

Vaginal delivery
    normal, 484
    uterine rupture complicating, 333
Vaginal hysterectomy, 412, 470
Valerian, 611
Valvular disease. *See* Aortic valve; Mitral *entries*
Variant (Prinzmetal's) angina (syndrome A), 95
Varicella-zoster virus infection, 334
Varices, gastrointestinal, bleeding from, 475
    treatment of, 475
Vascular disease
    atherosclerotic, 34, 94
    cerebral

Vascular disease *(Continued)*
    aneurysmal, surgery (clipping) for, 380
    ischemic, 77
    occlusive, 226, 242
    peripheral, 256
Vascular ring, around trachea and esophagus, 123
Venous air embolism, 400, 485
Venous thrombosis, deep, 106
Ventilation-perfusion scans, 629
Ventricle(s)
    of brain
        excess cerebrospinal fluid in, 170
        shunt of cerebrospinal fluid from, 487
    of heart
        defect in septum between. *See* Ventricular septal defect.
    single (common), 305
Ventricular bradyarrhythmias, 354
Ventricular fibrillation, 335, 354
Ventricular pre-excitation, 336
Ventricular septal defect, 337, 338
    congenital, 337, 486
        repair of, 486
    post–myocardial infarction, 338
Ventricular tachyarrhythmias, 339
Ventricular tachycardia, 340, 354
Ventriculoperitoneal shunt, 487
Verapamil, 508
Vertebrae. *See* Spine.
Vesicoureteral reflux, surgery for, 482
Viagra (sildenafil), 562
Viral hepatitis, 161, 162, 163
Visual loss
    as complication of anesthesia and surgery, 46
    as complication of glaucoma, 149
Vitamin B_2 (riboflavin), 559
Vitamin B_{12} (cyanocobalamin), 572
    deficiency of, 341

Vitamin D deficiency, 342
Vitamin K deficiency, 343
Vitamist (melatonin), 601
von Willebrand's disease, 344
V/Q scan (split lung function), 629

W

Waldenström's macroglobulinemia, 345
Warfarin (Coumadin), 24, 573
    toxicity of, 126
Weight. *See* Obesity.
Werner's syndrome (MEN I, multiple endocrine neoplasia I), 146, 228
Whipple procedure, 488
Whooping cough, 257
Wilms' tumor, 346
Window, aortopulmonary, 359
Wolff-Parkinson-White (WPW) syndrome, 336, 347
Wound botulism, 47
Wound coverage, with split-thickness skin graft, 462
WPW (Wolff-Parkinson-White) syndrome, 336, 347
Wrist, compression neuropathy at, 378

X

X-ray, chest, 616

Y

Yeast infection, 65

Z

Zafirlukast (Accolate), 500
Zileuton (Zyflo), 500
Zingiber officinale (ginger), 594
Zollinger-Ellison syndrome, 146
Zoster, 334
Zyflo (zileuton), 500